Occupational Therapy for Physical Dysfunction

THIRD EDITION

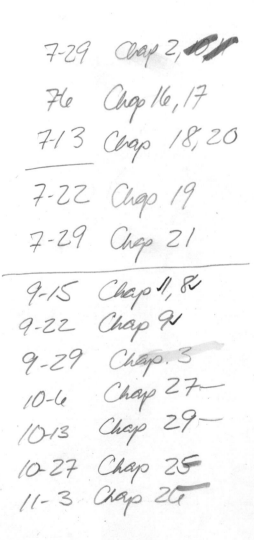

7-29   Chap 2, 10 11

76   Chap 16, 17

7-13   Chap 18, 20

7-22   Chap 19

7-29   Chap 21

9-15   Chap 1, 8

9-22   Chap 9

9-29   Chap 3

10-6   Chap 27

10-13 Chap 29

10-27 Chap 25

11-3   Chap 26

Occupational Therapy for Physical Dysfunction

THIRD EDITION

EDITED BY

Catherine A. Trombly, M.A., O.T.R., F.A.O.T.A.

Professor, Department of Occupational Therapy
Sargent College of Allied Health Professions
Boston University
Boston, Massachusetts

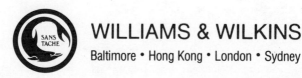

WILLIAMS & WILKINS
Baltimore • Hong Kong • London • Sydney

Editor: John P. Butler
Associate Editor: Linda Napora
Copy Editor: Lindsay E. Edmunds
Design: Norman W. Och
Illustration Planning: Raymond Lowman
Production: Theda Harris

Printed in the United States of America

First Edition, 1977
   Reprinted 1978, 1979, 1980, 1981, 1982
Second Edition, 1983
   Reprinted 1984, 1985, 1986, 1987

Library of Congress Cataloging-in-Publication Data
Occupational therapy for physical dysfunction.
Includes bibliographies and index.
1. Occupational therapy.   2. Physically handicapped—
Rehabilitation.   I. Trombly, Catherine Ann   [DNLM:
1. Handicapped.   2. Occupational Therapy.   WB 555 0143]
RM 735.033   1989   615.8'515   88-131
ISBN 0-683-08389-9

10   9   8   7   6   5   4   3   90   91   92   93

THIS BOOK IS DEDICATED TO

My Mother
(IN MEMORIAM)

My Father, and Christopher

———————————————

PREFACE
To the Third Edition

The original goals for writing this textbook are preserved in this edition. They were the transmission of currently published information on the evaluation and treatment of physically challenged adults and the presentation of the material within a conceptual framework rather than in a cookbook fashion. This orientation is based on our belief that the professional occupational therapist must be able to select and administer appropriate evaluation and treatment procedures for a *particular* patient. Since no two patients are alike, what is appropriate for one is not necessarily appropriate for another even when there is a similar diagnosis. Only by having a fund of factual knowledge *in combination with* a framework for decision making can the occupational therapist act as a professional rather than a technician.

Students learn the knowledge base relatively easily. The framework for decision making, or clinical-reasoning skill, is less easily acquired. Clinical reasoning is defined here as the ability to analyze patient behavior, to deduce the problem(s) manifested in that behavior, to synthesize these into problem and goal statements based on a theoretical rationale, and finally to translate the goal statements into therapeutic principles and procedures. New emphasis is being placed on this facet of professional education for occupational therapists as well as other health care professionals. We know that this skill is not acquired automatically as a logical extension of the knowledge base, nor is it acquired by rote memorization of formulas. We believe it results from practice in the application of a conceptual framework to clinical problems. Clinical-reasoning skill is a major objective of the internship phase of professional education, but the rudimentary bases for it must be developed in the university.

Our goals for the third edition of *Occupational Therapy for Physical Dysfunction,* then, reflect our original intent. Our first goal was to update each chapter so that the student's fund of knowledge would be current. Our second goal was to facilitate the clinical-reasoning process.

New material was incorporated into existing chapters from journals directly related to occupational therapy and from many articles only peripherally related but that contribute to the rationale for, or verification of, occupational therapy theory and practice. Several new topics have been added to the chapters. These include motor learning and skill acquisition; evaluation and treatment of dysphagia, industrial upper-extremity cumulative trauma injury, chronic back pain, and chronic obstructive pulmonary disease; the use of computers for treatment; and occupational therapy practice related to industry. Two new chapters have been added: (1) "Carr and Shepherd Approach: Motor Relearning Programme for Stroke Patients" and (2) "Cognitive and Perceptual Evaluation and Treatment."

The clinical-reasoning process has been addressed by clarifying and explicating the treatment planning process in Chapter 1. The decision tree has been edited to assist selection of appropriate evaluations and treatment goals for classes of patients. The evaluation chapters have been organized to lead the student from evaluation findings with a particular patient to development of appropriate treatment goals for that patient. The treatment approach chapters have been more clearly organized by goal to assist the student in moving from identification of a goal to translation of that goal into treatment principles and procedures. An attempt has been made to amplify the information given in all chapters to clarify its meaning. In the latter endeavor we are grateful to the students who use this textbook and who ask questions for clarification.

Study questions have been added to help the student focus attention on the most crucial pieces of information or issues that he or she needs to know initially. However, occupational therapy is learned in onion-like fashion, that is, in layers. Therefore, as the student acquires basic knowledge, he or she should go back and learn the next, more subtle layer of knowledge and so on. This process will take the student beyond this textbook and will continue throughout his or her professional life.

An instructor's manual to accompany this text has been written by Mary Ann Bush of the University of Western Michigan. This manual is available, on request, from the publisher; a student workbook also is available.

Faculty use this text in several courses within occupational therapy curricula. They have asked that I clarify which particular kinds of knowledge and skills are required before the different parts of the textbook can be used successfully by students at various levels of their education. Part Five, "Rehabilitation Approach," can be learned early in a student's program without prerequisite knowledge. Anatomy, physiology, kinesiology, and orthopedic clinical conditions are prerequisite to Parts Three, Four, and Seven. In addition, skill in construction techniques is required for making splints (chapter 14). Prerequisite to Parts Two and Six are courses in neuroscience and neurological clinical conditions. Part One, "Framework for Therapy," can and should be used in conjunction with each of these major divisions of knowledge.

Another point to be made is that whereas the same approaches and principles are used in the treatment of motor problems of pediatric physically challenged patients, this text is limited to adults. Pediatric occupational therapy evaluates and implements treatment using different tests and media and pays particular attention to the ongoing emotional, social, and cognitive development of children, all of which are beyond the scope of this text.

Again in the third edition, in order to simplify both the reading and the writing of this textbook, the **feminine** gender has been assigned to the **therapist** and the **male** gender to the **patient**.

Catherine A. Trombly

PREFACE
To the Second Edition

The purpose of this book is threefold: to compile evaluation and treatment procedures, to present the theoretical bases of these treatment procedures, and to challenge the clinician to research the effectiveness of his/her practice.

Accordingly, the book presents a compilation of evaluation and therapeutic procedures used in the practice of occupational therapy with physically disabled adults. Although a comprehensive compilation was attempted, it is not possible to include every procedure used in the practice of occupational therapy. Each therapist brings his or her own knowledge, perceptions, and unique creativity to his/her practice. Knowledge of the information in this textbook and development of skill in the procedures cited here will enable the beginning therapist to offer quality care to clients. Even the beginning therapist should not use this as a cookbook, however, without regard to the individuality of each patient and his or her unique response to any therapeutic procedure. The book, therefore, presents material in such a way as to help the student therapist begin to develop a process of thinking about the therapeutic process and its application. The book is organized into three approaches to treatment. For each approach, information from the basic sciences that form the theoretical bases for therapeutic procedures is presented in order that the student therapist may understand the rationale for therapeutic procedures and thereby gain flexibility in application of the procedures. Innovative treatment can be developed and treatment planning can be imaginative when the "whys" are known. Further, goal setting is the key to effective treatment. Within each approach, methods of identifying and implementing the goals are clearly stated. The reader is referred to the references listed at the end of each chapter for greater depth of knowledge, or specific directions for certain procedures, or for other points of view on specific issues.

Research on the effectiveness of therapeutic procedures is included. The research is sparse, although there has been a small increase since the last edition. Much more research is needed to identify what the minimally effective therapeutic dosages are, what the long-term effects of treatment are, and whether the effects of treatment are as expected on certain types of patients. All effectiveness research must eventually tell us what treatment, administered in what way, over what period of time improves the *function* of what type of patient. Clinicians are the source of this information. I look forward to including your studies in the next edition of this textbook!

Ideas for the present revision have been generated not only from our own experiences with using this book as a textbook, but also from clinicians, students, and educators who very kindly sent us constructive criticism. This revision is characterized by more examples in an attempt to help the student therapist translate theory into practice. Chapters on "Closed Head Injuries" and "Biofeedback as an Adjunct to Therapy" have been added as a reflection of increased involvement by OTRs with these issues. Published information was used primarily. In a few instances where important information was only available from workshops, theses, or verbal communication with experts, this is indicated.

We have assumed that student therapists who use this book have prerequisite knowledge of anatomy, physiology, neuroanatomy, neurophysiology, kinesiology, and orthopedic and neurological clinical conditions, and also prerequisite skills in use of tools and basic construction procedures used in splint-making.

To simplify both the writing and reading of this textbook, we have arbitrarily assigned the feminine gender to the therapist and masculine to the patient. It is not meant to assign value to either group of people.

Catherine A. Trombly

ACKNOWLEDGMENTS

Many people have contributed to the ongoing development of this textbook by providing constructive criticism, photographing or posing for photographs, arranging for photographs to be taken, and seeking or giving permission to use material published elsewhere. The textbook and its revisions could not have been produced without their help. To each of them, my sincere thanks and gratitude. They are:

Gail Bliss, M.O.T., O.T.R.
Berta Bobath, P.T.
Anita Bundy, Sc.D., O.T.R.
Mary Ann Bush, M.S., O.T.R.
John Butler, Senior Editor
Brian Despres, O.T.S.
Shelly Earley, M.O.T., O.T.R.
Mark Erickson
Anne G. Fisher, Sc.D., O.T.R.
Sam Fitzpatrick
Alice Follows, M.S., O.T.R.
Maureen Hayes Fleming, Ed.D., O.T.R.
Margaret Hayes, O.T.R.

Katherine Konosky, O.T.R.
Frederic J. Kottke, M.D.
Judith LaDrew
Lucia Grochowska Littlefield
Virgil Mathiowetz, M.S., O.T.R.
Linda Napora, Managing Editor
Lillian Hoyle Parent, M.A., O.T.R.
Lee Ann Quintana, M.S., O.T.R.
Deborah Yarett Slater, M.S., O.T.R.
Nancy Talbot, M.Ed., O.T.R.
Gayle M. Thompson, M.Ed., O.T.R.
Chistopher F. Trombly

Specific help has also been given by others to some of the contributing authors, who cite them at the end of the particular chapter.

CONTRIBUTORS

Patricia Weber Dow, M.S., O.T.R.
Private Practice, New Orleans, Louisiana.

Anne G. Fisher, Sc.D., O.T.R., F.A.O.T.A.
Assistant Professor, Department of Occupational Therapy, College of Associated Health Professions, University of Illinois at Chicago, Chicago, Illinois.

Beverly J. Myers, M.H.P.E., O.T.R./L.
Instructor, Department of Occupational Therapy, College of Associated Health Professions, University of Illinois at Chicago, Chicago, Illinois.

Lillian Hoyle Parent, M.A., O.T.R., F.A.O.T.A.
Coordinator of Education and Research, Department of Occupational Therapy, University of Texas Medical Branch, Galveston, Texas.

Cynthia A. Philips, M.A., O.T.R./L., A.S.H.T.
Hand Therapist and Chief of Occupational Therapy, Newton-Wellesley Hospital, Newton, Massachusetts.

Lee Ann Quintana, M.S., O.T.R.
Coordinating Therapist, Rehabilitation Medicine Unit, Catholic Medical Center, Manchester, New Hampshire.

Anna Deane Scott, M.Ed., O.T.R.
Associate Professor, Department of Occupational Therapy, Sargent College of Allied Health Professions, Boston University, Boston, Massachusetts.

Catherine A. Trombly, M.A., O.T.R., F.A.O.T.A.
Professor, Department of Occupational Therapy, Sargent College of Allied Health Professions, Boston University, Boston, Massachusetts.

Hilda Powers Versluys, M.Ed., O.T.R.
Assistant Clinical Professor, Department of Occupational Therapy, Sargent College of Allied Health Professions, Boston University, Boston, Massachusetts.

CONTENTS

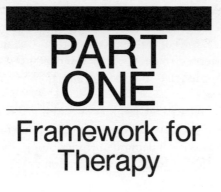

PART ONE
Framework for Therapy

The two introductory chapters of this book present ideas that underlie the practice of occupational therapy with the adult physically disabled. The first one identifies the reasoning processes that the author uses in making evaluation and treatment planning decisions. By identifying these processes I hope to assist the student occupational therapist to organize and utilize the information in the remainder of the book. With experience, the student therapist may develop his/her own organizational framework.

The second chapter specifically addresses the psychological needs and adjustments of a person who has become physically disabled. Hilda Versluys, M.Ed., O.T.R., has applied sound principles of psychiatric occupational therapy to the treatment of the unique emotional needs of the physically disabled. The emotional adjustment of the patient must be the foremost consideration when implementing planned therapy so that the patient may achieve his highest potential. The therapist must remain cognizant that the patient will be motivated by his primary concerns: his membership in his family and society.

The remainder of this book is organized according to my view that there are three treatment approaches from which the therapist may choose in attempting to assist the physically disabled person in reaching as high a level of independent functioning and life satisfaction as is possible for that person. These approaches are: neurodevelopmental, biomechanical, and rehabilitative.

The NEURODEVELOPMENTAL APPROACH is used for persons who have been born with a dysfunctional central nervous system or who have suffered trauma or disease to their central nervous system. This approach uses sensory input and developmental sequences to facilitate change in the sensorimotor organization of the central nervous system. The approach also includes use of cognitive information processing strategies to promote learning or relearning of movement control or perceptual or cognitive functional abilities.

If we respond negatively to the key question, "Does this person have an intact, fully matured central nervous system?", then we should select treatment based on neurophysiological, neurodevelopmental, and/or motor learning principles. The goal of the treatment is to effect an essential change in the physiological or behavioral organization of the central nervous system and thereby improve the overall functioning of the disabled person. Treatments developed as part of the neurodevelopmental approach are also appropriate for patients with an intact central nervous system because this approach capitalizes on and enhances the functioning of the central nervous system.

The BIOMECHANICAL APPROACH deals with increasing strength, endurance, and range of joint motion in patients who have an intact central nervous system but who have dysfunction in the peripheral nervous system or the musculoskeletal, integumentary, or cardiopulmonary systems. If we respond affirmatively to the key question, "Does this person have an intact, fully matured central nervous system?", then we would focus our attention on biomechanically oriented theories of treatment related to the specific problems of the disabled person. This approach is not appropriate, however, for the person with central nervous system dysfunction.

The REHABILITATIVE APPROACH aims at making the person as independent as possible in spite of residual disability that has resulted for any reason. If a person must live with a disability that decreases his independent functioning, then the occupational therapist will concentrate on helping him find ways to compensate for his losses by adapted techniques and/or equipment.

The neurodevelopmental and biomechanical approaches are used to remediate problems underlying an inability to be competent in life tasks. Treatment using these approaches precedes the use of the rehabilitative approach, which is used when remediation is complete or is not a possibility.

Beginning in October 1983, in an effort to contain geometrically increasing health care costs, Medicare started changing from a cost-based retrospective reimbursement system to a prospective payment system based on diagnosis-related groupings (DRGs). In the new system, expenses exceeding a set level of reimbursement are not paid. To make a profit, the expenses must be kept lower than the established cost.[1] Costs are reduced by discharging the patient quickly. This may mean that remediation of deficits may become less a part of practice and that the rehabilitative approach will become foremost in an effort to advance the patient most expeditiously toward independence. It is unfortunate that clinicians have not documented the value, in terms of eventual level of independence, of skills training preceded by remediation versus skills training alone. While continuing to believe that providing a base for development of skills is necessary, therapists may be forced to implement end-stage skills training without the opportunity to prepare the patient for generalized independence and true competency.

For each approach to treatment, there are evaluation procedures, treatment principles, and techniques related to the approach. The presentation of these is organized in this book so that student therapists can gain a conceptual knowledge of treatment of the physically disabled. Chapters on specific diagnoses are included not only to indicate the application of the treatment approaches, principles, and methods to classes of treatment problems shared among the diagnoses but also to describe the unique treatment problems presented by persons with these commonly seen diagnoses.

Because the philosophical base of occupational therapy is competency through occupation, whatever the treatment approach, activity is the treatment medium of choice for occupational therapists. Examples of therapeutic application of activity to treatment problems are presented throughout.

Knowledge and understanding are continually changing as a result of ongoing research. Consequently this compilation can only report currently acknowledged concepts with the expectation that they will change.

Reference
1. Henisee, P. A. An analysis of Medicare's DRG system. *Physical Therapy Forum,* 5(15): 1, 3, 1986.

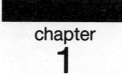

chapter

1

Treatment Planning Process

Catherine A. Trombly

Patients are referred to occupational therapy when they, or others responsible for their care, perceive that they are not adequately performing their daily activities. The therapist's first task is to develop a treatment plan for the particular patient.[1]

Treatment planning is problem solving applied to patient care. Methodology is similar to that used by scientists and businessmen to solve problems in their spheres of endeavor. Students need to learn the problem-solving process as well as the subject matter related to the problem situation.[2] Problem solving involves clearly stating the goal to be achieved, gathering information pertaining to achievement of the goal, analyzing and interpreting the meaning of that information, establishing specific subgoals and a plan to achieve them, implementing the plan, and reviewing the outcome. Every member of the treatment team utilizes this problem-solving process.

The team members must collaborate to plan an overall, nonconflicting program for the patient that enhances all of the patient's capabilities but does not overstress him. The composition of the team varies depending upon the particular problem and needs of the patient. In a rehabilitation center a core team of physician, nurse, occupational therapist, physical therapist, speech therapist, social worker, psychologist, and rehabilitation counselor are occasionally joined by the orthotist, prosthetist, rehabilitation nurse, teacher, and medical or surgical specialists, such as rheumatologists, cardiologists, etc. Each member is responsible for developing a treatment plan related to his or her own unique area of expertise.

The occupational therapy treatment planning process is the same whether it is applied to persons with physical, psychosocial, or cognitive-perceptual-motor disabilities. It is the process of *identifying the problem(s), establishing the goal(s),* and *and determining the approaches, principles, and methods* by which *this person* with *these problems* can reach *those goals*. The process can be further clarified by Figure 1.1.

Data Gathering

The occupational therapy treatment program is based on information concerning the present and predicted level of the patient's functioning in his occupational performance tasks. Information sought should include that specified in the Uniform Occupational Therapy Evaluation Checklist.[3,4] It is important to verify the consistency of data by obtaining multiple indicators of function.[5] Data can be obtained from the following sources, keeping in mind that "all evaluation methods shall be appropriate to the client's age, education, cultural and ethnic background, medical status, and functional ability"(p. 803).[4]

1. The *medical record* should yield demographic information concerning the person's diagnosis(es), date of onset, medical and surgical histories, precautions, medications, age, pertinent social and educational/vocational history, and discharge plan, as well as reports of the nursing staff about the disabled person's daily physical and psychological functioning.

2. *Observation of the disabled person* as he attempts to perform functional activities will allow the therapist to determine the person's present functional level as well as his sense of safety and judgment. These observations will also give the therapist a clue as to what is limiting the patient's functional performance so that appropriate evaluations may be selected to evaluate the sensorimotor limitations more objectively. For example, the disabled person may be unable to feed himself. By watching the person try to do this, the therapist observes that the patient can lift a heavy mug but cannot approach his mouth. The therapist concludes that the patient seems to have adequate strength but range of motion seems to be the limiting factor. The therapist will check out this observation by doing a cursory strength evaluation and, not finding a limitation here, a more detailed range of motion evaluation.

3. *Measurement* of the disabled person's *performance* to determine baseline performance. The thera-

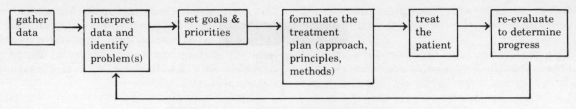

Figure 1.1 Treatment planning process.

pist, having observed the patient and knowing the implications of the diagnosis, makes an assessment plan based on a judgment about which capabilities to evaluate and which measurement procedures to use to elicit the necessary information regarding the strengths and limitations of the person. The assessment plan may be modified before the patient is actually seen based on information from records or staff about the patient's physical and psychological status.[5] Specifics of measurement are described in succeeding chapters of this book.

4. *Interview of the disabled person* should yield knowledge of his goals, feelings, readiness to participate in or to take responsibility for treatment, expectations for therapy, cognitive abilities such as memory, ability to sequence and organize information, orientation to time, place, and person, comprehension of directions, his perception of what he can do for himself, and his interests.

5. *Reports of other professionals* who are simultaneously gathering data in regard to the person relative to their particular service should be available from the medical record, be reported at team conferences, or be shared in other less formal ways. These reports will influence the development of the occupational therapy treatment plan.

6. *Interview of family members* should result in gaining knowledge of their goals for the disabled family member and their views about how the disability has affected the person, as well as how it has affected each of them and the family unit. Brain injury may cause changes in personality characteristics. The family is the source of information about the patient's premorbid personality.

7. It may be necessary for the therapist to *read resource material* regarding the classical symptoms, course, and prognosis of the person's disease(s) or to review the precautions and effects of the patient's medication before planning treatment.

Interpreting the Data and Identifying the Problems

A profile of strengths and limitations pertaining to the person's occupational functioning will emerge from results of evaluations and other data-gathering processes. To identify the problem(s) toward which the occupational therapy treatment plan will be directed, it is necessary to select the significant information. Significant information is that data and those scores that reflect limitations that decrease physical functioning, that limit the likelihood of return of function, and/or that lead to deformity or to maladaptive

personal-social functioning. Equally significant information that influences problem identification are the patient's goals for himself with respect to reality, his feelings, and his values.

Once the problems are identified, a problem list is developed. Each limitation or perception discrepant with reality constitutes a treatment problem.

Setting Goals and Priorities

Once the problems are identified, the goal related to each problem is listed. Because it is impossible to accomplish all goals at once, the goals are prioritized. There are two bases for establishing the particular order of priority. One is the client's (and his family's) view of what is most important. The other is the therapist's knowledge that some abilities must precede accomplishment of others. To help in setting priorities, therapists identify both long-term and short-term goals.

Long-term goals specify the end product of therapy. These are the type of goals cited by patient and family. They describe the expected level of functioning the patient will achieve by the termination of the therapy program. An example of this is: "although requiring a wheelchair for locomotion, the patient will be independent in self-care." Long-term goals are educated guesses that may need modification as the patient's progress is observed.

To achieve long-term goals, the therapist plans a series of short-term goals that are the mini-goals, the building blocks that lead to one or more long-term goals. For each problem to be addressed by occupational therapy, there is a short-term goal. Short-term goals imply sequencing and priority. They state which abilities must be developed before others. The sequencing is started from the point at which the patient is functioning successfully and stopped at the point where the long-term goal is achieved.

Several sequences of short-term goals may be ongoing concurrently. For example, in order to reach the long-term goal mentioned above, the patient must learn to (1) operate the wheelchair and (2) do self-care activities. If the person's disability is weakness, then one sequence of short-term goals will be to progress the person from one plateau of strength to the next. Concurrently, short-term goals related to self-care will be sequenced so that the person is taught to do those activities for which he has sufficient strength at any given time to assure successful experiences at each stage. In terms of priority, we see that activity to increase strength must precede each self-care task that requires greater strength and that certain aspects of self-care must be mastered before others that depend on a prior skill or are of a developmentally higher nature.

Labeling a goal "long-term" or "short-term" simply informs others that the goal is being aimed for eventually or is being worked on immediately. The labeling is not what is important in treatment planning; the establishment of a laddering of goals that the patient can successfully accomplish and by which he can succeedingly approach his final level of functioning is the essence of treatment planning.

Long-term goals must be established in collaboration with the person receiving therapy and other members of the rehabilitation team. Short-term goals are established by each professional and are specifically related to the expertise of that discipline. It is very important that the patient understand the relationship of each short-term goal to the long-term goals and how the activity implements the short-term goal.

Formulate the Treatment Plan for Each Short-Term Goal

In order to formulate the plan for a treatment program, the therapist must identify the treatment approach or approaches that are appropriate for the patient (see Fig. 1.3). Some patients may require one or more of the treatment approaches. Selection of the appropriate treatment approach at any given time depends upon the nature of the presenting problem, its causes, the state of recovery, and established priorities. For example, if the patient has a weak upper extremity secondary to a cerebral vascular accident, the therapist must choose from among three major therapeutic approaches: neurodevelopmental, biomechanical, or rehabilitative. A rehabilitative approach would be chosen if weakness were long-standing and apparently unlikely to improve. The therapist's reason for choosing this approach would be that teaching methods of compensation for the loss of the use of this extremity could help the patient be as independent as possible.

If recovery was hoped for, a biomechanical approach with its direct strengthening techniques involving maximal resistance might appeal to the therapist. However, this would be rejected in favor of the neurodevelopmental approach in answer to the key question, "Does this patient have an intact fully matured central nervous system?" This is because the patient who has suffered a cerebral vascular accident may lack voluntary control of his musculature, or his muscle tone may be altered due to lack of influence of the higher centers of the central nervous system: he would be unable to selectively strengthen certain muscles because he is probably only able to move in developmentally lower patterns of motion.

After identifying the treatment approach, the therapist must identify the principle of treatment to use for each of the problems. For example, using the above example, the neurodevelopmental approach having been chosen, the choice of principle within that approach depends on what is applicable to the patient at his particular stage of recovery. Our hypothetical therapist may select the principles of controlled sensory manipulation and retraining as a means of establishing voluntary control over the movement. The principle is the rationale for the treatment. It, along with the theoretical and empirical research that supports it, is the explanation or justification for the choice of a particular treatment. If a therapist is having the patient use highly textured threads in a finger weaving project, when asked to explain her reason, she will cite the principle of controlled sensory manipulation: that sensory input affects sensorimotor organization and motor output.

Once the principle is decided on, the method of implementing the principle must then be determined. The method is the means of translating the principle into a treatment form. The treatment principles of each approach and their methods for implementation are described in the remainder of this book.

Day[6] diagrammed a model for treatment planning as shown in Figures 1.2 and 1.3.

Treat the Patient

"Occupational therapy treatment refers to the use of specific activities or methods to develop, improve, and/or restore the performance of necessary functions; compensate for dysfunction, and/or minimize debilitation."[7] Purposeful activity may be used alone or in conjunction with adjunctive therapy such as splinting, adapted equipment, or biofeedback. The purposeful activity is presented to the person in such a way that he can concentrate on the process and goal of the activity and not the specific movements or muscle contractions desired. The activity should be one, whether adapted or not, that automatically calls forth the correct response.

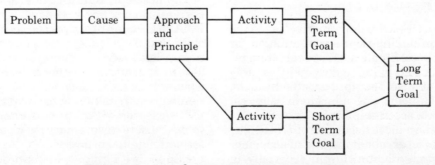

Figure 1.2 Day's[6] model for treatment planning.

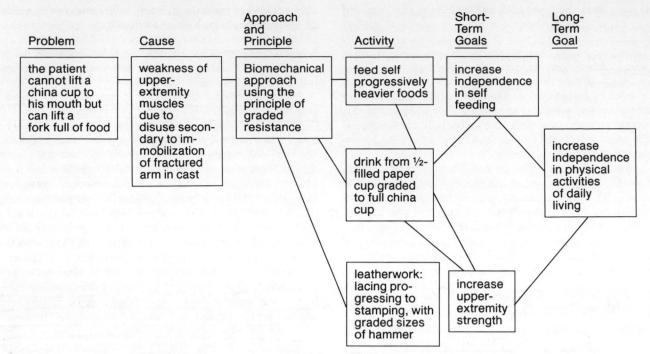

Figure 1.3 Flow chart of Day's[6] treatment plan applied to a problem.

Treatment is started at the point in a developmental or improvement sequence where the patient has to struggle but is able to achieve. The therapist observes the performance of the activity to determine whether the selected activity is challenging the patient's existing capabilities. If it is not, then the activity must be upgraded.

Fatigue of the person and safe use of the tools are monitored throughout the treatment period. Termination of the treatment period, rest, or further instruction may be necessary.

Reevaluation

Periodically, depending upon the course of the illness and the changes observed in the patient's performance or as a requirement of third-party payers, the therapist remeasures the parameters of performance. These data are compared to those of a prior evaluation to note changes. The problem list, goals, and treatment plan are adjusted to meet the person's rate of progress or new level of performance. The progress is recorded in the patient's medical record.

Recording

Graphing the changes is particularly motivating to the patient,[8] as well as providing clear documentation for administrative purposes. Single-subject evaluation research methods utilize graphing to document not only patient progress but also therapeutic effectiveness, thus providing the clinician with a mechanism for establishing therapeutic accountability.[9]

Problem-Oriented Medical Recording (POMR), developed by Weed,[10] is an excellent method of documentation and intrateam communication, especially in rehabilitation settings where many professionals con-

tribute to patient treatment.[11]. The POMR consists of four interconnected elements: (1) the data base; (2) the problem list; (3) the initial plan, which includes a short-term goal for each problem to be addressed and the treatment strategy for each goal; and (4) progress notes.[12] The first three elements appear in the initial note recorded in the patient's medical record. The progress note reports the outcome relative to each problem and any change in the problem list or plan. The student therapist, remembering that the medical record is a legal document, should write notes with precision and accuracy.

One Example of the Treatment Planning Process

DATA GATHERING

1. The medical record yielded the following information that will be used to plan treatment: quadriplegia secondary to fracture dislocation of C_{6-7}; incomplete lesion; C_6 functional level; no medical complications; cervical fusion and laminectomy performed on the day of the accident; multiple lacerations of both hands; currently in traction with tongs.

2. Observation of the patient led the therapist to conclude that there is slight movement in right toe; no motion in left lower extremity; sensory loss below T_4; is able to do teeth care, other light hygiene, and feeding when side-lying but is dependent in all else due to positioning requirements for cervical traction.

3. Measurement of the performance is too extensive to record here. A summary exists under significant information noted below.

4. Interview with the patient produced this information: He is 24 years old; is a high school graduate; is now

a computer operator; lives with his parents in a second floor apartment; has four siblings all married and living away from home; and is interested in sports and camping. He plans to return to work eventually and continue to live with his parents when accessible housing is located.

5. Reports of other professionals yielded the following: The patient has a very supportive family and many friends. He does not know the implication of spinal cord injury and expects to walk out of the hospital. Health is good.

6. Interview of the family (parents) informed the therapist that the patient will live temporarily with a married brother and sister-in-law, but will eventually live with the parents. The family does not yet know the implications of spinal cord injury.

7. The therapist had forgotten the effects of Dantrium and Decadron; when the *Physician's Desk Reference*[13] was consulted, it was learned that Decadron is a corticosteroid; the patient is on a low dosage so no adverse effects should occur (muscle weakness would be an adverse reaction). Dantrium is used to control spasticity of upper motor neuron origin. The adverse reactions that may occur during dosage regulation are weakness and drowsiness. Another adverse reaction that may occur is photosensitivity; therefore, the patient should not be exposed to strong sunlight. Persons taking Dantrium should not operate machinery or motor vehicles.

INTERPRETING THE DATA AND IDENTIFYING THE PROBLEMS

The significant information is: There is normal sensation of the upper extremities (UEs). Passive range of motion of the UEs is within normal limits. Muscles of the left shoulder, elbow, and forearm are adequate for function, being graded G to N (good to normal). The right upper extremity, including the wrist, is graded G to N. The left extensor carpi radialis (longus and brevis) is normal; the extensor carpi ulnaris is F+ (fair plus), and the wrist flexors grade F. The right finger muscles are stronger than the left; they grade P+ (poor plus) to G−, whereas the left finger muscles grade 0 except for T (trace) for the extensor digitorum and the flexor digitorum profundus 3,4. Thumbs: the left = 0; right grades range from 0 in the opponens and long flexor to F in the extensor pollicis longus. There are some muscles of the lower extremities that grade T.

The problems are:

1. Weakness of the left wrist.
2. Weakness of the fingers and thumbs bilaterally.
3. Spotty weakness (G) of proximal musculature.
4. ADL (activities of daily living) dependency.
5. Denial of meaning and/or permanency of the disability.

SETTING GOALS AND PRIORITIES

The long-term goal this patient has is to return to work as a computer operator and to be independent in his parents' home. To reach this goal, a plan must be de-vised. Shorter-term goals, each related to one or more of the problems, include the following:

a. Learn to prevent contractures at joints where muscles grade less than F (problems 1, 2, and 3).
b. Learn to protect the tenodesis function of the left wrist and hand (problem 1).
c. Increase strength of right hand muscles (problem 2).
d. Increase strength of left hand muscles (problem 2).
e. Increase strength of proximal muscles (problem 3).
f. Realize and accept that being independent will require use of a wheelchair (problems 4 and 5).
g. Determine need for, and skill in use of, other rehabilitation equipment needed for independence (problems 4 and 5).
h. Realize the need to move to accessible housing (problem 5).
i. Relearn to drive (problems 4 and 5).
j. Redevelop work capacity (problems 4 and 5).
k. Learn recreational skills for the wheelchair-bound (problems 4 and 5).
l. Learn to access the community as a wheelchair-bound person (problems 4 and 5).

Immediate short-term goals to achieve goal c are listed here in order from beginning to end. These would guide the portion of the daily treatment session that is devoted to this one goal. Many goals may be worked on within one session. For each goal, the therapist would have made such a list.

1. Increase strength of finger extensors from P+ to F−.
2. Increase strength of finger extensors from F− to F.
3. Increase strength of finger extensors increment by increment to normal or as much as possible.
4. Increase strength of finger flexors from F to F+.
5. Increase strength of finger flexors from F+ to G−.
6. Increase strength of finger flexors increment by increment to normal or as much as possible.
7. Increase strength of thumb extensors from F to F+.
8. Increase strength of thumb extensors from F+ to G−, etc.

FORMULATING THE TREATMENT PLAN FOR EACH SHORT-TERM GOAL

Immediate short-term goal 1 is to increase strength of the finger extensors of the right hand from P+ to F−. The approach to be used is biomechanical. The principle to be used is graded resistance in a gravity-eliminated plane. One method to be used is as follows: Patient is side-lying (due to cervical traction). The right arm is supported on a table with the forearm in midposition. A strap is placed around the fingers at the level of the proximal phalanges. A nylon fishline is attached to the strap, runs over a pulley attached to the edge of the table, and is attached at the other end to a 7-gm (½ oz.) weight. This amount of weight had been determined to be the weight that could be lifted 10 times through range.

This planning process is repeated for each short-term goal. The flow chart in Figure 1.4 has been de-

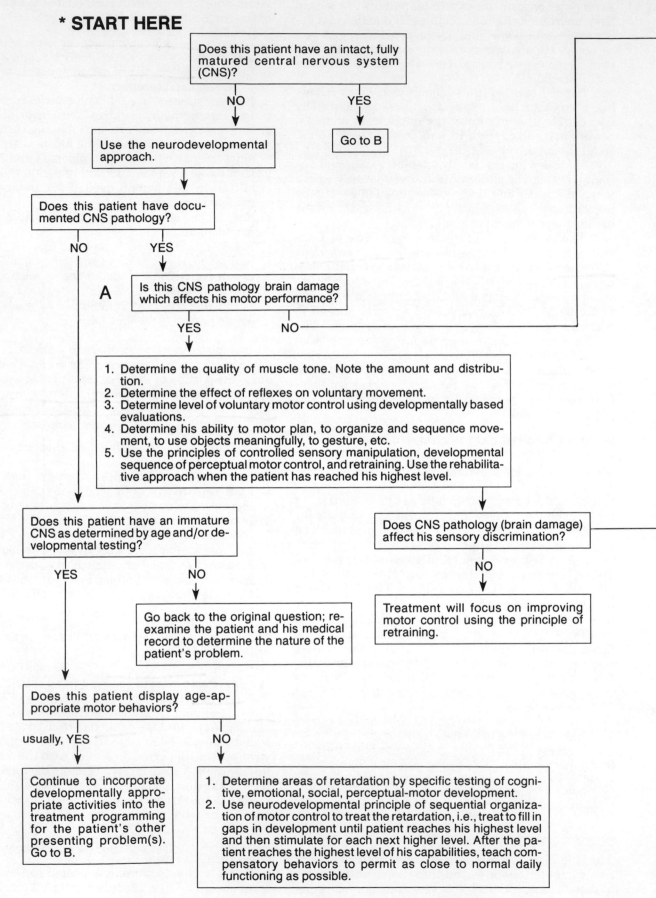

* START HERE

Does this patient have an intact, fully matured central nervous system (CNS)?

NO → Use the neurodevelopmental approach.

YES → Go to B

Does this patient have documented CNS pathology?

NO

YES →

A Is this CNS pathology brain damage which affects his motor performance?

YES →

NO ─────

1. Determine the quality of muscle tone. Note the amount and distribution.
2. Determine the effect of reflexes on voluntary movement.
3. Determine level of voluntary motor control using developmentally based evaluations.
4. Determine his ability to motor plan, to organize and sequence movement, to use objects meaningfully, to gesture, etc.
5. Use the principles of controlled sensory manipulation, developmental sequence of perceptual motor control, and retraining. Use the rehabilitative approach when the patient has reached his highest level.

Does this patient have an immature CNS as determined by age and/or developmental testing?

YES

NO → Go back to the original question; re-examine the patient and his medical record to determine the nature of the patient's problem.

Does CNS pathology (brain damage) affect his sensory discrimination?

NO → Treatment will focus on improving motor control using the principle of retraining.

Does this patient display age-appropriate motor behaviors?

usually, YES → Continue to incorporate developmentally appropriate activities into the treatment programming for the patient's other presenting problem(s). Go to B.

NO →
1. Determine areas of retardation by specific testing of cognitive, emotional, social, perceptual-motor development.
2. Use neurodevelopmental principle of sequential organization of motor control to treat the retardation, i.e., treat to fill in gaps in development until patient reaches his highest level and then stimulate for each next higher level. After the patient reaches the highest level of his capabilities, teach compensatory behaviors to permit as close to normal daily functioning as possible.

Figure 1.4 Treatment planning for patients with physical disabilities.

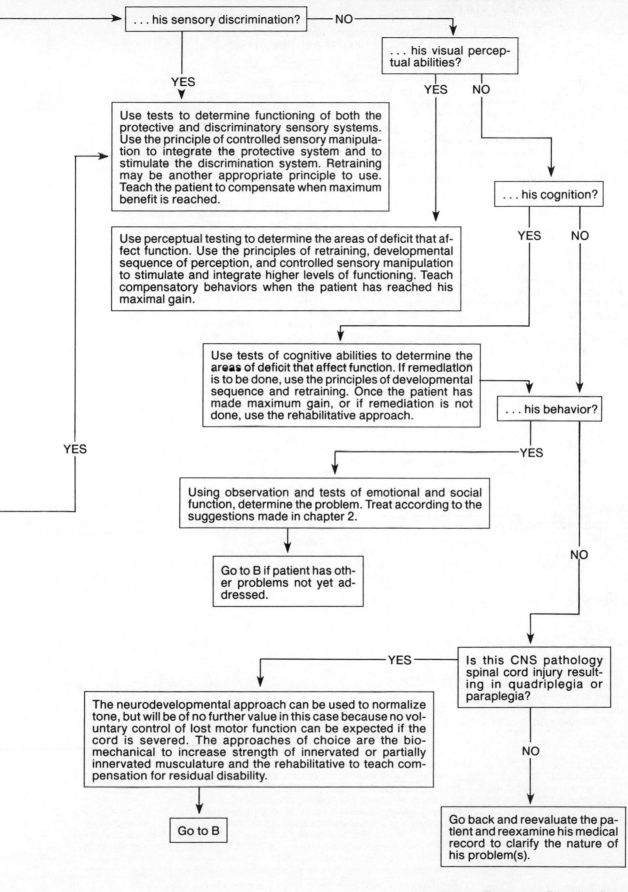

... his sensory discrimination? —NO—

... his visual perceptual abilities?

YES

Use tests to determine functioning of both the protective and discriminatory sensory systems. Use the principle of controlled sensory manipulation to integrate the protective system and to stimulate the discrimination system. Retraining may be another appropriate principle to use. Teach the patient to compensate when maximum benefit is reached.

YES   NO

... his cognition?

Use perceptual testing to determine the areas of deficit that affect function. Use the principles of retraining, developmental sequence of perception, and controlled sensory manipulation to stimulate and integrate higher levels of functioning. Teach compensatory behaviors when the patient has reached his maximal gain.

YES   NO

Use tests of cognitive abilities to determine the areas of deficit that affect function. If remediation is to be done, use the principles of developmental sequence and retraining. Once the patient has made maximum gain, or if remediation is not done, use the rehabilitative approach.

... his behavior?

YES

YES

Using observation and tests of emotional and social function, determine the problem. Treat according to the suggestions made in chapter 2.

NO

Go to B if patient has other problems not yet addressed.

YES

Is this CNS pathology spinal cord injury resulting in quadriplegia or paraplegia?

The neurodevelopmental approach can be used to normalize tone, but will be of no further value in this case because no voluntary control of lost motor function can be expected if the cord is severed. The approaches of choice are the biomechanical to increase strength of innervated or partially innervated musculature and the rehabilitative to teach compensation for residual disability.

NO

Go to B

Go back and reevaluate the patient and reexamine his medical record to clarify the nature of his problem(s).

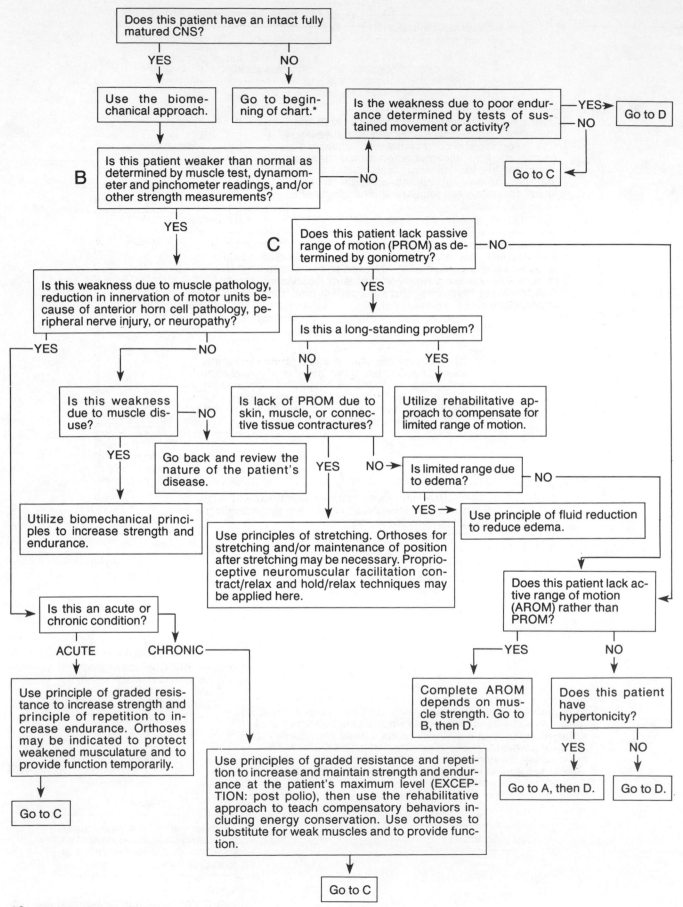

Does this patient have an intact fully matured CNS?

YES → Use the biomechanical approach.

NO → Go to beginning of chart.*

Is the weakness due to poor endurance determined by tests of sustained movement or activity?
- YES → Go to D
- NO → Go to C

B — Is this patient weaker than normal as determined by muscle test, dynamometer and pinchometer readings, and/or other strength measurements?
- NO → (to endurance question)
- YES →

Is this weakness due to muscle pathology, reduction in innervation of motor units because of anterior horn cell pathology, peripheral nerve injury, or neuropathy?

C — Does this patient lack passive range of motion (PROM) as determined by goniometry?
- NO
- YES → Is this a long-standing problem?
  - NO → Is lack of PROM due to skin, muscle, or connective tissue contractures?
  - YES → Utilize rehabilitative approach to compensate for limited range of motion.

YES → Is this weakness due to muscle disuse?
- NO → Go back and review the nature of the patient's disease.
- YES → Utilize biomechanical principles to increase strength and endurance.

Is lack of PROM due to skin, muscle, or connective tissue contractures?
- YES → Use principles of stretching. Orthoses for stretching and/or maintenance of position after stretching may be necessary. Proprioceptive neuromuscular facilitation contract/relax and hold/relax techniques may be applied here.
- NO → Is limited range due to edema?
  - YES → Use principle of fluid reduction to reduce edema.
  - NO →

Is this an acute or chronic condition?
- ACUTE → Use principle of graded resistance to increase strength and principle of repetition to increase endurance. Orthoses may be indicated to protect weakened musculature and to provide function temporarily. → Go to C
- CHRONIC → Use principles of graded resistance and repetition to increase and maintain strength and endurance at the patient's maximum level (EXCEPTION: post polio), then use the rehabilitative approach to teach compensatory behaviors including energy conservation. Use orthoses to substitute for weak muscles and to provide function. → Go to C

Does this patient lack active range of motion (AROM) rather than PROM?
- YES → Complete AROM depends on muscle strength. Go to B, then D.
- NO → Does this patient have hypertonicity?
  - YES → Go to A, then D.
  - NO → Go to D.

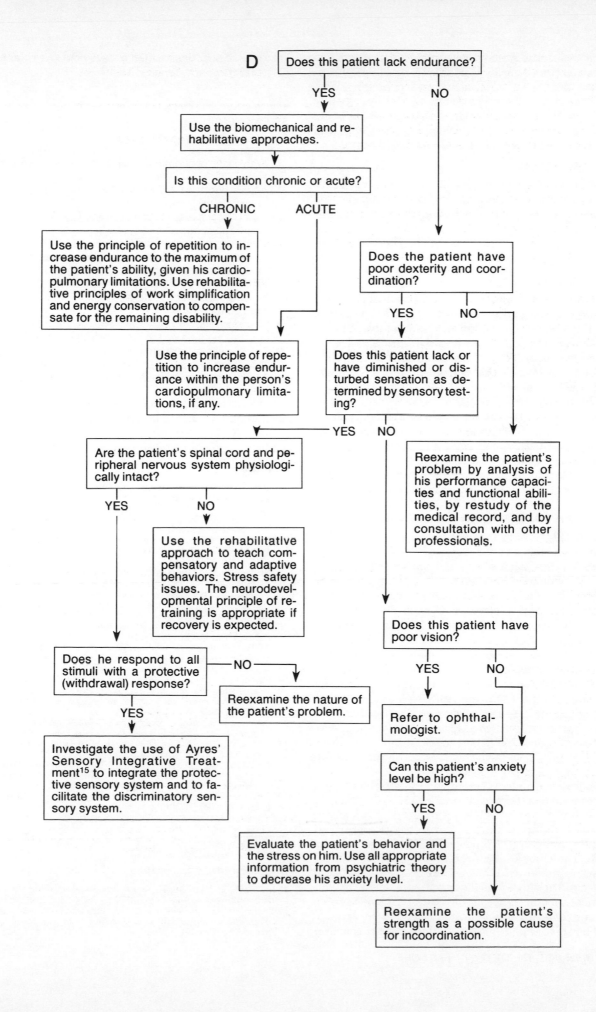

D Does this patient lack endurance?

YES → Use the biomechanical and rehabilitative approaches.

↓

Is this condition chronic or acute?

CHRONIC → Use the principle of repetition to increase endurance to the maximum of the patient's ability, given his cardiopulmonary limitations. Use rehabilitative principles of work simplification and energy conservation to compensate for the remaining disability.

ACUTE → Use the principle of repetition to increase endurance within the person's cardiopulmonary limitations, if any.

NO → Does the patient have poor dexterity and coordination?

YES → Does this patient lack or have diminished or disturbed sensation as determined by sensory testing?

NO → Reexamine the patient's problem by analysis of his performance capacities and functional abilities, by restudy of the medical record, and by consultation with other professionals.

YES → Are the patient's spinal cord and peripheral nervous system physiologically intact?

YES → Does he respond to all stimuli with a protective (withdrawal) response?

NO → Use the rehabilitative approach to teach compensatory and adaptive behaviors. Stress safety issues. The neurodevelopmental principle of retraining is appropriate if recovery is expected.

NO → Reexamine the nature of the patient's problem.

YES → Investigate the use of Ayres' Sensory Integrative Treatment[15] to integrate the protective sensory system and to facilitate the discriminatory sensory system.

Does this patient have poor vision?

YES → Refer to ophthalmologist.

NO → Can this patient's anxiety level be high?

YES → Evaluate the patient's behavior and the stress on him. Use all appropriate information from psychiatric theory to decrease his anxiety level.

NO → Reexamine the patient's strength as a possible cause for incoordination.

vised to assist the student occupational therapist to sort out a patient's physical problems and to select appropriate treatment approaches and principles. The chart does not include the detail of the therapeutic process (methods), which is the substance of this book, nor is it meant to take the place of the knowledge and professional judgment of an experienced therapist.

TREAT THE PATIENT

The patient lifts the weight through full range 10 times. Following a rest period, finger extension is used functionally by requiring the patient to extend his fingers to pick up larger and larger lightweight objects. This would combine treatment of the flexors and extensors, which is desirable.

REEVALUATION

Reevaluation would be carried out for each of the problems that are being addressed in therapy. In the case of the goal under consideration in this example, muscle strength would be remeasured, and progress, or lack of it, would be recorded. Treatment would be modified based on these results; that is if the patient's finger extensors had increased to F−, then short-term goal 2 would be next planned for and implemented. If they had not improved, treatment would be changed since it was not effective. The change may be in frequency (the number of treatments per day), duration (the amount of time spent doing one task within a treatment session), or intensity (the level of gradation according to the principle being used, e.g., increase resistance).

Flow Chart for Planning Treatment

The chart (Fig. 1.4) represents a series of choices that the therapist makes as a response to each question in working through each of the patient's problems. Because a patient may have several problems, it may be necessary to break into the chart at any of the questions designated by a letter (*A, B, C,* or *D*).

The chart reflects the author's bias that although neurodevelopmental principles may be effective for orthopedic patients, the biomechanical principles that focus primarily on force and motion of muscles and joints rather than nervous system function, per se, are not necessarily the best choice for developmentally immature patients nor those with brain damage. Biomechanical principles are appropriately applied to patients with orthopedic or cardiopulmonary disorders or patients who have regained motor control following a central nervous system lesion.

Therefore the chart is organized to help the student select the correct approach and principle within the approach for her particular patient. It is not a diagnosis-related reasoning process; therefore, it should be applicable to physically disabled patients in general. The chart is also designed to help the student therapist consider whether evaluation and treatment are needed for those basic capacities needed for performance, such as range of motion or muscle tone, or whether evaluation and treatment need to be aimed at higher levels of function that combine these capacities

into sets of abilities needed to carry out the roles of life: self-maintenance, leisure, and work.[14]

STUDY QUESTIONS:
Treatment Planning Process

1. What is the occupational therapy treatment planning process?
2. Where can data about the functioning of a patient be found?
3. How does a therapist decide on which evaluations to do for a particular patient?
4. Define *significant information*.
5. How does the problem list relate to the evaluation data?
6. How do the short-term goals relate to the identified problems?
7. What is the difference between long-term goals and short-term goals?
8. How does the occupational therapist choose the appropriate treatment approach for a particular patient?
9. What is a treatment principle?
10. Define occupational therapy treatment in your own words.
11. How do you know where to start treatment for a particular patient?
12. What is the purpose of reevaluation?
13. List the four components of Problem-Orientated Medical Recording.

References

1. Rogers, J. C. Eleanor Clarke Slagle lectureship–1983; Clinical reasoning: the ethics, science and art. *Am. J. Occup. Ther., 37*(9): 601–616, 1983.
2. May, B. J., and Newman, J. Developing competence in problem solving: a behavioral model. *Phys. Ther., 60*(9): 1140–1141, 1980.
3. Shriver, D., Mitcham, M., Schwartzberg, S., and Ranucci, M-H. Uniform occupational therapy evaluation checklist. *Am. J. Occup. Ther., 35*(12): 817–818, 1981.
4. Shriver, D., et al. Standard for practice for occupational therapy. *Am J. Occup. Ther., 37*(12): 802–804, 1983.
5. Rogers, J. C., and Masagatani, G. Clinical reasoning of occupational therapists during the initial assessment of physically disabled patients. *Occup. Ther. J. Res., 2*(4): 197–219, 1982.
6. Day, D. A systems diagram for teaching treatment planning. *Am. J. Occup. Ther., 27*(5): 239–243, 1973.
7. AOTA Commission on Uniform Reporting System Task Force. *Uniform Terminology for Reporting Occupational Therapy Services.* Rockville, MD: American Occupational Therapy Association, 1979.
8. Creed, C. L. Graph it up. *Accent on Living, 28*(2): 106–107, 1983.
9. Ottenbacher, K., and York, J. Strategies for evaluating clinical change: implications for practice and research. *Am. J. Occup. Ther., 38*(10):647–659, 1984.
10. Weed, L. L. *Medical Records, Medical Education and Patient Care.* Cleveland: Case-Western Reserve University Press, 1969.
11. Lynch, W. J., and Mauss, N. K. Brain injury rehabilitation: standard problem lists. *Arch. Phys. Med. Rehabil., 62*: 223–227, 1981.
12. De Weerdt, W. J. G., and Harrison, M. A. Problem list of stroke patients as identified in the problem orientated medical record. *Aust. J. Physiother., 31*(4): 146–150, 1985.
13. *Physicians' Desk Reference (34th edition).* Oradell, NJ: Medical Economics Co., 1980.
14. Standardized assessment being developed. *Occupational Therapy News,* January: 3, 1986.
15. Ayres, A. J. *Sensory Integration and Learning Disorders.* Los Angeles: Western Psychological Services, 1973.

Supplementary References

Cubie, S. H., and Kaplan, K. A case analysis method for the model of human occupation. *Am. J. Occup. Ther., 36*(10): 645–656, 1982.
Rothstein, J. M., and Echternach, J. L. Hypothesis-oriented algorithm for clinicians: a method for evaluation and treatment planning. *Phys. Ther., 66*(9): 1388–1394, 1986.

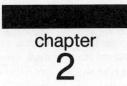

chapter

2

Psychosocial Accommodation to Physical Disability

Hilda Powers Versluys

The intent of this chapter is to help students understand their patients' emotional responses to disabling conditions. Psychosocial sequelae resulting from changes in health and loss of physical function prevent patients from maximizing potential or reengaging in life activities and also present barriers to successful discharge and a good quality of life within the community. The content of the chapter is planned to help students deduce their patients' psychosocial problems and to plan methods of treatment that will integrate physical and psychosocial treatment goals.

Despite excellent treatment programs and personal dedication, occupational therapists may encounter blocks to rehabilitation in that patients may remain passive, regressed, and depressed; seem unable to accept life-style changes; and fail to make the most of their assets. Psychosocial factors will influence the outcome of rehabilitation and these factors must be taken into account in the overall treatment programming for the patient. These psychosocial factors are described in the early sections of this chapter.

Some factors that influence rehabilitation are internal to the patient and some are external. Of the internal factors, some are developmental influences and others are related to a person's particular reaction to trauma, the way the individual copes with the disability (adaptive mechanisms), and the way that he adjusts over the long term (modes of accommodation). The occupational therapist needs to assess each patient regarding these factors in order not only to design a meaningful therapeutic program but also to know how to present the program to the patient in such a way that he wants to participate. Of the external factors, some are related to the patient's family and cultural background and others to the hospitalization experience. The degree to which these factors influence each individual patient varies, and this needs to be determined and incorporated into a holistic treatment plan.

In addition to the above factors that influence the patient's rehabilitation, specific diagnoses present particular problems of adaptation. Examples have been given of permanent neurological, chronic progressive, and invisible disabilities.

The treatment section provides theoretical rationales for treatment as well as concepts, methods, and techniques applicable in psychosocial intervention.

Psychological Considerations in the Rehabilitation of Physical Disability

Physical trauma and illness are devastating and cause disruptions in normal biological, physiological, and cognitive functioning. The developmental tasks, expectations, and plans of the adolescent and the lifestyle and goals of the adult may be arrested either temporarily or permanently. At the completion of the physical remediation program, the patient may be left with multiple disabilities that require adherence to different rules for living and influence the patient's ability to approach or continue in significant adult roles.[1-3]

Before experiencing disability or illness the patient, in most cases, has already developed a workable adaptation to life that represents an investment of time and personal commitment and that includes the development of an identity, life-style, and unique ways of achieving satisfaction from work, leisure, and social activities. Rapid and traumatic changes in the patient's ability to function and to experience life can precipitate an identity crisis because the recognizable self no longer exists.

The occupational therapy objective in rehabilitation of the disabled individual includes not only a restoration of maximum physical function but also the restoration of a sense of individuality and dignity and the determination of a life-style within society that provides enough satisfaction to motivate self-monitoring of physical and emotional health.[1,4,5]

This section on psychological considerations in rehabilitation describes those factors that influence the patient's ability to make effective use of rehabilitation opportunities. Such factors include the patient's developmental level, premorbid condition, position in the life cycle, reactions to trauma, and how all these factors affect the patient. Also discussed are problems related to dependency and depression, adaptive tasks and mechanisms, and different individual models of accommodation to the disability.

DEVELOPMENTAL INFLUENCES

Maturation with respect to psychosocial skills is necessary if individuals are to meet environmental demands for adult functioning. Psychosocial developmental stages are referred to in some occupational therapy literature as adaptive skills. Adaptive developmental-skill components are learned sequentially or simultaneously and must be integrated for mature functioning. The components of each adaptive developmental skill area are outlined in the references.[6,7]

Therapists will find that some patients have not matured psychosocially; they demonstrate a lack of learning or integration of skill components and are thus at risk for regression or loss of function developmentally. Other patients who have mature learned patterns of psychosocial adaptive behaviors have a difficult time maintaining their skills; for example, social and communication skills may atrophy in the environment of the long-term rehabilitation facility.

The following descriptions provide another way of viewing the loss of both psychological and physical developmentally achieved skills and the resulting impact on the patient. Traumatically injured patients, for example, risk losing physical functions such as motor ability, bowel control, and physical strength and developmentally achieved psychological functions such as autonomy and security. The patient's dependent position, invoked by hospitalization and medical care, can reawaken infantile conflicts including fears of abandonment and mutilation and may result in separation and castration anxiety. Although such fears may be symbolic, they also may be experienced in reality through loss of function or amputations due to injury, cancer, or diabetes.[2,8,9]

An evaluation of the patient's past and present developmental level provides information through which the patient's behaviors can be understood. Treatment goals to maintain or to develop adaptive developmental skills are an important part of the rehabilitation planning process.

PREMORBID CONDITIONS

The antecedent personality style, psychological and physical health, and preferred patterns of life are referred to as premorbid states or conditions. The patient's ability to adapt to disability is more certain when valued work, family and community roles, favorite activities, and membership in prized groups can be continued. Too great a variance between the premorbid and present life-styles may not be acceptable to the patient and will thus reduce intrinsic motivation to

identify acceptable alternative roles and to retain belief in personal competence. For example, some patients are cognitively oriented and enjoy intellectual and creative activities. Their interests more easily translate into career and vocational possibilities consistent with physical limitations.[10,11] Physically oriented people value strength, stamina, motor expression, and activities based on expression of these skills. For these people transition to more physically passive, functionally restrictive roles may be more difficult. These are generalizations, and much depends on the patient's range of interests, skills, past experiences, intelligence, and adaptability.[10]

The personality style of the patient influences his adaptive potential and the degree of internal stress he feels. To illustrate, the perfectionist has internalized high personal standards and often inflexible criteria of self-judgment. Thus slow, less-than-perfect achievement and a reduction in the ability to maintain valued personal standards will be threatening. The authoritative personality needs to be in control and has rigid perceptions about rules, values, and how things should be done, as well as the way people should live and behave. Adaptation to disability requires compromise, acceptance, and flexibility.

Certain personality patterns require special attention. Some patients have a deep fear of being abandoned and left helpless and thus require continual reassurances that the staff is concerned and understands their condition. Others rely on information from the staff to decrease their anxiety. Such patients benefit from clear, frequent explanations of their condition and the treatment plans. Some patients have a history of interpersonal problems and are phobic, and these patients find that the closeness of the rehabilitation environment provokes anxiety. They require special consideration and gradual inclusion into rehabilitation groups.

Compulsive work achievement, full independence, and high productivity are standards valued in our society and also can be compensatory ways of dealing with intrapersonal conflicts and low self-esteem. Diminished ability to adhere to these standards due to aging or disability may lead to feelings of worthlessness and helplessness and terminate in intractable depression. Some individuals have always had unrealistically high goals for themselves. Their pace of activity may cover unconscious feelings of guilt or a negative self-image, be a means of seeking approval, ward off depression, or provide satisfaction as they fill the role of the strong person who gives to others. A reduction in these individuals' ability to take significant roles, the need to accept help, or a reduction in their pace of activity is intolerable. They may see everything as lost and continue to define their worth in terms of the original abilities.[2,8,12,13]

Patients with borderline, antisocial, and passive-aggressive personality disorders are frequently encountered in mental health, medical, and rehabilitation practice. These individuals are often unmotivated and noncompliant; they demonstrate maladaptive responses to stress and have major social disabilities. Such patients distort reality and fail to take responsibility for their own lives. These patients find it difficult to tolerate the restrictions of hospitalization and the rules and procedures of medical treatment, such as casts, turning frames, or even splints. They fail to exercise good judgment and often exacerbate their dysfunctions by failure to comply with self-care procedures.[14]

The patient with a passive-aggressive personality disorder is defensive and aggressive and expresses hostility passively through stubbornness, procrastination, obstructiveness, and intended inefficiency. It is important, however, that the therapist discriminate between passive-aggressive behavior as a temporary effort to maintain control in response to trauma and the demands of rehabilitation and the entrenched personality disorder.[14]

Substance Abuse

Substance abuse behaviors are usually part of a preexisting premorbid pattern. Substance abusers can become physically disabled, and disabled patients can become substance abusers. The disabled individual runs a higher risk of exacerbating or developing substance abuse problems.[15] To illustrate, alcoholism, in terms of morbidity, is considered a major health problem today; and the disabled population is seen as particularly vulnerable to this form of substance abuse. Patients also may have easy access to prescription drugs because of their disability, pain, or other medical needs.[15,16]

Reasons predisposing disabled individuals to substance abuse problems can include a family and personal history; frustration and anxieties about being disabled; experiences with unproductive, unsatisfying, and dependent roles; functional inability to release tension; attendant motor and sensory deficits that accentuate the effects of alcohol; increased isolation; a lack of a sense of the ability to control events in their lives or to reach personal goals; and rejection experiences and other stressors related to loss and life-style changes. In addition, abuse of substances provides a way of avoiding the difficult and painful work of remediation.[15,16]

Therapists may fail to detect alcoholic problems as a secondary disability in their patients, so this condition may remain undetected, undocumented, and untreated. This lack of identification of alcoholism as a secondary disability can be due to a primary focus on the visible physical disability, lack of experience with signs and symptoms of alcoholism, or sympathy concerning drinking situationally to relieve stress.[16] The therapist should help the patient recognize the dangers of alcohol abuse, help relate the patient's medical, neurological, and psychosocial signs and symptoms to the abuse of alcohol, and encourage the patient to join a self-help group such as Alcoholics Anonymous and to seek specialized counseling from an alcoholism specialist or team.

Occupational therapy treatment for patients with alcoholic problems includes activities that focus on the mastery of skills such as improving planning and problem-solving abilities so that the patient gains a sense of competence and control and/or the development of strategies for coping such as increasing the ability to tolerate frustration and locating appropriate ways to relieve tension. Also important are a realistic identification of strengths and limitations and reality testing to reduce denial. Treatment programming can include stress reduction programs, assertiveness training, interpersonal skill development, and better ways to use spare time including the development of leisure time skills.[17]

During preparation for discharge it is important that therapists remain aware of the personal stress and anxiety that independence and responsibility within the community may pose for the patient with alcoholic problems. The therapists should monitor the patient's psychological health as it relates to exacerbation of drinking problems.[16,17]

A therapeutic community model program is described that provides treatment for the spinal cord-injured patient with alcoholic problems. Such patients require a treatment program that, besides being physically accessible, pays attention to the patient's adjustment to the disability and to the special medical problems connected with the injury.[18]

POSITION IN THE LIFE CYCLE

Each part of the life cycle has its specific developmental tasks, and personal role responsibilities. Each stage has specific psychological and social stresses that will influence the patient's ability to make adjustments and thus the rehabilitation process.

The adolescent period is a time of personal adjustment, turmoil, identity crisis, and concerns with separation, individuation, and appearance. When disability is superimposed over these normal but disruptive adolescent tasks and stresses, the developmental process is halted and prolonged, conflicts are intensified, and the potential for dependency is increased. For example, stress arises when the adolescent must live by different life-style rules, realizes his life span is shortened, is separated from the family experiences, and is frustrated at being different from peers.[2,19,20] Also influenced are the attainment of self and sexual identities, and the progression of normal life choices including vocational and career plans. Under these conditions adolescent rebellions may take place around compliance with medications, health rules, and rehabilitation programs.[21-23]

The middle-aged patient may be in the process of personal reappraisal that involves questions about the meaning of life, the recognition of physical decline, vocational disappointments, feelings of failure concerning original personal and career goals, and awareness of the shortening of time and inevitability of death. The patient at this stage of life may have major economic and personal responsibilities to children and parents. Family and career concerns provoke anxiety, and the patient may feel it is too late to start reshaping life patterns. These stresses are increased by the presence of physical and sensory losses, and the adjustment tasks facing the older client can be overwhelming. [2,12]

Rehabilitation is strengthened by the therapist's understanding of the tasks and stresses of each stage of development and by her sensitivity to multiple stressors at each life stage as they relate to disease and illness. Treatment goals should include experiences and activities related to the patient's normal developmental tasks and life stage concerns.

REACTIONS TO TRAUMA

Stress Reactions

This section uses crisis theory as a framework for understanding the intrapsychic process of responding to stress and those events that occur in rehabilitation that are particularly stressful to the patient. Crisis theory describes the needs for not only physiological homeostasis but also for social and psychological equilibrium. In a variety of crisis situations the patient will try to restore balance using his previous coping strategies and problem-solving techniques.

Coping strategies include all conscious and unconscious mechanisms used for adapting to environmental demands. The patient struggling for this stable condition also may use adaptive mechanisms such as denial, intellectualization, or obsessive-compulsive behaviors in trying to restore balance. If the crisis is too severe, adverse psychological reactions such as cognitive disorganization, disorientation, panic attacks, or somatization of anxiety may occur. Eventually a reappraisal takes place in which the individual patient subjectively assesses his ability to cope and continue with life. This period is significant for unless the patient can accept and integrate the disability into a framework for life he may fantasize about future potential, fail to adapt, retain maladaptive defenses, and remain at a lower level of life functioning. It is during this transition period that the patient is most receptive to external interventions and the therapist has an opportunity to influence the direction of adaptation.[24,25]

The patient under such traumatic physical, medical, and environmental conditions also may demonstrate behavior that parallels psychiatric conditions including anxiety disorders (neurosis) with hypochondriacal or obsessive-compulsive responses. Symptoms such as delusions, hallucinations, severe depression or regression, violence, and acting-out behaviors are usually reversible in formerly healthy patients as the medical status improves; the hospital milieu becomes less intense and threatening; the family network is stabilized; and the patient feels more in control, considers alternative ways to achieve satisfaction, understands the real boundaries of the disability, and sees possibilities for the future.[24-31]

Other crisis points in rehabilitation that are stressful to the patient include plateauing, making decisions about ambulation, using or buying adaptive equipment, waiting for and hearing a final diagnosis, the breakdown of denial, the family conference, and preparation for discharge. At these points the patient may again experience stress that may be less severe or tolerable, or may again require use of adaptive mechanisms.

The therapist should plan treatment interventions to meet the patient's special needs during such crisis periods. Stress reduction treatment is currently part of many occupational therapy programs. Treatment goals include increasing the patient's understanding of the nature of the stressors and treatment methods that use problem-solving techniques, relaxation exercises and activities, meditation, and imaging.

Anxiety

The arousal of anxiety can result in somatic preoccupation, sensitivity to pain, and a decrease in the motivation for learning new skills and reaching rehabilitation objectives. It is therefore an important concept for the occupational therapist to understand.

Anxiety is a normal response on the part of the patient to his medical condition. The patient's apprehension naturally increases in proportion to the threat to personal security, biological integrity, and self-esteem. In a mild form, anxiety causes discomfort for the patient; in a more severe form, it interferes with rehabilitation. Once anxiety has been aroused, it is slow to die down, and the effect spreads to all aspects of the patient's experience. Detecting the level of anxiety is important since a high level interferes with adaptation and learning. A very low or absent level of anxiety does not support motivation.[26]

Patients with a history of generalized anxiety disorder may be immobilized cognitively, emotionally, and physically. The resulting behavior is not always easy for the therapists to interpret. The patient may act in an unreliable, confusing manner; react to irrelevant cues; be unable to concentrate; be fearful, euphoric, or tense; and misinterpret events or develop false expectations. The staff may find that a patient has completely missed the point in discussions concerning his disability, the prognosis, or the goals of treatment. (This response may also result from denial.) In such cases the patient is not deliberately trying to confuse or sabotage but is attempting to deal with considerable anxiety and fear.[27,28]

Some patients respond to threat and the resulting anxiety by flights into activity. They may try to make radical changes in their lives (buying expensive items, engaging in fantasy plans). Such flight supports denial and temporarily eases anxiety but at the same time absorbs the economic, emotional, and energy resources needed for the rehabilitation effort. The patient also may be impractical, reckless, destructive, or rude and may abuse substances.[9,11,13,26,28,32]

The causes of anxiety are multiple. For example a posttraumatic stress syndrome is based on historical events and will mesh with, and exacerbate the emotional responses to, the present trauma. Acute anxiety and/or panic attacks occur when defenses and coping mechanisms are ineffective or when a premorbid generalized anxiety disorder is part of the personality structure. Cardiac symptoms of heart attack (nonorganic), catastrophic panic reactions, or severe regressions are examples of somatic and emotional reactions to anxiety.[14]

A therapist should anticipate that the patient will have strong emotions such as anxiety and hostility and recognize that while these issues remain unresolved, unidentified, and unexpressed the patient may not be successfully motivated for rehabilitation. Patients may be too anxious to understand what is causing the uncomfortable feelings. They may consider it weak to be afraid and, since adults have been taught to conceal fears, they may have little experience in verbalizing feelings. Treatment goals include helping patients recognize why they feel anxious, that problems are not as encompassing as believed, that they have some control over the direction of rehabilitation, and that planning for the future is possible.

Anger

Understanding the strong and negative emotions that may be described as hostility, hate, resentment, or rage is important, particularly because these feelings are generated by the intense but necessary relationships within the treatment environment. The development of strong feelings is often reciprocal among the patient, the family, and staff. The patient may be hostile toward staff who are physically intact, can leave the hospital, have freedom of movement, are in the position of authority, and who are present when the patient fails or struggles with seemingly unattainable tasks. Patients may deny their own residual disability and blame staff for incompetence or for not providing enough treatment time.[33]

Anger may be characterized as outward anger (expressed through controlling maneuvers, attack, sarcasm, glaring, or physical hitting) and inward anger (expressed by somatizing, depression, or suicide).[34]

In treating the patient, the occupational therapist is involved in his intimate areas of self-care and activities of daily living. For the patient this is a continual reminder of functional losses. The patient may not feel ready for reality testing generated by treatment aimed at improving self-care abilities, and expressions of hostility may be the result.

Patients do not always recognize or admit that they are angry and may have difficulty in expression of their anger because they need services from others. Unexpressed anger impedes treatment and may also cause development of physiological problems.

Therapists can recognize anger in the sabotage of treatment objectives, in withdrawal, in some forms of depression, in verbal attacks on staff, and in acting-out behaviors. The cause and remediation of the roots of such behaviors are important both for the patient's welfare and because their expression can cause rejection by the staff.[32-34]

The treatment goals include the reduction of anxiety and anger through clarification of feelings, helping the patient feel more in control, and encouraging safe avenues of both verbal and nonverbal expression of feelings. For example, the therapist can indicate that it is important to express such feelings and that it is normal to have them under the circumstances. The patient can be helped to feel that it is acceptable to verbally blow up, and the therapist can create the outlets for expression of strong feelings through activities and recreation. The reality is that severely injured patients may find expression threatening, and to verbalize strong feelings they would need reliable, proven, and strong support systems and relationships.

In general those patients who express strong affect such as aggression and anger make a better adjustment than the passive and denying patient. Anger becomes maladaptive when it prevents reality testing or distances staff, family, and personal-care attendants.

DEPENDENCY

Dependency is a major problem in the rehabilitation of the disabled patient, and the occupational therapist is concerned with counteracting the development of negative, intractable, dependent roles.[10,35] Dependency may be a predictable and acceptable response to helplessness and the hospital environment; may be part of a personality disorder or style and thus viewed as a premorbid condition; or may be latent in the patient and exacerbated by the situation. Dependency can also be understood as a condition that the patient must accept to some degree due to the need for treatment and attendant care assistance.

In the rehabilitation setting the patient is expected to comply with the medical regimen; to trust the staff to make important decisions concerning his health, life, and future; and to accept treatment in a system that may be efficient in meeting medical needs but neglectful in considering psychosocial aspects of adjustment. Faced with the integration of new realities about life and dealing with threatening implications about the future, the patient may not engage in rehabilitation or may develop dependent behaviors and fail to cope with community living upon discharge, necessitating frequent hospitalization.[3,10,11,36]

The following information discusses causes and types of dependency and provides treatment guidelines.

In the acute phase of illness the patient is unable to be independent, can function only with assistance, and must accept care from others. Such a situation feeds into a patient's sense of helplessness and may reinforce latent dependency needs and the underlying desire to be cared for by a strong parent figure. The patient with psychological problems may use the new patient role as a legitimate means of extracting the last ounce of attention and energy from his caretakers, as a means of avoiding personal responsibility, or as a weapon to demand love.[9,10,11,35]

The patient also may present with pseudoindependent behaviors that connote underlying dependency; hide anxiety, fear, and shame; and are a defense against vulnerability and dependency. Pseudoindependent behaviors include obstinacy, inappropriate confidence, inability to accept offers of assistance, and unrealistic goal setting. This type of coping mechanism is not successful over time since the patient ultimately needs the support and assistance of others. A breakdown in emotional functioning may be the result of collapse of denial or sudden reality experiences.[13]

There is also a danger that the patient's independent efforts and determination to influence treatment decisions will be seen by staff as interfering and difficult behaviors. Initially such behavior may be accentuated by an overlay of defenses and emotional responses to trauma and may be manifested as aggression. The patient may be labeled as a troublemaker and discouraged in his attempt to retain control over his own agenda.

The therapist needs to discriminate between these different types of dependent behavior and provide support or appropriate intervention. Those patients with latent dependency needs require a consistent staff approach to discourage the patient's passive role and encourage goal identification and collaboration in the treatment and decision-making process. The patient should be encouraged to maintain appropriate responsibility in personal and family roles and be provided with opportunities to make choices. Goals should be sequenced to arouse feelings of competence, success, and involvement.

Dependency also can be understood as a positive rather than a negative factor. A traumatically disabled patient may need to consider some aspect of a positive dependent role if maximum independence and an acceptable quality of life is to be achieved. A treatment goal would include helping the patient in understanding and accepting appropriate aspects of both independent and dependent roles. For example, the patient can be aided in recognizing that help with time-consuming skills relating to activities of daily living will free energy for involvement in more interesting and creative activities. Treatment goals are also focused to encourage patients to examine their values, to deal with personal feelings concerning accepting necessary help, to retain a positive self-view, to accent their competencies, to develop communication and interactive skills that help them tactfully direct others, and to engage in problem solving for maximum independence.[10,35]

DEPRESSION

In a rehabilitation setting one type of depression observed in patients is reactive depression, which appears when denial subsides. It is considered a normal response to functional loss, hospitalization, and recognition of life-style changes. In some cases, however, a patient may be affected by more than one type of depression, and recognition of this difference is critical information for treatment because unremitted depression prevents adaptation to the disability and reengagement with life tasks. This section discusses the multiple causes of depression, describes how depressive states affect rehabilitation, and suggests treatment approaches. Discrimination among the various types of depression ensures that the treatment approach is realistic and focuses on the real problem.

Why is depression so destructive, its treatment so essential, and its cause so important? Depressed patients require longer rehabilitation, have feelings of futility that block motivation, are often unable to make the mental effort to plan ahead, are more pessimistic about the future, show a lower level of self-care at discharge, have more mortality, and regress easily. Depressed patients also have difficulty with slow and less-than-perfect achievement and see this as a personal failure. These perceptual distortions influence their ability to feel pleasure in activities or skill mastery, to receive positive social reinforcement from others, or to reengage with life planning. Once the patient's concept of himself has changed permanently and he sees himself in a disabled, dependent, and helpless role, he may continue to function at a low level.[37,38]

Depressive states also are linked to the length of hospitalization and lack of preparation for discharge. Other precipitating causes are awareness of the loss of time, inability to meet work and family role obligations or to reach personal or career goals, and the inability to live up to personal standards or to the family and cultural values.[8,10,39-41]

Depressive states also are linked to the length of hospitalization and lack of preparation for discharge. Other precipitating causes are awareness of the loss of time, inability to meet work and family role obligations or to reach personal or career goals, and the inability to live up to personal standards or to the family and cultural values.[8,10,39-41]

Depressive states also can include major depressions or chronic depressive personality disorders, can be the result of organic diseases like cancers and viral infections, can be a reaction to medications, and can be a reaction to the disability and the symbolic meaning of loss.[14] Recently researchers have expressed a concern with lack of recognition of double depressive states. It is important, therefore, to recognize that an acute, reactive depressive condition can be superimposed on a premorbid chronic depressive condition (referred to as double depression) and influence recovery. Based on this previous pathology the expected remission of reactive depression does not occur, intervention fails to have a lasting impact, and there are continued relapses leading to entrenched states of depression.[38,42] Extended depression and grieving may be based on previous unresolved, intrapsychic conflicts, unconscious losses, and feelings of failure and self-hate.

diagnostic categories. In rheumatoid arthritic patients the symptoms of systemic disease such as fatigue, loss of appetite, decreased motivation, and diminished sexual drive are identical to those of depression.[37]

Reactive depression is a normal and expected response to loss and is associated with a specific external and observable trauma or medical event that precipitates the depressive condition. Examples of influential losses include familiar or pleasant sensations (sexual responses, running, active sports) or bodily functions that require lifelong catheterization or other daily care. Reactive depression is seen as normal at the beginning of the adjustment process and then periodically as the patient becomes discouraged or overwhelmed, is isolated, fails to progress in treatment, or remembers the losses in the form of an anniversary reaction.[8,10,13,38]

Treatment guidelines include: (1) encouraging the patient to express the sadness and loss and what this means personally, indicating that such feelings are appropriate, (2) clarifying values, (3) involving the patient in testing the real boundaries and influence of the disability, (4) facilitating identification of remaining assets and strengths, (5) establishing short-term and meaningful goals so that the patient can see the results, (6) helping the patient to examine alternative ways to fulfill adult role obligations and to engage in interests, (7) encouraging exploration of new life-style options, and (8) developing strategies to allow the patient to establish feelings of personal causation and control over events and the environment.

Therapists working with depressed patients must guard against the tendency to identify with the patient's mood (affect) and to become depressed themselves.

ADAPTIVE TASKS AND MECHANISMS

The Adaptive Tasks

The adaptive tasks required of the rehabilitant include coping with the hospital environment, isolation, pain, helplessness, and enforced dependency. The patient also must find a way to maintain a sense of individuality, self-worth, and relationships with family and friends and to interact successfully with the staff. The patient must deal with the adjustment demands of specific disabilities (paralysis, disfigurement, brain damage), with progressive illness (exacerbations, remission), with physiological or hormonal imbalances, or with the side effects of medications.

Coping mechanisms include the defenses used to cushion the trauma (i.e., denial, repression), the coping strategies employed to aid in emotional recovery (i.e., problem solving), and the patients' subjective understanding of their part in rehabilitation. Coping strategies are those mental and behavioral skills and techniques that include seeking information; using the intellect for problem solving; taking refuge in activity; requesting emotional support; setting concrete, realistic, and short-term goals; and involvement with support, educational, and therapeutic groups.[3,10,28,43,44]

Models of adaptation include the stage model, an outline of formal sequences of emotional and psychodynamic responses such as shock, denial, grief, and final acceptance. This stage-specific view is now considered instructional but too rigid and simplistic for use in therapy. Despite commonalities, each patient's accommodation to his physical and medical situation is highly individualistic. In reality adjustment is cyclical, fluctuates, overlaps, varies in order, and may not occur until much later in the recovery process. Note that life stresses, anniversary reactions, and sudden discovery of barriers to achievements or satisfaction may again stimulate depression, denial, mourning, and regression.[3,28,44-46]

All patients have emotional reactions, and such reactions are expected and normal. Accommodation is the most successful when the patient can acknowledge and experience the expected, normal feelings of anger, sadness, and loss and at the same time recognize and build on those aspects of life that are not affected by the disease.[2,11,13,37] The occupational therapist needs to understand the dynamics behind the behavior of her patients during the initial stages of recovery and the ongoing process of rehabilitation.

Adaptive Mechanisms

The term adaptive mechanisms has been selected to curb the tendency to label healthy and reasonable use of defense mechanisms in the process of adaptation to disability as maladaptive, neurotic, or pathological. Adaptive mechanisms are intrapsychic, unconscious, protective, and anxiety relieving. They aid in maintaining a normal state of emotional functioning.[14,46] Therapists need to be aware that such responses as denial, acting out, passive-aggressive behaviors, and destructive, rude, or hostile behaviors can represent the patient's inner and continual struggle to meet the new terms established by functional impairments. It is important to recognize that behaviors such as delusions or hallucinations, usually indicative of psychotic states, may be seen as situational, transitory stress reactions in patients who had sound coping skills originally. In some cases the signs of the adaptive process are repressed, displaced, delayed, or disguised so that the superficial clinical picture may suggest their absence, whereas careful observation generally reveals their operation.[8,9,13,28,46]

Denial. Denial is useful as a transient form of adaptation to trauma and protects the patient from full recognition of the prognosis while still vulnerable and incapacitated. As an emergency defense, denial reduces cognitive disorientation and despair and may prevent major depression or even psychosis. As an adaptive mechanism, denial allows the patient to integrate the realities of the disability at an individual and acceptable pace. Denial is usually present in cases of severe disability but varies in intensity; that is, the patient may be insightful at times but, when threatened by the overwhelming remedial task and made aware of barriers to life plans and satisfactions, may again become denying. At times denial may be necessary as a protective device to ward off depression and to cope with recognition of physical vulnerability. In other cases the patient may appear well motivated in the initial stages of treatment until a plateau in functional progress is reached. At this point hidden denial or intellectualization is confronted by the reality of the situation. The patient may suddenly become anxious, depressed, insistent that a cure is possible, regress, and/or become resistive to treatment.

Denial can be viewed as both positive and negative. In a positive sense denial reduces anxiety. For example, it can be calming to a myocardial infarct patient in intensive care or can allow a spinal cord patient time for those therapeutic interventions that focus on identification of remaining competencies and potential for achievement. In a negative sense denial leads to noncompliant behavior, refusal to sustain or seek treatment, and refusal to monitor or attend to health care responsibilities. It should be noted that patients who express a cheerful, instant, optimistic acceptance of their disability also may be denying and what appears as courage and flexibility may be a fragile and precarious adjustment. Such a patient may require psychiatric treatment to help him express the meaning of the loss and underlying sadness and grief.

Certain avoidance strategies are a kind of denial. The patient may avoid reality by displacement, an obsessive focus on concerns that appear inappropriate or flights into activities not related to remediation. As long as denial is not so excessive as to prevent engagement in the rehabilitation process, the therapist should not be concerned or surprised that the patient periodically or continually expresses a belief of the eventual return of function.

As the patient progresses toward clear, observable treatment goals, reality may be less threatening. The therapist can be supportive, assisting the patient in identifying and demonstrating competencies and exploring life goals within his capabilities. While the patient may not appear initially to commit to this approach, it has demonstrated value.

Patients may hold onto the belief that when they are discharged and in their own home, the dysfunction will lessen, and they will again be able to function in the usual manner. Thus patients may insist that training in activities of daily living is not necessary. When the patient rejects the need for treatment on this basis, the therapist can suggest that, while waiting for return, the patient learn skills for use now. In addition, a weekend pass or other reality experience may influence the patient to gradually accept the need to engage in treatment. Time and experience in the community may allow the patient to be more realistic, but he may wish to hold onto the hope of future functional return. The most successful approach may be to work around the patient's denial.

Prognosis is considered to be better when the patient faces the reality of the situation, becomes depressed, and mourns for a period of time rather than continuing to deny. As the patient begins to give up his denial, he feels the awful facts and enters a phase of depression and mourning.[38,43,47]

Regression. Regression is an emotional and physical retreat from adult standards of independence and self-determination to an earlier and less mature level of adaptation. Regressive behaviors include acting out in a childlike manner, persistent dependency, sabotage, lack of motivation, and passivity. Factors precipitating regressive behaviors may be the hospital environment, the control of the medical regimen, incontinence, enforced dependency, or the patient's anger about what has happened to his body. Regression may be precipitated by a therapist. A therapist who is too assertive and eager for results may push the patient too fast in treatment and miss the signs that he is becoming overwhelmed with the enormity of the rehabilitation tasks. During regressive periods, infantile fears may emerge and again become issues of conflict and crisis. The patient may again fear abandonment, destruction, and physical attack.[9,14] Some patients are able to regress adaptively in the service of their recovery in order to accept therapeutic services, while others regress maladaptively by denying problems and acting in ways that exacerbate their medical conditions.[9]

The therapist should identify the onset and presence of regression in the patient and intervene. Treatment approaches include reassurance, support, focus on short-term goals, identification of feelings, and realistic restructuring of treatment objectives. Regression cannot be overcome by willpower. Some patients may need time out from therapy, protection from an internal sense of failure, or an alternative therapeutic approach such as group work, adaptive play, or recreational experience. The therapist should maintain a relationship that is caring, realistic, and helpful. Some clinicians feel that management of the regressed patient requires a tolerant, gentle, but insistent push program.

Grief and Mourning. Grief, bereavement, and mourning are feeling states that occur as a consequence of loss. Anticipated losses also may be grieved for. Grief has been described as pain resulting from loss of physical functions, appearance, vocation, or relationships. Grieving may be an overwhelming and total experience. It may be demonstrated through acting-out behavior, hostility, profound sadness, or those behaviors associated with depression. A period of mourning may be seen as a time of personal disorganization, angry attempts to regain the lost object, pervasive ambivalence, and ever-changing feelings about the past, the loss, and the future. Grief can be such an intense experience that it may require a moratorium from the routine of living. Personal values can influence the severity of grief reactions, and values clarification is considered a useful intervention.[8,48-51]

Both the patient and family may begin acceptance and reality testing with initial reactions of disbelief and numbness, then sadness, grief, and mourning, expression of anger and hostility, and preoccupation with loss and ensuing changes, and then move to a reorganization of their values and perception of life possibilities.[32,52]

Because our culture values adequacy and strength, patients are sometimes criticized for the expression of their grieving reactions to what are frequently multiple losses. Asking such patients to behave as if nothing of significance has happened blocks the work of mourning, which can lead to future emotional difficulties.

The reestablishment of an acceptable self-identity requires that the patient relinquish some of his previous standards for evaluation of his self-worth and competence.[5,11,13,51] The patient is assisted in this process by a steady, understanding, and accepting therapeutic relationship. The therapist should be able to tolerate the patient's grief with empathy and refrain from prematurely cutting it off to relieve personal discomfort. Patients often need to verbalize feelings of loss and to discuss how it was before the accident, surgery, or illness. Provided the time span is reasonable, the process of mourning should be allowed to run its course.[48]

Treatment goals include facilitation of coping skills and identification of assets and potential. Treatment programs should include social and group activities and early mobilization. Intervention through psychiatric consultation can be made in cases of depression and mourning if in the judgment of the rehabilitation team the intensity or duration of these reactions is injurious to the patient.

Other Adaptive Mechanisms. Other adaptive mechanisms include intellectualization, in which the patient directs his attention away from his emotional reactions to focus on the disability. This full concentration on the facts and details of his condition can bypass feelings of pain or anxiety and can have a number of different outcomes. The patient may continue in this fashion with varying degrees of success; he may deal with the losses in an unobserved intrapsychic manner and manage quite well in the community. In other cases, some life event or evidence of the residual disability may suddenly force confrontation with reality, in which case the patient may experience a period of mourning and depression. Accommodation to this new reality must occur or the patient may continue in a maladaptive cycle of depression and mourning.

Somatization is a defense in which the patient's emotional responses never reach the conscious level but are expressed through physical symptoms like pain, headaches, or back problems. In the use of acting out as a defense, the patient translates his emotional feelings into action, for example into violent, verbal, and/or physical behavior. For some patients acting out and expressions of anger are more tolerable than feeling the disturbing emotions connected with loss.

Summary

In summary, strong emotional reactions and the use of various adaptive mechanisms are both expected and normal responses. Severe behavioral reactions may be reversible with a correct intervention such as support, change in the environment, family involvement, and psychosocial treatment. The concern is that patients will become fixed in maladaptive responses, which will then become techniques of resistance rather than ways to survive and progress.[9,13,14,24,25,27,51]

MODES OF ACCOMMODATION

The patient ultimately is confronted with the task of transcending the traumatic experience, reappraising reality, redefining personal values, and distinguishing between the loss of functions and those areas of life that are still viable. This requires giving up and letting go of things as they were and the recovery of belief and hope that life has interest and potential as it is.

Modes of accommodation to physical disability include both adaptive and maladaptive responses. Some patients never resolve their feelings about the physical limitations. Their maladaptive response is to desperately attempt to retain normal habits by pretending that they can do all their usual activities. Such patients act surprised when they cannot do everything that the nondisabled individual does. They tend to refuse the company of other disabled people and prefer to develop a group of nondisabled friends. They are committed to preventing the breakdown of their denial. This group of patients remains unaccepting and frustrated, and they continue to plan activities that they cannot carry out. Another group of patients seem eager to accept the limitations, even those that could be overcome. When treatment is successful for these patients and the physical limitations or effects of the disease are ameliorated, they continue to demonstrate deficits in the psychological and social spheres. Patients also may ignore their intact skills and abilities and become preoccupied with their predisability real or fantasized successes, making adaptation to their present situation more difficult. Other disabled individuals are able to accept the fact that they are still worthwhile and build a life on their unchanged assets, both physical and nonphysical. Such patients eventually accept the limitations of the disease and make the most of their lives.[11]

Modes of accommodation are influenced by unconscious conflicts and fears, by myths and beliefs that may be cultural, familial, or national, and by latent dependency needs. To illustrate: (1) The injury may be seen as confirmation of lack of self-worth and the patient becomes reconciled to a negative self-image. (2) The injury and deformity may relieve the patient of guilt for some real or imagined past act and lead to a sense of well-being or relief. (3) Physical illness and disability may satisfy security and dependency needs without stigmatizing the patient, since an invalid role is accepted by society and provides justification for dependent behavior. (4) The patient may wish to maintain security and financial support, for example, insurance or family assistance. In the case of work-related accidents, this has been termed compensation neurosis, and it can be unconscious. (5) The patient also may experience deep feelings of guilt and hold onto painful symptoms as a form of self-punishment. Guilt may be based on the patient's awareness that he used poor judgment, violated important rules, and failed to meet certain standards and thus was responsible for the accident. Patients also may feel responsible and guilty when they recognize the suffering, the extra work, and the worry caused others.[9,11,13,24,26,52]

In summary, adjustment to physical dysfunction and chronic illness is of long duration and continues after the patient is discharged. It is important during the vicissitudes of the rehabilitation process to remember that many patients make successful life-style adjustments despite the personal loss and disruption to their lives that the disability caused.

Ancillary Factors That Influence Rehabilitation

The following factors also influence the rehabilitation process. They include such things as restrictive environments, the therapist's role, family attitudes, and cultural and religious beliefs.

ENVIRONMENTAL DEPRIVATION

The hospital environment is alien to most people. It is impersonal, monotonous, and confining with unfamiliar rules of behavior. The lack of privacy, care by strangers, uncomfortable treatment procedures, and proximity and aversion to other patients and their families (habits, ethnicity, personalities) can increase the patient's stress. Patients with histories of avoidance or schizoid personality disorders, social phobias, different values, or cultural beliefs that distance them from the mainstream of society may experience excessive stress that is detrimental to treatment.[33,35,36,52,53]

The environmental influence within the hospital becomes critical as the acute stage of the illness subsides. The patient feels that he cannot influence his environment; he is given little opportunity for decision making, for using initiative, or for continuing a role of identity or responsibility. The patient is expected to yield control over his actions and personal decision making to those in authority, who do not know his skills or see him as an individual. Relationships with the staff may not be experienced at an adult level. Staff are often seen as authoritative and parental, and this encourages regressive and/or dependent behavior, which is antithetical to the goals of rehabilitation.[11,35,51,52]

The treatment procedures may cause social and sensory deprivation. The immobilization of the patient through traction, turning frames, or body casts in combination with decreases in stimulation of other senses can produce disorientation and even psychotic behaviors. Such observable behaviors include depression, panic, irritability, regression, hallucinations, or delusions.[53] Patients who have severe personality problems or who are impulsive or immature will have difficulty tolerating the restrictions of immobility and hospitalization and may present a management problem for the staff.

The type of injury, degree of functional loss, and the nature of the treatment of some medical and surgical conditions may result in a drastic reduction of the amount of everyday stimulation such as that found in work and social activities.[53] Also, a lack of fluency in English is isolating and contributes to misunderstandings, anxiety, and stress.

The occupational therapist should identify those patients at risk and discuss intervention recommendations based on evaluation findings with the rehabilitation team. Treatment programming might simply include the use of activities to provide sensory stimulation or opportunities for the patient to manipulate or change his environment. When possible, patients should be transported to social or task-oriented therapy groups and should be aided in resuming normal patterns of human interaction. Treatment in normalized environments reduces the negative impact of hospitalization and prepares the patient for successful discharge.

THE THERAPIST'S ROLE

This section discusses the therapist's role responsibilities, stressors that are inherent in the treatment of disabled patients, unconscious needs and attitudes that create problems for some therapists, and the importance of clear communication and a therapeutic relationship.

Working with the Patient

In general, working with physically challenged patients and their families is rewarding and challenging. It is also, at times, frustrating and stressful. The therapist is intimately involved with the patient for daily treatment procedures and thus is continuously in touch with his grief, depression, and bewilderment. Since the occupational therapist works with the patient in the area of self-care and other activities of daily living, she is in a position to help the patient test reality against his denial. In some cases the patient may continue to deny the permanence of functional loss and feel that his unchanging physical status is due to the therapist's incompetence, neglect, or to reduced treatment time.

Communication, an essential component of rehabilitation, can be hampered by the patient's and therapist's divergent viewpoints about treatment objectives. Such misunderstandings may stem from the therapist's lack of knowledge of the patient's subjective goals and priorities.

The therapist's role differs during each phase of rehabilitation. At one point the patient may need to have his regression understood and supported, and at another stage the therapist should encourage autonomy and personal decision making.

Problem Areas

Some individuals choose the helping profession because of personal interest or special skills, while others are partly influenced by unconscious motivation such as wanting to relieve others' suffering and thus expurgate their own, wanting an authoritative role with respect to others, or an excessive need to nurture. In addition therapists may have strong needs for lines of social division between patient and therapist, the need to control people and information, and judgmental attitudes concerning appropriate goals for certain patients.[54] These unconscious needs and attitudes of staff may impede the very process to which they are committed. Without conscious intent, therapists may encourage unrealistic rehabilitation goals based on the need to feel successful professionally (therapeutic ambitiousness) and to be liked by the patients and their families. When patients do not improve, therapists may feel anger, failure, guilt, and inadequacy and then reject the patient.[54] At times anger and disappointment are understandable, but therapists need to identify the basis for their emotional reactions so that they can empathize and be nonpunitive in their relationships with patients.[33]

Therapists working with the severely physically disabled may have unconscious fears of becoming disabled, of being helpless, or of regressing to an infantile state and being overwhelmed. Constant exposure to physical disability can be emotionally overwhelming and threatening to the therapist's own sense of intactness. Staff may feel guilty over good personal health and thus become self-protective by denying the extent of the patient's disability and the realistic reactive mourning of losses. Therapists are asked by the system to assume responsibility for patients and at the same time deal with conflicts concerning their own unresolved dependency needs and longing for care and affection. Support groups for therapists are helpful in retaining perspective.[4,8,9,24,25,53]

Treatment Focus

The relationship between the patient and the therapist is motivational when the therapist is consistent, maintains daily contact at least initially, acts as the patient's advocate, deals with concrete, real issues, tailors the treatment objectives to the patient's learning style, and clarifies reality by identifying those areas in which the patient can be proficient. Such a therapist shows respect for the patient and validates his individuality. She responds therapeutically but can also be firm and clear about important intervention objectives. She reality-tests with understanding and can help and guide without playing the authority role.[1,3,8,39,44,50]

What is important to patients is that the therapist understand their unique case, provide an opportunity for discussion of concerns, communicate helpful information about the implications of the injury, encourage experimentation and development of the patient's own ideas, and demonstrate concern about the quality of the patient's future life.[44,52,55]

The effective therapist structures the future for the patient by providing realistic hope. The future is characterized by a positive view of the work the patient needs to do and information about the means available for producing improved function and a satisfactory quality of life. It is important to remember that the principle investment is the patient's. The therapist can provide treatment, education, and guidance, but the motivation and effort must come from the patient.[4,5,44,50,54]

THE FAMILY

This section describes family responses to having a disabled or seriously ill family member, intrafamily dysfunctions, staff and family issues, and problems associated with discharge. The purpose is to identify those family situations that influence rehabilitation and in which intervention is important.

Family Responses

While many families have the coping and organizational ability to adapt to and deal with an intrafamily medical crisis, it is important for the therapist to recognize that the family may be as traumatized as the patient and requires support, education, patience, and understanding. The family, as well as the patient, uses adaptive mechanisms such as denial, intellectualization, and fantasies concerning restoration of function. This can be their temporary or long-term solution. Other family reactions include anxiety in dealing with the patient's behaviors (depression, hostility), distress at having to trust strangers to care for the patient, and a sense of powerlessness over their inability to influence the recovery process. At the plateau stage both patient and family face additional stressors. At this point in the rehabilitation process all hope for a complete recovery is gone, economic and emotional resources have worn thin, and future decisions must be made based on the realities of residual conditions of the patient.[32,52]

Therapists should be aware that families also may be disappointed at results that the therapist feels are very good, such as reconstructive surgery, burn treatment, use of adaptive eating equipment, or walking with braces.[32] Family frustration, fear, and worry over the patient's situation or suffering can be projected out at the staff in the form of anger, criticism, or hostility.

Family Dysfunctions

The prospect of caring for the disabled is, in some cases, threatening and can lead to instinctive withdrawal and increased alienation. Reacting to this threat, families may have difficulty making a steady commitment, may avoid discharge planning, may develop punitive behaviors toward the patient, and may assign another individual the patient's family roles on a permanent basis.

Therapists need to recognize the effect of the disability on the social and occupational activities of each particular family, as well as the family's current lifestyle and special needs.[52] It is unrealistic to expect families to deal with these problems unaided. Families vary in their ability to assess the patient's situation, to accept responsibility, and to make compromises in their plans. Families who are made to feel guilty about their perceived inadequacies may be driven away from any involvement with the patient.[52]

The additional stressors of the disability often accentuate existing marital and family problems. Although viable marital relationships may endure, other less committed marriages are likely to dissolve. Separation and divorce can influence the care and placement of the patient, who may need to make new living arrangements. In such a case, additional preparation for independence in the community will become a serious treatment objective.[11,52-57]

In addition, the patient may have been noncompliant for years in following medical and health care requirements (for example, in the case of a cardiac or diabetic condition), and the family is now faced with the care of a seriously disabled member. This produces anger and resentment.

Some family matters such as long-standing resentments, intrafamily control issues, and dysfunctional or dependent family constellations may absorb staff time and endanger the patient's emotional equilibrium and ability to concentrate on rehabilitation goals. Families may project their problems, feelings, and disorganization onto the staff or the patient, and they may become ill themselves and demand attention and care.[27,32,33] In addition, the patient can have the dilemma of dealing with his own personal adjustment, recognizing the long-term effects of the disability, and dealing with a family who is denying and anxious.[52]

Staff and Family Relationships

The staff and family relationships are important in the rehabilitation process, but they are also fragile. The family is cast in a new and unfamiliar role, and defensive reactions may last longer than the staff can accept. Families may find that they are in the way on the wards or in the treatment areas. Busy therapists may have little time or patience with questions. They may view the family effort to be involved as intrusive or troublesome. Staff can be critical and feel that some families are not interested or committed enough or that other families show the patient too much attention.

In other words the staff, while caring for the patient and understanding the process of his accommodation to disability, has a tendency to expect the family to show instant ability to cope with the problems and adjustment of having a disabled family member.[57] These staff attitudes can place the family in a no-win situation and reduce the opportunity for the staff and family to work together for the best interests of the patient. It is important that therapists evaluate the meaning behind family behaviors and that they aid the family in correcting misunderstandings and misperceptions and in identifying positive rehabilitation results.

Family Reactions To Discharge Time

The time of discharge can be anxiety provoking, and the family may resist taking the patient home by ne-glecting to make necessary arrangements or failing to seek suggested community resources or to order necessary equipment.

The modern family structure and the current demands on each individual member are sometimes incompatible with the patient's need for services within the home and community. It is clear that some families urged to take on major caretaker roles are not able to do so while simultaneously meeting other important obligations and retaining family stability. The family system and the health and welfare of its members can be threatened when the wife must seek employment for the first time and also care for a disabled husband, or a husband must work and care for a disabled wife and manage a home; or the children have to take over the household duties; or plans for the children's education are affected; and/or living accommodations must be changed.[11,52-57]

It is important to evaluate the family's ability to cope with the crisis of an injured member, to provide support that is useful to the patient, to retain the patient's family membership roles including his place in the family structure, and to assist in compliance with medical rules and procedures. Not all family systems are viable. Discharge plans will be influenced by the quality of family cohesion, the family's adaptive skills, their interest in the patient, and the presence or absence of family pathology.[52,55-58]

Interventions focused on the real source of the problem are important. Sometimes the patient is more independent than the family realizes, or the patient can play assistive roles in the family that should be identified and explored. The Independent Living Movement,[58] self-help groups, and other community resources offer support, training, education, and respite care. Families should be made aware of these services.

Because of prospective payment plans, with increased early discharge, more responsibility is disseminated to the family. It is important that the therapist resist a total emphasis on the patient's welfare and incorporate a broader view relative to the specific needs of each family unit for its successful survival.

CULTURE

This section examines the influence of culturally determined beliefs on the rehabilitation process and role change, the influence of the American culture, problems with racism, and the importance of language skills for clear communication.

The Effect of Culture

Cultural attitudes and values influence rehabilitation. Culturally determined beliefs affect the patient's understanding of the cause and meaning of the disability or illness, his trust of health professionals, his acceptance of the therapist's ability to treat him, and his personal priorities and decisions about continued involvement in rehabilitation. To illustrate, some patients may seek medical care but believe that they have offended evil spirits and that caused their illness. The patient may successfully internalize religious beliefs about the cause of the illness (sinning, evil spirits, magic) and may seek out treatment from spiritualists concomitantly with the medical or rehabilitation approach. In other cases cultural authority figures may direct decisions about rehabilitation, and the opinions of lay healers, friends, and family may carry more weight than those of the physician or rehabilitation team. Cultural background can influence attitudes toward types of therapy, for example, a distrust of psychotherapy, a discomfort with the expected collaborative relationship, and abhorrence toward crafts or manual activities, which may be seen as feminine or lower-class activities. The culture also determines the locus of family authority, the important people to be recognized in the patient's life, and who should be involved in all problem solving and decision making. A lack of awareness on the part of the staff of the difference in beliefs, priorities, and psychosocial needs, based on a cultural heritage, can evoke alienation and noncompliance in the family and the patients.[11,59-65]

Role Changes

Adult work, family, and personal-social roles may be culturally influenced. The loss of physical or cognitive performance skills may prevent the patient from continuing in previous work, family, or social roles or radically change the way in which these roles are carried out. In addition, the patient may need assistance to maintain certain work role functions and the authority of these roles may be compromised. For example, a mothering or homemaker role may require accepting the help of another and the person who carries out some of the role tasks may assume authority in that role and be viewed by others as having that role image.

Some cultures have strict demarcations between male and female roles. Thus options for compensatory role changes may be culturally limited and be viewed as departures from an acceptable way of performing an adult role. This may precipitate conflicts about personal and family values and pose rehabilitation problems. Examples of cultural and social influences on attitudes about adult role changes are the following: (1) Requirements for special, technical, or academic education for a new job or a redefined career goal may be outside the family and cultural experience and thus threatening. (2) A male parent may find his authority undermined by the disability, the wheelchair status, and/or his wife's return to work. These changes in the role of the male as provider and locus of authority in the family may result in loss of self-esteem, increased stress, marital difficulties, and depression. (3) Loss of physical abilities may precipitate a male patient's entry into roles that have been considered by tradition as feminine. This can include sedentary occupational roles or homemaker activities.

The Influence of American Culture

Cultural and national beliefs influence the rehabilitation philosophy of a country. Hence in the United States perceptions of important treatment goals are based on values of the American culture. Treatment goals, therefore, tend to stress the importance of being independent, having future plans and working toward objectives, being clean and on time, having good social and communication skills, and being physically and personally attractive. Cross-culturally these goals may not be seen as priorities or as valued.

In the American society, people often exclusively define themselves by their work roles with a strong emphasis on production and personal success. These goals are so internalized that not moving toward them can cause depression, self-blame, and hatred. Some patients, especially those in their middle years, may see the disability as a threat to their status both professionally and economically. If their personal worth continues to be defined in terms of the lost skills, roles, and concomitant self-image, and no value change takes place, the patient may never feel worthwhile or successful again.[11,12,66]

Racism

Racism can be destructive. Therapists must be clear on what their own values concerning ethnicity (race, religion, culture) are and remain free of misconceptions and prejudicial attitudes. Patients often assume that assignments of treatment time, availability of adaptive equipment, and inclusion in programs and plans for ongoing rehabilitation reflect prejudice. It is also important not to stereotype ethnic populations but to understand that even within cultural groups individuals have different heritages, customs, and values.[67,68]

Use of Language

A lack of proficiency in spoken English or in the primary language of a country is isolating for the patient, may prevent the patient from understanding all the facts of his medical condition or of the rehabilitation procedures, and may prevent collection of adequate evaluative information needed for treatment planning.

Therapists need to be aware that good pronunciation of English words used in general conversation may hide the fact that the patient may be understanding only a percentage of the actual conversation. A problem exists when information or directions are misunderstood or when the patient is unable to ask important questions. Under such circumstances it is easy for both the therapist and the patient to misread each other's meanings. A smile or a nod on the part of the patient may also cover lack of understanding and be based instead on a wish to please or on embarrassment. Both the patient and the family may fail to acknowledge that they do not comprehend the discussion with the therapist.

When a therapist recognizes that the patient has difficulty with the primary language or is hearing impaired she must speak clearly and directly and avoid idiomatic expressions. The therapist also should provide the time so that the patient can formulate what he wants to ask. Pressure and tension can reduce the ability to communicate in a less familiar language. Most hospitals list staff members who have language skills, and there are agencies that will supply interpreters with advance notice.

Religion

Religious taboos and beliefs influence patients and family attitudes and their understanding of the causes of the injury and/or disease. Historical beliefs that have come down through antiquity about the sources of disease are still deeply ingrained in the folklore and religion of cultural populations and have been integrated with current religious philosophies. During the Dark Ages misfortunes, including disease and disability, were blamed on witchcraft or evil spirits or were thought to be the evidence of sin and a punishment for wrongdoing. In some countries and cultures these beliefs still persist as valid reasons for ill health. The ancient Hebrews felt that illness was a punishment for sin, and the ancient Greeks looked on illness as a sign of inferiority. The early Christians saw sickness and pain as a way to salvation through suffering; during this same period, self-torture was thought to be the way to save and purify oneself. A parallel can be witnessed today in those patients who wear their disability with pride, feel especially selected by God for trial by suffering, or feel they were chosen due to their special qualities. The disability may give a purpose to their life. Such patients appear peaceful, uplifted, and superior. This latter attitude can be irritating to the therapist who is trying to treat their condition.

Stigma and negative attitudes toward physical and mental illness have been the result of the above historical beliefs, and it has been noted that such feelings are reproduced in modern man without much change. Unfortunately if the patient sees the disability as evidence of a sin he may decide to endure the punishment rather than be motivated toward treatment objectives. In some cases the family and the patient feel that prayer cures. When the expected result does not occur, patients may feel they have failed to atone for wrongdoing or that their faith is not great enough.[11,24,50,51]

Some patients believe in spiritualism and an invisible world of both good and evil spirits. They see the cause of their illness as their inappropriate activities or their failure to take protective measures against the evil spirits. Patients may feel powerless in the hospital because they do not have access to corrective artifacts or curative activities. Patients may also believe in folk healing, herbal medicines, the curative powers of special foods, prayer ceremonies, laying on of hands, the power of symbolic artifacts, and protective acts and signs to remove evil spirits.[64] In addition the disabled patient's personal faith and belief in a just universe where hard work, responsibility, and religious devotion are rewarded with justice and protection are violated.[25]

Occupational therapists treat patients with different religious beliefs and need to be sensitive to their unique perceptions of both the cause of disability and what is corrective. Their beliefs and ceremonies should be accepted as part of a treatment regimen when possible.

Disease-Specific Psychosocial Reactions

This section provides examples that will clarify the psychosocial accommodation demands of different diagnostic categories treated by occupational therapists. Illustrative examples include permanent functional disabilities such as spinal cord injury (SCI), cerebral vascular accident (CVA), and rheumatoid arthritis (RA). The complicated psychosocial effects of the invisible disabilities are also described. These disabilities include diabetes, renal disease, cardiac disease, and closed head injury.

SPINAL CORD INJURY

A physically and psychologically devastating disability, spinal cord injury results in the loss of both motor and sensory functions as determined by the level of the injury. (See chapter 28.) The patient faces major changes in such areas as occupational role, preferred life-style, expression of sexuality, and health maintenance since permanent physical/physiological changes will require vigilant, continual health compliance.

Psychosocial Consequences

Physical limitations in function and mobility restrict the patient's ability to physically express affection, cause him to feel vulnerable to attack from others, place him at a disadvantage when insisting on his rights during interpersonal encounters, and require him to deal with a nondisabled individual from a seated position. The patient's total expenditure of available mental and physical energy and daily time may be required to carry out basic activities of daily living. This limits activities of interest and choice.[4]

Physical dysfunction also alters the patient's ability to use familiar behaviors and actions to release tension, to externalize anger through physical action, to escape from unpleasant situations by moving away, or to gain pleasure from intrinsically satisfying action activities. Examples would be the thrill of running, the ability to leave an uncomfortable interpersonal situation, or to release tension physically through sports and recreation. To the SCI patient these losses and changes are not only continually frustrating but also threaten his developmental maturation and his sense of mastery and personal control over life events and the environment.[4,13,40]

In addition, long-term physical problems may reduce his involvement in work, school, and social and community activities. Examples are decubitus ulcers, incontinence, and muscle spasms. The patient who develops ulcers easily may need frequent bed rest to relieve pressure, and this is tedious and limiting. The incidents associated with incontinence are socially embarrassing, may require abrupt departure from social settings, and could foster permanent alienation from community activities. Muscle spasms are not within the patient's control, and they attract attention and accentuate differences.

In addition, the severely disabled patient tends to internalize hostility and negative feelings because the expression of these feelings may damage social relationships and prevent access to needed caretakers. This continual repression may find an outlet through passive-aggressive behavior (procrastination or sabotage), or the intolerable emotional stress may result in verbal explosions, acting-out behaviors, regression, and/or depression.[8,13,24,26]

Treatment Goals

The patient's psychosocial accommodation is a long-term major treatment goal. Patients may experience difficulty in accepting the need to be dependent in some living-skill areas and in retaining, at the same time, a sense of personal causation, mastery, and competence. The patient is helped to create opportunities for life satisfaction by redefining and refocusing occupational goals and by reappraising personal values. Also important are learning new ways to perform those skills (physical, process and planning, social, communication) that will maintain or create important family, social, and work roles.[40,44]

The development of avocational (leisure) skills is seen as important for providing meaningful activity, a satisfying use of time, and an opportunity to express creativity, increasing self-esteem, and creating opportunities for involvement with others. Treatment goals therefore also include the development and practice of hobbies and recreational or sports interests.[3,39,69-72]

CEREBRAL VASCULAR ACCIDENT

A cerebral vascular accident or stroke is a traumatic event with sudden loss of motor, sensory, and cognitive functions.[3,7,74] In stroke rehabilitation psychosocial sequelae were once considered unimportant or the result of neurological damage and thus of little significance in rehabilitation. A more current view recognizes that treatment goals directed toward the patient's psychosocial dysfunctions are an important component of rehabilitation.[75-78]

Emotional Reactions

Common emotional reactions after stroke are anxiety, denial, and depression. These responses are compounded by cognitive deficits that affect language, the ability to plan and to use logic, memory, and judgment, as well as perceptual and visual deficits. Resulting behaviors that can be witnessed in the patient include impatience, irritability, frustration, overdependence, insensitivity to others, and rigid, inflexible thinking. Poor social perception, due to the effects of the stroke, can cause aggravations that result in angry outbursts. Difficulties with communication can result in a buildup of annoyances and angry feelings. These behavioral reactions and misinterpretations of environmental events can lead to a breakdown in social and family relationships.[73-75]

Anxiety. Anxiety is a common problem and is experienced differently by different stroke patients due to the complex interweave of neurological, psychological, and emotionally reactive results of the stroke. Anxiety may be experienced as free floating, fixed on somatic preoccupation, as a general uneasiness, or as an extreme and prolonged anxiety arousal. In this latter arousal state the patient acts as if he were facing a series of catastrophes. Other causes of anxiety are the patient's inability to externalize concerns, his fear of a second stroke, obsessive thinking, or cognitive confusion.[73,74]

Denial. In the stroke patient the origins of denial can be organic, psychological, or a combination of both. The following examples provide descriptions of denial in the stroke patient: (1) the presence of the disability (paralyzed limb) is denied or is neglected; (2) the disabling condition is acknowledged, but the patient fails to accommodate to his condition; (3) the slightest change in function or spasm is interpreted as evidence that complete return will occur; (4) the patient insists that he can read but rationalizes his failure to do so (too small print or lack of glasses). In addition, the patient may deny the need for treatment, want to do things no longer possible such as drive a car or go immediately back to work, and may continue to work obsessively toward goals that are no longer possible. Years after the initial insult some stroke patients still appear bewildered about the presence of the disabling conditions and still insist that they can carry out tasks and activities that are no longer possible. Denying behaviors may also continue in those patients whose organic deficits have improved. While these descriptions are illustrative of the stroke patient, the information also pertains to patients with other kinds of cerebral trauma or neurological disease.[73,74]

Depression. Stroke patients may alternate between denial and depression. Depression is common in stroke survivors, has a strong psychosocial component, and is the result of a combination of losses. These losses include the suspension of those activities and roles that supported a sense of identity, belonging, and status and the inability or failure to reengage in social and community activities. Loss of previous social activities is seen as contributing significantly to the continuation of psychosocial dysfunctions including depression. It is thought that stroke patients even after a good recovery may still remain isolated and may be unable to be self-starting in the resumption of social, community, or avocational activities.[73-75,78]

Depressed patients with other physical disabilities often benefit from treatment approaches that encourage identification of abilities and resolution of losses through values clarification, discussion, and the development of other performance skills, interests, and roles. However, some stroke patients tend to perseverate both mood and affect and thus remain preoccupied with the somatic losses and changes in activities and life-style. The patient may be unable to shift his attention from the physical impairment and loss of competencies. He appears unable to focus on his remaining skills or positive rehabilitation gains.[73,75]

Social withdrawal and difficulties in resuming social patterns of life are also influenced by the residual neurological and physical dysfunctions. For some patients experiences with social interaction or with entering an unfamiliar environment are traumatic due to changes in body image, difficulty in communication and eating, cognitive disorientation, fatigue, or visual perceptual problems.[73,79] These problems, when possible, should be counteracted by an integrated treatment plan that encourages social and community experiences.

Treatment Goals

A holistic approach to the treatment of stroke patients should include not only treatment of neurological deficits, as described in other chapters of this text, but also treatment for psychosocial dysfunction. Psychosocial treatment goals for the stroke patient will be similar in concept to those cited for the SCI patient. Psychosocial goals will be integrated into the treatment plan and will include preserving a sense of mastery through maintenance of role performance skills when possible, increasing a positive self-concept by helping the patient resume social group activities, reinforcing activities of daily living in the community because of the patient's difficulty in changing environments, and adaptation of those leisure activities (one-handed if necessary) that are possible within the limitations of the dysfunctions.[40,78,79-88]

Although functional recovery may occur soon after the medical incident, some stroke patients can continue to develop and refine performance skills. They can learn and utilize problem-solving strategies that better integrate activities of daily living into a daily agenda and thus reduce psychosocial dysfunctions. Literature indicates that such skills continue to develop after discharge but require postdischarge programming including outpatient or home treatment services.[76,78,80,83]

The occupational therapist's role with the family of the stroke patient in education, training, support, and consultancy is considered valuable. In addition community support groups such as family and self-help groups are an important source of continued psychological, social, and educational intervention.[80,83,85-88]

RHEUMATOID ARTHRITIS

Rheumatoid arthritis is a chronic progressive systemic disease that follows an unpredictable course, involves multiple joints, is characterized by pain and inflammation, and has no known cause or cure to date.[89,90] Historically RA was thought to be the result of an arthritic personality that included traits of hostility, aggression, and rigidity. It was believed that all RA patients had similar premorbid personality constellations that precipitated the disease condition. However, early research was faulty and no evidence supports the contention that an arthritic personality pattern predates the disease or leads to an onset of symptomology. The negative personality traits noted in RA patients appear to be reactions to the chronic and uncertain nature of the disease. It is thought that psychosocial factors, including stress, play a precipitating role for some but not all arthritic patients.[40,89-91]

Psychosocial Problems

Psychosocial dysfunctions accompany RA because of the consequences of the disabling sequelae of chronic pain, immobility and fatigue, and the variable, unpredictable course of the symptomatology. The patient cannot make long-range plans because he never knows if physical function will be possible or when social plans or activities will have to be abandoned and important tasks left uncompleted. The effort of completing just the basic daily activities often diverts time and energy from more enjoyable pursuits. In addition it is difficult to maintain personal standards. The patient's sense of mastery is diminished. There is a reduction in life satisfaction.[89,92,93] Additional stressors include the reality of a chronic disease that sometimes requires radical changes in ingrained habits and family, work, social, and recreational roles and always requires consistent compliance with a regimen of health care.

Dependency. Dependency may be a reaction to the constellation of physical and psychosocial problems of the RA patient. Although dependency may not have been a personal characteristic of the patient before the onset of RA, it can become a way of life as the patient becomes more disabled and has difficulty in consistent functioning in his responsibilities and activities. Under these conditions the family may become overprotective and assume some or all of the patient's role responsibilities.[89,92]

Emotional Reactions. RA patients experience depression and body image distortions. Because of the effect of RA, patients have difficulty with flexible management of their lives and are often unable to see alternative ways to solve problems. Secondary responses to the course of the disease are overreaction to events, rigidity, conformity, perfectionism, and difficulty in expressing or dealing with hostility and aggressive feelings. The reduction of involvement in life activities including social events and interests leads to boredom and a decreased sense of personal causation, self-esteem, and mastery, and this precipitates discouragement and depression.[89,92,93]

The Family

The combination of physical dysfunction, changes in personal appearance, role losses, and personal and environmental stressors results in behaviors that are socially distancing and that hurt marital, family, and social relationships.[33,52,54,94] The exacerbation of arthritic symptoms may not be understood by the family. They may view the patient's inability to participate in family activities or personal activities of daily living on a regular basis as deliberate or malingering behavior. The patient's fluctuation in mood, irritability, and depression are difficult for family members to understand or tolerate. The impact of chronic disease on family life can be destructive.[90,91,93]

Psychosocial Treatment Goals

Treatment goals include the education of family members and the patient concerning the effects of RA, encouragement of interfamily communication, and increase of family and patient coping and problem-solving skills.[52,55,94]

Psychosocial goals include developing problem-solving strategies to help the patient maintain functional abilities and interests; clarifying values, including a lowering of expectations and standards for consistent performance; education in use of time, including rest periods, and in life management techniques. Self-control interventions, such as relaxation training, stress reduction programs, and biofeedback to increase pain tolerance, will foster a sense of personal control and mastery.[93]

It is important to recognize that the patient's participation in therapy is influenced by the degree of pain and discomfort present at a given time. In addition, his anxiety over the variability of the disease and its effect on his body may decrease his ability to listen to the therapist and to cooperate in the treatment session.[37]

Literature identifies group work as a supportive and successful milieu for the treatment of the RA patient. Group treatment goals include encouragement of social interaction, peer communication in sharing and solving common problems, identification of areas of strength and skills, exploration of alternative life activities and goals and encouragement of independence, an increase in self-acceptance and coping and problem-solving skills, and exploration of stressful events. In addition, group education and training in techniques of joint protection and energy conservation reinforce the importance of a consistent regimen.

INVISIBLE DISABILITY

Certain medical and neurological conditions like cardiac disease, diabetes mellitus, asthma, closed head injury, or the initial or remission stage of multiple sclerosis do not present visual evidence that sensitizes or clues the viewer to the condition of the disabled individual. The expectations of others are not altered because they see no visual signs. When the individual with an invisible disability does not participate in organized activities at school or in the community, his lack of participation may be viewed as malingering, passivity, lack of interest, noncompliant behavior, or rejection of activities planned by others. Medical requirements such as rest periods or special diets may be viewed as sissy or hypochondriacal behavior, may limit social acceptance, and may cause rejection. Misunderstandings can occur when others blame the need for consistent diet control on the rigidity of the individual or interpret the emotional response of mourning and depression precipitated by the illness as neurotic behaviors.[95]

It becomes the patient's responsibility to explain his hidden health problems, but unless his audience has some medical understanding they may show little change in attitude. The necessity for continual reinforcement of the facts of the illness requires confidence, social and communication skills, and persistence; such reinforcement is difficult for most patients. However, the patient with an invisible disability must continually let others know about his disease and lifestyle requirements or deal passively with the differences by withdrawal or elaborate avoidance schemes. Thus the development of the above skills are viewed as important psychosocial treatment goals.

Denial

The patient with a physical dysfunction reality-tests daily because of his limitations in the performance of activities. The responses of others, based on their observation of the disabling condition, provide social validation of the presence of the disability. The dynamics of adjustment of the obviously disabled patient and the patient with an invisible disability are very different. When the patient with an invisible disability feels well it is easy to deny, to intellectualize or rationalize, and to forget essential rules of health care. Patients who deny the presence of their illness may have frequent exacerbation of symptoms and endanger not only their health but their lives.[95]

Treatment Goals

A psychosocial treatment focus for the patient with an invisible disability includes examining with the patient the way in which the disease alters and influences his life patterns, personal standards, interests, and future plans, specifically his work, leisure, family, and community activities. Psychosocial goals should include the identification of work, personal roles, and interests consistent with the restrictions of the disability; lifestyle management techniques; and the development of social and communications skills to increase social involvement and also to aid the patient in informing others concerning the limitations posed by the disability. Treatment goals should also address learning new skills, including the development of interests that make adherence to health care rules more palatable, facilitate social interaction, and provide stimulation and satisfaction. These treatment objectives help to control depression and to increase self-esteem, feelings of competency, and mastery of life and the external environment. Treatment programs that include exercise, sports, and recreational experiences help to dispel the myth of invalidism.[95,96]

Treatment

THE OCCUPATIONAL THERAPY ROLE

Authentic occupational therapy practice has been defined as the science of eliciting adaptive responses and is characterized by the prescription of purposeful activities that are tangible, have demonstrable goals, and are representative of the patient's life requirements.[97] The therapeutic activity is chosen to elicit the active participation of the patient, whose conscious attention is impelled by the visible results of action, while simultaneously promoting adaptation to occur below the conscious level. Treatment programs consist of planned, sequenced experiences that aid the patient in the development of those performance skills and behaviors necessary for independence and personal adaptation. Such skills are practiced and reinforced in the simulated or real environment where they will be needed. Adaptation occurs when the patient is able to meet personal expectations, use adequate coping skills, and become personally involved in the restructuring of personal and life-style agendas.[40] An adaptive response becomes credible when the patient can consistently demonstrate it in daily activities, habits, and routines.[97,98]

The occupational therapist uses conceptual models to organize and guide treatment programming in keeping with the philosophy of the profession. The conceptual model identifies appropriate assessments and the focus of treatment and encourages consistent clinical problem solving for the individual patient's array of physical, psychological, family, and social problems.

CONCEPTUAL MODELS OF PRACTICE

This chapter can provide only an abridgment of practice models congruent with psychosocial practice in the treatment of the physically disabled. The intent is to influence clinical thinking and to direct the student to the study and review of the referenced literature.

The model of human occupation provides a holistic approach to the assessment and treatment of physical and psychosocial dysfunction. The components or subsystems of this model are arranged in a complex, hierarchical network of skills, roles, life patterns, and subjective life views. The subsystem hierarchy consists of the performance subsystem including the perceptual-motor, interactional-communication, and process (cognitive-problem solving and planning) skills; the habituation subsystem including habits, routines, and roles; and the volitional subsystem composed of the individual's personal goals, values, interests, feelings of personal causation, intrinsic motivation, temporal orientation (use and understanding of time), and standards for performance. The volitional subsystem thus influences the patient's feelings of control, competence, and mastery. Attention to the volitional area enhances the patient's remedial potential.[99,100]

The patient's lack of intrinsic motivation, failure to make good use of rehabilitation services, or retention of maladaptive responses can be based on undetected subsystem difficulties and a lack of understanding on the part of the therapist of the reciprocal and hierarchical nature of the human system as described by the model of human occupation. Dysfunction in one segment of this hierarchical organization can influence the other subsystems in both directions. Thus, a loss of performance skills can change the way in which a patient fulfills a work or family role and compromise his values concerning standards of performance. The treatment plan should acknowledge the interaction of

the performance, habituation, and volitional subsystems.[99,100]

Behavior therapy is based on a history of scientific research activities within the field of psychology. The behavioral theories represent a variety of models and approaches that include conditioning and social learning theories. The patient is viewed as an individual who is deficient in the necessary skills and behaviors required for adaptation to his social, physical, or cultural environment. The behavioral therapies are concerned with human learning, and treatment methods focus on teaching more adaptive skills, and behaviors and reducing stress and anxiety.[6,7,101,102]

The behavioral approach has had, at times, bad press because of overzealous interpretation and misuse of its concepts. This should not detract from the real value of a reasonable application of these theories to occupational therapy practice.

Most occupational therapists use behavioral techniques such as a social reinforcement, modeling, shaping of adaptive behavior, teaching and education, behavioral rehearsals, feedback, role playing, and structured practice sessions with experiential learning activities.[7,101-103]

Psychoeducational, assertiveness training, and stress reduction programs are all based on the behavioral learning theories. Those components of behavioral therapy most useful to occupational therapists include an identification of baseline performance that allows development of clear behavioral objectives and thus evaluation of progress; use of social and object reinforcement; identification of contingency events or situations that reinforce maladaptive behavior or are barriers to progress; and sequenced programming with identification of tangible, terminal goals.[101-103] These methods are considered useful with those patients who need to relearn activities of daily living, have difficulty learning new skills, are delayed developmentally, have residual or temporary cognitive deficits, or are depressed, self-defeating and/or noncompliant.

Knowledge of psychoanalytic theory helps the therapist understand the importance of the nonhuman environment to the patient, as well as his unconscious fears, conflicts, and use of adaptive mechanisms. The therapist's use of activities, media, and interactive group methods stimulates repressed, unconscious, or disregarded needs and provides a natural opportunity for the emergence, identification, and resolution of this symbolic material. The patients' understanding and expression of their feelings is considered important.[6,7,104,105]

Erikson's psychosocial developmental theory is an extension of the psychoanalytic theories but is more socially oriented. This approach provides a framework that elucidates the effect of trauma on the mastery and retention of developmental skills; provides an understanding of the reasons for, and effects of, regression; and aids in identification of the patient's original locus of psychosocial skills development. This developmental-stage theory has potential for guiding the choice of treatment activities and provides a structure for understanding the patient's acquisition of psychosocial skills.[106]

The hierarchy of human needs is considered part of Maslow's humanistic approach. According to this hierarchy there are five ascending levels of need: physiological balance, security, love and belonging, self-esteem, and self-actualization. To illustrate, the struggle to meet basic physiological needs (eating, health maintenance) consumes time and energy and prevents higher-level cognitive activity (learning, problem solving, planning) that aids the patient in developing or retaining significant roles or in reaching occupational goals. The need for safety and security is compromised by the patient's residual disability. For example, the patient's ability to influence the environment to exert control over important events, to protect the self, or to be financially secure may be initially or permanently changed, and these losses can stimulate catastrophic anxiety. Recognition of these dynamics as they influence the patient's rehabilitation is important. An understanding of this hierarchy provides guidelines for prioritizing goals for patient education, counselling, and choice of therapeutic activities.[2,6,70,107]

The Treatment Continuum

Effective treatment planning requires a clinical-reasoning process. The application of a conceptual framework ensures that treatment decisions will be made that are valid for the individual patient.

Evaluation. The focus of an interview or evaluation might include the patient's important work, personal or family roles, his view of change in these roles, what personal standards are important to him, the presence or absence of realistic future plans, his flexibility in reordering life goals, and the presence, change, or absence of those performance skills necessary to carry out life roles and to reach personal goals. The therapist should also observe, evaluate, and document all other behavioral, psychosocial, and psychodynamic dysfunctions that are part of the patient's condition and that are outlined in this chapter.[108-111]

Assessment is authentic under the following conditions. (1) Evaluation of dysfunction should not be drawn just from a textbook perspective but must be an analysis of just how the limitations, difficulties, and losses affect each particular patient's life, plans, and future.[108,109,112] (2) It is as important to identify strengths, assets, and skills as it is to identify dysfunctions. Their identification increases the patient's self-esteem and decreases feelings of despair and hopelessness. (3) It is important to identify the patient's personally held perspectives and subjective values that may block rehabilitation efforts. (4) It is important to determine the patient's previous or premorbid level of psychosocial adaptation. Some patients had mature adaptive skills that atrophied due to the injury, hospitalization, and a continued lack of opportunity to use the skills; whereas other patients may never have reached an age-appropriate developmental level. Treatment goals should reflect the patient's need to maintain and/or develop such skill.[36,39]

Goal Development. Treatment goals are action plans that enable a patient to understand his rehabilitation tasks and guide the treatment program. The therapist has the responsibility of guiding the patient in deciding the direction of his rehabilitation by providing him with adequate information and an opportunity to ask questions and to select treatment options. In this process the therapist follows a logical clinical problem-solving process, and moves from a problem list drawn from the assessment data to a set of prioritized, realistic, and obtainable goals. Therapists need to be aware that the development of attractive but unattainable goals based on the patient's, family's, or therapist's fantasies about what they would like to see happen only sets the stage for feelings of failure and depression. The therapist reassesses the feasibility of the treatment goals and the level of the treatment program when the patient regresses or appears unmotivated, defensive, or frustrated. Valued psychosocial treatment goals are seen as motivational.[108-116]

The patient's psychosocial goals should be integrated with the physical treatment goals. The following example illustrates this integration concept. The patient's treatment program includes a recreation and sports activity group. Treatment goals include increasing physical performance skills, such as strength and mobility, and practicing the use of adaptive equipment. Psychosocial goals include increasing feelings of personal control, self-esteem and mastery, and social and communication skills within an interactive team experience; developing recreational and hobby interests; and decreasing depression and dependency. Long-term treatment goals related to this activity group also include learning new performance skills to master the external environment by developing additional compensatory techniques, learning time management methods, and developing assertive social and communication skills.

The Treatment Plan. The therapist now considers those treatment methods that can be effectively combined in an individualized treatment plan. A treatment program plan, within the human occupation model, is organized on a developmental continuum that encourages the sequenced achievement of adaptive skills and behaviors. In the exploration phase of this continuum, performance skills are developed. The patient explores new interests, different life goals, and new roles. A treatment plan directed to the competence level encourages the combination of basic skills into more advanced activities, habits, and roles. These advanced skills allow the patient to feel greater control and mastery of the environment. At the achievement level, already existing performance skills and roles are maintained and skills are increasingly used and practiced in those environments where they will be required. The patient now becomes more independent and self-directed and chooses more advanced achievement goals based on personal values and interests.[111]

The following factors are significant considerations for the patient's ultimate success in rehabilitation. Motivation is influenced by the patient's premorbid characteristics and experiences and by those behavioral, psychodynamic, and personal factors described in this chapter. Sexuality and gender identity are primary concerns of the patient, and dysfunction in these areas may put the patient at risk for depression, diminished self-worth, and identity confusion. Treatment planning must consider these factors.

Motivation. Most patients make subjective estimates concerning the probability of their success in rehabilitation. Therefore, the patient's motivation and commitment to his treatment will depend on the value placed on the treatment goals; his assessment of the personal cost in effort, money, pain, and time; and his past experiences with failure. In addition, present or continuous failure to achieve treatment goals can have a damaging effect on the patient's intrinsic motivation.[26]

Motivation for rehabilitation may be influenced by the restriction of psychic energy caused by use of defense mechanisms like repression and denial, by the patient's inability to dispel tension motorically, and by distortions of body image. These factors help to explain the patient's reduced levels of cognitive activity, his temporal and cognitive disorientation, and his difficulty with appropriate psychosocial functioning. Under these conditions the patient may have difficulty with reality testing and with logical problem solving, including planning for discharge.[116]

Studies indicate that intrinsic motivation is enhanced by (1) therapist-patient codevelopment of acceptable, graduated, practical recovery goals; (2) a democratic therapeutic relationship; (3) opportunities for the patient to gauge his progress; (4) adequate frustration tolerance; and (5) the quality of the rehabilitation environment.[114] Finishing the treatment session with a task the patient can do well lessens stress, reinforces ability and function, and increases a sense of mastery.[37]

Motivation can be generated through planned individual and group activities and experiences where the patient can explore, learn to alter his environment, have fun, socialize, begin to feel good about himself, and be more in control of his own affairs. Competency, mastery, and social networking facilitate intrinsic motivation.[39,66,114,115]

Sexuality. A major concern of the patient after traumatic injury or the onset of medical-neurological disease is to maintain a gender identity and a continuing ability to function in sexual roles. A vital part of comprehensive medical and psychosocial rehabilitation is the provision of information on sexual issues and supportive counselling including the eradication of misinformation concerning sexual performance. Involvement at some level is natural for occupational therapists due to the developmental issues involved, the mandate to enable life satisfaction in all functional areas of the patient's life, and the patient's need for physical training for compensation and adaptation.[117-123] The therapist needs to obtain knowledge in this area as it pertains to each patient population to be treated.

The special concerns of patients regarding maintenance of sexual expressiveness and activity need to be anticipated and addressed. These concerns might include the loss of sexual interest (libido frequently returns with time and environmental change); worry about supposed reduction in male hormones (male characteristics are preserved); whether menstruation will resume or if fertility is preserved; and what alternative techniques and ways to experience sexual satisfaction are possible.[121] Patients of each diagnostic category have different concerns about sexuality, and their disabilities pose different adjustment and adaptive problems.[117]

Psychological, social, and environmental factors play a role in sexual readjustment. Such factors include difficulty with self-confidence, inadequate social and communication skills, barriers to meeting others socially, and fear of rejection. Also, the need for advance planning, including instructing others in order to engage in sexual activity, and values conflicts about alternate ways to achieve sexual satisfaction can be frustrating and limiting. Environmental barriers include inaccessible social meeting places and societal attitudes.[120,121,124]

Sexual education should include the eradication of myths and misinformation concerning sexual functioning. For example, patients who have had a myocardial infarct or a cerebral vascular accident may avoid intercourse out of fear of precipitating another episode. Their sexual partners often share these fears, or may lack information and have feelings of disgust or values conflicts concerning new procedures. This will influence the adjustment of both partners.

Psychosexual education is most successful within a comprehensive educational and counselling program before discharge. The responsibility for sexual education and counselling varies in different rehabilitation settings. It may be the sole responsibility of one department or disseminated among the services. The occupational therapist should be prepared to assume some professional responsibility for this aspect of the patient's rehabilitation by attaining a sound knowledge base, listening to the patient's concerns with sensitivity, assuming that all patients have questions that they may find difficult to ask, and by developing confidence in eliciting and responding to questions. The therapist also has the responsibility to help those patients who, out of fear of rejection and unfamiliarity with open discussion of intimate topics, may approach the subject in an obtuse manner. If another profession has the major responsibility in this area, the therapist should provide a referral while continuing to offer the patient support.

Gender Concerns. Professional attention has been directed to male sexual loss such as erection, ejaculation, and self-image, but women's special needs have only recently been considered. The rationale for this attitude was based on the belief that women were by nature passive and dependent, that they could still be involved sexually despite paralysis, and that they could more easily adapt to a reduction in sexual activity.

The facts, however, are different. For women the losses—including decreased mobility and sensation, changes in body image and appearance, and reduced opportunities to meet and attract compatible men—are difficult. Disabled women are also vulnerable to sexual abuse, are less apt to marry, and face more discrimination in the job market.[125]

Women's special concerns should be central when establishing treatment goals and planning their treatment programs. Women are concerned with retaining feelings of femininity, being able to dress attractively, express their individuality as women, date and establish relationships, continue their family roles, and establish vocational roles. Formation and continuation of family roles are important. Childbearing is possible; however, special attention must be taken before delivery due to paralysis, loss of sensation, and the danger of delivery without awareness.

Motherhood and child care may be an important focus for occupational therapy intervention. Adaptation of equipment and problem solving for child care activities are part of the therapist's responsibility.[125,126] (See chapter 18.)

Men have different concerns, fears, and difficulties during rehabilitation. Men are usually taught to value independence, strength, and competition. They may feel more demeaned by their disability, and their adjustment task can be complicated by their inability to maintain roles that make them feel adequate. Men may feel emasculated by role reversal with their wives or by losing identity-forming roles such as those related to work or their position in the family hierarchy. Before encouraging men to take on role sharing and home responsibilities in lieu of exterior work roles, it is important to be sure that this is a plan endorsed by the spouse and that the patient is prepared to accept. Treatment goals should be expressed in terms of masculine values and interests when possible.[127,128]

TREATMENT METHODS

Treatment methods chosen to address the patient's treatment goals are purposeful activity, including play and leisure activities, education and group work.

Purposeful Activity

Occupational therapists believe that change occurs and skills develop through planned action experiences that simulate or are actually activities of daily living. Such experiences are broadly defined and include not only basic living skills but activities related to leisure, play, recreation, community involvement, and social and family experiences. For example, effective treatment includes the use of purposeful activities as modalities to help the newly disabled patient to reduce stress and disorientation, to increase problem-solving

and coping responses, to restore temporal order, and to facilitate interaction with the expected environment.[129]

Adaptation is facilitated when the treatment program is designed to include activities and experiences that are real and relevant to the life of the patient. Purposeful activities should be chosen to meet multiple treatment goals simultaneously in order to provide efficient therapy, as well as enable the patient to sustain an interest in rehabilitation and feel self-directed toward a sense of satisfaction and accomplishment.[98,100,130,131]

Through the prescription of sequenced and self-reinforcing activities, patients can accomplish tasks and meet goals that they initially felt were beyond them. In the process of planning treatment the therapist must discuss with the patient why he is asked to engage in the activity and exactly how the activity relates to his long-term goals.

Play and Leisure. Treatment to develop leisure and recreational skills, including adaptation of activities so that the patient can participate, increases self-esteem, social confidence, and feelings of competency and mastery and decreases depression, discouragement, and apathy. Such activities facilitate the development of performance skills, physical mobility, exploration of the environment, and the mastery of equipment. They also provide an opportunity to externalize repressed anger and tension.[132-134]

Play and leisure activities are important in the integration of physical, cognitive, and psychosocial treatment goals. These activities provide the opportunity for motoric and psychosocial developmental experiences and facilitate adaptation to disability.[99,100,108]

The identification and development of the patient's avocational potential are primary treatment goals. Leisure interests provide opportunities for personal satisfaction and are useful to those patients who will be unable to assume full-time vocational roles. Participation in avocational activities will discourage a passive spectator role, encourage intercommunity involvement, and elevate the quality of the patient's life.[134]

Education

Educational curricula and teaching techniques are viewed as an important component of treatment programming. Programs in activities of daily living, self-help, and community reintegration are based on an educational format. Education programs are designed to simultaneously meet treatment goals and increase knowledge and skill in such areas as health and safety, time management, transportation, management of self-care attendants, repair of equipment, social assertiveness, stress reduction, and so on.[22,36,135-138]

A model of teaching-learning equates treatment with education and views the patient as an adult learner.[135,138] The therapist's responsibility within this model includes: (1) development of a teaching methodology consistent with the patient's learning style and previous knowledge; (2) relevant, individualized, reachable learning goals; (3) identification of learning readiness; (4) sequencing, timing, and assignment of learning tasks; and (5) identification and dissemination of information to the patient and family about the tasks the patient needs to perform.[138]

Group Work

Group work is an important and successful treatment modality for patients with physical and medical conditions. The use of groups in rehabilitation practice is seen as a superior method of comprehensive rehabilitation in which educational, behavioral, interactive, and dynamic components combine to help the patient gain the most from his treatment, resolve his losses, and learn to live realistically and comfortably with his disabilities. A well designed group provides a therapeutic environment wherein the patient's psychosocial dysfunctions can be identified and treated. Such a group also can provide experiences to stimulate, teach, and reinforce those social, problem-solving, and physical-adaptive skills the patient will need for successful discharge. The leader and group member interaction aids the patient in validating his strengths and skills, in reality testing, in planning around the disability, and in making changes in personal role taking and life plans.[1,39,139-145]

How Groups Integrate Goals. Group evaluation provides a more comprehensive opportunity to observe both positive and dysfunctional aspects of psychosocial functioning (interactive style, coping skills, adaptive mechanisms, performance skills) than evaluation of the patient alone, outside of the group. In addition, certain important personal qualities such as initiative, creativeness, persistence, cooperation, originality, values, and attitudes are more observable in the context of an interactive group.[140] Treatment goals related to social and communication skills are part of most occupational therapy groups.[113,141]

Group Activities. The group activity, whether educational or experiential, is an important component of rehabilitation group practice. It provides a focus for traumatized, anxious, and disoriented patients who often find the hospital experience, their painful feelings, and interaction with strangers threatening. A structured, planned group agenda that includes activity experiences, especially in the initial stages of group development, increases the comfort level for the patient and facilitates rehabilitation. The group activity component allows group members to learn from direct experience and the doing and experiential aspects of the group encourage development and retention of skills and behaviors that can be combined into new, continuing, and expanded role taking.[1,71,72,76,78,99,130,139,142,145]

Therapeutic Principles. Certain therapeutic principles are part of the dynamics of a treatment group, and they combat the social isolation of the rehabilitation experience and expand the patient's potential for life-style change. These therapeutic principles include the introduction of hope, a sense of universal-

ity or identification with others, catharsis or the opportunity to externalize painful feelings, the development and preservation of interactive skills, and a sense of cohesion or feelings of belonging. In addition, exploration of existential factors such as the lack of meaning in life, personal alienation, and fear of death are part of the dynamics of an interactive treatment group. These factors can emerge naturally within the group but also can be facilitated by the leader.[145-147]

Contributions of Group Work. The therapeutic value of rehabilitation group work is based on some of the following factors: (1) the group activity and group treatment plan can be adjusted and sequenced to allow the patient's participation at his current level of function; (2) the patient who becomes actively involved with other group members feels more confident, more in control, and more positive about his own ability to handle change; (3) group membership reduces social isolation and strengthens personal identity, counters the tendency to brood, and provides an opportunity to develop new friendships that may evolve into a community support network; (4) intermember problem solving promotes a useful exchange of ideas and a breadth of alternatives to encourage life-style changes; (5) family groups maintain family unity and relationships, encourage open communication, and aid the family in their adjustment and objectivity; (6) dependency on a single therapist is reduced; (7) peer support and interaction are motivational, and the group expands the patient's support system within the rehabilitation setting.

Occupational therapy process-oriented activity groups are a primary intervention method for the treatment of patients with physical disabilities.[1,39,140,142,143,145,148]

Summary

It is important that the rehabilitation effort not ultimately fail because of unrecognized and untreated psychosocial dysfunctions. Prevention includes expanding the patient's potential for independence and satisfaction by the integration of physical, psychological, and social goals into a comprehensive treatment program.

Treating patients with psychosocial dysfunction depends on knowledge and experience but also on the therapist's perception, warmth, sincerity, and responsiveness. Therapists should be personally capable in life skills, have developed mature skills of human interaction, and understand their own personal responses to stress. Therapists should be clear on when to support the patient, when to give more responsibility, when to be the patient's advocate, and when to encourage the patient to solve his own problems and initiate his own planning.

These concepts are not intended to convey the idea that a sound academic education in theory and treatment methods and techniques is not important. The above interpersonal attributes must be combined with a thorough understanding of physical, medical, and psychological sciences, as well as occupational therapy philosophy, theory, and models of practice.

STUDY QUESTIONS:

Psychosocial Accommodation to Physical Disability

1. Why is consideration of psychosocial issues in the treatment of all physically disabled individuals important?
2. Describe the importance of the patient's chronological and developmental age, that is, the life-cycle influence on disability. How does this information aid the occupational therapist in planning treatment?
3. What are the reactions and their behavioral manifestations, described in this chapter, that patients demonstrate as a result of traumatic illness or accident?
4. Identify, define, and describe the adaptive mechanisms. What is the occupational therapy role in intervention, and what are appropriate treatment goals?
5. What are some ancillary factors that can influence the rehabilitation outcome negatively, and how can the therapist minimize their effects?
6. Describe the negative aspects of staff and patient relationships. What are the underlying dynamics behind these interactional-communication problems? Describe the characteristics of a therapeutic relationship.
7. Describe probable major family concerns about having a disabled family member. What are both the negative and the positive factors that can exist within the patient and family relationship?
8. What are the typical psychosocial accommodation demands and reactions of patients with the major disease categories described in this chapter? What are the psychosocial goals for each?
9. Define authentic occupational therapy; identify and describe conceptual models of practice and their contribution to the treatment of psychosocial dysfunction in patients.
10. Describe group work practice as an intervention method and explain its contribution to the treatment of physically disabled patients. Cite treatment objectives that are facilitated by the group treatment approach.

References

1. Versluys, H. P. Community reintegration. The value of educational-action-training models. *Rehabil. Lit.,* 45(5-6): 138-145, 1984.
2. Stewart, T. D., and Rossier, A. B. Psychological consideration in the adjustment to spinal cord injury. *Rehabil. Lit.,* 39(3): 75-80, 1978.
3. Understanding psychosocial adjustment to disability through scientific research. *Rehab Brief.* Published by the National Institute of Handicapped Research. Office of Special Education and Rehabilitation Services, Washington, D.C. Vol. VII(10): 1-4, 1984.
4. Talbot, H. S. A concept of rehabilitation. *Rehabil. Lit.,* 45(5-6): 152-158, 1984.
5. Freed, M. M. Quality of life: the physician's dilemma. *Arch. Phys. Med. Rehabil.,* 65(3): 109-111, 1984.
6. Mosey, A. C. *Three Frames of Reference for Mental Health.* Thorofare, NJ: Charles B. Slack, 1970.
7. Briggs, A. D., Duncombe, L. W., Howe, M. C., and Schwartzberg, S. L. *Case Simulations in Psychosocial Occupational Therapy.* Philadelphia: F. A. Davis Co., 1979.
8. Tucker, S. J. The psychology of spinal cord injury: patient and staff interaction. *Rehabil. Lit.,* 41(5-6): 114-160, 1980.
9. Strain, J. J. *Psychological Care of the Medically Ill: A Primer in Liaison Psychiatry.* New York: Appleton-Century-Crofts, 1975.
10. Feldman, D. J. Chronic disabling illness: a holistic view. *J. Chronic. Dis.,* 27: 289-291, 1974.
11. Safilios-Rothschild, C. *The Sociology and Social Psychology of Disability and Rehabilitation.* New York: Random House, 1970.
12. McCranie, E. J. Neurotic problems in middle age. *Psychosomatics,* 19(2): 106-122, 1978.
13. Siller, J. Psychological situation of the disabled with spinal cord injuries. *Rehabil. Lit.,* 30(10): 290-296, 1969.
14. Kaplan, H. I., and Sadock, B. J. *Modern Synopsis of Psychiatry IV.* Baltimore: Williams & Wilkins, 1985.
15. Hepner, R., Kirshbaum, H., and Landes, D. Counselling substance abusers with additional disabilities: the center for independent living. *Alcohol Health Research World,* 5(2): 11-15, 1980/1981.
16. Alcoholism as secondary disability: the silent saboteur in rehabilitation. *Rehab Brief.* Published by the National Institute of Handicapped Research. Office of Special Education and Rehabilitation Services, Washington, D.C. Vol. V(6): 1-4, 1982.
17. Lindsay, W. P. The role of the occupational therapist: treatment of alcoholism. *Am. J. Occup. Ther.,* 37(1): 36-43, 1983.
18. Anderson, P. Alcoholism and the spinal cord disabled: a model program. *Alcohol Health Research World,* 5(2): 37-41, 1980/1981.
19. Mattsson, A. Long-term physical illness in children: a challenge to psychosocial adaptation. In *Coping with Physical Illness.* Edited by R. H. Moss. New York: Plenum Medical Book Co., 1977.
20. Zager, R. P., and Marquette, C. H. Developmental consideration in children and early adolescents with spinal cord injury. *Arch. Phys. Med. Rehabil.,* 62(9): 427-431, 1981.
21. Goldberg, R. T. Toward an understanding of the rehabilitation of the disabled adolescent. *Rehabil. Lit.,* 42(3-4): 66-73, 1981.
22. Haraguchi, R. S. Developing programs meeting the special needs of physically disabled adolescents. *Rehabil. Lit.,* 42(3-4): 75-78, 1981.
23. Blazyk, S. Developmental crisis in adolescents following severe head injury. *Social Work Health Care,* 8(4): 55-67, 1983.
24. Shontz, F. C. *The Psychological Aspects of Physical Illness and Disability.* New York: Macmillan Publishing Co., 1975.
25. Lilliston, B. A. Psychosocial responses to traumatic physical disability. *Social Work Health Care,* 10(4): 1-14, 1985.
26. McDaniel, J. S. *Physical Disability and Human Behavior.* New York: Pergamon Press, 1969.
27. Russell, R. A. Concepts of adjustment to disability: an overview. *Rehabil. Lit.,* 42(11-12): 330-338, 1981.
28. Moos, R. H., and Tsu, V. D. The crisis of physical illness: an overview. In *Coping with Physical Illness.* Edited by R. H. Moos. New York: Plenum Medical Book Co., 1977.
29. Counte, M. A., Bieliauskas, L. A., and Pavlou, M. Stress and personal attitudes in chronic illness. *Arch. Phys. Med. Rehabil.,* 64(6): 272-275, 1983.
30. Caplan, G. Mastery of stress: psychosocial aspects. *Am J. Psychiatry,* 138(4): 413-420, 1981.
31. Stensrud, R., and Stensrud, K. Interpersonal stress as a consequence of being disabled. *J. Rehabil.,* 47(2): 43-46, 1981.
32. Kaplan, D. M., Smith, A., Brodstein, R., and Fischman, S. E. Family mediation of stress. In *Coping with Physical Illness.* Edited by R. H. Moos. New York: Plenum Medical Book Co., 1977.
33. Gans, J. S. Hate in the rehabilitation setting. *Arch. Phys. Med. Rehabil.,* 64(4):176-179, 1983.
34. Thomas, M. D., Baker, J. M., and Ester, N. J. Anger: a tool for development of self awareness. *Am. J. Nurs.,* 70(12): 2586-2590, 1970.
35. Kutner, B. The social psychology of disability. In *Rehabilitation Psychology.* Edited by W. Neff. Washington, D.C.: American Psychological Association, 1971.
36. Kutner, B. Milieu therapy. *J. Rehabil.,* 34(2):14-17, 1968.
37. Melvin, J. L. *Rheumatic Disease: Occupational Therapy and Rehabilitation,* 2nd edition. Philadelphia: F. A. Davis Co., 1985.
38. Quigley, J. L. Understanding depression: helping with grief. *Rehabil. Gazette,* 19: 2-6, 1976.
39. Versluys, H. P. The remediation of role disorders through focused group work. *Am. J. Occup. Ther.,* 34(9): 609-614, 1980.
40. Kielhofner, G., Shepherd, J., Stabenow, C. A., Beledsoe, N., Furst, G., Green, J., Harlan, B. H., McLellan, C. L., and Owens, J. Physical disabilities. In *A Model of Human Occupation: Theory and Application.* Edited by G. Kielhofner, Baltimore: Williams & Wilkins, 1985.
41. Barris, R., Kielhofner, G., Neville, A. M., Oakley, F. M., Salz, C., and Watts, H. H. Psychosocial dysfunction. In *The Model of Human Occupation: Theory and Application.* Edited by G. Kielhofner. Baltimore: Williams & Wilkins, 1985.
42. Keller, M. B., and Shapiro, R. W. Double depression: superimposition of acute depression episodes on chronic depressive disorders. *Am. J. Psychiatry,* 134(4): 438-442, 1982.
43. Felton, B. J., and Revenson, T. A. Coping with chronic illness: a study of illness controlment and the influences of copying strategies of

psychological adjustment. *J. Consult. Clin. Psychol., 52*(9-10): 343-353, 1984.

44. Rogers, J. D., and Figone, J. J. Psychosocial parameters in treating the person with quadriplegia. *Am. J. Occup. Ther., 33*(7): 432-439, 1979.

45. Berry, J. L., and Zimmerman, W. W. The stage model revisited. *Rehabil. Lit., 44*(9-10): 275-277, 1983.

46. Vaillant, G. E. *Adaptation to Life.* Boston: Little, Brown and Co., 1977.

47. Malec, J., and Neimyer, R. Psychologic prediction of duration of in-patient spinal cord injury rehabilitation and performance of self-care. *Arch. Phys. Med. Rehabil., 64*(8): 359-363, 1983.

48. Simos, B. G. Grief therapy to facilitate healthy restitution. *Social Casework, 58*(6): 337-342, 1977.

49. Stewart, T., and Shields, C. R. Grief in chronic illness: assessment and management. *Arch. Phys. Med. Rehabil., 66*(7): 447-450, 1985.

50. Vargo, J. W. Some psychological effects of physical disability. *Am. J. Occup. Ther., 32*(1): 31-34, 1978.

51. Wright, B. A. *Physical Disability: A Psychological Approach,* 2nd edition. New York: Harper and Row, 1983.

52. Versluys, H. P. Physical rehabilitation and family dynamics. *Rehabil. Lit., 41*(3-4): 58-65, 1980.

53. Parent, L. H. Effects of a low stimulus environment on behavior. *Am. J. Occup. Ther., 32*(1): 19-25, 1978.

54. Leviton, G. The professional-client relationship. In *Rehabilitation Psychology.* Edited by W. Neff. Washington, D.C.: American Psychological Association, 1971.

55. Powers, P. W. Family coping behaviors in chronic illness: a rehabilitation perspective. *Rehabil. Lit., 46*(3-4): 78-83, 1985.

56. Versluys, H. P. Thuishulpcentrale: a Dutch model for practical family assistance. *Rehabil. Lit., 47*(3-4): 50-59, 1986.

57. Zisserman, L. The modern family and rehabilitation of the handicapped: a macrosociological view. *Am. J. Occup. Ther., 35*(1):13-20, 1981.

58. Frieden, L., and Cole, J. A. Independence: the ultimate goal of rehabilitation for spinal cord-injured persons. *Am. J. Occup. Ther., 39*(11): 734-739, 1985.

59. Low, S. M. The culture bias of health, illness and disease. *Social Work Health Care, 9*(11):13-23, 1984.

60. Guendelman, S. Developing responsiveness to the health needs of Hispanic children and families. *Social Work Health Care, 8*(4): 1-15, 1983.

61. Sanchez, V. Relevance of cultural values: for occupational therapy programs. *Am. J. Occup. Ther., 28*(1): 1-5, 1964.

62. Kunce, J. T. The Mexican-American: cross cultural rehabilitation counselling implications. *Interchange: World Rehabilitation Fund.* 400 E. 34th Street, New York, NY 10016. May 1983.

63. Ghali, S. B. Culture sensitivity and the Puerto Rican client. *Social Casework, 10:* 459-468, 1977.

64. Delgado, M. Puerto Rican spiritualism and the social work professional. *Social Casework, 10:* 451-458, 1977.

65. Szapocznik, J., Scoppetta, M. A., and Aranalde, M. A. Cuban value structure: treatment complications. *J. Consult. Clin. Psychol., 46*(5): 961-970, 1978.

66. Geis, H.J. The problem of personal worth in the physically disabled patient. *Rehabil. Lit., 33*(2):34-39, 1972.

67. Queralt, M. Understanding Cuban immigrants: a cultural perspective. *Social Work,* March-April, pp. 115-121, 1984.

68. Brantley, T. Racism and its impact on psychotherapy. *Am. J. Psychiatry, 140*(12): 1605-1608, 1983.

69. Green, B. C., Pratt, C. C., and Grigsby, T. E. Self-concept among persons with long-term spinal cord injury. *Arch. Phys. Med. Rehabil., 65*(12): 751-754, 1984.

70. Strach, P. L. Maslow's needs and the spinal cord injured client. *Rehabil. Nurs.,* September-October 1980, pp. 17-19.

71. Burnett, S. E., and Yerxa, E. J. Community-based and college-based needs assessments of physically disabled persons. *Am. J. Occup. Ther., 34*(3): 201-207, 1980.

72. Decker, S. D., and Schulz, R. Correlates of life satisfaction and depression in middle-aged and elderly spinal cord injured persons. *Am. J. Occup. Ther., 39*(11): 740-745, 1985.

73. Diller, L. Hemiplegia. In *Rehabilitation Practices with the Physically Disabled.* Edited by J. F. Barrett and E. S. Levine. New York: Columbia University Press, 1973.

74. Piotrowski, M. M. Body image after a stroke. *Rehabil. Nurs.,* January-February: 11-13, 1982.

75. Labi, M. L. C., Phillips, T. F., and Gresham, G. E. Psychosocial disability in physically restored long-term stroke survivors. *Arch. Phys. Med. Rehabil, 61*(12): 561-565, 1980.

76. Belcher, S. A., Clowers, M. R., and Cabanayan, A. C. Independent living rehabilitation needs of postdischarge stroke persons: a pilot study. *Arch. Phys. Med. Rehabil., 59*(9): 404-409, 1978.

77. Gresham, G. E., Phillips, T. F., Wolf, P. A., McNamara, P. M., Kannel, W. B., and Dawber, T. R. Epidemiologic profile of long-term stroke disability: the Framingham study. *Arch. Phys. Med. Rehabil., 68*(11): 487-491, 1979.

78. Feibel, J. H., and Springer, C. J. Depression and failure to resume social activities after a stroke. *Arch. Phys. Med. Rehabil., 63*(6): 276-278, 1982.

79. Anderson, T. P., and Kottke, F. J. Stroke rehabilitation: a reconsideration of some common attitudes. *Arch. Phys. Med. Rehabil., 59*(4): 175-180, 1978.

80. Marsh, M. A day rehabilitation stroke program. *Arch. Phys. Med. Rehabil., 65*(5): 320-323, 1984.

81. Binder, L. M. Current concepts of cerebrovascular disease. *Stroke, 18*(4): 17-21, July-August, 1983.

82. Goldberg, R. L., Wise, T. H., and LeBuffe, F. P. The stroke unit: psychological aspects of recovery. *Psychosomatics, 20*(5): 316-321, 1979.

83. Brinkmann, J. R., and Hoskins, T. A. Physical conditioning and altered self-concept in rehabilitated hemiplegic patients. *Phys. Ther., 59*(7): 859-865, 1979.

84. Dunn, S. A., Nelson, C. D., and Peterson, P. M. An education program about stroke. *Rehabil. Nurs.,* September-October 1984, pp. 27-29.

85. Wells, R. Family stroke education. *Stroke, 5*(May-June): 393-396, 1974.

86. D'Afflitti, J. R., and Weitz, G. W. Rehabilitating the stroke patient through patient-family groups. Edited by R. H. Moos. *Coping with Physical Illness.* New York: Plenum Medical Book Co., 1977.

87. Scanlon-Schilpp, A. M., and Levesque, J. Helping the patient cope with the sequelae of trauma through the self-help group approach. *J. Trauma, 21*(2): 135-139, 1981.

88. Evans, R. L., and Northwood, L. K. Social support needs in adjustment to stroke. *Arch. Phys. Med. Rehabil., 64*(2): 61-64, 1983.

89. Anderson, K. O., Bradley, L. A., Young, L. D., and McDaniel,L. K. Rheumatoid arthritis: review of psychological factors related to etiology, effects, and treatment. *Psychol. Bull., 98*(2): 358-387, 1985.

90. Spergel, P., Ehrlich, G. F., and Glass, D. The rheumatoid arthritic personality: a psychodiagnostic myth. *Psychosomatics, 19*(2): 79-86, 1978.

91. Zeitlin, D. J. Psychological issues in the management of rheumatoid arthritis. *Psychosomatics, 17-18*(8): 7-14, 1977.

92. Locker, D. *Disability and Disadvantage: The Consequences of Chronic Illness.* New York: Ravistock Publications, 1983.

93. Baum, J. A review of the psychological aspects of rheumatoid arthritis. *Semin. Arthritis Rheum., 11*(3): 352-360, 1982.

94. Power, P. W. Family coping behaviors in chronic illness: a rehabilitation perspective. *Rehabil. Lit., 46*(3-4): 78-82, 1985.

95. Flavo, D. R., Allen, H., and Maki, D. R. Psychosocial aspects of invisible disability. *Rehabil. Lit., 43*(1-2): 2-6, 1982.

96. Ben-Shlomo, L. S., and Short, M. A. The effects of physical conditioning on selected dimensions of self concept in sedentary females. *Occup. Ther. Mental Health, 5*(4): 27-46, 1985/1986.

97. Yerxa, E. J. Authentic occupational therapy. The 1966 Eleanor Clarke Slagle lecture. *Am. J. Occup. Ther., 21*(1): 1-9, 1967.

98. King, L. J. Toward a science of adaptive responses. The 1978 Eleanor Clarke Slagle lecture. *Am. J. Occup. Ther., 32*(7): 429-437, 1978.

99. Kielhofner, G., and Burke, J. P. Components and determinants of human occupation. In *A Model of Human Occupation: Theory and Application.* Edited by G. Kielhofner. Baltimore: Williams & Wilkins, 1985.

100. Kielhofner, G. Occupational function and dysfunction. In *A Model of Human Occupation: Theory and Application.* Edited by G. Kielhofner. Baltimore: Williams & Wilkins, 1985.

101. Stein F. A current review of the behavioral frame of reference and its application to occupational therapy. *Occup. Ther. Mental Health, 2*(4): 35-61, 1982.

102. Barris, R., Kielhofner, G., and Watts, J. H. Behavioral approaches. In *Psychosocial Occupational Therapy: Practice in a Pluralistic Arena.* Rockville, MD: Ramsco Publication Co., 1983.

103. Maslan, D. Rehabilitation training for community living skills: concepts and techniques. *Occup. Ther. Mental Health, 2*(1): 33-49, 1982.

104. Barris, R., Kielhofner, G., and Watts, J. H. Classical psychoanalysis. In *Psychosocial Occupational Therapy: Practice in a Pluralistic Arena.* Rockville, MD: Ramsco Publication Co., 1983.

105. Barris, R., Kielhofner, G., and Watts, J. H. The Neo-Freudians: Adler, Horney, Fromm, and Sullivan. In *Psychosocial Occupational Therapy: Practice in a Pluralistic Arena.* Rockville, MD: Ramsco Publication Co., 1983.

106. Zemke, R., and Grantz, R. R. The role of theory: Erikson and occupational therapy. *Occup. Ther. Mental Health, 2*(3): 45-63, 1982.

107. Barris, R., Kielhofner, G., and Watts, J. H. The existential-humanist bodies of thought. *Psychosocial Occupational Therapy: Practice in a*

Pluralistic Arena. Rockville,MD: Ramsco Publication Co., 1983.
108. Rogers, J. C., and Kielhofner, G. Treatment planning. In *A Model of Human Occupation: Theory and Application.* Edited by G. Kielhofner. Baltimore: Williams & Wilkins, 1985.
109. Rogers, J. C. Clinical reasoning: the ethics, science, and art. The 1983 Eleanor Clarke Slagle lecture. *Am. J. Occup. Ther., 37*(9): 601–616, 1983.
110. Cubie, S. H., and Kaplan, K. A case analysis method for the model of human occupation. *Am. J. Occup. Ther., 36*(10): 645–656, 1982.
111. Cubie, S. H., Kaplan, K. L., and Kielhofner, G. Program development: In *A Model of Human Occupation: Theory and Application.* Edited by G. Kielhofner, Baltimore: Williams & Wilkins, 1985.
112. Portnow, J. M. Complications of therapy. *Rehabil. Lit., 44*(9–10): 278–279, 1983.
113. Scott, A. H., and Haggarty, E. H. Structuring goals via goal attainment scaling in occupational therapy groups in a partial hospitalization setting, *Occup. Ther. Mental Health, 4*(2): 39–58, 1984.
114. Rabinowitz, H. S. Motivation for recovery: four social-psychological aspects. *Arch. Phys. Med. Rehabil., 42*(12): 799–807, 1961.
115. Burke, J. P. A clinical perspective on motivation: pawn versus origin. *Am. J. Occup. Ther., 31*(4): 254–258,1977.
116. Shontz, F. C., Fink, S. L., and Hallenbeck, C. E. Chronic physical illness as threat. *Arch. Phys. Med. Rehabil., 41*(4): 143–148, 1960.
117. Sidman, J. M. Sexual functioning and the physically disabled adult. *Am. J. Occup. Ther., 31*(2): 81–85, 1977.
118. Conine, T. A., Christie, G. M., Hammond, G. K., and Smith, M. F. An assessment of occupational therapists' roles and attitudes toward sexual rehabilitation of the disabled. *Am. J. Occup. Ther., 33*(8): 515–519, 1979.
119. Neistadt, M., and Baker, M. F. A program for sex counselling for physical disabled. *Am. J. Occup. Ther., 32*(10): 646–647, 1978.
120. Comarr, A. E., and Vigue, M. Sexual counselling among male and female patients with spinal cord and/or cauda equina injury. *Am. J. Phys. Med., 57*(3): 107–122, 1978.
121. Stewart, T. D. Sex, spinal cord injury and staff rapport. *Rehabil. Lit., 42*(11–12): 347–350, 1981.
122. Singh, S. P., and Magner, T. Sex and self: the spinal cord injured. *Rehabil. Lit., 36*(1): 2–7, 1975.
123. Sandowski, C. I. Sexuality and the paraplegic. *Rehabil. Lit., 37*(11–12): 322–326, 1976.
124. Goldman, F. Environmental barriers to sociosexual integration: the insiders' perspectives. *Rehabil. Lit., 39*(6–7): 185–189, 1978.
125. Thurer, S. L. Women and rehabilitation. *Rehabil. Lit., 43*(7–8): 194–197, 207, 1982.
126. Asrael, W. An approach to motherhood for disabled women. *Rehabil. Lit., 43*(7–8): 214–218, 1982.
127. Skord, K. G., and Schumacher, B. Masculinity as a handicapping condition. *Rehabil. Lit., 43*(9–10): 284–289, 1982.
128. Utrup, R. G. The male ego in the training kitchen. *Visual Impairment and Blindness,* October 1982, pp. 305–308.
129. Rosenfeld, M. S. A model for activity intervention in disaster-stricken communities. *Am. J. Occup. Ther., 36*(4): 229–235, 1982.
130. Fidler, G. S., and Fidler, J. W. Doing and becoming: purposeful action and self actualization. *Am. J. Occup. Ther., 32*(5): 305–316, 1978.
131. Rogers, J. D. Roles and functions of occupational therapy in long-term care. *Occupational Therapy News, March:* 8–9, 1983.
132. Kielhofner, G., and Miyake, S. The therapeutic use of games with mentally retarded adults. *Am. J. Occup. Ther., 35*(6): 375–382, 1981.
133. Gunn, S. L. Play as occupation: implications for the handicapped. *Am. J. Occup. Ther., 29*(4): 222–227, 1975.
134. Rogers, J. D., and Figone, J. J. The avocational pursuits of rehabilitants with traumatic quadriplegia. *Am. J. Occup. Ther., 32*(9): 432–439, 1979.
135. Lillie, M. D. and Armstrong, H. E. Contributions to the development of psychoeducational approaches to mental health services. *Am. J. Occup. Ther., 36*(7): 438–443, 1982.
136. Neistadt, M. E., and Narques, K. An independent living skills training program. *Am. J. Occup. Ther., 38*(10): 671–676, 1984.
137. Ogren, K. A living skills program in an acute psychiatric setting. *American Occupational Therapy Association Mental Health Special Interest Section Newsletter, 6*(4): 1–2, 1984.
138. Anderson, T. P. Educational frame of reference: an additional model for rehabilitation medicine. *Arch. Phys. Med. Rehabil., 59*(5): 203–206, 1978.
139. Spitz, H. I. Contemporary trends in group psychotherapy: a literature survey. *Hosp. Community Psychiatry, 35*(2): 132–142, 1984.
140. Mann, W., Godfrey, M. D., and Dowd, E. T. The use of group counselling procedures in the rehabilitation of spinal cord injured patients. *Am. J. Occup. Ther., 27*(2): 73–77, 1973.
141. Duncombe, L., and Howe, M. E. Group work in occupational therapy: a survey of practice. *Am. J. Occup. Ther., 39*(3): 163–170, 1985.
142. Fidler, G. S. The task-oriented group as a context for treatment. *Am. J. Occup. Ther., 49*(5): 43–48, 1978.
143. Donohue, M. V. Designing activities to develop a women's identification group. *Occup. Ther. Mental Health, 2*(1): 1–19, 1982.
144. Miller, D. K., Wolfe, M., and Spiegel, M. H. Therapeutic groups for patients with spinal cord injuries. *Arch. Phys. Med. Rehabil., 56*(3): 130–135, 1975.
145. Howe, M. C. and Schwartzberg, S. L. *A Functional Approach to Group Work in Occupational Therapy.* New York: J. B. Lippincott Co., 1986.
146. Yalom, I. D. *Theory and Practice of Group Psychotherapy,* 3rd edition. New York: Basic Books, 1985.
147. Power, P. W., and Rogers, S. Group counselling for multiple sclerosis patients: a preferred model of treatment for unique adaptive problems. In *Group Counselling and Physical Disability.* Edited by R. C. Lasky and A. E. Dell Orto. Duxbury, MA: Duxbury Press, 1979.
148. DeCarlo, J. J., and Mann, W. C. The effectiveness of verbal versus activity groups in improving self-perceptions of interpersonal communication skills. *Am. J. Occup. Ther., 39*(1): 20–27, 1985.

PART TWO
Neurodevelopmental Approach

This section includes the evaluation and restorative treatment procedures used for patients with sensorimotor, perceptual, and/or cognitive problems due to brain dysfunction. As a result of brain damage, a patient may lose basic cognitive and perceptual capacities and functional abilities. The patient's movement patterns may be immature and/or unduly controlled by sensory stimulation. He may lack the ability to voluntarily control the direction, speed, force, sequence, extent, or precision of his movements. Treatment to promote redevelopment of these abilities is based on principles derived from neurophysiology, neuropsychology, human development, cognitive psychology, and human movement science. Because the treatment of these losses follows a developmental sequence and the techniques reflect anatomical, functional, or behavioral reorganization of the central nervous system, this approach is entitled "neurodevelopmental."

Motor control, as well as perceptual or cognitive organization, depend on environmental sensory influences. Since this relationship is true for all humans, the neurodevelopmental approach is applicable to patients with and without brain injury. Its potential value for improving motor performance depends on the integrity of neural transmission. In a patient with spinal cord transection, sensation is lost below the level of the lesion and movements below that level cannot be voluntarily controlled. Sensations from the periphery can only produce reflex responses at segmental levels of the spinal cord with no lasting effect on motor function. In complete peripheral nerve lesions, sensations do not even travel to the spinal cord and are ineffective in influencing motor response. In brain injury, however, spinal cord and peripheral neural pathways are intact, and sensory stimulation can be transmitted to the brain with a potential for influencing voluntary motor control.

The neurodevelopmental approach is in the process of evolution. New information in the fields of neurophysiology and neuropsychology is being generated from research on primates and humans. Normal cognitive visuoperceptual, and perceptual motor processes are beginning to be better understood, enabling the emergence of more systematic evaluation and treatment procedures. Therapists are beginning to apply to brain-injured patients techniques that are used to teach motor skills to adults with normal sensory motor systems.

Occupational and physical therapy scholars and clinicians are researching the effectiveness of techniques used in clinical practice. However, two major detriments to the advancement of therapy exist. One is the current lack of valid, reliable, and sensitive standardized measuring instruments suitable for clinical use. The other is the unmet need to determine the controlling variables that operate to affect treatment outcome. Several such variables are assumed to affect outcome of neurodevelopmental treatment, e.g., age, time since onset of lesion, and location and extent of lesion. However, we do not yet know specifically what all the variables are or how they affect our therapeutic efforts. We do not know if each potentially controlling variable relates directly to outcome or if it relates only in combination with other variables to predict success or failure of a given treatment. This information is needed to increase the specificity of therapeutic intervention, which in turn would result in higher percentages of successful outcomes. Data to determine which variables are controllers exist in clinical records; clinicians with access to the records and researchers with knowledge of multivariate analyses need to collaborate to identify them. As all this new information is reported and integrated, practice will change.

Occupational therapists have primary responsibility for sensory, perceptual, and cognitive training of brain-injured patients. They share responsibility for motor retraining with physical therapists. The focus of physical therapy is to improve the patient's ability to move in a controlled way, whereas the focus of occupational therapy is to teach the patient to use movement to be competent in the occupations of his life roles. Ideally, physical therapy treatment would always immediately precede occupational therapy treatment for every patient so that the entire focus of occupational therapy could be application of the motor control just learned in physical therapy. That, however, does not occur, and occupational therapists find it necessary to do both the basic and applied aspects of motor control therapy.

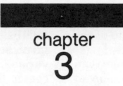

chapter

3

Evaluation and Treatment
of Somatosensory Sensation

Catherine A. Trombly and Anna Deane Scott

Occupational therapists are interested in how the person referred for treatment interacts with his environment for optimal occupational performance. The special and somatic sensory systems inform the person about the environment as well as about his own body and the interface between the two. The special sensory systems are auditory, gustatory (taste), olfactory (smell), vestibular, and visual. The somatosensory system includes the senses of touch, movement, temperature, and pain.

While aging may diminish the acuity and speed of perception of the special sensory systems, in young patients these systems rarely become nonfunctional due to trauma or disease. Information from these senses, especially visual, can therefore substitute for impairment of the somatosensory system.

The somatosensory system encompasses the receptors located within muscles, tendons, joints, ligaments, and the dermis of the skin; the peripheral nerves; the tracts in the spinal cord and brain stem; the thalamus; and the cortex. Damage to the receptors prevents stimuli from being appreciated. Disease or trauma to a peripheral nerve or the spinal cord will prevent or diminish the transmission of the sensory impulses to the brain for action. Damage to the brain centers will interfere with the interpretation and perception of the meaning of the sensory information and/or the integration of many bits of sensory information needed to produce coordinated movement and correct environmental interaction.

Because the sources of somatosensory dysfunction are multiple, it is a potential problem for many patients. Sensory testing, therefore, is a basic evaluation used by occupational therapists who specialize in treatment of the physically disabled.

Somatosensory Physiology

Briefly the physiology of the somatosensory system is as follows.

The somatosensory system consists of two subsystems: the primary and the discriminatory systems.

The primary system, formerly called the protopathic or protective system, receives and interprets simple sensations.[1] It is responsible for awareness of touch, including special touches such as tickling and itching; pain; and extremes of temperature. The primary system uses the spinothalamic route, specifically the lateral (pain and temperature) and anterior (light touch) spinothalamic tracts of the spinal cord, which transmit the sensory impulses to the lateral nucleus of the thalamus where primary interpretation of the meaning of the stimuli is made. This allows rapid motor adjustments to defend or protect the organism. The information is relayed to the somatosensory region of the cerebral cortex so that memories are stored and learning occurs.

The discriminative system, formerly called the epicritic system, is responsible for more complex, integrated sensory experiences such as location of touch, two-point discrimination, stereognosis (recognition of objects by touch alone), kinesthesia, and awareness of small temperature changes.[2] The function of this system is perceptual rather than purely receptive. The discriminative system projects, via the dorsal columns and medial lemniscal tract, to the cortex via the thalamus.[3] Several bits of sensory information are integrated into a perception of the meaning of the complex stimuli.[1] This interpretation involves memory of previous sensory experiences[4]; therefore, development or recalibration of the discriminative sensory function is a learning process.

Sensory receptors team with particular types of peripheral neural fibers that are classified according to size, myelination, and speed of adaptation. The small, unmyelinated group C fibers (for pain) conduct most slowly, whereas the large, myelinated group A fibers conduct rapidly. Cutaneous sensation is mediated by the group A-beta fibers.[3] Speed of adaptation of the combined receptor/fiber system determines the type of stimuli to which each will respond.[3] Quickly adapting A-beta fibers are associated with pacinian and Meissner's corpuscles to detect transient touch or vibration. Slowly adapting A-beta fibers are associated with Merkel's discs and respond to indentation of the skin.

Some sensory experiences are derived from more than one receptor/fiber system. Conscious appreciation of joint motion and joint position probably depends not only on input from joints[5] and muscle afferents[6] but also cutaneous sensation[7] and memory.[5,8]

Pathology of Sensation

Any type of disease process or injury that abolishes, interrupts, irritates, or deforms the receptors, the nerves, the spinal and brain stem transmission tracts, or the subcortical or cortical nuclei that receive and interpret the impulses will affect sensation. Burns, surgical removal of receptors secondary to joint replacement, lacerations from knife cuts or broken glass, accidental crush injuries, toxicity (e.g., lead poisoning), metabolic diseases (e.g., diabetes), excessively prolonged pressure on the nerve (e.g., from ill-fitting splints or slings, industrial cumulative trauma injury, wrong use of crutches, or inattentive leaning such as Saturday Night palsy), spinal cord injury, tumor or multiple sclerosis plaques in the spinal cord or supraspinal sensory centers, stroke, or other brain trauma can all result in sensory dysfunction. The dysfunction can be hyposensitivity ranging from partial to complete (anesthesia) loss, hypersensitivity, or inaccuracy. Causalgia, a specific instance of hypersensitivity, is described as a severe, burning type of pain, the severity of which is compounded by inactivity of the limb.[9]

Recovery of sensory function depends, of course, on the etiology, severity, and location of the lesion. Not all senses are recovered simultaneously. Sensory modalities subserved by the larger, myelinated fibers recover more slowly than those mediated by thinner, unmyelinated fibers.[4] One group of researchers suggest that the difference in pattern of sensory recovery mediated by the quickly and slowly adapting A-beta fibers is related to differences in regeneration of the receptors subserving the different sensory modalities.[4]

Recovery also may depend on learning to use alternate strategies to detect and interpret stimuli. Recovery of cortical sensation, such as stereognosis, may not occur following brain injury[1]; however, therapy to teach alternate strategies or substitutions may enable the patient to compensate for the loss.

Evaluation

A sensory evaluation involves presentation of stimuli appropriate to each sensory modality and observation of the patient's responses.

As with any evaluation, reliability of the scores is crucial. Reliability depends upon the skill and consistency of the tester in administering the tests and recording the results. It is important for institutional credibility that reliability of all evaluation procedures be determined within each occupational therapy department. By doing so, confidence can be placed in the scores as reported and in the progress noted for the patient. Therefore, estimating interrater reliability is an important administrative task. If interrater reliability falls below an acceptable level of at least 80–90% agreement, steps should be taken to decrease the sources of variability either by identifying and eliminating the controlling variable or by keeping it constant from test to retest. Potential variables are considered in three categories here.

Method

The type of stimulus and the manner of presentation should be standardized, such as described on the following pages for specific sensory modalities. Some general methodological issues to be considered are the following:

1. The test stimulus (S) should be presented randomly interspersed with nonpresentation trials and/or false presentation trials.

2. Multiple trials should be done for each modality and each area tested.

3. A time limit for the response to occur at each trial should be established. Time limit norms are established for few tests but those that are reported will be noted below with each specific test.

4. Learning trials should precede all tests.

5. Contralateral uninvolved areas of the body should be tested before the involved areas not only to assure that the patient understands the directions but also to establish what normal is for that patient. To date norms have been established for few sensory tests. When these exist, they should be used in conjunction with the norm for the particular patient in order to interpret the scores. For example, the norm for trunk and proximal body areas of the patient with cortical damage may be below the norms established for normal persons of comparable age because of bilateral innervation of these areas.[10]

6. Stimuli should be applied proximally to distally to determine the line of demarcation of normal versus abnormal sensation in spinal cord-injured patients and those with peripheral nerve injury.

7. Vision and hearing are powerful substitutes for sensory loss[10]; therefore, *the patient's vision must be occluded* for each trial, and auditory cues must be kept to a minimum. Vision can be occluded by asking the patient to keep his eyes closed, by using a blindfold, or by shielding the patient's view of his limb using a file folder or a screen (Fig. 3.1). If the patient closes his eyes or a blindfold is used, he is allowed to open his eyes in between each test procedure to prevent disorientation or inattention.

8. Scoring definitions and method of recording should be agreed upon by all therapists within a department. Responses are usually reported as follows: intact, indicating that the responses were quick and accurate; absent, indicating that no response was obtained; or impaired, indicating a delay of response, variable accuracy of response, or report of a sensation inappropriate to the stimulus.

9. Since both the accuracy of the response to the S condition and the speed with which the patient responds are noted, how accurate but delayed responses

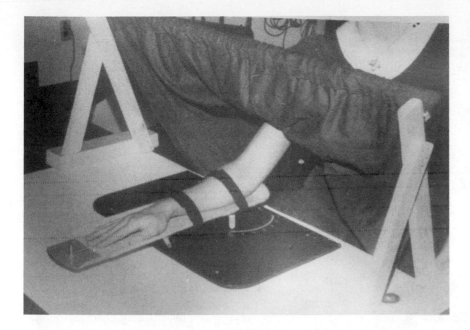

Figure 3.1 Use of a screen to occlude patient's vision of his arm, which is being tested.[27] (Reproduced with permission from Opila-Lehman, J., Short, M. A. and Trombly, C. A. Kinesthetic recall of children with athetoid and spastic cerebral palsy and of non-handicapped children. *Develop. Med. Child. Neurol., 27*: 223–230, 1985.)

will be interpreted needs to be considered. Patients who have delayed responses are considered by some to have abnormal sensation of the modality being tested.[1] However, delayed responses may indicate the patient is making a judgment about the S based on limited reception. Therefore, consistently accurate but delayed responses may point to a problem of information processing rather than one of primary sensory impairment. Further cognitive testing would need to be done to confirm this.

Environment

As in any evaluation, reliability of retest results increases if the same person retests under the same conditions. Use of the same quiet room with few extraneous stimuli is ideal. The environment should be conducive to full concentration on the testing process since attention is an important parameter of sensory recognition.

Patient State

Patient participation in sensory testing is a recognized variable influencing results. It is important that the patient understand the general purpose and the specific procedure of each sensory test; if he is unable to understand, he cannot be validly tested. He must actively participate and give full attention to the testing[11] as well as be able to communicate accurate responses. During testing, fatigue is avoided since it is a major source of error.[12]

TESTING PROCEDURES

Choice of which tests need to be administered to a particular patient is guided by the diagnosis, by the need to know certain information, and/or the knowledge that if primary sensory reception is lost, discriminatory sensation will be lost as well and therefore need not be tested.

Because the nature of the response required of the patient varies from test to test, some tests may need to

be adapted or eliminated due to the patient's other limitations such as expressive aphasia or apraxia. One adaptation is to allow the aphasic person to match or select his choice of response for stereognostic testing from an array of possible objects. The therapist should recognize, and record, that such an adaptation changes the task.[1]

Tests of Primary or Protective Sensation

The primary senses are tested to confirm that these basic sensations are present and to determine whether the spinothalamic tracts are intact. The results of these tests do not correlate with the ability to do precision grasp tasks,[3,13] nor do they yield precise information about damage to the somatosensory system.[1] In these tests, the patient has to process only one bit of information: present or absent.[1] Results of touch, pain, and temperature tests do not correlate perfectly ($\rho >$ 0.66); therefore, it is recommended that all three modalities be tested.[14]

Tactile Awareness (Light Touch). *Stimulus.* Lightly touch a small area of the patient's skin with cotton or the fingertip.[15,16]

Response. The patient says "now," "yes," or other indication each time the stimulus is felt. Nonverbal patients can squeeze the therapist's hand or change facial expression. The stimulus-response is repeated over those surfaces of the patient's skin expected to be dysfunctional according to the diagnosis.

Scoring. The score is the number of correct responses in relation to the number of S presentations. A score of 5/5, for instance, would indicate intact sense of touch, while a score of 3/5 would indicate impairment. A score is recorded for each area tested.

Pain. *Stimulus.* Using a safety pin, which has one sharp and one blunt end, the therapist applies mixed sharp and dull stimuli in a random pattern of presentation to verify accuracy of responses.

Response. The patient says "sharp" or "dull" or, if nonverbal, points to the end of the actual pin or a picture of a pin to indicate whether he felt the sharp or dull end. Again all appropriate surfaces are tested.

Scoring. The score is the number of accurate responses to the sharp stimuli in relation to the number of these presentations; dull stimuli are only used to require the patient to discriminate between touch and pain.[15,16]

Temperature. *Stimulus.* The patient's skin should be of normal temperature before testing begins. Capped test tubes, one with cold water and one with hot water, are applied in random order to the patient's skin. If metal test tubes are available, they are preferred because of metal's superior conduction property. Some therapists use metal spoons heated or cooled in water and dried to apply the stimuli. To prevent interpretation of the stimuli as painful, recommended approximate temperatures are 104° to 113°F (40° to 45°C) for hot and 41° to 50°F (5° to 10°C) for cold.[15] Knowing the temperature of the stimulus at the time of application is a problem. Stick-on temperature strips may be one solution; another may be use of the newly commercially available hot/cold discrimination units.

Response. After each presentation of a stimulus, the patient says "hot" or "cold." Again, appropriate skin surfaces are tested.

Scoring. The number of correct responses in relation to the total number of presentations is the score.

Tests of Peripheral Nerve Recovery

According to Dellon,[3,4,13] there is a sequence of recovery of sensation in the hand after suture of a peripheral nerve. As the nerve regenerates distalward, the lines of sensibility for each of the following modalities move distalward one after the other.

Pinprick. This test is described above as the test for pain. This, along with temperature sense, are the earliest senses to recover.[13]

Thirty Cycles per Second (cps) Vibratory Sense. *Stimulus.* A 30-cps tuning fork is activated by hitting the prongs and applying one of them to the skin surface to be tested.[3] The S presentations are randomized with false presentations in which the fork is not vibrating.

Response. The patient indicates when he feels the vibration. He also tells how it compares to the feeling in another finger and where he feels the sensation.[13]

Scoring. The score is the number of correct responses in relation to the total number of S presentations.

Moving Touch. The return of this sense quickly follows the return of 30-cps vibratory sense.[13]

Stimulus. The examiner strokes the finger using his own finger.

Response. The patient indicates whether he felt the S or not.

Scoring. None; the examiner notes the date to document the recovery.

Constant Touch/Pressure. *Stimulus.* The therapist uses a pressure aesthesiometer to apply a known level of firm pressure to the patient's skin.[15] The Semmes-Weinstein pressure aesthesiometer is one such tool.[17] (Fig. 3.2). This evaluation instrument consists of 20 graduated nylon monofilaments mounted in plastic rods.[17-19] Each monofilament is calibrated to exert specific pressures and is rated on a scale from 1.65 to 6.65, with the normal range being between 2.44 and 2.83.[18,19] The rod is held perpendicular to the skin to be tested. The monofilament is pressed against the skin until it just bends. Each filament bends according to its length and thickness and not according to the force exerted by the examiner.[17,19] When testing in the range of 2.44 to 4.08, it

Figure 3.2 Semmes-Weinstein pressure aesthesiometer.

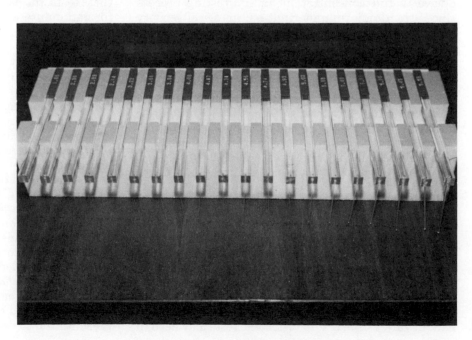

is recommended that the monofilaments be bounced off the skin.[18,19] Except for the heavy filaments, for which only one trial is given, three trials are given with each filament for each skin area under examination.[18,19]

Response. The patient indicates each time the stimulus is felt.

Scoring. The number of correct responses for each filament is the score for each area being tested.

256-cps Vibratory Sense. *Stimulus.* A tuning fork rated at 256 cps is used in the same way as described above for the test of low frequency vibratory sense. *Response* and *scoring* are the same as above.

Tests That Relate to Precision Use of the Hands

Weber Stationary Two-Point Discrimination (s2PD). The purpose of the two-point discrimination test is to determine if the person can distinguish between being touched by one or two points and at what distance this can be appreciated. The s2PD test measures the innervation density of the slowly adapting fiber/receptor system.[3,13] This test predicts the ability of the hand to do precision grip,[20] that is, to know how tightly to press to prevent dropping an object.[3,20] The patient who lacks perception of vibratory stimuli and of moving and constant touch will not be able to pass this test.[4]

Stimulus. The stimulus may be applied using a blunt-ended calibrated compass,[16,19] Boley gauge,[19] aesthesiometer, or paper clip (see Fig. 3.3). The two points, separated by 2 mm, are applied along the longitudinal axis in the center of the zone to be tested.[19] The two points are applied simultaneously and with equal, light pressure to the skin of the palmar surface of the palm and fingers. Heavy pressure invalidates the test by allowing the subject to perceive the two points when he would not be able to if correct pressure were used. One-point application trials are randomly interspersed with test trials. If the patient is unable to discriminate the two points at 2 mm, the separation between the two points is increased by 1 mm. This continues up to 10 mm on the fingers and to 20 mm on the palm. s2PD is considered absent beyond these points.[18]

Response. The patient says whether he felt "one" or "two" points. The nonverbal patient can hold up one or two fingers to indicate his response.

Scoring. The sensitivity at which the patient correctly discriminates more than 7 of 10 successive *S* presentations is the score.[3,12] Sensitivity increases from a low of 38-45 mm in the upper limb to 2.5 mm in the pads of the fingers,[12] although norms vary among researchers.[3] A score is recorded for each skin area being examined. Table 3.1 lists normative values for the volar surface of the hand according to Omer.[18,19] When using these norms to interpret the results, it should be noted that there is a large interperson variability within the normal population.[12,21] Kent[22] determined on a sample of 50 that test-retest reliability for adult hemiplegic patients was low. The correlation coefficients ranged from $r = 0.59$ to $r = 0.82$, depending upon the area of the body being tested. The unidentified source of variability probably is the reason why different researchers have found different normative values.

Moving Two-Point Discrimination Test[3,23] (m2PD). This is a test of the quickly adapting fiber/receptor system.[13,23] It relates to the ability to identify objects manipulated by the fingertips (tactile gnosis)[13] and predicts manipulatory skill.[20]

Stimulus. The two-pronged instrument used for s2PD can be used for this test also. The hand is supported on the table. The volar surface of the distal phalanges are tested by lightly but firmly moving the two points, applied equally, proximally to distally perpendicular to the majority of fingerprint ridges. The separation of the two points starts at 8 mm. Five test trials are done with one-point false presentations interspersed. If the patient passes 5/5 trials, the distance between the points is decreased to 6 mm, 4 mm, and then to 2 mm. If the patient fails some of the trials, the test continues until 10 *S* presentations have been made.

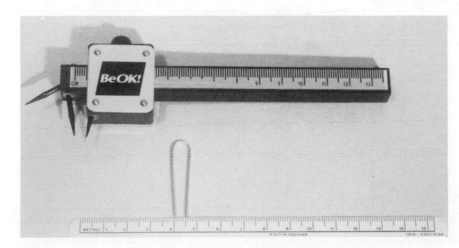

Figure 3.3 Two tools used for applying two-point discrimination stimuli: 3-point aesthesiometer and bent paper clip.

Table 3.1
NORMS FOR STATIONARY TWO-POINT DISCRIMINATION TEST (IN MILLIMETERS)[a]

	Normal	Impaired	Absent
Between tip and distal interphalangeal (DIP) joints	3–5	6–10	>10
Between DIP and proximal interphalangeal (PIP) joints	3–6	7–10	>10
Between PIP and metacarpo phalangeal joints	4–7	8–10	>10
Between web and distal palmar crease	5–8	9–20	>20
Between distal palmar crease and center of palm	6–9	10–20	>20
Rest of palm	7–10	11–20	>20

[a]Adapted and used with permission from Omer, G.E. Evaluation and reconstruction of the forearm and hand after acute traumatic peripheral nerve injuries. *J. Bone Joint Surg., 50-A*(7): 1454–1478, 1968.

Response The patient indicates whether he felt one or two points.

Scoring. In order to pass the test at a given sensitivity level, the patient must have been correct 7/10 times.[23] The score is the least number of millimeters the patient can discriminate. The normal m2PD is 2 mm at the distal finger tip.[23] Each finger is scored separately.

Moberg Picking-Up Test for Dexterity.[3,24] In 1958, Moberg introduced this test to relate sensation of the hand to hand function.[20] This static grip test correlates well with the Weber two-point discrimination test, both of which evaluate the slowly adapting A-beta receptor/fiber system.[3,20]

Stimulus A small box and several objects are placed on the table in front of the patient. The objects are several coins of different sizes, paper clip, safety pin, nails, and nuts and bolts of various sizes.

Response. With his eyes open, the patient is asked to pick these objects up as quickly as possible and drop them into the small container.[3,18,24] Two trials are done with each hand.

Scoring. A plus or minus is given for each object the patient can pick up and deposit into the box.[3] The score is the total items "passed." The score of the second trial is more reliable and is the one reported.

Modified Picking-Up Test for Sensation. In this test the subject is asked to identify what he is picking up, which prompts him to manipulate the object in his fingertips.[3] This test relates highly to m2PD and both evaluate the quickly adapting A-beta receptor/fiber system.[3,20]

Stimulus. Twelve small objects are placed on the table in front of the patient. The objects are listed in Table 3.2. The patient's ring and little fingers are flexed and taped to the palm to prevent their use.[3] A small box is placed 6 inches (15 cm) from the group of objects. The patient and therapist agree on the names of the objects; then his vision is occluded and he is asked to identify each object as it is placed on his thumb as a cue to prehend it. Two trials per hand are done; no more than 30 sec are allowed to identify any object.

Response. The patient names the object.

Scoring. Time required to identify each object is noted and recorded separately by item. The norms, based on a limited sample, are listed in Table 3.2. The score is the total time required to identify all objects on the second trial. Each hand is scored separately.

Other Tests of Discriminatory Sensation of the Hands and Upper Extremity.

Stereognosis. This is the ability to identify objects tactually. Astereognosis is the term used to designate an

Table 3.2
NORMS FOR MODIFIED PICKING-UP TEST (IN SECONDS)[a]

Object	Trial 1 Mean	Trial 1 Range	Trial 2 Mean	Trial 2 Range
1. Wing nut	1.7	1–3	2.0	1–3
2. Screw	1.4	1–2	1.5	1–2
3. Key	1.5	1–3	1.6	1–2
4. Nail	1.7	1–4	1.5	1–2
5. Large nut	1.8	1–3	1.4	1–2
6. Nickel	1.8	1–3	2.0	2
7. Dime	1.7	1–5	1.3	1–2
8. Washer	1.8	1–3	1.7	1–3
9. Safety pin	1.6	1–2	1.6	1–2
10. Paper clip	2.3	1–5	2.1	1–3
11. Small nut (hex)	2.1	1–3	1.6	1–3
12. Small nut (square)	1.6	1–3	1.6	1–3

[a]Reproduced with permission of Dellon, A. L. *Evaluation of Sensibility and Re-Education of Sensation in the Hand.* Baltimore: Williams & Wilkins, 1981.

absence of stereognosis. Several levels of ability can be tested, and the choice depends upon the patient's expected occupational performance status. The least discriminatory test stimuli are common objects used in self-care and home tasks, while the most discriminatory are closely similar objects made of the same material. In the latter case, the patient will be asked to tactually detect the difference in size, shape, weight, or texture of two objects. Since few patients return to jobs that require precision tactual discrimination, only the most common object test will be described here and the reader is referred to Roland's work[1] for a description of testing for greater discrimination.

Stimulus. With the subject's eyes closed, an easily recognizable object that he has not looked at previously is placed in the involved hand. Assistance in manipulation of the object may be required in the presence of paralysis.[22] Items commonly used include coins, key, safety pin, paper clip, pen, pencil, spoon, comb, toothbrush, bottle cap, etc. Some stimuli are deliberately chosen to be of the same material and approximately the same size to test fine discrimination.[3,15] Presenting the objects without previously showing them to the patient is a more critical test and is preferable; however, if the patient is unable to respond, all the items are shown to him first and it is ascertained that he knows their names.

Response. The patient names each object as it is identified. If the patient is aphasic, an array of some of the objects can be placed in front of him for his selection. The distractor objects can be very different or very similar depending upon the degree of discrimination being tested. Using this method changes the task to some degree.[1]

Scoring. The total number of objects correctly identified related to the total number of stimulus items presented is the score. Kent[22] found a test similar to this to be highly reliable on retest ($r = 0.97$) of 50 adult hemiplegics.

Proprioception (Position Sense). *Stimulus.*
The therapist holds the part laterally to avoid cutaneous input and slowly ($10°$ /sec)[25] passively positions the joint being tested. The subject is then asked to reproduce the position with the opposite extremity. When one side is involved, this side is positioned and the noninvolved side copies the position. Errors are attributed to impairment or loss of position sense on the involved side, i.e., the positioned side. Joints are tested singly and in combination. Large joints are tested separately from the wrist and finger joints. Proprioceptive memory, a higher level function, [26] can be tested by holding the terminal position at the end point for 2–4 sec while the patient concentrates on this position. The limb is returned to the start position, and the patient is asked to duplicate the stimulus posture[25].

Response. The patient imitates each posture with the opposite extremity or describes the position.

Scoring. The score is the total number of correct responses in relation to the number of *S* delivered. Each joint is scored separately.

Kinesthesia (Movement Sense). Two tests are presented here since they have been found to produce significantly different results and therefore are hypothesized to test two separate neural mechanisms.[25]

Test 1. Stimulus. The therapist holds the part laterally to reduce tactile input and moves the joint up or down at a slow steady rate of $5°$/sec. [25,27] Large and small amplitudes of movement are tested on large and small joints. In the upper extremity the shoulder, elbow, forearm, wrist, thumb, and index and little fingers are usually tested. If the patient fails to respond accurately at the slow speed, he may be able to detect motion if the stimulus movement is delivered rapidly. [5] The level of detection of kinesthesia is influenced by velocity: it is easier to detect brisk movement. [5,10]

Response. After each stimulus, the patient indicates whether the joint was moved "up" or "down."

Scoring. The number of correct responses in relation to the number of presentations for each joint is the score. Note is made of the pattern of responses: large versus small joints; gross versus fine movements.

Test 2. Stimulus. The patient's arm is positioned in a kinesthesiometer (see Fig. 3.1) that measures the angle of internal and external shoulder rotation with the elbow held at $45°$ of flexion.[27] The arm in the trough of the instrument is moved at $5°$/sec to a final point. The position is held at the end point for 2–4 sec, and the patient is told to concentrate on this position.

Response. After the arm is returned to $0°$, or other starting position, the patient is asked to reproduce the stimulus posture.[25] Several trials are given of both large and small excursion movements and of movements toward and away from the body.

Scoring. The difference, in degrees, between the stimulus end point and the reproduced end point is the score. The scores across trials are averaged for the final absolute error score.

Tactile Localization. Location of touch pressure may be tested separately or included with the test of constant touch.

Stimulus. The therapist touches the patient's skin with the aesthesiometer. Stimulus intensity and stimulus duration have been found to significantly influence the accuracy of response.[28]

Response. After each stimulation, the patient opens his eyes and places a finger or a pointed probe[19] on the spot touched. Accuracy is normally more precise in the hand and less so proximally.[16,28]

Scoring. The score is the distance in millimeters between the point of stimulation and the indicated point. This measure has been found to have high interrater reliability ($r = 0.98$).[28]

RECORDING THE RESULTS

The record of the results of the sensory evaluation should be specific enough to enable future comparison of progress and to communicate useful information to others.

Some centers have devised graphic methods of recording the findings of sensory evaluations.[4,29] In the case of peripheral nerve injury (PNI), the recording may be done on a diagram of the extremity using colors to designate different sensory modalities. In cases of spinal cord lesion, the losses may be marked on a full-body diagram of anterior and posterior views. Other centers prefer descriptive reports that relate each type of loss to a specific peripheral nerve distribution, in the case of PNI, or to a particular dermatomal level or body part such as nipple line or umbilicus, in the case of spinal cord injury. For cortical lesions the modalities affected in a particular body part are explicitly recorded.

Reporting that the patient has impaired stereognosis or kinesthesis, for example, does not communicate adequately. If, on the other hand, the report noted that the patient was able to identify 9/10 common objects but only 2/10 geometric shapes and that he was unable to detect rapid, small movements of less than 20° excursion in large or small joints, then documentation is clear and useful. Phrasing such a statement also helps the student therapist to determine where along the developmental continua treatment should begin.

INTERPRETING THE RESULTS

The occupational therapist approaches the evaluation data looking for specific pieces of information to guide treatment. The first question to be asked of the results is whether any or all primary sensations are intact, impaired, absent, or exaggerated. If these sensations are intact, the therapist would proceed to evaluate the discriminative sensory functions to determine if any are impaired or absent. If primary sensation is exaggerated, the patient will need a program of desensitization. If the primary sensations are impaired or absent, the patient is in jeopardy for further injury in the course of daily living. Therefore the next thing the therapist wants to know is what is the distribution of these abnormalities.

In the case of PNI, it is helpful to look at a chart of PNI distributions to determine which nerve is involved and to what extent (Fig. 3.4). Since recovery of function of peripheral nerves proceeds proximally to distally, it would be expected that in the proximal area where the nerve is normal, sensation would be intact; where the nerve is recovering, impaired sensation is expected; and where the nerve has not yet recovered, sensory loss is expected. Based on this knowledge, decisions can be made as to what modality would be retrained and at what location on the limb. Decisions about splinting and other protective measures are also made from this analysis.

In the case of complete anatomical or physiological spinal cord transection, sensory loss will occur in the dermatomes below the level of the lesion (Fig. 3.5). Recovery would not be expected and protective measures would be taught to protect the anesthetic skin. If there were any sensory reception below the diagnosed level

of lesion, partial damage to the spinal cord is indicated and the therapist would then help the patient recalibrate the meaning of those sensations as well as be attentive to returning muscle function that may follow.

Sensory impairment as a result of cortical dysfunction does not follow either the dermatomal distribution nor the peripheral nerve distribution. Damage to the sensory cortex results in total or partial loss of discriminative sensations. Retraining and/or compensation are the treatments that would be chosen.

Because distal limb parts have a larger representation in the sensory cortex than do proximal parts and because the distal parts are contralaterally represented cortically whereas proximal parts are represented bilaterally, there is more likelihood that a lesion would have a greater impact on distal parts. Therefore the therapist would look to the data from the discriminative tests in terms of possible differences between proximal and distal parts of the limb to help guide treatment of motor control. Additionally, the results of sensory evaluation are valuable in guiding treatment of motor control problems that bypasses defective sensory systems and utilizes intact ones[27] or in estimating rehabilitation outcome.[2]

Treatment

Treatment of sensory impairment involves education (recalibration) of touch sensation and/or protective and compensatory strategies to substitute for the losses. The mental status of the patient affects the choice of treatment. The treatment of choice for the confused patient with impaired sensation may be protective precautions taken by caretakers. Or treatment to increase sensory experiences via the intact senses[27] may be chosen to prevent further confusion and isolation.

HYPOSENSITIVITY: IMPAIRED SENSATION

Sensory retraining programs have the goal of recalibrating sensation, that is, of helping the patient to learn the meaning of the new sensation.[13] Developmentally, we learn to relate what we feel to our experiences in the environment. For example, after we have picked up and used a spoon many times, we come to expect the particular sensory experience we associate with the spoon whenever we use a spoon. Even in the dark we would know the object we held was a spoon because we learned to associate a certain feeling with the spoon. There is no objective, correct "spoon" sensation; everyone has his own sensation of a spoon using his own sensory system, the sensitivity of which varies from person to person.[12,21] Therefore, the task of the patient with impaired sensation is to learn what these new sensations mean in relation to his old sensory memories. The patient reteaches himself by interacting with the environment[30] under the guidance of the occupational therapist. Learning involves designation of a goal, active attention to task,[30] feedback, reinforcement, and practice.

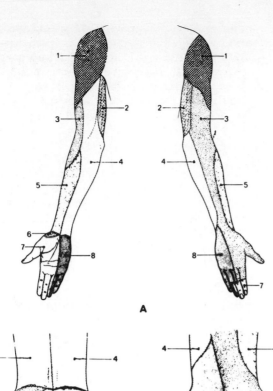

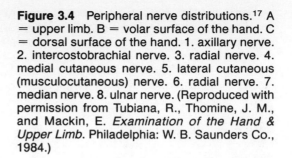

Figure 3.4 Peripheral nerve distributions.[17] A = upper limb. B = volar surface of the hand. C = dorsal surface of the hand. 1. axillary nerve. 2. intercostobrachial nerve. 3. radial nerve. 4. medial cutaneous nerve. 5. lateral cutaneous (musculocutaneous) nerve. 6. radial nerve. 7. median nerve. 8. ulnar nerve. (Reproduced with permission from Tubiana, R., Thomine, J. M., and Mackin, E. *Examination of the Hand & Upper Limb*. Philadelphia: W. B. Saunders Co., 1984.)

Sensory reeducation of PNI postrepair is geared to the specific stage in the recovery of sensation[4,13] as noted above. Early-phase reeducation starts when 30 cps vibratory sense and perception of moving touch have returned.[3] Early-phase reeducation involves the use of a pencil eraser to stroke the length of the area. The patient watches while stroking, then closes his eyes to concentrate on the feel of the stroking. He opens his eyes to reconfirm what is happening. Meanwhile, he verbalizes what he is perceiving throughout the process. A similar procedure is used to retrain localization of constant touch when awareness of this modality has returned.[3] At first the threshold of the applied touch is very high and a firm pressure is used. Late-phase reeducation begins when both moving and constant touch can be localized unambiguously[3] at the fingertips. This phase concentrates on tactile gnosis[3]

and object manipulation. Objects are graded in size from large to small and textures from diverse to same.

As an adjunct to the learning process, to heighten sensory awareness and attention, therapists sometimes use vigorous, generalized cutaneous stimulation, for example, rubbing the affected area briskly with terry toweling before having the patient use the limb. Another adjunct is cognitive cueing in which the patient and the therapist discuss the various qualities of the S in an attempt to help the patient to cognitively note the characteristics of it in order to recognize them on subsequent presentations. The stimuli are graded in such a way as to require only gross awareness or discrimination initially and more refined responses as the patient's accuracy improves.

Vision can compensate for impaired or lost sensation; therefore, it is occluded until the patient com-

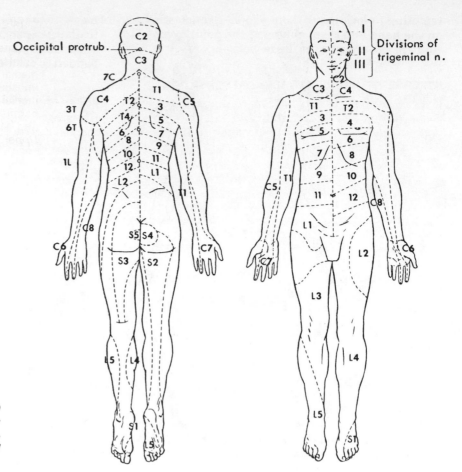

Figure 3.5 Sensory chart according to dermatomes. (Reproduced with permission from Gilroy, J., and Meyer, J. S. *Medical Neurology,* 3rd edition. New York: Macmillan, 1979.)

pletes each trial of the reeducation task. Then visual feedback confirms the accuracy of the response and reinforces the learning. Practice of this stimulus-response-feedback sequence continues until the patient demonstrates relearning or is unable to.

If the patient is unable to relearn, or the time required for a retraining process is not available, treatment becomes primarily aimed at teaching the patient to visually compensate for lost or impaired sensations to avoid injury and to improve motor performance.

Since peripheral sensation is a major source of feedback necessary for dexterous hand movement, loss of this feedback must be compensated for visually. Because the visuomotor transmission loop of the upper extremity is as much as two to three times as long as the somatosensory motor loop,[10] automatic reflex correction is lost. As a result, the patient will be limited in his ability to accurately do complex movement patterns such as buttoning a shirt; do long sequences of simple motor programs such as repetitive tapping; sustain force, for example, when using a tool; or learn new motor skills.[31] Visual compensation is also limited insofar as a patient with kinesthetic loss could not accurately use the involved limb in the dark.

Although vision is the primary means of compensation,[10] auditory compensation such as putting a bracelet or bell on the wrist may be a worthwhile way to remind the patient about an anesthetic limb's location.

Wynn-Parry[32,33] described a successful program of sensory retraining for patients following median nerve repair. The program concentrated on stereognosis and tactile localization, considered prerequisite to functional hand use. As soon as some appreciation of sensation had returned, the training began using blocks of different shapes and textures. The patient was blindfolded and was asked first to identify the shape of each block, attending to its characteristics (e.g., edges, weights, contours), in relation to other blocks. If he failed to identify the block, the blindfold was removed so that he could simultaneously see, feel, and describe the block. Once the shaped blocks were learned, then textures applied to blocks, followed by objects used in daily life, were used as stimuli. Because concentration is fatiguing, four 10-min sessions per day, rather than one longer session, was recommended. Retraining of localization of tactile stimuli followed object identification and used a technique similar to the first: attempting to localize, without vision, a touch stimulus on the hand and then looking at the point touched to confirm the accuracy of the response.

HYPERSENSITIVITY: EXAGGERATED SENSATION

Hypersensitivity is a condition characterized by extreme discomfort or irritability in response to normally nonnoxious tactile stimulation.[34] It disables the patient because he is unable to sustain contact with utensils or tools.

Treatment to decrease hypersensitivity is desensitization. Graded, tactile stimuli are used to desensitize. The stimuli are textured materials that are graded from soft to hard to rough. The force of application is also graded: from touch to rub to tap to prolonged contact. The textures and the force are graded in conjunction with each other. The desensitization program can be implemented by incorporating the gradation of textures and application force into activities of interest to the patient. For an example of a touching sequence, a patient could finger-feed marshmallows, then raw carrots, and then progress to pretzels. For an example of a rubbing sequence, the patient could pet the family cat, then finger-paint, and then build castles in the sand. For an example of a tapping sequence, the patient could juggle or toss cotton balls, then ping-pong balls, and then tennis balls. For an example of a prolonged contact sequence, the patient could search for an object hidden in a container filled with flour, then rice, then smooth kidney beans, and then shell macaroni. One example of a combination sequence in which the patient touches, rubs, taps, and contacts graded textures would be as follows: by the time the patient can pick up (touch) pine cones, he may be able to rub his body with a loofa sponge in the shower, tap soft cotton thread into place in a weaving project, and take handfuls (contact) of cotton balls to stuff a rag doll.

Due to the patient's anticipation of pain, a program of desensitization is best carried out by the patient himself under the direction of the therapist.[35]

One desensitization treatment program, as reported by Yerxa et al.[34] uses standard stimulation materials individually sequenced for the patient since each patient's tolerance for sensory stimuli differs. These sensory situations are used: dowel textures, which are different-textured materials ranging from moleskin to Velcro hook material mounted onto dowels sticks; contact textures, which range from cotton to sharp-edged plastic cubes in containers into which the hand is immersed; and vibration ranging from 23 to 100 cps. Each of these is graded for the individual patient into ten steps of degree of irritation. Treatment begins with exposure to a stimulus that is slightly irritating but tolerable, defined as contact for 10 min three or four times per day, and progresses along gradations as the patient learns to tolerate each successive level. The hierarchy established for each patient becomes the basis for use of the Downey Hand Center Hand Sensitivity Test to measure the effectiveness of this treatment for the particular patient.[34]

To compensate for hypersensitivity, objects can be padded to cushion the surface.

ANESTHESIA: SENSORY LOSS

Absence of sensation is a serious problem. Not only is the insensitive limb liable to be burned, cut, or abraded during the course of daily activities, but it can be seriously damaged due to prolonged pressure on the skin, particularly over bony prominences. Pressure greater than 30 mm Hg[36] to 32 mm Hg[37] reduces blood flow to the skin area, which deprives the tissue of oxygen and nutrients[38] thus causing necrosis of tissue in that area with subsequent ulceration. Excessive mechanical forces such as shear stresses, which twist or tear tissues and which occur when transferring without enough lift, or high-level forces concentrated in a small area, such as a thin handle on a heavy shopping bag, also cause tissue damage.[39] Moderate-level repetitive stress also can cause ulceration. It results in inflammation and later necrosis due to a chemical digestion of the deep tissue.[39]

The goal is to avoid hurt to the insensitive body area. Treatment is teaching the patient precautionary measures. The patient must learn to anticipate and avoid the danger. While obvious sources of danger may require little learning, pressure, an insidious source of severe danger, requires revision of habits. Habit training involves attention to the situation, problem solving, and large amounts of practice.

In patients with Hansen's disease, the hands and feet are particularly susceptible to pressure damage. Brand[39] offers practical suggestions for relief of localized pressure or mechanical stresses. Both changing shoes often during the day to change the pattern of pressure and reducing the amount of walking protect the feet. Cushioning or enlarging handles to distribute the forces over a larger surface, changing the shape of handles to avoid sharp edges, varying the tools used or changing which hand is used to do a job to change the pattern of stress, and wearing gloves are suggestions to protect the hands. To help the patient realize the threat of pressure, use of pressure-sensitive material developed by the staff at the United States Public Health Service Hospital at Carville, Louisiana is useful. Microcapsules of color are imbedded in the material and under pressure the capsules break to release a dye; the intensity of the color is proportional to the pressure exerted.[40] The material can be made into socks or gloves. The patient learns to avoid excessive pressure by adjusting his methods of performing tasks according to the intensity of dye released in a given area on the garment.[41] By discussing the reasons for these modifications with the patient, he will learn to adapt to situations encountered in the future.

The spinal cord-injured patient may be anesthetic over a large area of his body. He would need to have special pressure relief equipment installed in his bed and wheelchair as well as learn pressure relief techniques. All cushions are helpful in reducing pressure, but none reduce mean pressure to less than capillary pressure. Therefore, while use of a seat cushion is helpful, it must be accompanied by change of position and proper skin care.[36,37] Since the patient has lost awareness of the discomfort that arises from remaining in the same position for a long time, he must learn to remember to relieve the pressure by changing his body position at regular intervals. His memory can be jogged throughout the day by all personnel, but a method that promotes independence from others is to use an electronic timer or pressure-sensitive transducer to signal the time or need for doing a pressure relief maneuver. These maneuvers are detailed in chapter 17. He needs to learn to monitor the success of his daily efforts by visually inspecting, or supervising the inspection of, every inch of his skin, using mirrors if necessary. A reddened area forecasts potential future breakdown. Great care is taken to eliminate any pressure from such an area until it returns to normal color, indicating a reversal of the ulceration process.

Equipment used to relieve pressure in bed include sheepskins, foam mattresses, or such devices as alternating pressure pads that continually change the surface pressure. Many wheelchair cushions are available, and all types relieve some pressure on the ischial tuberosities and distribute pressure on the buttocks and posterior thighs, although none is universally superior for all patients. [42]

Seat cushions currently available are: (a) gel cushions that are filled with a substance that shifts to conform to the seat contour and thereby distributes pressure more evenly; (b) air or water-filled cushions that offer a surface that can shift to vary the support; (c) foam rubber cushions that absorb some pressure and are of a thickness and density that will not compress fully under the weight of the patient; (d) alternating pressure pads that have channels that fill with air and a compressor to shift the air in and out of the channels alternately to relieve and redistribute pressure.

Souther et al.[37] used a surface pressure manometer to compare ischial tuberosity pressure of subjects using 11 different cushions, including all types of commercially available cushions except the alternating pressure pad. Cushions with a mean pressure that was significantly less than the pressure obtained when sitting in a wheelchair with no cushion were the following: the Jobst Hydro-Float cushion ($P < 0.01$), the Jobst Hydro-Float pad ($P < 0.01$), the Bye-Bye Decubiti ($P\ 0.05$), and the 2-inch latex foam pad ($P < 0.05$).

DeLateur et al[43] studied the effects of seven different cushions on hyperemia of the skin by measuring the duration of the skin redness of paralyzed patients after they sat for 30 minutes on each of the cushions. There was no significant difference found among the cushions, and some hyperemia was found using all types of cushions. This study lent further support to the need for regular position change or push-ups several times

an hour as a supplement to the use of a wheelchair cushion. Footrest height was important to cushion effectiveness in both of these studies; footrests needed to be adjusted to distribute pressure evenly along the thighs and buttocks.

Ma et al[44] found that a cutout board placed under a 2- or 3-inch foam rubber or T-foam cushion reduced pressure over the ischial tuberosities significantly more than use of a foam cushion alone, although not below capillary pressure. The board is ⅝ inch plywood with a posterior cutout made to fit individual measurements. The ischial tuberosities must be cleared but without extra width so that weight can be distributed over a broad area of the buttocks and thighs. The posterior corners are notched to fit the back uprights of the wheelchair (Fig. 3.6). Measurements are taken with the patient lying prone on a firm, padded table. The height from the surface to the coccyx is measured between the legs, and 4 inches are added to determine the depth of the cutout. The lateral edges of the ischial tuberosities are found by palpation, and 2 inches are added to determine the width of the cutout. Seat depth and width are measured to determine the overall size of the board.

Garber et al. [45] used a Pressure Evaluation Pad with transducers that registered pressure that was displayed in a corresponding grid pattern on a lighted panel. Six cushions were evaluated with spinal cord-injured patients. The ROHO cushion and the Scimedics foam cushion with a "U"-shaped cutout registered the most pressure; the Temper Foam cushion registered the least pressure. Individual variation, however, was considerable.[45,46] Thin patients are noted

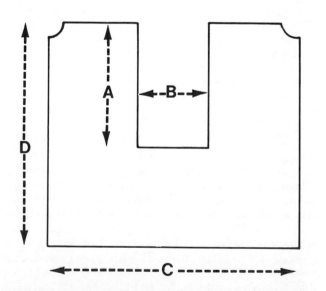

Figure 3.6 Cutout board to be placed under a foam cushion. See text for procedures to derive measurements for A, B, C, and D. (Reproduced with permission from Ma, D. M., Chu, D. S., and Davis, S. Pressure relief under the ischial tuberosities and sacrum using a cutout board. *Arch. Phys. Med. Rehabil., 57*: 352–354, 1976.)

to have higher pressures over bony prominences than average-weight or obese patients.[47] Evaluation of pressure should be used to select the best cushion for each patient.

Fisher et al.[48] studied the effect of various wheelchair cushions on skin temperature because an increase in temperature is a secondary factor contributing to tissue breakdown. Five cushions including foam rubber, gel, and the Jobst water flotation cushion were studied with normal subjects sitting for 30 minutes on each cushion. Surface temperature thermistors were taped under the ischial tuberosities and posterior thighs; graphic recordings and a printout of temperature readings were obtained. Skin temperatures decreased significantly on the water flotation cushion, remained the same on the gel cushions, and increased significantly on the foam rubber cushions. Fisher and Kosiak[49] studied the effectiveness of the ROHO cushion, a newer cushion not included in the previous studies. The ROHO cushion is lightweight, washable, and comfortably stable, but no significant difference in resting pressure or temperature change was found between the ROHO cushion and a 4-inch foam rubber cushion.

STUDY QUESTIONS:

Evaluation and Treatment of Somatosensory Sensation

1. What are the two subsystems of the somatosensory system?
2. What are the functions of each subsystem?
3. Patients with which types of disease or injuries will require sensory evaluation?
4. What are some variables that can affect the outcome of a sensory evaluation other than the condition of the patient?
5. Define the terms "intact," "absent," and "impaired" as they relate to sensory testing.
6. What is the sequence of recovery of sensation following surgical repair of a peripheral nerve?
7. How do s2PD and m2PD tests relate to hand function?
8. How should the results of the sensory test be recorded to clearly communicate the results?
9. Describe the sensory retraining process used for patients with impaired sensation.
10. Why is hypersensitivity so disabling?
11. Name two methods used by patients with anesthetic skin to decrease the likelihood of developing pressure sores and describe how these methods prevent ulceration.

References

1. Roland, P. E. Astereognosis: tactile discrimination after localized hemispheric lesions in man. *Arch. Neurol.*, 33: 543-550, 1976.
2. Anderson, E. K. Sensory impairments in hemiplegia. *Arch. Phys. Med. Rehabil.*, 52(7): 294-297, 1971.
3. Dellon, A. L. *Evaluation of Sensibility and Re-education of Sensation in the Hand*. Baltimore: Williams & Wilkins, 1981.
4. Dellon, A. L. Curtis, R. M., and Edgerton, M. T. Evaluating recovery of sensation in the hand following nerve injury. *Johns Hopkins Med. J.*, 130:235-243, 1972.
5. Newton, R. A. Joint receptor contributions to reflexive and kinesthetic responses. *Phys. Ther.* 62(1): 22-29, 1982.
6. Gandevia, S. C., Burke, D., and McKeon, B. The projection of muscle afferents from the hand to cerebral cortex in man. *Brain*, 107: 1-13, 1984.
7. Moberg, E. The role of cutaneous afferents in position sense, kinaesthesia, and motor function of the hand. *Brain*, 106: 1-19, 1983.
8. Barrack, R. L., Skinner, H. B., and Cook, S. D. Proprioception of the knee joint. *Am. J. Phys. Med.*, 63(4): 175-181, 1984.
9. Cailliet, R. *Hand Pain and Impairment*, 3rd edition. Philadelphia: F. A. Davis Co., 1982.
10. Jeannerod, M., Michel, F., and Prablanc, C. The control of hand movements in a case of hemianaesthesia following a parietal lesion. *Brain*, 107: 899-920, 1984.
11. Wolf, S. L., et al. Objective determinations of sensibility in the upper extremity. *Phys. Ther.* 57(10): 1132-1137, 1977.
12. Nolan, M. F. Two-point discrimination assessment in the upper limb in young adult men and women. *Phys. Ther.*, 62(7): 965-969, 1982.
13. Dellon, A. L. Functional sensation and its reeducation. *Clinics in Plastic Surgery*, 11(1): 95-99, 1984.
14. Harlowe, D., and Van Deusen, J. Evaluating cutaneous sensation following CVA: relationships among touch, pain, and temperature tests. *Occup. Ther. J. Research*, 5(1): 70-72, 1985.
15. De Jong, R. N. *The Neurologic Examination*, 3rd edition. New York: Harper & Row, 1967.
16. Alpers, B. J., and Mancall, E. L. *Essentials of the Neurological Examination*. Philadelphia: F. A. Davis Co., 1971.
17. Tubiana, R., Thomine, J. M., and Mackin, E. *Examination of the Hand & Upper Limb*. Philadelphia: W. B. Saunders Co., 1984.
18. Omer, G. E. Evaluating and reconstruction of the forearm and hand after acute traumatic peripheral nerve injuries. *J. Bone Joint Surg.*, 50-A(7): 1454-1478, 1968.
19. Werner, J. L., and Omer, G. E. Evaluating cutaneous pressure sensation in the hand. *Am. J. Occup. Ther.*, 24(5): 347-356.
20. Dellon, A. L. Touch sensibility in the hand. *Hand*, 9-B(1): 11-13, 1984.
21. Johansson, R. S., and Westling, G. Roles of glabrous skin receptors and sensorimotor memory in automatic control of precision grip when lifting rougher or more slippery objects. *Exp. Brain Res.*, 56: 550-564, 1984.
22. Kent, B. A. Sensory-motor testing: the upper limb of adult patients with hemiplegia. *J.A.P.T.A.*, 45(6): 550-561, 1965.
23. Dellon, A. L. The moving two-point discrimination test: clinical evaluation of the quickly adapting fiber/receptor system. *J. Hand Surg.*, 3(5): 474-481, 1978.
24. Moberg, E. Objective methods for determining the functional value of sensibility in the hand. *J. Bone Joint Surg.*, 40-B(3):454-459, 1958.
25. Barrack, R. L., Skinner, H. B., and Cook, S. D. Proprioception of the knee joint: paradoxical effect of training. *Am. J. Phys. Med.*, 63(4): 175-181, 1984.
26. Laszlo, J. l., and Bairstow, P. J. The measurement of kinaesthetic sensitivity in children and adults. *Dev. Med. Child Neurol.*, 22: 454-464, 1980.
27. Opila-Lehman, J., Short, M. A., and Trombly, C. A. Kinesthetic recall of children with athetoid and spastic cerebral palsy and of non-handicapped children. *Dev. Med. Child Neurol.*, 27: 223-230, 1985.
28. Sieg, K. W., and Williams, W. N. Preliminary report of a methodology for determining tactile location in adults. *J. Occup. Ther. Res.*, 6(4): 195-206. 1986
29. Moratz, V. A. Documentation with rubber stamps. *Am. J. Occup. Ther.*, 37(4): 268, 1983.
30. Herdman, S. J. Effect of experience on recovery following CNS lesions. *Phys. Ther.*, 63(1): 51-55, 1983.
31. Rothwell, J. C., et al. Manual motor performance in a deafferented man. *Brain*, 105: 515-542, 1982.
32. Wynn-Parry, C. B., and Salter, M. Sensory re-education after median nerve lesions. *Hand*, 8(2): 250-257, 1976.
33. Wynn-Parry, C. B. Management of peripheral nerve injuries and traction lesions of the brachial plexus. *Int. Rehabil. Med.*, 1(1): 9-20, 1978.
34. Yerxa, E. J., et al. Development of a hand sensitivity test for the hypersensitive hand. *Am. J. Occup. Ther.*, 37(3): 176–181, 1983.
35. Unpublished notes from course, "Hand Rehabilitation." Chapel Hill: University of North Carolina, 1968.
36. Peterson, M. J., and Adkins, H. V. Measurement and redistribution of excessive pressures during wheelchair sitting. *Phys. Ther.*, 62(7): 990-994, 1982.
37. Souther, S. G., Carr, D., and Vistnes, L. M. Wheelchair cushions to reduce pressure under bony prominences. *Arch. Phys. Med. Rehabil.*, 55: 460-464, 1974.
38. Krouskop, T. A., Noble, P. C., Garber, S. L., and Spencer, W. A. The effectiveness of preventive management in reducing the occurrence of pressure sores. *Journal of Rehabilitation R and D*, 20(1): 74-83, 1983.
39. Brand, P. W., Management of the insensitive limb. *Phys. Ther.*, 59(1): 8-12, 1979.

40. Brand, P. W., and James, E. A pain substitute pressure assessment in the insensitive limb. *Am. J. Occup. Ther., 23*(6): 470-486, 1969.
41 Wood, H. Prevention of deformity in the insensitive hand: the role of the therapist. *Am. J. Occup. Ther., 23*(6): 488–489, 1969.
42. Garber, S. L., and Krouskop, T. A. Wheelchair cushion modification and its effect on pressure. *Arch. Phys. Med. Rehabil., 65*:(10) 579-583, 1984.
43. DeLateur, B. J., Berni, R. B., Hongladarom, T., and Giaconi, R. Wheelchair cushions designed to prevent sores: an evaluation. *Arch. Phys. Med. Rehabil., 57*: 129-135, 1976.
44. Ma, D. M., Chu, D. S., and Davis, S. Pressure relief under the ischial tuberosities and sacrum using a cutout board. *Arch. Phys. Med. Rehabil., 57*: 354-543, 1976.

45. Garber, S. L., Krouskop, T. A., and Carter, R. E. A system for clinically evaluating wheelchair pressure-relief cushions. *Am. J. Occup. Ther., 32*(9): 565-570, 1978.
46. Garber, S. L. Wheelchair cushions for spinal cord-injured individuals. *Am. J. Occup. Ther., 39*(11): 722-725, 1985.
47. Garber, S. L., and Krouskop, T. A. Body build and its relationship to pressure distribution in the seated wheelchair patient. *Arch. Phys. Med. Rehabil., 63*(1): 17-20, 1982.
48. Fisher, S. V., Szymke, T. E., Apte, S. Y., and Kosiak, M. Wheelchair cushion effect on skin temperature. *Arch. Phys. Med. Rehabil., 59*: 68-72, 1978.
49. Fisher, S. V., and Kosiak, M. Pressure distribution and skin temperature effect of the ROHO wheelchair balloon cushion. *Arch. Phys. Med. Rehabil., 60*: 70-71, 1979.

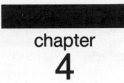

Evaluation of Motor Control

Catherine A. Trombly and Anna Deane Scott

Normal voluntary movement reflects the integrated functioning of several levels of motor control.[1] The segmental sensorimotor loop of the spinal cord keeps the muscles ready for action and for making quick adjustments to perturbations of movement. Groups of related spinal neurons cause phasic patterned movements in response to certain stimuli. Normally these patterned responses, or spinal reflexes, underlie automatic reciprocal movement patterns such as walking and are easily modified to allow adaptation to circumstances, e.g., walking on a rough or soft surface. The sensory tracts of the spinal cord transmit information from the periphery to higher centers to guide movement. The motor tracts of the spinal cord transmit signals from the brain stem, basal ganglia, cortex, and cerebellum to the interneuronal pool and anterior horn cells of the spinal cord and ultimately to the muscle fibers. The brain stem, in addition to being the locus of cranial nerve nuclei, mediates tonic patterned responses of the trunk and limbs in relation to the position of the head. In a person with a normal nervous system, these reflexes provide a background for posture and movement. The basal ganglia implement postural adjustments of the head in relation to the body, adjust body parts to maintain or regain balance, make anticipatory adjustments necessary to begin movement, and carry out the automatic execution of learned motor plans.[1,2] The cerebellum adjusts the number of motor units recruited and their sequence of firing to tailor the movement to the speed, force, and accuracy requirements of smooth movements.[3] The association cortex plans movement based on sensory information of the task at hand, the state of the body and the environment, and memories of the success of past movements in relation to the goal.[1] The motor cortex initiates movement.[1] It informs all the lower centers of the intent of the movement so each can be ready to participate and to monitor its own participation. The motor cortex also directly controls the recruitment of motor units of hand muscles.[4] Damage to any of these

levels of control results in abnormal postures or movements.

Normal movement also requires certain biomechanical integrity: the passive tissue elasticity and active contractile elements of muscle must be preserved[1]; the joints must be movable; and the skin and connective tissues must be intact.

Therefore, when evaluating a patient with central nervous system (CNS) dysfunction, all of these influences on coordinated voluntary movement must be considered. Specifically, evaluation of patients with CNS dysfunction includes estimation or measurement of passive range of joint motion, sensation, muscle tone as an indicator of muscle stiffness,[5] reflexes, level of maturation or recovery of motor milestones, level of voluntary control of acquired motor skills, ability to plan movement, ability to learn new motor skills, and ability to use objects meaningfully. Strength and endurance also are evaluated if the person has recovered voluntary control of isolated joint movement. These evaluations are found in Part Three.

Range of Motion

In CNS dysfunction passive range of motion is influenced by muscle tone. Passive range of motion is evaluated by moving each joint slowly through as full a range as possible in each of its motions. Slow movement is necessary in the case of spasticity to avoid eliciting the stretch reflex. If the stretch reflex is activated, resistance to movement will be felt. This resistance can be overcome by maintaining a steady, low force against the resistance until the hypertonic muscle relaxes and permits movement to continue. If muscle tone is decreased, the joints will be hypermobile and hyperextension may be found in joints that do not normally hyperextend. Chapter 8 describes the method of measuring and recording joint range of motion.

The affected shoulder of hemiplegic patients requires special attention. It is prone to subluxation and/or rotator cuff tear. Subluxation results from a combined weakness of the supraspinatus and stretching of the ligaments that support the superior capsule. In addition, downward rotation of the scapula with resultant relative abduction of the humerus "unlocks" the locking mechanism of the glenoid fossa, and gravity pulls the head of the humerus out of the fossa.[6] Rotator cuff tears occur when the head of the humerus is forced against the acromion process of the scapula. In stroke patients spasticity of the scapular adductors and downward rotators is common and prevents the scapula from upwardly rotating as it normally should during elevation of the arm above 90°. Attempts at elevating the humerus then squeeze the muscles between the bony points, resulting in torn muscle. Therefore, it is recommended that range of motion of the shoulder of the hemiplegic patient be done by approximating the head of the humerus into the glenoid fossa and moving the scapula and the slightly abducted humerus together (Fig. 4.1).

Sensation

The evaluation of sensation has been described in chapter 3. The importance of sensation to skilled motor performance has been thoroughly supported by research.[7]

Muscle Tone

Muscle tone refers to the stiffness or tension of the muscle. Normally the muscle is sufficiently stiff to react immediately and correctly when called upon. The tension is determined by the simultaneous combination of three factors: elastic properties of connective tissue, viscoelastic properties of muscle fibers, and motor unit activity.[8] Only the motor unit activity component is affected by CNS damage.[8] To review, a motor unit is one alpha motor neuron, its axon, and all muscle fibers attached to that axon. The stiffness of the muscle is estimated by noting the resistance it offers to passive stretch. If the resistance is greater than normal, the muscle is considered hypertonic; if less, it is termed hypotonic. A conceptual review of the physiology of tone is presented here because an understanding of it is basic to procedures of the neurodevelopmental approach.[5]

Normally when a muscle is stretched (elongated), it contracts (shortens) to resist the stretch. The force of the contraction is proportional to the speed of the stretch. Adjustments in the strength of muscle contractions depend on the number of motor units recruited voluntarily or reflexively. Recruitment to adjust suddenly applied loads (stretch) is reflexive via stretch reflexes involving a supraspinal loop that uses the information on length of muscle and velocity of change of length supplied by the muscle spindles.[5] The muscle spindles are length detector mechanisms located within the muscle and are normally kept at a "zero point" by impulses from supraspinal control centers. The zero point refers to the exact match of the spindle length to the length of the muscle fibers it is monitoring. CNS dysfunction disturbs this zeroing mechanism, altering muscle tone and affecting motor control. If too few supraspinal impulses are able to reach the spindle, it goes slack (hypotonic) and is unable to detect stretch of the muscle, and movement is absent or delayed. On testing, passive movement of the joint feels "mushy" or "loose." If too many supraspinal impulses are relayed to the spindle, it becomes too taut (hypertonic) and overreacts to slight stretches. Movement is curtailed in cases of spasticity because the spastic muscle, which is stretched during movement caused by an antagonist, automatically contracts, retarding the movement. On testing, the therapist will feel a "catch" at the point in range where the spastic muscle contracts. This is the stretch reflex. Spasticity is defined as hyperactive stretch reflexes.

There are two types of stretch reflexes: static and dynamic. The static or tonic stretch reflex is associated with posture, while the dynamic or phasic stretch reflex is associated with movement.

The muscle spindle, which derives its name from its shape, is mounted parallel to the muscle fibers so it can monitor their length. It is attached to extrafusal muscle fibers or tendons by a thread of connective tissue from each of its ends. Within each spindle are the mechanisms for both the static and dynamic stretch reflexes. Each spindle contains several nuclear chain fibers (static) and one to two nuclear bag fibers (dynamic).[9] These intrafusal muscle fibers get their names from the way their nuclei are configured. Each of these fibers has a noncontractile midportion and contractile polar portions.[10] When the contractile portions shorten, they pull on the midportion of the fiber, which causes that area to be stretched (internal stretch). The midportion also can be stretched me-

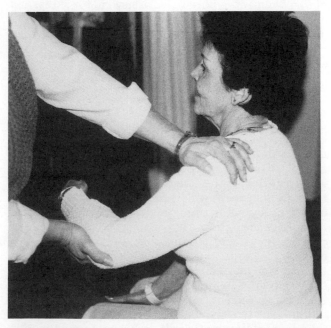

Figure 4.1 Method of doing range of motion of a hemiplegic shoulder to avoid rotator cuff tears.

chanically by stretching the whole muscle, and since the ends of the spindle are secured to the ends of the muscle, it too is stretched (external stretch) (Fig. 4.2)

The intrafusal muscle fibers contract when impulses reach them over a small motor neuron, the gamma efferent. The cell body of the gamma efferent is located in the anterior horn of the spinal cord just as the alpha motor neuron is. The alpha motoneuron is the large motor nerve to the extrafusal muscle fibers. The gamma efferent is activated by impulses descending from the reticular formation of the brain stem, from the cerebellum, and from other supraspinal centers, as well as by intersegmental spinal influences.

In cases of cortical or spinal cord damage, normal inhibition is lost. Therefore, too many impulses impinge on the gamma efferent, causing the intrafusal muscle fibers to be partially or fully contracted. Consequently, the central portions of the spindle fibers are on stretch, resulting in hypertonicity.[11] Cerebellar damage results in hypotonicity.

When the midportion of an intrafusal fiber is stretched, it generates a neural signal carried back to the spinal cord by afferent neurons. There are two types of afferent neurons: the primary (Ia) sensory fiber that serves the primary ending and the secondary (II) sensory fiber that serves the flower-spray ending. Tentacles of the primary ending coil or clamp around the midportions of both the bag fiber and the chain fibers.[9] The primary ending is velocity sensitive so its function is to detect dynamic change of length. The Ia endings have a low threshold for stretch: they respond to a single, brief stretch and to vibration.[12] The Ia afferent facilitates alpha motoneurons of the muscle in which it is located and reciprocally inhibits alpha motoneurons of the antagonist via an interneuron. Facilitation refers to a decrease of the threshold of the

cell, which increases the likelihood that the cell will fire. Inhibition is the opposite; the threshold of the cell membrane is increased, making firing less likely to happen.

The Ia ending around the bag fiber reacts to a single sudden stretch to produce a phasic muscle contraction,[12] while the Ia endings around the chain fibers react to repetitive small stretches to produce a sustained (tonic) response of the muscle.[13] The Ia afferent of the bag fiber has a monosynaptic connection to the alpha motor neuron of the muscle stretched. The knee jerk is an example of a monosynaptic Ia dynamic response.[12] The Ias of the chain fibers connect polysynaptically to alpha motor neurons. Whenever an interneuron is introduced into the chain of activation, there is increased opportunity of influence to the ongoing neural impulse from reverberating circuitry and/or other sources of neural impulses. The tonic vibratory reflex is an example of the polysynaptic Ia response. The strength of these reflexes can be altered by other conditions within the CNS such as effort to overcome resistance.[14]

The secondary endings spray out to either side of the central region of the nuclear chain fibers.[9] They are sensitive to length. The II afferents respond exclusively and proportionately to the amount of static or maintained length of the muscle.[12] The classical view on which some clinical procedures have been based holds that the IIs facilitate flexors and inhibit extensors, no matter in which muscle they are located.[5,15] According to this view, when an extensor muscle is lengthened the IIs of that muscle are activated, which inhibits the extensor muscle itself. Some hypothesize that this mechanism is the basis for the spinal flexor reflex patterns seen in some patients with CNS dysfunction.[13] This classical view is being challenged. It is now known that the II has both mono- and polysynaptic connections in the spinal cord.[15,16] The reflex response of the II endings varies for each type of reflex loop[15] and between patients. The monosynaptic response, like that of the Ia, facilitates the muscle in which it lies.[15-17] The predominant reflex action of the II afferent, however, is polysynaptic, mediated by interneurons whose activity is modified by supraspinal input.[15] The variable responses seen in patients may have to do with the differences in supraspinal input due to the location of the lesion.[15]

In spasticity there will be a range of free movement, and then a strong contraction of the muscle in response to stretch, followed by free movement when the muscle suddenly relaxes despite continued stretch. The sudden relaxation is termed the clasp-knife reaction[19] and has been attributed, in the lower extremity, to the effect of IIs in the extensor muscles.[18,19]

Regulation of muscle stiffness (tone) requires information about muscle tension as well as muscle length.[5] The Golgi tendon organs are receptors for change in muscle tension. They are located at the junction between the muscle fibers and the tendon.[18] They monitor changes in tension in individual muscle fibers of

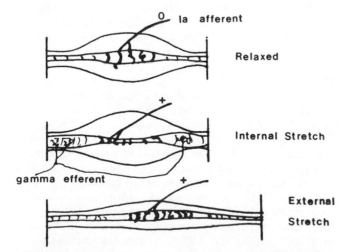

Figure 4.2 Schematic depicting two methods of causing stretch of muscle spindle, internal stretch and external stretch. (Modified from Twitchell, T. Normal motor development. In *The Child with Central Nervous System Deficit.* Washington, DC: U.S. Government Printing Office, 1965.)

different motor units.[18] Impulses from Golgi tendon organs are transmitted to the spinal cord via the Ib fibers, which synapse polysynaptically with alpha motor neurons.[18] Golgi tendon organs have low thresholds for tension created by muscle contraction, but they are also activated by tension generated when a muscle is stretched beyond the maximal length it normally has in the body.[19] When stimulated either by contraction or by excessive stretch, they inform the CNS about the amount of tension. The central control mechanisms then regulate muscle contraction or relaxation to meet environmental demands.[18]

EVALUATION OF MUSCLE TONE

Estimates of muscle tone are made in several ways. The most commonly used but least reliable method is to estimate the level of tone by moving the part quickly within available range of each motion. If tone is increased, the quick stretch elicits a Ia monosynaptic response that depolarizes the alpha motor neurons to cause the muscle to contract to resist the passive movement.[19,20] In flaccidity there is decreased resistance to passive movement. The extremity can be moved freely since the normal tension is absent.

The amount of tone is estimated for each muscle group and recorded as normal, absent (flaccidity), or increased (spasticity). Spasticity is further described as *mild* if the muscle can be lengthened quickly through most of its range of motion before the stretch reflex occurs in the last one-fourth of the range, *moderate* if the stretch reflex occurs midrange, and *severe* if it occurs in the initial one-fourth of the range. The distribution pattern of increased, decreased, and normal tone also should be recorded. The usual distribution pattern of tone in the upper extremities of brain-injured persons is increased tone in the flexor/adductor muscle groups and decreased tone in the extensor/abductor muscle groups and vice versa for the lower extremities.[20]

Other methods of estimating tone have been reported. Brennan[21] measured the "range of normal tonus," defined as the range of motion that is possible before resistance to movement is felt. To do so, he passively moved the part full range during a 1-sec time frame and documented the point of resistance using a goniometer. He averaged the goniometric reading of three trials as the recorded score. He also rated the degree of resistance offered to the first 10°–15° of passive movement beyond the point of resistance. It was graded from normal to intense, but the operational definitions of these terms were not given in his paper.

Bobath described a method of assessing the combined effects of tone and primitive reflexes.[22,23] The patient's limbs are moved in normal patterns of usage, and the adaptation of the different muscle groups to changes in position is evaluated. If reflex activity still dominates, tone in the limbs changes as body position changes. The nature of the resistance to movement of the limbs is noted. A quick, immediate adjustment of muscles to postural changes reflects normal tone. Undue resistance signifies hypertonicity, which is described as severe, moderate, or slight. Undue lack of resistance and hypermobility of joints denotes flaccidity. In athetosis, tone may fluctuate from increased to absent as the limb is moved. The evaluation procedure used by Bobath to evaluate tone in adult hemiplegia is described in chapter 6.

Pendulum testing of the spastic knee has been described and quantified by Bajd and Vodovnik.[24] An electric goniometer that records joint angle is fastened to the knee. The patient lies supine with the lower leg hanging free. The examiner brings the leg to the horizontal and allows it to fall freely. The goniometer tracks the degrees of pendular swing, the number of swings, and the speed of the swings. The goniogram can be used clinically to visually note changes in these parameters before and after treatment, or it can be analyzed mathematically for research purposes. In normal persons, no motor unit activity was detected during this process; therefore, it was determined to be a measure of the biomechanical and rheologic properties of tone.[25] In patients all three components of tone contribute to the goniogram.

Other instruments have been devised to precisely measure the effects of treatment on spasticity,[26] but none are commercially available. One developed by McPherson[27] is a spring-weighted scale used to assess that component of hypertonicity attributed to the viscoelastic property of muscle. The limb is passively moved to the normal rest position, which has been previously operationally defined, the scale is attached, and the limb is released. The force of the limb toward the abnormal resting position is registered on the scale and is recorded. This method was found reliable when evaluated using wrist and knee measurements.

There is a high variability in levels of spasticity from day to day in the same subject.[8,24,25] The test-retest reliability is affected by the speed of the passive test movement since the Ia response is velocity dependent.[19,20] Reliability is also affected by effort, emotional stress, temperature, changes in concurrent sensory stimulation, or head position, which activates brain stem reflexes[8,21]; these variables operate by changing the supraspinal input to the reflex loop.[14,20] Rigid standardization of the test procedure must be the rule; otherwise the findings may be quite misleading.[21] Therapeutic effectiveness may be obscured by poor evaluation techniques, which allow high test-to-test variability.[26]

Rigidity, another form of hypertonicity, is usually noted, but not measured per se. In rigidity tone is increased in both agonist and antagonist and resistance to movement is felt throughout the range of motion. In cogwheel rigidity, as seen in Parkinson's disease, tremor is superimposed on the rigidity, causing alternate contraction and relaxation throughout the range of the muscle being stretched.[28] Spasticity and rigidity may both be present in a muscle group. In moving the part through the range of motion, the resistance of rigidity will be felt initially and a stretch reflex will be added later in range.

Interpreting the Results and Treatment Planning

After the severity of tone in each of the muscle groups of the involved part has been graded, the therapist looks at the pattern of distribution of increased or decreased tone. The therapist devises treatment to inhibit hypertonic muscles and to facilitate hypotonic muscles in an effort to normalize the tone throughout the extremity. To prevent contractures, joints where the muscles are hypertonic should be protected by positioning or splinting into the direction opposite to the spastic forces.

Evaluation of Reflex Integration

A reflex is an involuntary, stereotyped response to a particular stimulus. Reflex responses to stimuli begin to develop in fetal life and continue to be clearly apparent in motor behavior in early infancy. In adults, they become apparent in motor behavior as a result of stress and/or fatigue.[23] Reflex motor patterns continue to underlie the organized voluntary movements used in daily activities and sports.[29]

Reflexes seen in the normal person differ in quality from those observed in persons with brain damage. The movement of the normal person is flexible; he can move in and out of reflex patterns while the stimulus remains in operation. The movement of a person with brain damage, however, is often obligatory; he cannot change posture while controlled by the stimulus. Obligatory primitive reflexes occur as a result of CNS damage[22] and indicate severe motor disability.[30]

Reflex testing is done by applying the appropriate stimulus in a standardized way and observing the response. Both the intensity and quality of the response are observed.[31] Intensity refers to the speed of the response and the degree of attitudinal changes. Quality refers to which components of the response are present under which conditions. If the reflex is weak the response may be a change of tone noted in the extremities rather than actual motion of the extremities.[32,33] To note tonal changes, the results of the evaluation of muscle tone completed under stimulus-neutral conditions are compared to a similar evaluation done under the stimulus conditions of the reflex being tested.

Reflexes can be tested with the person in any position as long as the stimulus can be applied in that position and the response can occur safely. The patient must be retested under the same conditions for reliability of scoring. If the response occurs, the reflex is *positive;* if the reflex does not occur, it is *negative.* Neither a positive nor negative rating can be equated with normal without considering what is normal for the age of the person being tested. No positive spinal or brain stem (primitive) reflexes are normal for adults.

Reflexes are tested according to developmental sequence. The time when each reflex is present in normal development is noted here to guide interpretation of the evaluation findings.

Innate Primary Reactions

Innate primary reactions are primitive reflexes found in newborns. They are indicative of severe brain damage if present beyond their usual time of disappearance. The adult patient with a closed head injury may manifest these reactions. Their absence on reevaluation is a sign of progress in recovery. Only those that can be tested in the adult are included here.

Placing Reaction of the Upper Limb. Birth to 6 months.[22,34]

Test Position. Place the adult patient in a sitting or supine position.

Stimulus. Brush the dorsum of one of the patient's hands against the under edge of a table or the edge of a stiff cardboard.

Response. Flexion of the arm with placement of the hand onto the table top.

Moro Reflex. Birth to 6 months.[22,32-34]

Stimulus. Several stimuli evoke the same response. A loud noise near the patient's head, sudden movement of the supporting surface, or dropping the patient backwards from a semisitting position may be used as the stimulus. If the patient is in a wheelchair it can be tipped backward. The Moro reflex as originally described was a response to the vestibular stimulation of being tipped off balance,[22] whereas the response to a noise was originally termed a startle reaction.[35] These are considered to be the same reaction in most neurology and developmental texts. By either name the response involves the total body, which differentiates it from the mature startle response to a loud noise seen in normal adults.

Response. Abduction, extension, and external rotation of the arms with abduction and extension of the fingers followed by flexion to the midline.

Grasp Reflex. Birth to 3 to 4 months.[34]

Stimulus. Apply pressure in the palm of the hand from the ulnar side.

Response. Finger flexion with a strong grip that persists and resists removal of the stimulus object.

Sucking Reflex. Birth to 3 to 4 months.

Stimulus. Place a finger on the patient's lips.

Response. Sucking motion of the lips.

Rooting Reflex. Birth to 3 to 4 months.

Stimulus. Stroke outward on the corner of the patient's mouth.

Response. The lower lip, tongue, and head move toward the stimulus.

Spinal Level Reflexes

These are phasic reflexes of total flexion or extension and are basic to mobility motor patterns.[22,33]

Flexor Withdrawal.[32,33] Birth to 2 months.

Test Position. The patient is supine or sitting with head in midposition and legs extended.

Stimulus. A quick tactile stimulus is applied to the sole of one foot. A stimulus therapists often use is to scrape the thumbnail from the heel to the ball of the patient's foot.

Response. Uncontrolled flexion of the entire leg.

Extensor Thrust.[22,32,33] Birth to 2 months.

Test Position. The patient is supine or sitting with head in midposition. One leg is in extension and the other leg is fully flexed.

Stimulus. Apply pressure to the ball of the foot of the flexed leg.

Response. Uncontrolled extension of the stimulated leg.

Crossed Extension.[32,33] Birth to 2 months.

Test Position. The patient is supine with head in midposition. One leg is in extension and the other leg is fully flexed.

Stimulus. Passively flex the extended leg.

Response. Extension of the opposite leg with hip adduction and internal rotation.

It is unsafe to test for this reflex while the patient is sitting. With a strong positive response, the patient could slide forward out of the chair. A patient with hemiplegia who can stand on both legs without exaggerated tone can be tested standing. The patient is asked to flex the noninvolved leg; a strong increase in extensor tone in the involved leg indicates a positive crossed extension reflex.[22] Guard the patient to prevent falling.

Brain Stem Reflexes

These are tonic or static reflexes that involve sustained changes in postural muscle tone affecting the whole body or more than one part of the body. They are precursors of stability motor patterns.[36] By changing the position of the head relative to the body or the position of the head (and body) in space, the proprioceptors located in the neck or in the vestibular apparatus are stimulated. The resultant changes in muscle tone are maintained as long as the stimulus is applied.[36]

Asymmetrical Tonic Neck Reflex (ATNR).[32,33,36] Birth to 4 months.

Test Position. The patient is supine or sitting[37] with arms and legs extended.

Stimulus. Passively or actively turn the head 90° to one side.

Response. Increase of extensor tone of limbs on the face side and flexor tone of limbs on the skull side.

Repeat the stimulus to the other side.

Evaluation in the quadruped position is more stressful, so a positive response will be more readily elicited in patients with minimal reflex responses than it would be in the supine or sitting positions. When the patient's head is rotated, the elbow of the skull side will flex, indicating a positive response. Alternately, the response can be reinforced by resisted grasp of the nonaffected extremity.[37]

Symmetrical Tonic Neck Reflex (STNR).[32,33] Birth to 4 or 5 months.

Test Position. The patient is sitting or placed in a quadruped position.

Stimulus 1. Flex the patient's head, bringing his chin toward his chest.

Response. Flexion of the upper extremities and extension of the lower extremities.

Stimulus 2. Extend the patient's head.

Response. Extension of the upper extremities and flexion of the lower extremities.

Tonic Labyrinthine Reflex (TLR)—Prone.[32,33,36] Birth to 4 months.

Test Position. The patient is prone with head in midposition.

Stimulus. The test position is the stimulus.

Response. Flexion of the extremities or increased flexor tone.

If there is severe extensor spasticity, there may still be extension in the prone position but with relatively weaker extensor tone than in a supine position.[22]

Tonic Labyrinthine Reflex—Supine.[32,33] Birth to 4 months.

Test Position. The patient is supine with head in midposition.

Stimulus. The test position is the stimulus.

Response. Extension of the extremities or increased extensor tone.

Positive Supporting Reaction.[22,23,32,33,36] Birth to 6 months.

Test Position. The patient is placed in an upright standing position if possible, or supine or sitting.

Stimulus. Firmly contact of the ball of the foot to the floor or footboard of the bed and dorsiflex the foot.[36]

Response. Extension of the lower extremity with cocontraction of flexors and extensors resulting in a stiff and rigid extension of the lower extremity.

Associated Reactions. Associated movements occur normally throughout life when a person is attempting strenuous activities. These are variable responses and may include such posturing as holding the tongue protruded to one side or fisting by the nongrasping hand. In central nervous system dysfunction, when there is increased tone,[38] associated reactions are stereotyped tonic reactions by which one extremity influences the posture of another extremity.[22,36] Associated reactions are abnormal; associated movements are normal.[23] The key difference is the variability and flexibility of the normal response in contrast to the tonic, obligatory nature of the abnormal response.

Test Position. May be tested in any position.

Stimulus. Resist any motion or have the patient squeeze an object with the unaffected hand.[29,33]

Response. The motion used as stimulus will be mimicked. If the stimulus is grasp, the response may be limited to grasp or increased flexor tone may be seen throughout the extremity.[22] In spastic hemiplegia associated reactions can also be elicited from one spastic extremity to the other spastic extremity on the same side of the body.[23,38]

Midbrain Reactions

These reactions permit the development of maturationally acquired motor milestones. The stimuli cause no abnormal tonal changes to occur; rather, the response is an active righting movement to bring the head and body into a normal relationship with each other in space.[33,39]

Neck Righting.[32,33] Birth to 6 months. This reflex orients the body in relation to the head.[39]

Test Position. The patient is supine with arms and legs extended.

Stimulus. Passively turn the head to one side and hold it in this position.

Response. The body rotates as a whole in the direction to which the head was turned.

The stimulus for neck righting is the same as that for the ATNR; therefore, the appearance of the neck righting reaction is heralded as a maturational step forward from brain stem level control to midbrain level control.

Labyrinthine Righting Acting on the Head.[32,33,39] These reactions orient the head in relation to space, gravity being the controlling influence. The importance of the labyrinths for orientation is less, compared to tactile and cortical influences, in mammals than in lower species.

Test Position. The patient is blindfolded. The adult patient cannot be tested; the small child is tested by holding him by the pelvis and suspending him in space.

Stimulus. The patient is tipped sideways so that his head is laterally flexed. Or he may be held suspended in a supine or prone position in space.

Response. The head is brought into the horizontal position.

Body Righting Acting on the Head.[39]

Test Position. The patient is blindfolded and placed first in a prone position, then in a supine position.

Stimulus. The asymmetric stimulation of the pressure sense organs on the anterior of the body surface as compared to the posterior surface.

Response. The head is brought into a face vertical position that orients it to the surface that the patient is in contact with.

The body righting reactions acting on the head enable the baby to raise its head when in prone or supine position. They indicate the integration of the TLR since the head raising is in a direction opposite to that dictated by the TLR.

Body Righting Acting on the Body.[22,32,33,39] Six months to 4 to 5 years.

Test Position. The patient is supine with arms and legs extended.

Stimulus. Passively or actively turn the head to one side.[10]

Response. Segmental rotation around the body axis so that the body rotates at the shoulder, then the trunk, and then the pelvis.

The stimulus for the neck righting and the more mature body righting acting on the body reactions is the same. The therapist observes the patient's response to determine his level of maturational control.

Basal Ganglia Level Reactions

Protective Extension (Parachute Reaction).[32,33] From 6 months throughout life.

Test Position. Whereas babies are tested by being held by the pelvis suspended upside down in the air, adults are tested in functional positions. Bobath lists detailed tests for evaluation of protective extension in the adult hemiplegic patient.[23] To test in a sitting position, the patient is positioned on a raised mat or in a wheelchair with removable arms. In the latter instance a chair is placed alongside the wheelchair on the patient's involved side.

Stimulus. Push the patient to the involved side with sufficient surprise and force that he believes his head will contact the mat or chair. The stimulus used to elicit protective extension is more forceful than that used to elicit equilibrium reactions. Guard the patient to protect him from actually falling.

Response. Extension of the arm with the fingers extended and abducted in an effort to break the fall in order to protect the head. The response should also be tested in kneel-standing and in standing positions. In these cases the person is pushed toward a wall.

The following equilibrium reactions are automatic responses to regain balance following disturbances of the center of gravity (COG). Equilibrium reactions are necessary for development of movement from posture to posture and for use of objects in the environment, which by their weight would pull the person off balance. These reactions are tested in the various developmental positions after the patient recovers voluntary control enough to be able to maintain the position. Recovery follows an orderly sequence, noted here.

Prone.[22,32,33] From 6 months throughout life.

Test Position. The patient is prone on an equilibrium board or a mat.

Stimulus. Unexpectedly tilt the board or mat to one side.

Response. The patient's head and upper trunk turn toward the raised side with abduction and extension of the extremities on the raised side and protective extension of the extremities on the lowered side.

Supine.[22,32,33] From 8 months throughout life.

Test Position. The patient is supine on a board or a mat.

Stimulus. Tilt the board or mat to one side.

Response. Same as for equilibrium reaction in the prone position.

Quadruped.[33] From 8 months throughout life.

Test Position. The patient is on his hands and knees on a flat surface.

Stimulus. Tilt the patient to one side by pushing against one side of his trunk.

Response. The patient will right his head and upper trunk. There will be abduction and extension of the extremities on the raised side with protective extension of the extremities on the side to which he was tipped.

Sitting.[22,23,32,33] From 10 to 12 months throughout life.

Test Position. The patient sits on a plinth (raised mat).

Stimulus. To test for lateral balance, tilt the patient to one side by pushing against one side of his trunk. To test for anterior-posterior balance, push the patient's shoulders forward or backward.

Response. Lateral balance is observed as the patient rights his head and upper trunk and abducts and extends the extremities on the raised side while protectively extending the extremities on the lowered side. Anterior balance is observed when the patient flexes his shoulders and hips and curves his trunk forward to regain his COG. The posterior balance reaction is an arching of the back and abduction and extension of the arms to regain COG.

Kneel-Standing.[33] From 15 months throughout life.[16]

Test Position. The patient is on his knees with his body upright.

Stimulus. Lateral balance is tested by tilting the patient to one side by pushing against one side of his trunk. Anterior-posterior balance are also tested.

Response. Lateral balance reaction involves righting of the head and upper trunk with abduction and extension of the extremities on the raised side and protective extension of the extremities on the side to which the patient was tipped. Anterior-posterior balance reactions are similar to those noted above.

Standing.[22,33,38] From 15 to 18 months throughout life.

Test Position. The patient is standing.

Stimulus. Tilt the patient to one side, holding him at the hips or around the upper trunk.

Response. Righting of the head and upper trunk with abduction and extension of the extremities on the raised side and protective extension of the extremities on the side to which the patient was tipped. Test anterior-posterior balance also.

Cortical Reactions

Optic Righting.[22,33,38] From 6 months throughout life.

Although these are righting reactions, they depend on the occipital cortex rather than the labyrinths and are therefore developmentally more advanced. The optic righting need not be tested if the labyrinthine righting reactions are positive because the responses cannot be differentiated. If labyrinthine righting is negative, however, the optic righting reaction should be tested since it can be used to compensate for the labyrinthine loss as a means of postural orientation.

Test Position. To test adults, position them prone or supine on a plinth or sitting with the head laterally flexed. The eyes are open.

Stimulus. The position of the head in relation to landmarks in space.

Response. The head is brought to a perpendicular position in line with environmental cues.

RECORDING REFLEX DEVELOPMENT AND PLANNING TREATMENT

Each reflex response can be recorded on a record similar to the sample form presented in Table 4.1. Scoring is done by indicating whether the response was positive or negative, although some forms have another column to indicate whether a response was normal or abnormal. The comment section on the form may be used to note any change from standard test position, the strength of the response, or other descriptions of the response. After recording the results of testing, the highest level of reflex control achieved is noted. If the level is age-appropriate then reflex development is normal, but if the level of control is lower than the normal expectancy for an adult, treatment is planned. Factors to consider in treatment planning include the strength of the primitive reflexes, the time since onset of damage to the CNS, and the extent of the damage. The sooner after the insult to the CNS occurs, the less severe the damage, and the weaker the reflex response, the greater are the chances that neurodevelopmental treatment will be effective.

When brain damage occurs early in development, as in cerebral palsy, development of control of voluntary movement may be delayed so that motor behavior is dominated by the spinal cord or brain stem reflexes beyond the age when these should have normally diminished. Therapy is aimed at establishing the higher level maturationally based normal motor patterns. A word of caution: for some patients with severe damage of long standing the primitive reflexes may be the person's only means of motor function. Treatment to inhibit these reflexes as a first step toward promoting higher level function may result in inhibition only and leave the person unable to function.

For adult patients who suffer generalized cortical damage, as in the case of closed head trauma, if improvement is expected, neurodevelopmental treatment is indicated. This involves preventing the primitive spinal cord and brain stem level reflex responses while applying the stimuli that we noted can elicit them or the higher level righting reactions. Later, the equilibrium responses are stimulated. If the results of the evaluation indicate that the person is stuck at one level of maturation, treatment involves activity and adjunctive treatment to move the patient to the next level of recovery. If the results indicate spotty maturation, then activity is designed to enable the patient to fill in the gaps.

When circumscribed cortical damage occurs in the adult, as in hemiplegia following a cerebrovascular accident, primitive reflexes released from higher inhibitory control also may be seen, especially under stress conditions. In therapy these patients will work toward relearning the higher level voluntary motor patterns they once had established. Therapy will be done in a nonstressful way to decrease the likelihood of evoking the primitive reflexes. With establishment of voluntary control it is expected that reflex responses will be less readily evoked.

The Influences of Reflexes on Voluntary Movement

Disturbances of reflex integration and tone produce stereotyped postures and movements in association with the person's voluntary attempts to move.

The influence of the positive supporting reaction is to increase extensor tone in standing, resulting in an

Table 4.1
REFLEX TESTING[a]

Name: Date:

                                                 Therapist:

	Pos.	Neg.	Comments
Innate Primary Reactions			
a. placing - upper extremity			
b. moro			
c. grasp			
d. sucking			
e. rooting			
Spinal Level Reflexes			
a. Flexor Withdrawal			
b. Extensor Thrust			
c. Crossed Extension			
Brain Stem Level Reflexes			
a. Asymmetrical Tonic Neck			
b. Symmetrical Tonic Neck			
c. Tonic Labyrinthine			
Supine			
Prone			
d. Positive Supporting Reaction			
e. Associated Reactions			
Midbrain Reactions			
a. Neck Righting			
b. Labyrinthine Righting Acting on the Head			
c. Body Righting Acting on the Head			
d. Body Righting Acting on the Body			
Automatic Movement Reactions			
a. Protective Extension			
b. Equilibrium Reactions			
Prone			
Supine			
Quadruped			
Sitting			
Kneel-standing			
Standing			
Cortical Reflexes			
a. Optic Righting			

[a]Adapted from Fiorentino, M. A. *Reflex Testing Methods for Evaluating CNS Development*, 2nd edition. Springfield, IL: Charles C Thomas, 1973.

inability to flex the lower extremities alternately in walking. The plantar flexion component of the positive supporting reaction places the weight on the balls of the feet and contributes to a lack of heel strike in the gait. However, when the lower extremities are flexed, as when changing to or from sitting and standing positions, the individual is unable to support his weight on the flexed extremity.

Once the positive supporting reaction is inhibited and a negative supporting reaction develops, the lower extremities can be flexed in walking. Extensor tone is modified to permit the slow relaxation required to raise and lower the body when rising from or assuming a sitting position, for ascending or descending stairs, and for reciprocal crawling.[22]

When the patient attempts to creep, the crossed extension reflex prevents reciprocal leg movement because the extended leg cannot be flexed.[33] The crossed extension reflex may combine with a positive supporting reaction in a standing position that reinforces extension of the affected extremity in spastic hemiplegia and prevents walking.[22]

The asymmetrical tonic neck reflex prevents rolling from supine to prone because the scapula retracts on the skull side extremity, preventing bringing that arm across. Also the arm on the face side extends in the direction toward which rolling is attempted[34] to further prevent it. In sitting, flexion of the extremities on one side due to the ATNR contributes to a loss of balance.[22] In a quadruped position the extremities on the skull side may collapse into flexion when the head is turned.[34] There may be an inability to maintain a standing position due to lack of stability resulting from flexion of the skull side lower extremity when the head turns. The ATNR may be so strong in patients with central nervous system damage that arm movement can be controlled only by turning the head. Contractures of the extremities, dislocated hip, and scoliosis may develop from an asymmetrical position maintained due to a strong ATNR response.

The symmetrical tonic neck reflex contributes to difficulty in maintaining a quadruped position. Flexion of the head causes the arms to flex and the patient collapses forward. Extension of the head causes the arms to extend and the legs to flex, and the patient sits back on the flexed legs.[22,34] This sitting position is often observed in young children with spasticity and "bunny hopping" in this position becomes their means of locomotion.

The tonic labyrinthine reflex prevents extension of the head in a prone position due to increased flexor tone. Strong extensor tone in a supine position prevents lifting the head in flexion and sitting up unassisted. If assisted to a sitting position the patient can remain sitting unless his head extends and increased extensor tone causes him to fall backwards.[22] When the patient is supine, the TLR prevents flexion of the trunk and extremities, and bilateral hand activities requiring bringing the hands together to midline cannot be accomplished. The TLR also prevents rolling over

from a supine position, and attempts to roll over increase extension to the extent that the back arches into hyperextension.[34]

The tonic reflexes interact to reinforce or negate each other so that observed abnormal motor behavior is most often the interaction of several reflexes rather than the domination of any one.[22]

Voluntary movements are supported by automatic postural patterns—righting and equilibrium responses. Righting and equilibrium reactions enable the individual to move against gravity, align the body, and maintain balance.[22,41] As these reactions develop, the dominance of the more primitive reflexes diminishes (reflexes are integrated).[22] In normal development integration of primitive reflexes is necessary for development of purposeful movements.[22]

When the body righting reflex develops to replace neck righting, the trunk follows the head with trunk rotation. With the development of the labyrinthine righting reaction the TLR is inhibited and the head can be lifted against gravity. The head can be extended in prone and the trunk then extends to a full prone extension position completely counteracting the influence of the TLR in prone. Flexion of the head in supine is also possible when the labyrinthine righting reaction develops, and supine flexion counteracts the influence of the TLR in supine[40,41] and indicates integration of the tonic reflex. The influence of body righting is also seen in the labyrinthine righting and optic righting reactions. When in an upright position, if the body is moved laterally, forward, or backward, the head rights itself to face vertical, and the trunk follows with a rotation component to align the trunk with the head. With a body righting reaction and inhibition of the tonic neck reflexes the individual can roll over to prone. A developmental sequence then follows in which the ability to roll over is combined with a labyrinthine righting reaction and inhibition of other tonic reflexes to a progression from rolling over to prone extension, on elbows, on hands and knees, to sitting and standing. Once a protective extension response develops, the arms extend to protect the individual from falling over, and support on the extended arms helps to maintain a position. Cocontraction of proximal muscles in the supporting extremities develops from weight-bearing positions. Balance in each developmental position is achieved by equilibrium reactions in which the postural muscles contract to maintain or regain an upright position when equilibrium is challenged. Equilibrium reactions and protective extension are usually seen together as normal reactions to threatened loss of balance.

Control of Voluntary Movement

Voluntary movement is a combination of maturationally acquired and learned motor patterns. The maturationally acquired patterns develop in this familiar sequence of motor milestones from lifting the head in a a supine position, to rolling over, to lifting the head in prone, to assuming and holding prone on elbows, to assuming and holding quadruped position, to sitting, to creeping on all fours, to kneel-standing, to standing, and to walking. The sequence of maturationally acquired patterns of hand function is given below. Learned motor patterns are elaborations of the maturationally developed patterns and depend on the integrity of the cerebral cortex for planning and commanding, of the cerebellum for smoothness and timing, and of the basal ganglia for automatic activation of supporting movements and postures and for execution of learned motor plans.[2] Coordination, a characteristic of learned skilled movement, is defined as the ability to control whole limb movements accurately and smoothly at whatever speed is necessary. Incoordination is a broad term for disabilities involving extraneous, uneven, or inaccurate movements.

COORDINATION TESTS OF CEREBELLAR FUNCTION

Incoordination may be caused by cerebellar dysfunction characterized by abnormalities of rate, range, or force of a movement; by abnormalities in timing (which reflect disturbed initiation of movement[42]); by abnormalities of the organization of complex movement; and by intention tremor.[43] Cerebellar disturbances and methods of evaluating them are as follows.

Tremor. Intention tremor occurs during voluntary movement and diminishes or is absent at rest.[28,44] The tremor can be observed during the performance of activities or by asking the patient to alternately touch his own nose and then the examiner's finger, which is held in front of him in various positions.[45] The tremor usually increases as the goal is approached.[46,47] Observe the joints involved; this tremor usually occurs proximally due to lack of stability.[47] Other tests are the finger to finger test in which the patient reaches out to touch first one of the examiner's fingers and then the other held a distance away.[48] The test is made more difficult by increasing the distance between the target points or by asking for a faster response. Note is made of the distance and the speed at which the patient is able to succeed.

Dysdiadochokinesia. Dysdiadochokinesia is the impaired ability to accomplish repeated alternating movements rapidly and smoothly.[28] When asked to perform alternate movements, a patient with this symptom will perform the movements slowly with an incomplete range of motion or may be unable to perform at all (adiadochokinesia). Tests include having the patient rapidly supinate and pronate the forearm or do grasp-release.[28] The number of alternations within a given time period is the score. Other tests include alternate rotation of the entire arm with the arms fully extended in front of the patient,[49] tapping the table with extended fingers,[46] or tapping one wrist with the index and middle fingers of the other hand.[49] Tests are performed bilaterally, and differences between the two extremities are determined by comparison.

Dysmetria. Dysmetria is an inability to control muscle length[50] resulting in overshooting or pointing past an object toward the side of the lesion.[51] For exam-

ple, if touching his face, a person might hit himself or if reaching for an object he might reach past the object. The finger to nose test (Fig. 4.3) or finger to finger test are used for evaluation, and the ability to prevent pointing past the targets is observed.[45,46] The test difficulty is increased by requiring the patient to reach forward with the proximal arm away from the stabilizing influence of the body or by increasing the speed.

Dyssynergia. Dyssynergia is a decomposition of movement. The lack of smoothness of movements occurs because the synergistic action or reciprocation between agonists and antagonists is impaired or lacking (asynergia).[46,47] In decomposition of movement each joint involved in a movement pattern functions independently so that the movement is broken up into its parts rather than being smooth and coordinated.[44,51]

Tests for other cerebellar functions also can provide an opportunity to observe dyssynergia. In tests of alternate movements, note whether there is loss of rhythm and regularity in performance or whether the arms drift out to the sides.[47] In the finger to nose test[45] or in reaching out to touch the examiner's finger in the finger to finger test,[47] note whether movements are jerky and broken up into parts.[46]

Ataxic Gait. Ataxic gait is a wide-based, unsteady, staggering gait with a tendency to veer toward the side of the lesion.[44,46] Observation of walking may suffice as an evaluation, or the patient may be asked to walk heel to toe along a straight line or to walk fast and turn quickly to elicit the symptoms.[46,47]

Rebound Phenomenon of Holmes. The Rebound Phenomenon of Holmes is the lack of a check reflex to stop a strong active motion to avoid hitting something in the path of the motion. To test for this phenomenon the examiner resists the patient's elbow flexion and then releases the resistance; the patient

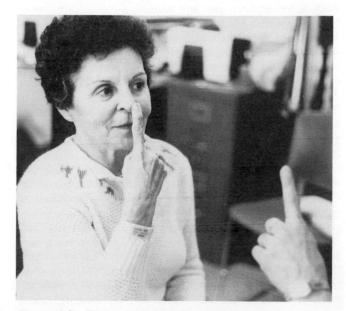

Figure 4.3 Finger to nose test.

may hit his own chest or shoulder if unable to check the motion.[46] The arm should be positioned to avoid having the patient hit his face.

Asthenia. Muscles are weak and tire easily.[51]

Hypotonia. Hypotonia is decreased muscle tone due to the loss of the cerebellum's facilitatory influence on the stretch reflex.[28] Granit[50] reports the results of many studies that lead to the conclusion that locomotor disturbances of cerebellar lesions suggest an absence of spindle control. After the removal of the cerebellum of a decerebrate cat there was reduction or loss of spindle stretch sensitivity, which is controlled by gamma motor neurons. With no organized gamma activity muscle spindles cannot measure or send messages regarding muscle length that would then influence control of muscle length. Destruction of the cerebellar link to alpha and gamma motor neurons could explain symptoms, such as dysmetria and adiodochokinesia.[50]

TESTS OF POSTERIOR COLUMN FUNCTION

Posterior column damage with loss of proprioception also results in incoordination due to misjudgment of limb position and balance problems. Coordination deficits from a loss of proprioception and methods of evaluation are as follows.

Ataxia. In this case the wide-based gait results from loss of position sense. The patient is able to correct if he watches the floor and the placement of his feet to visually compensate for the loss.[47] This ability differentiates posterior column dysfunction from cerebellar dysfunction and offers the therapist a clue to teaching the patient with this deficit to compensate for his loss.

Romberg Sign. The Romberg Sign is the inability to maintain balance in standing with the eyes closed. To test, the patient stands with his feet together and then closes his eyes; the test is positive if loss of balance occurs.[47] Guard to prevent falling.

In posterior column deficit the finger to nose test may show dysmetria or overshooting, but is distinguished from cerebellar dysfunction if the deficit is increased with the eyes closed.[47]

TESTS OF BASAL GANGLIA FUNCTION

The basal ganglia control automatic, rhythmical patterned movements[46] and the initiation of automatic (learned) movements. Lesions of the basal ganglia result in a "release phenomenon" in which the rhythmic movements are released from control[46] and by the lack of automatic movement or initiation of movement. One or more of the following abnormal rhythmical movements may be seen as a result of lesions.

Athetosis. Athetoid movements are characterized by slow, writhing, twisting, worm-like movements, particularly involving the neck, face, and extremities.[44] Athetosis is not present during sleep.[46] Muscle tone may be increased or decreased.[52,53] There is lack of controlled mobility in the neck, trunk, and proximal joints.[52] Movements are involuntary and exhibit excessive mobility from one limit of motion to the other. Observation should include notice of whether involvement is proximal or distal, which extremities are involved, whether motions are rotary or on an anterior-posterior plane of motion, whether tension is increased or decreased,[53] and what stimuli increase or decrease the abnormal movements or tone.

Dystonia. Dystonia is a form of athetosis in which increased muscle tone causes distorted postures of the trunk and proximal extremities.[28] Involuntary contractions of trunk muscles result in torsion spasms,[44] and there is increased lumbar lordosis.[28]

Chorea.[28,44,46] Choreiform movements are rapid, jerky, and irregular, primarily involving the face and distal extremities. The muscles are hypotonic. Chorea is related to degeneration of the putamen, as in Huntington's chorea, or may follow rheumatic fever, as in Sydenham's chorea. Chorea may occur in sleep.

Hemiballismus.[28,44] Hemiballismus is unilateral chorea in which there are violent, forceful, flinging movements of the extremities on one side of the body, particularly involving the proximal musculature. It is caused by a lesion of the subthalamic nucleus.

Tremors At Rest are characteristic of basal ganglia disease. The tremors stop at the initiation of voluntary movement but will resume during the holding phase of a motor task when attention wanes or is diverted to another task. Tremors at rest are fatiguing to the patient, and he needs to be taught compensatory methods of stopping them.

Bradykinesia means poverty of movement. Parkinsonian patients who have substantia nigra lesions have difficulty initiating slow movements.[42] The automatic movements such as arm swinging during walking or facial animation during talking are diminished or lost.

Patients with basal ganglia dysfunction are unable to carry out well-learned habitual motor patterns, such as walking over varied surfaces, without paying attention to the movement. There are no formal tests of these symptoms; they are simply documented from behavioral observation and described in enough detail to allow comparison of future patient behavior to note progression or regression.

In summary, evaluation of the subcomponents of coordination involves observation of the patient at rest and during activity to note the occurrence of any asynergic or involuntary movements as defined. Each problem of incoordination and its severity are noted. Involvement is often bilateral, but one side of the body may be more severely involved than the other. If cerebellar damage is unilateral, the ipsilateral extremities will show incoordination, whereas if basal ganglia damage is unilateral, the contralateral extremities will show symptoms.

Incoordination due to cerebellar or basal ganglia lesions is recorded by noting the absence or presence and the severity of the deficits. There is not a strong sense of success in restoring normal function to patients with cerebellar or basal ganglia lesions. Therefore, treatment focuses on compensation for the deficit(s).

Incoordination also may be apparent in patients with cortical lesions, due to their inability to control isolated joint movement. This incoordination can be expected to improve with treatment focused on promoting recovery of motor control. Motor control involves an interweaving of mobility (phasic movement) and stability (tonic postural) patterns. The earliest mobility patterns are random movements of the limbs; these become controlled movements after a base of proximal stability is established. Stability patterns develop in weight-bearing positions. Bilateral weight bearing distributes weight between the two extremities and because it is less demanding precedes unilateral weight bearing.[54] In each weight-bearing position, mobility and stability sequence from bilateral support (stability), to rocking in the bilaterally supported position (controlled mobility), to unilateral support (controlled stability), to using the extremity to accomplish a task (combination of controlled proximal stability and distal mobility).[54]

In patients with cortical lesions motor control redevelops progressively from mass patterns of movement to more selective, specific movements as the primitive reflex patterns are broken down into smaller units and reorganized into a wider choice of postures and movements.[55] Voluntary motor control develops from control of the posture and movements of the head and eyes, to that of the trunk, then the upper extremities, and finally the lower extremities.[35]

Evaluation of voluntary control of maturationally acquired patterns can be done using the evaluations of Rood, Bobath, or Brunnstrom described in chapter 6. The evaluations are used to determine, according to developmental sequence, the highest level of consistent control that the patient evidences. Therapy then focuses on establishing the next level of control.

DEVELOPMENT OF HAND FUNCTION

The ontogenetic development of sensory-motor control of hand function provides a basis for evaluation and treatment of adults who have suffered brain injury since the redevelopment of hand skill closely parallels normal development.

The development of the motor patterns involved in hand function as described by A. Jean Ayres[56] progresses as follows: (a) control of neck and eye movement; (b) trunk stability and balance; (c) scapular and shoulder stability and movement; (d) elbow motion; (e) gross grasp; (f) wrist positioning and movement; (g) release of grasp; (h) forearm supination and pronation; and (i) individual finger manipulation. Each stage in the progression overlaps the previous stage(s) in time so that one component is still being completed as the next begins.

The ontogenetic development of visually guided reaching and hand function depends upon the coordination of visual and sensorimotor mechanisms and includes the entire range of development from automatic to voluntary control of the head and eye through to digital release.[35,56] Prehension function involves reach, grasp, carry, and release.[56]

During the 18th prenatal week until the 16th to 24th postnatal week, grasping-type reflexes are evident.[56] The grasping reflex is assumed to be under subcortical control because the human cortex is probably not functioning appreciably at birth.[35] If a rod is placed in the hand of a newborn, he grasps it with strength enough to support his body weight.[35] Twitchell[57] refers to this as the traction response, the stimulus of which is stretch to the scapular adductors and the response includes not only grasping but also flexion at all the joints. Twitchell also identifies another reaction present at birth: the avoidance reaction. The hand withdraws or avoids (extension/abduction of the fingers) contact stimulation.[57] The effect of the avoidance reaction continues to contaminate hand function up to 5 or 6 years until controlled voluntary extension is learned.[56,57]

During the newborn period (0 to 2 months), an object placed in the hand will be reflexly grasped, but there is no reaction to an object held in view. At 4 weeks of age the true grasp reflex develops.[58] A contact stimulus moving out between the thumb and index finger elicits first an automatic adduction of these fingers, and then days later flexion is added to the response.[58]

The 3- to 4-month-old infant displays motor responses, however disorganized, in response to objects within the visual field.[35,57,58] The true grasp reflex, flexion and adduction of the fingers, is fully developed and stimulated by contact of an object moving distally along the medial aspect of the palm.[57] There is a catching phase and a holding phase.[58] When this reflex is fully developed, the traction response, with its attendant flexor synergy (flexion of all joints of the upper limb), can no longer be obtained. Fractionation of the grasp response occurs gradually. The first voluntary grasp to appear in the wake of the true grasp reflex is palmar grasp.[58] Palmar grasp does not include the thumb; it may be equated to hook grasp[57] and is the grasp used by adults to carry a suitcase.

At about 4 months, the sight of an object by the baby causes approaching movements of the digits and the entire upper extremity.[35] This visually triggered response does not seem connected to a desire to have the object. The approach is primitive and may be done with fisted or open hand. The instinctive grasp reaction is beginning to develop at this time also; in response to contact stimulation on the medial side of the hand, the forearm supinates to orient the hand toward the object.[57]

At 6 months, the child visually guides the hand toward an object with deliberateness once it is seen.[35] The child must give his undivided attention to securing the object, however, or the movement is interrupted. There is excessive extension of digits during the approach and too forceful a grasp on contact at first. The object is manipulated, once grasped. The grasp is crude with the thumb used incidentally.[56]

At about 8 months, reach involves rotation at the shoulder, rather than at the forearm, in order to orient the hand to objects. The elbow is more flexible[56] during reaching to secure close and far objects.

At about 9 to 10 months the child no longer must give full attention to approach and grasp of an object once he has seen it.[35] The wrist is more flexible.[56] The approach is still executed with excessive digit extension, which moderates with maturation.[41] The instinctive grasp reflex is fully developed: in response to contact stimulation, the hand gropes for and adjusts to grasp the object.[57,58] Scissors grasp (thumb flexion and adduction) becomes a crude pinch. Pincer grasp or opposition is achieved.[56,57] The index finger is able to poke, indicating that the grasp reflex is fully fractionated. If attended to, grasp can be released, indicating a beginning cortical control of finger extension. Voluntary finger extension occurs only after reaching and grasping have been perfected.[56]

Tasks that follow this developmental sequence can be used to evaluate hand function of adult brain-damaged patients. First observation is made of whether the patient has, and is obliged to use, the reflexes related to hand function: grasp reflex and avoidance reaction. The test for the grasp reflex was described earlier. The avoidance reaction is observed in response to contact of the hand with an object. This response is most clearly observed in patients with athetoid cerebral palsy. Although these reactions provide the reflex base for voluntary hand use, they are not functional of themselves. Voluntary hand function is sought. Evaluation consists of observing and documenting hand usage according to the stages of redevelopment. These are palmar (hook) grasp; forearm rotation to orient to an object; gross, uncontrolled (semireflex) finger extension in anticipation of picking up an object; lateral pinch; opposition; index, and later other fingers, used in nongrasp activities, for example poking, smoothing, raking, pointing, etc.; voluntary finger extension; release of opposition grasp; and greater and greater skill in the use of the fingers individually.

At 11 months there is release of pincer grasp.[56] Refinement of release continues for the next several years.[35,56] At 12 to 13 months supination comes under cortical control.[56] When the child reaches 12 to 14 years, all fine finger manipulation skills have developed.[56]

DEXTERITY TESTS

Dexterity is defined as the ability to manipulate objects with the hands. Accuracy and speed are the parameters of measurement. An estimation of manual dexterity can be made from observing whether the patient can do such functional tasks as thread a needle, button buttons, use scissors, pick up coins, write, or other similar tasks. The therapist would observe not only whether the patient could do the tasks, but also how easily, accurately, and quickly he did them. Timing his ability from treatment to treatment would document progress. However, if treatment is to be aimed at improving hand function, more standardized and sensitive measures of change, such as those reported below, should be used. The tests must be administered according to the standardized procedure in order to compare the patient's performance to the norms and to ensure reliability of reevaluation findings.

The Box and Block Test is a simply administered test of gross manual dexterity (Fig. 4.4). One hundred and fifty 1-inch (2.5-cm) blocks are used. The number of blocks transferred from one side of the box to the other within one minute is the score. Each hand is tested separately. A 15-sec practice trial precedes the actual test.[59] The construction details and standardized administration protocol have been published.[59] Validity established in relation to the Minnesota Rate of Manipulation placing subtest, a test actually validated on the performance of manual workers, was strong ($r = 0.91$).[60] That validation is based on use of 100 blocks, however. Norms have been established on 124 handicapped adults using 100 blocks[60] and 628 normal controls aged 20 to 94 years using 150 blocks.[59] Test-retest reliability was established at a six-month interval and found to be high: $r = 0.93$ and 0.97 for left and right hands, respectively.[59] The test can also be used to measure upper-extremity endurance by counting the number of blocks the patient is able to rapidly transfer before becoming fatigued.

The Nine-Hole Peg Test is a simple, quick test of finger dexterity.[61] The score is the time required to place nine 1 1/4-inch (3.2-cm) pegs in a 5-inch by 5-inch (12.7 cm) board and remove them.[61,62] The time is scored separately for each hand. A standardized administration procedure and norms based on 618 adults aged 20 to 75+ years have been published.[61] The test-retest reliability is modest ($r = 0.43$ for the left hand and $r = 0.69$ for the right hand), which probably reflects the learning effect from one administration to

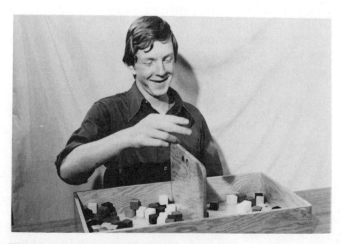

Figure 4.4 Box and block test.

the next. Administering several practice trials may improve its reliability as a measure of dexterity.

The **Jebsen Test of Hand Function**[63] is a seven-item test devised to evaluate a patient's functional capabilities. The test items are writing a specific sentence, turning over 3-inch by 5-inch cards, picking up small common objects and putting them in a container, stacking checkers, simulated eating, moving empty cans, and moving heavy cans. The method has been standardized, and the reader is referred to the original article for the details of administration. The test-retest reliability of subtests based on data from 26 patients with stable hand disabilities range from $r = 0.60$ to 0.99. Norms for the test derived from 300 adults aged 20 to 94[63] and further norms derived from 383 normal subjects aged 16 to 90[64] are published.

Some standardized dexterity tests, such as the Crawford Small Parts Dexterity Test, the Minnesota Rate of Manipulation Test, and the Purdue Pegboard have been validated on populations of persons employed in jobs requiring a known degree of dexterity. The normative data are therefore very useful, especially in prevocational testing.

The **Crawford Small Parts Dexterity Test** consists of pins, collars, screws, and a board with metal plates. One plate has 42 threaded holes and the other has 42 unthreaded holes to accommodate the screws and pins.[65] Six of each type of holes constitute practice trials; the actual test consists of 36 trials of both pins and screws. The pins and collars must be picked up and placed using tweezers. The screws are inserted to a certain depth using a screwdriver. The score for each subtest is the total time to complete the 36 trials. Split half reliabilities are, on average: pins $r = 0.86$ and screws $r = 0.92$.[65]

The **Minnesota Rate of Manipulation Test**[59,66] consists of a long frame (approximately 3 feet or 1 m long) having four horizontal rows of openings large enough to accommodate the 60 round blocks (approximately 1 1/2 inches or 3.8 cm in diameter). There are two subtests: Placing and Turning. Each is administered five times, the first being a practice trial. The score is the total time for four trials and is converted to a percentage (of the normal population) score using the table given.[66] Test-retest reliability ranges from $r = 0.84$ to $r = 0.91$.[59] The test has been adapted and standardized for the blind also.[67]

The **Purdue Pegboard** is a test of finger dexterity that was orginally designed to aid in the selection of adults for jobs requiring manual skill.[68,69] The test consists of a wooden board with two centered rows each with 25 small holes drilled in them and reservoirs for the pins, collars, and washers across the top. There are two subtests. In the first, the person being tested is required to put the metal pins into the holes as fast as he can after some practice. The number of pins inserted in 30 sec, averaged over three trials, is the score.[69] In the second subtest, the assembly task, the testee is required to place a washer, a collar, and a second washer on the pin once it is in position. The score is the number of parts assembled in one minute. Each completed assembly = 4 points. The score is an average of three trials. Norms for adults are published[69] but are incomplete.[68]

Other Observations

Since learning to control movement of a body changed due to paralysis is essentially new learning, it is important to note the patient's apparent ability to learn new motor skills. Quality of performance of habitual tasks that require use of the nonparalyzed limb such as brushing the teeth is contrasted to performance on novel tasks such as a craft or on functional tasks requiring the use of both limbs such as donning a shirt. If the patient is able to do habitual tasks with the intact extremity but not if the affected limb is involved, provide prompts to the patient to see if performance improves, indicating that the patient can learn by recalling old programs of movement. If the patient can do habitual tasks but cannot do novel tasks, again provide prompts and opportunity for practice to see if he can learn new motor programs. Specific procedures for evaluating the ability to plan movement and to use objects meaningfully are found in chapter 7.

STUDY QUESTIONS:

Evaluation of Motor Control

1. What is the relationship between voluntary motor control and reflexes?
2. What components of motor control are evaluated in a patient with CNS dysfunction?
3. Why should the shoulder of a hemiplegic patient be ranged in a particular way?
4. Compare the gamma motor neuron and the alpha motor neuron in terms of source(s) of excitation, location of cell body, type of motor fibers innervated, and involvement in stretch reflexes.
5. How is muscle tone rated?
6. Name the reflexes mediated by the following levels of control:
   a. Inborn reactions
   b. Spinal level
   c. Brain stem level
   d. Midbrain level
   e. Basal ganglia level
7. Name the motor milestones from supine to standing up.
8. How is voluntary motor control evaluated?
9. List the steps in the sequence of redevelopment of hand function.
10. Which is the most reliable dexterity test reported here? Which is the least reliable, and why might this be so?

References

1. Brooks, V. Motor control: how posture and movements are governed. *Phys. Ther.*, *63*(5): 664–673, 1983.
2. Marsden, C. D. The mysterious motor function of the basal ganglia: the Robert Wartenberg lecture. *Neurology, 32:* 514–539, 1982.
3. Flowers, K. Ballistic and corrective movements on an aiming task. *Neurology, 25:* 413–421, 1975.

4. Kuypers, H. G. J. M., and Brinkman, J. Precentral projections to different parts of the spinal intermediate zone in the rhesus monkey. *Brain Res., 40:* 117–118, 1972.
5. Scholz, J. P., and Campbell, S. K. Muscle spindles and regulation of movement. *Phys. Ther., 60*(11): 1416–1424, 1980.
6. Basmajian, J. V. *Muscles Alive: Their Functions Revealed by Electromyography,* 5th edition. Baltimore: Williams & Wilkins, 1985.
7. Granit, R., and Burke, R. E. The control of movement and posture. *Brain Res. 53:* 1–28, 1973.
8. Wyke, B. Neurological mechanisms in spasticity: a brief review of some current concepts. *Physiotherapy, 62*(10): 316–325, 1976.
9. Swash, M., and Fox, K. P. Muscle spindle innervation in man. *J. Anat., 112*(1): 61–80, 1972.
10. Kennedy, W. R. Innervation of normal human muscle spindles. *Neurology, 20:* 463–475, 1970.
11. Bishop, B. Spasticity: its physiology and management. Part II. Neurophysiology of spasticity: current concepts. *Phys. Ther., 57*(4): 377–383, 1977.
12. Matthews, P. B. C. *Mammalian Muscle Receptors and Their Central Actions.* Baltimore: Williams & Wilkins, 1972.
13. Kottke, F. J. Reflex patterns initiated by the secondary sensory fiber endings of muscle spindles: a proposal. *Arch. Phys. Med. Rehabil., 56*(1): 1–7, 1975.
14. Clarke, A. M. Effect of the Jendrassik manoeuvre on a phasic stretch reflex in normal human subjects during experimental control over supraspinal influences. *J. Neurol. Neurosurg. Psychiatry, 30:* 34–42, 1967.
15. Urbscheit, N. L. Reflexes evoked by group II afferent fibers from muscle spindles. *Phys. Ther., 59*(9): 1083–1087, 1979.
16. Kirkwood, P. A., and Sears, T. A. Monosynaptic excitation of motoneurones from secondary endings of muscle spindles. *Nature, 252* (November 15): 243–244, 1974.
17. Kirkwood, P. A., and Sears, T. A. Monosynaptic excitation of motoneurones from muscle spindle secondary endings of intercostal and triceps surae muscles in the cat. *J. Physiol., 245:* 64P–65P, 1975.
18. Moore, J. C. The Golgi tendon organ: a review and update. *Am. J. Occup. Ther., 38*(4): 227–236, 1984.
19. Lance, J. W., and Burke, D. Mechanisms of spasticity. *Arch. Phys. Med. Rehabil., 55*(8): 332–337, 1974.
20. Bishop, B. Spasticity: its physiology and management. Part III. Identifying and assessing the mechanisms underlying spasticity. *Phys. Ther., 57*(4): 385–395, 1977.
21. Brennan, J. B. Clinical method of assessing tonus and voluntary movement in hemiplegia. *Br. Med. J., 1* (March 21): 767–768, 1959.
22. Bobath, B. *Abnormal Postural Reflex Activity Caused by Brain Lesions,* 2nd edition. London: Heinemann Medical Books, 1971.
23. Bobath, B. *Adult Hemiplegia: Evaluation and Treatment,* 2nd edition. London: Heinemann Medical Books, 1978.
24. Bajd, T., and Vodovnik, L. Pendulum testing of spasticity. *J. Biomed. Eng., 6:* 9–15, 1984.
25. Vodovnik, L., Bowman, B. R., and Bajd, T. Dynamics of spastic knee joint. *Med. Biol. Eng. Comput., 22:*(1) 63–69, 1984.
26. Timberlake, W. H. Evaluation of hypertonia with the use of a gravity-driven ergograph. *Clin. Pharmacol. Ther., 5*(6): 879–882, 1964.
27. McPherson, J. J., et al. The reliability of spring-weighted scales in assessing hypertonicity. *Occup. Ther. J. Res., 2*(2): 118–119, 1982.
28. Bannister, R. *Brain's Clinical Neurology,* 4th edition. London: Oxford University Press, 1973.
29. Hirt, S. The tonic neck reflex mechanism in the normal human adult. *Am. J. Phys. Med.* (NUSTEP proceedings), *46*(1): 362–369, 1967.
30. Capute, A. J., et al. Primitive reflex profile: a pilot study. *Phys. Ther., 58*(9): 1061–1065, 1978.
31. Sieg, K. W., and Shuster, J. J. Comparison of three positions for evaluating the asymmetrical tonic neck reflex. *Am. J. Occup. Ther., 33*(5): 311–316, 1979.
32. Hoskins, T., and Squires, J. Development assessment: a test for gross motor and reflex development. *Phys. Ther., 53*(2): 117–126, 1973.
33. Fiorentino, M. A. *Reflex Testing Methods for Evaluating CNS Development,* 2nd edition. Springfield, IL: Charles C Thomas, 1973.
34. Fiorentino, M. A. *Normal and Abnormal Development.* Springfield, IL: Charles C Thomas, 1972.
35. McGraw, M. *The Neuromuscular Maturation of the Human Infant.* New York: Hafner Publishing Co., 1963.
36. Magnus, R. Cameron prize lectures on some results of studies in the physiology of posture. Part I. *Lancet,* September 11:531–536, 1926.
37. Warren, M. L. A comparative study on the presence of the asymmetrical tonic neck reflex in adult hemiplegia. *Am. J. Occup. Ther., 38*(6): 386–392, 1984.
38. Bobath, K., and Bobath, B. Cerebral palsy. In *Physical Therapy Services in the Developmental Disabilities.* Edited by P. H. Pearson and C. E. Williams. Springfield, IL: Charles C Thomas, 1972.
39. Magnus, R. Cameron prize lectures on some results of studies in the physiology of posture. Part II. *Lancet,* September 18:585–588, 1926.
40. Stockmeyer, S. A. Development from prone to upright posture. A slide-tape lecture. Boston: Instructional Resource Center, Sargent College, Boston University, 1971.
41. Ayers, A. J. *Sensory Integration and Learning Disorders.* Los Angeles: Western Psychological Services, 1972.
42. Brooks, V. B. Roles of cerebellum and basal ganglia in initiation and control of movements. *Can. J. Neurol. Sci., 2*(3): 265–277, 1975.
43. Hallett, M., Shahani, B. T., and Young, R. R. EMG analysis of patients with cerebellar deficits. *J. Neurol. Neurosurg. Psychiatry, 38:* 1163–1169, 1975.
44. Carpenter, M. Cerebellum and basal ganglia. In *Physiological Basis of Rehabilitation Medicine.* Edited by J. A. Downey and R. C. Darling. Philadelphia: W. B. Saunders, 1971.
45. DeJong, R. N., et al. *Essentials of the Neurological Examination.* Philadelphia: Smith Kline Corp., 1968.
46. Chusid, J. G. *Correlative Neuroanatomy and Functional Neurology,* 15th edition. Los Altos, CA: Lange Medical Publications, 1973.
47. Alpers, B. J., and Mancall, E. L. *Essentials of the Neurological Examination.* Philadelphia: F. A. Davis, 1971.
48. DeHaven, G. E., Mordock, J. B., and Loykovich, J. M. Evaluation of coordination deficits in children with minimal cerebral dysfunction. *Phys. Ther., 49*(2): 153–157, 1969.
49. Klingon, G. H. Motor and reflex testing. *J. Mt. Sinai Hosp., 33*(3): 225–235, 1966.
50. Granit, R. *The Basis of Motor Control.* London: Academic Press, 1970.
51. Noback, C., and Demarest, R. *The Nervous System: Introduction and Review.* New York: McGraw-Hill, 1972.
52. Guess, V. Central control insufficiency. II. Extraneous motion: a treatment approach. *Phys. Ther., 58*(3): 306–312, 1978.
53. Phelps, W. M. Classification of athetosis with special reference to the motor classification. *Am. J. Phys. Med., 35*(1): 24–31, 1956.
54. Stockmeyer, S. A. A sensorimotor approach to treatment. In *Physical Therapy Services in the Developmental Disabilities.* Edited by P. H. Pearson and C. E. Williams. Springfield, IL: Charles C Thomas, 1972.
55. Milani-Comparetti, A., and Gidoni, E. A. A pattern analysis of motor development and its disorders. *Dev. Med. Child Neurol., 9:* 625–630, 1967.
56. Ayres, A. J. Ontogenetic principles in the development of arm and hand functions. In *The Development of Sensory Integrative Theory and Practice.* Edited by A. Henderson et al. Dubuque, IA: Kendall/Hunt Publishing Co., 1974.
57. Twitchell, T. Normal motor development. In *The Child with Central Nervous System Deficit.* Washington, DC: U.S. Government Printing Office, 1965.
58. Twitchell, T. The automatic grasping responses of infants. *Neuropsychologia, 3:* 247–259, 1965.
59. Mathiowetz, V., et al. Adult norms for the box and block test of manual dexterity. *Am. J. Occup. Ther., 39*(6): 386–391, 1985.
60. Cromwell, F. S. *Occupational Therapist's Manual for Basic Skills Assessment: Primary Prevocational Evaluation.* Pasadena, CA: Fair Oaks Printing Co., 1965.
61. Mathiowetz, V., et al. Adult norms for the nine hole peg test of finger dexterity. *Occup. Ther. J. Res., 5*(1): 24–38, 1985.
62. Kellor, M., et al. *Technical Manual Hand Strength and Dexterity Tests.* Minneapolis: Sister Kenny Institute, 1977.
63. Jebsen, R. H. An objective and standardized test of hand function. *Arch. Phys. Med. Rehabil., 50*(6): 311–319, 1969.
64. Agnew, P. J. Hand function related to age and sex. *Arch. Phys. Med. Rehabil., 63*(6): 269–271, 1982.
65. Crawford, J. E., and Crawford, D. M. *Manual: Crawford Small Parts Dexterity Test.* New York: The Psychological Corp., 1956.
66. *Manual: Minnesota Rate of Manipulation Test.* Chicago: C. H. Stoelting Co., undated.
67. Bauman, M. K. A manual of norms for tests used in counseling blind persons. *American Federation of the Blind Research Series,* No. 6, 1958.
68. Mathiowetz, V., et al. The Purdue Pegboard: norms for 14- to 19-year olds. *Am. J. Occup. Ther., 40*(3): 174–179, 1986.
69. Tiffin, J. *Examiner Manual for the Purdue Pegboard.* Chicago: Science Research Associates, Inc., 1961.

Supplementary Readings

Bonder, B. Standardized assessments: ethical principles for use. *Am. J. Occup. Ther., 39*(7): 473–474, 1985.
Carlson, J. D., and Trombly, C. A. The effect of wrist immobilization on performance of the Jebsen hand function test. *Am. J. Occup. Ther., 37*(3): 167–175, 1983.

Dietz, V., and Berger, W. Normal and impaired regulation of muscle stiffness in gait: a new hypothesis about muscle hypertonia. *Exp. Neurol.,* 79(3): 680–687, 1983.

Erhardt, R. P. Sequential levels in development of prehension. *Am. J. Occup. Ther.,* 28(10): 592–596, 1974.

Hohlstein, R. R. The development of prehension in normal infants. *Am. J. Occup. Ther.,* 36(3): 170–176, 1982.

Morgan, M. H., Hewer, R. L., and Cooper, R. Intention tremor—a method of measurement. *J. Neurol. Neurosurg. Psychiatry, 38:* 253–258, 1975.

Potvin, A. R., et al. Quantitative methods in assessment of neurologic function. *CRC Crit. Rev. Bioeng., 6*(3): 177–224, 1981.

Van Deusen Fox, J., and Harlowe, D. Construct validation of occupational therapy measures used in CVA evaluation: a beginning. *Am. J. Occup. Ther., 38*(2): 101–106, 1984.

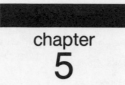

chapter

5

Motor Control
Therapy

Catherine A. Trombly

Sophisticated technology has led to an explosion of information about the generation, control, and acquisition of movement.[1] Neurophysiologists, neuropsychologists, and human-movement scientists contribute to this effort. In an attempt to impose order on the many pieces of information, they deduce models of control. These models are working hypotheses. Therapists extrapolate from the work of these scientists and apply the ideas to therapy. As the working hypotheses change, so does therapy. Neurorehabilitation treatment originally focused on peripheral control of movement by which therapists attempted to change motor output by controlling sensory input. Sensation was augmented and responses were channeled along developmental continua. The newer information places greater emphasis on the central control processes. In response, therapists are developing treatment regimes they believe use these central processes. These newer therapeutic procedures are derived primarily from research on motor learning and information processing within the central nervous system (CNS) of normal persons.

Research has brought another important fact to our attention; there is tremendous variability in the way normal persons use their muscles to accomplish the same goal, probably due to the complexity of central neural processing.[2] There is also variability, though of lesser degree, between how a normal person may use his muscles at one time versus another time to accomplish the same goal. This fact precludes our continued naive perception that an activity invariably uses certain muscles at certain levels of participation.

Treatment of the neurologically impaired patient has become extremely complex. There are no black-and-white rules to follow to treat these patients, not even those with the same diagnoses.[3] How then can a therapist possibly become competent in the treatment of such patients? The answer lies in continuing study and development of clinical-reasoning and psychomotor skills. The competent therapist is informed about the control and acquisition of normal movement and is able to look beyond each patient's neurological diagnostic label to discern what components of normal motor control are missing. This requires superb observational and reasoning skills developed through supervised practice. Then, additionally, the therapist develops evaluative and therapeutic skills through practice.

Normal Motor Control

Normal movement is the ability to interact with the environment in a flexible and adaptable way. It involves the generation of basic movement patterns for each limb and the coordination of these among the limbs; the adaptation of the strength and speed of the movement to suit the resistance and other sensory conditions of the task; and the maintenance of balance of the body despite changes in the center of gravity as the limbs move toward and away from the trunk.[4] The ability to move normally presumes the capabilities of sensing the environment, of processing the information to perceive the meaning of the sensed information, of remembering prior movement sequences, of selecting the appropriate response, and of implementing the appropriate motor response. An adaptive motor response results from an orchestration of all levels of the nervous system from the cortex down to the anterior horn cells in the spinal cord and beyond to the muscles themselves that effect the environmental interaction. Sensory feedback completes the control loop by confirming the precision of execution of both the postural stability and the skilled movements.[5]

One model of performance and learning of acquired motor skills that has been derived from basic science literature is depicted here. It is only one conceptualization that can be made. Until such time as knowledge of motor control is certain, each therapist is encouraged to devise a model that fits her understanding of published information and experience to guide practice.

One Model of Motor Control and Learning

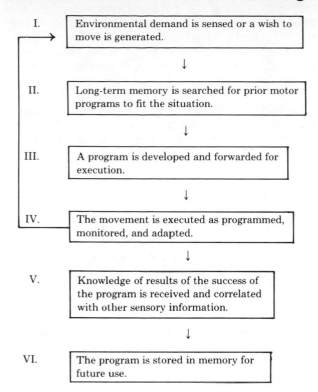

I. Environmental demand is sensed or a wish to move is generated.

II. Long-term memory is searched for prior motor programs to fit the situation.

III. A program is developed and forwarded for execution.

IV. The movement is executed as programmed, monitored, and adapted.

V. Knowledge of results of the success of the program is received and correlated with other sensory information.

VI. The program is stored in memory for future use.

Obviously this simple model is not useful unless the elaborations assumed under each major step are familiar to the therapist. Each step will be discussed conceptually. The reader is referred to the references listed at the end of this chapter for greater detail.

Environmental Demand Is Sensed or a Wish to Move Is Generated

Purposeful movement does not occur in the absence of a need to move.[6,7] This need is generated from within the person or as a response to external stimuli.[8] Vision is an especially powerful sensory input to stimulate voluntary movement.[6,9,10] The limbic system, as the seat of emotion and motivation, triggers movements from within.[11,12]

A movement is organized and planned prior to its initiation.[8,13] The plan takes into account not only environmental factors[8] but also the starting and ending positions of the body and its parts relative to each other and to the environment.[14]

Long-Term Memory Is Searched

All voluntary movement is based on previously acquired movement patterns.[6,15] The memories of how the effort to move felt and of the result that was achieved by the effort guide the present movement.[14] The idea to move, the "act of willing," simultaneously initiates search in long-term memory (LTM) for the memory trace of the planned movement and notifies the programming center to begin strategy development.[2,16-18] Whether the movement is urged from external stimuli or by an act of

willing, the same executive control mechanisms are likely to be employed.[6]

The motor plan is the concept of an action whose execution requires both the sequential operation of a number of simple motor programs[8] and some nonprogrammed components. Motor programs are an abstract representation of a movement pattern coded in a form that defines *relative* timing, amplitude, and force, but not specific muscles used or the amount of their activation.[19] They generate the postural adjustments and ballistic movements of the plan. The most practiced movements are the ones most imbedded in memory[19] and therefore available as programs for future use. Movements of everyday life are likely generated using generalized programs stored in symbolic memory; these are instantiated by supplying modifying features to produce the particular movement pattern required to fit the new situation. [8,16,19,20]

Motor memory can be accessed by concentrating on what it felt like to move for a particular purpose.[21] Access is facilitated by familiar temporal/contextual situations.[22]

A Program Is Developed and Forwarded for Execution

Some movements are more highly programmed than others, for example, walking[23] and writing.[12] An individual's signature is the same, or at least so similar that the difference would be detected if it were written by someone else, whether he writes it on paper using finger and wrist muscles or on the blackboard using shoulder muscles.[24] It is the plan of the act, which is stored in several programs that each specify a part of the plan, that is learned—not the strategy or exact use of particular muscles to do the specific task.[8,14,19] The chief characteristic of programmed movement involving intersegmental coordination (muscle linkage) is the temporal relationship between muscles involved in a particular skill; this temporal relationship is preserved invariantly over changes in the magnitude of muscle activity. [20,23,25,26]

Motor programs command the more automatic components of a motor skill[14] via all levels of control. The brain stem (in response to its input from vestibular receptors), the cerebellum, the cortex, and the basal ganglia all contribute to control of the automatic postural aspects of a program. [11,27,28] The programs are modified to fit the circumstances by strategies that specify the parameters of the movement in which the programs are to operate.[19,29] The parameters include the endpoint location,[30] and the speed, force, and timing of muscle contraction and relaxation.[12,18,31] The strategy can be thought of as a set of instructions of facilitation or inhibition to particular alpha and gamma[18] motor neurons and interneurons to fire at certain frequencies for certain periods of time.[14,32] If agonist and antagonist are to cocontract, the alpha motor neurons of both muscles must be excited, whereas for isotonic movements, the central program produces a triphasic muscle contraction pattern in which first the agonist contracts, then the antagonist to brake the movement, and then the agonist again to brake that countermovement.[33,34]

To support the voluntary movement, postural muscles must also contract bilaterally to provide a stable base from which movement may occur; the neurons of these muscles are activated automatically as part of the program.[6,18] Also as part of the program, the gamma motoneurons are programmed so that spindle sensitivity is exactly set, and accurate information concerning the length and speed of length change can be continually monitored.[27,35] Thus, the alpha motoneurons and the gamma motoneurons are coactivated.[36-38] This coactivation, or forwarding of program for execution, is initiated by the cortex as well as by centers in the brain stem.[39,40] Alpha and gamma coactivation is not invariable; either the alpha or gamma motor neurons can be activated separately for maximal flexibility.[37] Very fast movement, especially of distal muscles, may in fact be the responsibility of alpha motor neurons acting alone under cerebellar control via the motor cortex.[12,28]

Different types of movements and environmental factors require different control strategies.[12,14] Strategies also differ among people and between trials by the same person.[41]

The corticomotoneurons control the voluntary aspect of movement, the part toward which attention is focused.[28]

Movement Is Executed, Monitored, and Adapted

Evidence for two motor systems has been found.[42,43] One controls the gross body and limb movements, and the other controls skilled movements.[42] The system controlling gross movement is bilaterally represented in the brain and is responsible for integration of body and limb movements, upright posture, and independent movement of the extremities.[43] The other system controls the distal limb musculature and is especially concerned with isolated finger movements used in hand skills.[44] Both systems execute movement via the anterior horn cells, the final pathway of information to the effector muscles.

The anterior horn cell, or alpha motor neuron, connects via its axon to several muscle fibers within the muscle. This is known as a motor unit. Motor units are the basic units of muscular control. When the alpha motor neuron is depolarized and fires, all the muscle fibers of that unit contract.[45] The motor units fire asynchronously so that the contraction is smooth. When the muscle fatigues, greater and greater synchrony occurs until a tremor is noticeable.[46] The strength of a muscle contraction reflects both the *number* of motor units firing at the time and their *rate* of firing.[31,46,47] The number of motor units participating in a contraction are recruited according to the size principle.[48,49] The smallest are recruited first and the largest last. The order of recruitment is the same whether the units are volitionally or reflexively activated; one type of activation can enhance the recruitment of a unit only subliminally activated by the other type of activation.[50]

The small units are low-threshold, slow-twitch motor units with only a few muscle fibers served by each alpha motor neuron. These are usually tonic, or holding, type units. High-threshold, fast-twitch, phasic motor units are those with many muscle fibers served by one alpha motor neuron. Force of movement also is modulated by rate coding since increasing the frequency of firing of each recruited unit causes some to be activated at the same time as others, summating their effect to make a stronger contraction.[47,48] There is still enough asynchronous firing to result in a smooth contraction. Small muscles with limited numbers of motor units available for recruitment, especially if the motor units are small, rely more on rate coding to increase force than do large muscles.[47] Rate coding, while not efficient since fatigue soon ensues, represents the only means for further increases in force once all motor units of a muscle are recruited.

The proximal limb musculature system is more likely to be under open-loop control, while the distal system is under closed-loop control.

During fast movement (approximately 160 msec[51] or less) there isn't time to use fedback information for monitoring and correcting because the movement has ended before the feedback can be utilized. This type of control is termed open loop.[52] Open-loop movements are ballistic,[8] defined as fast movements whose termination is determined at the outset independent of current sensory information.[53] The muscle contractions are very energetic and completed before the limb has arrived at its destination.[8] Open-loop movements are the programmed[54] movements. Spontaneous movements, sequences of movements that no longer require attention,[12,17] and proximal limb movements that place the distal parts in position for skilled movement are examples of movements governed by open-loop control systems. In an open-loop system, knowledge of results compared with the sensation of how movement felt, although received late, is very important in the shaping of future similar motor acts.[15,55] When requirements of the motor act change—such as needing to increase speed of locomotion, walk on uneven surfaces, or turn—then sensory feedback is attended to and the motor act comes under closed-loop control.[56]

Closed-loop movements are not programmed ahead but are consciously or unconsciously controlled from moment to moment. Closed-loop movements are characteristically slow movements (approximately 650 msec or more[51]) or maintained postures, during which cutaneous input, visual and auditory cues, and ongoing proprioceptive input from the muscle spindle, Golgi tendon organs, joint receptors, and the otolith organs and semicircular canals of the vestibular apparatus[14,57] all feed back[8,16,58] to the cerebellum, basal ganglia, and cortex[14,27,36-38,59-61] to guide the movement. If the movement is sensed to be wrong, an adjustment is made while the movement is still in progress. Unlearned movements, the exact accuracy of end-point positioning, and skilled movement are examples of closed-loop movements. Skilled movement is defined as that which is attended to and which is usually monitored visually. Without visual feedback, closed-loop movements lack accuracy.[5,57,62]

You have experienced the relationship between program execution, monitoring, and adaptation of movement response many times. One example is if you have ever quickly grabbed a suitcase that you expected to be heavy but in fact was light. The necessary number of motor units in your agonist lifter muscles had been preprogrammed for a mighty lift to a certain final position. Your antagonist muscles also were preprogrammed to relax enough to allow the movement and then contract to brake the movement. The program specified the agonist/antagonist equilibrium relationship[63] needed to achieve the final position. Because the suitcase was lighter than programmed for, the number of motor units participating proved to be too many. You lifted much faster, higher, and with less precision than if your output matched the situation. In this case, the movement was completed before corrections could be made (open-loop control). Nonetheless your higher centers were speedily informed that the programmed movement exceeded the demand. The information returned to the CNS was probably a report from tendon organs of your "lifter" muscles that too many motor units were recruited, from the spindles of the stretched, noncontracting[64] antagonists that they had lengthened too fast to match the program, and from the spindles of the contracting muscles. Since the intrafusal muscle fibers of the spindles of the contracting muscles were still following the original program, but the extrafusal muscle fibers shortened faster than the program specified, the spindles of the contracting muscles slackened and decreased their firing, a signal that there was a problem. Attention became focused onto the movement and readjustment of final position was achieved under closed-loop control.

The opposite circumstance would be if you had expected, and so programmed for, a light suitcase, but in fact it was heavy. Then as the lift got under way, nothing happened at first because too few motor units were participating. The open-loop control then became closed loop as attention was directed to the error. Meanwhile, feedback caused reflex adjustments to be made[2] in the lifter muscles and in functionally related musculature.[65] Within 12 to 18 msec more alpha motor neurons were recruited via the monosynaptic stretch reflex.[24,37,64,66] Approximately 15 msec later more units were recruited via transcortical loop stretch reflexes, which are the primary basis for load compensation.[66-68] Finally, at about 120 msec a cerebellar-assisted cortically controlled adjustment in the program occurred to meet the sensed demand.[66,68]

It is important to understand what happened to bring about this flurry of activity during load compensation because it is the basis of some therapeutic procedures and illustrates the reason why active rather than passive movement is used in neurorehabilitation therapy. When movement is planned, the alpha and gamma motor neurons are coactivated. Both types of motor neuron, one driving the extrafusal muscle fibers and the other driving the intrafusal muscle fibers, receive the program and proceed to contract accordingly. When active movement is unexpectedly stopped, the extrafusal muscle fibers are mechanically prevented from shortening as programmed. They remain lengthened, held by the outside force that stopped the movement (extra-heavy suitcase, therapists's hand, or whatever). Meanwhile, the intrafusal fibers keep contracting as programmed. Soon the discrepancy between their length and the length of the extrafusal fibers is signalled to higher centers. Also, since the spindle is held in place by connective tissue related to the extrafusal muscle fibers, the spindle is mechanically prevented from shortening despite the intrafusal muscle contractions. These two types of stretch (external and internal) of the midportions of the spindle fibers add together, and the segmental and transcortical loop stretch reflexes are activated.[14] Therapists use this technique to enhance motor unit recruitment to increase the strength of muscle contraction.

Passive movement is only used in therapy to increase or maintain range of motion, never when improved motor control or learning is expected. There are central processing differences between active and passive movement. The cerebral readiness potential, which is an electric signal believed to reflect generalized motor cortex firing in preparation for movement,[8,54,69] can be recorded in conjunction with voluntary movement but does not exist for passive movement.[8] Not only is there a lack of reflex enhancement of passive movement because no coactivation had occurred in the first place, but also without the active attempt to move, no cortical planning takes place. There is no plan against which to match sensory feedback. Learning that requires the matching of correct sensory feedback to intent[70] does not occur. Additionally, sensory feedback is reduced because the spindles are not programmed to maintain their length in relation to the length of the extrafusal muscle fibers. Therefore when passive movement is stopped midcourse, no reflex enhancement occurs.

Knowledge of Results Is Received and Correlated with Other Sensory Information

A movement could be executed exactly as programmed and yet be inaccurate as far as accomplishing the goal.[52] Examples come readily to mind: a person throws a bowling ball with the goal of knocking over 10 bowling pins and fails to hit any; a person feeds himself candy while engrossed in reading and misses his mouth. These examples represent the type of voluntary movement that, once learned by matching knowledge of results with kinesthetic feedback, requires direct control and attention only if something goes wrong or to start the program as in sighting the ball to the bowling pins. Knowledge of results is awareness of the outcome of movement in relation to the goal. These open-loop movements were not always thus. They started as closed-loop movements in which attention was focused on the sensory input from the movement.

That sensory input was correlated to the outcome of the movement (knowledge of results) to guide and modify the performance of ongoing and future movements. This knowledge of results is crucial to motor learning even in the case of sensory deficits.[27,57]

The Program Is Stored in Memory for Future Use

Movements are generated from past experiences if success has been recognized.[14] Movement memories that have been successful are stored in LTM, which seems impervious to forgetting. "Successful" indicates that the sensory inflow generated by the movement matched the sensory outflow at the time the program was generated and accomplished the goal.[71] If attention is directed to the movement so that information concerning it remains in short-term memory (STM) for a time, then the memory becomes stored in LTM for future use. However, if the information is lost from STM, then it does not become part of LTM and learning does not take place.[19] The learned motor skill must be practiced to be retained at the same level of expertise.[14] Expertise is improved by practice with intention to improve. In other words, the person sets a more refined goal for himself and the process of motor control restarts at step 1 of the model.

Motor Dysfunction Due to CNS Deficits

CORTICAL LESIONS

Cerebral cortical areas have specific motor functions.[12] The primary motor cortex has the lowest-level control function: it is the executor of movement.[12,69] It translates program instructions from other parts of the brain into signals that specify which muscles should contract or relax when, and it informs the other centers of the intended movement so they can monitor themselves. Other cortical motor areas perform higher-order motor functions.[12] The supplementary motor area controls the programming of complex sequences of rapid discrete movements.[12,69] The premotor area is active in assembling new motor programs.[12] The posterior parietal areas direct attention to objects of interest in visual space, issue commands, form strategies[11] for eye and arm movements to these objects, and guide the arm movements in space.[12] The prefrontal cortex performs cognitive functions related to movement, e.g., STM processing.

The motor dysfunction that results from acquired cortical lesions depends on the site and extent of the lesion. Diffuse lesions such as may be seen after closed head injury can result in extensive damage to the surface and deeper structures of the brain. The motor dysfunction may then involve deficits in vital motor functions such as swallowing or breathing (brain stem injury); basic motor patterns such as righting and equilibrium responses (midbrain and basal ganglia injury) or coordination of movement (cerebellar injury); or motor planning and execution of voluntary goal-directed movements (cortical injury). Circumscribed cortical lesions, such as occur as a result of cerebrovascular accident, gunshot, or other penetrating injuries, result in dysfunctional planning or execution of goal-directed movement limited to the function and area controlled by the damaged tissue. The less voluntary movements are relatively spared. Although the patient may be unable to move a segment of a limb in isolation, he is often able to move the whole limb in a stereotyped way. However, even in those patients who seem to have similar lesions, dysfunction varies due to the complexity of the control options available to the CNS[3] and the way each individual uses them.

The motor deficits of cortical damage are both negative and positive. The negative deficit is the decreased ability to recruit sufficient motor units in the correct temporal relationship to perform normal movement. The positive deficits are those phenomena that are released from the inhibitory control of the cortex: exaggerated reflexes including the stretch reflex (spasticity). Until fairly recently the positive symptoms were considered to have the most devastating effect on the motor function of cortically damaged patients. It was also believed that the negative and positive symptoms were inextricably related—that until positive symptoms could be corrected, the negative deficit could not be improved. There is sparse but growing evidence to doubt this relationship, [72,73] and therapists are beginning to concentrate on remediation of the negative deficits.

Motor control is abnormal not only because of the motor deficits, but also because of deficits in sensation and cognitive and perceptual processing.

Cortical sensory deficits include the lack of awareness of a particular sensation or constellation of sensations[74] or the inability to localize and discriminate sensations. The patient with sensory loss will not use the limb spontaneously but can compensate for the loss using intact sensory systems when directed to do so.[74] The sensory loss will seriously affect the ability to sustain a constant level of force needed to hold an object or to maintain a posture. In the case of impaired sensation, movement is affected by the distortion[75,76] and the patient needs to relearn the meaning of the new sensations through active movement. No relearning occurs during passive movement, even if the patient watches the movement.[70]

Information processing related to motor control involves registration of the stimulus and manipulation within STM in which the stimulus data are attended to, coded, chunked to allow speedy transfer, rehearsed, and finally transferred to LTM.[77] The information in STM is labile and will rapidly decay unless attended to by a control process such as verbal rehearsal.[77] Left-brain-damaged (LBD) patients may be unable to attend or initiate control schemes to sustain information in STM long enough for it to be processed and transferred to LTM due to loss of language for self-rehearsal. Because of this, learning and executing manual sequences is especially affected in LBD patients.[78,79]

Reaction time (RT) tests are used as measures of cognitive processing[80] but in fact test the integrity of the input/output system as a whole. RT is defined as the time between onset of the "go" signal and the response. RT is made up of premotor time (PMT), the time from the "go" signal to the onset of electrical activity in the muscle, and motor time, the time from start of electrical activity to the beginning of actual movement.[80] In one study, patients with right brain damage (RBD) showed slower PMT in both hands as compared to controls, reflecting that the right hemisphere has a dominant role in the processing involved in simple RT tasks. The PMT of LBD patients was not significantly different from that of normal controls. Motor time was slower in the affected hands of both groups as compared to normal controls due to the paralysis.[81]

Apraxia, in one of its several forms, may be present in both RBD and LBD patients. LBD patients with ideomotor apraxia have been found to be deficient in motor learning compared to nonapraxic LBD patients. This seems to be due to the combined defect of both acquisition and retention.[82] Apraxic errors are characterized as omissions, disturbed order of submovements within a sequence, and perseveration. Movement is clumsy.[83] Apraxia is an inability to gesture or use objects correctly that cannot be accounted for by deficits in motor capacities per se, in comprehension of the act to be performed, or in recognition of the object to be used.[83]

CEREBELLAR LESIONS

The cerebellum specifies the movement parameters and initiates preprogrammed movement.[11] It programs patterns of muscle activity and organizes the temporal relationship between the agonist and antagonist in successive movements.[11,34]

Negative symptoms of cerebellar lesions are dysmetria, rebound phenomenon, and dysdiadochokinesia.[11,34] These deficits reflect timing abnormalities. The basis for these deficits is a combination of delayed initiation of preprogrammed patterns and delayed termination of agonistic muscular activity, which result in delayed or missing initiation of the antagonist.[11,34] These patients are able to carry out voluntary programmed movement of a limb but lack the fine adjustments needed for end-point accuracy. Intention tremor is a positive symptom of cerebellar lesion.

LESIONS OF THE BASAL GANGLIA

The major diagnosis involving basal ganglia lesions seen by occupational therapists is Parkinson's disease. Akinesia and bradykinesia are key negative symptoms of basal ganglia disease. There is a delay and slowness of initiating and carrying out movement. The slowness is not due to a simple overall increase in RT[53]; rather there is a differential increase in motor time, reflecting losses in the generation of movement.[8] There is no evidence of any selective impairment in speed of formulating or assembling a central motor program,[8] which would be reflected in an increase in premotor time. Although the pattern of activation is intact, the patient is unable to recruit the necessary number of motor units to produce the force of contraction sufficient to reach the target.[8] Instead, the patient approximates the target in small increments, using the available motor units to move bit by bit.

Patients with Parkinson's disease also show delay or failure to respond to external stimuli, especially those involved in automatic postural adjustments. Anticipatory postural reflexes (righting and protective reactions) are found to be grossly disturbed in patients with even mild Parkinson's disease.

The basal ganglia are responsible for "the automatic execution of learned motor plans."[8] It was once thought that they were responsible for slow ramp movements, that is, movements characterized by gradual smooth execution,[34,84] but it has now been demonstrated that patients with basal ganglia disease can do ramp movements but cannot do the ballistic components of movement.[8] With the loss of the ballistic component of movement, these patients lose a major advantage characteristic of ballistic movement: a reduced information load in the sensory motor system, since ballistic movement is preprogrammed and therefore not consciously attended to. This loss prevents the parkinsonian patient from doing two motor tasks at once, such as rising from a chair to greet a guest with an outstretched hand. As the patient changes his focus from standing up to preparing to shake hands, he is apt to fall back into the chair.[8] These patients have lost the use of learned programs of movement—a regression to the unskilled state, a reversal of the process of learning.[53] The agonist/antagonist/synergistic relationships of muscles, therefore simple motor programs, are preserved[8] since these relationships are governed by the cerebellum. The patient has trouble "calling up" or "running" the motor programs in a comprehensive motor plan in which programs are linked concurrently or sequentially. The patient with Parkinson's disease, having lost the ability to automatically run motor programs, must pay attention to each movement.

Rigidity, which is due to excessive and uncontrolled supraspinal drive to the alpha motor neuron, and tremors at rest are positive symptoms caused by other structures released from the inhibitory control of the basal ganglia. Positive symptoms do not indicate the function of a structure, other than its inhibitory function.

Recovery

Recovery occurs.[1] Recovery may be defined as attainment of a goal given that the organism was capable of accomplishing that goal immediately before but not immediately after neural injury.[85] Recovery can occur because of a takeover of function by spared tissue, by morphological reorganization, or by adaptive or learned changes in strategies for information processing. There is insufficient evidence to determine what exactly is responsible for recovery.[86,87] Recovery probably results from the collective contributions of several mechanisms acting together on the altered nervous system.[87] None of the physical or adaptive recovery mechanisms seem universal for type of lesion or species. People recover differently because no two brains are alike structually or functionally.[1]

Recovery from cortical lesions attributed to physical mechanisms usually follows a developmental sequence from reflex to voluntary control, from mass to discrete movements, and from proximal to distal control.[88] Recovery can stop at any level along the continua and this is not wholly predictable. The speed of early spontaneous recovery offers a clue to the ultimate level of function to be gained.[88]

Some believe that the amount of tissue damage is more disabling than specific sites of destruction because remaining healthy tissue can, with relearning, assume lost functions.[85] However, recovery is never complete.[89] Any cells in the brain that have been destroyed will not regenerate,[87] and the function for which they were responsible will be diminished by the loss. If all of the cells of the pyramidal tract are destroyed, thereby preventing the one means of control of discrete skilled movement of the contralateral side, especially that of the fingers, that function will not be regained. Functions served by bilateral systems may be preserved if the remaining system takes over the function.[1]

There is developing evidence that neuronal plasticity may continue throughout life and could be expected to occur in the remaining living cells[90-92] after trauma. Established neural circuits in mammals lack intrinsic plasticity; therefore, the neuronal plasticity that is seen is not due to respecification of the existing neural connections established during development,[93] but rather is due to the unique plastic properties of the dendritic spines whose growth is influenced by the environment.[93]

Diseases of the cerebellum or basal ganglia are degenerative, for the most part, and recovery due to neural changes is not expected. Any improvement, which is temporary as the disease proceeds and further incapacitates the patient, is probably due to functional compensation.

Functional recovery may occur through the substitution of a behavior similar to, but not the same as, the lost behavior.[89] Use of novel tactics,[85] i.e., learning new behavioral strategies to compensate for the loss, is one means (seemingly not dependent on neural reorganization) of recovering function.[85] Motivation plays a major role in functional recovery; without it, no recovery may occur,[1] probably because functional recovery is actually a relearning process. Without motivation and active goal setting on the part of the learner, behavioral changes (learning) do not take place. An example of functional recovery would be use of functions of the noninjured brain to process information. For example, the right brain specializes in visual information, which it processes spatially or globally. The left brain specializes in verbal information and processes it sequentially and logically. Patients can learn to use the processing style of the intact brain to process information that was previously the specialty of the other brain. If a visual stimulus is to be recognized, each characteristic of the stimulus can be described in words to enable recognition of it by the left brain. A patient who cannot decipher the tangle of his shirt in order to put it on may be able to do so if he names each part in sequence, finds it as he names it, and then put it on in a step-by-step fashion.

The passage of time alone has been found to be inadequate to account for recovery of motor function in monkeys.[94] Recovered abilities to do certain tasks require training that involves active interaction of the subject with the environment.[89] However, recovery has been found to be limited to the tasks practiced.[89,95] More research on the factors that promote transfer of learning among motor skills needs to be done.

The CNS seems to have tremendous recuperative potential. The reorganization that is induced by lesions of the CNS is a change in the "hard wiring" of the brain.[87] Patients with brain lesions have different neural connections than persons without brain damage.[87] Therapists need to discover how to use the potential of neural plasticity in rehabilitation of patients with CNS lesions.[87] Therapists are also in a position to contribute to the knowledge of recovery by carefully documenting the clinical course of recovery[186] in relation to possible controlling variables, especially the exact nature of the training experience.

The Acquisition of Movement

Normal movement is believed to have its origin in genetically wired configurations of neurons ("neuromotor synergies"[96]) that produce fairly stereotyped movements in response to certain stimuli.[56] Most innate motor systems are modifiable, which serves as the basis for development of acquired skills.[56] As the normal fetus/infant matures, the simple genetically based movement patterns become more elaborate, involving more complex "hard wired" circuits or functional linkages of muscles whose activities covary in order to accomplish a particular behavioral goal.[23] These neural circuits develop as the nervous system matures.[56]

The spinal reflexes, the most stereotyped movements, are the lowest level of control. They lose dominance as the brain stem reflexes emerge. This maturation continues as the reflexes are supplanted by the higher-level righting and equilibrium responses. As the righting reactions develop, the baby learns control of the head in space and automatic adjustments to keep the body and head aligned in relation to each other and the environment. Thus begin the ontogenetic motor milestones, starting with holding the head up and rolling over, that parents look for to document the child's ongoing development.

Reflex maturation proceeds caudocephaly; that is, spinal reflexes develop before those of the brain stem, which develop before those of the midbrain, etc. However, both reflex and voluntary control proceed cephalocaudally and proximally to distally; that is, the upper extremity exhibits a withdrawal reflex before the lower, voluntary head movement is learned before voluntary trunk movement, and shoulder control is learned before hand control. Learning occurs because throughout the developmental process not only is the normal baby always "practicing," but also the cortex is maturing so that organizational and decision-making capabilities increase to allow use of cognitive processes needed for the acquisition of complex skills.[29]

Movement and posture are intertwined developmentally. Phasic movement (mobility) is the lowest level of control. Early mobility patterns are largely without purpose or goal although they are temporally organized rather than being random.[25,97] The rhythmical movements of infants—spontaneous kicking, waving, banging, rocking, etc.—are carried out by fundamental functional muscle synergies that appear to be necessary for later skilled movement.[97] Mobility is in time replaced by "synchronous coactivation" of flexors and extensors,[97] which develops into the ability to hold a posture (stability). Stability develops from the neck down and from the midline out to the periphery. Equilibrium reactions become evident when the baby is able to regain his center of gravity if it is disturbed while he is holding a posture. The postures reflect the motor milestones. Development is not stepwise; that is, one milestone is not perfected before the next begins to develop. Development occurs spirally: as the baby learns to hold one posture, movement within the posture is attempted and beginning attempts toward assuming the next posture are made. The motor milestones bring the infant to an upright toddler. Full limb patterned movements give way to single joint movements from proximal to distal joints as cortical control adds speed and fractionation to movements.[42]

Visually directed reaching and hand function develop sequentially from visual regard of the hand during the asymmetrical tonic neck reflex stage to learning release of grasp (voluntary finger extension) and finally individual finger control later in childhood. These maturationally based sequences unfold replicably from person to person if the neuromuscular system is intact. Learned motor skills or purposeful goal-directed actions[7] used in self-care, work, and play are believed to be acquired by building on these maturationally acquired movement patterns.[6,15,56,98]

There is more variability from person to person in learned motor skills [1,99] than in the maturationally acquired motor patterns. For example, everyone has his or her own way of dancing, whereas walking—the maturational base of dancing—is fairly uniform among people as far as sequencing and timing of muscular actions. Although a person's performance may be different from that of another person's, as he practices and becomes skilled in a new motor task, the variability of his performance from one time to the next decreases. The decreased variability in the timing and pattern of muscle contraction and in the agonist/antagonist relationships among muscle groups are signs that motor learning has taken place.[41] Learned motor skills are characterized by automaticity; that is, large segments

of the skill are programmed and need not be attended to for correct execution. Automaticity is due to not only the physical capability of the performer but also the efficient operation of cognitive control processes, as well as a high level of learning of the movement.[9] Increased accuracy and speed are indicative of automaticity.

The current question of neurorehabilitation therapy is whether the therapist can best facilitate motor control through eliciting responses to specific stimuli to recapitulate the maturational sequence or through use of motor learning procedures, or a combination of the two.

Patients who have suffered brain damage need to reacquire previously learned motor skills. If they had progressed through ontogenetic motor development before brain damage, they had the genetic endowment that underlies the maturationally acquired patterns basic to motor learning. Their task becomes one of relearning to disassociate components of muscle linkages (also called synergies or associated reactions) and to recombine the components into voluntary response patterns.[99]

Treatment

GOAL: TO PREVENT LIMITATION OF RANGE OF MOTION

Although not related to restoration of motor control, per se, this goal must be included in therapy for patients with brain injury. It is important that range of motion be maintained so that if motor control recovers, movement is not limited by mechanical changes in the muscles and joints. Even if motor control does not recover, it is still important that the limb remain free of serious contracture so it will not become a functional or hygenic problem. For example, when a fixed flexion contracture of the fingers is allowed to develop, the skin can become severely macerated and only surgical release of the contracture will allow cleansing and healing to occur.

All patients who are unable to move their limbs to full range independently are in danger of developing contractures due to changes that occur in the viscoelastic properties of muscle and connective tissue when they remain in one position. Patients with CNS deficits are at risk not only due to their inability to move but also due to the excessive neural stimulation to the motor neurons as a result of loss of supraspinal inhibition.

Principle: Movement Through Full Range of Motion

Passive ranging is the method used to implement the principle of movement through full range of motion. Movement of the muscles and joints addresses both the viscoelastic etiology of contractures by preventing the structures from adhering and the neural etiology by counteracting the stretch receptor response.[100] Each joint of the limb is moved passively throughout full range at least once per day. Because tissue changes can occur rapidly, it is important that this treatment clearly be the responsibility of a designated person(s) so that it is faithfully carried out daily. The joint is moved very slowly from start position to end position as described in range of motion evaluation in chapter 8. Slow movement is used to prevent the activation of the dynamic stretch reflex. If the reflex is triggered, the therapist feels the limb "catch" or stop. The joint can be held still at that position until the reflex releases, and then the movement toward the full limit of motion is resumed. As tone becomes normalized due to recovery and treatment, the point in range where this "catch" occurs moves closer to the limit of motion. Review Figure 4.1 and the associated text for the technique to be used for ranging the shoulder of a hemiplegic patient.

Principle: Positioning

The principle of positioning is applied by placing the affected limb into position and holding it there by use of pillows, wedges, orthoses, or serial inhibitory casts.[101] This principle is aimed at counteracting the effects of the neural etiology of contractures by rebiasing the spindles of spastic muscles to a longer length, thereby decreasing their sensitivity.

The position in which the limb is placed is exactly opposite to that in which the limb would tend to go due to the pattern of actual or anticipated hypertonicity. In the upper limb the typical pattern is one of flexion, adduction, and internal rotation (including pronation); therefore, the position of choice is extension, abduction, and external rotation, which lengthens those muscles typically kept too short by the hypertonicity. The typical pattern in the lower limb is extension, adduction, and internal rotation.

The degree to which the limb is counterpositioned depends on several factors: degree of hypertonicity, alternate unacceptable outcome, number of joints served by the hypertonic muscles, and pain. Counterpositioning a severely hypertonic limb at all joints and in full opposition to the typical pattern may be necessary, whereas for a mildly hypertonic limb, a position slightly away from typical position on one dimension may be adequate to reduce the tone of the whole limb. For example, external rotation at the shoulder may result in a decrease in elbow flexor tone that allows the elbow to be left free for relearning of active movement. The therapist determines, by reevaluating muscle tone as described in chapter 4, whether the amount of counterpositioning effectively reduces the abnormal neural input to muscles.

Positioning the limb in the opposite direction can result in an equally unacceptable outcome because of the viscoelastic etiology of contractures by which holding in any position results in cellular changes of connective tissue. Therefore, the degree of counterpositioning may need to be kept to a minimum, while the hypertonicity is treated more directly. One example is the knee of a hemiplegic patient; if a contracture developed in the counterposition of flexion, future ambulation would be jeopardized. Therefore, the knee is just barely flexed in an attempt to break up the extensor pattern, but not cause harm.

Joints served by multiarticular muscles must be positioned so that the effects of hypertonicity are not shunted to one of the joints that is served by the muscles but that seemingly is in normal position at the time of evaluation. An example of this is the case where the wrist is flexed due to hypertonia but the fingers are extended. If the wrist is positioned into extension by use of a wrist cock-up splint, soon the fingers will develop flexor contractures. Both the wrist and the fingers must be included in the splint. It is also important to be sure the splint does not aggravate hypertonicity by causing tactile stimulation of the spastic muscles.

Pain also guides the degree of positioning. The limb must be positioned within a pain-free range, even if that range is less than the limit of motion. Pain causes facilitatory changes to the neurons of stretched and related musculature that can undermine the value of positioning. To increase the point in range where pain-free positioning can occur, the source of pain needs more direct treatment.

The limb is positioned whenever it is not being used for functional activity or in treatment to relearn motor control. It is held in that position by the least restrictive means that is effective. Propping by pillows or wedges is least restrictive; casting is the most restrictive. The minimal amount of time the positioning should be maintained has not been determined and probably varies for each individual. One study of 10 brain-damaged subjects found that 2 hours of inhibitory splinting caused a decrease, although not a significant one, in muscular activity in 7 patients but an increase in muscular activity in the other 3.[102]

GOAL: TO NORMALIZE TONE

Some therapists think that normalization of tone must precede treatment for reacquisition of movement control.[103] Others think that once voluntary movement control is regained, tone will automatically normalize. The actual situation may be that abnormal tone and lack of motor control are independent manifestations of the CNS deficit that are not causally related to each other, although they each are related to CNS deficit. If they are independent symptoms, then treatment to address both deficits simultaneously may be ideal. Lack of clinical research on these hypotheses is a serious detriment to the advancement of effective and efficient therapy. The assumptions on which normalization of tone is based are the following. A certain level of tone is necessary to enable movement and posture.[103] If there is too much tone, movement by the antagonist muscle(s) is prevented. If there is too little tone, then signals to the anterior horn cells are ineffective since there is not enough subliminal depolarization of these cells to support their firing. The goal is to achieve a normal balance of tone in agonist and antagonist muscles of each joint throughout the limb by increasing or decreasing the tone of opposing muscles through the use of peripheral stimulation.[100,103]

Principle: Controlled Sensory Manipulation

The neural component of tone can be affected by the number and nature (electrical charge) of impulses that impinge on the motor neurons all at once (spatial summation) or in quick succession (temporal summation). Sensory input is manipulated in a controlled manner to enhance or reduce the electrical charge on interneurons or motor neurons, making them more or less likely to fire when stimulated by supraspinal impulses.

It is assumed that the sign of the electrical charge can be manipulated by controlling the kind and amount of sensory input. Some sensory stimuli are termed facilitatory and some inhibitory. Facilitatory stimuli generally are arousing, whereas inhibitory stimuli are soothing and relaxing. Facilitation refers to the state of readying neurons to depolarize. Small subthreshold depolarizations occur as each facilitatory impulse arrives at a neuron, but these must summate to cause the impulse to be propagated by the neuron.[21,27] Some of the impulses that arrive at the neuron are inhibitory; that is, they hyperpolarize the cell membrane to decrease the likelihood of propagating the impulse.[36] The neuron sums algebraically; if there are more facilitatory than inhibitory impulses, then the neuron depolarizes and the impulse is propagated along to the next synapse. If the inhibitory influences are greater, no impulse is propagated. The effects of input of similar type (facilitatory or inhibitory) summate to cause an enhanced response. Stimuli of different types act antagonistically to reduce the effect of any one type of stimulus. For example, if neutral warmth, an inhibitory stimulus, were being administered in a busy, stimulating environment, the treatment might be ineffective to decrease spasticity.

Facilitatory stimuli are applied directly to hypotonic muscles. Hypertonic muscles may be inhibited generally, directly, or reciprocally. Immediately after injury, affected limbs are usually hypotonic due to the shock to the nervous system. As the shock subsides, tone may develop in the typical distribution. Typically tone is increased in the flexors and adductors and decreased in the extensors and abductors. Because therapists fear that facilitation of the flexors will result in too much flexor tone (via treatment and normal recovery) and that the patient will become "stuck" in flexion, they avoid facilitation of the flexors/adductors altogether or they very carefully integrate flexor facilitation with facilitation of the extensors.

The distribution of changes in tone may be atypical, or the several muscles of one functional group may not be equally affected by changes in tone. The location of application of sensory stimuli will be determined for each patient by his particular needs.

When applying the stimuli, it cannot be assumed that because a particular technique worked for one patient that it will work in the same way for another.[3,104,105] Although it seems like a simple research project to apply stimuli and measure the results to determine the therapeutic effects, in reality, with the possible exception of stretch, no stimulus seems to be universally facilitating or inhibiting.[105] The effect that any sensory stimulus has on any individual is different from its effect on any other individual. Each patient's response is determined by his own central regulator, not by the peripheral stimulus per se.[36,38,49,106] The type of response to a particular stimulus on repeated stimulation is usually the same for a particular individual,[105] although the strength of the response at any given moment depends on the state of the CNS, or more specifically the spinal interneurons, at the time of stimulation.[36,49] According to the Law of Initial Values, if a "standard dose" of excitatory stimulus from the periphery arrives at excited central neurons, the effect of that dose of stimulus may add little to the state of excitation and the response may well be less than anticipated. On the other hand, if the "standard dose" of excitatory stimulus arrives at inhibited neurons, the response will be greater than expected.[107] The same applies to inhibitory stimuli arriving at already inhibited or facilitated neurons. When the CNS is in an excessive state of either excitation or inhibition, the response may be paradoxical, that is, the opposite of what is expected.[107] No one can predict from known outward signs what the overall state of excitation of the CNS is. It is therefore important when using controlled sensory manipulation therapeutically to know what response is expected, to apply the chosen stimulus with care, and to observe the reactions of the patient, however minute, in response to the stimulation. If the patient does not react as expected, the intensity or duration of application is changed.

Subgoal: To Increase Tone. Facilitatory sensory stimuli are used to provoke movement or to enhance weak ongoing muscle contraction. Movement is provoked as a reflex response to sensory stimuli, whereas enhancement of muscle contraction is achieved by increasing the participation of the motor units of the muscle(s) responsible for the movement. Only the absolute minimal amount of stimulation that is needed to produce the desired response is ever used, and the patient is weaned from the external stimulation as soon as he recovers enough control to move successfully without it. Stimuli used to evoke reflex responses are the first to be deleted from treatment because they are the most primitive means of controlling movement.

Motor unit recruitment is increased by an imposed external stretch or by internal stretch in which the sensitivity of the muscle spindles is biased so that any added stretch or supraspinal command will activate additional motor units. The spindles are biased through sensory stimulation that is directed to the gamma motor neurons through the reticular activating system.

Tactile Stimulation. Cutaneous sensation is extremely important in motor control[36,66]; therefore, stimulation of tactile receptors provides an important avenue to modify the motor response. Tactile stimulation involves the application of a gentle, moving stimulus over the skin to provoke a spinal-level phasic withdrawal reflex response or a sustained tonic response of a particular muscle group. The rationale for this latter usage stems from research that showed that tactile stimulation (light pinching) of the skin over the flexor or extensor muscles of cats was found to facilitate the alpha motor neurons of the muscle beneath and inhibit the motor neurons of its antagonist.[108] The same was found to be true for gamma motor neurons,[109] indicating that tactile stimulation works via the reticular activating system,[103,110] as well as directly through a segmental loop.[103]

A tactile stimulus is applied by stroking or brushing the skin over the muscles that are being treated[108] with a piece of cotton or a soft paint brush. A quick swipe of the stimulus is used to elicit a phasic response, and sustained, highly repetitive brushing is used to elicit a tonic response. The effect is immediate,[103,110,111] not delayed as previously thought.[112] Therefore, tactile stimulation should be applied at the time that movement is demanded and the patient is making the effort to move. Since the stimulus is believed, but not proven, to have a bilateral effect, stimuli applied bilaterally ought to be more effective than if only applied unilaterally to the affected extremity.

Orthokinetics is a technique that may be considered tactile stimulation, although it is reported to stimulate the proprioceptors of muscles and tendon also. A band of rubber-reinforced elastic bandage is made to fit around the limb at the area of the belly of the muscle to be stimulated. Several layers of bandage are used. The active part that is to be placed directly over the muscles to be stimulated is left free and stretchy; the remainder of the band, the inactive part, is sewn back and forth over and over to make it relatively inelastic. The cuff fits snugly but not tightly around the limb with the active field placed exactly over the muscles to be stimulated(Fig. 5.1). As the patient exercises, especially by using reciprocal movements, or as he goes about his daily activities, the contraction and relaxation of muscles that lie under the cuff push the skin against the orthokinetic cuff, and the elastic part stimulates the skin by small pinches. Although the effectiveness has not been definitely established,[113,114] it is an intriguing idea deserving of more controlled study. The idea of the orthokinetic cuff can be incorporated into a spasticity-reduction spint; the plastic splint material provides the inactive, inhibitory field and wide, fuzzy straps or elastic bandage used as straps provides the active, facilitatory field.[115]

Thermal Stimulation. The brief application of ice to the skin in the palm of the hand or on the soles of the feet is used to provoke a phasic withdrawal reflex response. Application of the ice for several seconds on the skin over the muscles being treated is expected to result in a sustained contraction although this lacks documentation. Icing is thought to work both segmentally and through the reticular activating system, as touch does,[103] but the rationale for the effects of ice in facilitating tone is not stated in the literature.

One study reports the use of prolonged (30-min) icing by immersion of the limb in 10° to 12°C ice water

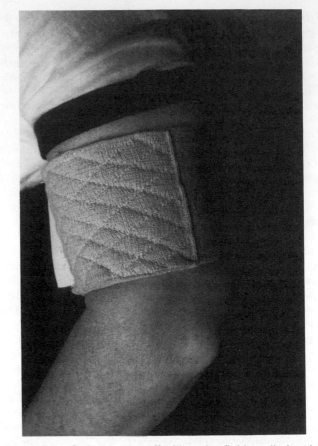

Figure 5.1 Orthokinetic cuff with active field applied to the triceps of a hemiplegic patient's affected arm.

to increase strength during the posticing recovery phase.[116] Prolonged icing is thought to be an inhibitory stimulus (see below). No adverse effects were reported in the normal young adult subjects used in this study; however, since both warmth and cold produce autonomic nervous system effects such as changes in blood flow in the limb and since icing may elicit a major sympathetic response, including cardiorespiratory changes, caution must be observed when using thermal stimuli on patients with cardiovascular disease or whose central nervous systems are already under stress from disease or trauma.

Two beneficial uses for icing in the neurorehabilitation of adult patients are (1) to elicit a phasic swallowing response in patients who drool by swiping the skin over the sternal notch in an upward direction and (2) to elicit a breathing (inspiration) response in patients with partially paralyzed diaphragms by swiping the ice over the skin along the border of the rib cage in an upward direction.

Vestibular Stimulation. These stimuli are used to evoke an automatic movement pattern or to enhance tone. Specifically, vestibular stimulation is used to challenge equilibrium responses as described in chapter 4 or to facilitate tonic extensor tone. The labyrinth has two types of receptors, the semicircular canals and the otolith organ (utricle and saccule).[117] These receptors are stimulated by rotary and linear movements, especially the acceleration and deceleration phases of these movements, and by head position. The otolith organ is primarily concerned with detection of linear acceleration[49] and static head position. The semicircular canals are primarily concerned with angular acceleration (rotary movements).[49]

The tonic labyrinthine inverted (TLI) posture in which the head is upside down[118] uses the effects of otolith organ stimulation to increase tone in the postural extensor muscles. The upside-down position causes maximum stimulation of the sensory hairs to which the otoliths are attached.[49] The effect is to increase extensor tone via the vestibulospinal tract. The TLI posture was found to facilitate extensor tone, whereas the upright posture was found least facilitatory to extensor tone, as hypothesized.[119] Intermediate postures were found to produce intermediate effects on extensor tone.[119] Interestingly, the most pronounced effect of the TLI posture was observed in the distal muscles (extensor carpi radialis and ulnaris, flexor carpi radialis and ulnaris, soleus and tibialis anterior); whereas the least effect was evident in the proximal muscles (deltoid and gluteus maximus), although the proximal muscles are more responsible for antigravity postural responses. In the above study, the stimulus was administered to adult subjects by rotating them into all positions from upright to upside down while they were lying on a flat surface. A partial TLI posture can be achieved in the clinic by placing a person over a large inflatable pillow or ball, a cable spool, or a barrel so that the head is down. The response is immediate and lasts only as long as the stimulus is applied.

Caution should be observed to detect unwanted changes in blood pressure in any patient, but especially in a stroke patient. Of course the TLI posture should not be used for any head-injured or stroke patient for whom increased intracranial pressure is contraindicated. Because of this limitation, the TLI posture is rarely used in treatment of adults.

Linear and rotary acceleration and deceleration stimulate equilibrium responses as well as increased extensor tone. Acceleration and deceleration can be achieved by swinging or twirling the patient on a swing or in a net hammock suspended from one hook in the ceiling that encloses the person within the hammock and gives him a feeling of safety, by placing the person prone on a scooter board or skateboard and letting him roll down an incline (Fig. 5.2), or by pulling on a rope attached to the scooter board. The patient on a skateboard or scooter board lifts his limbs in order to get a better ride, which combines attention to the goal with the effects of vestibular stimulation. A scooter board is a flat board large enough to support the patient from midchest to hips that has free-wheeling universal casters at each corner. An equilibrium board can be used to elicit equilibrium responses in supine-lying, prone-lying, sitting, quadruped, and kneeling. The equilibrium board is a large (3 feet × 5 feet), flat board

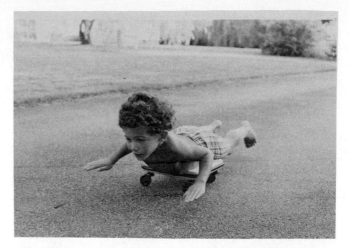

Figure 5.2 Scooter board on an incline eliciting the pivot prone position and providing vestibular stimulation.

mounted on low rockers located at the short ends. The board is tilted rapidly to the degree that is required to challenge the patient's balance, but within recoverable limits. The patient must be guarded to prevent falling. Again, use of these devices with adults is limited. Alternate choices to stimulate equilibrium responses are the use of a rocking chair or a game of catch in which the patient, seated on a raised mat, attempts to catch a large colored ball or balloon that is thrown to him from various directions. This activity requires that he move his head to attend to the ball and move the top of his body to reach to catch the ball, both of which stimulate the labyrinths.

Proprioceptive Stimulation. Propricoceptive stimuli include the brain stem reflexes and stretch reflexes. These stimuli are used to evoke movement, to enhance ongoing movement, or to increase awareness of movement.

The brain stem reflexes, the stimuli for which have been described in chapter 4, are used by some therapists to evoke movement or postural responses when the patient is otherwise unable to initiate these responses or has little to no tone.[120] Other therapists believe this to be a detrimental treatment.[121] There are no data to support the validity of either point of view. Stimulation of the reflexes is discontinued once the patient has begun to move with volition.

Although reflexes are known to be the basis of voluntary motor patterns, [122,123] the development of reflex movement per se is not appropriate because reflex movement does not automatically become voluntary movement in brain-injured patients. Voluntary control of reflex-generated movement is encouraged by providing tasks for the patient to do that inherently demand movement similar to the reflex response. The reflex is elicited as the patient attempts to move purposefully. His attention is focused on the intent to do the task rather than on the actual step-by-step process of moving or the reflex response.

The stretch reflex is a component of every functionally organized movement, volitional or automatic, meaning that during normal movement the muscles opposite to those that are contracting are being stretched.[36] In therapy the stretch reflex is used to enhance the contraction of a muscle.

Quick, light, passive stretch is the best stimulus to use to elicit a response from the primary (Ia) afferent of the spindle, which monosynaptically facilitates a dynamic response of the same muscle being stretched.[124] Repeated, brief, light, short stretches are delivered by tapping the free end of the limb in the direction opposite to the pull of the muscles to be stimulated (Fig. 5.3) or by firmly tapping on the muscle belly or the tendon[37] with the ends of the four fingers held together (Fig. 5.4). The speed and amplitude of the stretch controls the level of response, [103] which is a brief, unsustained contraction of the stimulated muscle.

Firmer stretch or placing the muscle in a lengthened position is used to differentially elicit a response from the secondary (II) afferents of the muscle being stretched. Because it once was thought that the IIs always inhibit extension and always facilitate flexion no matter in which muscle they are located, therapists have learned, before asking for a movement, to place a limb in a position considered most advantageous for the weaker muscles. For example, to give the weaker extensor an advantage, the joint is extended at the start of movement,[125] which means that the extensor muscle is in its shortened range and its IIs are not activated. Current information is that the effect of stimulating the IIs more probably results in autogenetic excitation[37,126] depending on the thresholds of the interneurons to which the IIs connect as set by the CNS to serve the moment-to-moment needs of the organism.[37,38,106]

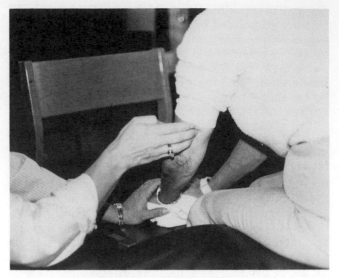

Figure 5.4 Facilitating the triceps by firmly tapping the tendon and muscle belly.

Because passive, or external, stretch of a muscle evokes only a monosynaptic tendon jerk, no learning occurs because there has been no coactivation of the alpha and gamma motor neurons. Therefore, when the muscle is externally stretched passively in the absence of a goal to move or maintain a posture, none of the process described on page 75 involving long loop stretch reflexes occurs. Neither is the response supported by the gamma motor system. Therefore, when using stretch as a facilitatory method, the therapist focuses the patient's attention on the goal, such as keeping the elbow straight when using the arm for weight bearing. To further augment the otherwise momentary, singular effect, the patient also may be asked to resist the obtained goal movement.

As described previously, resistance is a form of stretch that recruits motor units to overcome the imposed load. Resistance also causes cocontraction of muscles around the resisted joint. Too much resistance can cause abnormal movement by stressing the CNS, which responds by regressing to lower levels of behavior. The abnormal movement may be characterized by primitive reflexes or by synergistic responses caused by the overflow of excitation. Synergy refers to two or more muscles working together to accomplish a movement or posture or combination of these. For example, the wrist extensors and the finger flexors are normally synergistic in that the wrist extensors contract during grasp to add tension to the flexors and to prevent dropping the object held. Some synergies reflect primitive reflex coalitions of muscles that originally may have been useful to phylogenetically lower species, but are not useful for the skilled movement of humans. One is the flexor synergy, which is a withdrawal response in which the hand or foot is pulled away from the stimulus by contraction of all or most flexors/adductors within the limb. Another is the extensor synergy, which is a

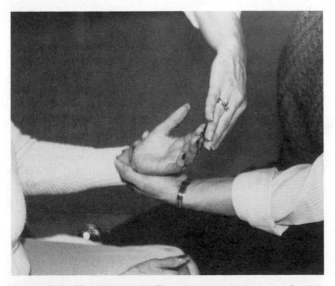

Figure 5.3 Facilitating the finger extensors by use of quick, light stretch by tapping the dorsal surface of the fingers.

supportive response in which the limb is stiffened and straightened in response to a stimulus. These synergies reappear in brain-injured patients and are detrimental to voluntary movement if they persist.

Another way that a stretch stimulus can be implemented is by the use of a vibrator, which delivers a series of stretches that produce a sustained (tetanized) response.[127,128] Such a response is desired to facilitate the extensor (antigravity) tonic muscles that are responsible for posture.[129]

Vibration has been well documented to selectively stretch the Ia afferents of the nuclear chain fibers, not the II endings.[37] The tonic vibration reflex (TVR) is a polysynaptic stretch reflex that depends not only on spinal pathways, but also on supraspinal pathways. Vibration is used to enhance an ongoing postural effort and to increase awareness of limb posture.

When a TVR is elicited, the tension within the muscle slowly increases. There is a rise time of 20[128] to 30[129] sec in normal subjects depending on the amount of initial relaxation of the muscle, before the response reaches its maximum; this may take longer in patients with a damaged CNS.[128] Because the primary afferents on the nuclear chain fibers respond to each small stretch delivered by the vibrator, the frequency of the vibrator is the most crucial paramenter of the stimulus application; it must be greater than 50 Hz. The most effective frequency range to elicit the TVR in humans is 100–200 Hz.[130] The amplitude of the vibrator determines the amount of stretch and therefore the number of receptors activated; 1–2 mm excursion produces a maximum TVR.[130]

Application of the vibrator to the tendon is more effective[127,128] than application to the muscle belly because more spindles are accessed. This choice is especially good for patients with a heavy-set body build in whom deeply located spindles may not get stimulated. On the other hand, in a very thin person, to limit the spread of the stimulus to antagonist muscles, the vibrator can be applied to the muscle belly. The choice of tendon or belly, although guided by these considerations, depends on the response of the individual patient.

The vibrator should be applied for at least 30 sec but not more than 1 or 2 min in any one place because the heat of friction produced by the vibrator may be uncomfortable.[125] Preferably, the vibrator is moved slowly over the area. The response lasts only as long as the stimulus is applied.[125] However, repeated short periods of vibration cumulatively increase the response to approach the maximum the muscle can exert.[37]

The strength of the TVR can be enhanced by lengthening the muscle at the time vibration is applied,[127,131] which combines the effects of the II stimulation of stretch with the TVR response. The TVR is even more greatly enhanced by voluntary contraction than by passive lengthening[127] especially if the muscle is isometrically contracted in the shortened range,[127,131] which activates most motor units. However, vibration applied to a muscle that is voluntarily maximally contracted adds nothing more to the response[127] because all motor units are engaged. Combining the TVR with a voluntary goal is the only way in which the reflex response can become incorporated into voluntary motor control (Fig. 5.5).

Vibration is an extremely effective method to increase the stretch sensitivity of tonic muscles and to inhibit antagonistic phasic muscles[127,128]; however, the results seen in patients with a damaged CNS can differ from those results seen in subjects with a normal CNS. In spastic patients, synergistic muscles acting on neighboring joints may show a sustained reflex contraction even if they are not vibrated. Even antagonists, usually reciprocally inhibited, sometimes have been found to be facilitated.[132] In patients with cerebellar disorders, vibration either aggravated their condition or had no effect.[125] As a general rule, vibration should not be applied if it accentuates a patient's motor disorder. Spastic muscles are never vibrated; their antagonists are vibrated.

Subgoal: To Decrease Tone. The difference between treatment to inhibit and that to facilitate is in the mode of application rather than the kind of stimuli used. Inhibition is also brought about indirectly through reciprocal inhibition, a neurophysiological organizing principle of the CNS in which the antagonist muscle is automatically inhibited when the agonist is facilitated.[36,125,131] Care must be exercised that an inhibitory response is actually occurring because recip-

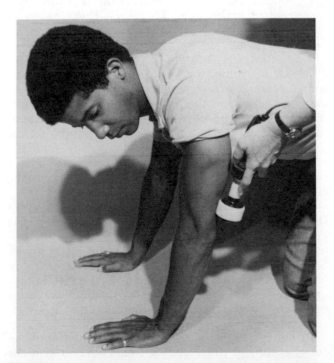

Figure 5.5 Vibration of triceps tendon contracted in a shortened range to assist achievement of full elbow extension in a weight-bearing position.

rocal inhibition may be faulty in persons with spasticity.[133]

Tactile Stimulation. Rood has identified a particular type of tactile stimulus for inhibition: slow stroking over the sensory distribution of the posterior primary rami. The effect is a general inhibition possibly due to a calming influence on the sympathetic chain since the autonomic nervous system is known to affect gamma firing.[134] The person lies prone in a quiet environment. The therapist uses the palm of her hand or extended fingers to apply firm pressure over the skin of the back alongside the spine from the occiput to the coccyx in a slow, rhythmical manner. Inhibition should occur within minutes.

Thermal Stimulation. Prolonged icing of more than 3 minutes' duration inhibits muscle contraction[103,135,136] for generally 30 to 60 min; however, the response differs for every patient.[104] It is used in therapy by applying an ice cube or ice pack over the muscle group or by immersing the limb in ice water. The precautions cited earlier relative to icing apply here also. Additionally after removal of the ice and as the muscle warms, there may be a rebound effect in which greater tone[137] or increased strength[116] is exhibited.

One group[138] has had some success with the use of prolonged icing of the extensor muscles of patients with intention tremor; they did not report seeing the rebound phenomenon. The tremor was decreased for as long as the ice was used and in some cases up to 30 min posttreatment. To further test the results, the researchers cooled the flexor muscles and also warmed the extensor muscles; they found that the tremor was increased in both cases. Therefore, they concluded that prolonged icing of extensor muscles decreased intention tremor.

Vestibular Stimulation. Very slow rhythmical movement is inhibiting. A general decrease in hypertonicity should be seen within minutes. Any apprehension on the part of the patient concerning the treatment will cancel its effectiveness; therefore, the stimulus must be applied in a way that is comfortable for the patient. The stimulus can be delivered by manually rolling the patient from side lying to supine and back repetitively or by use of a hammock, swing, or rocking chair.

Proprioceptive Stimulation. Slow stretch is the best stimulus to directly relax a given muscle or muscle group.[103] Stretch, prolonged over several minutes during which the patient's limb is not moved, results in an adjustment of the intrafusal muscle fibers to a new longer length.[139] The therapist can feel this "letting go" of the hypertonic muscle. Greater range of motion is gained by stretching in this manner increment by increment.

Prolonged stretch provides the rationale for use of serial casting in which spastic limbs are casted at the end of easily obtainable range. The cast is left on 7 to 10 days, and then is changed to one that holds the limb in a new, slightly improved position of correction. Cast changes continue until the amount of range desired has been achieved; then the bivalved cast is used only at night so that the limb is left free during the day to relearn active movement control.[101]

Prolonged stretch, applied as pressure maintained for 10 sec on a tendon, has been shown to be immediately effective in normal subjects in reducing alpha motor neuron excitability. However, since the effect only lasted 5 to 30 sec,[140] its use is limited.

Vibration is reciprocally inhibitory when it is applied to the weaker antagonist of the spastic muscle.

Resistance can be used to inhibit or damp movement in persons with ataxia by applying weight cuffs to the wrist or ankle. There is an optimal weight for each person, determined by trial and error, and to exceed that amount voids the effect of weighting.[141,142] Unfortunately, this treatment is limited to those ataxic patients who are strong enough to be able to move against the amount of weight necessary to dampen their involuntary movement.

GOAL: TO REACQUIRE MATURATIONALLY BASED POSTURAL AND MOVEMENT PATTERNS

Maturationally based motor patterns are those that have been genetically inscribed in the nervous system and that manifest themselves through the developmental process witnessed in normal children. These patterns form the basis for acquired motor skills[17,25,123,143]; therefore, if they are deficient it is hypothesized by some,[111,120,121] but not all,[144] that they must be reacquired before normal skilled movement can be expected.

Treatment principles to be used to implement this goal reflect each patient's particular problems as determined by neurodevelopmental evaluation. If the patient's motor behavior is dominated by primitive reflexes (asymmetrical tonic neck reflex, tonic labyrinthine reflex, associated reactions, etc.), then the principle to be used in treatment is integration of primitive reflexes. If the patient manifests automatic postural adjustments, indicating integration of the lower-level reflexes, but is unable to carry out ontogenetic postural and movement patterns, the principle used becomes recapitulation of ontogenetic developmental sequence.

Patients whose lesions occur in adulthood presumably developed movement control normally at one time, indicating that these innate programs existed. Since the lesion may not have actually destroyed the program, but only memory of it,[19,78,145] or sensory access to it,[57] the patient may be able to recover these patterns through use of motor learning methodologies.

Principle: Integration of Primitive Reflexes

Although the spinal and brain stem reflexes are the earliest building blocks of motor skill development, they need to be prevented from dominating the motor output of the patient. The tonic brain stem reflexes, evident in non-brain-damaged persons when they are working under great stress (excess resistance or at the limits of endurance),[122] are all the more evident in the motor behavior of brain-damaged patients whose nervous system, already distressed, has limited capacity for coping with additional stress.[146] Stressful conditions that occur in therapy include fatigue, fear of falling, excessive effort to overcome gravity or resistance, demand for a motor response beyond the current capability of the patient, or the complexity of the activity used as the medium.[146] In the adult cerebrovascular-accident patient, as in normal subjects, primitive reflexes are not demonstrable under nonstressed conditions.[146]

Integration of the primitive reflexes means that although they remain available as program components when extra effort is needed, they do not appear readily. When integration has occurred, the stimuli evoke the more mature righting responses that are needed for voluntary ambulation and interaction with the environment rather than these reflexes. The procedure to integrate the reflexes in stroke patients or others with circumscribed lesions is to avoid stressful situations in which these reflexes would manifest themselves and immediately decrease the stress when the primitive reflexes appear. As the CNS heals and as motor control improves with training, more task complexity can be required without precipitating the stress reaction. In patients with diffuse cortical damage, the reflexes may occur when little exogenous stress is apparent. Treatment to integrate the reflexes may include (1) positioning of the spastic limbs opposite to the position they would assume in response to the stimulus to decrease the tone in hyperactive muscles through prolonged stretch and (2) stimulation of the righting, then later the equilibrium, reactions while manually preventing the lower-level reflex-bound response from occurring and simultaneously helping the patient to move into the correct righting response.

Some therapists believe the patient's attention should not be focused on the response since righting and equilibrium reactions are automatic stimulus-response mechanisms mediated by the basal ganglia below conscious awareness and acquired by normal infants and animals when the wiring in their CNS matures enough to allow the response. These therapists believe that by assisting the patient to move repetitively into the higher-level responses when the stimulus is given, the automatic stimulus-response mechanism will be reactivated. Others believe that because the CNS is different after a lesion, the wiring is disrupted; therefore, relearning—the components of which are attention, feedback, and practice—is required. Much research is needed to determine if one point of view is more valid than the other. Meanwhile, the student therapist may want to incorporate ideas from both practices by demanding a simple, yet meaningful, motor goal that uses the stimulus that could either evoke a reflex or righting reaction while manually guiding the patient to shape the correct response. A simple activity to evoke the neck righting reaction would be to have the patient, while supine in bed, turn his head to look at something on the bedside table and attempt to reach for it with the hand opposite to the location of the table. This would require him to roll over and would counter the asymmetrical tonic neck reflex. Manual guidance would be needed to start the roll over and perhaps to begin the arm moving toward the table.

Integration of primitive reflexes has been particularly addressed by the Bobaths in their treatment of children with cerebral palsy, and it is also used by therapists to treat adult patients with diffuse cortical damage. See chapter 6 for an overview of their method.

Principle: Recapitulation of Developmental Sequence

Recapitulation of developmental sequence is believed basic to redevelopment of voluntary motor control in which acquired motor skills are based on the "hard wired" or innate postural and movement programs.[123] This preadaptive phase of motor control appears automatically as the infant matures.[123] No motor learning theories address the redevelopment of these innate components of movement since theory development is currently limited to understanding how normal subjects, in whom these components are intact, acquire motor skills. Therapists know that movement can be learned without this base, but it is done in a task-by-task fashion and lacks the flexibility characteristic of true skilled motor performance. Therefore, therapists attempt to help the patient reacquire this base of control.

Recapitulation starts at the point where the patient has control. Several developmental sequences intertwine, so a specific treatment must take each into consideration. One sequence is based on direction of development of control (cephalocaudal; proximodistal; ulnar [power] to radial [precision]). The proximal-to-distal control sequence is still currently used in treatment, although it has been challenged by evidence that muscles of these regions are subserved by two separate control systems [42] and that control of the motor functions of these areas may be independent in children.[147,148] Another sequence reflects the motor milestones seen in children and reviewed in chapter 4. Another is based on types of muscles and movements (flexion and adduction precede extension and abduction, which precede rotation; withdrawal responses precede maintained contact responses). Yet another developmental sequence is the interaction of control of movement and posture, the two motor patterns that interweave to accomplish the motor tasks of life. The sequence of development of control is as follows: Spontaneous movement (mobility) occurs first, followed by learning to hold a limb in a posture anywhere within range (stability). Then moving in a controlled way within range is learned. Finally being able to combine proximal stability with distal movement, the essential requirement of skilled use of the extremity, is learned.[137]

Mobility. For the patient who is unable to move, movement is evoked by any means including eliciting reflex responses singly or in combination. Controlled sensory facilitation is used to provoke the withdrawal reflex, the tonic neck and labyrinthine reflexes, or associated reactions. The reflex is evoked in combination with a demand for voluntary effort to accomplish a goal that is developmentally appropriate for the patient's abilities. The flexor/adductor muscles are facilitated first. Removing the counterforces of gravity and resistance by supporting the arm in the therapist's hand placed under the elbow, on a "skate" (Fig. 5.6), or in a mobile arm support allows the limb to move as a result of the stimulus. Once the response occurs, it is reinforced by adding resistance to the evoked movement to recruit more motor units and to cause a central reprogramming of the motor units, which is essential for learning. Other sensory stimuli are added to enhance the ongoing movement. The patient gets somatosensory and visual feedback because of the movement. As the pattern is learned through repetition, the facilitation is deleted from treatment, starting with the stimuli that cause the most primitive responses. Variations of the newly learned response are practiced and used functionally. Once gross spontaneous reciprocal movements are possible, stability responses are sought.

Stability. A stability response requires a tonic contraction of muscles evoked through appropriate sensory stimulation, a demand for a holding response in developmental sequence, and repetition to learn it. Stability refers to cocontraction of the agonist and antagonist muscles around a joint to maintain a posture against gravity. Controlled sensory facilitation is used to enhance the antigravity extensor/abductor (tonic) muscles because they need facilitation to achieve cocontraction with the flexors, which are usually hypertonic in cases of cortical damage. The flexors of the upper extremities in humans are the antigravity muscles in the upright posture[149]; therefore, whether this reasoning holds for the upper extremities needs study. The stimuli used are those that cause a tonic response, for example, highly repetitive tactile stimulation, vibration, or repeated tapping of the muscle belly or tendon.

Sensory facilitation is applied as the patient attempts to (has the plan to) hold a weight-bearing posture. The adult patient can do these postures in a modified way rather than get into the exact developmental posture, which may feel undignified to him. One modification is to place the arm in a weight-bearing posture while sitting on a raised mat or to lean forward on the elbows or outstretched arm while engaged in a game or holding down something being worked on by the other hand. Weight-bearing postures are used because they evoke cocontraction responses,[137] as long as the person is not balancing in the posture using only his ligaments and articular surfaces. Electromyographic evidence has shown that if the parts are lined up, one on top of the other, no muscle output occurs in normal subjects.[46,150,151] As soon as the person is off balance or must take a greater part of the weight distribution on that limb, the muscles do contract in response to the demand to regain the balance and maintain the posture.[151] Therefore, the therapist

must be sure the activity requires the limb to be in a position other than perpendicular to the surface so that the muscles will be activated. Unilateral weight bearing in which the limb must support more of the body weight in a more precariously balanced position also activates the muscles. In the beginning the patient will need to attend especially to keeping the joint steady, and the therapist will need to facilitate the extensor muscle(s) serving that joint. The patient should concentrate on the kinesthetic feedback when he has successfully achieved the posture. The posture is practiced by holding it for increasing amounts of time while attention is diverted.

Combined Mobility and Stability. When the patient has learned to hold a posture for 1 to 2 min, the next step would be for him to move within that posture by rocking his weight onto and off the limb while stabilized distally either against a surface or by tightly grasping something. For example, if the patient is developing control of the upper extremity, he can be seated on a raised mat with the affected arm used as a support while he reaches with the other arm to move game pieces or other task materials from one side of the mat to the other or to a table placed in front, slightly toward the involved side. In the process, the weight of the upper body first comes over the arm and then is removed. He learns control by moving slightly away from the stable position in all directions as the need to reach is changed by the therapist, who controls the placement of the materials. The patient concentrates on controlling the movement of the proximal joint for greater and greater precision. When precise

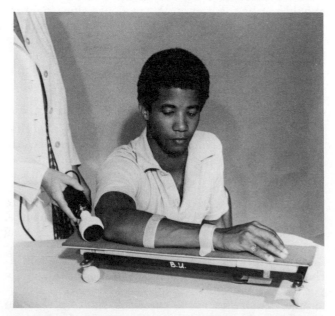

Figure 5.6 The affected arm is supported on a therapeutic skate; elbow extension is sought and facilitated by vibrating the triceps.

control of the proximal segment has been learned, the next step is for the patient to learn to automatically activate the scapular and shoulder muscles as required to place the hand in space. This is ordinarily the programmed part of upper-extremity skilled movement. Programmed movements are typically ballistic patterns controlled as open-loop systems. Open-loop control of motor performance develops first under closed-loop conditions in which the person plans the movement, attends to and appreciates the sensory feedback, and relates this to the outcome (knowledge of results) repeatedly until the feel of the movement is learned and attention need no longer be focused on it. Attention is then freed for learning of skilled movement of the hand.[152]

An example of integrating these sequences may clarify the therapist's task in designing a particular treatment session. For example, assume that the evaluation reveals that the patient is able to maintain a prone-on-elbows position when placed (has stability), but is unable to assume it or move within it (lacks controlled mobility) and is unable to hold a quadruped position (the next ontogenetic motor milestone). This indicates that control has progressed cephalocaudally through to the upper trunk but not to the lower trunk and is developing in the scapular girdle but not yet in the pelvic girdle or in the elbows. Controlled movement within the prone-on-elbows posture is the immediate goal to be addressed. Controlled movement requires agonist and antagonist muscles to contract and relax alternately; therefore, the therapeutic activity must demand this response. Once the patient can control shoulder and scapular movement within this posture, the next immediate goal can either be to develop control of the lower trunk and pelvic girdle (cephalocaudal developmental sequence) or to develop elbow control (proximodistal developmental sequence). If development of elbow control is chosen on the basis of need to develop functional use of the upper extremity, this would start with learning to position the elbow anywhere in range by simultaneous contraction of the flexors and extensors (stability). If the adult patient demonstrated head and trunk balance in sitting, he could be seated to work on this goal. The activity would demand the elbow-holding response; perhaps by holding something that the noninvolved or lesser-involved hand would work on or (if the patient had distal motor control, a developmental oddity sometimes seen) by holding the affected limb in a certain position in space, using elbow cocontraction, while manipulating a tool for the skilled aspect of the activity. If the response becomes maladaptive (increased tone; incoordinated, reflexive, synergistic movement) because the demand exceeds the patient's capabilities, the patient is stopped or allowed to continue in a lower developmental posture.[76] Patients should be warned that regression to unwanted reflex motor patterns is a normal sign of stress in the CNS and should be taught how to deal with the situation.[86]

GOAL: TO ACQUIRE OR REACQUIRE SKILLED VOLUNTARY MOVEMENT

Reacquisition of skilled voluntary movement is based on (1) principles of recapitulation of developmental sequences of control and (2) relearning of acquired skills in which new movement builds on previously learned movement. Whereas early voluntary movement is based on a background of maturational responses,[88] later skilled movement is a refinement[8,53,100,143] or a recombination of previously learned skills.[143,153]

Principle: Learning or Relearning

Theories of how persons with normal central nervous systems learn motor skills are in their beginning stages of testing; extrapolation to persons with CNS deficits is based on almost no data as to what differences exist between how normal persons and CNS-damaged patients control movement, learn new motor skills, or relearn formerly know motor skills. Skill acquisition is hierarchical[123] and consists of three stages. The first is the cognitive-motor stage. Cognitive processes or strategies are much more involved than previously realized in the acquisition of complex motor behaviors.[29,154] In this stage, the learner formulates a plan about the skill to be learned and develops control strategies that include the contractile patterns for the action and sensory interactions relating the action to the environment.[151] The plan is defined in terms of coordinative structures, the fundamental unit of control, defined as a group of muscles operating synergistically over one or more joints that act as a single unit.[123,155,156] The coordinative structure provides a control system with one degree of freedom control over a unit containing many possible degrees of freedom.[156] New synergies or coordinative structures are constructed from basic reflexive synergies, previously learned synergies, or trial-and-error experimentation. Learning focuses on temporally organizing the contractions of the agonist and antagonist, that is, developing strategies.

In the fixation stage, cognitive-perceptual-motor integration occurs, and the new program is stabilized. The sensory motor integration of temporal and spatial patterns of movement replace cognition as the controlling variable in the execution of the skill.[157] A sign of this is that the patient can do two actions at once. In this stage the movement also is refined by reducing both the number of motor units recruited in a synergy and the frequency of cocontraction and associated movements, all signs of immature motor skill.[46]

Automation occurs in the third stage, in which parts of the synergy become stored as program modules for use ad lib and are available to be recombined subcortically to meet novel environmental demands.

Automaticity refers to tasks performed quickly, effortlessly, and autonomously. Automaticity does not equate to skill,[158] which is defined as harmonious coordination of component movement elements organized in time and space to achieve a desired goal.[156] For movement to be skillful it must be purposeful, efficient, and adaptable.[156] Both skill and automaticity are acquired only through practice.[158]

The important components of motor learning are attention, feedback, knowledge of results, and practice. Each will be considered separately but are applied in combination to each stage of learning.

Attention. Initiating corrective movements demands attention, whereas monitoring feedback does not.[159] The goal of the second stage of learning is to advance from conscious control to feedback control. An inexperienced performer requires active and conscious participation to learn a task, whereas conscious involvement is uncharacteristic of an experienced individual's performance.[159]

Voluntary control of a muscle under direct consciousness provides the basis for development of an automated pattern or engram.[143] Without conscious attention to movement, learning will not take place.[9,15] Conscious control is limited to one motion, muscle action, or position at a time. A normal person can shift attention only two to three times per second; therefore, the activity to be learned must be limited in complexity and performed very slowly compared to the rate of performance of normal automatic activity.[143]

Feedback. In the first phase of learning when the perceptual trace (or reference) for the movement has to be developed, feedback is essential. The reference or template specifies the value that the sensors should detect for a particular movement so that when the sensation is fed back, it can be compared to this reference for error detection and correction if necessary.[155] Information necessary to control movement is provided by a combination of the visual sense of eye position with respect to surrounding surfaces, the vestibular sense of head orientation in inertial-gravitational space, and the somatic sense of body segment positions in relation to one another and to the support surface.[151]

Lack of precise sensory feedback in the early stages of learning interferes with proper development of the perceptual trace. A deficit in flow of proprioceptive and/or exteroceptive sensory information after the trace is formed causes disturbed skilled motor performance. Because the patient needs to receive reliable information concerning the movement, visual and auditory feedback may need to be substituted for unreliable proprioceptive feedback.[160,161] In cases of "vague sensory feedback" augmented feedback can provide better information about movement and therefore increase learning.[162]

Teaching the patient not only to attend to feedback but to structure the interpretation of the input improves the patient's chance of getting the full meaning of the information and reduces the cortical processing space requirements[29] by increasing the processing capacity. If a patient can process information faster, he can do movement sequences faster. Effective methods to help the person improve these information-processing abilities have not yet been published.

Knowledge of Results and Knowledge of Performance. The single most important variable governing learning of motor skills is knowledge of results.[163] Precise knowledge of results, up to an optimal level, increases learning; beyond that level it exceeds the information-processing capacity and learning is detrimentally affected.[154,164] To help the patient notice that he missed a target by a certain distance rather than just noting that he failed to hit it is an example of increasing the precision of the knowledge of results. The interval after knowledge of results must be long enough to allow processing of the information; the more precise the knowledge of results, the greater the interval needed[165,166] before making the next attempt to do the action.

The ability to use more precise knowledge of results (up to an optimal level) increases with age and increasing information-processing capabilities of the developing brain.[154] Changes in the information-processing ability accounts for a significant proportion of the variance in improved performance associated with development.[166] The greater the capacity of the system, the greater the amount of information that can be included in each chunk to be processed; therefore, the faster the processing. Small children process slower due to ineffectual strategies for moving information within the memory system.[166] Elderly persons process slower than younger adult subjects on cognitive processing tasks because they use the slower serial processing mode rather than faster simultaneous (parallel) processing mode; no differences between the groups were found on those tasks for which serial processing was approriately used.[167]

Knowledge of results represents information about what happened relative to the outcome of response, not how the action was completed.[163,165] Knowledge of performance provides information about the movement itself.[71,163,165] Focusing on knowledge of performance may most effectively assist learning skills in which the movement pattern is supposed to match an externally imposed criterion (diving, gymnastics, crutchwalking).[165] Knowledge of performance is best used when the action is to be invariant and when the learner is trying to increase consistency.[168] Knowledge of results is used when variable actions can meet the same goal (feeding, throwing at a target).[168] Knowledge of performance can be developed by use of videotape replay and verbal cueing by which the person's sense of how the movement felt is related to the model. The effectiveness of these teaching tools depends on the skill level of the performer. Beginners need much verbal cueing along with the videotape to direct their attention to key points or to sort out the information given on the videotape.

Practice. Once a correct response is elicited, it must be repeatedly practiced correctly for learning to occur. Practice is repetition with the intention to improve.[19] Practice brings organization and consistency to muscle interactions of learned synergies to produce a fixed pattern.[123]

Automatic neuromuscular control is the highest level of motor learning.[6,143] An automatic response is characterized by decreased variability and speed. Automatic control of postures and movements indicates that patterns of muscle contraction have become programmed. Practice is necessary for an automatic programmed level of control. It is believed that repetitious use of the same synaptic pathways results in development of an engram[92,143] that enhances the likelihood of that pathway activating as a whole when the appropriate stimulus is encountered.[15] Hundreds[156] or thousands[143] of repetitions are needed to begin to form an engram. Millions are needed to perfect it.[143] Sufficient practice is indicated when measured improvement reaches a plateau.

If a skill is not practiced sufficiently for it to become automatic, then performance level will swiftly decline when attention and feedback are withdrawn.[86,162]

The whole response of which the patient is capable should be practiced using as close to normal timing as possible. Once the whole response is developing, perfection of each part can be stressed separately.[19] Practice should occur using the implements and in the environment that is natural for the response.[19] This idea, used in athletic training, is most appropriate for brain-damaged patients. For transfer of training to occur, practice must include variability.[154]

Practice sessions that distribute rest periods between bouts of practice have been found most effective in athletic training.[19] Practice sessions can be continuous with brief rests or alternately can be organized into periods of brief practice and extended rest. Practice should not produce fatigue because performance deteriorates with fatigue.

Mental rehearsal of the sequence of the motor task is helpful[18] because it holds the information in short-term memory long enough to be transferred to long-term memory.[77] Mental rehearsal of movement sequences activates the cortical area responsible for programming of skilled movement.[69] It should not be assumed that patients with CNS damage can use mental rehearsal, but some may be able to do so to their benefit. Mental rehearsal can be verbal (sequential) or nonverbal (imagery of concrete objects).[169] Imagery enhances memory more than verbal rehearsal alone.[169] Individual differences have been found in normal subjects in the vividness of their imagery; more vivid imagers were able to reproduce movement more accurately.[169]

Teaching Process. In the cognitive-motor stage, the learner must understand the task in terms of the goal, the movement necessary to reach the goal, and the strategy that will work best to produce the desired movement. It is unhelpful to instruct a person via tactical details,[13] that is, which muscles to contract or relax. The learner can discover the strategies himself by trial and error by referring to similar patterns within his repertoire or can be guided in selecting strategies. Imposing a strategy on the learner with a normal nervous system will help him achieve initial skill acquisition faster, but only a self-initiated strategy will enable transfer of the learning to new situations.[170] Therefore, it is best to teach the learner what the strategies are and how to use them. We only have beginning evidence at this time that some patients with cortical damage may lack basic strategies, whereas these are preserved in other types of brain damage.[151]

The simplest potentially successful level for most deficient patients would be practice of prime mover control; however, if the patient has correct simple engrams these can be combined into more complex units.[143] Each component should be practiced before chaining it into more complex patterns.[143] Subdividing the activity into units simple enough for the patient to be able to do successfully at his current level of coordination has been used with good results. This part-to-whole learning was used to teach activities of daily living to a patient with cortical damage due to cerebral anoxia.[171] Complex motions (eating, writing) were analyzed and segmented into smaller isolated chronological component steps, which were then presented sequentially as an exercise program. The patient practiced these motions and eventually built each step into an automatic whole motion.[171]

The trainer can facilitate learning in the cognitive-motor stage in the following way. The learner is encouraged to feel competent enough to do the task. The learning experience is structured so that the patient has complete understanding of the task to be performed.[14,143] He is helped to attend selectively to instruction given orally and visually. The patient can be instructed by demonstrating the performance to him or by passively manipulating his limbs. Instruction can also be given through use of movies or videotapes of expert performance or provision of videotape feedback. Videotapes are useful in that they can show the skill at normal and slow motion, and close-ups can be included to emphasize the key elements for efficient performance. Each videotape should be limited to one skill and be short to avoid overload.[157] Instruction should include a description of the implements to be used insofar as they are absolutely necessary to do the task. Instruction is presented immediately before performance.[157] The level and amount of information are kept within the processing capacity of the patient because success depends on the effectiveness of the information-processing system. The amount of formal instruction given to the patient also depends on his familiarity with the skill.

The patient should do the task slowly, precisely, and effortlessly under direct conscious control and no resistance should be offered.[143] The therapist should manually assist if necessary to prevent excessive contraction of antagonists or synergists.[143] Precise control can be exerted through the pyramidal system only when the patient is relaxed, the effort is low and attention is directed to the activity being attempted.[143] The person is cued to attend to specific somesthetic feedback in relation to the outcome of the movement.[18,19,71]

His attention is directed to the kinesthetic feedback more than therapist's guidance because the former is perceived faster (500 msec) than the latter (2 to 5 sec).[143]

In the fixation[157] or kinesthetic stage, the trainer is most helpful by structuring the consistency of the environment and the schedule of practice and rest and by cueing the person to attend to specific sensations, which helps him develop knowledge of performance.[19,21,71] The goal of this stage is to develop consistency of performance over trials.[71]

The goal of the third stage of learning is automaticity characterized by attention reduction. The patient is given the opportunity to do the action repetitively without having his attention called to the process of moving by the therapist. Paying attention to automatic movement performance, such as describing the steps as they occur or noticing the correctness of a component, destroys the automaticity of the behavior.[159]

Once the person with CNS deficit has developed an ability to move each joint of the limb independently of others, an indication of normal voluntary control, then the treatment goals become those of increasing coordination and dexterity, that is, improving the accuracy (end point control) and the speed. The principles described for the biomechanical approach to increase strength and endurance would also be appropriate.

Effectiveness

The effectiveness of neurodevelopmental therapy to restore functional movement control lacks definitive documentation.[86] Although anecdotal reports from therapists attest to the effectiveness of some of the methods, small-group research has failed to date to support major effectiveness.[172,173] The truth may be that certain methods of this approach are differentially effective for some patients but not others. The need to identify the variables that invariantly control outcome to enable more specific application of the methods to appropriate patients has reached crisis levels with the introduction of the prospective payment system, which limits the patient's hospital stay. Neurodevelopmental treatment as it is now practiced requires an extensive time commitment and without adequate demonstration of its success is in jeopardy of continuing as a treatment option.

A few limited studies have even begun to raise doubts about the validity of some of the assumptions on which neurodevelopmental therapy is based. For instance, the ideas that proximal control must precede distal control[147,148] or that function improves as a consequence of increased motor unit activity[174] have not been supported. These studies need replication and other studies must be done until all the assumptions are tested.

For those persons prevented from receiving this treatment due to financial regulations, or those unable to benefit from this approach, the only treatment option that remains is the compensatory Rehabilitation Approach, by which patients are taught to be as independent as they can be despite their disability. Competency in life tasks is the essential goal of occupational therapy.

Summary of General Concepts of Motor Control Therapy

1. The demands made of the patient for posture and movement must be within his capability so he can receive the reward of accomplishment.
2. The demands follow the sequences in which posture and movement develop.
3. The patient's effort is enhanced with peripheral stimulation.
4. A reflex response is evoked only in conjunction with volition so that the patient learns to control the evoked response.
5. A correct response is practiced repeatedly in varied functional activities until it becomes an automatic, flexible motor pattern.
6. The demand is upgraded by gradually requiring the posture to be held slightly longer or the movement to be done slightly more precisely.
7. When the patient begins to lose control, the demand is lessened to again be within his control.
8. When the patient's motor behavior becomes reflexive, a sign of distress, the source of stress on the patient is removed.

STUDY QUESTIONS:

Motor Control Therapy

1. What are the various capabilities that contribute to a person's ability to move normally?
2. List the six steps of the Model of Motor Control and Learning in order to describe the process of motor performance and learning.
3. What are the differences between open-loop movements and closed-loop movements?
4. How is the concept of alpha and gamma motor neuron coactivtion used in therapy?
5. Describe negative and positive motor deficits seen in patients with CNS dysfunction.
6. What are the mechanisms of recovery after brain damage?
7. What are the principles related to the goal of preventing limitation of range of motion?
8. How does controlled sensory manipulation affect motor output?
9. List the sensory stimuli that are used therapeutically to increase tone. Describe the responses expected for each.
10. What precautions have been cited regarding the use of thermal, vestibular, and proprioceptive stimulation?
11. What does "integration of primitive reflexes" mean?
12. In using the principle of recapitulation of developmental sequence, what are the various developmental sequences that must be considered in each treatment session?
13. Why might the motor behavior of a patient with brain damage regress to unwanted reflex motor patterns?
14. What are the three stages of motor learning? What teaching processes are used in each?
15. What are the important components of motor learning?

References

1. Moore, J. C. Recovery potentials following CNS lesions: a brief historical perspective in relation to modern research data on neuroplasticity. *Am. J. Occup. Ther.,40*(7): 459-463, 1986.
2. Johansson, R. S., and Westling, G. Roles of glabrous skin receptors and sensorimotor memory in automatic control of precision grip when lifting rougher or more slippery objects. *Exp. Brain Res., 56*: 550-564, 1984.
3. Scholz, J. P., and Campbell, S. K. Muscle spindles and the regulation of movement. *Phys. Ther, 60*(11): 1416-1424, 1980.
4. Nashner, L. M., and Wollacott, M. The organization of rapid postural adjustments of standing humans: an experimental-conceptual model. In *Posture and Movement.* Edited by R. E. Talbott and D. R. Humphrey. New York: Raven Press, 1979.
5. Sanes, J. N., Mauritz, K.-H., Evarts, E. V., Dalakas, M. C., and Chu, A. Motor deficits in patients with large-fiber sensory neuropathy. *Proc. Natl. Acad. Sci. USA, 81*: 979-982, 1984.
6. Granit, R. *The Purposive Brain.* Cambridge, MA: MIT Press, 1977.
7. Connolly, K. The nature of motor skill development. *J. Human Movement Studies, 3*: 128-143, 1977.
8. Marsden, C. D. The mysterious motor function of the basal ganglia: the Robert Wartenberg lecture. *Neurology, 32*: 514-539, 1982.
9. Klein, R. M. Attention and movement. In *Motor Control: Issues and Trends,* Edited by G. E. Stelmach. New York: Academic Press, 1976.
10. Adams, J. A., Gopher, D., and Lintern, G. Effects of visual and proprioceptive feedback on motor learning. *J. Motor Behavior, 9*(1): 11-22, 1977.
11. Brooks, V. B. Roles of cerebellum and basal ganglia in initiation and control of movements. *J. Neurol. Sci, 2*(3): 265-277, 1975.
12. Cheney, P. D. Role of cerebral cortex in voluntary movements: a review. *Phys. Ther., 65*(5): 624-635, 1985.
13. Miller, G. A., Galanter, E., and Pribram, K. H. *Plans and the Structure of Behavior.* New York: Henry Holt & Co., 1960.
14. Brooks, V. B. *The Neural Basis of Motor Control.* New York: Oxford University Press, 1986.
15. Gardner, E. B. The neurophysiological basis of motor learning. *Phys. Ther., 47*: 1115-1222, 1967.
16. Adams, J. A. Issues for a closed-loop theory of motor learning. In *Motor Control: Issues and Trends.* Edited by G. E. Stelmach. New York: Academic Press, 1976.
17. Rosenbaum, D. A., Inhoff, A. W., and Gordon, A. M. Choosing between movement sequences: a hierarchical editor model. *J. Exp. Psychol. [Gen.], 113*(3): 372-393, 1984.
18. Keele, S. W., and Summers, J. J. The structure of motor programs. In *Motor Control: Issues and Trends.* Edited by G. E. Stelmach. New York: Academic Press, 1976.
19. Schmidt, R. A. *Motor Control and Learning: A Behavioral Emphasis,* 2nd edition. Champaign, IL: Human Kinetics Publishers, 1988.
20. Schmidt, R. A. The 1984 C. H. McCloy research lecture: the search for invariance in skilled movement behavior. *Res. Q. Exerc. Sport, 56*(2): 188-200, 1985.
21. Pribram, K. H. The neurophysiology of remembering. *Sci. Am., 220*: 73-86, 1969.
22. Atkinson, R. C., and Shiffrin, R. M. The control of short-term memory. *Sci. Am., 225*: 82-90, 1971.
23. Kelso, J. A. S., Southard, D. L., and Goodman, D. On the nature of human interlimb coordination. *Science, 203*(March 9): 1029-1031, 1979.
24. Merton, P. A. How we control the contraction of our muscles. *Sci. Am., 226*(5): 30-37, 1972.
25. Thelen, E., and Fisher, D. M. From spontaneous to instrumental behavior: kinematic analysis of movement changes during very early learning. *Child Dev. 54*: 129-140, 1983.
26. Jeannerod, M. The timing of natural prehension movements. *J Motor Behavior, 16*(3): 235-254, 1984.
27. Granit, R., and Burke, R. E. The control of movement and posture. *Brain Res., 53*: 1-28, 1973.
28. Evarts, E. V. The third Stevenson lecture: changing concepts of central control of movement. *Can. J. Physiol. Pharmacol., 53*: 191-201, 1975.
29. Singer, R. N. Cognitive processes, learner strategies, and skilled motor behaviors. *Can. J. Appl. Sport Sci. 5*(1): 25-32, 1980.
30. Polit, A. and Bizzi, E. Characteristics of motor programs underlying arm movements in monkeys. *J Neurophysiol. 42*(1): 183-194, 1979.
31. Stein, R. B. Peripheral control of movement. *Physiol. Rev., 54*(1): 215-243, 1974.
32. Gazzangia, M. Sensory motor control mechanisms. In *The Bisected Brain.* Edited by M. Gazzangia. New York: Appleton-Century-Crofts, 1970.
33. Sanes, J. N., and Jennings, V. A. Centrally programmed patterns of muscle activity in voluntary motor behavior of humans. *Exp. Brain Res., 54*: 23-32, 1984.
34. Hallett, M., Shahani, B. T., and Young, R. R. EMG analysis of patients with cerebellar deficits. *J. Neurol. Neurosurg. Psychiatry, 38*: 1163-1169, 1975.
35. Vallbo, A. B. Discharge patterns in human muscle spindle afferents during isometric voluntary contractions. *Acta Physiol. Scand., 80*: 552-566, 1970.
36. Granit, R. The functional role of the muscle spindle—facts and hypotheses, *Brain, 98*: 531-556, 1975.
37. Matthews, P. B. C. *Mammalian Muscle Receptors and Their Central Actions.* Baltimore: Williams & Wilkins, 1972.
38. Moore, J. C. The Golgi tendon organ: a review and update. *Am. J. Occup. Ther., 38*(4): 227-236, 1984.
39. Lawrence, D. G., and Hopkins, D. A. The development of motor control in the rhesus monkey: evidence concerning the role of corticomotoneuronal connections. *Brain, 99*: 235-254, 1976.
40. Evarts, E. V. Brain mechanisms in movement. *Sci. Am., 224*: 96, 1973.
41. Abend, W., Bizzi, E., and Morasso, P. Human arm trajectory formation. *Brain, 105*: 331-348, 1982.
42. Lawrence, D. G., and Kuypers, H. G. J. M. Pyramidal and nonpyramidal pathways in monkeys: anatomical and functional correlation. *Science, 148*(May 14): 973-975, 1965.
43. Freund, H.-J., and Hummelsheim, H. Premotor cortex in man: evidence for innervation of proximal limb muscles. *Exp. Brain Res., 53*: 479-482, 1984.
44. Haaxma, R., and Kuypers, H. Role of occipito-frontal cortico-cortical connections in visual guidance of relatively independent hand and finger movements in rhesus monkeys. *Brain Res., 71*: 361-366, 1974.
45. Buller, A. J. The neural control of the contractile mechanism in skeletal muscle. *Endeavor, 29*: 107-111, 1970.
46. Basmajian, J. V., and De Luca, C. J. *Muscles Alive: Their Functions Revealed by Electromyography,* 5th edition. Baltimore: Williams & Wilkins, 1985.
47. De Luca, C. J., LeFever, R. S., McCue, M. P., and Xenakis, A. P. Behaviour of human motor units in different muscles during linearly varying contractions. *J. Physiol., 329: 13-128, 1982.*
48. Henneman, E. The Size Principle: How the Dimension of Motoneurons Influence their Properties and Those of the Muscle Fibers They Supply. Keynote Address. International Society of Electrophysiological Kinesiology, Boston, August 1979.
49. Eyzaguirre, C., and Fidone, S. J. *Physiology of the Nervous System,* 2nd edition. Chicago: Yearbook Medical Publishers, 1975.
50. Ashworth, B., Grimby, L., and Kugelberg, E. Comparison of voluntary & reflex activation of motor units. *J. Neurol. Neurosurg. Psychiatry, 30*: 91-98, 1967.
51. Russell, D. G. Spatial location cues and movement production. In *Motor Control: Issues & Trends.* Edited by G. E. Stelmach. New York: Academic Press, 1976.
52. Schmidt, R. A. The schema as a solution to some persistent problems in motor learning theory. In *Motor Control: Issues & Trends.* Edited by G. E. Stelmach. New York: Academic Press, 1976.
53. Flowers, K. Ballistic and corrective movements on an aiming task. *Neurology, 25*: 413-421, 1975.
54. Libet, B., Gleason, C. A., Wright, E. W., and Pearl, D. K. Time of conscious intention to act in relation to onset of cerebral activity (readiness-potential). *Brain, 106*: 623-642, 1983.
55. Hoffer, J. A. Central control and reflex regulation of mechanical impedance: the basis for a unified motor-control scheme. *The Behavioral and Brain Sciences, 5*: 548-549, 1982.
56. Grillner, S. Neurobiological bases of rhythmic motor acts in vertebrates. *Science, 228*(April 12): 143-149, 1985.
57. Rothwell, J. C., Traub, M. M., Day, B. L., Obeso, J. A., Thomas, P. K., and Marsden, C. D. Manual motor performance in deafferented man. *Brain, 105*: 515-542, 1982.
58. Kelso, J. A. S., and Stelmach, G. E. Central and peripheral mechanisms in motor control. In *Motor Control: Issues & Trends.* Edited by G. E. Stelmach. New York: Academic Press, 1976.
59. Eldred, E., and Hagbarth, K.-E. Facilitation and inhibition of gamma efferents by stimulation of certain skin areas. *J. Neurophysiol., 17*: 59-65, 1954.
60. Millar, J. Joint afferent fibers responding to muscle stretch, vibration, and contraction. *Brain Res., 63*: 382, 1973.
61. Freeman, M. A. R., and Wyke, B. Articular contributions to limb muscle reflexes. *Br. J. Surg., 53*: 66, 1966.
62. Prablanc, C., Echallier, J. F., Komilis, E., and Jeannerod, M. Optimal response of eye and hand motor systems in pointing at a visual target. I. Spatio-temporal characteristics of eye and hand movements and their relationships when varying the amount of visual information. *Biol. Cybern., 35*: 113-124, 1979.
63. Bizzi, E., Chapple, W., and Hogan, N. Mechanical properties of muscles: implications for motor control. *Trends in Neuroscience,* November 1982, pp. 395-398.

64. Gottlieb, G. L., and Agarwal, G. C. The role of the myotatic reflex in the voluntary control of movements. *Brain Res., 40*: 139-143, 1972.

65. Cole, K. J., Gracco, V. L., and Abbs, J. H. Autogenic and non-autogenic sensorimotor actions in the control of multiarticulate hand movements. *Exp. Brain Res., 56*: 582-585, 1984.

66. Evarts, E. V. Motor cortex reflexes associated with learned movements. *Science, 179*: 501-503, 1973.

67. Marsden. C. D., Merton, P. A., and Morton, H. B. Is the human stretch reflex cortical rather than spinal? *Lancet,* April 7: 759-761, 1973.

68. Conrad, B., Matsunami, K., Meyer-Lohman, J., Wiesendanger, M., and Brooks, V. B. Cortical load compensation during voluntary elbow movements. *Brain Res., 71*: 507-514, 1974.

69. Lassen, N. A., Ingvar, D. H., and Skinhoj, E. Brain function and blood flow. *Sci. Am., 232*: 62-71, 1978.

70. Held, R. Plasticity in sensory-motor systems. *Sci. Am., 213*: 84-94, 1965.

71. Gentile, A. M. A working model of skill acquisition with application to teaching. *Quest, 17*: 3-23, 1972.

72. Nwaobi, O. M. Voluntary movement impairment in upper motor neuron lesions: is spasticity the main cause? *Occup. Ther. J. Res., 3*(3): 131-140, 1983.

73. Nashner, L. M., Shumway-Cook, A., and Marin, O. Stance posture control in select groups of children with cerebral palsy: deficits in sensory organization and muscular coordination. *Exp. Brain Res., 49*: 393-409, 1983.

74. Jeannerod, M., Michel, F., and Prablanc, C. The control of hand movements in a case of hemiaesthesia following a parietal lesion. *Brain, 107*: 899-920, 1984.

75. Opila-Lehman, J., Short, M. A., and Trombly, C. A. Kinesthetic recall of children with athetoid and spastic cerebral palsy and of non-handicapped children. *Dev. Med. Child Neurol., 27*: 223-230, 1985.

76. Mercer, L., and Boch, M. Residual sensorimotor deficits in the adult head-injured patient. *Phys. Ther., 63*(12): 1988-1991, 1983.

77. Diller, L., and Weinberg, J. Differential aspects of attention in brain-damaged persons. *Percept. Mot. Skills, 35*: 71-81, 1972.

78. Jason, G. W. Hemispheric asymmetries in motor function. I. Left-hemisphere specialization for memory but not performance. *Neuropsychologia, 21*(1): 35-45, 1983.

79. Kimura, D. Acquisition of a motor skill after left-hemisphere damage. *Brain, 100*: 527-542, 1977.

80. Siegel, D. Information processing abilities and performance on two perceptual-motor tasks. *Percept. Mot. Skills, 60*: 459-466, 1985.

81. Nakamura, R., and Taniguchi, R. Reaction time in patients with cerebral hemiparesis. *Neuropsychologia, 15*: 845-848, 1977.

82. Heilman, K. M., Schwartz, H. D., and Geschwind, N. Defective motor learning in ideomotor apraxia. *Neurology, 25*: 1018-1020, 1975.

83. Roy, E. A. Current perspectives on disruptions to limb praxis. *Phys. Ther., 63*(12): 1998-2003, 1983.

84. Kornhuber, H. H. Motor functions of cerebellum and basal ganglia: the cerebellocortical saccadic (ballistic) clock, the cerebellonuclear hold regulator, and the basal ganglia ramp (voluntary speed smooth movement) generator. *Kybernetik, 8*: 157-162, 1971.

85. Laurence, S., and Stein, D. G. Recovery after brain damage and the concept of localization of function. In *Recovery from Brain Damage: Research & Theory.* Edited by S. Finger. New York: Plenum Press, 1978.

86. Craik, R. L. Clinical correlates of neural plasticity. *Phys. Ther., 62*(10): 1452-1462, 1982.

87. Bishop, B. Neural plasticity. Part 4. Lesion-induced reorganization of the CNS. *Phys. Ther., 62*(10): 1442-1451, 1982.

88. Twitchell, T. E. The restoration of motor function following hemiplegia in man. *Brain, 74*: 443-480, 1951.

89. Herdman, S. J. Effect of experience on recovery following CNS lesions. *Phys. Ther., 63*(1): 51-55, 1983.

90. Stenevi, U., Bjorklund, A., and Moore, R. Y. Morphological plasticity of central adrenergic neurons. *Brain Behav. Evol.* 8:110-134, 1973.

91. Lynch, G. G., Smith, R. L., and Cotman, C. W. Recovery of function following brain damage: a consideration of some neural mechanisms. In *Neurophysiologic Aspects of Rehabilitation Medicine.* Edited by A. A. Buerger and J. S. Tobis. Springfield, IL: Charles C Thomas, 1976.

92. Eccles, J. C. *The Understanding of the Brain,* 2nd edition. New York: McGraw-Hill, 1977.

93. Bishop, B. Neural plasticity. Part 2. Postnatal maturation and function-induced plasticity. *Phys. Ther., 62*(8): 1132-1142, 1982.

94. Goldman, P. S. The role of experience in recovery of function following orbital prefrontal lesions in infant monkeys. *Neuropsychologia, 14*: 401-412, 1976.

95. DeLateur, B., et al. Isotonic versus isometric exercises: a double shift transfer-of-training study. *Arch. Phys. Med. Rehabil.,*53(5); 212-216, 1972.

96. Lee, W. A. Neuromotor synergies as a basis for coordinated intentional action. *J. Motor Behavior, 16*(2): 135-170, 1984.

97. Thelen, E., and Fisher, D. M. The organization of spontaneous leg movements in newborn infants. *J. Motor Behavior, 15*(4): 353-377, 1983.

98. Thelen, E. Simplifying assumptions: can development help? *Behavioral and Brain Sciences, 8*(1): 165-166, 1985.

99. Michels, E. Associated movements and motor learning. *Phys. Ther., 50*(1): 24-33, 1970.

100. Harris, F. A. Muscle stretch receptor hypersensitization in spasticity. *Arch. Phys. Med., 57*(1): 16-28, 1978.

101. Booth, B. J., Doyle, M., and Montgomery, J. Serial casting for the management of spasticity in the head-injured adult. *Phys. Ther., 63*(12): 1960-1966, 1983.

102. Mills, V. M. Electromyographic results of inhibitory splinting. *Phys. Ther., 64*(2): 190-193, 1984.

103. Harris, F. A. Facilitation techniques in therapeutic exercise. In *Therapeutic Exercise,* 3rd edition. Edited by J. V. Basmajian. Baltimore: Williams & Wilkins, 1978.

104. Urbscheit, N., Johnston, R., and Bishop, B. Effects of cooling on the ankle jerk and H-response in hemiplegic patients. *Phys. Ther., 51*(9): 983-988, 1971.

105. Cohen, L. Manipulation of cortical motor responses by peripheral sensory stimulation. *Arch. Phys. Med. Rehabil.,* 495-506, 1969.

106. Hagbarth, K.F., Wallin, G., and Lofstedt, L. Muscle spindle responses to stretch in normal and spastic subjects. *Scand. J. Rehab. Med., 5*: 156-159, 1973.

107. Wilder, J. Basimetric approach (Law of Initial Value) to biological rhythms. *Ann. N.Y. Acad. Sci. 98*(article 4): 753-1326, 1962.

108. Hagbarth, K.-E. Excitatory and inhibitory skin areas for flexor and extensor motoneurones. *Acta Physiol. Scand., 27*: 129-160, 1952.

109. Eldred, E., and Hagbarth, K.-E. Facilitation and inhibition of gamma efferents by stimulation of certain skin areas. *J. Neurophysiol., 17*: 59-65, 1954.

110. Matyas, T. A., and Spicer, S. D. Facilitation of the tonic vibration reflex (TVR) by cutaneous stimulation in hemiplegics. *Am. J. Phys. Med., 59*(6): 280-287, 1980.

111. Spicer, S. D., and Matyas, T. A. Facilitation of the tonic vibration reflex (TVR) by cutaneous stimulation. *Am. J. Phys. Med., 59*(5): 223-231, 1980.

112. Rood, M. S. The use of sensory receptors to activate, facilitate, and inhibit motor response, autonomic and somatic, in developmental sequence. In *Approaches to the Treatment of Patients with Neuromuscular Dysfunction..* Edited by C. Sattely. Dubuque, IA: Wm. C. Brown Book Co., 1962.

113. Blashy, M., and Fuchs, R. Orthokinetics: a new receptor facilitation method. *Am. J. Occup. Ther., 13*: 226, 1959.

114. Whelan, J. Effect of orthokinetics on upper extremity function of the adult hemiplegic patient. *Am. J. Occup. Ther., 18*(4): 141-143, 1964.

115. Kiel, J. L. Making the dynamic orthokinetic wrist splint for flexor spasticity in hand and wrist. In *Sensorimotor Evaluation and Treatment Procedures for Allied Health Personnel,* 2nd edition. Edited by S. D. Farber and A. J. Huss. Indianapolis, IN: University Foundation, 1974.

116. Oliver, R. A., et al. Isometric muscle contraction response during recovery from reduced intramuscular temperature. *Arch. Phys. Med. Rehabil., 60*(3): 126-129, 1979.

117. Carpenter, M. B. *Human Neuroanatomy,* 7th edition. Baltimore: Williams & Wilkins, 1976.

118. King, T. I. Brief: use of the tonic labyrinthine inverted positon to facilitate extensor tone: a pilot study. *Occup. Ther. J. Res., 3*(3): 176-177, 1983.

119. Tokizane, T., Murao, M., Ogata, T., and Kondo, T. Electromyographic studies on tonic neck, lumbar, and labyrinthine reflexes in normal persons. *Jpn. J. Physiol., 2*: 130-146, 1951.

120. Brunnstrom, S. *Movement Therapy in Hemiplegia.* New York: Harper & Row, 1970.

121. Bobath, B. The neurodevelopmental approach to treatment. In *Physical Therapy Services in Developmental Disabilities.* Edited by P. Pearson and C. Williams. Springfield, IL: Charles C. Thomas, 1972.

122. Hirt, S. The tonic neck reflex mechanism in the normal human adult. *Am. J. Phys. Med.* (NUSTEP Proceedings), 46: 362-369, 1967.

123. Bressan, E. S., and Wollacott, M. H. A prescriptive paradigm for sequencing instruction in physical education. *Human Movement Science, 1*: 155-175, 1982.

124. Stuart, D. G., et al. Selective activation of Ia afferents by transient muscle stretch. *Exp. Brain Res., 10*: 477-487, 1970.

125. Bishop, B. Vibratory stimulation. Part III. Possible applications of vibration in treatment of motor dysfunctions. *Phys. Ther., 55*(20): 139–143, 1975.

126. Matthews, P. B. C. A critique of the hypotheses that the spindle secondary endings contribute excitation to the stretch reflex. In *Advances in Behavioral Biology, Vol. 7: Control of Posture and Locomotion.* Edited by R. B. Stein, K. G. Pearson, R. S. Smith, and J. B. Redford. New York: Plenum Press, 1973.

127. Eklund, G., and Hagbarth, K.-E. Normal variability in tonic vibration reflexes in man. *Exp. Neurol., 16*: 80–92, 1966.

128. Johnston, R., Bishop, B., and Coffey, G. Mechanical vibration of skeletal muscles. *Phys. Ther., 50*:(4): 499–505, 1970.

129. Lance, J. W., DeGail, P., and Neilson, P. D. Tonic and phasic spinal cord mechanisms in man. *J. Neurol. Neurosurg. Psychiatry, 29*: 141, 1966.

130. Curry, E. L., and Clelland, J. A. Effects of the asymmetric tonic neck reflex and high-frequency muscle vibration on isometric wrist extension strength in normal adults. *Phys. Ther., 61*(4): 487–495, 1981.

131. Hagbarth, K. E., and Eklund, G. Motor effects of vibrating muscle stimuli in man. In *Muscular Afferents and Motor Control: Nobel Symposium I.* Edited by R. Granit, New York: John Wiley & Sons, 1966.

132. Hagbarth, K. E., and Eklund, G. The effects of muscle vibration in spasticity, rigidity, and cerebellar disorders. *J. Neurol. Neurosurg. Psychiatry, 31*: 207–213, 1968.

133. Kenny, W. E., and Heaberlin, P. C. An elecytomyographic study of the locomotor pattern of spastic children. *Clin. Orthop., 24*: 139–151, 1962.

134. Hunt, C. C. The effect of sympathetic stimulation on mammalian muscle spindles. *J. Physiol., 151*: 332–341, 1960.

135. Miglietta, O. Action of cold on spasticity. *Am. J. Phys. Med., 52*: 198–205, 1973.

136. Hartviksen, K. Ice therapy in spasticity. *Acta Neurol. Scand., 38*(Suppl 3): 79–84, 1962.

137. Stockmeyer, S. An interpretation of the approach of Rood to the treatment of neuromuscular dysfunction. *Am. J. Phys. Med.* (NUSTEP Proceedings), *46*(1): 900–956, 1967.

138. Chase, R. A., Cullen, J. K., and Sullivan, S. A. Modification of intention tremor in man. *Nature, 206*:485–487, 1965.

139. Herman, R., and Schaumburg, H. Alterations in dynamic and static properties of the stretch reflex in patients with spastic hemiplegia. *Arch. Phys. Med. Rehabil., 49*(4): 199–204, 1968.

140. Kukulka, C. G., et al. Effect of tendon pressure on alpha motoneuron excitability. *Phys. Ther., 65*(5): 595–600, 1985.

141. Morgan, M. H. Ataxia and weights. *Physiotherapy, 61*: 332–334, 1975.

142. Hewer, R. L., Cooper, R., and Morgan, M. H. An investigation into the value of treating intention tremor by weighting the affected limb. *Brain, 95*: 579–590, 1972.

143. Kottke, F. J. From reflex to skill: the training of coordination. *Arch. Phys. Med. Rehabil., 61*(12): 551–561, 1980.

144. Carr, J. H., and Shepherd, R. B. *A Motor Relearning Programme for Stroke.* Rockville, MD: Aspen Systems Corp., 1988.

145. Brodal, A. Self-observations and neuroanatomical considerations after a stroke. *Brain, 96*: 675–694, 1973.

146. Warren, M. L. A comparative study on the presence of the asymmetrical tonic neck reflex in adult hemiplegia. *Am. J. Occup. Ther., 38*(6): 386–392, 1984.

147. Loria, C. Relationship of proximal and distal function in motor development. *Phys. Ther., 60*(2): 167–172, 1980.

148. Wilson, B. N., and Trombly, C. A. Proximal and distal function in children with and without sensory integrative dysfunction: an EMG study. *Can. J. Occup. Ther., 51*(1): 11–17, 1984.

149. Ashby, P., and Burke, D. Stretch reflexes in the upper limb of spastic man. *J. Neurol. Neurosurg. Psychiatry, 34*: 765–771, 1971.

150. Zimny, N. *Effect of Position and Sensory Stimulation on Scapular Muscles.* Master's thesis. Boston: Sargent College of Allied Health Professions, Boston University, 1979.

151. Nashner, L. M., and McCollum, G. The organization of human postural movements: A formal basis and experimental synthesis. *Behavioral and Brain Sciences, 8*: 135–172, 1985.

152. Bushnell, E. W. The decline of visually guided reaching during infancy. *Infant Behavior and Development. 8*: 139–155, 1985.

153. Bruner, J. S. Organization of early skilled action. *Child Dev. 44*: 1–11, 1973.

154. Goodgold-Edwards, S. A. Motor learning as it relates to the development of skilled motor behavior: a review of the literature. *Physical & Occupational Therapy in Pediatrics, 4*(4): 5–18, 1984.

155. Mulder, T., and Hulstyn, W. Sensory feedback therapy and theoretical knowledge of motor control and learning. *Am. J. Phys. Med., 63*(5): 226–244, 1984.

156. Clark, J. E. The role of response mechanisms in motor skill development. In *The Development of Movement Control and Co-ordination.* Edited by J. A. S. Kelso and J. E. Clark. New York: John Wiley & Sons, 1982.

157. Gonnella, C., et al. Self-instruction in a perceptual motor skill. *Phys. Ther., 61*(2): 177–184, 1981.

158. Logan, G. D. Skill and automaticity: relations, implications, and future directions. *Can. J. Psychol., 39*(2): 367–386,1985.

159. Stelmach, G. E., and Larish, D. D. A new perspective on motor skill acquisition. *Res. Q. Exerc. Sport, 51*(1): 141–157, 1980.

160. Harris, F. A. Exteroceptive feedback of position and movement in remediation for disorders of coordination. In *Behavioral Psychology in Rehabilitation Medicine: Clinical Applications.* Edited by L. P. Ince. Baltimore: Williams & Wilkins, 1980.

161. Lee, D. N., Lough, F., and Lough, S. Activating the perceptuo-motor system in hemiparesis. *J. Physiol. 349*: 28P, 1984.

162. Talbot, M. L., and Junkala, J. The effects of auditorially augmented feedback on the eye-hand coordination of students with cerebral palsy. *Am. J. Occup. Ther., 35*(8): 525–528, 1981.

163. Salmoni, A. W., Schmidt, and Walter, C. B. Knowledge of results and motor learning: a review and critical appraisal. *Psychological Bulletin, 95*(3): 355–386, 1984.

164. Gill, D. L. Knowledge of results precision and motor skill acquisition. *J. Motor Behavior, 7*(3): 191–198, 1975.

165. Newell, K. M., and Walter, C. B. Kinematic and kinetic parameters as information feedback in motor skill acquisition. *J. Human Movement Studies, 7*: 235–254, 1981.

166. Thomas, J. R. Acquisition of motor skills: information processing differences between children and adults. *Res. Q. Exerc. Sport, 51*(1): 158–173, 1980.

167. Cowart, C. A., and McCallum, R. S. Simultaneous-successive processing across the life span: a cross sectional examination of stability and proficiency. *Exp. Aging Res., 10*(4): 225–229, 1984.

168. Wallace, S. A., and Hagler, R. W. Knowledge of performance and the learning of a closed motor skill. *Res. Q., 50*(2): 265–271, 1979.

169. Hall, C. R. Imagery for movement. *J. Human Movement Studies, 6*: 252–264, 1980.

170. Singer, R. N., and Pease, D. Effect of guided vs. discovery learning strategies on initial motor task learning, transfer, and retention. *Res. Q., 49*(2): 206–217, 1978.

171. DeLisa, J. A., Stolov, W. C., and Troupin, A. S. Clinical note: Action myoclonus following acute cerebral anoxia. *Arch. Phys. Med. Rehabil., 60*(1): 32–36, 1979.

172. Stern, P. H., et al. Effect of facilitation exercise techniques in stroke rehabiliation. *Arch. Phys. Med. Rehabil., 51*(9): 526–531, 1970.

173. Trombly, C. A., et al. Clinical study of effectiveness of therapy to improve finger extension in stroke patients. *Am. J. Occup. Ther., 40*(9): 612–617, 1986.

174. Trombly, C. A., and Quintana, L. A. Differences in responses to exercise by post-CVA and normal subjects. *Occup. Ther. J. Res., 5*(1): 39–58, 1985.

Supplementary Reading

Gowitzke, B. A., and Milner, M. *Understanding the Scientific Bases of Human Movement,* 2nd edition. Baltimore: Williams & Wilkins, 1980.

Linder, K. J. Transfer of motor learning: from formal discipline to action systems theory. In *Psychology of Motor Behavior: Development, Control, Learning & Performance.* Edited by L. Zaichkowsky and Z. Fuchs. Ithaca, NY: Mouvement Publishers, 1986.

Matyas, T. A., Galea, M. P., and Spicer, S. D. Facilitation of the maximum voluntary contraction in hemiplegia by concomitant cutaneous stimulation, *Am. J. Phys. Med., 65*(3): 125–134, 1986.

Sage, G. H. *Motor Learning and Control: A Neurophysiological Approach.* Dubuque, IA: Wm. C. Brown Publishers, 1984.

Schwartz, R. K. *Therapy as Learning.* Dubuque, IA: Kendall/Hunt Publishing Company, 1985.

Shimizu, H. Brief: Prediction of motor performance using a replacement learning mathematical model. *Occup. Ther. J. Res., 6*(1): 49–51, 1986.

Stein, R. B. What muscle variable(s) does the nervous system control in limb movements? *Behavioral and Brain Sciences, 5*:585–577, 1982.

Umphred, D. A., editor. *Neurological Rehabilitation.* St. Louis: The C. V. Mosby Company, 1985.

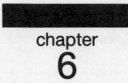

chapter
6

Neurophysiological and Developmental Treatment Approaches

Five programs of treatment for patients with motor control problems due to brain damage have been developed:

1. Rood Approach
2. Bobath Neurodevelopmental Approach
3. Brunnstrom Approach: Movement Therapy
4. Proprioceptive Neuromuscular Facilitation (PNF) Approach
5. Carr and Shepherd Approach: Motor Relearning Programme for Stroke Patients

Each approach is described as it is presented in the literature. Additional information is available to those who attend training workshops. Primary sources of information have been supplemented by the writings of others to present as complete a description of each approach as possible.

The approaches are more similar than divergent, which is not surprising, because each has the goal of improved motor control for patients with brain damage and because each is based on information about the same central nervous system. Similarities include the importance of sensation to movement and the importance of repetition for learning. The differences have to do with whether conscious attention should be directed toward the movement itself or only toward the goal of the movement, whether spinal and brain stem reflexes should or should not be used to elicit movement, and whether or not it is necessary for the patient to redevelop motor control in an ontogenetic sequence. The Brunnstrom and PNF approaches as well as the Motor Relearning Programme for Stroke Patients focus the patient's attention on the movement, whereas both the Rood and Bobath approaches emphasize the importance of eliciting goal directed movement subcortically.

The Brunnstrom approach utilizes primitive reflexes to elicit movement when the patient is otherwise unable to move, whereas the Bobath approach actively inhibits the appearance of these reflexes. The first four approaches assist the patient to redevelop movement and posture in developmental sequence, but the developers of the Motor Relearning Programme do not concur with the importance of this principle. None of the approaches addresses methods of developing skilled movement; all emphasize the development of basic movement and postures that underlie skill.

There must be collaboration among members of the rehabilitation team when these approaches are used because all the stimulation offered the patient during each day will affect his motor control and because goals must be coordinated. For example, if the goal of one therapy is to inhibit associated reactions, treatment given by other therapies should not be directed toward facilitating them.

Although the reader is encouraged to develop his or her own treatment approach based on a sound rationale of neurophysiology, motor learning, and motor development, he or she may decide to eclectically choose procedures from several of the approaches presented in this chapter as those procedures fit his or her own theoretical framework at his or her level of understanding. Every procedure, whether proposed by others or originated by the reader, must be clinically tested for effectiveness.

STUDY QUESTIONS:

Neurophysiological and Developmental Treatment Approaches

1. What are the points of agreement and disagreement among the theorists who have developed treatment approaches for the patient with central nervous system dysfunction?
2. What point is not addressed by any of the approaches? (See also questions after each section.)

A/Rood Approach

CATHERINE A. TROMBLY

Margaret Rood was both an occupational and a physical therapist. Her major contributions to the treatment of persons with brain damage included emphasis on controlled sensory stimulation, the use of ontogenetic sequence, and the need to demand a purposeful response through the use of activity. Rood spent many years studying and clinically testing treatment methods that she devised based on her readings. She interpreted the data derived from basic neurophysiological and movement-development research and attempted to bridge between what she learned from this basic research to the treatment of brain-injured patients. Her treatment was originally designed for cerebral palsy, but she believed it was applicable to any patient with motor control problems.[1]

Rood shared her ideas with others through clinical and classroom teaching but published very little. Because she so rarely wrote, some of the ideas reported here are based on interpretations of her method by three other knowledgeable therapists: Joy Huss, A. Jean Ayres, and Shirley Stockmeyer, who have helped clarify for other therapists the procedures and their rationale. It is sometimes difficult to identify where Rood's thinking leaves off and the other therapists' begins.

Rood's basic premise was[2]:

> Motor patterns are developed from fundamental reflex patterns present at birth which are utilized and gradually modified through sensory stimuli until the highest control is gained on the conscious cortical level. It seemed to me then, that if it were possible to apply the proper sensory stimuli to the appropriate sensory receptor as it is utilized in normal sequential development, it might be possible to elicit motor responses reflexly and by following neurophysiological principles, establish proper motor engrams.

There are four major components of Rood's theory, which are included in each treatment:[3,4]

1. The normalization of tone and evocation of desired muscular responses is accomplished through the use of appropriate sensory stimuli. Correct sensory input is necessary for the development of correct motor responses. Controlled sensory input is used to evoke muscular responses reflexively,[5] which Rood believed is the earliest developmental step in gaining motor control.

2. Sensorimotor control is developmentally based, and therefore therapy must start at the patient's level of development and progress him sequentially to higher and higher levels of sensorimotor control according to sequences Rood has identified. Muscular responses reflexively obtained are used in developmental patterns[5] in an effort to develop surpraspinal control of those responses.

3. Movement is purposeful. Rood used activity to demand a purposeful response from the patient in order to subcortically elicit the desired movement pattern. The responses of agonists, antagonists, and synergists are reflexively programmed according to a purpose or plan.[5] When the cortex commands "pick up the glass," for example, all the subcortical centers involved in motor performance cause facilitation or inhibition of muscles as appropriate for that program to allow the accomplishment of the motion[4] in a coordinated manner. The cortex does not direct each muscle individually.[5] The patient's attention is drawn to the end-goal or purpose, not the movement. Sensation that occurs during movement is basic to motor learning. In this way, the patient is helped to gain control over movement that has been elicited reflexively.[5]

Purposeful movement cannot be invariably used; it may not be possible for a severely involved patient to respond in this way. It is, however, important to use this method when possible.[4] It is especially applicable when the focus of treatment is the trunk, lower extremities, or the proximal segments of the upper extremities, all of which are more or less subcortically controlled.[4,5] If the focus of treatment is development of skill in the distal segments of the upper extremities, then the attention of the patient must be on the movement of these parts which are more directly cortically controlled.[4,5]

4. Repetition of sensorimotor responses is necessary for learning.[4,6] Activities are used to provide not only purposeful response but also repetition.

Controlled Sensory Input

Rood has determined certain methods of influencing motor responses from trial and error in clinical practice, based on the results cited in studies of the effects of stimuli on animals. The following methods have been found to be facilitating or inhibiting as described. However, the reader is reminded that the actual response each patient will exhibit will be an algebraic summation of all internal and external stimuli he is experiencing. Therefore, as in any therapeutic procedure, the response of the patient is carefully monitored and the stimuli changed as necessary to elicit the desired response. The effects of the tonic labyrinthine reflex (TLR) and the tonic neck reflex (TNR) may assist or retard the effects of the applied stimulus, and therefore the positioning of the patient during stimulation is important.[6]

FACILITATION METHODS

Tactile stimulation is offered in two ways: fast brushing and light stroking. Fast brushing refers to brushing of the hairs[7] or the skin over a muscle[5] by the use of a soft camel hair paint brush that has been substituted for the stirrer of a hand-held battery-powered cocktail mixer[8,9] (Fig. 6.1) and is now commercially available as a battery-powered brush. The revolving brush is applied on each skin area over the muscles to be stimulated.[5,6] Fast brushing of the skin over the distribution of the posterior primary rami of the peripheral nerves, which innervate the muscles and skin of the back,[10] facilitates the tonic, deep muscles of the back; whereas fast brushing of the skin over the rest of the body, supplied by the anterior primary rami,[10] facilitates a tonic response of the superficial muscles.[5] Brushing is done on the skin of the dermatome (Fig. 3.5) served by the same spinal segment as those muscles in which the therapist is attempting to sensitize the muscle spindles.[5] This area usually corresponds to the skin located over the muscle. Brushing of the dermatome is done for 5 sec for each area.[11] If there is no response to the brushing after 30 sec, the brushing of each area should be repeated three to five times.[5,6] Fast brushing is thought to stimulate the C-size sensory fibers, which discharge into polysynaptic pathways that influence the background gamma efferent activity of muscles[5,12,13] involved in the maintenance of posture.[5] Spindles so biased respond more readily to added external or internal stretch.[5] High threshold receptors, of which the C fiber is an example, are difficult to stimulate and require a high-intensity stimulus.[5] Fast brushing is classified as a high-intensity stimulus because of the high rate of revolutions of the brush and the duration of application.[5]

Rood hypothesized that the effect of fast brushing is nonspecific, has a latency of 30 sec, and reaches its maximum 30 to 40 min after stimulation due to the enhancement of the reticular activating system into which the C fibers feed.[5,7,14] In controlled studies of normal and poststroke persons, however, it was demonstrated that although fast brushing produced a significant immediate facilitatory effect,[13,15] the postapplication effect lasted only 30[16] to 45[13,15] sec. The facilitatory effect was seen only in the lower extremity, not in the upper extremity in normal subjects.[15] The upper extremity was not tested in the stroke patients.[13] These researchers also found that brushing produced a greater effect in hemiplegic patients than in normal subjects.[13]

Rood stated that the first manifestation of effects may be on the opposite side of the body, especially in the lower extremities[6]; therefore, brushing applied to both the nonaffected and the affected sides would probably be beneficial.[6,9]

There are some precautions to be observed in relation to fast brushing. Fast brushing of the pinna of the ear stimulates the vagus nerve, which influences cardiorespiratory functions. The vagus nerve is part of the parasympathetic section of the autonomic nervous system. Activation of this nerve slows the heart, produces bronchial constriction, and bronchial secretion.[17] Fast brushing over the posterior primary rami of L_{1-2} will cause voiding; over S_{2-4} will cause bladder retention (improve incontinence).[5]

Light touch or stroking of the skin activates the low threshold A-size sensory fibers to activate a reflex reciprocal action of the superficial phasic or mobilizing muscles.[5-8] Low threshold receptors are easily stimulated and effect a fast, short-lived response. Light stroking of the dorsum of the webs of the fingers or toes, or of the palms of the hands or the soles of the feet, elicits a phasic withdrawal motion of the stimulated limb.[5] Repetitive use of this stimulus to these areas will result in a crossed extensor reflex pattern.[5]

As soon as the patient is able to voluntarily control movement, stroking (brushing) is no longer an effective[6] or appropriate treatment.

Thermal facilitation or icing is thought to have the same effects as brushing and stroking through the same neural mechanisms[5,7]; however, icing has been found to be significantly less effective in hemiplegic patients than fast brushing for recruitment of motor units.[13] A convenient way to administer icing is by the use of plastic popsicle molds, which gives the therapist a handle to hold while icing.[8] "C-icing" is a high threshold stimulus used to stimulate postural, tonic responses via the C-size sensory fibers.[5] Icing to activate the C fibers is done by holding the ice cube pressed in place for 3 to 5 sec,[5] then wiping away the water. The skin areas to be stimulated are the same as noted for fast brushing with the exception of the distribution of the posterior primary rami along the back, which is avoided because it may cause a sympathetic nervous system response.[5,11] The ice, a noxious stimulus, when applied over the sympathetic chain causes a protective response of that system.[17]

"A-icing" is the application of quick swipes of the ice cube to evoke a reflex withdrawal, similar to the response of light touch, when the stimulus is applied to the palms or soles or the dorsal webs of the hands or

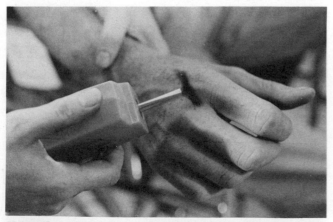

Figure 6.1 Battery-operated brush applied to facilitate finger extension.

feet.[5] When the reflex response occurs, resistance to the movement is usually given[8] to reinforce it and to help develop voluntary control over it.

Quick icing is for use with "flaccid-placid types only."[5] A-icing of the upper right quadrant of the abdomen in the dermatomal representation for T_{7-9} will result in stimulation of the diaphragm.[5] Touching the lips with ice opens the mouth (a withdrawal response), but ice applied to the tongue and inside the lips closes the mouth.[5]

There is a rebound effect to icing which occurs approximately 30 sec after stimulation[5] in which the muscles so stimulated become temporarily inhibited. It is not clearly stated whether this rebound effect occurs with both types of icing.

Precautions about icing are similar to those for brushing. Icing of the pinna causes autonomic vagal responses.[5] Ice to the trunk at the level of L_2 causes voiding and to S_{2-4}, urinary retention.[5]

The effectiveness of the controlled sensory input advocated by Rood has been meagerly tested. In one study,[18] a statistically significant ($P = .01$) increase was found following a 2-week period of treatment in the strength of the triceps of children with bilateral upper-extremity flexor spasticity and those who had normal upper extremities. Treatment consisted of brushing, stroking, rubbing, icing, and squeezing of the triceps. Strength was measured by the amount of weight the subject's triceps could lift. The study design provided control against the testing procedure itself accounting for the increase in strength. There was also an increase in strength of triceps of both groups in the unfacilitated upper extremity, but this increase never exceeded the effect of direct stimulation. There was a significant mean decrease in strength of both elbow extensors of both groups following a 2-week period of no facilitation.

The remainder of the stimuli to be discussed are proprioceptive stimuli; the effects of which last only for as long as the stimulus is applied.

Heavy joint compression is hypothesized to facilitate cocontraction of muscles around a joint, although one study calls this into question.[19] Heavy compression refers to resistance greater than body weight[5] that is applied so that the force is through the longitudinal axes of the bones whose articular surfaces approximate each other.[4] Resistance greater than body weight is that which is more than the weight of the body parts usually supported by the joint. This type of stimulus is thought to activate high-threshold joint receptors.[4] The stabilizing muscles need to go through a stage of holding against resistance in a shortened position before they are asked to cocontract as a response to heavy joint compression.[8] Weight-bearing positions of prone on elbows, prone on hands, quadruped, and standing can offer heavy joint compression if the patient lifts one or two extremities and bears weight on the other, weaker ones. Or weights can be added: a hat or crown that incorporates a ring filled with buckshot increases neck joint compression, thereby improving head control.[14] Weighted bags, lead x-ray aprons, etc., can be placed on the shoulders, hips, or backs of patients to increase joint compression.

Quick, light stretch of a muscle is a low-threshold stimulus that activates an immediate phasic stretch reflex of the same muscle stretched and inhibits its antagonist.[5]

Tapping of the tendon or the belly of the muscle to be facilitated is essentially the same phenomenon as quick stretch.[4] The therapist percusses the area using the fingertips (see Fig. 5.4).

Pressure on the muscle belly similarly elicits a stretch response by placing a stretch on the spindles.[4] It is done by manually pressing on the muscle or by the use of equipment which presses on the muscle.

Secondary stretch is a maintained stretch at the end of range used to facilitate the secondary (II) afferent fibers of the spindle. Secondary stretch of the heavy work muscles, the physiological extensors and abductors, was hypothesized to facilitate their antagonists, the flexors and adductors, at the same time that these muscles are in the shortened range[4,5] and not facilitated by their own IIs. This was thought to be the mechanism underlying flexor participation in cocontraction. In light of newer research evidence concerning the role of the secondary afferents, clinical research is needed to verify whether secondary stretch actually facilitates a cocontraction response.

Stretch to the intrinsic muscles of the hand or foot was hypothesized to facilitate cocontraction of the proximal stabilizer muscles.[4,8] Forcefully grasping handles of tools is used to obtain this response, especially if the handles have been modified to be cone shaped with the widest part of the cone at the ulnar border of the hand or to be spherical, both of which increase intermetacarpal stretch. If such activities can be combined with weight-bearing positions, the proximal stabilizers are believed to be further facilitated through the demand placed on them for cocontraction. For example, to develop shoulder cocontraction, a patient can lean on his elbow in a modified prone-on-elbows position while using an electric drill to drill holes in a vertically placed project. Whether shoulder cocontraction is actually improved using these methods needs study; in one electromyographical study of the scapulohumeral muscles of normal adults, the prone-on-elbows position used in combination with resisted grasp evoked only a low level of response from these muscles.[19]

Resistance is a form of stretch in which many or all of the spindles of a muscle are stimulated.[9] The spindle, of course, cannot know whether the discrepancy it senses is due to being stretched by a moving force or by resistance that is preventing the extrafusal muscle fibers from shortening as it shortens as programmed. The discrepancy causes the spindle to fire impulses in order to get more extrafusal muscle units firing. The electrical activity of the interneuronal pool is consequently high, and more and more motor units are more easily recruited to fire, a phenomenon called overflow.

Resisting a phasic contraction is hypothesized to activate stretch reflexes and to prevent immediate inhibition due to the effect of the Golgi tendon organs (GTOs) of the contracting muscles.[8] Resistance applied to muscles contracted in a shortened range stretches the spindles to activate more motor units; this method is hypothesized to be the way to bias spindles of the deeper, more tonic limb muscles used for posture that cannot be stimulated by C fibers, which are effective in activating a tonic response of peripheral muscles only.[5]

A shortened, held, resisted contraction (SHRC) used in combination with the pivot prone position is thought to be an important preparation for weight-bearing postures. Pivot prone is a position in which the person lies prone and extends upper trunk and head; abducts, extends, and externally rotates his shoulders; and extends his hips and knees off the surface so that he rests on the pivot point at approximately the level of T[10] (Fig. 5.2 and 6.2). The spindles of the muscles responsible for this posture are programmed, along with the extrafusal muscle fibers, to hold this position. The resistance of gravity exerts a constant force against holding the position, which not only causes the CNS to reprogram more and more motor units but also causes

recruitment of more units through the stretch reflex servo-assist mechanisms. It is reasoned that immediately following a SHRC in prone extension (pivot prone), the spindles of the extensor/abductor muscles are biased short and are therefore very responsive to small increments of stretch. If the person moves into prone-on-elbows or quadruped position, the shoulder and hip extensor/abductor muscles are stretched relative to their new shortened range and are facilitated to contract through the servo-assist mechanism. The flexor part of the cocontraction around the hips and scapulohumeral joints was thought to be due to secondary stretch, as mentioned above, but more probably is brought about by central programming commands to maintain the posture.

Eccentric contraction against resistance provides a great amount of both internal and external stretch to spindles that maximally activates the primary afferents to produce stretch reflex responses.

Pressure on bony prominences has both facilitatory and inhibitory effects during normal purposeful movement.[4] For example, pressure over the lateral aspect of the calcaneus facilitates the medial dorsiflexors while inhibiting the calf muscles to allow dorsiflexion. Pressure on the medial aspect of the calcaneus facilitates the lateral dorsiflexors.[4]

Rood utilized stimuli to special senses to facilitate or inhibit the skeletal musculature generally or that involved in vital functions more specifically. Stimuli from all cranial nerves feed into the reticular formation,[5,7] the alerting mechanism. Olfactory and gustatory stimuli are facilitating or inhibiting through their influence on the autonomic nervous system. Unpleasant or potentially dangerous stimuli elicit a sympathetic "fight or flight" reaction, and pleasant stimuli evoke a parasympathetic response that inhibits the sympathetic reaction.[5] The therapist should be aware that these stimuli will produce an emotional response as well as a physical response.[5]

Auditory and visual stimuli can be used to generally facilitate or inhibit the central nervous system of the patient. Music with a definite beat would be facilitatory; soft, lullaby music would be inhibitory. A noisy, raucous clinic will be stimulating and may affect the performance of the patient with central nervous system dysfunction. The therapist's voice and manner of speech (fast and staccato vs. slow and calming, for example) may also affect the patient's performance. A drab, dull, colorless, and uninteresting environment will promote sleep and loss of tone.[7] A colorful, lighted, multistimuli environment will have a generalized facilitatory effect. Different colors may be more facilitating than others for each patient.

In summary, facilitation of phasic responses is done when no movement exists or following development of tonic responses. A-brushing and icing, quick, light stretch, and muscle or tendon tapping are used. Resistance to the movement is added after it starts in order to reinforce it. Tonic responses are facilitated when there is too much movement or to develop postural sta-

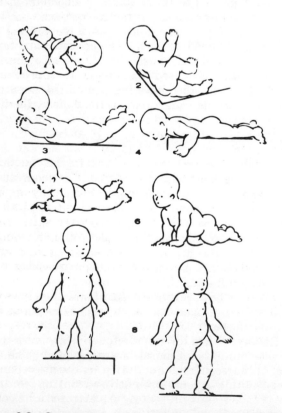

Figure 6.2 Ontogenetic motor patterns according to Rood. (1) Supine withdrawal; (2) Roll over; (3) Pivot prone; (4) Neck cocontraction; (5) On elbows; (6) Quadruped; (7) Standing; (8) Walking. (Reproduced with permission from *Occupational Therapy,* 3rd edition. Edited by H. S. Willard and C. S. Spackman. Philadelphia: J. B. Lippincott, 1963.)

bility. C-brushing and icing, secondary stretch, repetitive tendon or muscle belly tapping, heavy joint compression, and resistance are used to facilitate tonic responses.

INHIBITION METHODS

To inhibit muscle output, stimuli that inhibit directly are used or stimuli that facilitate the antagonist muscle are used to cause reciprocal inhibition. The difference between inhibition and facilitation is in the mode of application rather than the kind of stimuli.

Light joint compression, also called joint approximation, can be used to inhibit spastic muscles.[4] This is used to relieve shoulder pain seen in hemiplegic patients due to spastic muscles. The method is to grasp the patient's elbow and, while holding the humerus abducted to about 35° to 45°, gently push the head of the humerus into the glenoid fossa and hold it there; the spastic muscles will relax.[4,14]

Rood identified a particular type of tactile stimulation for inhibition: slow stroking over the distribution of the posterior primary rami. The effect is probably through calming of the output of the sympathetic chain; the autonomic nervous system is known to affect gamma motorneuron firing.[20] The person lies prone in a quiet environment. The therapist uses the palm of one hand or extended fingers to apply firm pressure along the vertebral musculature from occiput to coccyx, at which time the therapist's other hand starts at the occiput and progresses likewise to the coccyx. This slow, rhythmical stroking using alternating hands is done for about 3 to 5 min[6,9] or until the patient relaxes.[6]

Slow, rhythmical movement is inhibiting,[11] that is, relaxing. Slow rolling is done similarly to fast rocking except much more slowly. The patient is slowly rolled from supine to side-lying by the therapist, who holds the patient's shoulder and hip. A decrease in hypertonicity should be seen within minutes. Slow rocking in a rocking chair is a variation. Self-administered rocking must be carefully monitored because if it develops into fast rocking it will be facilitatory.

Neutral warmth refers to maintaining the body heat by wrapping the specific area to be inhibited, or the area served by the posterior primary rami for a general effect, in a cotton blanket or down pillow or comforter for 10 to 20 min.[4,11] Neutral heat is used because if heat greater than body temperature is used a rebound effect may occur in 2 to 3 hours, which means the inhibited muscles become as facilitated as they were before this treatment or even superfacilitated.[5]

Pressure on the tendinous insertion of a muscle inhibits that muscle through the receptors located under the tendinous insertions, the Pacinian corpuscles.[4,8,11] The extrinsic flexors of the hand may be inhibited by applying constant pressure over the entire length of the long tendons.[8] Grasp of enlarged, firm, or hard adapted handles of tools would provide this stimulation. Grasp also facilitates proximal cocontraction, as was stated previously.

A maintained stretch or maintenance of a lengthened position for a period of time ranging from several minutes to several weeks rebiases the spindle to the longer position. The lengthened muscle's spindles are rebiased longer and will not react to stretch as briskly at shorter ranges following this procedure. On the other hand, if a muscle is positioned in the shortened range, the muscle's spindles will be rebiased shorter and will react briskly to stretch beyond that shortened range. The balance of tone between agonists and antagonists will be disturbed if prolonged positioning is allowed. A contracture may ensue. Sometimes prolonged positioning is desired; e.g., when a spastic flexor muscle is held into a lengthened range by a cast or splint for several weeks, its spindles reset to the longer position and it is therefore less spastic. It has been demonstrated that a decrease of tone in the flexors of the hand and wrist, with a corresponding reciprocal increase of tone in the extensors, results.[17] A very weak muscle's spindles can be biased shorter to increase tone in this passive way, although some of the more direct facilitatory methods that have been described that bias the spindle and increase internal stretch sensitivity are faster. Unresisted contraction can be used to inhibit the agonist by way of the low-threshold GTOs; this would reciprocally facilitate the antagonists. To inhibit tight (spastic) muscles, Rood recommended that the patient be requested to contract maximally (brief, intense contraction[8]) before moving the limb into a lengthened position.[5] The brevity and intensity of the contraction is thought to activate a large number of GTOs at once, which was believed to produce an overriding autoinhibition instead of the facilitation that is seen when resistance is added gradually during an on-going contraction.[8]

Sequences of Motor Control

Rood has identified several sequences that she used interrelatedly but that will be presented separately here for clarity. One sequence was already mentioned earlier, when the components of the Rood method were listed. To reiterate: a muscular response is first evoked reflexively using sensory stimulation, then responses so obtained are used in developmental patterns, and finally the patient uses the response purposefully to gain control over it.

Two more sequences that Rood identified have to do with differences in muscle types and motor patterns. One difference is the distinction between the responses of light-work and heavy-work muscles due to their anatomical design. Light-work muscles lie superficially, laterally, or distally and have a tendinous origin and insertion.[5] They are multiarthrodial; they are under more voluntary control and do phasic work.[5] They are activated by light stretch or low-threshold exteroceptor stimulation and inhibited by unresisted contraction. Rood identified the light-work or mobilizing muscles as primarily the flexors and adductors, but multiarthrodial finger and wrist extensors are included in this category also. These muscles are termed physiological flexors[17] even though their action is extension of the finger, thumb, or wrist joints. Heavy-work muscles are deep, lie close to the joint, and are uniarthrodial. In the body, they are located proximally and medially. Heavy-work muscles are tonic stability muscles capable of prolonged, sustained contraction.[17] They are under greater reflex control and are activated by heavy resistance or maintained stretch and high-threshold receptor stimulation. These are primarily the trunk and proximal limb extensors and abductors,[5] but also include such muscles as the interossei of the hands and feet.

The other difference reflects the type of muscle response. Rood believed that neuromuscular integration was most normal if each muscle learned to contract first as it would normally be used phylogenetically and ontogenetically. Flexion precedes extension; adduction precedes abduction; ulnar patterns develop before radial ones; and rotation develops last.[11] She believed that if the normal first response of a muscle was a stabilizing contraction, it should be facilitated to contract in this manner and not in a mobilizing pattern. However, there is no convenient listing of what the original phylogenetic or ontogenetic function of each muscle was to guide this aspect of treatment. Therapists are guided by Rood's definitions of heavy-work (tonic, stabilizing) muscles and light-work (phasic, mobilizing) muscles in planning treatment. Therapeutic movement should be planned to be most advantageous to the particular muscle group being facilitated. It was recommended that phasic flexors be positioned so that their motion started from the lengthened range, i.e., at the farthest point toward extension that could be easily achieved, because it was believed that flexors are facilitated by both their Ia and II afferents and the lengthened range would activate the IIs.[8,9] It was further recommended that tonic extensors not be started in their lengthened range due to the inhibitory effects of their own II afferents, but should rather start their contraction in the mid to shortened range.[8,9] Because of the uncertainty of the effects of stimulation of the II afferents, as mentioned in the previous chapters, these suggestions need to be clinically tested. In the process of strengthening a muscle's responses, treatment must continue until the muscle is able to work strongly in all positions and the spindles exhibit a normal bias in all positions for voluntary motor control to be considered complete.

Another sequence that Rood identified has to do with the levels of developing motor control. There are four phases.

1. Muscles contract through their range with reciprocal inhibition of the antagonists.[4,5] Stockmeyer[8] terms this the Mobility phase. Movement first appears as phasic, reciprocal shortening and lengthening contractions of muscles that cause movement that subserves a protective function.[4,5] The stimulus for this type of response is quick, light stretch or stroking of the distal parts or other low-threshold, A-fiber type of stimulation. The movement of the neonate, waving his extremities back and forth in unresisted motion, typifies phasic movement.

2. Muscles around the joint contract simultaneously (cocontraction) to provide stability.[4,8] This tonic, holding contraction is next to develop and is the basis for maintaining proximal posture to allow exploration of the environment and development of skill by the distal segments of the body.[4] Development of stability should precede work on developing phasic, skilled movement.[6] The stimuli for stability responses are high-threshold stimulation: joint compression; stretch, especially of the intrinsic muscles of the hands and feet; fast brushing and other C-fiber stimulation; as well as resistance.[5] Maintained sensory input is necessary for a maintained response.[5,8]

3. Proximal muscles contract to do heavy work superimposed on distal cocontraction.[4,5] "Mobility superimposed on stability" is Stockmeyer's way of designating this level of motor control[8] in which the distal segment is fixed and the proximal segment moves. This phase is used to develop controlled mobility of the proximal joints. Sensory stimuli from high-threshold spindle and joint receptors are involved in this response.[8] An example of this kind of motion occurs when an infant learns to assume the quadruped position but has not learned to move in that position yet: he rocks back and forth with his knees and hands planted firmly on the floor.

4. *Skill.* At this level of motor control, the proximal segment is stabilized and the distal segment moves.[4,5] Examples of this level include walking, crawling, and use of the hands. Occupational therapists who are tempted to start therapy at this level are cautioned against it.[4]

These four levels of motor control are developed as the patient is paced through the skeletal developmental sequences which Rood referred to as ontogenetic motor patterns (Fig. 6.2). These eight patterns will be described, then the interrelationship may be studied using Table 6.1.

1. *Supine withdrawal,*[5] also called supine flexion, is a position of total flexion toward the vertebral level of T_{10}.[5,8] The upper extremities cross the chest, and the dorsum of the extended hands touch the face. The lower extremities flex and abduct. This posture, which demands heavy work of the trunk and proximal parts of the extremities and light work of the distal parts of the limbs,[5] is used to obtain flexor responses when the patient has no movement or is dominated by extensor responses or to develop reciprocal phasic movement through normal range. It is also used to integrate the TLR[5] by requiring a voluntary contraction of the flexors in spite of reflex facilitation of the extensors.

To elicit the withdrawal motor pattern, Rood used this method[5]: First, the low back and the dermatomes of C_{1-4} posterior primary rami distribution were fast brushed. Second, a small wedge pillow was placed under the head and another under the pelvis to slightly statically stretch the short extensors of the back, which was expected to facilitate the trunk flex-

Table 6.1
INTEGRATION OF ONTOGENETIC MOTOR PATTERNS WITH LEVELS OF MOTOR CONTROL[a]

Level I: Mobility[8]		Level II: Stability		Level III: Mobility on Stability[8]		Level IV: Skill	
Skeletal	Vital	Skeletal	Vital	Skeletal	Vital	Skeletal	Vital
1. Supine withdrawal	1. Inspiration	4. Pivot prone (held)	5. Phonation[b]	6. Neck cocontraction (orient head in space)	4. Swallow fluids	9. Prone on elbows (head is doing skilled movement and one arm is free for skilled use; belly crawling)	5. Phonation
2. Roll over	2. Expiration	5. Neck cocontraction	3. Sucking	8. Prone on elbows, (shift from side to side, push backward and pull forward, unilateral weight bearing)	6. Chewing	12. Quadruped (one arm free for skilled use; creeping, trunk rotation and reciprocal movement, crossed diagonal)	8. Speech
3. Pivot prone (assume the position)		7. Prone-on-elbows		11. Quadruped (rocking, shifting, unilateral weight bearing)	7. Swallow solids	15. Standing and walking	
		10. Quadruped		14. Standing (weight shift, unilateral weight bearing)			
		13. Standing					

[a] The steps are numbered sequentially, but they blend together, i.e., one step is not completely mastered before the next begins at the most basic level.
[b] Although out of sequence, phonation is facilitated in the pivot prone position.[8]

ors via the secondary endings of the extensors. Third, the neck flexors and abdominals were put in a shortened position to cause them to rebias their spindles to a shorter length, which was believed to make them more sensitive to stretch and therefore more apt to contract if the patient reverted to a trunk extended position due to the influences of the TLR. And finally, after the heavy-work response of the trunk was obtained, a light-work response of the limbs was then elicited by stroking or A-icing the sole or palm and immediately providing an activity that demanded the light-work flexion/adduction pattern of the limbs. An activity with some resistance was used to reinforce the ongoing movement because an unresisted contraction was believed to inhibit the muscle group responsible for the movement. Note that the force of the activity should be toward flexion/adduction, even though reciprocal movement may be involved. Some examples are tetherball, squeezing a toy accordion, using a cylindrical balloon blower, or playing ping-pong (forehand shot), and stirring batter in a counter-clockwise direction using the right arm or in reverse direction using the left.

If the extensor response in supine was too strong to permit flexor movement, Rood recommended starting treatment with the patient in a side-lying position.[5]

According to Rood,[5] this motor pattern also helps develop bowel and bladder function, eye convergence, and respiratory patterns.

2. *Roll over*, in which the arm and leg on the same side flex[5] as the trunk rotates. This pattern is appropriate for patients who are dominated by the primitive tonic reflexes, need mobilization of the extremities, or activation of lateral trunk musculature. Attempts at rolling over integrate the TNR since the topmost limbs, in this case the skull side limbs, flex and adduct proximally and tend to extend at the elbow and knee, which is opposite to the typical asymmetrical tonic neck reflex skull side response. Activity examples: roll over to reach an attractive or needed object, roll down an incline, or turn to look at something enticing. To elicit a response subcortically, move the object the person is looking at around to the side, thereby causing the patient's head to turn to maintain visual contact with it; the body will reflexively follow the head if the righting reactions are developing.

3. *Pivot prone*,[5] also called prone extension,[8] involves extension of the neck, trunk, shoulders, hips, and knees, abduction and external rotation of the shoulders, and elbow flexion. This is the first postural or stability pattern, on which all others depend. Assumption of the position is a phasic, reciprocal movement. Holding the position involves an SHRC of the extensor muscles that biases their spindles shorter so they are more sensitive. This facilitates extensor tone preparatory to weight bearing. When this position can be maintained, it indicates that the symmetrical tonic neck reflex (STNR) and TLR are integrated and the righting reactions are developing. Prone extension is a chain response of the labyrinthine righting reaction.

The process of therapy to achieve the whole pattern will be described although this is adapted to a limited or modified pattern in which the patient is not actually placed fully prone for use with adult patients who have trunk control. The patient is placed prone on a firm, padded surface large enough to support the trunk only. If not contraindicated for the patient, the tonic labyrinth inverted (TLI) posture can be imposed while the patient's abdomen and pelvis are supported on a treatment ball (Fig. 6.3), a small stool, or a bolster. The area over the deep back extensors is C-brushed, taking care to avoid L_{1-2} and S_{2-3} areas. The skin over the posterior deltoid, latissimus dorsi, trapezius, proximal hamstrings, and gluteus is C-brushed and iced. Simultaneously with the activity demand, vibration is applied to the deep back and neck extensors and other extensor muscles involved in the pattern starting at the midline. The pivot prone pattern is held for gradually increasing periods of time, until the patient can hold it for at least 1 to 2 min. An activity is presented to demand and resist the response. Activity suggestions are pulling back on the string of a talking doll or toy, pulling back on an elastic-propelled plane in preparation for shooting it, using a sling shot (unilateral pattern),[8] riding prone on a scooter board (see Fig. 5.2), playing with a "button-on-string" toy, rowing, tearing apart strips of cloth preparatory to weaving rag rugs, or stirring batter in a clockwise direction with the right arm or in the opposite direction with the left. Note that the force of the activity is in the direction of the prone extension pattern although other movements are also involved in the activity.

4. *Neck Cocontraction* is the pattern used to develop head control and is first activated in the prone position. Prior to putting the person prone, it is necessary to activate the flexors[6] if they are not already active. The short neck flexors are activated first by C-brushing the dermatomal distribution of C_2. Next, the long neck flexors, the sternocleidomastoids, are activated. The person is then placed prone and is asked to raise his head against gravity. The labyrinth righting reaction stimulates the person to align his head so that his eyes are parallel and his nose is perpendicular to the surface on which he is lying. As the head then bobs into flexion, the neck and trunk extensors are stretched and thereby facilitated to contract and neck extension is again sought. As the patient attempts to maintain neck extension, the upper trapezius is facilitated to maintain the extension by C-brushing and repetitive muscle tapping.[6] Activities that require the person to look up while lying prone are used to demand the neck cocontraction pattern. Sucking a resistive liquid through a straw or playing games in which a small object is picked up by sucking on a straw are activities that result in reflexive cocontraction of the neck muscles.[5,8]

5. *On elbows*,[5] also called prone on elbows,[8] is a pattern of vertical extension, which inhibits the STNR.[4] When the shoulders are brought into forward flexion so that the patient can bear weight on his elbows, the extensor muscles of the proximal upper extremity are stretched relative to the pivot prone position in which they are held shortened in extension and abduction. They are therefore facilitated to cocontract with the flexors and adductors at the shoulder in this position. A normal infant can be observed assuming the pivot prone position just prior to going into a prone-on-elbows position, as if to "prime" his system. The child will progress to pushing backwards then forwards, like a marine belly crawling, and in time will progress to a prone position in which the arms are extended with the hands bearing the weight.

A procedure to achieve on elbows pattern is as follows: The back and neck extensors are C-brushed. The glenohumeral extensors and abductors are C-brushed and iced. The patient is asked to assume the pivot prone position, or an activity that demands pivot prone is used, and resistance is added manually by pushing the thighs and upper trunk toward the supporting surface. Then the patient is placed in the prone-on-elbows position so that there is good joint compression at the shoulder. Pressure and vibration are applied to the extensor/abductor muscles of the glenohumeral joint as needed to gain cocontraction. An activity that demands resisted grasp is introduced to obtain reinforcement of shoulder cocontraction. One suggestion is for a child to shoot water pistols at a target placed in front of him. Another activity example: the person lies on the floor to watch TV, which is placed so that the person must extend his neck and upper trunk to look at it. Other activities include playing board games or doing crafts while prone lying.[19] These activities begin to combine the static bilateral position with unilateral positioning and reaching. Unilateral weight bearing is more advanced than bilateral weight bearing. The activities could progress to involve some crawling, which is a higher-level response (see Table 6.1). Treatment of adults is more likely to involve a modified prone-on-elbows position in which the seated patient leans with his elbow on the table or laptray. Activities are easy to devise for this modified posture and usually involve use

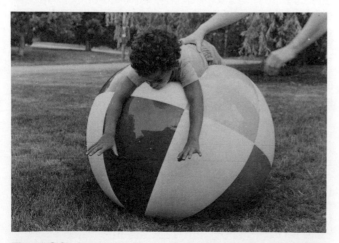

Figure 6.3 Large beach ball illustrating its use to elicit equilibrium reactions in prone and protective extensor thrust.

of the less-affected limb for the skilled activity while the more-affected limb is leaned on to provide stability to the trunk or to hold down the object being worked on. Stockmeyer believes that it is unnecessary for the patient to actually be prone or that the activity be bilateral.[8]

6. *The all-fours* pattern,[5] also called quadruped,[8] occurs when the neck and upper extremities have developed stability; this position helps the trunk and lower extremities develop cocontraction. At first, the quadruped position is static; later the person is able to shift weight backwards and forwards, from side to side, and diagonally, and then is able to lift one or two of the points of support, i.e., one arm and one leg. Finally these activities develop into crawling.[5,8] A suggested procedure to develop the all-fours pattern is as follows: The back and neck extensors are C-brushed. The glenohumeral and hip extensors and abductors and the elbow extensors are C-brushed and iced. The patient assumes and holds the pivot prone position while resistance is added. Then the patient is placed into the all-fours position so that there is good joint compression at the elbows, shoulders, and hips. An activity that demands that the patient maintain the actual quadruped position or a modified version of it is offered. Activity examples include holding a sling shot prepared to shoot (unilateral pattern while upright), weaving on a large loom adapted to resist elbow extension (while upright), holding wood in place while sawing it with the other hand, painting a large mural on the floor, or playing with a toy truck. While the activity is ongoing, repetitive stretch, muscle tendon tapping, and/or vibration are applied to the muscles listed above as needed to maintain the posture.

7. *Standing* is first done as a static bilateral posture, then progresses to shifting weight and to a unilateral posture.[5] Activity suggestions include doing craft activities while standing at a high table or writing on a wall blackboard. Playing ball[18] or throwing bean bags help develop balance while standing.

8. *Walking* is the skill level of standing. It consists of stance, push off, pick up (swing through), and heel strike.[5]

Rood's method underwent continual evolution as she encountered and processed neurophysiological information. Although Rood never recorded her most recent thinking, she did present these ideas at a symposium in Boston in July, 1976. They appeared to amplify rather than negate the previous information. Specifically, she renamed the two major developmental motor patterns that precede development of the more differentiated patterns associated with skilled motor performance.[1]

Pattern I, "toward pattern," is a phasic flexion pattern elicited by a light touch to the upper lip at midline (cranial nerve V area). Pattern I seems to be equivalent to the first mobility response, the supine flexion or withdrawal pattern. The patient's hands reach toward the mouth in response to this stimulus. The elbow and shoulder flex while the wrist and fingers extend. In a child, the legs also flex. In an adult, the legs flex only if the patient is touched on the abdomen near the umbilicus. Pattern I has a longer latency between stimulus and response than does pattern II. If no response is seen in supine, the patient should be positioned sidelying with the moving arm uppermost. This eliminates the contact stimulus to the extensor surface of the body and decreases the influence of the TLR which facilitates extension. For young children and occasionally with adults, the light touch to the upper lip is followed by a maintained touch to the same area in order to balance the phasic response with a tonic response. A more discrete flexion pattern is elicited by applying the touch stimulus peripherally.[1]

Pattern II, "away from pattern," is a tonic extensor pattern elicited by stimulation of the labyrinths, stretch receptors in muscle, and fast repetitive stimuli, such as fast brushing, which, Rood stated,[1] has the effect of eliminating the stretch reflex in phasic muscles. She reiterated that she believed fast brushing should precede all other stimulation, since it requires 30 min to become maximally effective. The labyrinths are stimulated by use of the TLI posture, although in adult hemiplegics, the patient is not inverted below horizontal due to the increase in cranial blood pressure that occurs when the head is dependent. The stretch receptors are stimulated by vibration; the midline deep back muscles are stimulated first before the more superficial, peripheral extensor muscles. A demand for extension against resistance is made on the patient through the use of activity.[1] Pattern II seems to be the first stability pattern, equivalent to prone extension or pivot prone.

Treatment Programming

Rood evaluated the patient to determine what the distribution of muscle tone was and to determine what level of motor control, according to her developmental sequences, the patient had achieved. She started therapy by facilitating the patient's muscles needed to effect the pattern desired. Stimulation involved use of the appropriate type of stimuli to facilitate the desired response (tonic or phasic). If necessary, the patient was assisted into the desired pattern, and a purposeful activity that demanded the movement and/or position and was within the capability of the patient, was immediately presented. The motor pattern chosen to be worked on was the one that the patient could do, but not easily. Then the patient was progressed through the sequences as he mastered each new level. As he was working on perfecting a lower-level skill, he would also begin to learn a higher-level skill. In Table 6.1 the steps are numbered sequentially for both the skeletal and vital function sequences, indicating the order used for evaluation and treatment planning.

The point at which the patient was easily able to do the task represented his highest level of development. Treatment started at the point where the patient had to struggle to do the pattern.

In an attempt to illustrate treatment planning using Rood's sequences, this example may be helpful. The evaluation of an hypothetical poststroke patient indicated that he has some voluntary elbow flexion but his shoulder begins to abduct simultaneously with elbow flexion. He is able to grasp, but unable to release objects. He is able to roll over in bed and rotate his trunk while sitting. In sorting this data out, the therapist notes that the elbow flexors, probably primarily light-work muscles, are contracting in that capacity, but the shoulder abductors, which are heavy-work muscles, should be contracting in a tonic pattern first not in a phasic pattern as they are. If they were stabilizing, it would prevent the reflex phasic abduction seen during elbow flexion. It is also noted that flexion has developed at the elbow and, knowing the developmental sequence, the therapist knows that extension is the next movement to be sought at that joint. The therapist also knows that prone extension would be the next ontogenetic pattern to work for since rollover is already within the patient's repertoire. Therefore, treatment of this patient would begin with controlled sensory stimulation of the tonic physiological extensors of the shoulder and scapula and an activity to demand a static prone extensor response at least unilaterally of the affected side and would proceed to prone-on-hands or quadruped position to develop elbow extension as the patient was able to progress.

Rood suggested this plan for a post-cerebrovascular-accident (CVA) patient whose tonic muscles do not work well: 30 to 40 min before treatment, C-brush the tonic muscles of the unaffected side first, then those on the affected side. At treatment time, elicit pattern I (flexion) for feeding by touching the midline above the lip, which will cause the hand to move to the mouth. The patient is either back- or side-lying during this procedure.[1]

Joy Huss suggests some other treatment planning guidelines[9,18].

1. Hypotonia ("floppy baby syndrome," upper motor neuron flaccidity) is treated by overall general stimulation, especially swinging, rolling, spinning in all planes for labyrinth stimulation, and specific exteroceptive and proprioceptive stimulation for specific muscle stimulation. Activities are used to elicit specific motor patterns in sequence.

2. Hypertonia (spasticity which may be seen in spastic cerebral palsy, CVA, and multiple sclerosis patients, for example) is treated using neutral warmth for relaxation. Exteroceptive and proprioceptive stimulation of the antagonists of the spastic muscles is done. Activity is used in developmental sequence to reinforce normal movement.

3. Hypertonia (rigidity such as seen in Parkinson's disease) is treated using neutral warmth for relaxation. Reciprocal movement patterns are stimulated and reinforced using activity.

4. Hyperkinesis (uncontrolled movement such as seen in athetosis, chorea, ataxia) is treated by slow stroking for relaxation. Maintained holding patterns are stimulated at first and then patterns that involve keeping the distal segment stabilized while the proximal segment moves are used. When control is developed, the patient is progressed to movement patterns such as crawling and creeping.

Treatment goals relate to identified problems. Subgoals may need to be achieved before the more obvious goal is able to be pursued. For example, for hypotonic or weak physiological extensors, the goal is to increase the strength of contraction of these muscles. Since these are the tonic stability muscles, a holding response is sought. The key posture for developing holding responses of physiological extensors is pivot prone; therefore, facilitation of the pattern becomes the first goal of treatment. For a weak flexor response, or more likely for excessive extensor tone, supine flexion (withdrawal) response or rollover pattern is sought. Supine flexion is not used for most patients because flexor tone is usually strong or readily activated. For this reason, patients start in the rollover pattern, which can easily be incorporated into functional activities. If the patient lacks movement due to rigidity (Parkinson's disease), the goal is development of reciprocal gross movement through use of supine flexion or rollover patterns. If the patient lacks movement due to hypertonicity secondary to cortical damage (CVA; head injury), reciprocal gross movement, starting with rollover pattern, is also the first goal. If the patient has intention tremor, a simplistic interpretation is that he lacks movement control. The goal is to develop controlled mobility. The subgoals of developing spindle bias of the extensor muscles through the pivot prone pattern or developing cocontraction responses through weight bearing may need to be accomplished first. If the patient has poor head control, nystagmus, and/or poor swallow and sucking, the goal is to develop neck cocontraction.

VITAL FUNCTION DEVELOPMENTAL SEQUENCE[11]

Functions involving food intake, respiration, and a combination of these two that are used for speech, compose this sequence, which is related to the skeletal sequence (see Table 6.1). Both sequences are handled concurrently in treatment, if appropriate. The vital function developmental sequence precedes speech. Therefore, the occupational therapist, who facilitates this sequence with the goal of decreasing dysphagia as part of a feeding program, collaborates with the speech pathologist to achieve mutual goals. The sequence of development of speech mechanisms is:

1. Inspiration, which is effected reflexively at birth.[5]

2. Expiration, which is dependent on the depth of inspiration. The depth of inspiration is dependent on patterns set in the withdrawal pattern: cocontraction of the deep neck flexors and extensors and cocontraction of the low back musculature with the rectus abdominus.[5] The depth of inspiration can be further increased by icing the upper right quadrant of the abdomen to stimulate the diaphragm.[6] Crying, sneezing, and coughing are all expiration-type phenomenon; asking the patient to attempt to increase the force of coughing is used to improve expiration function.

3. Sucking. "Heavy work sucking is produced by the basic activation of cocontraction of the neck with the stabilizing influence of the infra- and suprahyoid muscles of the tongue, of cocontraction of facial muscles against the orbicularis oris above and below the mouth. Respiration and feeding depend on heavy work sucking."[5] If pressure is applied to the tip of the tongue, then sucking will ensue after five to seven repetitions of the pressure.[1] Resisted sucking facilitates neck cocontraction, which in turns facilitates sucking.

4. Swallowing liquids may be activated by cutaneous stimulation of the mucous membranes of the palate, tongue, and uvula[6]using a long, cotton-tipped applicator stick. Rood believed that the obicularis oris was the key to swallowing because she thought that it activated, by direct stretch, the buccinators and superior constrictor of the pharynx[5]; therefore, in therapy the obicularis oris muscle is facilitated by tapping and brushing. Care is taken that the chin is not brushed or stroked because this will cause the patient to be unable to keep his mouth closed to swallow, resulting in drooling. Slow stroking of the cutaneous distribution of the posterior primary rami is used to relax the voluntary neck muscles preceding stimulation of the muscles involved in the swallowing or sucking reflexes.[6]

5. Phonation, defined as babbling, is controlled expiration as opposed to reflexive expiration of sneezing, coughing, or crying. Reflex motor abilities precede voluntary motor abilities.

6. Chewing.

7. Swallowing solids.

8. Speech, defined as production of recognizable words.

Conclusion

Rood's methods are used eclectically by both occupational and physical therapists in the United States and other countries; however, controlled research on the effectiveness of this approach is extremely limited. As theses projects, some graduate students have conducted limited studies of isolated aspects of the approach on normal persons and patients with central nervous system deficits. However, the accessibility of their theses is limited. Other written case reports of successful results using this therapy are seemingly nonexistent. There is a need for therapists to document the success of this approach to effect more mature motor responses in patients if it is to survive as a treatment methodology.

STUDY QUESTIONS:

The Rood Approach

1. What is the premise on which Rood based her treatment approach?
2. What are the four components of Rood's theory that are included in each treatment?
3. What are the facilitation methods used to evoke a mobility (phasic, movement) response?
4. What facilitation methods are used to evoke a stability (tonic, holding, cocontraction, postural) response?
5. What facilitation or inhibition procedures have a generalized effect and which have an effect localized to the muscle(s) being treated?
6. What Is the sequence of muscle activation, according to Rood?
7. What are the differences between light-work and heavy-work muscles?
8. What are the four phases of development of motor control used in this approach?
9. What are the eight ontogenetic motor patterns of Rood?
10. Why is pivot prone considered a key developmental step?
11. How are patients evaluated using the Rood Approach?
12. How is therapy carried out using the Rood Approach?
13. What is the sequence of development of vital functions?
14. Think of one activity, appropriate for adults, that can be used for each of the ontogenetic patterns.

B/Bobath Neurodevelopmental Approach

CATHERINE A. TROMBLY

Dr. and Mrs. Bobath, English neurologist and physiotherapist, respectively, have devised methods of evaluation and treatment for persons with cerebral palsy and hemiplegia. They believe the methods would be effective for any patient having central nervous system deficit resulting in abnormal patterns of movement.[21]

The premises on which the Bobaths based their treatment approach are as follows. Sensations of movements are learned, not movements per se. Basic postural and movement patterns are learned that are later elaborated on to become functional skills. Every skilled activity takes place against a background of basic patterns of postural control, righting, equilibrium, and other protective reactions (such as the parachute reaction of the arms), reach, grasp, and release.[22]

When the brain is damaged, abnormal patterns of posture and movement develop that are incompatible with the performance of normal everyday activities. The abnormal patterns develop because sensation is shunted into these abnormal patterns. The law of shunting refers to a phenomenon the Bobaths describe as afferent inflow being

> short circuited either temporarily (the athetoid patient) or more permanently (the spastic patient) into patterns of abnormal coordination released from higher inhibitory control . . . . A patient with abnormal motor output who moves abnormally in response to motivation and normal sensory input will still only experience and memorize the sensation of his abnormal movements, of excessive effort and lack of co-ordination. He will, therefore be unable to develop and lay down the memory of normal sensorimotor patterns.[22] (p. 837)

The abnormal patterns must be stopped, not so much by modifying the sensory input, but by giving back to the patient the lost or undeveloped control over his motor output in developmental sequence. The basic patterns of posture and movement, the righting and equilibrium responses, are elicited by providing the appropriate stimuli while the abnormal patterns are inhibited. In this way, the patient experiences normal motor patterns. The sensory information from these correct motor patterns is absolutely necessary for the development of improved motor control. This assumption that correcting the motor responses will result in correct sensory feedback to the CNS in those with damaged central nervous systems needs verification. In one study,children with cerebral palsy were found to be significantly more inaccurate in their estimations of limb positions based on kinesthetic feedback of passive movement compared to normal children.[23] In other words, the children with cerebral palsy misperceived the location of their arms much more than did normal children and therefore could not be expected to be developing "correct" motor response capabilities. This study, however, did not address the issue of whether somatosensory feedback can be recalibrated in patients with defective systems by using vision to match the perceived sensation with the movement. It may be this recalibration process to which the Bobaths refer when they speak of teaching the patient how correct movement feels.

Evaluation and Treatment of Cerebral Palsy

An overview of the procedures used in the evaluation and treatment of children with cerebral palsy is included in this textbook because of the potential usefulness in the treatment of the severely brain-damaged or traumatic head-injured adult.

Evaluation is an integral part of treatment.[21] The whole evaluation is not completed before treatment begins. It is designed in developmental sequence; once the patient's highest level of consistent performance is ascertained, treatment begins to develop the next level of control. Within each treatment session the patient's progress is evaluated. Some measurable change should occur at every session; if it does not, treatment must be modified.[24] As part of the developmental evaluation the extent and distribution of hyper- and hypotonus are determined, as well as the effect hypertonus in one

part of the body has on other parts of the body. Tonus is estimated while placing the patient into developmentally sequenced postural patterns rather than testing at each joint.[21,24] The therapist looks for the immediacy of adjustment of muscles to new positions (normal), for undue ease of placement and hyperextensibility (hypotonia), or for undue resistance to the test movement (hypertonia). The degree and pattern of abnormal tone are noted.

The Cerebral Palsy Assessment Chart and directions for administering the evaluation that was devised by Semans et al.[25] is included here (Table 6.2) because the book in which it was originally published is now out of print.

Throughout the testing, the therapist should ensure maximal freedom from emotional and physical tension through proper handling. In all tests, the therapist should first place the patient in the test position. Physical manipulation to reduce tension (a reflex-inhibiting pattern [RIP]) should be used if spasticity interferes with placement. If the therapist is unable to place the patient because of inability to relax tension or the presence of contractures or structural deviations, there are indicated on the form. Secondly, after being placed, the patient is asked to stay in the test position. As a third step, he is asked to move into the test position independently.

GRADING KEY FOR CEREBRAL PALSY ASSESSMENT CHART

A grading system with values from 0 to 5 is used as follows:

0—Cannot be placed in test posture.

1—Can be placed in test posture, but the position cannot be held.

2—Can hold test posture momentarily after being placed.

3—Can assume an approximate test posture unaided, in any manner.

4—Can assume and sustain test posture in a near normal manner (note any abnormal detail).

5—Normal.

SPECIFIC INSTRUCTIONS FOR ADMINISTERING THE TEST ITEMS

Each item in the test represents necessary postural control for various functional activities. It is helpful to keep in mind the functional significance of each test while administering it in order to observe the most critical aspects contributing to the test score. The following groups are arranged in the approximate order of normal developmental sequence.

Supine

Test 1. Purpose—To test freedom from extensor hypertonus in the supine position. Emphasis in this test is on proximal joints.

Bring the knees, one after the other, to the chest with enough external rotation at the hips to point the knees toward the axillae. This is needed to get complete flex-

Table 6.2
CEREBRAL PALSY ASSESSMENT CHART BASIC MOTOR CONTROL[a]

Name:_____ Birthdate:_____ Diagnosis:_____

Test Postures and Movements	Examiner:	Name: Date	Remarks	Name: Date	Remarks	Name Date	Remarks
Supine 1. Hips and knees fully flexed, arms crossed, palms on shoulders.							
2. Hips and knees fully flexed. (a) Extend right leg. (b) Extend left leg.		R. L.		R. L.		R. L.	
3. Head raised.							
Prone 4. Arms extended beside head. Raise head in midposition.							
5. Arms extended beside body, palms down.							
6. (a) Flex right knee, hips extended. (b) Flex left knee, hips extended.		R. L.		R. L.		R. L.	
7. Trunk supported on forearms, upper trunk extended, face vertical.							
8. Trunk supported on hands with elbows and hips extended.							
Sitting erect 9. Soles of feet together, hips flexed and externally rotated to at least 45°.							
10. Knees extended and legs abducted; hips 90°–100°.							

Table 6.2—*continued*

Name:_____ Diagnosis:_____ Birthdate:_____

Test Postures and Movements	Examiner:	Name: Date	Remarks	Name: Date	Remarks	Name: Date	Remarks
11. Legs hanging over edge of table. (a) Extend right knee. (b) Extend left knee.		R. L.		R. L.		R. L.	
Kneeling 12. Back and neck straight (not hyperextended). (a) Weight on knees. (b) Weight on hands.		a b		a b		a b	
13. Side sitting, upper trunk erect, arms relaxed: (a) On right hip. (b) On left hip.		R. L.		R. L.		R. L.	
14. Kneeling upright, hips extended, head in midposition, arms at sides.							
15. (a) Half kneeling: weight on right knee. (b) Half kneeling: weight on left knee.		R. L.		R. L.		R. L.	
Squatting 16. Heels down, toes not clawed, knees pointing in same direction as toes, hips fully flexed, head in line with trunk.							
Standing and components of walking 17. Standing, correct alignment.							
18. Pelvis and trunk aligned over forward leg. Both knees extended. (a) Right leg forward. (b) Left leg forward.		R. L.		R. L.		R. L.	
19. Bear weight on one leg in midstance. (a) Shift weight over right leg. (b) Shift weight over left leg.		R. L.		R. L.		R. L.	
20. Heel strike. Rear leg extended and externally rotated, heel down. Both knees straight: (a) Right heel strike. (b) Left heel strike.		R. L.		R. L.		R. L.	

[a]Reprinted with permission from Semans et al. A cerebral palsy assessment chart. In *The Child with Central Nervous System Deficit*. Children's Bureau Publication No. 432, U.S. Government Printing Office, 1965.

ion; if not attained, there is probably not full range of hip flexion. Steady the knees in position with your body while placing the patient's arms as follows: Pull the arms forward at the shoulders, abducting the scapulae, and fold them across his chest so that his open palms cup his shoulders; the arms should be up, away from the chest wall; the head should remain in a neutral position; feet should be relaxed in plantar flexion. If the patient assumes the position except for dorsiflexed feet or incompletely relaxed hands, grade 4 should be given.

Test 2.   Purpose—To test ability to flex or extend one leg at a time through full range.

Starting with hips and knees fully flexed and arms across chest or relaxed at side, bring the right leg down to the table into an extended position, avoiding internal rotation. The back should not arch. Return to starting position and repeat with left leg.

Test 3.   Purpose—To test ability to raise head.

Place in a symmetrical supine position with legs extended and arms at sides. Raise the patient's head by flexing the neck. The shoulders should remain relaxed. If the patient can raise the head but protracts the shoulder, a grade of 3 is given.

Prone

Test 4.   Purpose—To test freedom from flexor hypertonus in prone position.

Place the patient prone, lift under the shoulders to free the arms; place the arms overhead one after the other, elbows and wrists extended, palms down, legs extended and relaxed. The head is raised in midposition. Replace the arms below shoulder level before asking the patient to move into the test position.

Test 5.   Purpose—To test freedom of arms and shoulders from flexor hypertonus in prone position.

Place the patient prone, arms externally rotated beside the body, palms down. Place the hands out a short distance from the body so that the arms are not pressed against the thorax. Before asking the patient to assume the position actively, place the patient's arms at shoulder level or above. Note any change of tension resulting from turning the head from one side to the other.

Test 6.   Purpose—To test selective control of hip and knee.

Place the patient prone, arms relaxed beside head or at his sides. Flex right knee to 90° without flexion at hip. The foot should not dorsiflex and the other leg should remain relaxed. Repeat with the left leg. For grade 4 or 5, there should be no appreciable motion in the hip.

For the next postures to be successfully performed, righting reactions are required. Equilibrium and protective extension reactions are evaluated in each of the test postures also. The righting reactions have to do with orienting the head relative to the body, or the body relative to the head and neck, or maintaining the head in a normal position in space. The equilibrium re-

sponses are automatic responses to a disturbance in balance by which the organism makes covert or overt motor adjustments to regain balance over his center of gravity. The protective extension patterns are automatic patterns of the upper extremities that cause the person to reach out in an attempt to break a fall and to protect the head from injury. The Bobaths attempt to elicit these responses at all developmental levels in their handling of the patient.

Test 7.   Purpose—To test postural control in spinal extension. This is important for beginning locomotion (crawling), erect sitting, and beginning use of the hands.

Place the patient prone, extend the thoracic spine, and place the arms one after the other in at least 90° shoulder flexion with slight abduction so that the patient is supported on his forearms. The arms should point straight ahead with the hands open. The head is raised with face vertical.

Test 8.   Purpose—To test ability to support weight on extended arms. This position is often difficult to attain, but it is necessary for creeping.

Start from test position 7. Lift the patient's head, giving gentle traction on the cervical spine so that he supports himself on extended arms and the heel of his open hand; the entire spine and the hips are fully extended. An alternate method to achieve this position is to lift the patient to position from under his shoulders or under his chest.

Sitting Erect

Test 9.   Purpose—To test control of hips in flexion, abduction, and external rotation.

Place the patient in erect sitting position with hips abducted, flexed, and externally rotated to at least 45°, with the soles of the feet together and the arms relaxed. For grades 3 to 5, start in any sitting position on a flat surface.

Test 10.   Purpose—To test erect sitting with legs straight.

Place the patient in erect sitting position with thighs abducted without internal rotation and with knees extended; flexion angle at hip should be 90° to 100°. The arms should be relaxed.

Test 11.   Purpose—To test selective control of hip and knee.

Place the patient in an erect sitting position with the flexion angle at the hip 90° to 100° and the legs hanging vertically. Extend one knee fully without further extension of the hip. The other leg and arms should remain relaxed. (a) Right knee extended; (b) left knee extended.

Kneeling

Test 12.   Purpose—To test weight-bearing and balance control on knees and heels of open hands.

Start in four-point kneeling (quadruped), with the back and neck straight (not hyperextended), legs parallel, elbows extended, hands pointing forward. (a) The patient takes the weight predominantly on his knees; (b) the patient takes the weight predominantly on his hands.

Test 13. Purpose—To test ability of the trunk to adapt to gravitational changes.

Place the patient in side sitting from four-point or upright kneeling by lowering the hips to one side of the feet. The head and upper trunk should be erect and the arms free. (a) The patient first sits on right hip; (b) then on left hip.

Test 14. Purpose—To test anterior-posterior control of pelvis and trunk on thighs.

Place the patient in upright kneeling (kneel standing) position, with the hips extended, legs parallel, trunk and head erect, head in midposition and arms relaxed.

Test 15. Purpose—To test control of rotation at the hip. Place the patient in a half-kneeling position from upright kneeling. The other foot is placed on floor in front and to the side for adequate supporting base. The hip, knee, and ankle of the forward leg are positioned at 90°, toes not clawed. The pelvis and trunk face forward with the knee angled slightly outward.

Squatting

Test 16. Purpose—To test control of extensor spasticity.

Place from squat sitting, i.e., legs and hips fully flexed and outwardly rotated, feet flat on floor, toes not clawed, knees pointing in same direction as toes, arms forward for balance. Shift weight forward over feet into squatting position. Adult patients can be placed from a low stool. It is easier to assume this position if the legs are spread wide apart.

Standing and Components of Walking

Test 17. Purpose—To test normal distribution of tone in standing.

Place the patient in a standing position with the body segments in normal alignment with relation to the line of gravity in midcoronal and midsagittal planes, i.e., the weight evenly distributed over both feet, legs in midposition of rotation, and so on. Points of control might be the hip of one side and the knee of the opposite side, or the hip and opposite arm. A lift may be used to equalize leg length.

Test 18. Purpose—To test the ability to shift weight forward onto the stance leg with the rear leg extended for push off.

Place the patient in forward step position. Shift weight over the forward leg with the trunk, pelvis, thigh, and leg correctly aligned over the foot. The rear leg should be extended, outwardly rotated at the hip, and resting on the normal, roll-off point (the head of the first metatarsal); the arms should be relaxed. For grades 2 to 5, the therapist may steady the patient by holding one of his hands.

Test 19. Purpose—To test the ability to support the body over one leg (absence of Trendelenburg sign).

From a symmetrical standing position, shift the patient's weight laterally over one leg and lift the other free of the floor, as for the swing phase of walking. The trunk should remain erect. For grades 2 to 5, the therapist may steady the patient by holding one hand.

Test 20. Purpose—To test heel strike.

One foot is advanced in dorsiflexion and the heel is placed on the floor. Body weight is supported mainly on the rear leg, with the hip extended and both knees straight. Ankles remain at approximately 90°. Arms should be relaxed. For grades 2 to 5, the therapist may steady the patient by holding one of his hands.

Guiding questions that should be considered by the therapist during the evaluation include the following:[26]

1. Are the patient's motor abilities arrested at one level of development or are his abilities scattered in several different stages of development? The answer to this question will identify the gaps that must be filled in between the patient's lowest and highest levels of performance.

2. What abnormal postures does the patient exhibit and how do they interfere with his activities? The answer to this question indicates which patterns have to be inhibited in order to facilitate the normal patterns.

3. Does the patient have any abnormal postural patterns or persistent asymmetries that may in time develop into contractures and deformities? Treatment must be aimed at preventing deformities.

4. What is the distribution of abnormal tone? How does tonus change with stimulation or effort? Is there abnormal tone only in certain positions and not others? Does movement affect tone? The answers to these questions will guide the design of reflex-inhibiting patterns and the selection of other treatment techniques.

Treatment for the patient with generalized brain injury concentrates on handling the patient in such a way as to inhibit abnormal distribution of tone and abnormal postures while stimulating or encouraging active motion in the next level of motor control. The abnormal postures and tone are controlled at key points using reflex-inhibiting movements or patterns called RIPs. If the patient lacks tone, sensory stimulation or "tapping" is used while the RIP is applied so that the sensory inflow will not shunt into abnormal patterns. The Bobaths believe that once the patient can move easily in and out of normal basic patterns of posture and movement he will automatically be able to elaborate on these patterns to learn more skilled activities required in daily living.[22,24,26,27]

Early treatment is considered ideal and necessary if true gains are to be made and fixed abnormal patterns, or contractures, avoided.[24,28]

Treatment principles include the following:

1. Developmental progression is followed. For children with cerebral palsy or for adults with traumatic head injury, that progression refers to the development, or redevelopment, of basic static and dynamic

postural responses may be preserved, the progression may be limited to redevelopment of limb control from mass to discrete movement, from proximal to distal control, and/or from isometric to eccentric to concentric movement control.

2. Normal integration of both sides of the body is sought while associated reactions are avoided.

3. Abnormal tone is always inhibited concurrently with elicitation of normal reactions.

4. Normal responses, once elicited, are always repeated. Opportunity is given to practice the new ability in functionally meaningful ways.

5. Voluntary control of normal responses is encouraged.

REFLEX-INHIBITING PATTERNS

RIPs are used to inhibit patterns of abnormal muscle tone, such as those caused by the influence of predominating primitive tonic reflexes (tonic neck and tonic labyrinthine reflexes) so often seen in children with cerebral palsy and other brain-injured patients. RIPs are partial patterns opposite to the typical abnormal patterns of postural tone that dominate the patient. The RIPs prevent shunting of the sensory inflow into abnormal patterns and redirect it into normal ones. As tone becomes more normal the patient can learn to control the abating tonic reflex activity.[27] Inhibition of abnormal tone is always used concurrently with facilitation of the righting and equilibrium reactions. Severely involved patients, or older children, who have not been successfully treated previously, may need to be inhibited for a long time before a period of relative normalcy occurs during which they can actively move.[26,27] Even these patients are moved passively when postural tone decreases to begin stimulation of the righting reactions.[26] RIPs are designed by examining the patient in all patterns of posture (during the evaluation) to determine which distribution of abnormal tone is typical. By holding a key part of the patient in an opposite pattern, the inhibiting pattern is tested to see if it tends to redistribute the tone of the whole patient more normally as it should if it is to be used for treatment.[26] Key points of contacting the patient are changed to allow the patient to develop flexible control over his own movements and postures. Key points are usually proximal parts of the body (head, neck, shoulder girdle, pelvic girdle or trunk) from which abnormal reflexes seem to originate,[26] but may also be distal (fingers, thumbs, toes). Semans et al.[25] advises that one should not yield to the temptation to start the RIP where the spasticity is most obvious. If the therapist chooses the key point of control where hypertonus is greatest, the patient will not be able to move that part and cannot develop control. Full body RIPs are not used because the tone is liable to be shunted into a reverse pattern.[26] Rather, a key point is chosen that allows the full pattern of tone to be broken up during the handling[26] by the least restrictive RIP.

A few examples of RIPs will be listed here. However, the RIPs must be individualized for each person following a careful analysis of the patient's problems. These examples can be used as models. Raising the head into hyperextension facilitates extensor tone of the rest of the body and inhibits flexor tone.[26] Flexion of the head encourages flexion of the rest of the body and inhibits extensor hypertonicity.[21] Internal rotation of the limb inhibits extension, whereas external rotation inhibits flexion. Horizontal abduction or diagonal extension of the humerus inhibits flexion in the neck, arms, and hands. Elevation of the arms inhibits flexor hypertonus[26] and facilitates extension of the hips and trunk.[27] Flexion of the hip and knee combined with abduction of the hip inhibits extensor tone of the trunk and head and limbs. Symmetrical extension of the limbs, with the head in midline to rule out the influences of the asymmetrical tonic neck reflex, inhibits flexor spasticity of the arms. Rotation of the trunk between the shoulder and pelvic girdles inhibits both flexor and extensor hypertonus.

HANDLING

The Bobaths term their manner of control of the patient through RIPs and their movement of him to elicit righting and equilibrium responses, "handling."[27] This simulates handling of the normal infant by his mother. Handling is used to influence postural tone; to regulate coordination of agonists, antagonists, and synergists; to inhibit abnormal patterns; and to facilitate normal automatic responses. At first the therapist handles the patient to move him passively in correct patterns of posture or movement while the patient is encouraged to cooperate and help as he can. The therapist withdraws guidance and support as the patient is able to take over more and more initiative to move in correct patterns.

The handling is constantly changing to inhibit the undesired and to facilitate the desired responses in the dynamic treatment situation in which the patient's responses are changing due to the therapist's stimulation. It requires constant attention to the demands to be made of the patient, to the stimulation to be offered, and to the patient's responses to each. Abnormal tone or movement is prevented from happening at the first sign. The patient is not allowed to exert effort because tone increases with effort and may become shunted into the abnormal patterns. Once the first normal reaction has occurred, it is repeated to establish new sensorimotor patterns and to make the reaction quicker and more reliable.[21]

RIGHTING AND EQUILIBRIUM REACTIONS

RIPs are inhibitions imposed from the outside; true inhibition of primitive patterns can be gained only through elicitation of the righting and equilibrium reactions. Righting reactions and equilibrium responses (including protective extension patterns) are elicited for each posture and movement that is being used in therapy. Many postures and movements are used during a treatment sequence to help the patient develop dynamic control and to mimic normal development which occurs spirally; as one motor task is being elaborated on, others are beginning to enter the patient's repertoire. "The movements (used in therapy) are the fundamental motor patterns that normal children develop during the first two years of life."[28]

The neck righting reaction and the body righting reaction on the body are evoked to assist the patient to move from supine to prone, to on-elbows, to quadruped, to kneel-standing, and finally to standing. The patient is moved in and out of the positions which are within his developmental capabilities using these reactions. He is moved to these postures in a variety of ways. For example, he does not always turn to the right when moving supine to prone but alternates moving toward the left. He is moved slowly at first, then with increasing speed as he is able to respond. When eliciting neck righting and body righting acting on the body the head is used as the key point. This may be contraindicated in some patients, however, and the patient's neurologist should be consulted before using the head as a key controlling point. When eliciting labyrinthine righting reactions the key points used are scapulae or shoulders, and the head is left free to automatically adjust to the stimulus. When facilitating movements from the head and neck, the therapist places one hand lightly under the patient's chin and the other against the back of his head. When facilitating movements from the shoulder girdle the therapist places her hands under the patient's axillae, spreading the fingers over the scapulae in order to control the shoulder girdle. The patient may be moved through a whole sequence of postures using these key points, or each segment of the whole process may be done separately for reinforcement. The patient is not moved into postures he is not developmentally ready to assume.

Equilibrium reactions are elicited by displacing the person's center of gravity while he is in one of the developmental postures and can maintain that posture against gravity. The person is moved in all directions within each posture: backward and forward, side to side, and obliquely. The therapist must withdraw support to the point that the patient feels the need to recover his own balance but not so much as to instill in him a fear of falling. Abnormal tone would increase due to fear of falling.[26] Elicitation of equilibrium responses is at first done slowly and gently; then the speed and range of displacement are increased as the patient is able to adjust. When moving the person, the therapist "taps" him off balance in one direction and then catches him with the other hand and taps him back to midline in the opposite direction. Or the patient can be held by his hips or shoulders so his arms and head are left free to adjust the balance just as a tightrope walker does. For more advanced patients these responses may be elicited on mobile surfaces, such as an equilibrium board, which is a flat surface on rockers; a very large beach ball (Fig. 6.3); or inflatables, which are large, rectangular, inflated plastic pillows that tip from side to side and back to front but less so than the ball. However the therapist can exert more control moving the person rather than the surface.

Protective responses can be elicited at the same time as equilibrium reactions. The patient is held in an RIP using the arm on the side opposite to the one on which the response will be elicited. He is pushed to the side or forward slowly at first and later with more speed. He should respond by protecting himself by outstretching the free arm to meet the surface.

SENSORY STIMULATION

Sensory stimulation is used for hypotonic patients and others that appear to be "weak" when the abnormal tone is inhibited, or those who have a sensory disturbance. Sensory stimulation is never done unless the patient is in an RIP in order to shunt the inflow into desired channels. Sensory stimulation is done very carefully and stopped if the response becomes abnormal or hyperactive. It is aimed at local responses, and widespread associated reactions are avoided. The kinds of sensory stimulation advocated by the Bobaths include the following:

1. Weight bearing with pressure and resistance is used to elicit increased postural tone and to decrease involuntary movements. This is especially good for ataxic and athetoid patients who need to develop static postures and slow movements within small ranges. Spastic patients need active movement; therefore, weight bearing is done in such a way that weight transfer is allowed;[26] that is, weight is shifted on and off the limb(s) being treated so that the limb intermittently bears weight. Use of added resistance may be contraindicated in cases of spasticity if it increases abnormal posturing.

2. Placing and Holding.[24,26] Placing refers to the ability to arrest a movement at any stage automatically or voluntarily. At first the therapist moves the limb to various positions as the patient assists in this. The patient then holds the position without assistance once the limb is placed. Later, the patient places his own limb and holds it at various intermediate ranges within the limits of motion.

3. Tapping has several meanings. (a) Pressure tapping (joint compression) is used to increase tone for maintenance of an acceptable posture. (b) Inhibitory tapping is used to activate muscles that are weak due to reciprocal inhibition by spastic antagonists. The method used is to release the body part and to catch it as it falls a very small distance, thus stimulating the stretch reflexes. (c) Alternate tapping is used to stimulate balance reactions and is done by pushing the person using light "taps" towards and away from upright position. (d) Sweep tapping is used to activate synergic patterns of muscle function and is done by the therapist sharply sweeping his hand over the desired muscles in the direction of the desired movement.

"Only those techniques which bring about an immediate improvement of tone and active movement in any one treatment session should continue to be used."[29]

TREATMENT PROGRAM

An example of combining an RIP with elicitation of a righting reaction and then equilibrium reactions is as follows: starting in supine, the neck is flexed to inhibit the extensor tone, then rotated to elicit the neck-righting reaction, which is log roll to prone. The head is held in extension to inhibit flexor tone. If the patient is on an equilibrium board it is tipped to elicit a recovery response. (See chapter 4 for descriptions of normal equilibrium responses.)

To progress, with the neck again extended to inhibit flexor tone, a gentle upward movement of the head prompts the patient to assume an on-elbows position. Again he is tipped or pushed off balance to elicit equilibrium responses once he can hold the posture. Then to progress, the neck is flexed and is combined with backward pressure against the top of the head to encourage flexion of the hips and assumption of a quadruped position. Or, to alternately facilitate sitting up, the patient's head is lifted and rotated to one side. Then, before he reaches a side-lying position, pressure is exerted backward against the top of the head to flex the spine and hips while continuing with rotation of the spine. This results in sitting. Equilibrium responses would be elicited when the patient had control of each posture. Detailed directions concerning the use of righting reactions to attain each developmental posture are available in Bobaths' publications.

The occupational therapist will want to combine these suggestions for therapy with activity ideas to both motivate the patient and to encourage practice in functional situations. For example, handling the patient from supine to prone could be combined with the patient's interest in looking at something or need to reach to the side. Eventually, the therapist could use an enticing activity to stimulate the person to move in this pattern without the therapist handling him. To encourage maintenance of the prone-on-elbows posture, activities such as watching TV, reading a magazine, or playing a board game such as chess can be used. Prone-on-hands posture can be encouraged by moving the stimulus object higher, which then encourages the patient to raise himself up to be able to continue to look at the object. Holding an object steady with the more affected arm so that the more skilled hand can work on it requires the patient to use a modified prone-on-elbows posture if sitting at a table or a modified prone-on-hands posture if standing at a table. From an on-hands position, side-sitting may be encouraged by having the person reach toward the back of himself to get an object such as game parts. Once side-sitting is achieved, the person can support himself on his affected extremity to develop postural supporting reactions in that limb.

From a side-sitting position, the quadruped position can be achieved by requiring that the person throw something using the limb that was supporting him, in order to build up momentum that is directed toward the quadruped position. To practice development of equilibrium reactions in quadruped, the patient could be presented with the need to reach for objects placed in front or to the side of him, or to move within the position. From quadruped, kneel-standing can be achieved by making a demand for the person to reach up for an object. Of course activity demands must be within the capability of the patient. Excess effort produces tension, which shunts into abnormal postures.

Although the sequential steps are presented as a whole here, the student therapist should realize that many treatment sessions will need to be spent in trying to help the patient gain control of each step. Since progress is slow, both patient and therapist need to note small improvements to sustain motivation. Daily progress should be documented in terms of level of posture achieved, time during which it could be held, ease of moving from one posture to another, and/or functional achievements made possible by the improvements in control.

Evaluation and Treatment of the Adult Hemiplegic[25]

THE PROBLEM AND RATIONALE

Instead of righting reactions, equilibrium responses and automatic adaptation of antigravity muscles to changes of posture seen in a normal person, a person with a lesion of the upper motor neuron exhibits static and stereotyped movement patterns (abnormal postural reflexes), spasticity, and exaggerated cocontraction that prevents free, coordinated movement. The abnormal postural reflexes that the hemiplegic patient most commonly exhibits are a symmetrical tonic neck reflex, the positive supporting reaction, and associated reactions. Associated reactions are not the normal, co-ordinated associated movements of the opposite side of the body often seen in children and new learners. They are tonic reflex movements of the affected side of the body which may outlast the duration of the stimulus. The stimulus for these abnormal postural reflexes is forceful tonic contraction of the muscles of the sound side, which occurs during excessive effort or in response to fear of falling. Therefore, these situations are avoided in the treatment of the stroke patient. Demands for too complex a movement or the use of an activity requiring too highly skilled a response also causes the patient to regress to more primitive motor behavior.[30]

Also contributing to the hemiplegic person's problem in initiating and performing movement is disturbed sensation and perception. Normally, movement is performed in response to perceived environmental stimuli. If the reception or perception of that stimuli is defective, then the motor response will also be defective. In the case of sensory loss or impairment, the two sides of the body present the patient with different sensations. It may seem to him that he is divided into two halves with no interplay between the sound and affected sides, which can lead to negation of the affected side and complete orientation to the sound side.[31]

Bobath treatment is "based on the view that spasticity is caused by the release of an abnormal postural mechanism which results in exaggerated static function at the expense of dynamic postural control. The aim of treatment is to help the patient gain control over the patterns of spasticity by inhibiting the abnormal reflex patterns." Spasticity underlies the abnormal reflex patterns and is reduced by counteracting these patterns. Inhibition is combined with techniques of handling to elicit movement patterns of righting and equilibrium responses that underlie normal function and to elicit increasingly selective and less stereotyped movement patterns.[31] Emphasis of treatment is on changing the motor output, thereby influencing sensory inflow necessary for learning of normal movement, as opposed to "putting in" sensory stimuli, which are believed to be shunted by the lesion into the stereotypical patterns of spastic hemiplegia.

EVALUATION

Sensation is evaluated because a persistent loss of sensation indicates a poor prognosis for regaining motor control. Specifically, loss of kinesthesia, proprioception, localization of pressure and light touch, and stereognosis predict poor recovery of motor control.[24] Functional improvement of the hand has been found possible only in those with little or no sensory deficit.[31]

Evaluation and treatment are interwoven; that is, the postures used in evaluation are used as treatment goals. The evaluation stops and treatment begins at the point where the patient cannot control the test posture.

The strength and distribution of spasticity is assessed in patterns. The limb is moved by the therapist in exactly the movement patterns that the patient must eventually learn but that are at first interfered with by spasticity. As the therapist moves the limb, the patient's adaptation to the normal patterns of posture and movement imposed on him is assessed. Normal adaptation means that the person actively controls the weight of the limb; a holding response is immediately seen if the limb is left alone at any stage of the movement. Spasticity causes resistance if the movement is away from the pattern of spasticity or uncontrolled assistance to the passive or guided movement into the direction of the spasticity. Flaccidity causes the limb to feel heavy and abnormally relaxed and no active adjustment of the muscles to changes in posture and gravity and no holding of a position against gravity are felt.

Due to spasticity, the postural patterns are usually restricted to one or two stereotyped patterns; therefore, testing involves estimation of the level of control of patterns contrary to these synergistic responses. Note is made of which functional patterns exist and the degree of selectivity of those patterns. By observing the patient's attempts to move, abnormal patterns that may interfere with function are noted. Finally, as control develops, the patient's use of the extremity to accomplish a given skill is analyzed to determine which motor patterns necessary to do the skill correctly are still missing.

The patient's ability to perform specific movements is evaluated using two groups of tests: I. Tests for the Quality of Movement Patterns; and II. Tests for Balance and Other Automatic Protective Reactions. Test I has three grades of tasks, each more difficult than the previous one. The items within each grade are also arranged according to difficulty. Tests for balance and other automatic protective reactions are used for patients with slight disability only.

Equilibrium (balance) reactions are tested by displacing the patient's center of gravity or by asking him to lift the unaffected limb while in a weight-bearing position, which automatically and naturally displaces the weight of his body onto the affected side and demands an automatic equilibrium adjustment. Note is made of whether he can do this and how he responds when equilibrium reactions are elicited. These reactions are tested when the patient is prone, sitting, on all fours, kneel-standing, kneeling on one knee, standing with one foot in front of the other, and standing on one foot (first the unaffected, then the affected). The patient is tested only in those positions that he can safety maintain.

Protective extension of the affected arm is also tested in all these positions by pushing the patient off balance, while holding the patient by the unaffected hand with the arm held in extension and external rotation to facilitate extension of the affected arm and hand. Note is made whether he responds to each stimulus by reaching out to prevent a fall. The student is referred to the original source for greater detail concerning the administration of these tests.

The test forms pertaining to the quality of movement of the upper extremity are reproduced here, with permission (Table 6.3). The wording on the form and the description of administration of the evaluation are not entirely clear as written. Although there is space to grade the patient's response while supine, the description of the test posture appears to have been developed for the upright posture. The role of gravity changes between supine and upright and interpretation of the results due to this difference is not clearly addressed in the original source.

In planning treatment, the therapist identifies from the evaluation (1) whether to increase, decrease, or stabilize tone; (2) which abnormal patterns need to be inhibited and which normal ones need to be facilitated; and (3) which functional skills the patient will need to relearn and the order of learning. The therapist then devises a "teaching plan" for these.

TREATMENT

Bobath believes that compensatory rehabilitation (activities of daily living and gait training) results in increased spasticity and inactivity of the involved side and should be postponed until patients naturally enter the treatment process, which should concentrate on restoration of control of basic postural and movement patterns. However "everything done in treatment

Table 6.3
TEST FORMS FOR THE QUALITY OF MOVEMENT OF THE UPPER EXTREMITY

I. Tests for the Quality of Movement Patterns

Tests for arm and shoulder girdle (to be tested separately in supine, sitting, and standing, as the result will be different in these positions.)

	Supine		Sitting		Standing	
Grade 1	Yes	No	Yes	No	Yes	No
a. Can he hold extended arm in elevation after having it placed there?						
With internal rotation?						
With external rotation?						
b. Can he lower the extended arm from the position of elevation to the horizontal plane and back again to elevation?						
Forward-downward?						
Sideways-downward?						
With internal rotation?						
With external rotation?						
c. Can he move the extended abducted arm from the horizontal plane to the side of his body and back again to the horizontal plane?						
With internal rotation?						
With external rotation?						
Grade 2						
a. Can he lift his arm to touch the opposite shoulder?						
With palm of hand?						
With back of hand?						
b. Can he bend his elbow with his arm in elevation to touch the top of his head?						
With pronation?						
With supination?						
c. Can he fold his hands behind his head with both elbows in horizontal abduction?						
With wrist flexed?						
With wrist extended?						
Grade 3						
a. Can he supinate his forearm and wrist?						
Without side-flexion of trunk on the affected side?						
With flexed elbow and flexed fingers?						
With extended elbow and extended fingers?						
b. Can he pronate his forearm without adduction of arm at shoulder						
c. Can he externally rotate his extended arm?						
(i) in horizontal abduction?						
(ii) by the side of his body?						
(iii) in elevation						
d. Can he bend and extend his elbow in supination to touch the shoulder of the same side? starting with:						
(i) arm by side of his body?						
(ii) horizontal abduction of the arm?						

Tests for wrist and fingers	Yes?	No?
Grade 1		
a. Can he place his flat hand forward down on table in front?		
Can he do this sideways when sitting on plinth?		
With fingers and thumb adducted?		
With fingers and thumb abducted?		
Grade 2		
a. Can he open his hand to grasp?		
With flexed wrist?		

Table 6.3—_continued_

	Yes?	No?
With extended wrist?		
With pronation?		
With supination?		
With adducted fingers and thumb?		
With abducted fingers and thumb?		
Grade 3		
a. Can he grasp and open his fingers again?		
With flexed elbow?		
With extended elbow?		
With pronation?		
With supination?		
b. Can he move individual fingers?		
Thumb?		
Index finger?		
Little finger?		
2nd and 3rd finger?		
c. Can he oppose fingers and thumb?		
Thumb and index finger?		
Thumb and 2nd finger?		
Thumb and little finger?		

II. Tests for Balance and Other Automatic Protective Reactions[a]

Balance reactions.	Yes?	No?
Patient in prone-lying, supporting himself on his forearms.		
a. His shoulder girdle is pushed toward affected side. Does he remain supported on affected forearm?		
b. His sound arm is lifted forward and up, as when reaching out with one hand. Does he immediately transfer his weight toward the affected arm?		
c. His sound arm is lifted and moved backward, and he is turned to his side, support on affected arm. Does he remain supported on affected arm?		
Patient sitting on the plinth, his feet unsupported.		
a. He is pushed toward the affected side. Does he stay upright?		
Does he laterally flex his head toward the sound side?		
Does he abduct his sound leg?		
Does he use the affected forearm for support?		
Does he use the affected hand for support?		
b. He is pushed forward.		
Does he bend affected hip and knee?		
Does he extend his spine?		
Does he lift his head?		
c. Both his legs are lifted up by the therapist, knees flexed.		
Does he stay upright?		
Does he move affected arm forward?		
Does he support himself backwards with affected arm?		
Patient in four-foot kneeling.		
a. His body is pushed toward the affected side.		
Does he abduct the sound leg?		
Does he remain on all fours?		
b. His sound arm is lifted and held up by the therapist.		
Does he keep affected arm extended?		
c. His sound leg is lifted.		
Does he keep affected leg flexed and transfer weight on to it?		
d. His sound arm and affected leg are lifted.		
Does he keep affected arm extended?		

[a]In order to test these reactions the patient must be able to assume and hold the test position. He should react with specific movements in order to regain his balance or protect himself against falling when being moved or pushed unexpectedly.

Table 6.3—*continued*

	Yes?	No?

    e. His affected arm and his sound leg are lifted.
        Does he remain on affected flexed leg?
    f. His sound arm and leg are lifted.
        Does he transfer his weight toward the affected side and maintain position?

Patient in kneel-standing.
    a. He is pushed toward the affected side.
        Does he abduct the sound leg?
        Does he bend head laterally toward the sound side?
        Does he use his affected hand for support?
    b. He is pushed toward the sound side.
        Does he abduct the affected leg?
        Does he extend the affected arm sideways?
    c. He is pushed backward and asked not to sit down.
        Does he extend the affected arm forward?
    d. He is pushed gently forward, his sound arm held backward by the therapist.
        Does he use affected arm and hand for support on the ground?
        Does he lift affected foot off the ground?

Patient half-kneeling, sound foot forward. (He should not use sound hand for support.)
    a. His sound foot is lifted up by the therapist.
        Does he remain upright?
    b. His sound foot is lifted by the therapist and placed sideways.
        Does he remain upright?
        Does he show balance movements with his affected arm?
    c. His sound foot is placed from the above position back to kneel-standing.
        Does he keep upright?
        Does he keep affected hip extended?

Patient standing, feet parallel, standing base narrow.
    a. He is tipped backward and not allowed to make step backward with sound leg.
        (Therapist puts her foot on his sound one to prevent step.)
        Does he step backward with affected leg?
    b. He is tipped backward and not allowed to make steps with either leg.
        Does he dorsiflex toes of affected leg?
        Big toe only?
        Dorsiflex ankle and toes of affected leg?
        Does he move affected arm forward?
    c. He is tipped toward sound side.
        Does he abduct affected leg?
        Does he abduct and extend affected arm?
        Does he make steps to follow with affected leg across sound leg?
    d. He is tipped toward the affected side.
        Does he abduct the sound leg?
        Does he bend head laterally towards the sound side?

Patient standing on affected leg only. (He is not allowed to use sound hand for support.)
    a. His sound foot is lifted by the therapist and moved forward as in making a step, extending his knee.
        Does he keep the heel of affected leg on the ground?
        Does he keep the knee of the affected leg extended?
        Does he assist weight transfer forward over affected leg with extended hip?
    b. His sound foot is lifted by the therapist and moved backward as in making a step backward.
        Does he keep the hip of affected leg extended?
        Does he assist weight transfer backward over affected leg?
    c. His sound foot is lifted by the therapist and held up while he is *pushed* gently sideways toward the affected side.

Table 6.3—*continued*

	Yes?	No?
Does he follow and adjust his balance, moving the foot of the affected leg sideways by inverting and everting his foot alternately?		
The same maneuver is done *pulling* him toward the affected side. Does he follow and adjust his balance by moving his foot as above?		

Protective extension and support of the arm

When testing these reactions the patient's sound arm should be held by his hand, so that he cannot use it. It is advisable to hold the sound arm in extension and external rotation because this facilitates the extension of the affected arm and hand.

	Yes?	No?
a. The patient stands in front of a table or plinth. His sound arm is held backward and he is pushed forward toward the table.		
Does he extend his affected arm forward?		
Does he support himself on his fist?		
On the palm of his hand?		
His thumb adducted?		
His thumb abducted?		
b. The patient stands facing a wall, at a distance which allows him to reach it with his hand. He is pushed forward against the wall, his sound arm held backward.		
Does he lift his affected arm and stretch it out against the wall?		
Does he place his hand against the wall, fingers flexed, thumb adducted?		
Fingers open, thumb abducted?		
c. The patient is sitting on the plinth. His sound arm is held sideways by the therapist. He is pushed toward the affected side.		
Does he abduct the affected arm and support himself on his forearm?		
On his extended arm?		
Does he support himself on his fist?		
On his open palm?		
Thumb and fingers adducted?		
Thumb and fingers abducted?		
d. The patient stands sideways to a wall, at a distance which allows him to reach it with his affected hand.		
Does he abduct and lift the affected arm?		
With flexed elbow?		
Does he reach out for the wall with extended elbow?		
Does he support himself with his fist against the wall?		
With his open hand?		
With adducted thumb and fingers?		
With abducted thumb and fingers?		
e. The patient lies on the floor on his back. His sound hand is placed under his hip so that he cannot use it. The therapist takes a pillow and pretends to throw it towards his head.		
Does he move his affected arm to protect his face?		
With flexed elbow?		
With extended elbow?		
With internal rotation?		
With external rotation?		
With fisted hand?		
With open hand?		
Can he catch the pillow?		

should serve as a direct preparation for specific functional use."[31]

Treatment consists of reflex-inhibiting patterns, sensory stimulation, weight bearing, and holding (postural control) and placing (movement).

Spasticity must be prevented by use of the special techniques of handling that counteract the abnormal patterns of tonic reflex activity, called reflex-inhibiting patterns. The therapist changes the abnormal patterns by using the key points previously mentioned to reverse the most important part of the pattern, which results in spasticity reduction throughout the body or limb. RIPs are designed for the individual patient and involve the least restrictive control necessary to obtain relaxation of spasticity. In the hemiplegic, RIPs are used to counteract the typical distribution of flexor spasticity in the upper extremity and trunk and extensor spasticity of the lower extremity.

The main RIP used to counteract flexor spasticity of the arm is extension and external rotation of the shoulder with elbow extension. Extension of the wrist with supination of the forearm and abduction of the thumb may be added. Flexor spasticity of the upper trunk can be counteracted by neck and spine extension alone or in combination with arms overhead. Rotation of the shoulder girdle in relation to the pelvis reduces trunk and/or limb flexor or extensor spasticity. To counteract flexor or extensor spasticity of the lower extremity, the pattern used is hip abduction and external rotation combined with extension of the hip and knee. Further reduction of extensor spasticity can be achieved by adding dorsiflexion of the ankle and toes and abduction of the great toe. Slight knee flexion also will counteract extensor tone in the lower limb; care must be taken that a knee flexor contracture does not develop.

Sensory stimulation (tactile and proprioceptive) is used for flaccid patients while the limb is held in an RIP to prevent development of tone in the pattern of spasticity. See the description of tapping given above.

Although manipulation of tone is one aspect of treatment, the major goal of therapy is to provide the patient with the feeling of many different normal automatic and voluntary patterns of movement so that he learns (stores in memory) the sensation of movement. As can be seen on the evaluation form, which also serves as a guide to treatment, introduction of movement follows the developmental progressions of mass to isolated movement and proximal to distal control.

An introductory summary of treatment techniques used for the upper extremity will be presented here. The reader is referred to the original source, *Adult Hemiplegia: Evaluation and Treatment* (2nd edition), and to the short courses offered by the Bobaths and their associates for detailed knowledge of the whole treatment program and to develop skill under supervision.

Treatment during the Initial Flaccid Stage

The stages are labeled according to expected levels of recovery; however, treatment described for the flaccid stage may be ongoing into the next "spastic stage."

In the flaccid stage, tone is primarily absent, but spasticity is developing and appears as intermittent reactions to stretch. Because treatment for this stage occurs in the patient's bed, it requires cooperative effort between therapists and nursing personnel. Treatment focuses on positioning and movement in bed to avoid the typical postural patterns of hemiplegia by reversing these patterns. The typical pattern in the upper extremity is as follows: the scapula is retracted and depressed; the shoulder is adducted and internally rotated; the elbow, wrist and fingers are flexed; the forearm is pronated; the wrist is ulnarly deviated; and the fingers are adducted. In the leg, the hip, knee, and ankle are simultaneously extended and the foot inverted; the thigh is inwardly rotated; and the pelvic girdle is rotated backward. The lateral flexors of the trunk and neck on the affected side are shortened.

Positioning. The patient should be encouraged to lie on either side for a time each day in order to be out of the supine position, which encourages extensor tonus. The position of choice to inhibit the development of flexor tone in the upper extremity and extensor tone in the lower extremity, which is the usual picture in hemiplegia, is as follows: side-lying on the sound side with the head laterally flexed away from the affected side, the lateral trunk flexors lengthened, and the affected arm propped on a pillow in front of the patient in order to bring the scapula forward from its retracted position. The elbow is extended. The affected leg should lie in a normal semiflexed position and not touch the foot of the bed, which would elicit the positive supporting reaction (Fig. 6.4).

While the patient is lying supine, the head should be laterally flexed away from the affected arm to counteract the tendency of the head to be drawn toward the affected side. There should be a pillow under the arm to pull the scapula forward and one under the knee to

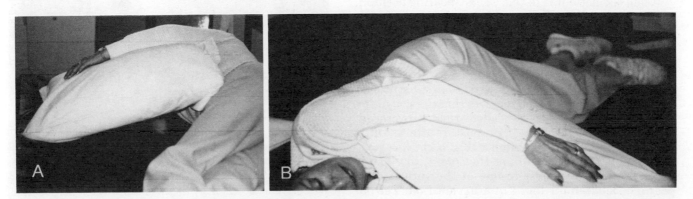

Figure 6.4 A and **B:** Two views of a hemiplegic patient positioned to counteract the typical distribution of hypertonus.

break up the lower extremity extension pattern. If the patient lacks extensor tone or has a tendency for flexor spasticity of the lower extremity, no pillow is used under the knee. Flexor contractures of the hip and knee and plantar flexor contractures must be avoided so that future ambulation will not be jeopardized.

Movement in Bed. The patient must relearn segmental rolling over in bed to either side. The movement should be done passively at first if necessary. Frequent passive turning is done by nurses to prevent deformity and decubiti. Turning of patients unable to move ought to be done segmentally, as one normally would turn, so the patient will get the correct sensory input.[21] Then, to begin to learn to turn over actively, the patient must be able to clasp his hands with the fingers interlocked and elbows extended (a RIP), and move the arms to a forward flexion or overhead position. To allow full shoulder movement without pain, the retracted, depressed scapula needs to be mobilized into protraction and upward rotation. To mobilize the scapula, the therapist supports the patient's arm against her body with the elbow extended and the shoulder externally rotated. Then, while holding along the vertebral border of the scapula with one hand and under the glenoid fossa (axilla) with the other (Fig. 6.5), the therapist slowly and rhythmically moves the scapula upward, forward, and downward (but not backward into retraction). This rotary movement is done until the scapula feels mobilized or free as evidenced by the patient's ability to raise the humerus above the horizontal. Once the patient, using the strength of the unaffected arm, can do so he then moves his outstretched and raised arms from side to side, building momentum to finally enable him to roll over onto his side (Fig. 6.6). At first he may need help to rotate the pelvis and flex the hip and knee to move the leg into position.

Once the patient can roll over to side-lying, he can learn to bear weight on his elbow. The patient is encouraged and helped to use the affected arm for support as early as possible because weight bearing facilitates normalization of tone. By bearing weight on the elbow of the affected limb, it is believed that postural control of the glenohumeral joint and scapula is developed, which is prerequisite to holding and placing.

When the patient is in this weight-bearing position, he can do an activity that would require him to repeatedly release and reapply the weight onto the affected upper extremity. Reaching back to get puzzle or craft pieces that are used to do a task in front of him accomplishes this goal.

Holding and placing begins with the first pattern on the evaluation form, which requires that the scapula be kept well forward and the extended arm held overhead. The patient tries to maintain the posture after the limb has been placed by the therapist (Fig. 6.7). Once he is able to control the posture at that point, the limb is lowered by the therapist to one of the various midpostures between the limits of arm elevation. The patient needs to learn to hold each midposture because before he can move against gravity, he must be able to

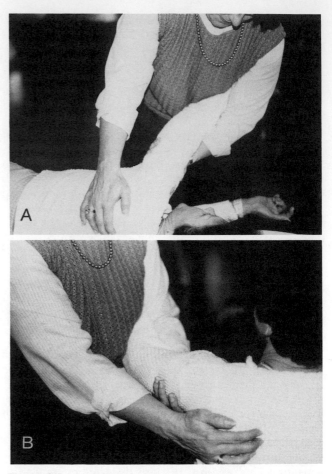

Figure 6.5 Mobilization to allow upward rotation and protraction of the scapula needed for elevation. **A,** side-lying; **B,** sitting.

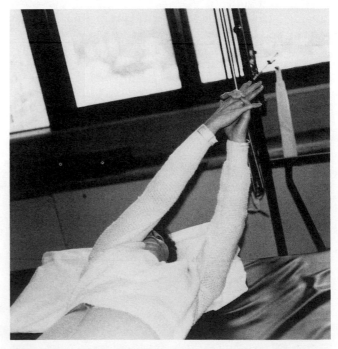

Figure 6.6 Arms outstretched and raised in preparation to rolling over.

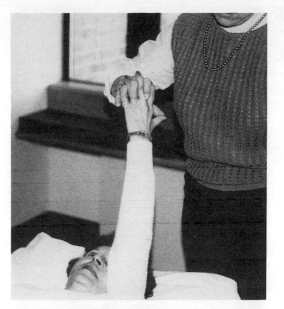

Figure 6.7 Patient attempts to hold after the limb is placed by the therapist. Note reflex-inhibiting pattern.

hold him limb against gravity. To facilitate the holding, tapping as described previously is used to increase tone in weak muscles if necessary.

Treatment continues with the arm being placed as described in evaluation test I for arms and shoulder girdle grade 1 (Table 6.3). *Associated reactions are steadfastly avoided* by keeping the demands within the patient's capabilities. As the patient learns to maintain the placed posture (isometric contraction), he is asked to actively lower the limb slightly (eccentric contraction) to a new position. When he is able to move the limb eccentrically, he should be able to reverse the movement (concentric contraction). If he cannot control the movement (eccentric or concentric), the arm is placed close to the last controlled position, and an isometric response is requested. Eccentric and concentric contractions are then again sought.

The next level of control of movement in bed is to learn to sit on the edge of the bed preparatory to learning dressing and/or transferring activities. The person rolls onto his side as described above and rests on his forearm with his hands still clasped if possible because finger and thumb abduction is a RIP used to control spasticity in the limb. He then lifts his head to vertical while he simultaneously pushes down with the arm(s) to get his trunk upright and brings his legs over the side of the bed. In the beginning, he will need help with each step of this procedure and will find it easier to sit after rolling to his sound side, although it is more therapeutic for him to sit after rolling to the affected side.

While sitting, the affected arm should be used for weight bearing to gain balance that reduces the fear of falling, so the patient will learn to feel safe when bearing weight on the affected side. Also, by positioning the arm in extension, external rotation, and abduction of the shoulder, extension of the elbow, and supination of the forearm, flexor spasticity is inhibited and the ex-

tensor muscles are facilitated in a functional postural pattern preparatory to learning holding and placing involving control of the elbow. At first it may be necessary for the arm to be placed to the back of the person to get maximal external rotation and therefore greater inhibition of flexion. Later weight bearing on the arm can be done with the arm to the side, then in front of the person (Fig. 6.8). At that point, the person should be able to use the arm increasingly in the non-weight-bearing mode without reverting to excess flexion. Holding and placing using grade 2 movements are then done.

Treatment during the Spastic Stage

This stage is characterized by hypertonicity. The spasticity develops slowly with a predilection for the muscles involved in the typical hemiplegic posture described above, and the spastic patient tends to move in total patterns. Treatment at this stage is a continuation of that in the previous stage. The goal is to break down the total patterns by developing control of the intermediate joints. Treatment demands correspond to the movements described in the evaluation test I for grades 2 and 3 (Table 6.3). These movements start while the patient is supine but progress to upright positions as soon as possible. Distal RIPs are used as necessary.

To learn, the patient must be given time to adjust to each new movement ability and to try it out and to experiment with it under different conditions.[31] Activities that incorporate these movements while offering a purposeful goal provide this opportunity. Eggers[32] has devised clever, simple activities that correspond to each phase of recovery and reflect Bobath treatment principles.

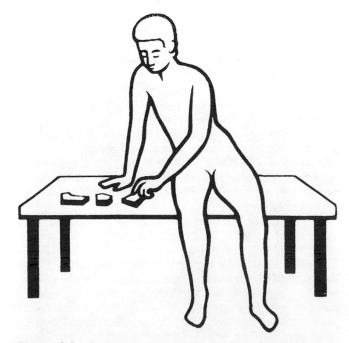

Figure 6.8 Patient bears weight on the affected limb in preparation for placing and holding of the elbow.

Treatment during the Stage of Relative Recovery

Not all patients reach this level of recovery. During this stage, spasticity is slight. The patient is able to walk unaided and use the upper extremity for support and gross grasp. Treatment in this stage aims at improving the quality of gait and use of the affected hand. Treatment in the second stage overlaps with that of the third stage. Bobath sees the occupational therapist active in the patient's therapy to utilize the obtained movements in daily living and to provide bilateral and repetitive therapeutic tasks that reinforce the learned movements (Fig. 6.9). Activities are illustrated in the original source and in the book by Eggers.

Bobath cautions that the occupational therapist must also avoid letting the patient experience stress, which reverts movement to spastic patterns. The therapist should provide opportunities for the patient to move automatically without having to think about the movement, e.g., gestures, moving in rhythm with music, or movement while speaking or counting (Fig. 6.10).

Simple movements of the hand, following developmental sequence, should be practiced before they are combined with the actual use of the hand in daily tasks. Bobath cites the hand skills of a 9- to 10-month-old child as examples of these simple movements: scratch,

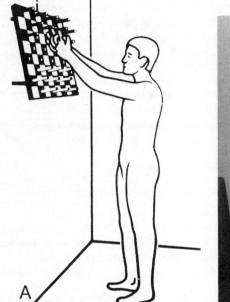

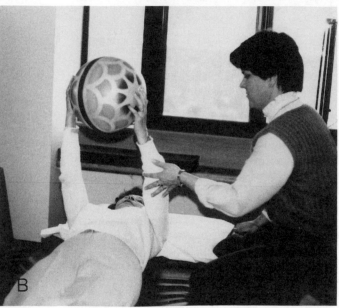

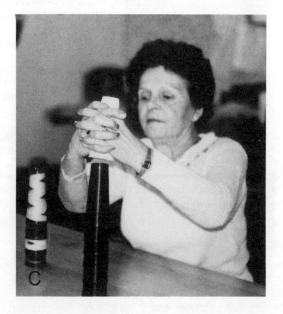

Figure 6.9 A, B, and **C:** Bilateral repetitive therapeutic tasks.

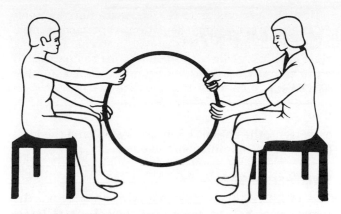

Figure 6.10 Task involving rhythmical, automatic movement. From Eggers, O. *Occupational Therapy in the Treatment of Adult Hemiplegia*. London: William Heinemann Medical Books, 1983.

rake with fingers, poke with the index finger, pincer grasp, pull, push, wave, pat, throw, and release objects. He can transfer objects between his hands, and play hand games such as "patty cake." These same motions can be incorporated into adult games and activities.

The patient needs to learn to use whatever function is regained in the hand independent of the positions of the proximal segments of the limb.

Bobath suggests that the occupational therapist uniquely contributes to the treatment of the adult hemiplegic in the areas of hand function and sensory retraining.

Effectiveness

The effectiveness of neurodevelopmental therapy (NDT) for patients with cerebral palsy has been more frequently studied than any other approach. However, most of those studies are anecdotal and lack the controls needed in order to unequivocally attribute any gains to the treatment. The majority of these reports do not clearly support NDT as an effective therapeutic procedure. A major problem contributing to this failure may be the lack of measures sensitive to small changes in movement, postural tone, or automatic responses.[31]

In one very well done, but limited, model study of four infants, each acting as his own control, NDT was compared to nonspecific play therapy over a 5-week period (eight treatments). The nonspecific play sessions controlled for those aspects of therapeutic intervention not necessarily part of NDT, i.e., touch, general movement, and interaction with the therapist. Pre- and posttest sessions were videotaped and rated by using goal criteria established for each child by the treating therapist. The conclusion reached was that NDT did not significantly improve the motor behavior of these children more than nonspecific play did.[33]

A quantitative review of nine research reports on the effectiveness of NDT with handicapped infants and children did demonstrate a quantifiable treatment effect for NDT versus no therapy. The result suggested that the average subject who received NDT or a combination of NDT and some relative therapy performed better on developmental scales than about 62% of subjects in comparison groups who did not receive therapy.[34]

Except for one abstract, there does not appear to be any effectiveness studies of the Bobath NDT approach applied to the hemiplegic population. French clinicians noted in the abstract that in their experience, the treatment was effective only for "benign" hemiplegia in that it helped the patient to acquire better postural reactions and to improve quality of movement, but that the functional results were about the same as with every technique.[35]

STUDY QUESTIONS:

Bobath Neurodevelopmental Approach

1. What are the premises on which the Bobaths based their treatment approach?
2. What components of motor control are evaluated during the use of the Cerebral Palsy Assessment?
3. Define "reflex-inhibiting pattern" and name a pattern used to inhibit flexor tone of the upper limb.
4. List the treatment principles of the Bobath Approach.
5. What is the relationship between RIPs and elicitation of the righting and equilibrium reactions?
6. What types of sensory stimulation do the Bobaths suggest?
7. Differentiate between associated reactions and associated movements. Which of these should be avoided?
8. What components of motor control are evaluated during use of the Test for the Quality of Movement Patterns?
9. What is the relationship of the Test for the Quality of Movement Patterns to treatment?
10. What comprises the treatment of hemiplegic patients according to the Bobath Approach?
11. What is the typical distribution of spasticity in the upper and lower extremities of the hemiplegic patient? What are the RIPs commonly used to counteract this spasticity?
12. How should a hemiplegic patient be positioned while in bed?
13. What is the value of weight bearing on an affected limb?
14. In which order should the patient learn the following types of contractions: concentric, eccentric, isometric?
15. Think of activities, appropriate to adults, that give the patient the opportunity to use the movements he is learning.

C/Brunnstrom Approach: Movement Therapy

CATHERINE A. TROMBLY

Signe Brunnstrom, a physical therapist, was particularly concerned with the problems of patients with hemiplegia. Brunnstrom carefully noted the conditions under which motor responses and spontaneous willed movements occurred in recovering hemiplegic patients. She experimented by applying, in a trial-and-error fashion, procedures that she derived from the literature or from observations of patients. She attended to the patient's motor and verbal reactions to each procedure, interpreted those reactions in light of her neurophysiological knowledge, and adjusted the procedure accordingly. Successful procedures were replicated patient to patient. The principles of this approach and the evaluation and treatment procedures presented in this section are summarized and adapted from *Movement Therapy in Hemiplegia*[36] in which Brunnstrom described her approach in detail.

The premises of this approach are as follows. In normal persons, as development progresses, spinal cord and brain stem reflexes become modified and their components rearranged into purposeful movement through the influence of higher centers. Since reflexes and whole-limb movement patterns represent normal stages of development, they may be considered "normal" when the CNS has reverted to an earlier developmental stage as it does in hemiplegia. Brunnstrom believed that no reasonable training method should be left untried. She stated[37]: "It may well be that a subcortical motion synergy which can be elicited on a reflex basis may serve as a wedge by means of which a limited amount of willed movement may be learned." Therefore, reflexes can and should be used to elicit movement when none exists as part of a normal developmental sequence. Proprioceptive and exteroceptive stimuli also can be used therapeutically to evoke desired motion or tonal changes.

The stereotyped whole-limb movement patterns of the limbs of hemiplegic patients are called limb synergies. Synergy, in thise sense, refers to patterned flexion or extension movements of the entire limb in response to a stimulus or to voluntary effort. The spastic hemiplegic patient is unable to move except in these patterns. Recovery proceeds in sequence from these mass, stereotyped movement patterns to movements that combine features of the two patterns, and finally to discrete movements of each joint at will. Newly produced, correct motions must be practiced in order to learn them. Practice within the context of daily activities enhances the learning process.

Evaluation

Evaluation identifies the tonic reflexes and associated reactions that may be used to influence the patient's movement, the patient's sensory status, and the level of recovery of voluntary motor control.

TONIC REFLEXES

The primitive reflexes that may be present include the symmetrical and asymmetrical tonic neck reflexes, tonic labyrinthine reflexes, and tonic lumbar reflexes. With the exception of the tonic lumbar reflexes, the evaluation of these reflexes has been previously described in chapter 4.

In the tonic lumbar reflexes, changes in the position of the upper trunk in relation to the pelvis influence tone of the muscles of the extremities. For example, rotation of the upper trunk to the left facilitates flexor tone in the left upper extremity and extensor tone in the left lower extremity. Conversely, there is increased extensor tone in the right upper extremity and increased flexor tone in the right lower extremity, the side opposite to the direction of rotation.

ASSOCIATED REACTIONS

Associated reactions are involuntary movements or reflexive increases of tone that are observed in the involved extremities of hemiplegic patients when other parts of the body are resisted during movement. These reactions are more easily elicited when spasticity is present. Some associated reactions are influenced by tonic neck reflexes, but resistance must be added in addition to the neck movements to gain the summation of sensorimotor influences that would elicit an associated reaction. Examples of associated reactions in patients with hemiplegia include the following: Resistance to shoulder elevation or elbow flexion of the noninvolved upper extremity can cause a flexor synergy of the involved upper extremity. Similarly, resistance to horizontal adduction or pronation of the noninvolved upper extremity evokes an extension syngery of the involved upper extremity. Conversely, in the lower extremity, resistance to flexion of the noninvolved extremity causes extension of the involved extremity, and resistance to extension on the noninvolved side causes flexion of the involved extremity. Resisted grasp by the noninvolved hand causes a grasp reaction in the involved hand.

The interdependence of the upper and lower extremities on one side of the body is called homolateral synkinesis: a response in one extremity facilitates the same response in the other extremity. For example, flexion of the involved upper extremity facilitates flexion of the involved lower extremity.

Raimiste's phenomena are associated reactions of hip abduction or hip adduction, named for the French neurologist who described them. Resistance to hip abduction or adduction of the noninvolved extremity evokes the same motion of the involved extremity. There is a similar phenomenon in the upper extremities affecting shoulder horizontal adduction.

BASIC LIMB SYNERGIES

Limb synergies may be elicited as associated reactions or as voluntary movements in the early stages of recovery when spasticity is present. When the patient initiates a movement of one joint, all muscles that are linked in a synergy with that movement automatically contract, causing a stereotyped movement pattern.

In the upper extremity, the flexor synergy is composed of scapular retraction and/or elevation, shoulder abduction and external rotation, elbow flexion, and forearm supination. Position of the wrist and fingers is variable. Elbow flexion is the strongest component of the flexion synergy and the first motion to appear. Shoulder abduction and external rotation are weak components. Shoulder hyperextension may be seen when abduction and external rotation are weak, although it is not considered part of the flexion synergy.[38]

The extensor synergy of the upper extremity is composed of scapular protraction, shoulder adduction and internal rotation, elbow extension, forearm pronation, and variable wrist and finger motion, although wrist extension and finger flexion may be seen. The pectoralis major is the strongest component of the extension synergy; consequently, shoulder adduction and internal rotation are the first motions to appear. Pronation is the next strongest component. Elbow extension is a weak component.

The upper-extremity flexion synergy usually develops before the extensor synergy. When both synergies are developing and spasticity is marked, the strongest components of flexion and extension combine to produce the typical upper-extremity posture in hemiplegia: The arm is adducted and internally rotated with the elbow flexed, forearm pronated, and the wrist and fingers flexed.

The lower-extremity flexor synergy is composed of hip flexion, hip abduction and external rotation, knee flexion, dorsiflexion, and inversion of the ankle, and dorsiflexion of the toes. In this synergy hip flexion is the strongest component, whereas hip abduction and external rotation are weak components.

The lower-extremity extensor synergy is composed of hip extension, hip adduction and internal rotation, knee extension, plantar flexion and inversion of the ankle and plantar flexion of the toes. Hip adduction, knee extension, and plantar flexion of the ankle with inversion are all strong components. Weak components of this synergy are hip extension, hip internal rotation, and plantar flexion of the toes. Note that ankle inversion occurs in both lower extremity synergies.

The lower-extremity extensor synergy is dominant in a standing position, due to the strength of this synergy combined with the influences of the positive supporting reaction and stretch forces against the sole of the foot that elicit plantar flexion.

SENSATION

The results of a sensory evaluation provide necessary information for treatment planning. The patient's ability to recognize movements of the affected arm and to localize touch in the hand are especially noted. Results of the sensory evaluation also guide choice of facilitation modalities that may benefit the patient and alert the therapist as to whether the patient needs to substitute visual feedback for lost movement or position senses. The reader is referred to chapter 3 for evaluation procedures.

RECOVERY STAGES

Tables 6.4 and 6.5 list the six stages of recovery that are used to guide the evaluation and treatment planning processes. Recovery proceeds sequentially but may stop at any stage depending on the severity of the cortical damage.

Not appearing in the tables is the recovery sequence for the wrist. When the arm begins to develop movements deviating from synergy, the wrist begins a sequence that progresses from wrist stability during active grasp, with the elbow both flexed as well as extended; to wrist flexion and extension with the fist closed; to wrist radial and ulnar deviation progressing to wrist circumduction.

TESTING PROCEDURE

The patient is made physically and psychologically comfortable. The sensory evaluation precedes the motor evaluation. The sequential aspects of the motor evaluation (see Table 6.6) are used to determine the patient's level of motor control; no movements beyond the patient's capabilities are demanded. No facilitation is used during the evaluation. Each motion is demonstrated to the patient, and he does it with his unaffected extremity before he attempts it with his affected one. Instructions should be given in functional terms. For example, to test the flexion synergy of the upper extremity, say "touch behind your ear"; or for the extension synergy, "reach out to touch your [opposite] knee." The patient's ability to do the requested movement is recorded according to the percentage of range of motion that he completed. For example, when asked for a flexor synergy response, if the patient is only able to bring the hand as far as his mouth rather than to his ear, the therapist may observe that he has complete elbow flexion (100%), about 45° of shoulder abduction (50%), supination to midrange (50%), and minimal external rotation (25%). When the patient's response is incomplete, as in this example, it may be necessary to observe the patient's repeated attempts to determine the specific weak areas of the synergy or movement pattern and to decide on the rating.

A patient is reported to be in the stage at which he is able to accomplish all motions specified for that stage. Since progress is gradual, there will be instances when the patient is in transition between stages. If he has completed one stage but is just beginning to be able to do the motions of the next stage, many therapists would record his level as "2 going on 3" or "3 going on

Table 6.4
RECOVERY STAGES OF THE UPPER EXTREMITY

Stage: Arm	Stage: Hand
1. Flaccidity—no voluntary movement	1. Flaccidity
2. Synergies developing—flexion usually develops before extension (may be a weak associated reaction or voluntary contraction with or without joint motion); spasticity developing	2. Little or no active finger flexion
3. Synergies performed voluntarily Increased spasticity which may become marked	3. Mass grasp or hook grasp No voluntary finger extension or release
4. Some movements deviating from synergy: a. Hand behind body b. Arm to forward-horizontal position c. Pronation-supination with elbow flexed to 90°; spasticity decreasing	4. Lateral prehension with release by thumb movement Semivoluntary finger extension (small range of motion)
5. Independence from the basic synergies: a. Arm to side-horizontal position b. Arm forward and overhead c. Pronation-supination with elbow full extended; spasticity waning	5. Palmar prehension Possibly cylindrical and spherical grasp (awkward) Voluntary mass finger extension (variable range of motion)
6. Isolated joint movements freely performed with near normal coordination Spasticity minimal	6. All types of prehension (improved skill) Voluntary finger extension (full range of motion) Individual finger movements

4," etc. The upper and lower extremities as well as the hand may all be in different stages of recovery at a given time.

Brunnstrom's evaluation is valid in that it reflects observations made by Twitchell[39] of the recovery process of 118 patients who had suffered strokes, onset of which ranged from 5 days to 5 years before observation. No data exist concerning the reliability of the evaluation, but the reliability can be assumed to be low because the rating scales are not operationally defined. To improve reliability, Brunnstrom recommended that a standard procedure be adopted by therapists. One such system was developed by Fugl-Meyer et al.[40] Fifty details of joint motion across the six levels of recovery were operationally defined. The Fugl-Meyer Motor Test uses an ordinal level scoring system in which each

Table 6.5
RECOVERY STAGES OF THE LOWER EXTREMITY

Stage:
1. Flaccidity
2. Minimal voluntary movements
3. Hip flexion, knee flexion, and ankle dorsiflexion performed as a combined motion in sitting and standing
4. In sitting: Knee flexion beyond 90° Ankle dorsiflexion with the heel on the floor
5. In standing: Isolated knee flexion with hip extended Isolated ankle dorsiflexion with knee extended
6. Hip abduction in standing Knee rotation with inversion and eversion of the ankle in sitting

detail is rated 0 (cannot be performed), 1 (can be partly performed), or 2 (can be performed faultlessly). Total scores can range from 0 (flaccidity) to 100 (normal motor function).

Treatment

The focus of treatment is the recapitulation of normal movement developmentally from its reflexive base to voluntary control of individual motions that can be used functionally.

TREATMENT PRINCIPLES

Treatment progresses developmentally. When no motion exists, movement is facilitated using reflexes, associated reactions, proprioceptive facilitation, and/or exteroceptive facilitation to develop muscle tension in preparation for voluntary movement. Reflex responses elicited in this way combine with the patient's voluntary effort to move which produces semivoluntary movement. In this way, "the patient experiences the sensation and satisfaction that accompanies a voluntary muscle contraction."[36]

Proprioceptive and exteroceptive stimuli assist in eliciting the synergies. Resistance (a proprioceptive stimulus) promotes a spread of impulses to other muscles to produce a patterned response (associated reaction), whereas tactile stimulation (exteroceptive) facilitates only the muscles related to the stimulated area.

When voluntary effort produces or contributes to a response, the patient is asked to hold (isometric) the contraction. If successful, he is asked for an eccentric (controlled lengthening) contraction and finally a concentric (shortening) contraction. When even partial movement is possible, reversal of movement from flexion to extension is stressed within each treatment session.

Table 6.6

HEMIPLEGIA—CLASSIFICATION AND PROGRESS RECORD: UPPER LIMB—TEST SITTING

Name _____ Age _____ Date of Onset _____ Side Affected _____

Date	Stage
_____	1. No movement initiated or elicited. Flaccidity.
_____	2. Synergies or components may be elicited. Spasticity developing. Note extent of response:

Flexor synergy _____

_____

_____   Extensor synergy _____

_____

_____   3. Synergies or components initiated voluntarily. Spasticity marked.

Flexor synergy   % Active Joint Range

Date	Component	% Active Joint Range
_____	Shoulder girdle elevation	_____
_____	retraction	_____
_____	Shoulder joint abduction	_____
_____	external rotation	_____
_____	Elbow flexion	_____
_____	Forearm supination	_____

Remarks: _____

_____

_____

Extensor synergy   % Active Joint Range

Date	Component	% Active Joint Range
_____	Shoulder girdle protraction	_____
_____	Shoulder joint adduction and internal rotation (pectoralis major)	_____
_____	Elbow extension	_____
_____	Forearm pronation	_____

Remarks: _____

_____

_____

_____   4. Movements deviating from basic synergies. Spasticity decreasing.

                                               % Range of Motion (ROM)

Date	Movement	% Range of Motion (ROM)
_____	a. Hand behind back	_____
	b. Raise arm to forward-horizontal	_____
_____	c. Pronation-supination, elbow at 90°	_____

Remarks: _____

_____

_____

Table 6.6 *Continued*

Date	Stage	
	5. Relative independence of basic synergies. Spasticity waning.	
		% Range of Motion (ROM)
_____	a. Raise arm to side-horizontal	_____
_____	b. Raise arm forward overhead	_____
_____	c. Pronation-supination, elbow extended	_____
_____	6. Movement coordinated and near normal. Spasticity minimal.	
	Wrist	**Describe Motion**
_____	4. Wrist stabilization for grasp	
	a. Elbow extended _____	
	b. Elbow flexed _____	
_____	5. Wrist flexion and extension, fist closed	
	a. Elbow extended _____	
	b. Elbow flexed _____	
_____	6. Wrist circumduction _____	
	(stabilize forearm)	
	Digits	
_____	1. Flaccidity. No voluntary movement	
_____	2. Little or no active finger flexion	
_____	3. Mass grasp or hook grasp	
_____	4. a. Lateral prehension; release by thumb movement	
_____	b. Semivoluntary mass extension-small ROM	
_____	5. a. Palmar prehension	
_____	b. Voluntary mass extension-variable ROM	
_____	c. Spherical grasp (awkward)	
_____	d. Cylindrical grasp (awkward)	
_____	6. a. All types of grasp with improved skill	
_____	b. Voluntary finger extension-full ROM	
_____	c. Individual finger movements (do dexterity tests)	

Facilitation is reduced or dropped out as quickly as the patient shows evidence of volitional control. Facilitation procedures are dropped out in order of their stimulus-response binding. Reflexes, in which the response is stereotypically bound to a certain stimulus, are the most primitive and are dropped out of treatment first. Responses to exteroceptive stimulation are least stereotyped and therefore tactile stimulation is eliminated last. *No* primitive reflexes, including associated reactions, are used beyond stage 3. Emphasis is placed on willed movement to overcome the linkages between parts of the synergies.

Correct movement, once elicited, is repeated to learn it. Practice should include functional activities to increase the willed aspect and to relate the sensations to goal-directed movement.

Training Procedures

TRUNK CONTROL

Some patients with hemiplegia may have poor trunk control and may require training to enable them to bend over to retrieve an object from the floor or to dress their lower extremities. The patient is gently pushed in forward, backward, and side-to-side directions to elicit balance responses. At first emphasis is given to a push toward the involved side to promote contraction of trunk muscles on the noninvolved side; then the patient is pushed toward the unaffected side. The patient is pushed only to the point where he is able to hold the position and then regain upright posture. Training then progresses to promote trunk flexion, extension, and then rotation. Practice in forward flexion of the trunk is assisted. The patient crosses his arms with the noninvolved hand under the involved elbow and the noninvolved forearm supporting the involved forearm. The therapist, sitting facing the patient, supports the patient under the elbows and assists in trunk flexion forward, avoiding any pull on the shoulders. Some pain-free shoulder flexion is accomplished during this forward movement. The patient is concentrating on trunk control and shoulder movement occurs without conscious awareness. Return from trunk flexion is performed actively by the patient. Then, while sitting without back support and with the affected arm supported as described above, the patient is pushed backward and encouraged to actively regain upright posture.

Forward flexion in oblique directions is then done to incorporate more scapular motion with the shoulder flexion already achieved.

Trunk rotation is then practiced with the patient supporting his involved arm and the therapist guiding trunk motion. Trunk rotation can be combined with head movements in the opposite direction of the trunk rotation, so that the tonic neck and tonic lumbar reflexes can be utilized as one way to begin to elicit the shoulder components of the upper extremity synergies. The arms and trunk move in one direction while the head turns in the opposite direction. Head and trunk movements are combined with increasing ranges of movement of the shoulder, enabling pain-free shoulder and scapular abduction and adduction to be accomplished during trunk rotation.

UPPER EXTREMITY: STAGES 1 TO 3

In stages 1 to 3 the goal of treatment is to promote voluntary control of the synergies and to encourage their use in purposeful activities. All movements occur in synergy patterns, but with increasing voluntary initiation and control of these patterns. To move the patient from stage 1 (flaccidity) to stage 2 (beginning synergy) the basic limb synergies are elicited at a reflex level using as many reflexes, associated reactions, and facilitation procedures as are necessary to elicit a response. The effects of these procedures combine to produce a stronger response. The patient tries to move as facilitation is used.

The flexor synergy is the first to develop. Within that synergy, the strongest component, elbow flexion, is the first motion that can be elicited. Once elbow flexion is seen, the therapist turns concentration from elbow flexion to the proximal components of the synergy with the goal of enabling the patient to "capture the synergy," that is, bring it under voluntary control (stage 3).

Since many patients with hemiplegia have difficulty achieving shoulder movements; experience pain with passive range of motion and/or experience shoulder subluxation, the shoulder and scapula are given special attention. Efforts to achieve voluntary control of the flexor synergy begin with scapular elevation. Lateral flexion of the neck toward the involved side can be used to initiate scapular elevation because the upper trapezius does both motions although it may have "forgotten" how to elevate the scapula. With the patient's arm supported on a table in shoulder abduction with elbow flexion, resistance is given simultaneously to the head and shoulder while the patient is asked to "hold" the head and not let it be moved away from the shoulder. When the trapezius is felt to respond, both the patient's effort and the therapist's resistance emphasize shoulder elevation when lateral flexion of the neck is repeated. Once elevation begins active contraction

may be promoted by an associated reaction: as the patient attempts bilateral scapular elevation, resistance is given to the noninvolved scapula. If the involved scapula elevates as a result of an associated reaction, resistance is then added on the involved side as the patient is asked to "hold."

Unilateral scapular elevation of the involved arm is attempted next and may be achieved as a result of the previous procedures. If the patient is unable to accomplish the motion, the therapist supports the patient's arm and assists the patient to elevate the scapula. Percussion or stroking over the upper trapezius will facilitate muscle contraction. The patient is then told to hold, "Don't let me push your shoulder down." After repeated holding with some resistance added, the patient does an eccentric contraction to let the shoulder down. Then a concentric or shortening contraction is attempted when he is told, "Now pull your shoulder up toward your ear." Active scapular elevation evokes other flexor components and tends to inhibit the pectoralis major. The patient repeats scapular elevation and relaxation as the therapist gently abducts the shoulder in increasing increments. Shoulder external rotation and forearm supination are then included in the movement. Reversal of movements into the opposite direction begins to develop some components of the extensor synergy.

The extensor synergy tends to follow the flexor synergy and may need to be assisted in its initiation. Contraction of the pectoralis major, a strong component of the extensor synergy, can be elicited by an associated reaction similar to Raimiste's phenomenon. To elicit this phenomenon, the therapist supports the patient's arms in a position between horizontal abduction and adduction, instructs the patient to bring his arms together, and resists the noninvolved arm just proximal to the elbow. As contraction occurs bilaterally the patient is instructed, "Don't let me pull your arms apart." Then he attempts to bring his arms together voluntarily.

Because of the predominance of excess tone in the elbow flexors and relative weakness of elbow extensors, elbow extension is usually more difficult to obtain but can be assisted by the following methods.

Bilateral "rowing" is the procedure used to initiate elbow extension. In the rowing procedure, movements toward extension combined with pronation are resisted (Fig. 6.11) and movements into flexion combined with supination are guided (Fig. 6.12). Rowing is done with the therapist and patient seated facing each other; the therapist's arms are crossed so that she and the patient grasp right hand to right hand and left hand to left hand.

First, elbow extension is elicited as an associated reaction by resisting the noninvolved arm as it moves into extension and assisting the involved arm into extension toward the noninvolved knee. Once the affected limb is felt to contract, resistance is offered bilaterally. "Hold after positioning" is used to reinforce voluntary effort. When the patient's arm is positioned in extension synergy with the elbow in nearly full extension, he is asked to "hold" against resistance. To fa-

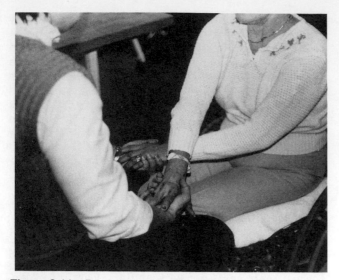

Figure 6.11 Rowing to encourage elbow extension: resistance to elbow extension combined with pronation.

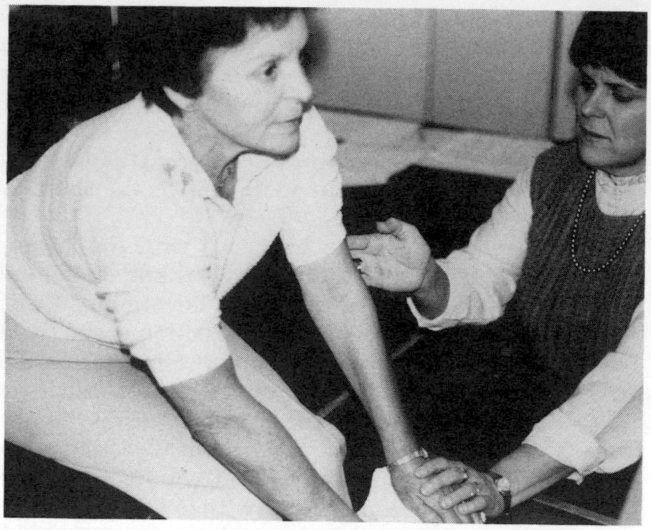

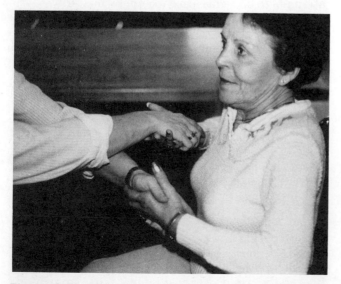

Figure 6.12 Rowing to encourage elbow extension: guided reversal of motion into elbow flexion and supination. Note the support given to the wrists.

cilitate the extensors, quick stretcher are applied to the involved arm by lightly pushing back toward elbow flexion.

When the extensor synergy is seen to come under active control, it is further developed through use of bilateral weightbearing. The patient leans forward onto his extended arms supported by a low stool placed in front of him. (Fig. 6.13). The patient uses the noninvolved hand to position the involved hand on a sandbag, pillow, or towel placed on the stool. Vigorous stroking of the skin over the triceps or tapping is done as the patient attempts to bear his weight on both outstretched arms (See Fig. 5.4). Once he is successful, weight is shifted so that the noninvolved extremity attempts to

Weight bearing on the affected upper extremity.

Figure 6.13 Weight bearing on the affected upper extremity.

support the weight of the upper trunk. Again tapping and tactile stimulation may be useful. Unilateral weight bearing can be used functionally to hold objects while they are being worked on by the other hand, e.g., holding a piece of wood while sawing, hammering, or painting it; holding a package steady while opening it, addressing it, or fastening it; supporting body weight while polishing or washing large surfaces such as a table or floor.

To encourage active extensor movement, once the triceps is activated via rowing and weight bearing, unilateral resistance is offered to the patient's attempts to move into an extension pattern. Resistance gives direction to his effort and facilitates a stronger contraction. Other means that may be used to facilitate extension movement include use of supine position (tonic labyrinthine reflex); having the patient watch his extremity, which requires head turning and pulls in the asymmetrical tonic neck reflex; working with the forearm pronated, which is a strong component of the extensor synergy; or rotating the trunk toward the noninvolved side to facilitate extension of the involved arm via the tonic lumbar reflex.

As the synergies come under voluntary control, they should be used in functional activities. The extensor synergy can be used to stabilize an object to be worked on by the other side or to push the arm into the sleeve of garments. The flexor synergy can be used functionally to assist in carrying items, such as a coat, handbag, or briefcase. Bilateral pushing and pulling activities reinforce both synergies. Sanding, weaving, and ironing are activities which use the flexor and extensor synergies alternately and repeatedly.

To promote movement deviating from synergy, motions that begin to combine components of synergies in small increments are encouraged as a transition from stage 3 to stage 4. For example, as the patient begins to extend his arm consistently in response to the unilateral resistance given by the therapist, the therapist guides the direction of movement toward shoulder abduction in conjunction with elbow extension to break up the synergistic relationship of shoulder adduction to elbow extension. When the triceps and pectoralis major are disassociated, the synergies no longer dominate.

UPPER EXTREMITY: STAGES 4 AND 5

In stages 4 and 5 the goal of treatment is to "condition the synergies," that is, to promote voluntary movement that combines components of the two synergies into increasingly varied combinations of movements that deviate from synergy. Proprioceptive and exteroceptive stimuli are still used in this phase of training, but tonic reflexes and associated reactions, appropriate in the earlier stages when reflex behavior was desriable, are no longer used; willed movement with isolated control of muscle groups is the desired goal.

Stage 4 Motions

The first out-of-synergy motion is hand behind the body, which combines relative shoulder abduction (flexor synergy) with elbow extension and forearm pronation (extensor synergy). This motion requires that the strongest components of each synergy be subdued. To assist in getting the hand behind the body, a swinging motion of the arm combined with trunk rotation is helpful; if balance is good, this can be done more easily when standing. As the hand reaches the back of the patient, he uses a stroking motion of the dorsum of the hand against the body to help complete the arm-behind-the-back movement. Stroking the dorsum of the hand on the back is thought to give direction to the attempted voluntary movement. If the patient is unable to do the motion actively, the therapist passively moves the patient's arm into position and strokes the dorsum of the patient's hand against his sacrum. The patient is then assisted into and out of the pattern, which gradually becomes voluntary with practice. Practice, using functional tasks as much as possible, continues until the motion can be freely accomplished.

The second-out-of-synergy motion is shoulder flexion to a forward-horizontal position with the elbow extended. If the patient is unable to actively flex the shoulder forward even with the therapist providing local facilitation and guidance of movement, then the arm is brought passively into position. While tapping over the anterior and middle deltoid muscles, the therapist asks the patient to "hold" the position. If hold after positioning is accomplished, active motion in small increments is then sought starting with lowering of the arm followed by active shoulder flexion. This continues until the full forward flexion motion can be done. Stroking and rubbing of the triceps is used to assist in keeping the elbow straight as the arm is raised.

The third motion sought in stage 4 is pronation and supination with the elbow flexed to 90°. Supination would not be expected to be a problem unless the pronators retained some spasticity. The problem would be to combine pronation of the extensor synergy with elbow flexion of the flexor synergy. Initially, pronation can be resisted with the elbow extended, and gradually the elbow can be brought into flexion as the resistance to pronation is repeated. When resistance is no longer required and the patient can supinate and pronate with the elbow near the trunk, this motion has been achieved and indicates the patient is ready to enter stage 5 training.

Stage 5 Motions

Therapy at this stage involves active attempts by the patient to move in patterns increasingly away from synergy. Excess effort is avoided, however, so that the limbs will not revert back to stereotyped movements. The attempts are bolstered by use of quick stretch and tactile stimulation. Each new motion is incorporated into functional activities.

The first motion sought in stage 5 is arm raised to side-horizontal, which combines full shoulder abduction with elbow extension. When this can be accomplished disassociation of components of the synergies has occurred. When the muscles are still under the influence of the synergies, the arm will drift toward horizontal adduction when the elbow is extended or the elbow will flex when the shoulder is abducted.

The second motion of stage 5 is arm overhead. To achieve it, the scapula must upwardly rotate. The serratus anterior must be specifically retrained to do this. If the scapula is bound by spastic retractors, passive mobilization may need to be done before seeking an active response. Passive mobilization of the scapula is done by grasping the vertebral border and rotating it as the arm is passively moved into an overhead position. Once mobilized, the serratus is activated in its alternate duty of scapula protraction by placing the arm in the forward-horizontal position and asking and assisting the patient to reach forward. It is helpful to rehearse this motion with the patient using the noninvolved extremity. Quick stretches are applied by pushing backward into scapular retraction and the patient is asked to "hold." Once activated, a holding contraction of the serratus is sought. These procedures continue, moving the arm in increments toward the arm overhead position.

The third motion sought in stage 5 is supination and pronation (external and internal rotation) with the elbow extended. The best way to achieve this control is by using both hands in activities of interest to the patient that involve supination and pronation in various arm positions. One activity that can be used is grasping a large ball with the arms outstretched and then rotating it so the affected arm is on top (pronated) and the unaffected arm is on the bottom (supinated) and vice versa. To improve supination, the elbow is at first kept close to the trunk and gradually extended. There are no special treatment procedures recommended to assist in developing disassociation of supination and elbow flexion.

All actions of stages 4 and 5 should be reinforced by use in meaningful and interesting activities. Examples of activities requiring placing the involved hand behind the back are tucking his shirt tail into trousers, bathing the back, and tying a belt around the waist.

Raising the arm to forward-horizontal is involved in any vertically mounted game such as tic-tac-toe or checkers (using Velcro tabs to secure the pieces). Sponge painting is repetitive and essentially nonresistive and can be mounted vertically on an easel to practice the same motion.

Certain activities that require turning objects such as a knob, a screwdriver, or a dial use supination and pronation. Resistance to supination or pronation depends on the direction in which the major force is exerted. Woodworking projects involving sanding of curved edges or assembly with screws can be used. Some games like Skittles are knob operated and require rotary motions, as do card games that require turning the cards over. Wall checkers can be adapted by the use of threaded dowels that must be turned to remove and replace them for each move on the checkerboard. In stage 4 where resistance to pronation is suggested, first with the elbow extended and then with increasing amounts of elbow flexion, block printing could be positioned to resist pronation with gradual changes in the amount of elbow flexion. Activities to encourage side-horizontal movement can employ placement of project pieces or materials on a high table to the side of the patient. The table can be gradually moved to require more and more horizontal abduction and elbow extension. The patient would use the materials on a project to be done in front of him. Sanding on an inclined plane is an example of an activity requiring a forward push with an increasing range of movement in scapular protraction and rotation and shoulder flexion.

Patients who recover comparatively rapidly after a stroke may spontaneously achieve stage 6; however, many hemiplegic patients do not achieve full recovery. Twitchell,[39] stated that patients who reached stages 3 and 4 within 10 days after stroke recovered completely. Patients who failed to respond to proprioceptive facilitation did not recover willed movement at all. The longer the duration of the flaccid stage, the less likely was recovery.

HAND AND WRIST

Training techniques for return of function in the hand are presented separately because the hand may be in a different stage of recovery than the arm. Hand motions require the most direct cortical control; therefore, full recovery may not occur if the corticospinal tract was involved in the stroke, as it commonly is.

If the patient is unable to initiate active finger flexion (stage 1) or mass grasp (stage 2), the traction response in which stretch of the scapular adductors produces reflex finger flexion or an associated reaction to resisted grasp by the nonaffected hand may be used in combination with voluntary effort.

In hemiplegia, wrist flexion usually accompanies grasp initially so stability of the wrist in extension must be developed. It is easier for the patient to stabilize the wrist in extension when the elbow is extended; therefore, training starts with the elbow extended and the wrist supported by the therapist. The wrist extensor muscles are facilitated, and the therapist directs the patient to do a forceful grasp by commanding, "Squeeze." Grasp promotes normal synergistic contraction of the wrist extensors. This is repeated until the wrist extensors are felt to respond, allowing the therapist to remove her support from the wrist with the command, "Hold." Tapping on the wrist extensor muscles facilitates holding. Once wrist extension and grasp are possible with the elbow extended, the process of positioning, percussion, and hold is repeated in increasing amounts of elbow flexion. Emphasis in training is on wrist stability, although wrist flexion and extension and circumduction may then be practiced.

To move from stage 3 (flexion) to stage 4 (semivoluntary mass extension) spasticity of the finger flexors must be relaxed using a series of manipulations. The therapist reflexively releases the patient's grasp by holding the thumb into extension and abduction. Still holding the thumb, the forearm is slowly and rhythmically supinated and pronated. Cutaneous stimulation is given over the dorsum of the wrist and hand while the forearm is supinated. These continue until a release of flexor tension is seen by some relaxation of the flexed position. If relaxation is incomplete, further manipulations are done. With the forearm still supinated, rapid repeated stretch stimuli are applied to the dorsum of the fingers by rolling them toward the palm with a rapid stroking motion to stretch finger extensors (see Fig. 5.3). When flexor tension is relaxed, the forearm is pronated and the arm elevated above horizontal (Souque's phenomenon). Stroking over the dorsum of the fingers and forearm continues as extension is attempted, but effort exerted should be minimal to avoid a buildup of tension. Imitation synkinesis, in which the normal side performs a motion that is difficult to achieve on the involved side, may be observed when the patient attempts finger extension. After the fingers can be voluntarily extended with the arm raised, the arm is gradually lowered. If there is an increase of flexor tension reflected by decreasing range in extension, it is necessary to repeat the manipulations that inhibit flexion and facilitate extension.

The second motion sought at stage 4 is lateral prehension and release. The patient attempts to move the thumb away from the index finger to gain release of lateral prehension while the therapist percusses or strokes over the abductor pollicis longus tendon to facilitate this motion. Once the patient has some active release, functional use of lateral prehension is then encouraged. Activities are selected to encourage voluntary finger and thumb extension in nonprehensile and prehensile patterns.

Once the patient is able to voluntarily extend the fingers to release objects, advanced prehensile patterns (stage 5) are encouraged through activities. Musical instruments (tambourine, drum, claves, cymbal, tomtom, etc.) provide motivating opportunities for gross use of various hand patterns.[41] As the patient progresses, activities are chosen to reinforce particular prehensions at more precise levels. Holding a pencil or paint brush encourages palmar prehension. Spherical grasp is used to pick up round objects, and cylindrical grasp is used when holding the handles of tools.

Individual finger movements (stage 6) may be regained in rare instances. The patient should be given a home program of activities to encourage more and more individual finger use and to increase speed and accuracy of hand movements, but he should also be cautioned about expecting 100% recovery.

LOWER EXTREMITY

Gait patterns, principles used in preparation for walking, and ambulation training are also described by Brunnstrom; these principles and procedures fall under the primary responsibility of the physical therapist.

STUDY QUESTIONS:

Brunnstrom Approach: Movement Therapy

1. What is a synergy?
2. What is an associated reaction and how is it elicited?
3. Describe the flexor synergy of the upper extremity and state which component(s) is strongest.
4. Describe the extensor synergy of the upper extremity and state which component(s) is strongest.
5. List in order the six recovery stages of the upper extremity.
6. List in order the six stages of hand recovery.
7. Name the treatment principles of the Brunnstrom Approach.
8. How is the flexor synergy initiated in the upper extremity when the patient is flaccid?
9. How is elbow extension developed?
10. Describe therapeutic activities appropriate for a patient in stage 4 of the recovery of the upper limb.
11. How is finger extension developed?
12. Describe what activities of daily living a patient can be expected to do if he is in stage 5 of upper-limb recovery and stage 4 of hand recovery.

D/Proprioceptive Neuromuscular Facilitation (PNF) Approach

BEVERLY J. MYERS

PNF embodies broad concepts of human motion derived from normal development. As such, PNF has value to occupational therapists in evaluating and enhancing motor performance. PNF has been defined as "a method of promoting or hastening the response of the neuromuscular mechanism through stimulation of the proprioceptors."[42] Various techniques are superimposed on patterns of movement and posture with attention to the sensory stimulation from manual contacts, visual cues, and verbal commands so as to bring as many favorable influences as possible to bear on the patient.

Applying PNF to the treatment of patients in occupational therapy requires that the therapist understands the concepts, learns the motor skills, and then incorporates the approach into activities that meet the individual patient's needs. This introduction presents the principles of PNF and some examples of application in occupational therapy (OT). To learn the motor skills, the patterns and techniques must be performed under the supervision of a knowledgeable instructor. Learning by practicing with other students develops the feeling of how normal balanced antagonistic muscle groups respond in different developmental positions. Then learning may proceed to application and repeated use with patients.

History

Herman Kabat, Ph.D., M.D., neurophysiologist and physician, developed the method of proprioceptive neuromuscular facilitation at the Kabat-Kaiser Institute during the years 1946 to 1951. Sherrington's physiology and philosophy provided the foundation for many of the techniques. Some of the other experimenters who influenced the PNF approach were Gellhorn, a neurophysiologist who studied proprioception and cortically induced movement; Gesell, who studied the development of motor behavior and patterned movement; McGraw, who studied the development of behavior as it relates to the maturation of neural structures; Hellebrandt, who studied combinations of movements and mass movements, finding that one can circumvent fatigue or speed recovery by changing the combination used; and Pavlov, who studied the mechanisms of learning and formation of habit patterns.

The diagonal patterns, PNFs unique feature, were the last aspect to be identified. Specific combinations of motion were carefully analyzed in 1951. Dr. Kabat found that when topographically aligned groups of muscles were stretched they produced a movement in a diagonal direction. Observation of functional movement and sport skills revealed the same spiral and diagonal characteristics.

Kabat began his work in the early 1940s in treating patients with cerebral palsy and multiple sclerosis. However, by the early 1950s PNF had been applied to the treatment of patients with all diagnoses, from those with central nervous system deficits to orthopedic conditions, arthritis, and peripheral nerve injuries.

In 1956, the first edition of the PNF textbook was written by two physical therapists who worked with Dr. Kabat, Margaret Knott and Dorothy Voss. The book was revised in 1968 and 1985[42] and translations are available in seven different languages. OTs used PNF as evidenced by the related articles published during the 1950s.[43-48] Ayres' series of three comprehensive articles [44] on PNF and application to OT were published in 1955. Voss also contributed a significant article on the same topic in 1959.[46]

No courses or workshops were offered for OTs until 1974 when Voss taught the first PNF course for OTs at Northwestern University. This course was cosponsored by the curriculum in OT, University of Illinois. Continuing education in the form of 1- and 2-week courses and 1-day workshops continues to be offered for occupational therapists.

Principles

In developing the PNF method, Dr. Herman Kabat relied on authorities in the fields of neurophysiology, motor learning, and motor behavior. The basic principles of PNF, as stated in 1966 by Voss, encompass the developmental concepts as drawn from these fields. The 11 principles follow.

1. *All human beings have potentials that are not fully developed.*[49] This first principle is a statement of philosophy. It provides the base for an attitude toward treating patients. The patient's abilities and potentials become the means to reduce his inabilities. When the patient's progress declines, the idea that the patient has reached a plateau is the last factor to be acknowledged. The cause may not be due to the patient's natural limitations, but rather due to the lack of experience and skills of the therapist, the lack of coordination with the rehabilitation team and the patient's family, the lack of time for appropriate treatment, or the lack of funds. PNF does not disregard the fact that some persons may reach a limit beyond which no further learning may occur. However, the emphasis is on bringing as many favorable influences to bear as possible on developing a patient's potential. Consider the common reaction of a person watching a tennis game for the first time. "Oh, I could never do that," he might exclaim. But after a few lessons, that same person may have channelled his potential and abilities to perform a skill that he previously thought was impossible. This philosophy, inherent in the PNF approach, is compatible with that of occupational therapy, where emphasis is placed on ability rather than disability.

Also, this philosophy underlies the approach of PNF in using the patient's stronger movement patterns to strengthen the weaker motions. Thus, an indirect approach results. In treatment, when the superior region

is intact, as in a person with paraplegia, the movements of the head, neck, upper trunk, and upper limbs are used to facilitate and reinforce movements in the weaker lower extremities. When the patient has one involved upper extremity, as in the person with a frozen shoulder, the motions of the intact upper extremity and inferior region are emphasized in bilateral combinations and total patterns to reduce the pain and increase movement in the affected arm.

2. *Normal motor development proceeds in a cervico-caudal and proximodistal direction.*[49] In treatment, this direction is heeded with attention given first to the development of motion in the head and neck, then in the trunk, and last in the extremities. For example, with the patient who is comatose, treatment would not begin by quietly performing range of motion on the hand but rather by first directing sensory stimuli to the head, as in greeting and talking to the patient, touching his face or head while talking, or providing other tactile input to the facial region. Positioning the patient in a total pattern, such as side-lying, would follow and would stimulate rotation of head, neck, and trunk. Then, if indicated, passigve range of motion of the extremities could be administered.

As the head and neck lead the rest of the body in embryonic differentiation and reflex development,[50] so too the position of the head and neck influences the movement of the body's total pattern throughout life. For example, in standing when the head is quickly rotated to one side, the body weight shifts to that side. In treatment, this principle is applied when facilitating weight bearing. When a patient rises to stand from a wheelchair or bed, if weight is not equally distributed, asking the patient to look toward the inefficient side may promote a shift of weight toward that side. Likewise, when working on developing stability of the affected side of the patient who has hemiplegia, positioning the activity on the hemiplegic side will increase a weight shift toward the involved leg or arm, thus facilitating weight bearing on that side.

The development of movement and stability in the limbs proceeds in a proximodistal direction. In therapy, developing the function of the head, neck, and trunk precedes developing the function of the extremities, and that of the shoulder girdle before developing the fine motor skills of the hand. However, coordinated movement proceeds in a distal to proximal direction. When reaching for the telephone on a desk, the shoulder and elbow do not lead the movement; rather, the hand opens and reaches to grasp the phone. The rest of the arm supports and follows the movement of the hand.

3. *Early motor behavior is dominated by reflex activity. Mature motor behavior is reinforced or supported by postural reflex mechanisms.*[49] In other words, the reflexes present in the newborn do not disappear completely but become integrated into the child's nervous system as he matures. For example, the asymmetric tonic neck reflex (ATNR) supports rolling, the symmetric tonic neck reflex (STNR) supports the assump-

tion of the hands-knees posture, and the body-on-body righting reflex supports the assumption of side-sitting from prone. In the adult, reflexes are available when needed to support movement. Evidence of this exists frequently in sports or when the body performs under stressful conditions. For example, head and neck extension in the STNR reinforces extension of the arms in pushing a heavy object, such as a bed or box.

Recognizing reflex responses in humans requires good observation skills, as the reflex response may not be complete. Tonus changes and partial movements are common. Hellebrandt et al.[51] studied the effect of the tonic neck reflex in the normal adult. An adaptation of one of her experiments can be easily performed with a partner. One person assumes a hands-knees position and the other person tests the triceps strength unilaterally four times. The first time, the person on hands and knees dorsiflexes her head and maintains this position. The tester waits 15 sec, allowing for the latency of the tonus change, and then resists the triceps by attempting to passively flex the elbow. This procedure is repeated with the head ventroflexed, rotated away from the arm, and rotated towards the arm being tested. One would expect stronger responses when elbow extension is supported by the STNR, head dorsiflexed, and by the ATNR, head rotated towards the resisted arm. In treatment, application occurs when a patient with weakness on one side has difficulty assuming a hands-knees posture. Directing the patient to turn his head toward the weaker side will elicit the support of the ATNR to reinforce elbow extension.

4. *The growth of motor behavior has cyclic trends as evidenced by shifts between flexor and extensor dominance.*[49] For example, in the development of the sitting posture, the first cycle is flexion. The newborn child is positioned in sitting and with assistance, or with support of arms, remains sitting in a flexor-dominant posture. The next cycle is one of extension. Sitting is assumed independently, but usually with extension from prone to hands and knees and then with rotation to side-sitting and long-sitting. Finally, the cycle shifts to flexion again as the child learns to assume sitting symmetrically from supine.

Interaction between movements of flexion and extension is necessary for functional movement. In the action of rising to stand, one begins by flexing the superior region forward to shift weight onto the feet. Extension of the body follows as the upright position is attained. The normal child facilitates this interaction by rocking alternately from flexion to extension in various postures.[52] Gesell describes this process as reciprocal interweaving in which relationships of opposed functions are established.[53] These reciprocal relationships provide the basis for development of stability and balance of postures.

In treatment, the therapist applies this principle in observing the patient's movements. If flexor tone dominates, then extensor-dominant activities and methods of assumption will be selected. Likewise, if extensor tone is dominant, activities stimulating flexor domi-

nance will be chosen. Care should be taken when stimulating flexion responses, as flexor reflexes are more primitive than extensor reflexes and may become dominant, creating an imbalance. Emphasis of treatment is rarely limited to one dominance, as an interaction between balanced antagonistic movements is sought.

5. *Goal-directed activity is made up of reversing movements.*[49] Early motor behavior occurs in random fashion through full range of motion. The spontaneous limb movements of the newborn usually fluctuate from extremes of flexion to extension. Yet the movements are rhythmic and reversing, qualities which continue throughout life. The act of eating is reversing movement of the arm and jaw. Reversal of a total pattern is commonly found in removing a can of soda from the refrigerator. Initially the action includes walking forward to open the door and reaching forward to grasp the can. Reversal of direction follows to remove the can from the shelf and walk backward to close the door. If a patient cannot reverse directions, his functional ability will be limited. The rhythmic reversing of direction then becomes a goal of treatment, as reversing movements help to reestablish the balance and interaction between antagonists.

6. *Normal movement and posture are dependent upon "synergism" and a balanced interaction of antagonists.*[49] This principle encompasses the previous three and states the main goal in the PNF approach: to develop a balance of antagonists. A continual adjustment in reflex activity, dominance, and reversing or antagonistic movements is required for the constant changes of movement and posture that occur in functional activity. For example, getting dressed demands interaction in all of these areas. Without a balance of antagonists, the quality of performance decreases, becoming more deliberate and losing its smooth and rhythmical characteristics. Thus, in treatment, prevention and correction of imbalances between antagonists is an objective.[49]

7. *Developing motor behavior is expressed in an orderly sequence of total patterns of movement and posture.*[52,54] The concept of recapitulating the developmental sequence is followed in treatment. The developmental sequence is considered a universal experience, common to all normal human beings. Thus, if a person, such as a child with cerebral palsy, has not experienced these total patterns, he has need to do so. With the patient who has developed normally and then becomes disabled, this sequence of developmental positions will have meaning to him.[49] In occupational therapy, the developmental sequence has direct application, as functional activities can be performed in a variety of postures. Thus, the patient not only experiences total patterns that facilitate the use of and integration of postural reflexes, but frustration is reduced. For example, his ability to dress is built through the total patterns of rolling, lower trunk rotation, bridging, and assumption to sitting, rather than through practice of inadequate or unstable sitting and standing positions.

The developmental sequence also includes the "combining movements" of the extremities as they interact with the head, neck, and trunk in total patterns (Table 6.7). The upper or lower extremity movements occur in an olderly sequence.[52,54] First to appear are bilateral symmetrical patterns, then bilateral asymmetrical and bilateral reciprocal patterns, and lastly unilateral patterns. When the upper and lower extremities move together, they begin in an ipsilateral pattern, then progress to alternating reciprocal, where contralateral extremities move in the same direction one at a time, while opposite contralateral extremities move in the opposite contralateral extremities move in the opposite direction one at a time. For example, an infant beginning to creep uses an ipsilateral pattern. Later, the child uses an alternating reciprocal pattern, moving one extremity at a time. As coordination and rate of movement increase, the child progresses to the most advanced combination, diagonal reciprocal. This combination is similar to alternating reciprocal with only one difference: contralateral extremities move in the same direction at the same time, while the other contralateral extremities move in the opposite direction at the same time, as in normal creeping or walking.

Table 6.7
COMBINED MOVEMENTS OF UPPER AND LOWER EXTREMITIES[a]

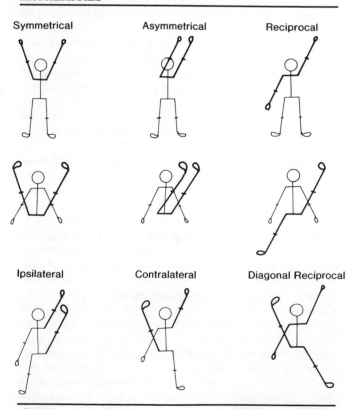

Symmetrical   Asymmetrical   Reciprocal

Ipsilateral   Contralateral   Diagonal Reciprocal

[a]Courtesy of D. E. Voss, Northwestern University Medical School, Chicago, IL. Figures redrawn by Julie A. Livingston (Class of 1973).

In occupational therapy, these combining movements may be used to assess a patient's level of performance or to design a treatment activity for stimulation of a response in the total pattern. For example, standing in a bilateral symmetrical combination will facilitate head, neck, and trunk flexion and extension. Swinging a bat or racquet in a bilateral asymmetrical combination will facilitate head, neck, and trunk rotation. On the other hand, performing a reciprocal combination, such as throwing a ball or reaching for an item on a high shelf, promotes stability of head, neck, and trunk.

Direction of movement also develops in an orderly sequence. Gesell observed that the child follows a significant pattern in developing the ability to use a crayon. The strokes move from scrawl, to vertical, to horizontal, to circular, and then to oblique or diagonal. Comparable sequences of direction have been demonstrated in visual behavior eye-hand coordination, vocalization, percept-concept formation, and postural behavior.[55] Thus, the diagonal direction or pattern of movement is a combination of the previous three movements, and is the most advanced. Voss,[49] in citing Gesell, pointed out that in PNF, total patterns of movement are performed in a diagonal direction, as well as in forward, backward, sideward, and circular directions. A cerebrovascular-accident (CVA) patient may be able to creep forward and backward. However, difficulty may occur when changing direction in circular and diagonal creeping. Thus, facilitation of circular and diagonal patterns of creeping can be goals of treatment.

8. *Normal motor development has an orderly sequence but lacks a step-by-step quality. Overlapping occurs.*[49] In treatment, a patient does not remain in sitting until perfection of balance is achieved before attempting to stand. The order of the developmental sequence aids the therapist in finding a posture or a place to begin when treating the patient. A posture in which the patient is stable and can move successfully becomes a place to begin. The developmental sequence provides a direction in which to progress. However, the overlapping quality occurs as the patient may benefit from working on activities in postures above and below his level of ability.

Performing activities in developmental postures will enhance a person's adaptive response to the task or movement. However, the activity must be graded in keeping with the physical demands on the patient. If the physical demands are high, the activity must be simple. If the physical demands are low, the activity may be more complex. For example, a patient with brain damage may need to develop balance in kneeling and standing and improve his writing skills. In treatment, activities in kneeling may include simple gross motor activities, such as playing tic-tac-toe on the blackboard or sanding on an inclined board. However, when the patient practices writing, a fine motor activity, a more stable posture such as sitting is required. Besides kneeling and sitting the patient may engage in standing activities, walking to and from each activity, and gait training in physical therapy. Thus, overlapping of postures occurs in treatment during an individual therapy session or throughout the day.

9. *Improvement of motor ability is dependent upon motor learning.*[49] The concepts of motor learning that PNF applies to therapeutic exercise are similar to those used by occupational therapists in functional activity training. These concepts will be reviewed briefly with specific emphasis on the PNF approach.

Motor learning extends from the conditioning of responses to the learning of complex voluntary motor acts.[56] Harlow and Harlow[57] classified the conditioning of responses as the simplest form of learning. Proprioceptive feedback as received from receptors in the muscles, tendons, joints, and labyrinths plays a significant role in simple conditioned responses.[56] In addition, stress promotes maturation.[58] Levine[58] studied infant rats and their responses to the stresses of handling and electric shock. The rats who received either form of stress developed into normal active adults. Those rats that were not subjected to stress defecated and urinated more frequently and did not explore their environment. Thus, motor learning is facilitated by appropriate stress coupled with sensory and environmental stimulation.

As maturation occurs, more complex acts may be learned. The sequence begins with conditioned responses progressing to an ability to discriminate between objects, to an ability to transfer learning from one problem to another, and then to the ability to solve complex problems requiring concept formation. Learning complex tasks can be facilitated by the use of "step-wise procedures," as demonstrated in Harlow's studies.[57] In PNF, the therapist helps the patient to learn many complex motor acts, such as transfers and other self-care skills. By selecting and providing appropriate sensory cues and through the use of techniques of facilitation, the demands of a task or parts of the task that the patient is unable to perform independently may be made more appropriate. PNF emphasizes the step-wise procedures of a task, yet allows the patient to complete the whole task. Thus, by training with repetition, the conditioning of responses occurs and leads to the achievement of the whole task.

Sensory cues include visual, auditory, and tactile stimuli. Vision and hearing give direction to movement.[59] Vision may lead movement or follow the movement. For example, in lifting an object up to a shelf, the person will look to the shelf first, then lift the object. Thus, if a patient is not engaging the movement with his eyes, he has a need to do so. Following the movement visually will enhance the motor performance.

Verbal commands increase sensory stimulation and may facilitate movement. Tone of voice may influence the quality of the muscle response. A loud, sharp command will yield a quick response and recruit more motor units. A soft, low command will produce a slower response. In the presence of pain, soft commands are always used to avoid stimulating jerky movements and further increasing the pain.[49]

Verbal mediation[60] occurs when the patient speaks aloud to direct his movements. For example, a patient who has difficulty preparing the wheelchair in a transfer may say, "I am going to lock the brakes, put my feet on the floor, and move the footrests away." Expressing the movement verbally, as the task is performed, enhances the organization, memory, and execution of the task.

Tactile cues in PNF are mainly provided by the therapist's manual contacts, which facilitate movement or promote relaxation. Also, stretch and resistance may be applied by opposing the patient's effort and yet becoming part of his effort.[49] Additional tactile stimulation may be provided by adjuncts to treatment, such as vibration and cold.

Thus, motor learning is enhanced by tracking sensory cues. One may track a visual stimulus, the sound of a voice, or a touch. Tactual tracking is more efficient.[61] In cybernetics research, movement with visual tracking was discovered to be less accurate than movement with tactual feedback. In treatment, an application of tracking may occur when a patient reaches for an object and is unable to complete the range of movement. A light touch on the back of the patient's hand, guiding him toward the object, may be the only cue he needs to achieve the goal. Another example may occur when a patient with unilateral weakness in the upper limb attempts to wipe the table with a sponge. The performance may quickly deteriorate with the patient complaining of fatigue. With a light touch on the back of the patient's hand from the therapist hand or with self-touch from the patient's uninvolved hand, the patient's movement becomes less deliberate, endurance improves, and the task is completed. In summary, the application of motor learning concepts in PNF becomes one of combining as many favorable influences as possible to achieve the desired response.

10. *Frequency of stimulation and repetition of activity are used to promote and for retention of motor learning and for the development of strength and endurance.*[49] Patients, as well as any child or adult learning a new skill, require frequent stimulation and opportunity to practice in order that the task being learned may be retained. Motor learning has occurred when the movement is repeated enough to become integrated into the body's repertoire of movements and can be used automatically. In treatment, repetition cannot be overemphasized. Activity has an inherent advantage over exercise because during activity repetition occurs naturally.

11. *Goal-directed activities, coupled with techniques of facilitation, are used to hasten learning of total patterns of walking and of self-care activities.*[49] Facilitation techniques or exercise alone are not as meaningful as when they are coupled with an activity. Activity that directs attention away from the motor aspects of the task and toward a purposeful goal enhances neurological

integration.[62] Likewise, purposeful activity alone is not enough. It is necessary but not always sufficient to meet the patient's needs. Therapists need to relate the facilitation techniques to activity.[62]

Evaluation

Assessment becomes an ongoing process in the PNF approach. Following the initial evaluation, a treatment plan is established using selected procedures and techniques. Modifications in the plan occur as the needs of the patient change or as the therapist observes a change in the patient's performance.

As PNF encompasses concepts that may be applied to many diagnoses, the evaluation is general in nature. Forms for evaluation, analysis, and planning treatment programs in physical therapy were developed by Voss[63] in 1967 and 1969. Descriptions of the evaluation process have been presented in detail in the literature.[42,59] The evaluation reflects the developmental sequence, proceeding from a proximal to distal direction. A brief summary of the evaluation process is presented here.

Vital and related functions of the body are considered first. Functions of respiration, swallowing, voice production, and facial and tongue motions are evaluated with impairments, weakness, or asymmetry noted. Also, movements in response to visual, auditory, and tactile stimuli are elicited to determine which sensory cues may be used to reinforce movement and posture.

Head and neck patterns, the key to upper trunk patterns, receive the next consideration. Observation of head and neck position is made during the performance of developmental and functional activities. The following are noted: dominance of tone (flexor or extensor), alignment (midline or asymmetrical), and stability vs. mobility (balanced or deficient in one or both areas).

Combinations of diagonal patterns of the extremities are next in the evaluation sequence. The patient is asked to perform bilateral symmetrical, bilateral asymmetrical, and bilateral reciprocal combinations. The following areas are assessed: influence of head, neck, and trunk; range of motion, remembering that rotation is not complete in any pattern; quality of movement, such as smooth and rhythmical; and normal timing, with the distal component leading in coordinated movement.

Developmental postures are observed by asking the patient to assume and maintain positions in the developmental sequence. These total patterns are assessed to determine how muscle groups function in relation to each other in a given pattern. Previous evaluation centered on individual segments and functions. During observations of total patterns a central problem or imbalance may be identified. For example, is more stability or mobility needed? Is there a dominance rather than a balance of flexor or extensor tone? And does the patient have difficulty shifting from one dominance to another?

Functional activities, as performed in self-care tasks and transfers, are observed finally to determine any discrepancies between the patient's ability to perform individual and total patterns and his ability to combine these movements in performance of a functional task.

Treatment Procedures

DIAGONAL PATTERNS

For every major part of the body: the head, neck, trunk, and extremities, two pairs of diagonal patterns of movement exist. Each pair of antagonistic patterns consists of three motion components. Flexion or extension is always present as the major component. These flexion and extension components are combined with rotation, either external or internal, and with abduction or adduction. For example, in diagonal one (D1) flexion of the upper extremity, flexion combines with adduction and external rotation. In diagonal two (D2) flexion, flexion combines with abduction and external rotation. These diagonal patterns are described in the book by Voss et al.[42] according to shoulder motion components, the original designation by Kabat. The briefer designations of diagonal one and diagonal two were introduced by Voss.[49] In development, the diagonal patterns appear in the functional movements of rolling and prone locomotion. Diagonal one is derived from rolling and diagonal two from crawling on the belly.

Five factors support the use of diagonal patterns in treatment. First, the patterns agree with the spiral and diagonal characteristics of normal functional movement. Most muscles, by virtue of their attachments and alignment of their fibers, support this movement. Second, scientists who have studied integrative function of the brain support the concept that voluntary movement consists of mass movement patterns rather than individual muscle action. Hughlings Jackson[64] was one of the first to stimulate specific areas of the motor cortex and discovered that mass movement patterns were produced. Third, Gesell noted that diagonal movement occurs last in the normal development of direction and is the most advanced motion.[55] Thus, diagonal movements are combinations of the three pairs of antagonistic motions of flexion or extension, abduction or adduction, and external or internal rotation. Fourth, all diagonal patterns cross the midline, thereby facilitating interaction between two sides of the body, which is important to perceptual motor and sensory integrative functioning. Fifth, the diagonal patterns always incorporate a rotation component. As rotation is one of the last movements to develop, it is usually the first to be lost following an injury or with aging.[49] Use of diagonal patterns in therapy reinforces the component of rotation, necessary to the performance of functional tasks. Placing an activity in a diagonal direction will elicit a diagonal pattern and the desired rotation. Range of motion may also be performed in diagonal patterns. Rotation is incorporated with each limb motion. This method is more efficient than the traditional range of motion performed in anatomical planes. Figures 6.14 through 6.43 are arranged to show the two extremes of the bilateral patterns

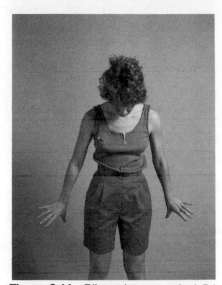

Figure 6.14 Bilateral symmetrical D1 extension, shortened range; bilateral symmetrical D1 flexion, lengthened range: shoulders extend, abduct, and internally rotate; elbows extend (intermediate joint, the elbow, may flex or extend), forearms pronate; wrists extend toward ulnar side; fingers extend and abduct; and thumbs extend and abduct.

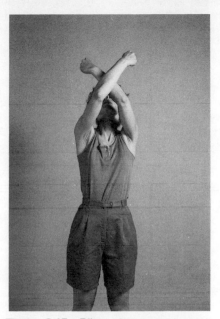

Figure 6.15 Bilateral symmetrical D1 flexion, shortened range; bilateral symmetrical D1 extension, lengthened range: shoulders flex, adduct, and externally rotate; elbows flex (intermediate joint, the elbow, may flex or extend), forearms supinate; wrists flex toward radial side; fingers flex and adduct; and thumbs flex and adduct.

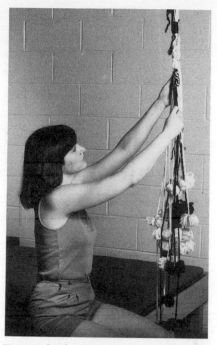

Figure 6.16 Bilateral asymmetrical flexion to the left to macramé. Left arm is in D2 flexion; right arm in D1 flexion.

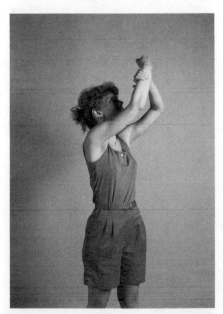

Figure 6.17 Bilateral asymmetrical pattern with limbs in contact, as in "chopping." A chop to the right begins with the right arm in D1 flexion, and the left hand grasping the dorsum of the right wrist.

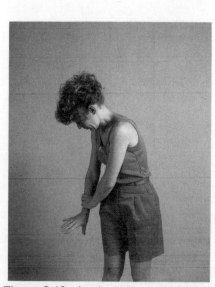

Figure 6.18 In chopping to the right, the right arm moves in D1 extension, with the left arm assisting in D2 extension.

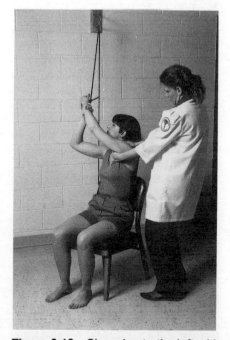

Figure 6.19 Chopping to the left with pulleys. Left arm will move into D1 extension. Right arm will assist in D2 extension. Note rotation of head, neck, and trunk. Therapist resists scapular movement.

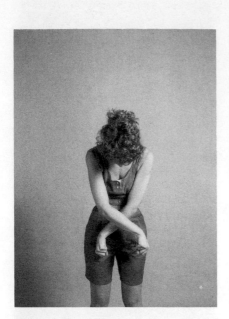

Figure 6.20 Bilateral symmetrical D2 extension, shortened range; bilateral symmetrical D2 flexion, lengthened range: shoulders extend, adduct, and internally rotate; elbows flex (intermediate joint, the elbow, may flex or extend); forearms pronate; wrists flex toward ulnar side; fingers flex and adduct; thumbs in opposition.

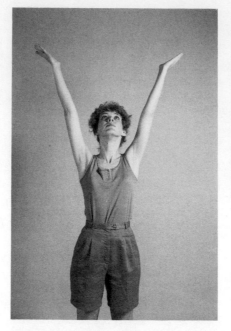

Figure 6.21 Bilateral symmetrical D2 flexion, shortened range; bilateral symmetrical D2 extension, lengthened range: shoulders flex, abduct, externally rotate; elbows extend (intermediate joint, the elbow, may flex or extend); forearms supinate; wrists extend toward radial side; fingers extend and abduct; thumbs extend and adduct.

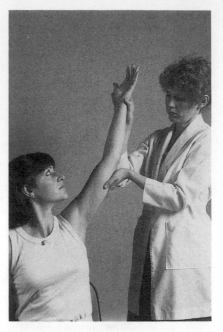

Figure 6.22 Range of motion in D2 flexion. Therapist's manual contacts are on the extensor surface to facilitate wrist and elbow extension in the D2 flexion pattern. Contacts will switch to flexor surfaces as the patient reverses the pattern in D2 extension.

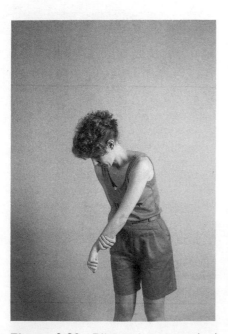

Figure 6.23 Bilateral symmetrical pattern with limbs in contact, as in "lifting." A lift to the left begins with the left arm in D2 extension and the right hand grasping the volar surface of the left wrist.

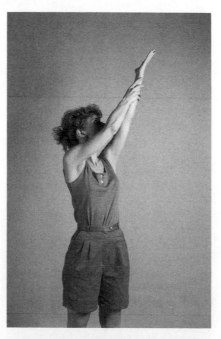

Figure 6.24 In lifting to the left, the left arm moves in D2 flexion, with the right arm assisting in D1 flexion.

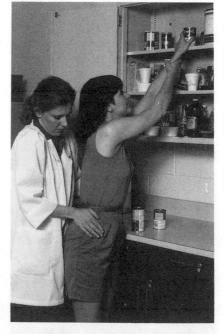

Figure 6.25 Lifting to the left to place groceries on the shelf. Therapist approximates at the pelvis.

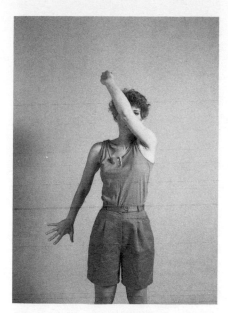

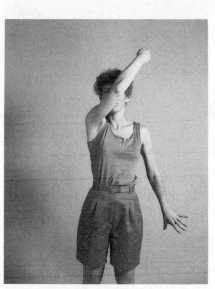

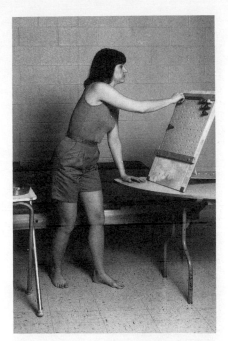

Figure 6.26 Bilateral reciprocal D1, lengthened range. Left arm begins in D1 flexion. Right arm begins in D1 extension.

Figure 6.27 Bilateral reciprocal D1, shortened range. Left arm moves in D1 extension. Right arm moves in D1 extension.

Figure 6.28 Bilateral reciprocal D1 in a palmar prehension activity. Note the simultaneous static and dynamic position, with the left arm weight bearing (static) in D1 extension and the right arm moving (dynamic) in D1 flexion.

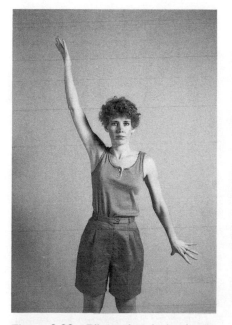

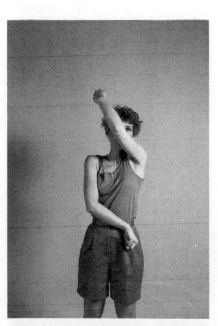

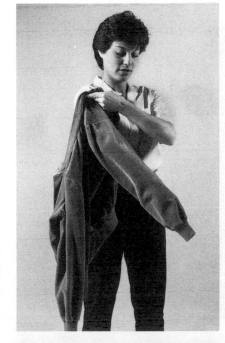

Figure 6.29 Bilateral reciprocal combined diagonals, lengthened range. Right arm begins in D2 flexion. Left arm begins in D1 extension.

Figure 6.30 Bilateral reciprocal combined diagonals, shortened range. Right arm moves in D2 extension. Left arm moves in D1 flexion. Head and neck may rotate, diagonally flex and extend, or remain in midline.

Figure 6.31 Bilateral reciprocal combined diagonals in donning a jacket. Right arm moves through the sleeve in D2 extension. Left arm pulls the jacket over the right arm in D1 flexion.

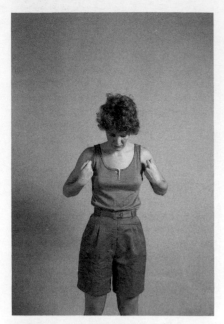

Figure 6.32 Bilateral symmetrical D1 ulnar thrust, lengthened range; shoulders extend, abduct, and internally rotate; elbows flex; forearms supinate; wrists flex toward radial side; fingers flex and adduct; thumbs flex and adduct.

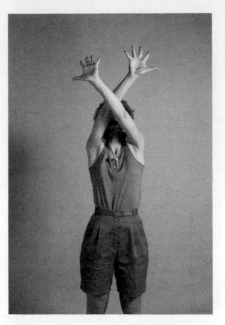

Figure 6.33 Bilateral symmetrical D1 ulnar thrust, shortened range; shoulders flex, adduct, and externally rotate; elbows extend, forearms pronate, wrists extend toward ulnar side, fingers extend and abduct, thumbs extend and abduct.

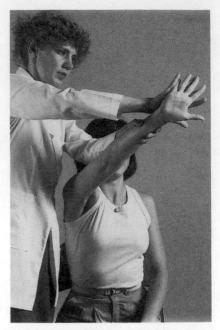

Figure 6.34 Unilateral D1 ulnar thrust to the left. Therapist resists wrist extension using the technique of repeated contractions.

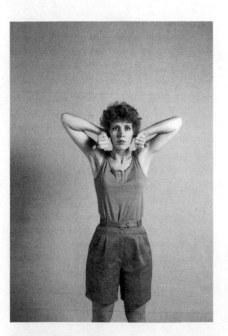

Figure 6.35 Bilateral symmetrical D2 radial thrust, lengthened range; shoulders flex, abduct, and externally rotate; elbows flex; forearms pronate; wrists flex toward ulnar side; fingers flex and adduct; thumbs in opposition.

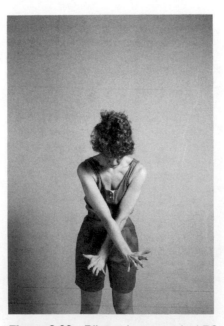

Figure 6.36 Bilateral symmetrical D2 radial thrust, shortened range; shoulders extend, adduct, and internally rotate; elbows extend; forearms supinate; wrists extend toward radial side; fingers extend and abduct; thumbs extend and abduct.

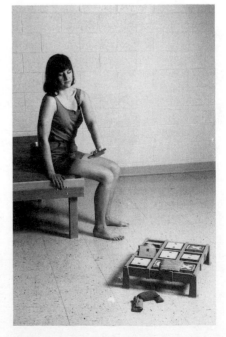

Figure 6.37 Unilateral D2 radial thrust to the right in a beanbag toss. Thrusting facilitates hand opening with elbow extension.

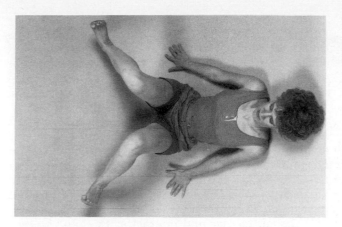

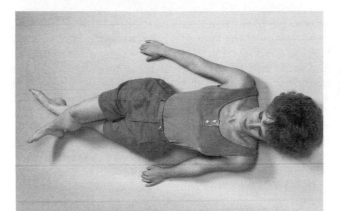

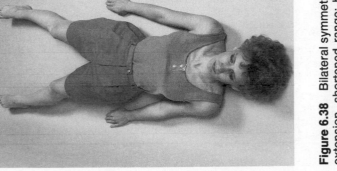

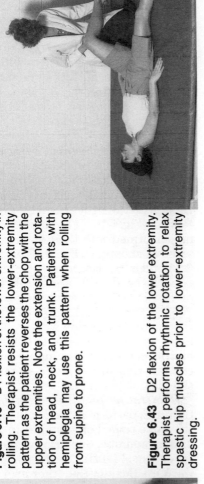

Figure 6.38 Bilateral symmetrical D1 extension, shortened range; bilateral symmetrical D1 flexion, lengthened range: hips extend, abduct, and internally rotate; knees extend (intermediate joint, the knee, may flex or extend), ankles and feet plantar flex and evert; and toes flex and adduct.

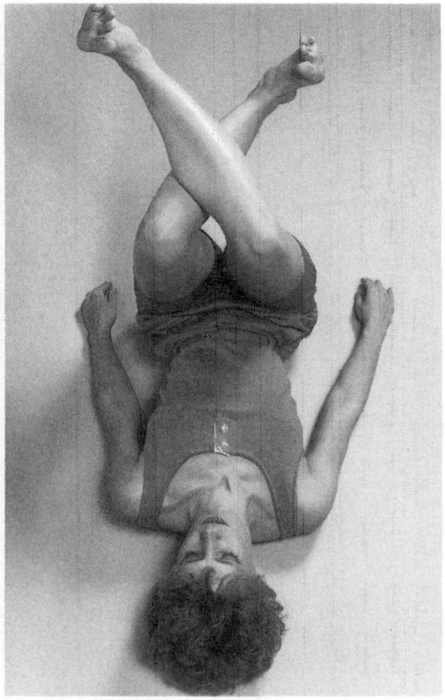

Figure 6.39 Bilateral symmetrical D1 flexion, shortened range; bilateral symmetrical D1 extension, lengthened range: hips flex, adduct, and externally rotate; knees flex (intermediate joint, the knee, may flex or extend), ankles and feet dorsiflex and invert; toes extend and abduct.

Figure 6.41 Bilateral symmetrical D2 extension, shortened range; bilateral symmetrical D2 flexion, lengthened range: hips extend, adduct, and externally rotate; knees extend (intermediate joint, the knee, may flex or extend); ankles and feet plantar flex and invert; toes flex and adduct.

Figure 6.42 Bilateral symmetrical D2 flexion, shortened range; bilateral symmetrical D2 extension, lengthened range: hips flex, abduct, and internally rotate; knees flex (intermediate joint, the knee, may flex or extend); ankle and feet dorsiflex and evert; toes extend and abduct.

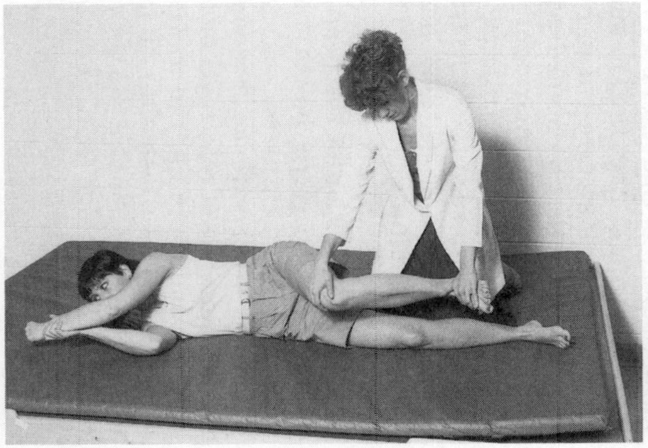

Figure 6.40 D1 flexion of the lower extremity in rolling. Therapist resists the lower-extremity pattern as the patient reverses the chop with the upper extremities. Note the extension and rotation of head, neck, and trunk. Patients with hemiplegia may use this pattern when rolling from supine to prone.

Figure 6.43 D2 flexion of the lower extremity. Therapist performs rhythmic rotation to relax spastic hip muscles prior to lower-extremity dressing.

along with a treatment application of the particular pattern.

Bilateral symmetrical patterns occur where paired extremities perform like movements at the same time. These combining movements are the first to develop; therefore, they are often the easiest to learn. Also, as they influence head, neck, and trunk flexion and extension, they play an important role in facilitating a reciprocal relationship between flexor and extensor dominance. Bilateral symmetrical patterns of the upper extremities (Fig. 6.14 and 6.15, Fig. 6.20 and 6.21) are commonly observed in the daily activities of riding a bicycle, putting a roast in the oven, and removing a pullover shirt overhead. Bilateral symmetrical patterns of the lower extremities (Fig. 6.38 and 6.39, Fig. 6.41 and 6.42) are seen in the postures of standing and sitting.

Bilateral asymmetrical patterns occur when paired extremities perform movements toward one side at the same time. The limbs may move together free from contact as in bilateral asymmetrical flexion to the right, with the right arm in D2 flexion and the left in D1 flexion (Fig. 6.16). The combining movement may also be performed with the arms in contact, as in the patterns of chopping (Fig. 6.17 and 6.18) and lifting (Fig. 6.23 and 6.24). Bilateral asymmetrical patterns influence the head, neck, and trunk movements in patterns of flexion with rotation or extension with rotation. When the arms perform in contact, the range of trunk flexion and extension with rotation increases. Swinging a baseball bat is an example of a bilateral asymmetric pattern in the upper extremities. The same combination in the lower extremities is found in the side-sitting position.

Bilateral reciprocal patterns occur when paired extremities perform movements in opposite directions at the same time. For example, in reciprocal movements of diagonal one, one arm begins in D1 extension, the other arm in D1 flexion. Fig. 6.26 As one arm moves toward D1 flexion, the other arm moves toward D1 extension. Fig. 6.27 Less flexion and extension of head, neck, and trunk are present in reciprocal motions as compared to other combined patterns. Rotation of head, neck, and trunk may occur, but the range is incomplete. When antagonistic patterns of both diagonals are performed at the same time, as in a reciprocal combination in combined diagonals with one arm in D1 extension and the other arm in D2 flexion, the movement of the head, neck, and trunk continue to decrease. The position of the head remains in midline. The reciprocal patterns have a stabilizing influence on head, neck, and trunk because one extremity flexes while the other extends, producing stability in the trunk. Examples of reciprocal movements are walking, running, and swimming the crawl stroke. They are also seen in activities which place an increased demand for equilibrium reactions on the body, such as in reaching for an item on a high shelf, or performing a lay-up shot during a basketball game.

Unilateral patterns in developing motor behavior emerge from the bilateral patterns. The motions of the unilateral diagonal patterns are the same as those described in the bilateral symmetrical patterns (Fig. 6.14 and 6.15, 6.20 and 6.21). In skilled tasks the two diagonals may interact or one may dominate. Diagonal one in the upper extremities is observed in the basic activities of feeding and washing the face, right side with left hand. Diagonal two is seen in the self-care activities of zipping a front-opening zipper and winding a watch. Diagonal one in the lower extremities is observed in pushing one foot through a pant leg and in crossing one leg to don a sock. Diagonal two is seen in hurdling and in swimming the breast stroke.

Diagonals change and interact as the hand crosses the midline of the face and body. They also interact when the pattern crosses the horizontal plane that transverses at the shoulders. An example occurs when waving goodbye. The right arm begins in extension on the same side of the body in D1 extension. When the arm raises above the shoulder to wave goodbye on the same side, it moves into D2 flexion with elbows flexed. Another example of the two diagonals interacting occurs in washing the face (Table 6.8). When the right hand contacts the left face, it is moving into D1 flexion. When the right hand washes the right side of the face, it is moving toward D2 flexion with elbow flexion.

In all of the above bilateral and unilateral patterns, the intermediate joints, the elbow and the knee, may flex or extend. While the intermediate joints may change, the motions of the proximal and distal joints are consistent with each other. In the upper extremity, the consistency between the proximal and distal joints changes in a variation of the diagonal pattern called *thrusting* (Fig. 6.32 and 6.33; 6.35 and 6.36).

Table 6.8
ACTIVITY FOR ANALYSIS: PRIMITIVE[a]
WASHING OF FACE AND NECK[b]

Hand(s)	Side(s) of Face	Diagonal and Sequence[c]	Combined Diagonals[d]
R	L, then R	D1, then D2	
L and R	Both sides	D1, then D2	BS
L contacts R wrist	L, then R	L, D2, then D1 R, D1, then D2	BA, chop and lift
R contacts L wrist	R, then L	L, D1, then D2 R, D2, then D1	BA, chop and lift

[a]Primitive: Using hands and running water, without washcloth.
[b]Reprinted with permission from D. E. Voss, unpublished data.
[c]Diagonals change and interact as hand crosses midline of face, nose, or mouth.
[d]BS, both hands use *bilateral* symmetry, same diagonal; BA, one hand uses one diagonal as other hand uses the second, or other diagonal. Hands placed in contact as for "chopping and lifting" permits one hand to guide or "track" the other. This *bilateral asymmetrical* combination of diagonal patterns may be useful with hemiplegic patients among others.

The two pairs of upper extremity thrusting patterns are the ulnar thrust, D1, and the radial thrust, D2. In diagonal one flexion, external rotation is consistent with supination. In the D1 ulnar thrust, the shoulder remains the same, but the forearm is counterrotated in pronation, and the hand opens to the ulnar side. In diagonal two extension, internal rotation is consistent with pronation. In the D2 radial thrust, the shoulder remains the same, but the forearm is counterrotated in supination, and the hand opens to the radial side. All bilateral combinations can be performed with the thrusting patterns. In the lower extremities, mass extension of hip and knee is a powerful thrusting movement. Thrusting patterns represent primitive patterns of protection, defense, reach, and grasp. The movement of thrusting occurs more forcefully than motions in other diagonal patterns. In treatment, thrusting is a good pattern in which to retrain elbow extension with wrist extension.

The diagonal patterns provide OTs with a framework from which to assess and train functional movements. If a patient performs an incomplete hand-to-mouth pattern, the D1 flexion pattern is weak. Thus, treatment activities to facilitate a stronger D1 flexion pattern are designed. For example: pulleys in chopping pattern (Fig. 6.19), grasp and release activity in reciprocal D1 using simultaneous static-dynamic position (Fig. 6.28), and resisting the D1 pattern using the techniques of slow reversal-hold and repeated contractions.

TOTAL PATTERNS

PNF has been described as a developmental approach by Knott and Voss. In the course of normal motor development, total patterns of movement precede individual patterns.[65] Each total pattern requires interaction of component patterns of the head, neck, and trunk with those of the extremities. When movement in a forward or backward direction is combined with movement in a lateral direction, the diagonal patterns of facilitation become evident. In treatment, performance of total patterns is used to develop the ability to perform diagonal patterns. In PNF, the techniques of facilitation are superimposed upon total patterns of movement and posture. The total pattern provides the base for all other movement.

The sequence and procedures for assisting patients into the developmental postures were developed by Voss in 1971. A videotape was made in 1972 and revised in 1973.[66] In 1981 the sequence and procedure for use in OT were produced by Myers.[67] In this sequence of total patterns, the therapist elicits reflex support in order to assist the more severely involved patient. With reflex support the assumption of postures may be achieved with minimal effort on the part of the therapist and patient. One procedure, assisting a patient from prone to prone on elbows, will be described in detail with application to activities.

Prone on Elbows

The prone-on-elbows posture may be used in daily living to watch TV or read on the floor. In *active assumption* prone on elbows is a symmetrical movement that is extensor dominant. The tonic labyrinthine prone reflex must be overcome, while the optical and labyrinthine righting reflexes support the assumption. The pattern begins with head, neck, and upper trunk extension followed by adduction of shoulders with forearms pronated and wrist and fingers extended.

To assist a patient from prone to prone on elbows (Fig. 6.44), the *preparatory maneuvers* include placing the lower extremities in symmetrical extension and placing the head in a symmetrical position or turned to one side for comfort. Head, turned to one side, will be more difficult for the therapist to control as the shoulder toward which the head is turned will be elevated, with the other depressed against the mat. The upper extremities are placed in symmetrical D2 flexion with elbows flexed, fingers pointing to the nose. The *therapist positions* herself astride the patient if the patient is on the mat, or to one side if he is on a bed or cart. The therapist's hips and knees should be flexed.

Manual contacts, with the hands in a mitt-like position and fingers and thumbs relaxed, apply stretch and assistance or resistance. The hands, placed over the pectoral region with fingers pointing toward the umbilicus, stimulate a muscle response in the shoulder adductors that lends stability to the posture (Fig. 6.45). Hands should be placed medially to allow the patient's arms to assume a vertical position.

Auditory commands are "When I say three, look up. One, two, three, *look up!*" Simultaneously with the word, "up," the therapist leans backward, so that the

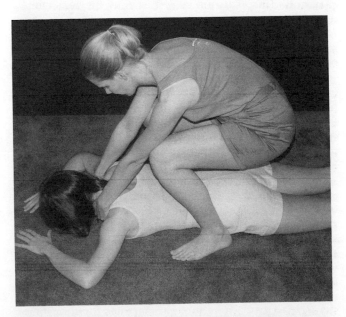

Figure 6.44 The position of the patient and the therapist for assisting a patient from prone to prone on elbows.

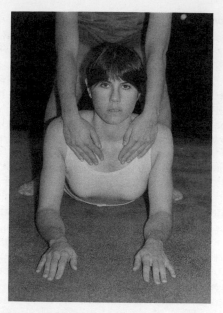

Figure 6.45 The manual contacts in assisting a patient from prone to prone on elbows. Hands are placed over the pectoral region with fingers pointing toward the umbilicus.

patient's superior region is elevated with forearms falling into place.

In *application to activity* prone on elbows provides a good position in which to work for control of head and neck extension with weight bearing to facilitate stability in the scapulohumeral joint. Also, any patients who need to spend time prone for healing or prevention of decubiti or to maintain muscle tone will need to be able to assume and maintain this posture to perform self-care activities. Various activities may be performed, depending on the patient's ability.

In level one, practicing assumption, rocking, raising and lowering the head, and depressing the scapula may be all that the patient can perform.

In level two, the patient is able to maintain an adequate posture for longer periods of time. Straw or mouth stick activities may be used. Margaret Rood has demonstrated that sucking and swallowing facilitate cocontraction of neck muscles and reinforce head and neck extension.[68] Control of the tongue may be enhanced in this primitive posture.

In level three, the patient will begin to perform manual activities with the elbows immobile and bearing weight. The activity will be confined to a small area as with a drawing or a tile project. Eating finger foods is another facilitatory activity. The tongue receives a stretch stimulus in this position. With flaccidity or marked weakness, food may drop out of the mouth unless lip closure is maintained and the tongue is functional. The tongue and lips do not work as hard in the sitting posture. If a patient can perform for short periods in prone, his performance in sitting may improve faster.

In level four, the patient is able to decrease the support needed to maintain the posture and lift one extremity from the surface, as in playing a table game, typing one-handed, or combining one's hair. A brief outline of other sequences for assisting patients into developmental postures follows.

Position of therapist: On side toward which patient will move

Manual contacts: Scapula and pelvis

Commands: "Look here!" Patient is assisted to side-lying.

Application to OT: Patients who must attend therapy on a cart may be positioned in side-lying. Also side-lying, a very stable posture, may be a "place to begin" treatment for the severely involved patient.

Examples of activities are: Use of a skateboard, stabilizing or rolling a ball, macramé, grasping and releasing objects in diagonal patterns, sliding the hand on the wall in various directions, and writing on the wall.

Side-Lying to Side-Sitting

Reflex support: Body on body righting

Preparatory maneuvers: Position legs in asymmetric flexion, and arms in asymmetric flexion at shoulder level.

Position of therapist: Behind patient's hips

Manual contacts: Shoulder girdle

Commands: "On the count of three, look back at me. One, two, three, *look* at me!" Patient is assisted to side-sitting.

Application to OT: Side-sitting is useful for increasing trunk rotation, facilitating equilibrium reactions, and movement of the free arm, while the supporting arm is stable with compression of joint surfaces and cocontraction of antagonistic muscle groups. Examples of activities are: table buffer exercises, stacking cones (reaching behind body to pick them up), turning pages of newspaper or magazine, playing chess, watching television, eating a snack, and rug punching where the frame is stabilized in a vise. Response of supporting arm may be enhanced by vibration of elbow extensors.

Variation: The patient may move from side-lying to leaning on one elbow before progressing to side-sitting. Side-lying on elbow is often used by patients with paraplegia or quadriplegia during eating and hygiene activities performed on a cart or in a bed.

Supine to Long-Sitting

Reflex support: Labyrinthine righting, optical righting

Preparatory maneuvers: Place legs in symmetrical extension and abduction.

Position of therapist: Astride patient at knees

Manual contacts: Dorsum of wrists

Commands: "On the count of three, look at your feet and sit up. One, two, three, *look* at your feet!" Patient is assisted to long-sitting.

Alternate sequence: Side-sitting to long-sitting

Preparatory maneuvers: Assist to side-sitting.

Position of therapist: Behind patient

Manual contacts: Shoulder girdle, one anteriorly, the other posteriorly

Commands: Tell patient to look in direction of turn and reach over for support with moving arm. Assist patient to rotate, distributing weight on both hips.

Application to OT: Long-sitting improves sitting balance and provides stability for dressing lower extremities in bed. It is easily applied to a variety of one-handed or two-handed activities. Some activities are: One-handed—Stack cones in a diagonal pattern, play checkers, throw bean bags, hit ball with stick, sanding project positioned on incline board, painting. Two-handed—Pull putty, throw and catch ball, roll ball around body, macramé, leather stamping, throw and mold clay, mix ingredients in a bowl, prepare vegetables.

Variation: Small lap board with legs placed over patient's legs provides a hard working surface and expands type of activities that can be done in this position.

Prone to Hands-Knees

Reflex support: STNR (head midline), or ATNR (head rotated)

Preparatory maneuvers: Position inferior region so that hips are flexed and thighs are vertical to floor.

Position of therapist: Astride patient holding hips securely between the therapist's knees

Manual contacts: Pectoral region

Commands: "On the count of three, look up. One, two, three, *look* up!" Patient is assisted to hands-knees.

Application to OT: Hands-knees posture promotes or enhances balance and stability in hips and shoulders. Initially activity may include use of rhythmic stabilization following or preceding rocking in different directions—forward, backward, sideward, and diagonally to left and right. Simultaneous static/dynamic activity, *i.e.,* stacking cones, sanding, hammering, placing tiles in trivet, and figure eight board may follow as appropriate. Functional activities usually performed in this posture may be used, such as: washing and waxing floor, cleaning under bed, picking up item on floor, cleaning low shelves or oven, or working in garden.

Kneeling

Reflex support: Labyrinthine and optical righting, and equilibrium reactions

Procedure: Varies depending on method of assumption, *i.e.,* from heel-sitting, hands-knees, side-sitting.

Application to OT: Kneeling provides opportunity to develop upper-extremity function for free standing, as well as hip extension, and hip extension with knee flexion necessary for gait. Activities will vary according to the patient's ability. Begin with both hands in contact with a supporting surface, as in rocking in various directions. Follow with a surface contact activity, such as sanding or dusting. Later, with both arms free, catching and throwing a ball, writing on a blackboard, or cooking may be tried. Kneeling is the only position other than sitting and standing where both arms can be used free of the supporting surface.

Hands-Knees to Plantigrade

Reflex support: Labyrinthine and optical righting and equilibrium reactions

Preparatory maneuvers: Assist to hands-knees posture.

Position of therapist: Behind patient

Manual contacts: Pelvis

Commands: "Straighten your knees" or "Bring one foot forward and place it flat on the floor, then the other."

Application to OT: Plantigrade posture has minimal application to OT. However, a modified plantigrade posture with feet flat on the floor and hands or elbows resting on a supporting surface is easily used in many occupational therapy activities. A few are: washing dishes, wiping table, making bed, painting, grasping and releasing objects, playing cards with card holder, throwing bean bags in a game of "toss-a-cross," getting out of bathtub.

Assisting the patient into various postures helps him to experience functional movements with normal environmental and sensory stimulation to the total body. For example, the patient in the wheelchair, with lower limbs supported on footrests, is essentially suspended above the ground in a flexed posture. The sensory cues provided by gravity, body in contact with the ground, will be limited. If activities must be performed in a wheelchair, placing feet on the floor will facilitate a better response from the total pattern.

SELECTED PROCEDURES AND TECHNIQUES

Techniques for facilitation and inhibition include a battery of procedures that may be used singly or in combination, according to the abilities and needs of the patient. All techniques are superimposed on patterns of movement and posture.[49]

Sherrington described three principles of neurophysiology from which Kabat[69] developed many of the PNF techniques. *Irradiation,* the facilitation of one voluntary motion by another, is not haphazard but spreads in a specific pattern of muscle groups. The stimulus for irradiation is generated by tension in contracting muscles and related structures. In treatment, resistance coupled with stretch, as in repeated contractions, may elicit irradiation for the purpose of using the motions of the stronger muscle groups to facilitate the weaker motions of a pattern. *Successive induction* is also a process of facilitating one voluntary motion by another. However, the stronger antagonist facilitates the weaker agonist, as in resisted reversals of antagonists. In treatment when techniques of slow reversal and slow reversal-hold are used, a contraction of the stronger muscle groups is elicited first to more effectively facilitate the weaker muscle groups. If a muscle imbalance is present, this procedure carries the risk of increasing the imbalance. *Reciprocal innervation* is a process of inhibiting reflexes by voluntary motion. At the time that the agonist is facilitated or contracted against resistance the antagonist lengthens and provides control as the agonist contracts so that smooth movement is achieved. In treatment a slow reversal-hold-relax technique may be used to relax spastic or tight muscle groups. Relaxation of spastic antagonists can also be achieved by facilitation of the agonist through patterns of irradiation, stretch, and supporting reflexes.[69]

Techniques of *positioning, manual contacts,* and *verbal commands* may be used to promote a mobility or a stability response. Since these all have been discussed previously in this chapter, other techniques will be described. *Stretch* may be used as a stimulus to initiate movement or to initiate voluntary motion within the pattern and to increase strength and timing of a weak response.

When applied as a stimulus, stretch is the positioning of a body part in the extreme lengthened range of a pattern to the point of tension. All motion components are stretched, especially rotation, as it is the rotary component that elongates the muscle fibers in a given pattern.

The stretch reflex can be superimposed on a pattern in two ways. One occurs after the position for stretch stimulus has been achieved. The body part is quickly and smoothly taken past the point of tension, just before the initiation of movement by the patient. The second application occurs in repeated contractions where stretch stimulates isotonic contractions through increased range or strength of a pattern.

Repeated stretch, followed by assisted or voluntary motion, can be an effective technique for patients with little or no voluntary control. For example, repeated stretch of the D2 bilateral reciprocal pattern in the C6 quadriplegic patient may stimulate the pectoral muscles. The increased adductor tonus contributes to functional use of hands at and across the midline, which is important in dressing and feeding.

Traction, separating joint surfaces, stimulates joint receptors to promote movement. Traction is maintained throughout the active range of motion.[42] *Approximation* also stimulates joint receptors by compressing joint surfaces. In treatment, approximation promotes stability and postural responses. Application in treatment occurs prior to demanding a voluntary contraction of muscle groups by the patient. In sitting, with arms extended and bearing weight, pressure may be applied in a downward direction over the shoulders. The pressure occurs in the form of a sustained push or as repeated pushes. The expected result is increased extensor tone in the arm and trunk, which promotes strength and endurance for activity in the posture. Approximation repeated quickly may be contraindicated for the patient with pain and with ataxia as seen in multiple sclerosis.[42]

Maximal resistance is probably the most misunderstood PNF technique. It does not refer to the maximal effort of the therapist, but rather to the maximal resistance that the patient can receive and still move smoothly through the full range of the pattern or maintain an isometric contraction. Manual contacts must be specifically applied over the agonists to facilitate a maximal response. For some patients, maximal resistance may only be a light touch, as resistance is graded to elicit the patient's maximal response. In treatment, maximal resistance is provided by the therapist on motions before and during activity or by equipment, such as pulleys and weighted tools.[42]

Two techniques directed to the agonist are repeated contractions and rhythmic initiation. *Repeated contractions* are used to increase range and endurance in weaker components of a pattern through a technique of emphasis. For example, if a patient is unable to reach his mouth for eating, he would be instructed to "hold," with an isometric contraction of all components at the point where the active motion decreases in power. Then the patient is asked repeatedly to "pull again" towards his mouth, shifting from isometric to isotonic contractions. *Rhythmic initiation* is used to improve the ability to initiate movement. This technique involves passive rhythmic motion, followed by active motion. Resistance may be gradually imposed as the patient's response increases. For example, a patient may lack the ability to initiate reaching for a glass on the table, due to rigidity from Parkinson's disease or severe spasticity. The therapist would ask the patient to relax and "let me move you." Then the therapist moves the part through the available range, until relaxation is felt. The patient is directed to begin moving actively in the direction of the agonistic pattern with the command. "Now help me move you." As the patient's response increases, resistance may be added to reinforce the movement. The patient is then asked to move actively by himself and complete the task.[42]

The reversal of antagonists techniques, based on the principle of successive induction, include slow reversal, slow reversal-hold, and rhythmic stabilization. These reversal techniques are primarily used for strengthening or gaining range of motion. Either isotonic, isometric, or a combination of both types of contractions may be used. *Slow reversal* is an alternating isotonic contraction of antagonists. The procedure begins by asking the patient to perform the weaker agonistic pattern. In this example, D2 flexion will be the agonist. Manual contacts with maximal resistance are applied to determine the patient's response. The patient then performs the antagonistic pattern D2 extension by the therapist. *Hold-relax* includes an isometric contraction of the antagonist, relaxation, then active movement of the agonist by the patient. *Slow reversal-hold-relax* includes as isotonic contraction followed by an isometric contraction of the antagonist, relaxation, then active movement of the agonist.[42] If the patient has the ability to move the agonist, slow reversal-hold-relax is used.

Application to Occupational Therapy

PNF can be used in OT to (1) evaluate motion, (2) facilitate motor function, (3) prepare and position a patient for an activity, and (4) enhance the performance of an activity. As the evaluation process was presented previously, (p. 00), the emphasis in this section will be on the application of PNF in five selected problems of patient care. Then one sample treatment procedure will be explained.

The *first problem* is commonly seen in patients with C5 quadriplegia. During the initial recovery the upper extremities have poor muscle strength. The motion of raising the hand to the mouth and the repetition of that movement to complete a meal are problems that limit independence in self-feeding. Often, mobile arm supports are required to assist the arm against gravity. To facilitate feeding without support, the arm needs to be strengthened.

Diagonal one is known as the feeding pattern because the necessary motions of shoulder flexion, elbow flexion, and supination are present in the D1 flexion pattern. Therefore, to strengthen these movements, the D1 pattern is resisted with manual contacts on the wrist and shoulder. The techniques of stretch in the lengthened range of D1 flexion, slow reversal-hold, and repeated contractions can be used.

The *second problem* is often found in a person with right hemiplegia from a CVA. Spasticity is present with beginning isolated movement in the hand. Grasp and release occur, but coordination of the intrinsic hand muscles is poor. For example, this patient is unable to coordinate palmar abduction of thumb with finger extension to remove the right hand from a drinking glass. Therefore, frequent spilling occurs when the glass is returned to the table.

The diagonal pattern is the optimal pattern for the abductor pollicis brevis and the extensor digitorum. The D1 extension pattern is resisted using techniques of slow reversal-hold, repeated contractions, and rhythmic stabilization with manual contacts on the thumb and finger. The shortened range of D1 extension is emphasized for two reasons: (1) the patient can initiate abduction of the thumb in the lengthened range but has difficulty maintaining the contraction in the shortened range; and (2) the patient has spasticity in the flexor muscles. By working in the shortened range of D1 extension, the influence of the spastic flexors is minimized. In one patient, four repetitions of extension facilitated voluntary release of the glass with coordinated thumb abduction and finger extension.

against maximal resistance. The agonistic pattern is now repeated, with an increase in power or range of motion expected due to the law of successive induction. Resistance must be graded to facilitate a strong contraction of the antagonist followed by maximal range of motion in the weaker agonist. Activities performed with the assist of a pulley automatically use the slow reversal technique. The pulley assists the gravity-resisted agonist and then resists the antagonistic movement. *Slow reversal-hold* proceeds in the same manner; however, an isometric contraction follows the completion of the isotonic contraction. Directions for a slow reversal-hold in the second diagonal would be: "Push your arm up and out toward me, and hold. Now, pull your arm down and across, and hold.[42]

Rhythmic stabilization is the simultaneous isometric contraction of antagonists, which results in cocontraction if the isometric contraction is not broken. This technique promotes stability by eliciting a more balanced response between antagonistic muscle groups. Relaxation is often achieved following the stabilization. As repeated isometric contractions are performed, circulation may increase. Also, the patient may hold his breath. Thus, only three or four repetitions are used.

This technique has numerous applications in therapy to provide increased stability and endurance for performance of a task. Rhythmic stabilization cannot be incorporated into an activity as it is an isometric exercise. However, it is used before an activity to enhance performance, during activity as the performance weakens, and after activity to prevent and correct imbalances built up during the activity.

This technique is contraindicated for patients with cardiac problems who are advised not to perform isometric contractions by their physician. Also rhythmic stabilization may be impossible for some patients, such as those with ataxia, who are unable to perform isometric contractions. These patients may be taught to stabilize by using the technique of slow reversal-hold through decrements of range until no motion occurs.[42]

Relaxation techniques include passive rotation, slow reversal-hold relax, contract-relax and hold-relax. *Rhythmic rotation* coupled with range of motion is an effective technique used prior to dressing or splinting a limb in which the muscles are shortened or spastic (Fig. 6.43). Place manual contacts on the intermediate and distal joints and perform range of motion. When restriction occurs, repeat rotation of all components of the pattern at the point of limitation, moving slowly and gently. As relaxation is felt, movement may continue through further range.

The procedures for the remaining three relaxation techniques follow the same sequence. Since only the stronger pattern of motion is resisted, a danger of creating further imbalances exists. These techniques rely upon the principle of reciprocal inhibition and can be effective when used appropriately. *Contract-relax* includes an isotonic contraction of the antagonist, relaxation, then passive movement of the agonist pattern

A *third problem* is frequently seen in patients with multiple sclerosis who exhibit ataxia. Fine motor tasks such as eating, writing, and applying make-up become difficult due to the incoordination. Several PNF concepts and techniques can be applied.

The first priority is to select a stable posture in which the patient can perform the activity. In sitting, the arms are positioned close to the body with elbows and forearms resting on a lapboard or table. Other stable postures include side-lying, prone on elbows, and kneeling with both hands in contact with an elevated surface, such as a bench or chair. Rhythmic stabilization, with manual contacts on shoulders or shoulders and pelvis, is used to reinforce the patient's ability to maintain the posture. Then the movements of rocking in different directions are resisted with slow reversal-hold and repeated contractions to build strength and control.

After these preparatory techniques, the patient is ready to perform an activity, such as writing or use of make-up. Self-touching or simultaneous static-dynamic positioning[70] may enhance control. For example, the patient may hold the wrist of the dominant hand while eating (self-touching) or bear weight on one arm (static arm) while writing with the other arm (dynamic arm). Another technique, move and stop, can facilitate control in middle range. For example, as the patient raises her arm to apply make-up, stopping at midrange enables her to gain control of the movements in the remainder of the range. Sometimes more than one stop during the range of motion is needed.

A *fourth problem,* found in a variety of neurological disorders, is difficulty with oral motor function such as sucking, chewing, and swallowing. The patient with dysarthria from a stroke (CVA) has problems of poor tongue control, drooling, inadequate lip closure, and may pocket food between teeth and cheek. Application of the techniques: stretch, slow reversal, slow reversal-hold and repeated contractions can facilitate a stronger response in the affected muscles prior to eating. The reader is referred to *Proprioceptive Neuromuscular Facilitation: Patterns and Techniques* (third edition)[42] for an illustrated presentation of specific techniques.

A *fifth problem* occurs in patients with limited shoulder motion due to joint disease, such as arthritis. Reaching overhead to dress or comb one's hair becomes difficult and often unsuccessful.

Both diagonals are used in combing hair. The combing arm demonstrates D2 flexion when the shoulder abducts to reach the back of the head. D1 flexion occurs as the shoulder adducts to comb the front and opposite side of the head. Bilateral patterns for combing are common as one hand combs and the other adjusts and smoothes the hair. In treatment, bilateral combinations of the upper extremities can be resisted with slow reversals, slow reversal-hold-relax, rhythmic stabilization, and repeated contractions to gain range of motion and strength.

The patient can be taught to apply the techniques of stretch and reversing movement. For example, instead of struggling to move the arm in a partial range from lap level to the head, the motion is reversed. The patient extends the arm in the antagonistic pattern (D1 extension). Then stretch is applied by pushing the arms back and down toward the floor. Immediately the hands reach toward the head in D1 flexion. The patient can use bilateral symmetrical or asymmetrical combinations to seek reinforcement from the trunk and a more normal interaction of body segments.

Sequences of PNF treatment procedures vary according to the diagnosis and the individual patient's needs. The sample treatment sequences in this section provide guidelines for application of PNF. Adaptations may be required for the specific patient's age, medical status, and level of ability.

The first sequence outlines treatment activities for a patient with a shoulder-hand syndrome due to trauma (Table 6.9). The main goals of treatment include (1) reduction of pain and edema, (2) increase in range of motion, (3) restoration of a balance between antagonistic movements, and (4) increase in strength and endurance for functional activity.

Steps 1–8 are examples of the indirect approach. The therapist does not directly touch the affected hand or arm. However, the patient experiences a variety of movement patterns that facilitate control and range of movement. Proprioceptive stimulation is applied through weight-bearing activities and resistance to unaffected extremity and trunk.

With success in the preceding steps, the patient is ready for a more direct approach. The affected hand, wrist, elbow, and shoulder are resisted directly in pattern. Stronger components of the pattern are used to reinforce weaker motions. Initiation of motion is emphasized in the lengthened range, while strengthening is resisted toward the shortened range of the pattern. The performance of functional and work-related activities follows. Specific movement problems are analyzed and facilitated as necessary.

A home program would include: (1) self range of motion using the chopping and lifting patterns; (2) active range of motion, incorporating the distal component of forearm rotation with opening and closing of the hand; (3) grasp and release activities that involve reaching diagonally in a developmental position; (4) using door pulleys for chopping and lifting patterns; and (5) functional activities in which the patient incorporates the facilitated pattern into his daily routine. For example, after bathing, the patient may dry the shower wall with a tower using D1 and D2 patterns. Prior to morning hygiene, the patient may rock in modified plantigrade position while weight bearing at the sink. Then the patient could reach to grasp the toothpaste and comb from the bathroom shelf in a D1 pattern.

Research

Research to support the effectiveness of the PNF treatment approach is limited. The majority of the research reported in the last 10 years analyzed the response of able-bodied subjects to selected techniques

Table 6.9.
SAMPLE SEQUENCE OF TREATMENT FOR THE PATIENT WITH SHOULDER-HAND SYNDROME

Preparatory Procedures and Techniques[a]	Patient Position	Manual Contacts
1. Breathing techniques	Sitting	Sternum and dorsal spine
2. Rhythmic stabilization	Sitting	Shoulders
3. Proprioceptive disturbance of balance with resisted recovery	Sitting	Shoulders

Note: Breathing techniques and rhythmic stabilization also are used during treatment when the patient fatigues or the motor response deteriorates.

Activities	Patterns	Patient Position	Technique	Manual Contacts
4. Grasp and release	Chopping or lifting	Sitting or rolling	Resist unaffected arm Resist scapula of unaffected side, then affected side	Shoulders and wrist Scapula
5. Weight bearing	Bilateral symmetrical D1, D2	Modified plantigrade Hands-knees Sitting with elbows extended Sitting-leaning forward on flexed elbows	Rhythmic stabilization	Shoulders or shoulders and pelvis

Note: If the patient is unable to bear weight with the wrist fully extended, a push-up block or soft beanbag may be used under the hand to decrease the degree of wrist extension.

Activities	Patterns	Patient Position	Technique	Manual Contacts
6. Rocking	Bilateral symmetrical Bilateral asymmetrical D1, D2	Same as #5	Stretch, resistance Slow reversal Slow reversal-hold Repeated contractions	Shoulders, pelvis, or shoulders and pelvis
7. Surface contact, i.e., washing table sanding, figure-of-8	D1,D2	As above	Light touch or self-touch	Back of hand and wrist
8. Free active movement	D1, D2	Modified plantigrade Sitting	Simultaneous static and dynamic	

Note: Examples of activities are grasp and release tasks or games, writing with a marker (built-up as necessary) or a one-handed craft such as a rug punch. Activities can be placed on an elevated surface to increase shoulder range of motion and reduce edema in the hand.

by recording electromyographic (EMG) activity. Studies that support the principles and techniques are summarized briefly.

Holt et al.[71] tested the isometric strength of elbow flexion using EMG and dynamometer readings. Six subjects participated, three able-bodied and three with cerebral palsy. Four muscle contractions were measured with: (1) the head in anatomic position; (2) the head turned right; (3) the head turned left; and (4) a prior contraction of the antagonists. The results indicated that the reversal of antagonists was superior to the other independent variables in facilitating strength.

Tanigawa[72] compared the effects of the PNF hold-relax procedure and passive mobilization on tight hamstring muscles. He used a mathematical method to measure the angle of passive straight leg raising on 30

able-bodied male subjects. The results showed that subjects receiving the PNF hold-relax procedure increased their range of passive straight leg raising to a higher degree and at a faster rate than the subjects receiving passive mobilization.

Markos[73] compared the effects of the PNF procedures of contract-relax on active hip flexion in 30 able-bodied female subjects. The range of motion increased significantly more in subjects in the contract-relax group, both in the exercised and in the unexercised lower extremities. The author presented application of each technique to treatment, suggesting that contract-relax applied ipsilaterally may prevent disuse atrophy in specific muscles of the contralateral lower extremity.

Sullivan and Portney[74] monitored four shoulder muscles on 29 able-bodied subjects to confirm that each muscle tested would exhibit maximal EMG activity in an optimal diagonal pattern. The anterior deltoid demonstrated maximal activity in the D1 flexion pattern; the middle deltoid in the D2 flexion pattern; the posterior deltoid in the D1 extension pattern; and the sternal portion of the pectoralis major in the D2 extension pattern. The authors also reported that performing the patterns with elbows straight, flexing, and extending changed the amount of shoulder muscle activity. This study is of practical value to occupational therapists in that it confirmed the optimum diagonal patterns for four specific shoulder muscles. This may aid the therapist in selecting a place to initiate a treatment program given a particular shoulder limitation.

Pink[75] measured EMG activity in three muscles of the nonexercised upper extremity. The results from 10 able-bodied female subjects indicated that the following muscles do become active in the nonexercised limb. The sternal portion of the pectoralis major produced similar EMG activity during D1 flexion and extension of the contralateral limb. The infraspinatus was more active during D1 flexion, while the latissimus dorsi was more active during D1 extension. The author stated that these results could be used in treatment programs for patients who are unable to exercise one of their upper extremities.

In 1960 Mead[76] reported on a 6-year evaluation of PNF techniques. The author compared an experience using traditional therapeutic exercise to treat patients with poliomyelitis from 1948 to 1953 in a university physical medicine clinic to an experience using PNF to treat patients with varied diagnoses from 1954 to 1960 at the California Rehabilitation Center in Vallejo. Although a controlled study with statistical analysis was not done, the author found that the PNF approach was more effective than the traditional approach. Mead described the therapy program at Vallejo, and concluded that PNF techniques have application to all diagnoses.

Nelson et al.[77] examined the effects of PNF and weight training on muscular strength and performance in 30 healthy college women. Subjects were tested for changes in knee and elbow extension strength, throwing distance, and vertical jump following an 8-week training program. Results indicated the PNF-trained group had the greatest increases in all of these areas as compared with the weight-trained and control groups. The authors suggest this may be attributed to PNF's "incorporation of the theories of irradiation, spatiotemporal summation and stretch reflex." They also conclude that "PNF might be superior to weight-training for athletic training programs and injury rehabilitation."

Studies that question the principles and procedures are summarized as follows:

Arsenault[78] reviewed the literature and reported that success in using PNF techniques to treat neurological disorders was not universally true. Thus, he questioned the acceptance of using mass patterns of movement based on the lack of scientific support. Arsenault reviewed several studies on quadricep function with conflicting results on the effects of PNF irradiation patterns. Toe, ankle, and hip movements made no difference in the augmentation of quadriceps activity. Therefore, further research must be done to confirm the use of the PNF irradiation patterns.

Arsenault and Chapman[79] studied the effects of movement patterns used to promote quadriceps activity in seven able-bodied subjects over an 8-week period. No consistent response was found. In general, the D1 flexion pattern of the lower extremity increased the activity of the rectus femoris, but not the vastus medialis. The D2 flexion pattern produced a decrease of rectus femoris activity. The findings confirmed D1 flexion as the optimal pattern for the medial portion of the rectus femoris and disputed D2 flexion as the optimal pattern for the lateral portion of the rectus femoris. Either a proximal or distal resistance provided the ipsilateral overflow to the quadriceps. However, it is not clear whether precise PNF manual contacts and procedures were employed.

Synder and Forward[80] compared the sequential EMG activity in selected muscles of the lower limb during flexion and extension of the knee. Ten able-bodied female subjects performed active range of motion in the sagittal and diagonal planes of movement. An electrogoniometer was used to monitor the degree of knee flexion. The findings showed that selected muscles were more active in the sagittal plane than in the diagonal plane. Also, the authors observed the interaction of antagonists during fast and slow movements and following transiently induced pain in the semisquat position. They concluded that the assumption of increased activity in a diagonal plane of movement appears unjustified.

Surburg[81] studied the effects of maximal resistance with PNF patterns upon reaction, movement, and response time. Fifty able-bodied subjects participated for 6 weeks in one of three training programs: weight training, PNF patterning without resistance, and PNF patterning with maximal resistance. Analysis revealed no significant differences among the training groups.

In summary, scientific studies of the effectiveness of the PNF approach are limited to only one aspect of the approach. Research on the effect of total patterns and combining movements with functional application still needs to be done.

Acknowledgment. The author thanks Dorothy E. Voss, Associate Professor Emeritus of Rehabilitation Medicine, Northwestern University Medical School, Chicago, Illinois, for her assistance and support in developing and reviewing this chapter. Also, the author is grateful to Mary Herbin, O.T.R./L., Kathy Knutson, O.T.R./L., and Cindy Shanker, O.T.R./L., for their time and technical skill in posing for the illustrations, and to Laura M. Kearny, O.T.R./L. for her contribution to updating the review of research, introduction to total patterns, and study questions.

STUDY QUESTIONS:
Proprioceptive Neuromuscular Facilitation (PNF) Approach

1. Discuss 4 of the 11 principles of PNF.
2. From which developmental activities are diagonals one and two derived?
3. What is the advantage of giving passive range of motion in the diagonal patterns?
4. Distinguish the difference between bilateral symmetrical, bilateral asymmetrical, bilateral reciprocal, and unilateral patterns. Give an example of a functional activity where each of these patterns may be observed.
5. Given a patient with a shoulder-hand syndrome, select a therapeutic activity and PNF patterns and techniques that could facilitate more range of motion.
6. Discuss three of the five factors that support the use of diagonal patterns in treatment.
7. Which PNF technique provides increased stability and endurance for performance of a task through a simultaneous isometric contraction of antagonists?
8. List a contraindication for the use of stretch, traction, or approximation during patient treatment.
9. Discuss the importance of the therapist's positioning, appropriate manual contacts, and verbal commands when assisting a patient to a developmental posture.
10. What bilateral asymmetrical pattern could a hemiplegic patient use to put his flaccid arm through the sleeve of a shirt?
11. In a child with cerebral palsy who exhibits a spastic right upper extremity, drooling, and poor sitting balance, which problem would you address first during treatment? What relaxation technique would you use to decrease spasticity in the arm?
12. What is the effect on head, neck and trunk during bilateral symmetrical D1 extension? Bilateral D2 extension: Which pattern elicits the greatest amount of flexion?

E/Carr and Shepherd Approach: Motor Relearning Programme for Stroke Patients

CATHERINE A. TROMBLY

The *Motor Relearning Programme (MRP)* [82,83] was developed by Janet Carr and Roberta Shepherd, Australian physical therapists, from their clinical experience and extensive review of contemporary motor control and motor learning literature. One of their goals in developing this program was to promote among therapists higher expectations for outcomes for stroke patients; they felt that up to now therapists have been settling for a level of recovery that included residual motor deficits. Another goal was to offer an alternative to current therapy, which the authors believe not only delays active treatment in very early stage poststroke patients by concentrating on positioning but also emphasizes concepts that do not apply to the adult stroke patient. Specifically, in their opinion, neither exercise therapy nor stimulus-response based neurorehabilitation treatment is adequate for the treatment of post stroke patients. Therefore, the program does not aim at increasing muscle strength nor the activation of a maximum number of motor units but at helping the patient learn to control the muscle activation needed for a particular function. The therapy is expected to trigger previously known motor programs by involving the patient cognitively in remembering the movements and activities he was able to do prior to the stroke.

Carr and Shepherd believe that treatment directed toward active training of motor control relevant to daily activities is to be preferred and should begin as soon as the person's medical condition is stable. The program emphasizes practice of specific everyday activities through cognitive control over the muscles and movement components of these activities and conscious elimination of unnecessary muscle activity. Their approach is nondevelopmentally based.

Theories of learning and motivation as well as research in the areas of human-movement science and motor skill acquisition form the foundations on which the program is based. Which learner-initiated strategies are most relevant and effective for learning, retention, and transfer of psychomotor tasks is yet to be determined in normal subjects[84] or patients with CNS deficits. It appears, however, that cognitive processes are much more involved in the acquisition of complex motor behaviors than previously realized.[84] This program, using available information pertaining to how normal persons learn skills, proposes a method of helping the poststroke patient reestablish the cognitive processes associated with functional movement. As such, it changes the focus of treatment from subcortical elicitation of movement to conscious involvement of the patient in movement control.

Spasticity is not addressed directly by this program. The authors believe that what is called spasticity is unnecessary muscle activity that has become habitual, and the goal is for the patient to learn to control this excess muscle activity as part of the relearning process. It is expected that early involvement in MRP will lessen the chance that unwanted motor habits will be learned. The program requires the patient to concentrate and use his cognitive abilities to suppress excess muscle activity as well as to perform desired movements. Patients' abilities to concentrate and to cognitively control motor output have been seen to improve in clinical practice. The goal is to train patients to activate muscles in exactly the way the muscles perform in normal everyday activities. The therapist monitors the patient's performance to correct errors as they occur to ensure that only correct motor responses are practiced.

The *Motor Relearning Programme* assumes that the brain has the capacity for reorganization and adaptation. The program aims at stimulating or making the best use of these processes. It also assumes that three factors known to be essential for learning of motor skills in normal persons apply to the stroke population as well. Those factors are the abilities to eliminate unnecessary muscle activity, to use feedback to modify motor output, and to benefit from practice.

Learning a complex motor skill involves two major components: identification of what is to be learned and organization of the information into correct sequences to carry out the task. Both of these are cognitive in nature. Guided by the therapist, the patient concentrates and uses his cognitive abilities to eliminate all extraneous muscle activity and to control muscle contraction in order to learn the movement components of activities. A well-documented characteristic of the early phases of motor skill learning is that undivided attention of the performer is required to process the information needed to perform.[85] Each performer has a limited information-processing capacity and if this capacity is exceeded, performance will break down.[85] The therapist must keep the demands within the capability of the patient by introducing small variations in movements as the patient progresses toward the goal of accomplishing functional activities. Concentration and cognition, used in early training, are expected to be replaced by a more automatic processing of information and level of control in the later stages of skill acquisition.

The therapist gives immediate, specific feedback. Only a successful performance, not merely a good attempt, is rewarded by praise so that the patient knows exactly what is correct. If the performance is unsuccessful, the therapist says so and offers a suggestion to correct it on the next attempt. For example, "this time make sure you keep your elbow straight." This type of feedback also helps the patient to focus on the important movement components of the activity.

Feedback about performance, whether self-generated or externally provided, serves several functions: It helps to regulate ongoing behavior to adapt the behavior to situational demands, to modulate emotions, or to form the basis for self-evaluation of performance.[84] In early learning, response-produced feedback appears to be relatively unimportant, whereas knowledge of results (KR) appears to be the important information-processing activity. This emphasis may not be true for later stages of learning.[86] This program emphasizes visual KR on the part of the patient and verbal KR provided by the therapist. Biofeedback can be used for adjunctive practice sessions; however, the authors feel that it does not replace the learning possible when feedback is given by a skilled therapist. This may be true because the therapist offers the patient strategies to correct his performance, whereas the biofeedback machine merely signals correct and incorrect responses and the patient must then figure out how to move more correctly if in error.

Basic, common, real-life specific activities, not exercises, are practiced. Skill (activity developed by practice) is made up of movement components that, when linked together, allow smooth, controlled movement.

The program trains the patient to perform key components of movement that are missing and then follows that with practice of the entire activity. This follows a behavioral-psychology philosophy, which is that one cannot expect complex behavior to emerge "full blown"—correct in all details—but rather it must be shaped through a series of stages progressing from a crude approximation toward an ultimate goal.[87] "The *essential* features of an activity must be taught before the *refinements* or final polishing are attended to."[87] The patient should experience success even if his first performance requires considerable manual guidance from the therapist. No incorrect response should be repeated.

The environment is organized to include motivation, positive attitudes, reinforcement from relatives and friends, consistency of feedback, and consistency of practice. These things are not left to chance or goodwill.

There are four steps to the MRP, each of which is included in every treatment:

1. Analysis of function (evaluation)
2. Practice of missing components
3. Practice of activity
4. Transference of learning

Each will be briefly described here. The reader is referred to the original source for details of all the evaluation and treatment procedures.

STEP 1: ANALYSIS OF FUNCTION

Immediately poststroke, the patient is unable to move. Evaluation involves placing the patient in the optimal position to encourage muscle activation and actively searching for even the slightest amount of muscle activity. The patient is encouraged to concentrate on his muscle activity although it is barely detectable and attempt to increase it. When the patient is able to move, evaluation involves observation of his attempts to perform an activity, e.g., use a fork, and comparison of his performance to normal movement. Using her knowledge and/or the guide provided, the therapist analyzes the attempt and notes the missing components. Analysis involved identification of any anatomical, biomechanical, physiological, or behavioral factors that mechanical, physiological, or behavioral factors that limit the patient's ability. The therapist selects, from among those movement components that are missing, those that are essential to the activity; that is, those that are biomechanical necessities or the determinants of movement. The most essential components are targeted for retraining first.

The essential components for different activities have been listed in the original source. For example the major functions of the hand are grasp, release, and manipulation of objects. The essential components for these functions are radial deviation combined with wrist extension, wrist extension while holding an object, thumb opposition, finger opposition, extension of the metacarpophalangeal (MP) joints while the interphalangeal (IP) joints are in some flexion, and supination of the forearm while holding an object. The difficulties in hand function most commonly seen poststroke, to continue the example, are as follows: grasping with wrist in extension and radial deviation, extending the MP joints with the IP joints in some flexion to position the fingers to grasp and release an object, opposing the thumb for grasp and release, and cupping the hand. Other motor control deficits include the inability to release an object without flexing the wrist, uncontrolled finger and thumb extension on release, a tendency to pronate whenever the fingers flex, the inability to hold objects while moving the arm, and excessive ulnar deviation while using the hand.

Step 1 continues throughout the rest of the program; the therapist continually analyzes and reevaluates the patient's responses to assess progress. Errors in analysis are frequently the cause of ineffective therapy.

STEPS 2 AND 3: PRACTICE OF MISSING COMPONENTS AND PRACTICE OF ACTIVITY

Principles that guide these stages of treatment are as follows: Arm movements, including movements of the hand, must be stimulated early following stroke. Activity should be elicited in the position of greatest advantage for the muscle. If a muscle does not contract under a particular set of conditions, the conditions are varied. If the flexor activity cannot be overcome by conscious control, extensor activity will need to be encouraged reflexively. As soon as isolated muscle action is elicited, this must be incorporated into meaningful activities that allow the patient to gain control of the muscle in increasing ranges of movement and in its different roles. Recovery does not take place from proximal to distal; it is not necessary to have shoulder control before attempting to regain control of the hand. All muscle activity unnecessary to the movement being attempted must be eliminated through conscious effort. The support given to the limb by the therapist when there is insufficient muscle activity is changed to guidance as soon as possible. Passive movement should be avoided except to help the patient understand the movement being sought. Muscles must not be allowed to contract incorrectly. The patient should not be allowed or encouraged to practice movements that are part of an abnormal synergy and that have no func-

tional significance. Gross patterns of movements of the upper extremity should be avoided because they mask minimal muscle activity present in underactive muscles and encourage the overactive muscles. The therapist should not think in terms of strengthening muscles; the objective is to stimulate muscle activity and to train the patient to control this activity for function. Bilateral movements should be avoided until the patient regains control over the affected limb.

Techniques include the following:

1. Explanation and demonstration of the component movement are given to the patient, who must understand the importance of the component to the overall activity. By immediately using the component in practice of at least part of the activity that he is preparing for, the patient should be motivated to learn the component. Practice of the entire activity with manual guidance may trigger movement memory. Once he has the idea of the movement he can concentrate on practicing components to become skilled. Passive movement must not persist beyond one or two demonstrations. It is important that the patient move actively at least for part of the movement. Brief verbal or gestured instructions are given to guide the patient and to trigger movement. For example, to stimulate supination, the patient holds a cylindrical object and tries to supinate the forearm. The therapist gives these directions: "try to turn your palm so it faces upwards—don't worry about holding the object—I'll help you".

2. The patient gains visual feedback firsthand by paying attention to his movements.

3. Verbal feedback is brief, relevant, concise, and continuous. It is given during and after performance to provide both knowledge of performance and knowledge of results.

4. Certain points that are common errors made by the patient or therapist are checked. The points to be checked are listed in the original source for each goal. For example, a point to be checked when the patient attempts to supinate is the tendency to flex and ulnarly deviate the wrist.

5. Manual guidance or physical monitoring is done throughout performance. For example, the therapist would hold the patient's fingers around the object and help stabilize the wrist if necessary. This leaves the patient free to attend to supination.

The patient should not waste time practicing what he can already do. During step 3, as he develops skill, the patient makes a transition from the cognitive phase of learning to the automatic phase of learning. The patient should practice at peak performance and be progressed to his limits as soon as he has some control. Manual guidance and feedback are decreased as the patient improves in his ability to control his own movements. Practice is done under conditions that offer variety with different objects and in demands of direction, speed, and/or accuracy. Developmental sequence is not followed as these therapists believe developmental progression is a false assumption on which to base treatment of the adult stroke patient. Neither is he progressed from passive movement to resisted movement, which is the basis of the biomechanical approach.

STEP 4: TRANSFERENCE OF LEARNING

Practice under various environmental and task conditions allows the patient to transfer the learning from therapy to daily living. The patient works with the therapist to solve problems of activities encountered in daily life. In this way he learns the problem-solving process that he can use outside of therapy. A great deal of practice is required to learn a motor skill. Both physical and mental practice may be used.

Effectiveness

The effectiveness of the MRP depends on the individual therapist's knowledge of movement and motor control and her problem-solving ability. The therapist must be able to recognize and analyze the motor problem, select the most essential missing component, effectively teach the patient the required movement, monitor the patient's response, give meaningful feedback, and create an environment that promotes a drive toward recovery and relearning. Although the authors have written the techniques for each goal very specifically, their books are not cookbooks. Each attempt of each patient will be different, and the therapist must be skilled enough to detect the nuances of the ongoing performance and knowledgeable enough to direct the patient to the next stage of movement control.

Clinical experience has found this approach to be successful, although studies documenting the effectiveness of this approach have not yet appeared. The authors see the documentation of effectiveness as very important and consider their detailed description of the MRP to be the first step in researching it. They invite clinicians to assist in the effort.

STUDY QUESTIONS:

Carr and Shepherd Approach: Motor Relearning Programme for Stroke Patients

1. How does the MRP differ from the other approaches described in this chapter?
2. What is the emphasis of this program?
3. What is the therapist's role in this approach?
4. What is one characteristic of early motor learning?
5. What is the nature of the feedback that the therapist gives to the patient?
6. What is a movement component? How does it relate to a skill?
7. What are the four steps of the MRP?
8. What are the principles of this approach?
9. How is transfer of a learned motor skill encouraged?

References

A/Rood Approach

1. Rood, M. S. The Treatment of Neuromuscular Dysfunction: Rood Approach. Notes taken by C. Trombly at lecture delivered in Boston, Mass., July 9-11, 1976.

2. Rood, M. S. Neurophysiological reactions as a basis for physical therapy. *Phys. Ther. Rev., 34:* 444-449, 1954.
3. Curran, P. A study toward a theory of neuromuscular education through occupational therapy. *Am. J. Occup. Ther., 14:* 80-87, 1960.
4. Ayres, A. M. Integration of information. In *The Development of Sensory Integrative Theory and Practice.* Edited by A. Henderson *et al.* Dubuque, IA: Kendall-Hunt Publishing Co., 1974.
5. Rood, M. S. The use of sensory receptors to activate, facilitate, and inhibit motor response, autonomic and somatic, in developmental sequence. In *Approaches to the Treatment of Patients with Neuromuscular Dysfunction.*/Edited by C. Sattely. Dubuque, IA: Wm. C. Brown Book Co., 1962.
6. Rood, M. S. Neurophysiological mechanisms utilized in the treatment of neuromuscular dysfunction. *Am. J. Occup. Ther., 10:* 220-225, 1956.
7. Harris, F. Control of gamma efferents through the reticular activating system. *Am. J. Occup. Ther., 23:* 403-408, 1969.
8. Stockmeyer, S. An interpretation of the approach of Rood to the treatment of neuromuscular dysfunction. *Am. J. Phys. Med.* (NUSTEP Proceedings), 46 (1): 900-956, 1967.
9. Huss, J. An introduction to treatment techniques developed by Margaret Rood. In *Neuroanatomy and Neurophysiology Underlying Current Treatment Techniques for Sensorimotor Dysfunction.* Edited by S. Perlmutter. University of Illinois, Division of Services for Crippled Children, undated, pp. 89-94.
10. Carpenter, M. B. *Human Neuroanatomy,* 7th edition. Baltimore: Williams & Wilkins, 1976.
11. Huss, J. Sensorimotor treatment approaches. In *Occupational Therapy,* 4th edition. Edited by H. S. Willard and C. S. Spackman. Philadelphia: J. B. Lippincott, 1971.
12. Harris, F. A. Facilitation techniques in therapeutic exercise. In *Therapeutic Exercise,* 3rd edition. Edited by J. V. Basmajian. Baltimore: Williams & Wilkins, 1978.
13. Matyas, T. A., and Spicer, S. D. Facilitation of the tonic vibration reflex (TVR) by cutaneous stimulation in hemiplegics. *Am. J. Phys. Med., 59*(6): 280-287, 1980.
14. Ayres, A. J. Occupational therapy directed toward neuromuscular integration. In *Occupational Therapy,* 3rd edition. Edited by H. S. Williard and C. S. Spackman. Philadelphia: J. B. Lippincott, 1963.
15. Spicer, S. D., and Matyas, T. A. Facilitation of the tonic vibration reflex (TVR) by cutaneous stimulation. *Am. J. Phys. Med., 59*(5): 223-231, 1980.
16. Mason, C. R. One method for assessing the effectiveness of fast brushing. *Phys. Ther., 65*(8): 1197-1202, 1985.
17. Eyzaguirre, C., and Fidone, S. J. *Physiology of the Nervous System,* 2nd edition. Chicago: Year Book Medical Publishers, 1975.
18. Rider, B. Effects of neuromuscular facilitation on cross transfer. *Am. J. Occup. Ther., 25:* 84-89, 1971.
19. Zimny, N. *Effect of Position & Sensory Stimulation on Scapular Muscles.* Master's thesis. Boston: Sargent College of Allied Health Professions, Boston University, 1979.
20. Hunt, C. C. The effect of sympathetic stimulation on mammalian muscle spindles. *J. Physiol., 151:* 332-341, 1960.

B/Bobath Neurodevelopmental Approach

21. Semans, S. The Bobath concept in treatment of neurological disorders. *Am. J. Phys. Med.* (NUSTEP Proceedings), *46:* 732-985, 1967.
22. Bobath, K., and Bobath, B. The importance of memory traces of motor efferent discharges for learning skilled movement. *Dev. Med. Child Neurol., 16:* 837-838, 1974.
23. Opila-Lehman, J., Short, M.A., and Trombly, C.A. Kinesthetic recall of children with athetoid and spastic cerebral palsy and of non-handicapped children. *Dev. Med. Child Neurol., 27:* 223-230, 1985.
24. Bobath, B. *Adult Hemiplegia: Evaluation and Treatment,* 2nd edition. London: William Heinemann Medical Books, 1978.
25. Semans, S., et al. A cerebral palsy assessment chart. In *The Child with Central Nervous System Deficit.* Childrens Bureau Publication No. 432, U.S. Government Printing Office, 1965.
26. Bobath, B. The neurodevelopmental approach to treatment. In *Physical Therapy Services in Developmental Disabilities.* Edited by P. Pearson and C. Williams. Springfield, IL: Charles C. Thomas, 1972.
27. Bobath, K., and Bobath, B. The facilitation of normal postural reactions and movements in the treatment of cerebral palsy. *Physiotherapy, 50:* 3-19, 1964.
28. Bobath, B. The very early treatment of cerebral palsy. *Dev. Med. Child Neurol., 9:* 373-390, 1967.
29. Bobath, B. Motor development, its effect on general development and application to the treatment of cerebral palsy. *Physiotherapy, 57:* 1-7, 1971.
30. Warren, M. L. A comparative study on the presence of the asymmetrical tonic neck reflex in adult hemiplegia. *Am. J. Occup. Ther., 38*(6): 386-392, 1984.

31. Bobath, B. Treatment of adult hemiplegia. *Physiotherapy, 63:* 310–313, 1977.
32. Eggers, O. *Occupational Therapy in the Treatment of Adult Hemiplegia,* London: William Heinemann Medical Books, 1983.
33. DeGangi, G. A., Hurley, L., and Linscheid, T. R. Toward a methodology of the short-term effects of neurodevelopmental treatment. *Am. J. Occup. Ther.,* 37(7): 479–484, 1983; 37(12): 849–850, 1983.
34. Ottenbacher, K. J., et al. Quantitative analysis of the effectiveness of pediatric therapy. *Phys. Ther.,* 66(7): 1095–1101, 1986.
35. Arne, L. Eyssette, M., and Held, J. P. Potential and limitations of rehabilitation in hemiplegia. *France Annals Med. Phys.,* 23(2): 242–247, 1980. [In French]

C/Brunnstrom Approach

36. Brunnstrom, S. *Movement Therapy in Hemiplegia.* New York: Harper & Row, 1970.
37. Brunnstrom, S. Associated reactions of the upper extremity in adult patients with hemiplegia. *Phys. Ther. Rev., 36:* 225–236, 1956.
38. LaVigne, J. M. Hemiplegia sensorimotor assessment form. *Phys. Ther.,* 54(2): 128–134, 1974.
39. Twitchell, T. The restoration of motor function following hemiplegia in man. *Brain, 74:* 443–480, 1951.
40. Fugl-Meyer, A. R., Jaasko, L., Leyman, I., Olsson, S., and Steglind, S. The post-stroke hemiplegic patient. I. A method for evaluation of physical performance. *Scand. J. Rehabil. Med., 7:* 13–31, 1975.
41. Cofrancesco, E. M. The effect of music therapy on hand grasp strength and functional task performance in stroke patients. *J. Music Ther.,* 22(3): 129–145, 1985.

D/Proprioceptive Neuromuscular Facilitation (PNF) Approach

42. Voss, D. E., Ionta, M. K., and Myers, B. J. *Proprioceptive Neuromuscular Facilitation: Patterns and Techniques,* 3rd edition. New York: Harper & Row, 1985.
43. Kabat, H., and Rosenberg, D. Concepts and techniques of occupational therapy neuromuscular disorders. *Am. J. Occup. Ther.,* 4(1): 6–11, 79, 1950.
44. Ayres, A. J. Proprioceptive facilitation elicited through the upper extremities. Part I. Background 9(1)1–9. Part II. Application 9(2)57–62. Part III. Specific application 9(3)121–126. *Am. J. Occup. Ther.,* 1955.
45. Cooke, D. M. The effects of resistance on multiple sclerosis patients with intention tremor. *Am. J. Occup. Ther.,* 12(2): 89–94, 1958.
46. Voss, D. E. PNF: application of patterns and techniques in occupational therapy. *Am. J. Occup. Ther.,* 8(4): 191–194, 1959.
47. Whitaker, E. W. A suggested treatment in occupational therapy for patients with multiple sclerosis. *Am. J. Occup. Ther.,* 4(6): 247–251, 1950.
48. Carroll, J. The utilization of reinforcement techniques in the program for the hemiplegic. *Am. J. Occup. Ther.,* 4(5): 211–213, 239, 1950.
49. Voss, D. E. Proprioceptive neuromuscular facilitation. *Am. J. Phys. Med.,* 46(1): 838–898, 1967.
50. Hooker, D. Evidence of prenatal function of the central nervous system in man. In *Scientific Bases for Neurophysiological Approaches to Therapeutic Exercise: An Anthology.* Edited by O. Payton et al. Philadelphia: F. A. Davis, 1977.
51. Hellebrandt, F. A., Schade, M., and Carns, M. L. Methods of evoking the tonic neck reflexes in normal human subjects. *Am. J. Phys. Med., 41:* 90–139, 1962.
52. McGraw, M. B. *The Neuromuscular Maturation of the Human Infant.* New York: Columbia University Press, 1945. New York: Haftner Press, reprinted edition, 1963.
53. Gesell, A. Reciprocal interweaving in neuromotor development. In *Scientific Bases for Neurophysiologic Approaches to Therapeutic Exercise: An Anthology.* Edited by O. Payton et al. Philadelphia: F. A. Davis, 1977.
54. Gesell, A., and Amatruda, C. S. *Developmental Diagnosis,*2nd edition. New York: Paul B. Hoeber, 1947.
55. Gesell, A. Behavior patterns of fetal infant and child. *Genetics, (Proc. Assoc. Res. Nerv. Mental Dis.),* 33: 114–123, 1954.
56. Buchwald, J. S. Basic mechanisms of motor learning. *J.A.P.T.A.,* 45: 314–331, 1965.
57. Harlow, H. F., and Harlow, M. K. Principles of primate learning lessons from animal behavior. In *Little Club Clinics in Developmental Medicine No. 7,* The Spastics Society, Ch. 5. London: William Heinemann Medical Books, 1962.
58. Levine, S. Stimulation in infancy. *Sci. Am.,* 202(5): 80–86, 1960.
59. Voss, D. E. Proprioceptive neuromuscular facilitation: the PNF method. In *Physical Therapy Services in Developmental Disabilities.* Edited by P. Pearson and C. Williams. Springfield, IL: Charles C. Thomas, 1972.
60. Loomis, J. E., and Boersma, F. J. Training right brain-damaged patients in a wheelchair task: case studies using verbal mediation. *Can. J. Physiotherapy, 34:* 204–208, 1982.

61. Smith, K. U. Cybernetic foundations for rehabilitation. *Am. J. Phys. Med.,* 46(1): 379–467, 1967.
62. Ayres, A. J. Integration of information. In *Approaches to the Treatment of Patients with Neuromuscular Dysfunction.* Study Course VI, 3rd International Congress WFOT. Dubuque, IA: William C. Brown Book Co., 1962.
63. Voss, D. E. Teaching materials presented during short term courses and undergraduate curriculum at Northwestern University Medical School Programs in Physical Therapy. Evaluation Forms: Introduction and Sections 1–3, 1969.
64. Jackson, J. H. *Selected Writings,* vol. 1. Edited by J. Taylor. London: Hodder and Staughton, 1931.
65. Hooker, D. *The Prenatal Origin of Behavior.* Lawrence, Kansas: University of Kansas Press, 1952.
66. Voss, D. E. Assistance in the Assumption of Total Patterns of Posture, PNF Approach (videotape). Chicago: Northwestern Medical School Program in Physical Therapy, 1973.
67. Myers, B. J. Assisting to Posture and Application in Occupational Therapy Activities (videotape). Chicago: Rehabilitation Institute of Chicago, 1981.
68. Stockmeyer, S. A. An interpretation of the approach of Rood to the treatment of neuromuscular dysfunction. *Am. J. Phys. Med.,* 46(1): 900–956, 1967.
69. Kabat, H. Proprioceptive facilitation in therapeutic exercise. In *Therapeutic Exercise,* 2nd edition. Edited by S. Licht. New Haven: Elizabeth Licht, 1961, pp. 327–343.
70. Hellebrandt, F. A., Houtz, S. J., Hockman, D. E., and Partridge, M. Physiological effects of simultaneous static and dynamic exercise. *Am. J. Phys. Med., 35:* 106–117, 1956.
71. Holt, L. E., Kaplan, H. M., Okita, T. Y., and Hoshiko, M. The influence of antagonistic contraction and head position on the responses of agonistic muscles. *Arch. Phys. Med. Rehabil.,* 50(5): 279–291, 1968.
72. Tanigawa, M. C. Comparison of the hold-relax procedure and passive mobilization on increasing muscle length. *Phys. Ther.,* 52(7): 725–735, 1972.
73. Markos, P. D. Ipsilateral and contralateral effects of proprioceptive neuromuscular facilitation techniques on hip motion and electromyographic activity. *Phys. Ther.,* 59(11): 1366–1373, 1979.
74. Sullivan, P. E., and Portney, L. G. Electromyographic activity of shoulder muscles during unilateral upper extremity proprioceptive neuromuscular facilitation patterns. *Phys. Ther.,* 60(3): 283–288, 1980.
75. Pink, M. Contralateral effects of upper extremity proprioceptive neuromuscular facilitation patterns. *Phys. Ther.,* 61(8): 1158–1162, 1981.
76. Mead, S. A six-year evaluation of proprioceptive neuromuscular facilitation technics. *Phys. Med.,* 373–376, 1960.
77. Nelson, A. G., Chambers, R. S., McGown, C. M., and Penrose, K. W. Proprioceptive neuromuscular facilitation versus weight training for enhancement of muscular strength and athletic performance. *The Journal of Orthopedic and Sports Physical Therapy,* 7(5): 250–353, 1986.
78. Arsenault, A. B. Techniques of muscle re-education: analysis of studies on the effect of techniques of patterning and neuromuscular facilitation. *Physiother. Can.,* 26(4): 190–194, 1974.
79. Arsenault, A. B., and Chapman, A. E. An electromyographic investigation of the individual recruitment of the quadriceps muscles during isometric contraction of the knee extensors in different patterns of movement. *Physiother. Can.,* 26(50): 253–261, 1974.
80. Synder, J. L., and Forward, E. M. Comparison of knee flexion and extension in the diagonal and sagittal planes. *Phys. Ther.,* 52(12): 1255–1263, 1972.
81. Surburg, P. R. Interactive effects of resistance and facilitation patterning upon reaction and response times. *Phys. Ther.,* 59(13): 1513–1517, 1979.

E/Carr and Shepherd Approach

82. Carr, J. H., and Shepherd, R. B. *A Motor Relearning Programme for Stroke.* Rockville, MD: Aspen Systems Corp., 1983.
83. Carr, J. H., and Shepherd, R. B. *A Motor Relearning Programme for Stroke,* 2nd edition. Rockville, MD: Aspen Systems Corp., 1986.
84. Singer, R. N. Cognitive processes, learner strategies, and skilled motor behaviors. *Can J Appl Sport Sci.* 5(1): 25–32, 1980.
85. Marteniuk, R. G. Motor skill performance and learning: Considerations for rehabilitation. *Physiother. Can.,* 31(4): 187–202, 1979.
86. Marteniuk, R. G. Information processes in movement learning: capacity and structural interference effects. *J Motor Behavior,* 18(1): 55–75, 1986.
87. Harris, F. A. Muscle stretch receptor hypersensitization in spasticity. *Am. J. Phys. Med.,* 57(1): 17–28, 1978.

Supplementary Reading

Bobath, B. The treatment of neuromuscular disorders by improving patterns of coordination. *Physiotherapy, 55:* 18–22, 1969.

Brunnstrom, S. Motor behavior of adult hemiplegic patients. *Am. J. Occup. Ther., 25*(1): 6–12, 1961.

Brunnstrom, S. Training the adult hemiplegic patient: orientation of techniques to patient's motor behavior. In *Approach to the Treatment of Patients with Neuromuscular Dysfunction.* Edited by C. Sattely. Dubuque, IA: Wm. C. Brown Book Co., 1962, pp. 44–48.

Brunnstrom, S. Motor testing procedures in hemiplegia. *.A.P.T.A., 46*(4) :357–375, 1966.

Delaney, F. Y. The geriatric patient with central nervous system dysfunction. *Phys. Occup. Ther. Geriatrics, 2*(3): 5–25, 1983.

Duncan, P. W., Propst, M., and Nelson, S. G. Reliability of the Fugl-Meyer assessment of sensorimotor recovery following cerebrovascular accident. *Phys. Ther., 63*(10): 1606–1610, 1983.

Goff, B. The application of recent advances in neurophysiology to Miss M. Rood's concept of neuromuscular facilitation. *Physiotherapy, 58:* 409–415, 1972.

Hughes, E. Bobath and Brunnstrom: comparison of two methods of treatment of a left hemiplegia. *Physiother. Can., 24*(5): 262–266, 1976.

Kabat, H. Neuromuscular dysfunction and treatment of athetosis. *Physiotherapy, 46*(5): 125–129, 1960.

Knott, M. Report of a case of Parkinsonism treated with proprioceptive facilitation technics. *Phys. Ther. Rev., 37*(4): 229, 1957.

Knott, M. Bulbar involvement with good recovery. *J.A.P.T.A., 42*(1): 38–39, 1962.

Knott, M. Neuromuscular facilitation in the treatment of rheumatoid arthritis. *J.A.P.T.A., 44*(8): 737–739, 1964.

Kukulka, C. G., et al. Effect of tendon pressure on alpha motoneuron excitability, *Phys. Ther., 65*(5): 595–600, 1985.

Perry, C. E. Principles and techniques of the Brunnstrom approach to the treatment of hemiplegia. *Am. J. Phys. Med.,* (NUSTEP Proceedings), *46*(1): 789–812, 1967.

Safranek, M. G., Koshland, G. F., and Raymond, G. Effect of auditory rhythm on muscle activity. *Phys. Ther., 62*(2): 161–168, 1982.

Sodring, K. M. The Bobath concept in treatment of adult hemiplegia. *Scand. J. Rehab. Med., 7*(Suppl): 101–105, 1980.

Voss, D. E., and Knott, M. The application of neuromuscular facilitation in the treatment of shoulder disabilities. *Phys. Ther. Rev., 33*(10): 536–541, 1953.

Wolff, P. H., Gunnoe, C. E., and Cohen, C. Associated movements as a measure of development age. *Dev. Med. & Child Neurol., 25:* 417–429, 1983.

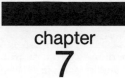

chapter

7

Cognitive and Perceptual Evaluation and Treatment

Lee Ann Quintana

Following brain injury the patient is often left with various degrees of cognitive and perceptual dysfunction as well as the more obvious motor and sensory deficits. The medical field has expended much energy developing knowledge and techniques regarding the physical/medical sequelae of brain injury and is now beginning to realize the impact of residual cognitive/perceptual deficits and to focus on them. Cognitive deficits[1,2] and visual perceptual deficits[3,4] have been found to be significantly related to eventual independence in self-care and discharge disposition. Occupational therapists, therefore, need to focus attention on the evaluation and restoration of these abilities as prerequisites to the overall goal of occupational therapy, which is to help the patient function as independently as possible. However, in a survey of occupational therapy evaluation forms used for stroke patients, it was found that less than 50% included visual perception or cognitive functions as part of the evaluation.[5] Further, it has been suggested that there has been a lack of emphasis in the area of visual perception as compared to motor performance and that occupational therapists must consider the role played by visuospatial deficits in the successful rehabilitation of the stroke patient.[3] Their impact on the patient's activities of daily living (ADL) skills sometimes outweighs that of the physical deficit (Table 7.1).

With this increasing interest in the importance of cognitive/perceptual deficits, there has developed an overlap of services among psychologists, speech/language pathologists, and occupational therapists. A survey of various hospital and rehabilitation settings revealed that the primary responsibility for cognitive rehabilitation therapy fell on psychology in 55% of those responding, speech/language pathology in 40%, occupational therapy in 20%, and other disciplines in 14% (some respondents indicated more than one discipline, which is why the total is greater than 100%).[6] Obviously all those involved in the treatment of the brain-injured patient must concern themselves with

these deficits to some degree. The emphasis today is on the team approach with all members concerned about the total rehabilitation of the patient. These team members work together, but the occupational therapist's role in cognitive rehabilitation may vary depending on the team with which she works.

Cognition refers to the ability of the brain to process, store, retrieve, and manipulate information.[7] Perception refers to the integration of sensory impressions into psychologically meaningful information.[8] For a deficit in perception to be identified, the primary senses must be intact. For example, a person who has poor visual acuity cannot necessarily be said to have a deficit in visual perception when he is unable to match objects, whereas the patient with good acuity who is unable to match objects may be said to have a perceptual deficit.

In the literature there is much overlap and blurring of definitions of the various cognitive and perceptual deficits seen after brain injury. For the purposes of this chapter, general evaluation and treatment guidelines will be discussed and then specific guidelines will be given for the following perceptual deficits: body scheme, including right/left discrimination, body part identification, finger agnosia, and anosognosia; unilateral neglect; spatial relations/position in space; topographical orientation; figure-ground discrimination; constructional apraxia; dressing apraxia; motor apraxia; and the following cognitive deficits: attention, orientation, memory, and problem solving.

Contrary to standards of good practice, occupational therapists have tended to do only a cursory evaluation in the areas of perception and cognition. Standardized measures are not used; there is a tendency to gather information on a subjective level.[5] Standardized quantitative assessment tools must be used, when available, if treatment success is to be documented in measurable terms. When standardized tests are not available, the occupational therapist can present and score the evaluation materials in a consistent manner.

Table 7.1

DEFINITIONS AND DESCRIPTIONS OF COGNITIVE/PERCEPTUAL DEFICITS

Deficit	Definition	Functional Description
Body scheme	Awareness of body parts, position of body and its parts in relation to themselves and objects in the environment	May result in dressing apraxia; may not recognize body parts or relationship between them; transfers may be unsafe
Right/left discrimination	Deficit in ability to understand the concepts of right and left. Right brain damage (RBD): may be due to visuospatial deficits; left brain damage (LBD): in aphasics due to a language deficit; in non-aphasics due to general mental impairment	May have difficulty dressing; understanding directions that include right and left
Body part identification	Difficulty identifying parts on self and/or others	Patient may respond incorrectly when told to move a specific body part
Finger agnosia	Difficulty naming or being able to name fingers touched	May have difficulty with fine dexterity
Anosognosia	Unawareness or denial of deficits	Functional activities are unsafe; unable to teach compensatory techniques
Unilateral neglect	Nelgect of one side of the body or extrapersonal space	Patient shaves one side of face, dresses one side of body; eats half of his plate of food; reads half of a page; deletes half of a drawing; transfers and functional mobility are unsafe; bumps into door jambs and objects on one side
Position in space	Difficulty with concepts of over/under, above/below, etc.	Difficulty moving through a crowded area; difficulty with dressing; difficulty following directions using these terms
Spatial relations	Difficulty perceiving self in relation to other objects	As above; transfers unsafe
Topographical orientation	Ability to find one's way from one place to another	Patient has difficulty finding his way from his room to therapy or from one room to another
Figure-ground	Difficulty distinguishing foreground from background	Patient unable to find object in cluttered drawer, white wash cloth on white sheet, brakes on wheelchair, food in the refrigerator
Constructional apraxia	Deficit in constructional activities: graphic and assembly RBD: drawings are complex but exhibit disorganized spatial relations and poor orientation in space; felt to be result of visuospatial deficits LBD: drawings tend to be oversimplified with decreased number of details; felt to be an executive or conceptual deficit	May result in dressing apraxia, difficulty setting a table, making a dress; wrapping a gift, arranging numerical figures for mathematial processing, making a sandwich, assembling a craft project from a kit, etc.
Apraxia	Inability to carry out purposeful movement in the presence of intact sensation, movement, and coordination	May experience difficulty with functional tasks involving objects, as patient doesn't know how to use objects or attempts to use wrong object (e.g., uses knife to eat soup); may have difficulty writing, knitting, etc.

Table 7.1 *continued*

Deficit	Definition	Functional Description
Dressing apraxia	Inability to dress oneself	Patient attempts to put clothes on inside out, backwards, in the wrong order; dresses only one half of the body
Attention	The ability to focus on a specific stimulus without being distracted	Patient exhibits inability to follow directions, to learn; may appear lethargic; may have difficulty in group situations
Orientation	Oriented times three refers to knowledge of person, place, and time	Unable to answer orientation questions; may ask simple questions over and over; may be easily agitated due to disorientation
Memory	The registration/encoding, consolidation/storage, and recall/retrieval of information	Appears disoriented; will forget names, schedule, etc.; decreased ability to learn or to follow directions
Problem solving	The ability to manipulate fund of knowledge and apply this information to new or unfamiliar situations	Patient has difficulty with routine self-care and household chores, e.g., routine shopping, planning a meal, etc.; may be socially inappropriate; exhibit poor judgment; difficulty ordering or sequencing information, e.g., organizing his time, work, etc.

Evaluation of cognitive deficits is generally carried out by the psychologist or neuropsychologist using psychometric tests. The occupational therapist's role is to evaluate the patient's functional cognitive deficits.[9] As the brain-injured patient often performs better in a structured testing situation used by the psychologist, his performance in a functional situation provides important information for the team. Therefore, while the occupational therapist specifically evaluates for various cognitive deficits, the effects of these deficits are observed during functional activities.

The occupational therapist may do an initial screening of the various cognitive and perceptual deficits with her patients and then, depending on the patient's life-style and goals, might pursue a specific area in more depth. For example, if the patient has had a stroke, is 35 years old, and works as a mechanic, the therapist might evaluate his constructional abilities in more depth; whereas if the patient is 75 years old, retired, and spends his time reading and watching television, in-depth evaluation of constructional abilities may not be indicated. This idea is carried over into treatment as well. The 35-year-old mechanic will need a higher level of constructional skills than would the 75-year-old man. In addition, the therapist may find that the patient performs adequately on a test, but he has difficulty in a functional situation. This would indicate the need for further evaluation.

Treatment generally takes one of three forms: compensation, substitution, or retraining.[7] Compensation is the method by which a particular deficit is circumvented. For example, a log/diary may be used for someone with memory problems. Substitution refers to teaching a new method of response (e.g., use of verbal sequencing skills when map skills are lost). Retraining is the attempt to reorganize and improve the area of deficit. It requires repetitive exercises that place demands on the patient to perform the impaired skill.[10]

Barriers to overcome in treatment of these disorders in brain-damaged patients include problems in attention, learning, and integration.[11] If a patient has difficulty attending, it is difficult to obtain either a valid assessment or cooperation with various retraining techniques. The patient must not only be able to pay attention to the stimulus offered during evaluation and treatment, but he must also be able to retain and learn what is taught to him. Finally, he needs to be able to integrate the various techniques and processes taught to him so that he can generalize these to everyday life.

Almost any activity can be adapted for use in the treatment of a variety of deficits. Things to consider when choosing an activity include (1) the activity must demand a response that involves the impaired skill; (2) the level of difficulty must be variable so that the demand can start within the patient's capabilities and progress to higher levels; (3) progress should be quantifiable and objective; (4) the patient should receive immediate feedback; and (5) the activity should be such that the patient is prevented from making an inordinate number of errors.[12] Activities can be varied in many ways, including speed of presentation; modality of presentation (auditory, visual, tactile); speed of response required; number of items presented at one time; number of spatial dimensions included (two- or three-dimensional); concreteness of directions; and amount of supplementary information available from other sensory modalities.[13]

Patients must be shown the relevance of treatment to daily life. The more relevance they see, the more likely they are to become involved in their treatment and use the techniques taught to them. Our goal is to improve the patient's daily living skills. Only by relating our treatment to activities of daily living will we and the patient know we are on the right track. Studies being done now often show improvement on specific skills but either do not relate them to functional tasks or report little carryover into daily living skills. These researchers are becoming more aware of the need to carry out treatment in a variety of functional situations.

Group treatment is frequently used in cognitive rehabilitation as a supplement to individual treatment. Groups generally meet on a daily basis. Goals of these groups can include reality orientation, improvement of organizational skills, increased awareness of behavior and encouragement of self-monitoring, improved judgment, and increased socialization.

Computers are increasingly being used as a method for cognitive and perceptual retraining. In centers with cognitive rehabilitation programs, 73% reported the use of computer-assisted therapy.[6] Their acceptance has been due to novelty, flexibility, availability, and public acceptance.[14] Because much of cognitive rehabilitation consists of repetitious drills, a computer is a good way to provide these repetitive activities. In addition, the computer can give more precise feedback and provide the therapist and the patient with objective measures of the patient's performance. However, the computer is a tool and, like any therapeutic activity, its usefulness with a particular patient must be continually monitored.

Various types of commercial software are being used, including arcade games and educational software, as well as specific cognitive rehabilitation programs. A listing of resources can be found in the *Computers Information Packet* available from the American Occupational Therapy Association.[15] Although use of computers is increasing, there have been few controlled studies into their effectiveness in cognitive rehabilitation.

Evaluation and treatment of the brain-injured patient may vary depending on the side of lesion. There are certain general characteristics of patients following damage to either the right or left hemisphere that may influence the manner in which evaluation and treatment are carried out (see Table 7.2).

Generally the left hemisphere is dominant for language, and the right hemisphere is dominant for visuospatial tasks. The left hemisphere processes information by breaking it down into details and storing it as verbal symbols on the basis of conceptual similarities. The right hemisphere processes information visually or spatially and on the basis of structural similarities.[8] For

Table 7.2
DIFFERENCES IN RIGHT AND LEFT HEMISPHERES[8,16,17,19]

Left Hemisphere	Right Hemisphere
Dominant for language	Dominant for visuospatial tasks, face recognition
Analyzer, breaks down into details	Synthesizer, looks at the whole
Organizes data in conceptual similarities	Organizes data in structural similarities
Reason, attention to detail	Intuition, imagination
Verbal memory	Figural memory

Following Damage	
Aphasia	Aprosodia
Catastrophic reaction	Indifference reaction
Difficulty processing information in auditory modality; profit more from non-language-related cues, pantomime, gestural demonstration, and use of visual images	Difficulty processing information in visual modality; profit more from language-related cues and verbal elaboration

example, the left hemisphere sees an apple and a peach as alike because they are fruit, whereas the right hemisphere sees them as alike because they are round.

These differences have a definite impact on treatment. Patients with left brain damage (LBD) have difficulty processing information in the auditory modality, whereas patients with right brain damage (RBD) have difficulty processing information in the visual modality.[16] As a result, LBD patients generally respond better to visual demonstration, and RBD patients generally respond better to verbal instructions.

Aphasia, a language disorder that has been well described and researched, generally occurs after LBD. In recent years a similar disorder of affective language called aprosodia has been described as a sequela of RBD.[17,18] Prosody is the coloring, melody, and cadence of speech. The aphasic patient may not understand the phrase "I'm happy" because he does not understand the words. The patient with aprosodia may only understand the phrase, but miss the real meaning if it is spoken in a sad voice. Such a patient's use and appreciation of gestures may be disturbed as well.

After brain damage, different emotional reactions, depending on the side of lesion, are generally described. RBD patients frequently deny their deficits and appear indifferent and euphoric. Their reaction is termed an indifference reaction. LBD patients are generally said to show a catastrophic reaction often characterized by depression, agitation, and restlessness.[19] These descriptions are being challenged. The label of indifference reaction in RBD patients may be the result of their difficulty with affective language. For the

RBD patient, a more accurate assessment of his emotional state would be a verbal report of his feelings rather than a judgment based on nonverbal behavior.

Evaluation and Treatment of Perceptual Deficits

Comprehensive perceptual evaluation requires selection of various subtests for specific deficits that are put together by the therapist to form the test battery for a specific patient. There is one test battery available, however, that evaluates visual perception as a whole; that is the *Motor-Free Visual Perception Test* (MVPT). The MVPT, which was originally designed for children, measures spatial relations, visual discrimination, figure-ground perception, visual closure, and visual memory. It has been adapted for use with brain-damaged adults and standardized on a normal adult population.[20] The test was adapted by adding a time factor and interpretational guidelines designed to determine lack of compensation for visual field deficits and/or unilateral neglect. If a patient underresponds to test items directed to one side of the body, a field defect is suspected and this side is not used to determine the patient's perceptual ability. Interpretation of severity of unilateral visual neglect must be made cautiously, as mild functional unilateral visual neglect does not consistently correlate with underresponding on this test. The score on this test gives an overall measure of visual perception and is not meant to be differentiated into the various areas tested. Please refer to the adult test manual for specific administration instructions.[20]

BODY SCHEME

Body scheme is the awareness of body parts and position of the body and its parts in relation to themselves and objects in the environment. Related deficits include right/left disorientation, impaired body part identification, finger agnosia, anosognosia, and unilateral neglect.

Disorders of body scheme as measured by body part identification and right/left discrimination are more frequently observed in LBD patients.[21-23] However, failure can be the result of several problems: (1) verbal, (2) sensory, (3) conceptual, or (4) visuospatial. Therefore, patients may exhibit deficits in body scheme under one test condition, but not under a different condition.[23] For example, a RBD patient may have no difficulty indicating right/left or body part on self, but be unable to indicate right/left on a confronting person or to imitate right/left movements due to a visuospatial problem.

MacDonald[24] describes a test of body scheme that includes finger agnosia, right/left discrimination, body part identification, and body revisualization. Scores on this test by neurologically impaired and nonneurologically impaired adults were significantly different at the 0.001 level of probability.

The goal of treatment of body scheme disorders is to increase the patient's awareness of his body and decrease his disorientation. Treatment starts in a low-stimulation environment. As the patient becomes less disoriented, treatment can be expanded to the clinic. Marmo[25] suggests a sensory integrative approach to treatment of body scheme disorders that includes controlled sensory stimulation and developmental motor patterns administered under conditions of decreased stress to help the patient in reorganizing his body scheme. She recommends beginning with tactile rubdowns, progressing to rolling over, followed by prone-on-elbows posture. There is no documentation of the effectiveness of this treatment approach.

Right/Left Discrimination

Right/left (R/L) discrimination denotes an ability to understand the concepts of right and left. R/L disorientation to one's own body is uncommon in nonaphasic patients.[21,26] However, RBD patients exhibit difficulty identifying body parts of a confronting person. Nonaphasic LBD patients tend to perform adequately on R/L tasks. It appears that poor R/L discrimination in aphasic LBD patients is due to a language problem,[22] whereas the deficit seen in RBD patients is most likely due to visuospatial deficits.[23] Nonaphasic patients with general mental impairment also exhibit deficits in this area, most probably due to a conceptual problem.[23]

Evaluation. Tests of R/L discrimination usually include orientation to one's own body (e.g., "touch your left ear"), orientation to a confronting person (e.g., "touch my left hand"), or a combination of both. The complexity is increased by requiring double uncrossed tasks (e.g., "touch your right knee with your right hand") or double crossed tasks (e.g., "touch your right knee with your left elbow").

Benton et al.[26] present a standardized 20-item test that requires the patient to point to lateralized body parts on command and takes about 5 min to administer (see Table 7.3). A total score of less than 17 is considered defective. Performance patterns can be classified as normal (score of 17–20, no more than one error on the first 12 "own body" items); generalized defect (score of less than 17, more than one error on the first 12 "own body" items); confronting person defect (score of less than 17, no more than one error on "own body" items) and no more than two errors on the remaining items); specific "own body" deficit (more than one error on the 12 "own body" items) and systematic reversal (score of 17–20 when performance is scored in reverse fashion, no more than one error on "own body" items).

Treatment. Boone and Landes[22] observed that they were unable to retrain aphasics in R/L discrimination (no information is given as to what the training included). If the patient is unable to regain automatic knowledge of the difference between right and left, he may have to learn to compensate cognitively (e.g., use

Table 7.3
RIGHT-LEFT ORIENTATION TEST[a]

1. Show me your *left* hand.
2. Show me your *right* eye.
3. Show me your *left* ear.
4. Show me your *right* hand.

5. Touch your *left* ear with your *left* hand.
6. Touch your *right* eye with your *left* hand.
7. Touch your *right* knee with your *right* hand.
8. Touch your *left* eye with your *left* hand.
9. Touch your *right* ear with your *left* hand.
10. Touch your *left* knee with your *right* hand.
11. Touch your *right* ear with your *right* hand.
12. Touch your *left* eye with your *right* hand.

13. Point to my *right* eye.
14. Point to my *left* leg.
15. Point to my *left* ear.
16. Point to my *right* hand.

17. Put your *right* hand on my *left* ear.
18. Put your *left* hand on my *left* eye.
19. Put your *left* hand on my *right* shoulder.
20. Put your *right* hand on my *right* eye.

[a]Form A; reprinted with permission from Benton, A. L., Hamsher, K. deS., Varney, N. K., and Spreen, O. *Contributions to Neuropsychological Assessment—A Clinical Manual.* New York: Oxford University Press, 1983.

the ring on his left hand as a cue for the left side). If "right" and "left" only confuse the patient, it would be useful to avoid using these words during treatment.[9,22]

Treatment can include activities that stress right and left (e.g., using "right" and "left" in directions), or use of increased cutaneous or proprioceptive input to one extremity.[9] For example, the therapist may have the patient wear a weight cuff on one arm during treatment to provide increased proprioceptive input while calling his attention to that side. It is important to consistently apply the input to the same side.

Body Part Identification

The ability to identify body parts on self and others is referred to as body part identification. Boone and Landes[22] found that RBD patients perform better than LBD patients in pointing to body parts. When analyzing the errors made by both RBD and LBD patients, they found that the majority were on items where the dimension of right and left was added. They concluded that although occasional hemiplegic patients have difficulty recognizing body parts, the more prevalent disorder is a deficit in R/L discrimination.

Evaluation. Evaluation consists of the same items as used for R/L discrimination. Testing should include requests to identify body parts both separately and in combination with R/L tasks; a patient with a deficit in body part identification would have difficulty on all phases of the test, whereas a patient with only R/L discrimination deficits will score well on the "pure" body part identification tasks.[22]

Treatment. Anderson and Choy[27] report a program to increase awareness of body image, space perception, and unilateral neglect. To increase body awareness, they suggest the following activities: the patient verbally identifies parts of the body as they are touched; the therapist names a part followed by the patient rubbing the area; the patient mimics the therapist, who moves her head and limbs in different positions.

Finger Agnosia

Finger agnosia denotes an inability to identify one's own fingers, difficulty naming fingers, or being able to indicate which finger was touched. This deficit is not usually seen as a single entity, but in combination with either an aphasic disorder or mental impairment.[23]

Evaluation. Evaluation generally consists of requiring the patient to name fingers that have been touched, identifying a finger named by the examiner, and/or imitating the finger movements of the examiner.[9,21] Goodglass and Kaplan[28] describe a test of finger agnosia that includes naming, finger-name comprehension, visual-visual matching, and visual-tactile matching. The reader is referred to the reference for further description of the test.

Treatment. Fox[29] found that using pressure and cutaneous stimulation improved finger agnosia in hemiplegic patients. This treatment consists of stimulation using a corduroy-covered, padded wooden stimulator that is applied to one or more of the following areas: dorsal surface of forearm, hand, and fingers and the ventral surface of fingers. In addition, grasp of a rough-surfaced cardboard cone is used to provide pressure to the volar surface of the hand. This stimulation should feel comfortable to the patient to avoid a protective response; therefore, the area of stimulation depends on the patient's response. These two types of stimulation should be done for a minimum of 2 min each, although the rubbing and pressure can be alternated (30 sec each).[9]

Anosognosia

Anosognosia refers to an unawareness of hemiplegia. The extent of this awareness of self can vary greatly among patients and can range from an unawareness of hemiparesis to lack of concern to total denial. It is most often seen in RBD patients.[30,31] It is usually seen immediately after an acute lesion, persisting for a few days, and then ameliorating to milder forms of denial. Initially, the patient may deny that the hemiplegic limbs belong to him and insist that nothing is wrong; later, he may admit that they are his limbs, but still refer to them in the third person.

Evaluation. There are no formal tests for anosognosia. Observation should be made of how the patient positions the hemiplegic limbs, the manner in which the patient refers to his limbs (does he refer to them in the third person, or indicate that they belong to someone else?), and whether he spontaneously complains about the loss of function of one side.[32]

Treatment. If the patient denies he has a problem, little can be done to teach him to compensate for it.[9] As the patient begins to recover and denial lessens, efforts must be made to make the patient aware of his deficit. (See Chapter 2 for a discussion of denial as a defense.)

UNILATERAL NEGLECT

Unilateral neglect is referred to by a variety of names including hemiinattention, hemispatial neglect, and unilateral spatial agnosia. It is manifested by a failure to respond or orient to stimuli presented contralateral to a brain lesion.[32] It is observed functionally in the patient who only eats the food on half of his plate, shaves only one side of his face, etc. It is most commonly caused by lesion in the right hemisphere, although it does occur following LBD; however, the deficit after LBD is usually of a lesser degree.[31,33-35]

It was found that when given a task, both LBD and RBD patients were apt to scan only homolateral space and fail to attend to the whole task. However, if the task demanded active exploration, LBD patients were more able to complete the task, whereas RBD patients continued to scan only homolateral space.[36] Furthermore, they found that if the patients' attention was directed to the fact that the task was not completed, LBD patients were able to find the errors, but the neglect persisted in the RBD patients. Functionally, tasks such as reading or eating from a tray require active exploration and would prove more difficult for the RBD patient with unilateral neglect.

Initially, it was felt that unilateral neglect was due to defective sensory input superimposed on altered mental function[37] or deficits in body scheme.[38] More recently it has been attributed to a deficit in arousal and attention.[39-42] In a study of normal subjects, it has been found that the right hemisphere attends to stimuli presented on either the right or left sides, whereas the left hemisphere responds mainly to stimuli presented on the right.[39] It was proposed that following RBD, neglect is more severe because the left hemisphere is unable to attend to ipsilateral stimuli, whereas following LBD the right hemisphere is able to process stimuli presented ipsilaterally to some degree.

Unilateral neglect is generally either mild or severe. In the mild case, the neglect may not be apparent during functional tasks, but can be elicited in testing situations.[43] The patient may be able to respond to unilateral stimuli, but exhibit difficulty with bilateral simultaneous stimulation[32] or difficulty with tasks in which cognitive demands are more extensive.[44] Severe neglect has been associated with functional deficits in self-care, reading, and writing.[4,43,45] In this case the patient presents the classical case of being able to read only one-half of the page and being unaware of or unable to compensate for this deficit.

Unilateral neglect is frequently seen in combination with visual field deficits, but either condition can occur independently of the other.[46] In fact, if the neglect is severe, it may not be possible to determine accurately whether there is in fact a field cut. The question remains: is the deficit due to a field cut, or is the patient just neglecting that side?

Unilateral neglect tends to be most pronounced immediately after brain damage, but may continue for a long time. Recovery tends to be slow and often incomplete.[32]

Evaluation. Unilateral neglect is evaluated in a variety of ways including drawing tasks,[9] cancellation tasks,[43] crossing-out tasks,[46] and line bisection.[33,47] In all such tasks the therapist looks for omissions and errors concentrated on one side.

Schenkenberg et al.[33] designed a line bisection test that consists of 20 lines. Eighteen of the lines are organized so that six lines are primarily on the left side of the page, six lines on the right, and six lines in the middle (the top and bottom lines are used for instructions to the patient and deleted from the score). The lines are of varying lengths and the patient is told to cut each line in half by placing a pencil mark through the center (Fig. 7.1). The patient is told to make only one mark on any line and is not allowed to move the paper (when necessary it can be taped to the table directly in front of him). The difference between the true center and the patient's mark is measured in millimeters. They found that this test differentiated between patient groups and that RBD patients were likely to totally neglect two or more of the lines.

Van Deusen[47] presented normative data from 93 adults using the Schenkenberg line bisection test. Using the standardized method of scoring [percent deviation = [(measured left half − true half)/true half] × 100], an average percent deviation score was obtained for the six left-placed lines and for the six left-placed

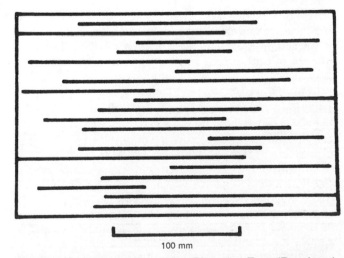

100 mm

Figure 7.1 Schenkenberg Line Bisection Test. (Reprinted with permission from Schenkenberg, T., Bradford, D. C., and Ajax, E. T. Line bisection and unilateral visual neglect in patients with neurologic impairment. *Neurology, 30:* 509–517, 1980.)

lines plus the six center-placed lines for each subject. The mean and standard deviations were determined (Table 7.4). The patient's standard deviation can be determined by the following formula: (patient mean − normal mean)/normal standard deviation = patient standard deviation. Van Deusen[47] suggests that a standard deviation of ±1 be considered slight neglect, ±2 moderate, and ±3 severe neglect.

Another method of evaluation frequently used is that of cancellation tasks. These usually consist of a sheet of paper with several lines of typed letters, and the patient is asked to mark a specific stimulus letter that is scattered randomly throughout. Scoring is determined by the number of omissions (target letters that are not marked), number of commissions (cancellation of letters other than the target letter), and time.[48] In addition, note is taken on what area of the page these errors are made. The greater the number of errors, the greater the visual scanning deficit. Errors on one side of the page are generally indicative of unilateral neglect; random errors throughout are generally due to an attention problem. The patient with neglect may complete this task either very rapidly because he only attends to a portion of the page and makes no attempt to compensate; or if he is aware that he has a deficit, he may take a long time because in his attempt to compensate he keeps going over the same lines gradually finding more letters on the left side (although usually not all of them). When cancellation tasks are used for training, level of difficulty can be increased, for example, by requesting two target letters, decreasing the spacing between letters, or decreasing the size of the letters. Gordon et al.[49] presented means and standard deviation scores on this test derived from a group of RBD patients. Comparison to these scores, however, does not allow interpretation of the score obtained from a patient in relation to normal expected performance.

Albert[46] presented a test in which 40 lines were drawn in an apparently random manner on a sheet of paper, but actually consisted of six rows of six lines and one row of four lines. The examiner draws over each of the 40 lines, in a random manner, with a red pencil. The patient is asked to cross out all the lines on the page. This test was standardized on a group of normal subjects who made no errors.

Treatment. Fox[50] noted three approaches to treatment: learning theory approach (shaping behavior with feedback and positive reinforcement), neurological approach (reestablishing awareness of unilateral body and space), and adaptation of the environment.

Weinberg et al.[43] developed a training program for left neglect that included reading, writing, and calculation activities. They used the principles of anchoring (supplying a cue on the impaired side to indicate starting position), pacing (controlling speed), density (facilitating response by increasing the distance between stimuli), and offering immediate feedback and found that after training RBD patients improved on tests of academic skill.

This training program was later expanded to include training to increase sensory awareness and spatial organization.[51] The new tasks included practice in identification of locus of touch on the back and estimation of gross size of objects. They found that the two phases of training combined were even more effective with regard to improving reading and math skills than just the initial phase. They further suggested that these training principles (anchoring, pacing, etc.) could be applied to ADL tasks. They also provided a description of their training program, and the reader is referred to the reference for further details.[48]

Later, a third phase was added to this training program that was aimed at improving complex visual perception.[44] These three training modules (scanning, somatosensory awareness and size estimation, and complex visual perception) were combined into one program. Improvements in basic scanning functions and complex visual perceptual skills were found after this program, but generalization of skills was not as extensive as with the previous two phases.[52] To increase generalization, they suggested providing a wider range of stimuli in which the patient must use his newly learned compensatory strategies (e.g., always use an anchor on the left whether dressing, eating, walking down the hall, etc.).

The Thinking Skills Workbook: A Cognitive Skills Remediation Manual for Adults[53] consists of exercises designed to retrain visual scanning, visual-spatial, and time judgment ability in adult patients. It contains a pretest to determine which sections of the book the patient needs to work on and a posttest. Training using this workbook resulted in significantly ($P < 0.005$) higher improvement in test scores by acute stroke patients as compared to a control group of similar patients.[54]

Anderson and Choy[27] reported improvement in unilateral neglect in hemiplegic patients with the use of tactile stimulation and icing. This treatment included having the therapist stroke the patient's involved arm as the patient watched; the therapist initially uses her hand and progresses to rough cloth, brush, or ice to the degree necessary for sensory appreciation of the stimulus. The patient may be asked to stimulate himself in the manner described above. This method may serve to increase arousal and attention to the neglected side. Fox[50] recommended the use of brushing and icing to the nonspastic muscles of the involved upper extrem-

Table 7.4
MEAN AND STANDARD DEVIATION NORMS FOR LINE BISECTION TEST[a]

	Left Lines	Left Plus Center Lines
Mean	−0.48	−0.59
Standard deviation	5.55	4.35

[a]Reprinted with permission from Van Deusen, J. Normative data for ninety-three elderly persons on the Schenkenberg line bisection test. *Phys. Occup. Ther. Geriatrics, 3*(2): 49–54, 1983.

ity followed by gross visual perceptual activities (e.g., block design or copying tasks) requiring orientation of the head and uninvolved arm toward the involved side as far as possible to focus the patient's attention on the neglected side. She further indicated that instructions be kept to a minimum. The use of visual perceptual tasks and decreased verbal stimulation are recommended as it has been suggested that verbal stimulation can increase left neglect by increasing arousal asymmetries, whereas perceptual stimuli may lessen neglect by activating the right hemisphere.[55]

Adaptation of the environment includes such things as arranging the patient's bed so that his uninvolved side is toward the activity in the room, or always interacting with the patient on his uninvolved side.[32] Although adapting the environment might be a good idea initially to evaluate the patient and to keep him from harming himself, it does nothing to help the patient overcome his deficit. It is therefore recommended that treatment based on the learning theory and neurological approaches be used along with clinical observation of the results.[50]

POSITION IN SPACE/SPATIAL RELATIONS

A patient with a deficit in position in space has difficulty with concepts such as over, front, back, below, etc., whereas a patient with a deficit in spatial relations has difficulty perceiving himself in relation to other objects or objects in relation to himself. These two deficits are sometimes referred to as visual spatial agnosia.[38] Functionally a patient with a deficit in these areas might run into objects due to difficulty judging distance; may exhibit topographical disorientation, becoming easily lost; or may exhibit dressing apraxia.

Evaluation. The *Space Visualization Test*, a subtest of the *Sensory Integration and Praxis Tests*,[56] and the *Spatial Relations* and *Position in Space* subtests[57] of Frostig's *Developmental Test of Visual Perception* are sometimes used for evaluation. These tests are standardized for children only. Other methods of evaluation include the Bender *Visual Motor Gestalt Test*,[58] the cross test, and positioning blocks.[9] The *Visual Motor Gestalt Test* consists of nine patterns that the patient is asked to copy. Scoring depends not only on the form of the reproduced figures, but on their relationship to each other. Positioning blocks consists of using two blocks and asking the patient to describe their position in relation to each other (e.g., in front of, behind, on top, etc.)

Treatment. Siev et al.[9] suggested various table top activities in which the patient is given the opportunity to practice discriminating different orientations in space by copying designs set up by the therapist or from pictures using blocks, pegs, puzzles, or matchsticks. A functional activity such as organizing a closet can require use of the concepts of position in space. This type of activity can be graded from simple to complex. To improve spatial relations, the patient can be asked to navigate his body through a maze or to follow a path through an obstacle course. If the patient has poor body scheme, he may experience difficulty perceiving himself in relation to other objects. If this is the case, treatment to increase the patient's awareness of his body, such as a sensory integrative approach is indicated.

TOPOGRAPHICAL ORIENTATION

The patient with a deficit in topographical orientation exhibits difficulty finding his way from one place to another. This difficulty in route finding may be due to a variety of causes and is usually associated with other visual spatial problems.[38,59,60] Left neglect of external space may be present so that the patient shows a preference for turns in one direction over another.

Topographical memory is the ability to visualize familiar scenes and describe familiar routes. This loss is usually independent of other forms of visual disorientation and loss of memory for object.[38]

Evaluation. Topographical orientation is not generally evaluated on a formal basis. Reports from staff and/or the patient himself may indicate that the patient is having difficulty finding his way to therapy, around the hospital, etc. Problems with memory or mental confusion must be ruled out to arrive at a diagnosis of topographical disorientation.[9] There are no specific tests for this deficit, although some researchers base their diagnosis on the patient's ability to draw a map of familiar places or ability to describe familiar routes, as well as on how the patient performs functionally.[38,59] If the patient does not exhibit topographical disorientation functionally, difficulty with map drawing may be due to other reasons such as constructional apraxia or deficits in spatial relations, etc.

Treatment. Siev et al.[9] suggest several methods of treatment including rote practice and memorization of routes. As a means of compensation, markers could be used to mark a route and these markers could gradually be removed.[61] It would also seem appropriate that if it is determined that the basis for the difficulty in topographical orientation is left neglect, spatial relations, etc., then treatment should be aimed at the more basic visual perceptual skills.

FIGURE-GROUND PERCEPTION

Figure-ground perception is the ability to distinguish the foreground or figure from the background. A deficit in this area can be seen functionally in the patient who is unable to find a white washcloth on the bed, the brakes on his wheelchair, or eyeglasses in a cluttered drawer.

Deficits in figure-ground perception have been seen after lesions to any area of the brain. Aphasic LBD patients perform significantly worse on tests of figure-ground perception than RBD patients and RBD patients perform significantly worse than nonaphasic LBD patients.[62,63]

Evaluation. Evaluations most frequently used are the *Figure-Ground Perception Test*, a subtest of the *Sensory Integration and Praxis Tests*,[56] and the Frostig *Figure Ground Test*,[57] a subtest of the *Developmental*

Test of Visual Perception, both of which were developed for use with children. One study found that the *Frostig Figure Ground Test* did not correlate with other figure-ground tests, although it did correlate with a constructional apraxia test.[9] On this basis, it was indicated that this test may not be an appropriate test for figure-ground abilities of adult brain-damaged patients. Further research is needed.

The *Figure-Ground Perception Test*[56] presents the patient with a design consisting of three overlapping objects or geometric designs. The patient is asked to choose the three correct figures from six choices, and the test is discontinued after the fifth error. This test is easy to administer, and the patient's response can be either motor (pointing) or verbal (by name of object or number of the answer). Petersen and Wikoff[64] administered this test to 100 normal adult men aged 19 to 57. They changed the method of scoring such that points were given for each correctly identified figure through the design in which the fifth error is made (all correct responses for the design are scored, rather than immediately stopping upon making the fifth error). The scores they obtained had a range of 15 to 48, a mean of 29.72, and a standard deviation of 8.83. They also found that the scores were not related to age, education, or socioeconomic status. Their scoring procedure should be followed when using their mean and standard deviation as norms.

Treatment. Treatment can include several types of activities for practice. Activities such as word search games (finding words embedded in a group of letters) are commonly found in crossword puzzle books. Scanning activities, such as having the patient find certain objects within pictures taken from magazines or from a random scattering of objects, can be used and graded from easy to difficult as the patient improves. Treatment can include compensation techniques. One example is that in the hospital, compensation arrangements could include using washcloths/towels of a color other than white and keeping the environment as simple and uncluttered as possible.

CONSTRUCTIONAL APRAXIA

Constructional apraxia "denotes an impairment in combinatory or organizing activity in which details must be clearly perceived and in which the relationships among the component parts of the entity must be apprehended if the desired synthesis of them is to be achieved."[65] This deficit emerges in tasks where individual parts must be arranged in a given spatial relationship to form a unitary structure.[66] Patients with constructional apraxia have difficulty with copying, drawing, and constructing designs in two and three dimensions. It can be seen functionally as difficulty with such activities as setting a table, making a sandwich, making a dress, or any mechanical activities in which parts are to be combined into a whole. It is one of the causes of dressing apraxia.

Constructional apraxia can be found in both RBD and LBD patients. It has often been found to be more frequent and more severe in RBD patients.[67-70] There is some question about whether this finding may have been due to a bias introduced by exclusion of more involved LBD patients from studies due to aphasia and their subsequent failure on intelligence tests. Other researchers when attempting to control for these factors have found no difference in the incidence of constructional apraxia between RBD and LBD patients.[71,72]

In general, drawings of RBD patients tend to be more complex, show disorganized spatial relationships, and decreased orientation in space (Fig. 7.2). Drawings of LBD patients tend to be oversimplified and have a decreased number of details (Fig. 7.3).[67,70,73] Due to these qualitative differences noted in the performance of RBD and LBD patients, some researchers feel that the basis underlying constructional apraxia differs according to the side of the lesion.[65,67] Constructional apraxia in RBD patients is felt to be the result of visuospatial deficits, whereas that in LBD patients is felt to be due to an executive or conceptual disorder.

Evaluation. Benton[65] suggests two types of constructional activities: (1) graphic and (2) assembly tasks, and that both types should be included in an evaluation of constructional apraxia. The most frequent type of graphic tasks are copying tasks. These include copying geometric shapes (from simple to complex) and drawing without a model (e.g., house, clock, flower).

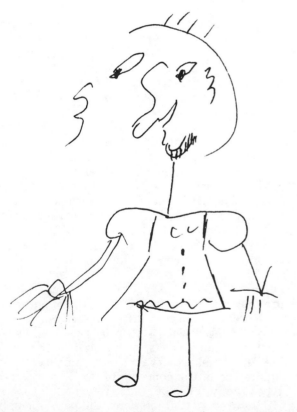

Figure 7.2 Drawing of a person by a patient with right-brain damage.

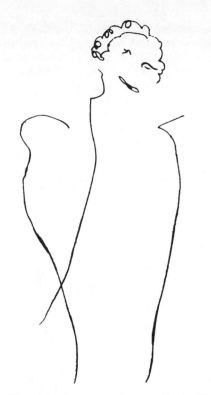

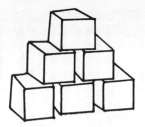

Six cubes (2.5 cm x 2.5 cm x 2.5 cm)

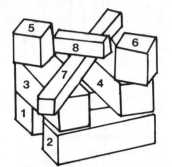

1-4 = 7.5 cm x 2.5 cm x 2.5 cm
5-6 = 2.5 cm x 2.5 cm x 2.5 cm
7 = 15 cm x 1.25 cm x 1.25 cm
8 = 3.75 cm x 1.25 cm x 1.25 cm

Figure 7.3 Drawing of a person by a patient with left-brain damage.

Assembly tasks include such activities as stick arrangement and three-dimensional block designs. Common errors on stick arrangement include selecting sticks of incorrect length, failure to reproduce parts of the model (especially lateral), making lines more oblique than the model indicates, a tendency to remove part of the model to make the copy, and a "crowding in" phenomenon in which the patient's copy rests on top of or touching the model.[30] Assembly tasks can be varied in numerous ways to test more subtle deficiencies by changing these aspects: copying from a model (representational or actual) may be easier than constructing from memory; providing the patient with the correct number and type of blocks/sticks structures the task and makes it simpler than requiring the patient to choose the correct pieces from a large number of blocks/sticks.

In general these tasks are not standardized and rely on subjective judgment of the results. It is important to note the patient's method of completing the task, the patient's comments, any emotional display, hesitancy, indecision, and change of mind, as well as the type of errors made.[30]

Benton et al.[26] present a standardized three-dimensional block construction task. There are two forms to allow for retesting and comparison of the patient's performance on successive occasions. This test consists of three block models that are presented one at a time (Fig. 7.4). The patient is asked to construct an exact replica, selecting blocks from an assortment of 29 blocks (Fig. 7.5). Time taken to complete each model is

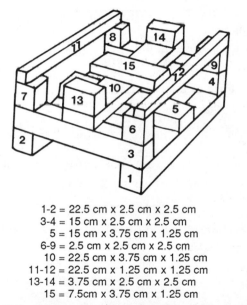

1-2 = 22.5 cm x 2.5 cm x 2.5 cm
3-4 = 15 cm x 2.5 cm x 2.5 cm
5 = 15 cm x 3.75 cm x 1.25 cm
6-9 = 2.5 cm x 2.5 cm x 2.5 cm
10 = 22.5 cm x 3.75 cm x 1.25 cm
11-12 = 22.5 cm x 1.25 cm x 1.25 cm
13-14 = 3.75 cm x 2.5 cm x 2.5 cm
15 = 7.5cm x 3.75 cm x 1.25 cm

Figure 7.4 Schematic representation of block designs (Reprinted with permission from Benton, A. L., Hamsher, K. deS., Varney, N. K., and Spreen, O. *Contributions to Neuropsychological Assessment—A Clinical Manual.* New York: Oxford University Press, 1983.)

recorded in seconds, with a maximum of 5 min allowed. The score is obtained by crediting one point for each correctly placed block (29 possible points). The types of errors (omissions, additions, substitutions, and displacements) are recorded. If the total time taken to construct the three models is greater than 380 sec, two points are subtracted from the score. Of the normal

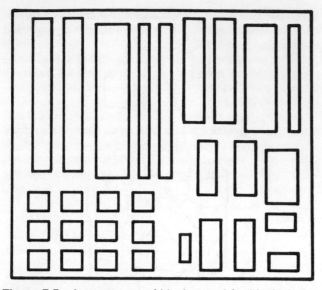

Figure 7.5 Arrangement of blocks used for block design test. (Reprinted with permission from Benton, A. L., Hamsher, K. deS., Varney, N. K., and Spreen, O. *Contributions to Neuropsychological Assessment—A Clinical Manual*. New York: Oxford University Press, 1983.)

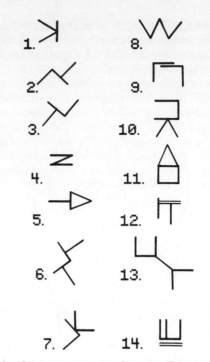

Figure 7.6 Stick construction figures. (Reprinted with permission from Goodglass, H., and Kaplan, E. *The Assessment of Aphasia and Related Disorders*. Philadelphia: Lea & Febiger, 1972.)

controls, 78% had errorless performances, 12% made one error, and 10% made three to five errors.

Goodglass and Kaplan[28] describe three tests, as part of their parietal lobe battery, for evaluation of constructional difficulties. These include drawing to command, stick construction from memory, and three-dimensional block designs. Drawing to command includes having the patient draw a clock, daisy, elephant, cross, cube, and house (for scoring criteria, see Table 7.5). Stick construction from memory consists of 14 designs (Fig. 7.6) that are assembled by the therapist

before the patient, who is then allowed to view each one for 10 sec. The design is then swept away, and the patient is asked to reproduce the design. The wooden sticks are ¼ inch square by 3 inches long. The patient receives one point for each correct item. These authors also describe a three-dimensional block construction task that involves copying ten block designs presented for the patient to reproduce.

Table 7.5
SCORING CRITERIA FOR DRAWING TO COMMAND[a]

Shape	Instruction	Scoring
Clock	"Draw the face of a clock showing the numbers and the two hands."	0 to 3. One point each for approximately circular face, Symmetry of number placement, and correctness of numbers
Daisy	"Draw a daisy."	0 to 2. One point each for general shape (center with petals around it) and symmetry of petal arrangement
Elephant	"Draw an elephant."	0 to 2. One point each for general shape (legs, trunk, head, body) and relative proportions correct
Cross	"You know what the Red Cross looks like? Draw an outline of it without taking your pencil off the paper."	0 to 2. One point each for basic configurations and ability to form all corners adequately with a continuous line
Cube	"Draw a cube-shaped block in perspective, as it would look if you could see the top and two sides."	0 to 2. One point each for grossly correct attempt and correctness of perspective
House	"Draw a house in perspective, so you can see the roof and two sides."	0 to 2. One point each for grossly correct features of house and accuracy of perspective

[a]Reprinted with permission from Goodglass, H., and Kaplan, E. *The Assessment of Aphasia and Related Disorders*. Philadelphia: Lea & Febiger, 1972.

Treatment. Although much research has been done on the incidence, severity, and mechanisms underlying constructional apraxia, little has been written regarding treatment. It has been found that LBD patients benefitted from the use of landmarks on a drawing task.[74] With LBD patients, attempts should be made to determine whether their performance is improved by the use of landmarks on simple designs. If this is the case, the number of landmarks is gradually reduced and treatment progresses to more complicated designs.[9] Both RBD and LBD patients benefitted from visual cues on a block design task.[75] Training[70] and provision of a model[67] also have been found to benefit the performance of LBD patients, but not necessarily that of RBD patients.

Treatment can take the form of having the patient copy simple block designs, beginning with three blocks and gradually increasing the number of blocks and complexity of the design.[27] It can begin with plain wooden cubes, proceed to colored cubes (which adds another dimension, specifically color), and finally to blocks of various sizes and shapes. The patient can be required to transfer a two-dimensional design to three-dimensional, as when copying a block design from a photograph or pattern on paper. Stick designs and pegboard designs can be used in a similar fashion.

DRESSING APRAXIA

Dressing apraxia refers to an inability to dress oneself. Brain[38] attributed it to an underlying visuospatial disorganization. It can be seen in patients both with RBD and LBD and can be the result of constructional apraxia, unilateral neglect, and/or body scheme disorders.[30,60] Research has supported the link between constructional apraxia and dressing apraxia.[4,76-79] In the case of constructional apraxia, the deficit "shows itself in the total disarray, whereby garments are put on in the wrong order . . . , or at the wrong end . . ."[30] If the basis is unilateral neglect, the patient may put clothes on in the proper order, but leave one half of his body undressed. Other patients may exhibit problems with right/left, determining top from bottom, etc. Warren[80] found that a test of body scheme was a better predictor of dressing performance than a constructional apraxia task, although both significantly correlated with dressing performance. She felt that both body scheme and constructional apraxia jointly contribute to dressing apraxia.

Evaluation. Dressing apraxia is generally evaluated functionally by observing the patient dressing himself. To better determine the cause of the dressing apraxia, the evaluation should also include evaluation of constructional apraxia, unilateral neglect, and body scheme.

Treatment. Little is written specifically regarding treatment for dressing apraxia. In one study, initial scores on body scheme and design copy were correlated with final dressing scores.[80] The patients all "received the same amount and type of dressing and perceptual training commonly provided." This training was not described nor was it stated whether there was a difference on scores of body scheme or design copying upon discharge.

If the basis for the dressing apraxia is found to be constructional apraxia, unilateral neglect or body scheme disturbances, treatment is aimed at ameliorating those deficits.[27]

Treatment generally consists of teaching the patient a pattern of dressing. Cognitive cues, such as using the label to tell front from back or talking himself through the steps of the activity as he attempts to put on his shirt, are used and the patient eventually learns through practice.[9]

APRAXIA

Apraxia is the inability to carry out purposeful movement in the presence of intact sensation, movement, and coordination.[28,81,82] Apraxia is generally seen in patients with LBD.[28,82,83] In patients who have use of both arms, the impairment can be demonstrated to be bilateral.[28,83] There are two types of motor apraxia: ideomotor and ideational. These are brought about by disruption of higher level motor processes, specifically in impaired selection of elements that make up a movement and impaired sequencing.[82]

Ideomotor apraxia is generally exhibited only under testing situations, as the patient is able to carry out an activity spontaneously, but fails on verbal command.[82] For example, the patient is able to brush his teeth in the morning, but when asked to "show me how you brush your teeth," he is unable to perform the movement adequately. The movement will be awkward but still bear a resemblance to the intended movement.[81] Heilman[84] found that patients with ideomotor apraxia, although able to use objects, are clumsy.

Ideational apraxia is seen as difficulty with sequencing motor acts and is thought to be a disturbance in the conceptual organization of movements. This is a more serious deficit and apparent during functional activities. For example, the patient may experience difficulty with eating, not knowing how or which utensil to use. Performance of a task may be more skillful than seen in a patient with ideomotor apraxia, but be conceptually wrong.[81]

Evaluation. Evaluation for apraxia usually includes both transitive gestures, those involved in manipulation of objects ("show me how you comb your hair"), and intransitive gestures, those meant to express ideas or feelings ("show me how you wave good-bye"). Use of objects are thought to highlight deficits in ideational apraxia, whereas intransitive gestures are considered a convenient measure of ideomotor apraxia.

Although apraxia usually affects all modalities, there may be a disruption of gestures in one modality (visual, verbal, tactile), but not another.[85] Testing is usually done initially by verbal command. Since apraxia is often associated with aphasia, requests for movements presented in the visual modality might be appropriate with severe aphasics. Visual presentation can take the form of providing a model for the patient to imitate or placing the object out of reach and asking the patient to pantomime its use. Testing is carried out in the tactile modality by having the patient handle the object while blindfolded and have him show how to use it.

Goodglass and Kaplan[28] describe a test of apraxia in which the patient is asked to perform common movements (Table 7.6). In this test, the patient is first asked to perform the movement on command (e.g., "show me how you use a screwdriver"). If unable to do this, he is asked to imitate the examiner. If unable to do this, he is then given a screwdriver. Apraxic patients frequently use body part as object when asked to perform a movement. For example, when asked to "show me how you brush your teeth," the patient may use the index finger as the brush. If this occurs, the patient is asked to try again as if holding the object. Use of body part as object

is rare in normal adults.[28] There are no norms for this evaluation. Scoring is subjective: normal—patient performed most tasks correctly on verbal request; impaired—patient performed most tasks correctly only when given the actual object; and severely impaired—patient was unable to perform the tasks even when given the actual object.[9]

Treatment. Poeck[82] states that there is a strong tendency for spontaneous recovery in apraxia and that treatment is usually not necessary with ideomotor apraxia, as the patient is able to use the limbs spontaneously.

Some treatment activities suggested include gross motor activities involving interpretation and use of tactile, kinesthetic, and proprioceptive stimulation to influence motor patterns; manual contact or guiding

Table 7.6
TEST OF APRAXIA[a]

Movements to Oral Command	Movements to Imitation	Movements with Real Object
Buccofacial		
1. Cough	If failed to command	Does not apply
2. Sniff	If failed to command	If failed to command
3. Blow out a match	If failed to command	If failed to command
4. Suck through a straw	If failed to command	If failed to command
5. Puff out cheeks	If failed to command	Does not apply
Intransitive Limb		
1. Wave good-bye	If failed to command	Does not apply
2. Beckon "come here"	If failed to command	Does not apply
3. Finger on lip for "shsh"	If failed to command	Does not apply
4. Salute	If failed to command	Does not apply
5. Signal "stop"	If failed to command	Does not apply
Transitive Limb[b]		
1. Brush teeth	If failed to command	If failed to command
2. Shave	If failed to command	If failed to command
3. Hammer	If failed to command	If failed to command
4. Saw board	If failed to command	If failed to command
5. Use screwdriver	If failed to command	If failed to command
Whole Body		
1. How does a boxer stand?	If failed to command	Does not apply
2. How does a golfer stand?	If failed to command	Does not apply
3. How does a soldier march in place?	If failed to command	Does not apply
4. How do you shovel snow?	If failed to command	Does not apply
5. Stand up, turn around twice, and sit down.	If failed to command	Does not apply

Serial Actions (with real objects only)

1. Provide box of matches and pack of cigarettes.
   "Take a cigarette and light up."
2. Provide paper, envelope, and penny stamp.
   "Put the paper in the envelope, seal it, and stamp it."
3. Provide candle, candlestick, box of matches.
   "Put the candle in the holder, light it, and blow it out."

[a]Reprinted with permission from Goodlglass, H., and Kaplan, E. *The Assessment of Aphasia and Related Disorders.* Philadelphia: Lea & Febiger, 1972.
[b]In items 2–5, for female subjects, say, "How would a man . . ."

of the apraxic extremity through the task; backward chaining; and use of the real object (personal communication, Lisen Cameron, O.T.R., Braintree Hospital, Braintree, MA, 1981). Therapists should keep verbal commands to a minimum and ask the patient to perform activities in the environment in which they would normally be done. Also, the patient can be asked to visualize the movement before attempting to carry it out.[9] The therapist may need to break down the activity into component parts and teach each part separately; then, as these are learned, the parts are integrated into two- and three-part activities.[27]

Evaluation and Treatment of Cognitive Deficits

"Cognitive disturbances are difficulties in information processing due to brain damage, which alter the ways in which the person experiences and responds to stimuli and interfaces with everyday life."[11] Attention, orientation, and memory are the basic processes upon which are built the higher cognitive functions. Higher cognitive functions include fund of knowledge, ability to manipulate old knowledge (e.g., calculations), social awareness and judgment, and abstract thinking.[86] These higher cognitive functions are a measure of the patient's reasoning and problem-solving skills, and deficits in these areas will be exhibited by the patient's inability to function effectively in the environment. These deficits can still be a significant problem years after trauma.

ATTENTION

Attention refers to the ability to focus on a specific stimulus without being distracted.[86] The patient's ability to sustain attention must be established before evaluation of more complex functions; if inattentive and distractible, the patient will be unable to assimilate information presented in the evaluation.

Alertness, a more basic arousal process, refers to a state in which the patient is able to respond to stimuli in the environment.[86] A patient who is attentive is alert. The opposite is not necessarily true; the patient may be alert, but unable to screen out extraneous stimuli in order to attend to the test stimulus.

Three aspects of attention are vigilance, distribution, and selection.[87] Vigilance is the ability to sustain attention over a long period of time; 30 sec is required for the purposes of a mental status exam.[86] Distribution of attention may vary from concentrated to diffuse. For example, the patient whose main concern is walking may be able to focus his attention during gait training in physical therapy, but his attention may be more diffuse when presented with a perceptual task that has no functional connection to walking for him. Lastly, attention can be selective; the patient may focus on one aspect of a task while ignoring others (e.g., if being asked to scan and tell what is happening in a picture, his attention may focus on one detail and he'll miss the story in the picture.)

Three operations are required in moving attention from one stimulus to another: disengagement of attention from current focus, moving attention to another location, and engaging attention at the new location.[88] Functionally, perseveration in an activity may indicate difficulty with the ability to disengage attention, while distractibility may indicate a failure to engage attention on a stimulus.

Evaluation. Attention is generally evaluated using the digit repetition test. Numbers are presented at a rate of one per second in groups of gradually increasing lengths. When the patient fails twice at one length, the test is stopped. Normally a person is able to repeat five to seven digits without difficulty; less than five is indicative of a deficit.[86] Reverse digit span (the patient is asked to repeat digits in reverse order), as well as serial addition and subtraction (e.g., "count backwards from 100 by 3's"), is used to determine the patient's ability to divide his attention.[89]

The random letter test is used as a test of vigilance.[86] This test consists of a series of letters that contain a target letter occurring with more than random frequency (Fig. 7.7). The letters are read to the patient at the rate of one letter per second. The patient indicates when he hears the target letter by tapping the table with a pencil. Common errors include omissions (failure to indicate a target letter), commissions (indicating any other than the target letter), and perseveration (failure to stop tapping after presentation of a target letter). Although the test is not standardized, the patient should be able to complete this task without error.

Treatment. As the environment has an effect on attention, treatment should begin in a quiet, uncluttered environment. When ability to attend improves, treatment can progress to a more normal environment. Be aware of the patient's emotional status, as this too will affect his ability to attend.

The patient who has difficulty attending is usually poorly oriented, his gaze is not focused on the task, and he may appear passive and uninvolved. The therapist may have to prepare the patient for the task. This is done by (1) focusing the patient's gaze and attention on the task (i.e., verbally calling his attention to the task and using items that are provocative—bright, colorful, etc.), (2) activating the patient (stating what is to be done and if necessary, physically moving the patient's hand, for example, to start the activity), and (3)

```
L T P E A O A I C T D A L A A

A N I A B F S A M R Z E O A D

P A K L A U C J T O E A B A A

Z Y F M U S A H E V A A R A T
```

Figure 7.7 Random letter test. (Reprinted with permission from Strub, R. L., and Black, F. W. *The Mental Status Examination in Neurology.* Philadelphia: F. A. Davis Company, 1977.)

engaging the patient's interest in the activity (may involve some sort of "pep talk").[90]

In a small study of two patients, contingent token reinforcement (tokens, which could be exchanged for a reward, were given to the patient when he exhibited attention to task behavior) was found to significantly improve attention in one patient, and improve attention, although not significantly, in the other patient.[91] In a further study of four patients, token reinforcement was linked to training in tasks of auditory and visual attention. A significant improvement in attention to task behavior was exhibited following training, but the improvement in attentional behavior did not translate into improvement on performance on tests of auditory recall memory. The author felt this may have been due to the small sample size, insufficient training, or presence of other cognitive deficits. Computer programs may be beneficial for treatment of attentional deficits. Further research into their effectiveness is needed.

ORIENTATION

After brain injury, the patients are frequently disoriented as to person, place, and/or time. The patient may be unable to state where he is and may wander away and get lost. He may be unable to identify others or himself. One study found that RBD patients tend to be more impaired on orientation tests than LBD patients; however, patients with aphasia were excluded from this study, which may have biased the results.[92]

Evaluation. Orientation to person is determined by asking the patient such questions as: What is your full name? How old are you? When is your birthday? etc. Assessment of orientation to place usually includes questions as to the name and location of the hospital/center where the patient is being tested. It might include the type of place and possibly directions between that location and his home.

Temporal orientation is generally assessed by asking: What is today's date? What day of the week is it? What time is it now? Five responses are scored: the stated day of the week, day of the month, month, year, and time of day (Table 7.7).[26]

The *Test of Orientation for Rehabilitation Patients* (TORP) is currently in research form.[93] This test, designed for use with inpatients, contains 48 items divided into five areas: person, place, time, schedule, and temporal continuity. The TORP is intended to develop into a standardized test with normative data for use with brain-injured and neurologically impaired patients without aphasia.

The *Galveston Orientation and Amnesia Test* (GOAT) is a rating scale that measures disorientation and amnesia after closed head injury.[94] It evaluates orientation, posttraumatic amnesia, and retrograde amnesia. It consists of 10 questions. A perfect score is 100; the defective range is a score below 66. It is designed to be used serially, on a daily basis. The serial scores have been found to be predictive of long-term outcome after acute head injury.[94]

Table 7.7
TEST OF TEMPORAL ORIENTATION[a]

Administration

What is today's date? (The patient is required to give month, day, and year.)
What day of the week is it?
What time is it now? (Examiner makes sure that the patient cannot look at a watch or clock.)

Scoring

Day of week: 1 error point for each day removed from the correct day to a maximum of 3 points.
Day of month: 1 error point for each day removed from the correct day to a maximum of 15 points.
Month: 5 error points for each month removed from the correct month with the qualification that, if the stated date is within 15 days of the correct date, no error points are scored for the incorrect month (for example, May 29 for June 2 = 4 error points).
Year: 10 error points for each year removed from the correct year to a maximum of 60 points with the qualification that, if the stated date is within 15 days of the correct date, no error points are scored for the incorrect year (for example, December 26, 1982 for January 2, 1983 = 7 error points).
Time of day: 1 error point for each 30 minutes removed from the correct time to a maximum of 5 points.

Interpretation

The total number of error points constitutes the patient's obtained score.

Normal: score of 0 to 2	Moderately defective: score of 4 to 7
Borderline: score of 3	Severely defective: score of 8 or more

[a]Adapted from Benton, A. L., Hamsher, K. deS., Varney, N. K., and Spreen, O. *Contributions to Neuropsychological Assessment —A Clinical Manual.* New York: Oxford University Press, 1983. Used with permission.

Treatment. Treatment is often compensatory. The patient uses cue cards, calendars, rehearsal, and other such techniques to remember these facts. One mode of treatment was described in which groups met daily to practice skills related to goals set by the group.[95,96] One such group defined seven behavioral objectives related to orientation to time, locale, identity of group members and staff, general facts, personal facts, and episodic information. Members of the group were rated daily by one of the group leaders on each of the behavorial objectives. This information was combined over a week and used to reflect the patients' development of dynamic cognitive skills over time rather than the acquisition of individual skills in a serial manner.[96] Although more research is needed to determine the effectiveness of this treatment, this type of daily monitoring of cognitive skills provides a means of justifying further treatment. If the therapist can objectively show that the patient is progressing, it is easier to justify treatment rather than basing continued need for treatment on a subjective description that the patient is "improving."

Table 7.8
MEMORY TERMS[a]

Type of Memory	Definition
Immediate memory	Memory held in conscious awareness, usually less than one minute
Short-term memory (STM)	Memory held temporarily; period of slightly longer than one minute elapses between stimulus and recall. Sometimes called primary memory.
Long-term memory (LTM)	Memory that involves an interval of more than a few minutes between stimulus and recall. Sometimes called secondary memory.
Working memory	Temporary storage and manipulation of information needed to perform a task.
Recent memory	Usually corresponds to long-term memory, includes memory from hours to months after stimulus presentation.
Remote memory	Very long term memory; memory for past events as from childhood.
Episodic memory	Memory of one's personal history (i.e., what you had for breakfast this morning, etc.).
Semantic memory	Personal knowledge of the world (i.e., that horses are big and ants are small, etc.).
Retrograde amnesia	Loss of ability to recall events prior to trauma.
Anterograde amnesia	Decreased memory of events occurring after trauma.
Posttraumatic amnesia	Period following trauma during which the patient is confused, disoriented, and seems to lack the ability to store and retrieve new information.

[a]This table was based on information from several sources.[8,87,97–100]

MEMORY

The abilities to process, store, and retrieve information depend on intact memory systems. There are several forms of memory and their definitions are often overlapping (Table 7.8). Memory processes include registration/encoding, consolidation/storage, and recall/retrieval of information. Any of these processes can be disrupted by brain damage. Memory deficits are a common sequelae of brain injury and their effects may continue for years posttrauma.[97]

If a patient has a decreased attention span and/or poor concentration, he will have difficulty getting the information to encode to begin with; therefore, it is important to distinguish between memory deficits per se and problems of concentration/attention. For instance, you may find that the patient does poorly on a formal memory test presented in a noisy and/or visually stimulating room, but performs adequately in a quiet room. Functionally, the patient may have difficulty remembering a one-handed shoe tying technique taught in a busy clinic, yet remember a more complicated dressing technique taught in a quiet room.

In studies on head-injured patients it has generally been found that although there are deficits in both short-term memory (STM) and long-term memory (LTM), LTM exhibits the major deficit.[101,102] This may be due to the fact that STM is felt to be equally represented in both hemispheres and therefore less affected by unilateral lesions.[92]

Verbal memory is generally thought to be located in the left hemisphere and figural/spatial memory in the right hemisphere.[98] LBD patients exhibit impaired verbal memory whether the information is presented visually or auditorily, whereas RBD patients show impaired verbal memory when material is presented visually.[103]

Evaluation. The most commonly used evaluation for memory is the *Wechsler Memory Scale*,[104] which is generally administered by psychologists and neuropsychologists. Occupational therapists generally do a screening of memory skills that includes estimation of immediate memory, STM, and LTM. Therapists need to know the status of these memory levels to plan any relearning program for the patient.

Digit repetition is generally used as an indicator for immediate memory. This was described earlier in the Attention section.

A measure of STM and LTM is to ask the patient to remember four words (e.g., brown, honesty, tulip, and eyedropper), and then test his immediate recall and recall after 5 min, 10 min, and 30 min.[86] If the patient is unable to recall any of the four words, verbal cues can be used to get an indication if there was any memory storage: semantic cues (e.g., "one word was a color"); phonemic cues (e.g., "eye . . . , eyedrop . . . , eyedropper); contextual cues (e.g., "A common flower in Holland is a _____"). If the patient is unable to profit from these cues, the therapist may ask the patient to choose from several examples (e.g., "Was the color red, brown, yellow, or green?"). A person should be able to remember all four words after a 10-minute delay, and after 30 minutes at least three of the four should be recalled.[86] This quiz could also be used to assess visual memory by pointing to four objects in the room and having the patient recall them immediately, after 5 min, and at the end of the session.[105]

Treatment. Treatment can focus on retraining and improvement of lost skills or on compensatory inter-

Table 7.9
COMPENSATORY MEMORY AIDS[a]

Technique	Description
Rehearsal	Patient repeats out loud or to self information to be remembered.
Visual imagery	Patient consolidates information to be remembered by making a mental picture that includes the information (e.g., to remember the name Barbara, patient pictures a barber holding the letter A).
Semantic elaboration	Patient consolidates information by making up a simple story (e.g., if patient is to remember the words lawyer, game, and hat, he develops a sentence such as "The lawyer wore a hat to the game").
First letter mnemonics	Patient consolidates information to be remembered by using the first letter of each word to make up a word or phrase to be remembered (e.g., to remember a shopping list of salt, ham, olives, peanut butter, pickles, ice cream, napkins, and grapes, he uses the word SHOPPING to help recall the items).
PQRST	A rehearsal method in which the patient: 1. Preview—skims the material for general content. 2. Questions—asks questions about the content. 3. Read—actively reads to answer the questions. 4. State—rehearses or repeats the information read. 5. Test—patient tests himself by answering the questions.
Establish motor routines and environmental predictability	Patient develops habits (e.g., if he cannot remember where he puts his watch, he sets up a routine in which he always places the watch in the same place when undressing and learns to associate that place with "Where is my watch?").

[a]This table was based on information from several sources.[108-111]

ventions. The use of computer-assisted cognitive rehabilitation programs is an example of retraining. In a study using computer programs for memory retraining, patients made significant gains from the first to last (12 total) session, but this gain was not maintained when retested 15 days later.[106] Another study, conducted on an acute medical rehabilitation unit, used a general memory retraining program consisting of visual imagery, verbal mediation, and other techniques. The researchers found no change in memory after 12 sessions and indicated that it may be more appropriate in the acute stage to work on attention/concentration deficits, rather than memory deficits.[107]

There are various compensatory techniques that can be used with patients who have memory deficits. These include both internal and external aids. For an explanation of various internal aids, see Table 7.9. External memory aids include storage devices (e.g., diaries, notebooks, lists, calculators, computers), cueing devices (e.g., alarm watches, bell timers), and structured environments that reduce memory load (e.g., labelling and/or color coding of drawers, cupboards, etc.).[112] The patient may require special training to use an external aid. For example, if the patient is using a notebook, he may have to be trained to consult the notebook on a regular basis, or how to construct meaningful cues in the notebook (or he may not understand the meaning of what he wrote at a later time). These aids, as well as others that the therapist can develop, can be applied to specific functional problems the patient is experiencing.

In determining which strategy to use, it is important to understand the patient's strengths and weaknesses.

If the patient has difficulty with writing and reading, he may benefit more from imagery than first-word mnemonics, or from the use of pictures in conjunction with words rather than words alone. When using imagery with a patient with RBD, more involved images that require mediation may be easier than simple images.[108]

It is also important that the patient and his family be involved in developing and using these strategies.[111] The patient may initially require cueing to use the techniques learned, and the family must know the techniques and how to assist the patient when at home and in the community.

PROBLEM SOLVING

Problem solving requires both an intact fund of knowledge and the ability to manipulate and apply this information to new or unfamiliar situations.[86] Problem solving generally consists of three stages: preparation—understanding the problem; production—generating possible solutions; and judgment—evaluating the solutions generated.[87] When solving a problem, a person may cycle repeatedly through these stages. A deficit in problem solving will affect all phases of the patient's daily life. He may exhibit difficulty ordering or sequencing information and thus be unable to figure out what bus to take or how to plan a meal. He may experience difficulty in social situations, being unable to figure out what to do.

Evaluation. An evaluation of problem solving frequently used is that of proverb interpretation. Proverbs are presented in ascending order of difficulty and scored on the basis of whether the response is concrete,

Table 7.10
PROVERB INTERPRETATION AND SCORING[a]

1. Rome wasn't built in a day.

0–concrete	"It took a long time to build Rome."
	"You can't build cities overnight."
1–semiabstract	"Don't do things too fast."
	"You have to be patient and careful."
	"You can't learn everything in one day."
2–abstract	"Great things take time to achieve."
	"If something is worth doing, it is worth doing carefully."
	"It takes time to do things well."

2. A drowning man will clutch at a straw.

0–concrete	"Don't let go when you're in the water."
	"That guy will grab anything."
1–semiabstract	"Self-preservation is important."
	"Nobody wants to die."
2–abstract	"A man in trouble tries anything to get out of it."
	"If sufficiently desperate, a man will try anything."

3. A golden hammer breaks an iron door.

0–concrete	"Gold can't break iron!"
	"Hammers can break down doors."
1–semiabstract	"Money wins everything."
	"The harder something is, the more you have to work to get it."
2–abstract	"Virtue conquers all."
	"If you have sufficient knowledge, you can accomplish even the most difficult."

4. The hot coal burns, the cold one blackens.

0–concrete	"Hot coals will burn you and leave it black."
	"Hot coals get black when they're cold."
1–semiabstract	"You can get trouble from both."
	"Getting burned and dirty are both bad."
2–abstract	"Extremes of anything can be bad."
	"There may be bad aspects to things that appear good."
	"One should be careful and not impetuous in any situation."

[a]Adapted from Strub, R. L., and Black, F. W. *The Mental Status Examination in Neurology.* Philadelphia: F. A. Davis Company, 1977. Used with permission.

semiabstract, or abstract (Table 7.10). This test is not standardized, but the average person should provide abstract interpretations to at least two proverbs and semiabstract to the remaining proverbs; any concrete response is suggestive of impairment.[86]

Social awareness is usually evaluated by responses to questions concerning environmental situations (e.g., "What should a person do if he sees smoke in a building?").[86] Social judgment concerns the patient's actual response in a real situation and is therefore difficult to assess in a testing situation. Information from family and staff must be used to determine his performance in day to day events.

Verbal similarities require the patient to describe the similarity between two objects or situations. The patient is presented with the following pairs of words, one set at a time: turnip-cauliflower; desk-bookcase; poem-novel; horse-apple. The responses are scored 0 to 2, 2 being the correct response. An average person is expected to obtain a score of at least 4; any concrete (0 points) answer or score of less than 4 is indicative of a deficit.[86]

Conceptual series completion is a test of verbal abstraction, problem solving, and reasoning (Table 7.11). The response is either correct or incorrect and the average person should be able to complete two of the four examples.[86]

The ability of the patient to solve math problems also is evaluated. These are presented both orally and in written form.

Treatment. Treatment may include exercises such as anagrams, puzzles,[9] analysis of proverbs, categorization exercises, or functional problem-solving tasks.[113] The patient is given different problems to solve. The therapist observes his manner of doing so and provides him with different strategies, as needed, to complete the task. These might include chaining (or breaking the activity down into its component parts), having the patient do the problem one step at a time, having the patient check for errors, providing the pa-

Table 7.11
CONCEPTUAL SERIES COMPLETION[a]

Test Items	Correct Response
1. 1 4 7 10 ____	13
2. AZ BY CX D ____	W
3. tote to snow on spun up stab ____	at
4. elephant 87654321 plant 5732 lap ____	735

[a]Reprinted with permission from Strub, R. L., and Black, F. W. *The Mental Status Examination in Neurology.* Philadelphia: F. A. Davis Company, 1977.

tient with external cues, or having the patient write down the steps to increase memory of them.[9]

Group treatment is frequently used. As the patient's deficits in higher level cognitive skills become readily apparent in a functional situation, this type of treatment provides a means of interaction and generalization to everyday life. It is a means for the patient to become more aware of his strengths and weaknesses, his social interactions, and the importance of compensatory strategies, as well as providing the opportunity to use the skills he has learned. Goals of these groups can vary according to the patient population. Goals of the group may be to provide strategies for problem solving and memory storage,[95] training in attention/concentration and abstract reasoning,[113] or reality orientation.[96]

STUDY QUESTIONS

Cognitive and Perceptual Evaluation and Treatment

1. Define cognition.
2. Define perception.
3. Name and define three approaches or types of treatment used for cognitive or perceptual deficits.
4. What are the factors to be considered when choosing an activity to treat cognitive perceptual deficits?
5. What are the differences in processing between the right hemisphere and the left hemisphere and why are these differences important for an occupational therapist to know?
6. What deficits are more likely to be seen in left-brain-damaged patients?
7. What deficits are more likely to be seen in right-brain-damaged patients?
8. What functional deficits could be ascribed to constructional apraxia? (The student should learn what functional deficits could be expected for each perceptual deficit.)
9. Compare and contrast ideomotor and ideational apraxia.
10. How might memory deficits be treated?

References

1. Eiben, C. F., Anderson, T. P., Lockman, L., Matthews, D. J., Dryja, R., Martin, J., Burril, C., Gottesman, N., O'Brian, P., and Witte, L. Functional outcome of closed head injury in children and young adults. *Arch. Phys. Med. Rehabil., 65:* 168-170, 1984.
2. Forer, S. K., and Miller, L. S. Rehabilitation outcome: comparative analysis of different patient types. *Arch. Phys. Med. Rehabil., 61:* 359-365, 1980.
3. Kaplan, J., and Hier, D. B. Visuospatial deficits after right hemisphere stroke. *Am. J. Occup. Ther., 36:* 314-321, 1982.
4. Lorenze, E. J., and Cancro, R. Dysfunction in visual perception with hemiplegia: its relation to activities of daily living. *Arch. Phys. Med. Rehabil., 43:* 514-517, 1962.
5. Ottenbacher, K. Cerebral vascular accident: some characteristics of occupational therapy evaluation forms. *Am. J. Occup. Ther., 34:* 268-271, 1980.
6. Cognitive rehabilitation survey results. *Cognit. Rehabil., 2*(6): 12-15, 1984.
7. Prigatano, G. P., and Fordyce, D. J. Cognitive dysfunction and psychological adjustment after brain injury. In *Neuropsychological Rehabilitation After Brain Injury.* Edited by G. P. Prigatano. Baltimore: John Hopkins University Press, 1986.
8. Lezak, M. D. *Neuropsychological Assessment.* New York: Oxford University Press, 1976.
9. Siev, E., Freishtat, B., and Zoltan, B. *Perceptual and Cognitive Dysfunction in the Adult Stroke Patient.* Thorofare, NJ: Slack Inc., 1986.
10. Bracy, O. L. Cognitive rehabilitation: a process approach. *Cognit. Rehabil., 4*(2): 10-17, 1986.
11. Ben-Yishay, Y., and Diller, L. Cognitive deficits. In *Rehabilitation of the Head Injured Adult.* Edited by M. Rosenthal, E. R. Griffith, M. R. Bond, and J. D. Miller. Philadelphia: F. A. Davis, 1983.
12. Golden, C. J. *Diagnosis and Rehabilitation in Clinical Neuropsychology.* Springfield, IL: Charles C Thomas, 1978.
13. Diller, L. A model for cognitive retraining in rehabilitation. *Clin. Psychol., 6:* 13, 1976.
14. Bracy, O., Lynch, W., Sbordone, R., and Berrol, S. Cognitive retraining through computers: fact or fad? *Cognit. Rehabil., 3*(2): 10-17, 1985.
15. American Occupational Therapy Association. *Computers Information Packet.* Rockville, MD: American Occupational Therapy Association, 1985.
16. Diller, L., and Weinberg, J. Differential aspects of attention in brain-damaged persons. *Percept. Mot. Skills, 35:* 71-81, 1972.
17. Ross, E. D., and Mesulam, M.-M. Dominant language functions of the right hemisphere? *Arch. Neurol., 36:* 144-148, 1979.
18. Ross, E. D. The aprosodias. *Neurology, 38:* 561-569, 1981.
19. Ruckdeschel-Hibbard, M., Gordon, W. A., and Diller, L. Affective disturbances associated with brain damage. In *Handbook of Clinical Neuropsychology.* Edited by S. Filskov and T. Boll. New York: John Wiley & Sons, 1986.
20. Bouska, M. J., and Kwatny, E. *Manual for Application of the Motor-Free Visual Perception Test to the Adult Population.* Philadelphia: Manual, P.O. Box 12246, 1983.
21. Sauguet, J., Benton, A. L., and Hecaen, H. Disturbances of the body schema in relation to language impairment and hemispheric locus of lesion. *J. Neurol. Neurosurg. Psychiatry, 34:* 496-501, 1971.
22. Boone, D. R., and Landes, B. A. Left-right discrimination in hemiplegic patients. *Arch. Phys. Med. Rehabil., 49:* 533-537, 1968.
23. Benton, A. Body schema disturbances: finger agnosia and right-left disorientation. In *Clinical Neuropsychology.* Edited by K. M. Heilman and E. Valenstein. New York: Oxford University Press, 1985.
24. MacDonald, J. C. An investigation of body scheme in adults with cerebral vascular accidents. *Am. J. Occup. Ther., 14:* 75-79, 1960.
25. Marmo, N. A. A new look at the brain-damaged adult. *Am. J. Occup. Ther., 28:* 199-206, 1974.
26. Benton, A. L., Hamsher, K. deS., Varney, N. K., and Spreen, O. *Contributions to Neuropsychological Assessment—A Clinical Manual.* New York: Oxford University Press, 1983.
27. Anderson, E. K., and Choy, E. Parietal lobe syndromes in hemiplegia. *Am. J. Occup. Ther., 24:* 13-18, 1970.
28. Goodglass, H., and Kaplan, E. *The Assessment of Aphasia and Related Disorders.* Philadelphia: Lea & Febiger, 1972.
29. Fox, J. Cutaneous stimulation—effects on selected tests of perception. *Am. J. Occup. Ther., 18:* 53-55, 1964.
30. Critchley, M. *The Parietal Lobes.* New York: Hafner Publishing Company, 1966.
31. Denes, G., Semenza, C., Stoppa, E., and Lis, A. Unilateral spatial neglect and recovery from hemiplegia. *Brain, 105:* 543-552, 1982.
32. Heilman, K. M., Watson, R. T., and Valenstein, E. Neglect and related disorders. In *Clinical Neuropsychology.* Edited by K. M. Heilman and E. Valenstein. New York: Oxford University Press, 1985.
33. Schenkenberg, T., Bradford, D. C., and Ajax, E. T. Line bisection and unilateral visual neglect in patients with neurologic impairment. *Neurology, 30:* 509-517, 1980.
34. Gainotti, G., Messerli, P., and Tissot, R. Qualitative analysis of unilateral spatial neglect in relation to laterality of cerebral lesions. *J. Neurol. Neurosurg. Psychiatry, 35:* 545-550, 1972.

35. Plourde, G., and Sperry, R. W. Left hemisphere involvement in left spatial neglect from right-sided lesions. *Brain, 107*: 95-106, 1984.

36. Colombo, A., DeRenzi, E., and Faglioni, P. The occurrence of visual neglect in patients with unilateral cerebral disease. *Cortex, 12*: 221-231, 1976.

37. Battersby, W. S., Bender, M. B., Pollack, M., and Kahn, R. L. Unilateral "spatial agnosia" ("inattention") in patients with cerebral lesions. *Brain, 79*: 68-93, 1956.

38. Brain, W. R. Visual disorientation with special reference to lesions of the right cerebral hemisphere. *Brain, 64*: 244-272, 1941.

39. Heilman, K. M., and Van Den Abell, T. Right hemisphere dominance for attention: The mechanism underlying hemispheric asymmetries of inattention (neglect). *Neurology, 30*: 327-330, 1980.

40. Riddoch, M. J., and Humphreys, G. W. The effects of cueing on unilateral neglect. *Neuropsychologia, 21*: 589-599, 1983.

41. Mesulam, M.-M. A cortical network for directed attention and unilateral neglect. *Ann. Neurol., 10*: 309-325, 1981.

42. Caplan, B. Stimulus effects in unilateral neglect? *Cortex, 21*: 69-80, 1985.

43. Weinberg, J., Diller, L., Gordon, W. A., Gerstman, L. J., Lieberman, A., Lakin, P., Hodges, G., and Ezrachi, O. Visual scanning training effect on reading-related tasks in acquired right brain damage. *Arch. Phys. Med. Rehabil., 58*: 479-486, 1977.

44. Weinberg, J., Piasetsky, E., Diller, L., and Gordon, W. Treating perceptual organization deficits in nonneglecting RBD stroke patients. *J. Clin. Neuropsychol., 4*: 59-75, 1982.

45. Anderson, E. K. Sensory impairments in hemiplegia. *Arch. Phys. Med. Rehabil., 52*: 293-297, 1971.

46. Albert, M. L. A simple test of visual neglect. *Neurology, 23*: 658-664., 1973.

47. Van Deusen, J. Normative data for ninety-three elderly persons on the Schenkenberg line bisection test. *Phys. Occup. Ther. Geriatrics, 3*(2): 49-54, 1983.

48. Diller, L., Weinberg, J., Piasetsky, J., Ruckdeschel-Hibbard, M., Egelko, S., Scotzin M., Couniotakis, J., and Gordon, W. *Methods for the Evaluation and Treatment of the Visual Perceptual Difficulties of Right Brain Damaged Individuals.* Monograph No. 67. New York: New York University Medical Center, 1980.

49. Gordon, W. A., Ruckdeschel-Hibbard, M., Egelko, S., Diller, L., Simmens, S., Langer, K., Sano, M., Orazem, J., and Weinberg, J. *Evaluation of the Deficits Associated with Right Brain Damage: Normative Data on the Institute of Rehabilitation Medicine Test Battery.* New York: New York University Medical Center, 1984.

50. Fox, J. Unilateral neglect: evaluation and treatment. *Phys. Occup. Ther. Geriatrics, 2*(4): 5-15, 1983.

51. Weinberg, J., Diller, L., Gordon, W. A., Gerstman, J., Lieberman, A., Lakin, P., Hodges, G., and Ezrachi, O. Training sensory awareness and spatial organization in people with right brain damage. *Arch. Phys. Med. Rehabil., 60*: 491-496, 1979.

52. Gordon, W. A., Hibbard, M. R., Egelko, S., Diller, L., Shaver, M. S., Lieberman, A., and Ragnarsson, K. Perceptual remediation in patients with right brain damage: a comprehensive program. *Arch. Phys. Med. Rehabil., 66*: 353-359, 1985.

53. Carter, L. T., Caruso, J. L., and Languirand, M. A. *The Thinking Skills Workbook: A Cognitive Skills Remediation Manual for Adults,* 2nd edition. Springfield, IL: Charles C Thomas, 1984.

54. Carter, L. T., Howard, B. E., and O'Neil, W. A. Effectiveness of cognitive skill remediation in acute stroke patients. *Am. J. Occup. Ther., 37*: 320-326, 1983.

55. Heilman, K. M., and Watson, R. T. Changes in the symptoms of neglect induced by changing task strategy. *Arch. Neurol., 35*: 47-49, 1978.

56. Ayres, A. J. *Sensory Integration and Praxis Tests.* Los Angeles: Western Psychological Services, 1987.

57. Frostig, M. *Developmental Test of Visual Perception.* Palo Alto, CA: Consulting Psychologist Press, 1966.

58. Bender, L. *Instructions for the Use of Visual Motor Gestalt Test.* New York: American Orthopsychiatric Association, 1946.

59. Paterson, A., and Zangwill, O. L. Disorders of visual space perception associated with lesions of the right cerebral hemisphere. *Brain, 67*: 331-358, 1944.

60. McFie, J., Piercy, M. F., Zangwill, O. L. Visual-spatial agnosia associated with lesions of the right cerebral hemisphere. *Brain, 73*: 167-190, 1950.

61. Charness, A. *Stroke/Head Injury: A Guide to Functional Outcomes in Physical Therapy Management.* Rockville, MD: Aspen Systems Corporation, 1986.

62. Teuber, H.-L., and Weinstein, S. Ability to discover hidden figures after cerebral lesions. *Arch. Neurol. Psychiatry, 76*: 369-379, 1956.

63. Russo, M., and Vignolo, L. A. Visual figure-ground discrimination in patients with unilateral cerebral disease. *Cortex, 3*: 113-127, 1967.

64. Petersen, P., and Wikoff, R. L. The performance of adult males on the Southern California Figure-Ground Visual Perception Test. *Am. J. Occup. Ther., 37*: 554-560, 1983.

65. Benton, A. L. Constructional apraxia and the minor hemisphere. *Confin. Neurol., 29*: 1-16, 1967.

66. DeRenzi, E. Constructional apraxia. In *Disorders of Space Exploration and Cognition.* New York: John Wiley & Sons, 1982.

67. Piercy, M., Hecaen, H., and Ajuriaguerra, J. Constructional apraxia associated with unilateral cerebral lesions—left and right sided cases compared. *Brain, 83*: 225-242, 1960.

68. Benton, A. L., and Fogel, M. L. Three-dimensional constructional praxis. *Arch. Neurol., 7*: 347-354, 1962.

69. Arrigoni, G., and Deranzi, E. Constructional apraxia and hemispheric locus of lesions. *Cortex, 1*: 170-197, 1964.

70. Warrington, E. K., James, M., and Kinsbourne, M. Drawing disability in relation to laterality of cerebral lesion. *Brain, 89*: 53-82, 1966.

71. Arena, R., and Gainotti, G. Constructional apraxia and visuoperceptive disabilities in relation to laterality of cerebral lesions. *Cortex, 14*: 463-473, 1978.

72. DeRenzi, E., and Faglioni, P. The relationship between visuo-spatial impairment and constructional apraxia. *Cortex, 3*: 325-342, 1967.

73. Gainotti, G., and Tiacci, C. Patterns of drawing disability in right and left hemispheric patients. *Neuropsychologia, 8*: 379-384, 1970.

74. Hecaen, H., and Assal, G. A comparison of constructive deficits following right and left hemispheric lesions. *Neuropsychologia, 8*: 289-303, 1970.

75. Hadano, K. On block design constructional disability in right and left hemisphere brain-damaged patients. *Cortex, 20*: 391-401, 1984.

76. Baum, B., and Hall, K. M. Relationship between constructional praxis and dressing in the head-injured adult. *Am. J. Occup. Ther., 35*: 438-442, 1981.

77. Bradley, K. P. The effectiveness of constructional praxis tests in predicting upper extremity dressing abilities. *Occup. Ther. J. Res., 2*: 184-185, 1982.

78. Kowalski-Lundi, M. H., and Mitcham, M. D. The relationship of constructional praxis to an upper extremity dressing task. *Occup. Ther. J. Res., 4*: 311-313, 1984.

79. Williams, N. Correlation between copying ability and dressing activities in hemiplegia. *Am. J. Phys. Med., 46*: 1332-1340, 1967.

80. Warren, M. Relationship of constructional apraxia and body scheme disorders to dressing performance in adult CVA. *Am. J. Occup. Ther., 35*: 431-437, 1981.

81. DeRenzi, E. Methods of limb apraxia examination and their bearing on the interpretation of the disorder. In *Neuropsychological Studies of Apraxia and Related Disorders.* Edited by E. A. Roy. Amsterdam: North-Holland Elsevier Science Publishers, 1985.

82. Poeck, K. Clues to the nature of disruptions to limb praxis. In *Neuropsychological Studies of Apraxia and Related Disorders.* Edited by E. A. Roy. Amsterdam: North-Holland Elsevier Science Publishers, 1985.

83. Kimura, D., and Archibald, Y. Motor functions of the left hemisphere. *Brain, 97*: 337-350, 1974.

84. Heilman, K. M. A tapping test in apraxia. *Cortex, 11*: 259-263, 1975.

85. DeRenzi, E., Faglioni, P., and Sorgato, P. Modality-specific and supramodal mechanisms of apraxia. *Brain, 105*: 301-312, 1982.

86. Strub, R. L., and Black, F. W. *The Mental Status Examination in Neurology.* Philadelphia: F. A. Davis Company, 1977.

87. Bourne, L. E., Dominowski, R. L., and Loftus, E. F. *Cognitive Processes.* Englewood Cliffs, NJ: Prentice-Hall, 1979.

88. Nissen, M. J. Neuropsychology of attention and memory. *J. Head Trauma Rehabil., 1*(3): 13-21, 1986.

89. Mack, J. L. Clinical assessment of disorders of attention and memory. *J. Head Trauma Rehabil., 1*(3): 22-33, 1986.

90. Ben-Yishay, Y., and Diller, L. Cognitive Remediation. In *Rehabilitation of the Head Injured Adult.* Edited by M. Rosenthal, E. R. Griffith, M. R. Bond, and J. D. Miller. Philadelphia: F. A. Davis, 1983.

91. Wood, R. L. Rehabilitation of patients with disorders of attention. *J. Head Trauma Rehabil., 1*(3): 43-53, 1986.

92. Wang, P. L., Kaplan, J. R., and Rogers, E. J. Memory functioning in hemiplegics: A neuropsychological analysis of the Wechsler Memory Scale. *Arch. Phys. Med. Rehabil., 56*: 517-521, 1975.

93. Deitz, J. C., Thorn, W. D., and Beeman, C. I. Assessing orientation in brain-injured patients: a new test. Presented at the 66th Annual Conference of the American Occupational Therapy Association, 1986.

94. Levin, H. S., O'Donnell, V. M., and Grossman, R. G. The Galveston Orientation and Amnesia Test: a practical scale to assess cognition after head injury. *J. Nerv. Ment. Dis., 167*: 675-684, 1979.

95. Lundgren, C. C., and Persechino, E. L. Cognitive group: a treatment program for head-injured adults. *Am. J. Occup. Ther., 40*: 397-401, 1986.

96. Corrigan, J. D., Arnett, J. A., Houck, L. J., and Jackson, R. D. Reality orientation for brain injured patients: group treatment and monitoring of recovery. *Arch. Phys. Med. Rehabil., 66*: 626-630, 1985.

97. Schacter, D. L., and Crovitz, H. F. Memory function after closed head injury: a review of the quantitative research. *Cortex, 13*: 150-176, 1977.

98. Russell, E. W. A multiple scoring method for the assessment of complex memory functions. *J. Consult. Clin. Psychol., 43*: 800-809, 1975.

99. Lewisohn, P. M., Danaher, B. G., and Kikel, S. Visual imagery as a mnemonic aid for brain-injured persons. *J. Consult. Clin. Psychol., 45*: 717-723, 1977.

100. American Rehabilitation Educational Network. *Head Trauma: Managing Memory Through Cognitive Rehabilitation.* Pittsburgh, PA: American Rehabilitation Educational Network, 1985.

101. Brooks, D. N. Long and short term memory in head injured patients. *Cortex, 11*: 329-340, 1975.

102. Roth, D. L., and Crosson, B. Memory span and long term memory deficits in brain-impaired patients. *J. Clin. Psychol., 41*: 521-527, 1985.

103. Schwartz, R., Shipkin, D., and Cermak, L. S. Verbal and nonverbal memory abilities of adult brain-damaged patients. *Am. J. Occup. Ther., 33*: 79-83, 1979.

104. Wechsler, D. A standardized memory scale for clinical use. *J. Psychol., 19*: 87-95, 1945.

105. Bigler, E. D. *Diagnostic Clinical Neuropsychology.* Austin: University of Texas Press, 1984.

106. Kerner, M. J., and Acker, M. Computer delivery of memory retraining with head injured patients. *Cognit. Rehabil., 3*(6): 26-31, 1985.

107. Fussey, I., and Tyerman, A. D. An exploration of memory retraining in rehabilitation following closed head injury. *Int. J. Rehab. Res., 8*: 465-467, 1985.

108. Wilson, B. Success and failure in memory training following a cerebral vascular accident. *Cortex, 18*: 581-594, 1982.

109. Malec, J., and Questad, K. Rehabilitation of memory after craniocerebral trauma: case report. *Arch. Phys. Med. Rehabil., 64*: 436-438, 1983.

110. Glasgow, R. E., Zeiss, R. A., Barrera, M., and Lewisohn, P. M. Case studies on remediating memory deficits in brain-damaged individuals. *J. Clin. Psychol., 33*: 1049-1054, 1977.

111. Milton, S. B. Compensatory memory strategy training: a practical approach for managing persistent memory problems. *Cognit. Rehabil., 3*(6): 8-15, 1985.

112. Glisky, E. L., and Schacter, D. L. Remediation of organic memory disorders: current status and future prospects. *J. Head Trauma Rehabil., 1*(3): 54-63, 1986.

113. Carberry, H., and Burd, B. The use of psychological theory and content as a media in the cognitive and social training of head injured patients. *Cognit. Rehabil., 3*(4): 8-10, 1985.

Supplementary Reading

Annett, J. and Sparrow, J. Transfer of training: a review of research and practical implications. *Programmed Learning & Educational Technology: Journal of the Association for Programmed Learning, 22*(2): 116-124, 1985.

Billig, N. et al. Assessment of depression and cognitive impairment after hip fracture. *J. Am. Geriatr. Soc., 34*(7): 499-503, 1986.

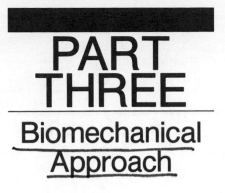

PART THREE
Biomechanical Approach

The principles and methods that are presented in this section are appropriate for patients who have problems that directly affect their range of motion, strength, or endurance necessary to perform daily life tasks, but who have voluntary control of specific movements and/or motor patterns.

The biomechanical approach to treatment applies the mechanical principles of kinetics and kinematics to movement of the human body. Historically, the biomechanical approach preceded development of the neurodevelopmental approach. Physical activity for therapeutic exercise was used by occupational therapists in the 1940s and was then termed kinetic occupational therapy to signify its restorative rather than diversional goal. Exercise techniques were borrowed from other disciplines either directly or combined with activities. Restorative efforts focused on specific diseases or disability categories and emphasized the application of these techniques to particular problems without recognizing common or underlying principles.[1] Activity was prescribed based on assumptions about therapeutic effects for particular conditions. Some of these assumptions, e.g., exclusive recruitment of prime movers during activities requiring rapid, phasic movements, have since been called into question.[2,3] Despite these shortcomings, biomechanical treatment regimens have been effective in restoring skills needed for function. Information is now becoming available from studies that use sophisticated instrumentation to measure movement parameters and muscle participation in movement to allow greater precision in activity prescription. So, although biomechanical treatment has a long history, it is a dynamically developing approach to which research of many disciplines contributes by identifying effective techniques and the precautions to be observed and by isolating variables that control outcome.

References
1. Mosey, A. C. Occupational therapy—historical perspective. Involvement in the rehabilitation movement—1942–1960. *Am. J. Occup. Ther.* 25(5): 234–236, 1971.
2. Trombly, C. A., and Cole, J. M. Electromyographic study of four hand muscles during selected activities. *Am. J. Occup. Ther.,* 33(7): 440–449, 1979.
3. Trombly, C. A., and Quintana, L.A. Activity analysis: electromyographic and electrogoniometric verification. *J. Occup. Ther. Res.,* 3(2): 104–120, 1983.

Evaluation

Catherine A. Trombly and Anna Deane Scott

Procedures for evaluation of range of motion, edema, muscle strength, and endurance are described in this chapter. The clinical measures most commonly used by practicing therapists are presented in detail.

Sensation

Patients with conditions that may also affect peripheral sensation must be evaluated to determine the extent and distribution of sensory loss or dysfunction. The procedures described in chapter 3 are used for this evaluation.

Range of Motion

Each joint is potentially able to move in certain directions and to certain limits of motion due to its structure and the integrity of surrounding tissues. Trauma or disease that affects joints or surrounding tissues can alter the amount of motion at the joint. When there is alteration of joint motion, evaluation and treatment of this problem are indicated. Because it is the responsibility of the occupational therapist to document the effectiveness of treatment to increase range of motion, the therapist must be skilled in the measurement of joint range of motion. If you treat it, measure it!

The most widely used method of measuring joint motion is the system using the universal goniometer. Every goniometer has a protractor, an axis, and two arms. The stationary arm extends from the protractor on which degrees are marked. The other arm is termed the movable arm and has a center line or pointer to indicate the degrees of the angle measured. The axis is the point where these two arms are riveted together. Goniometers vary in size; large goniometers most accurately measure large joints and small goniometers most accurately measure small joints. A full-circle goniometer that measures degrees from 0° to 180° in each direction permits measurement of motion in both directions, i.e., flexion and extension, without repositioning the tool. Half-circle goniometers are also useful, and a small half-circle goniometer is preferred for measuring the forearm, wrist, and hand. When using a half-circle goniometer it is necessary to position the protractor opposite to the direction of motion for the indicator to remain on the face of the protractor. A finger goniometer is of special design with a short movable arm and flat arm surfaces that fit comfortably over the finger joints (see Fig. 8.1).

In using the goniometer to measure joint motion, care must be taken when placing the axis and the two arms to ensure accuracy and reliability. The axis of the goniometer is placed over the axis of joint motion, which is the point around which the motion occurs. The axis of motion for some joints coincides with bony landmarks, whereas for other joints the axis of motion must be found by observing movement of the joint to determine the point around which motion occurs. Because it is not always possible to center the axis of the goniometer over a specific anatomical landmark, pri-

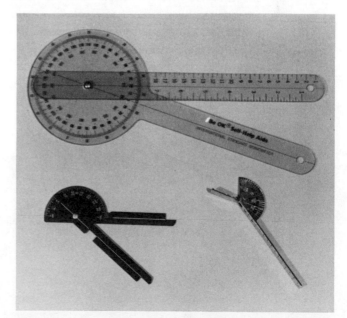

Figure 8.1 Full-circle, half-circle, and finger goniometers.

mary attention is focused on aligning the two arms of the goniometer correctly, which in turn assures correct placement of the axis.[1] When the two arms of the goniometer are placed correctly they will intersect at the axis of motion. The stationary arm is positioned parallel to the longitudinal axis of the part proximal to the joint; the movable arm is positioned parallel to the longitudinal axis of the part distal to the joint. Which arm of the goniometer is used proximally and which is aligned with the moving part is not as important for accuracy of measurement as is correct alignment of the arms. In shoulder flexion, for example, the axis at the beginning of the motion is located below the acromion process, but at the end of the motion the arm position has changed to the extent that the original axis position of the goniometer is no longer accurately placed over the joint. Because the anatomical landmark that corresponds to the axis of motion shifts during the movement, measurements are taken at the beginning and again at the end of the range of motion. These two measurements represent the limits of motion.

There are many factors of the test situation that influence accuracy and reliability. Care must be taken to reduce the effect of these factors. The tester supports both the body part and the goniometer in a way that does not interfere with movement of the joint, i.e., supports proximally and distally to the joint leaving the joint free to move. Because clothing may interfere with full movement of a joint and can obstruct the correct alignment of the goniometer, the patient's clothing is removed as necessary, but feelings of modesty are respected. In addition, accuracy and reliability can be influenced by environmental and patient-related factors. Environmental variables include the time of day, the temperature and atmosphere of the room, the kind of goniometer used, and the experience and rigor of the tester. Therefore, original and retest measurements must be taken at the same time of day by the same person using the same kind of goniometer and technique in the same or similar setting. Patient-related factors include reaction to pain and fatigue and feelings of fear, tension, or stress. Every effort is made to make the patient physically and emotionally comfortable. With careful adherence to technique in the use of the goniometer, measurements taken at different times by the same tester are accurate to within 3° to 5°.[2,3] Those taken by different testers, using standard technique, are accurate to within 5° for the upper extremity, not including the hand, which was not studied, and 6° for the lower extremity.[3] Interrater reliability, determined from measures made by four therapists at four different test sessions, has been reported to be $r = 0.86$ for upper-extremity motions and $r = 0.58$ for lower-extremity motions.[3] Intrarater reliability was $r = 0.89$ for upper-extremity and $r = 0.80$ for lower-extremity motions.[3] These levels of reliability have also been found when tested clinically.[4]

RANGE OF MOTION MEASUREMENT TECHNIQUE

If there is no limitation in active range of motion (AROM) as determined by observation of the patient's ability to move or no limitation in passive range of motion (PROM) as determined by passively moving each joint to the limits of motion, a detailed measurement is not needed. Range of motion can be noted to be within normal limits (WNL) as determined by observation. Detailed measurements of joints that have limitations are taken and recorded to objectively identify problems, to assist in treatment planning, and to document improvement following treatment.

Measurement of joint range may be done actively or passively. PROM indicates the amount of motion at a given joint when the joint is moved by the therapist. Measurement of AROM indicates the amount of motion at a given joint achieved by a patient using his own muscle strength. If AROM is less than PROM this is a problem of muscle weakness or tendon integrity in hands. (See Chapter 25.) AROM measurement is used as a supplement to muscle testing to indicate fine gradations of change in weak muscles. When joint limitation is the problem being evaluated, PROM must be done.

Measurements of the upper extremities are given in more detail here than those for the lower extremities because daily life tasks involve more refined upper-extremity movement and necessitate more detailed consideration of hand function.

Some clinics still use a 180° starting position, that is, anatomical position is 180° and motion occurs toward zero by this method. In the International SFTR (sagittal, frontal, transverse, rotation) Method the zero starting position is used, and ranges are recorded in terms of anatomical planes.[5]

A Neutral Zero Method for measuring and recording is recommended by the Committee on Joint Motion of the American Academy of Orthopaedic Surgeons[6] and is generally used. In this method anatomical position is considered to be zero, or if a given starting position is different from anatomical position, it is defined as the zero starting position. Extension is the term used for the natural motion opposite to flexion, and hyperextension is used only when the motion is unnatural, as occasionally seen, for example, in the elbow or knee joints. Ranges are compared to the noninvolved extremity or to average ranges expected for each motion. The average ranges that have been stated by the Committee on Joint Motion are estimates rather than documented norms and are included below with the instructions for measurement and on the recording form.

Recording Range of Motion

Each measurement is accurately recorded on a range of motion form. The therapist must date and sign each evaluation and indicate whether measurements represent AROM or PROM. A sample form is provided here, although each treatment facility may have its own form (see Table 8.1). Some facilities use forms with graphic representation, in which case each range of motion is shaded on a diagram of the movement. Whether the recording is numerical or graphical, the starting and end-

Table 8.1
RANGE OF MOTION

AROM _____
PROM _____

Patient's Name _____

Left			Date of Measurement		Right	
			Tester's Name			
			SHOULDER			
			Flexion	0-180		
			Extension	0-60		
			Abduction	0-180		
			Horizontal Abduction	0-90		
			Horizontal Adduction	0-45		
			Internal Rotation	0-70		
			External Rotation	0-90		
			Internal Rotation (Alternate)	0-80		
			External Rotation (Alternate)	0-60		
			ELBOW and FOREARM			
			Flexion-Extension	0-150		
			Supination	0-80		
			Pronation	0-80		
			WRIST			
			Flexion	0-80		
			Extension	0-70		
			Ulnar Deviation	0-30		
			Radial Deviation	0-20		
			THUMB			
			CM Flexion	0-15		
			CM Extension	0-20		
			MP Flexion-Extension	0-50		
			IP Flexion-Extension	0-80		
			Abduction	0-70		
			Opposition	cm.		
			INDEX FINGER			
			MP Flexion	0-90		
			MP Hyperextension	0-45		
			PIP Flexion-Extension	0-100		
			DIP Flexion-Extension	0-90		
			Abduction	No Norm		
			Adduction	No Norm		

ing positions (limits of motion) for each movement are included.

If starting position cannot be achieved due to a limitation, measurement is taken as close to starting position as possible and again at end position or as close to end position as possible. The limits thus obtained are recorded to indicate limitations in movement.

Examples using elbow flexion:

> 0° to 150°—No limitation
> 20° to 150°—A limitation in extension
> 0° to 120°—A limitation in flexion
> 20° to 120°—Limitations in both flexion and extension

Some therapists indicate a limitation in extension by recording the limitation negatively, for example, −20° of extension or lacks 20° of extension or −20° to 150°. On the other hand, some therapists record −20° to 150°

to indicate that there are 20 degrees of hyperextension in a joint where hyperextension is not normally present. If hyperextension as an unnatural motion is recorded as a separate measurement as recommended by the American Academy of Orthopaedic Surgeons then the elbow range would state 0° to 20° of hyperextension and 0° to 150° of flexion and would fully describe the available range of motion without confusion, while eliminating the use of unclear negative recordings. According to the American Academy of Orthopaedic Surgeons the following notations of range would be used to describe these elbow measurements:

> 0° to 150° of flexion
> 150° to 0° of extension
> 0° to 20° of hyperextension, if present

A recording of 20° to 150° of flexion would be termed a 20° flexion deformity.[6] Since these notations vary in

Table 8.1—*continued*

	MIDDLE FINGER			
	MP Flexion	0-90		
	MP Hyperextension	0-45		
	PIP Flexion-Extension	0-100		
	DIP Flexion-Extension	0-90		
	Abduction (radially)	No Norm		
	Adduction (ulnarly)	No Norm		
	RING FINGER			
	MP Flexion	0-90		
	MP Hyperextension	0-45		
	PIP Flexion-Extension	0-100		
	DIP Flexion-Extension	0-90		
	Abduction	No Norm		
	Adduction	No Norm		
	LITTLE FINGER			
	MP Flexion	0-90		
	MP Hyperextension	0-45		
	PIP Flexion-Extension	0-100		
	DIP Flexion-Extension	0-90		
	Abduction	No Norm		
	Adduction	No Norm		
	HIP			
	Flexion	0-120		
	Extension	0-30		
	Abduction	0-45		
	Adduction	0-30		
	Internal Rotation	0-45		
	External Rotation	0-45		
	KNEE			
	Flexion-Extension	0-135		
	ANKLE			
	Dorsiflexion	0-20		
	Plantar Flexion	0-50		
	Inversion	0-35		
	Eversion	0-15		

Comments:

their meaning, it is important to clarify the intended meaning and to ensure consistency within the same treatment facility.

In a fused joint the starting and end positions will be the same with no range of motion. This is recorded as fused at *x* degrees. If a joint that normally moves in two directions is unable to be moved in one direction, this range of motion is recorded as *None*. For example, if wrist flexion is 15° to 80° with a 15° flexion contracture, the wrist cannot be positioned at zero or moved into extension. Wrist extension is therefore *None*.

If range of motion is limited by pain or other abnormalities, such as edema or adipose tissue, the reason for the limitation should be clearly indicated on the range of motion recording form.

Interpreting the Results

The recording of range of motion is reviewed to identify which joints are limited. A significant limitation is one that decreases function or may lead to a deformity. Some causes of range of motion limitations are joint disease or injury, edema, pain, spasticity, skin tightness, muscle and tendon shortening due to immobilization, or muscle weakness. With the significant limitations and underlying causes in mind, the short-term goals necessary to achieve the long-term goal of increased range of motion can be identified. Treatment goals will reflect the identified problem. For example, if skin, joint, and/or muscle tissue has become shortened due to immobilization, the goal will be to increase range through stretching these tissues. If the limitation is due to edema, pain, spasticity, or muscle weakness, the primary goal is to reduce or correct the underlying problem, and the secondary goal is to prevent loss of range of motion due to the immobility imposed by the primary condition.

MEASUREMENT OF THE UPPER EXTREMITY

For the measurements given here, the patient is seated with trunk erect against the back of an armless straight chair. The measurements may be taken with the patient standing or supine, if necessary, unless otherwise noted.

Shoulder Flexion

Movement of the humerus anteriorly in the sagittal plane (0 to 180°, which represents both glenohumeral and axioscapular motion).

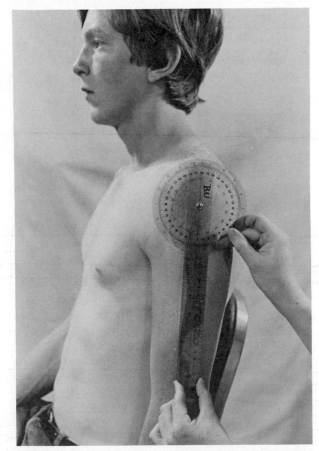

Figure 8.2 Starting position: Arm at side in midposition.

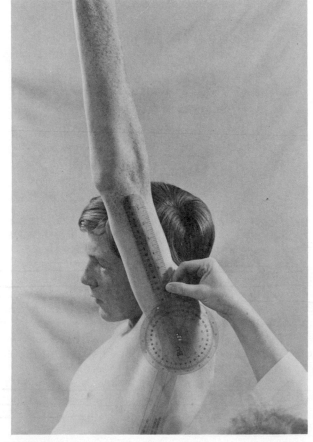

Figure 8.3 End position: Arm overhead in midposition.

Goniometer Placement

Axis. A point through the lateral aspect of the glenohumeral joint around which motion occurs, located approximately 1 inch below the acromion process.

Stationary Arm. Parallel to the lateral midline of the trunk.

Movable Arm. Parallel to the longitudinal axis of the humerus on the lateral aspect.

Possible Substitutions. Trunk extension, shoulder abduction.

✗ Shoulder Extension

Movement of the humerus posteriorly in a sagittal plane (0° to 60°).

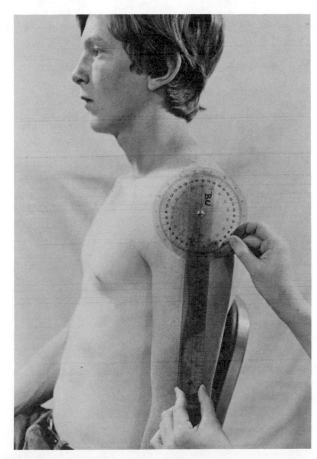

Figure 8.4 Starting position: Patient seated at the edge of the chair so there is no restriction behind humerus. Arm at side in internal rotation.

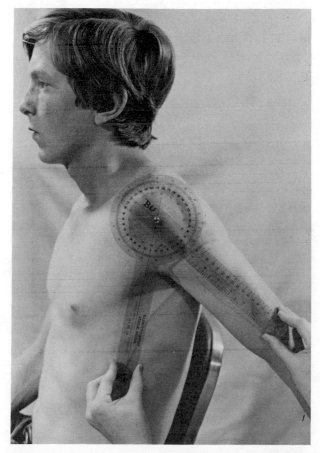

Figure 8.5 End position: Arm backwards at limit of motion.

Goniometer Placement

Axis. A point through the lateral aspect of the glenohumeral joint around which motion occurs, located approximately 1 inch below the acromion process.

Stationary Arm. Parallel to the lateral midline of the trunk.

Movable Arm. Parallel to the longitudinal axis of the humerus on the lateral aspect.

Possible Substitutions. Trunk flexion, scapular elevation and downward rotation, shoulder abduction.

Shoulder Abduction

Movement of the humerus laterally in a frontal plane (0° to 180°, which represents both glenohumeral and axioscapular motion).

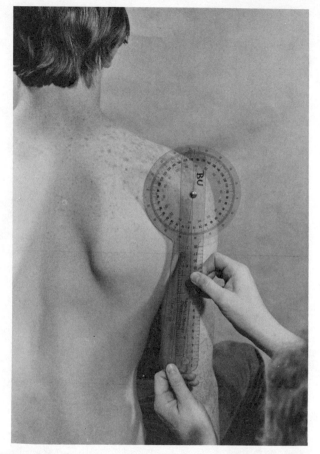

Figure 8.6 Starting position: Arm at side in external rotation, which allows the humerus to clear the acromion process.

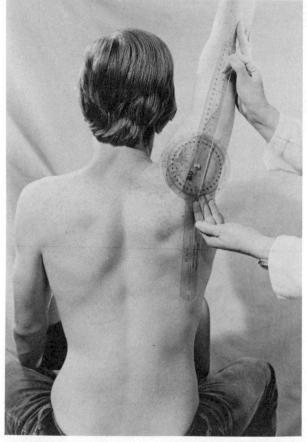

Figure 8.7 End position: Arm overhead with palm facing opposite side.

Goniometer Placement

Axis. A point through the anterior or posterior aspect of the glenohumeral joint. Some people consider measurement from the anterior aspect safer, since the patient's back can be supported against the chair, but it is preferable to measure adult female patients from the posterior aspect.

Stationary Arm. Laterally along the trunk, parallel to the spine.

Movable Arm. Parallel to the longitudinal axis of the humerus.

Possible Substitutions. Lateral flexion of trunk, scapular elevation, shoulder flexion or extension.

Horizontal Abduction

Movement of the humerus on a horizontal plane from a position of 90° of shoulder flexion to a position of 90° of shoulder abduction and to the limit of motion (0° to 90°).

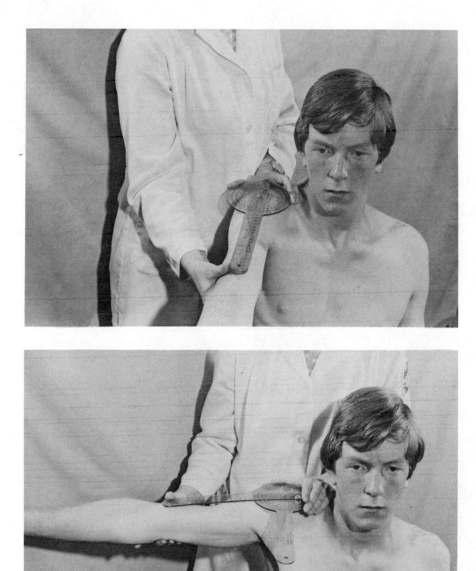

Figure 8.8 Starting position: Arm internally rotated and at 90° of shoulder flexion.

Figure 8.9 End position: Arm at 90° of shoulder abduction.

Goniometer Placement

Axis. On top of the acromion process.

Stationary Arm. To start, this arm is parallel to the longitudinal axis of the humerus on the superior aspect and remains in that position, perpendicular to the body, although the humerus moves away. (An alternative position of the stationary arm is across the shoulder, anterior to the neck, and in line with the opposite acromion process. In this alternate position the goniometer would read 90° at the start, and this must be considered when recording.)

Movable Arm. Parallel to the longitudinal axis of the humerus on the superior aspect.

Possible Substitution. Trunk rotation.

Horizontal Adduction

Movement of the humerus on a horizontal plane from a position of 90° of shoulder abduction through a position of 90° of shoulder flexion, across the trunk to the limit of motion. The 90° of return motion from horizontal abduction is not measured. The motion is measured from a position of 90° shoulder flexion across the trunk (0° to 45°).

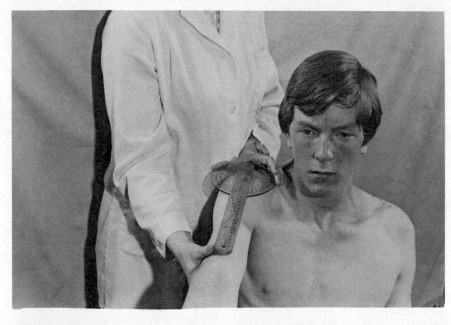

Figure 8.10 Starting position: Arm internally rotated and at 90° of shoulder flexion.

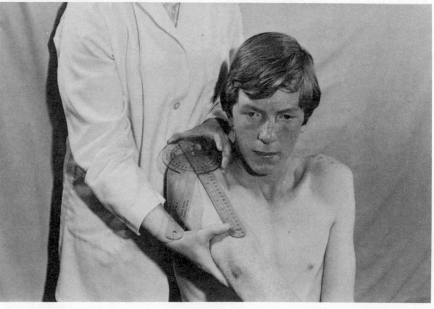

Figure 8.11 End position: Arm across trunk at limit of motion.

Goniometer Placement

Axis. On top of the acromion process.

Stationary Arm. Parallel to the longitudinal axis on the superior aspect of the humerus in starting position and remains perpendicular to the body, although the humerus moves away. The alternative placement given for horizontal abduction also applies in this case.

Movable Arm. Parallel to the longitudinal axis of the humerus on the superior aspect.

Possible Substitution. Trunk rotation.

Internal Rotation

Movement of the humerus in a medial direction around the longitudinal axis of the humerus (0° to 70°).

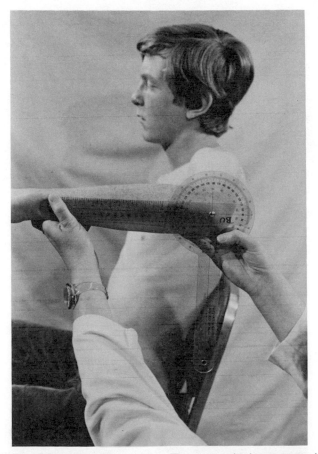

Figure 8.12 Starting position: The extremity is supported in a position of 90° of shoulder abduction and 90° of elbow flexion with the forearm pronated and parallel to the floor.

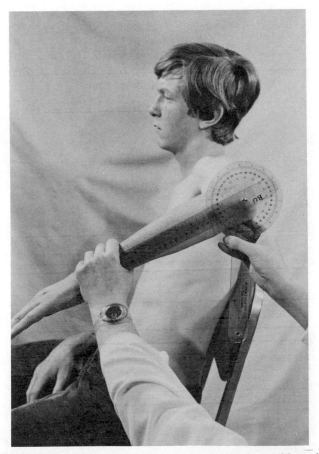

Figure 8.13 End position: The extremity is in a position of 90° of shoulder abduction and 90° of elbow flexion; forearm and hand have moved toward the floor to the limit of motion.

Goniometer Placement

Axis. Olecranon process of ulna.

Stationary Arm. Perpendicular to the floor, which will be parallel to the lateral trunk if the patient is sitting up straight with his hips at 90°. The goniometer will read 90° at the start, and this score must be deducted from the final score when recording range of motion.

Movable Arm. Parallel to the longitudinal axis of the ulna.

Possible Substitutions. Scapular elevation and downward rotation, trunk flexion, elbow extension.

Note. In the supine position with the shoulder abducted to 90° and the elbow flexed to 90° the stationary arm is perpendicular to the floor with the movable arm along the ulna. The goniometer will read 0° at the start.[1]

External Rotation

Movement of the humerus in a lateral direction around the longitudinal axis of the humerus (0° to 90°).

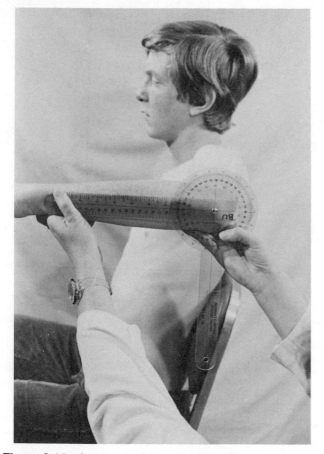

Figure 8.14 Starting position: The extremity is supported in a position of 90° of shoulder abduction and 90° of elbow flexion with the forearm pronated and parallel to the floor.

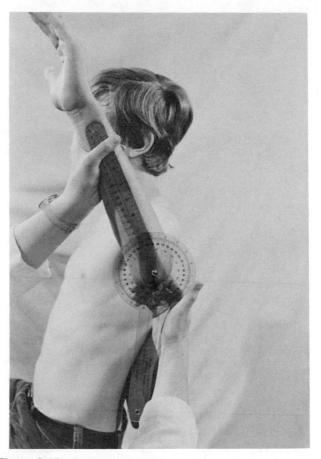

Figure 8.15 End position: The extremity is in a position of 90° of shoulder abduction and 90° of elbow flexion; forearm and hand have moved toward the ceiling to the limit of motion.

Goniometer Placement

Axis. Olecranon process of ulna.

Stationary Arm. Perpendicular to the floor. The goniometer will read 90° at the start, and this must be considered when recording range.

Movable Arm. Parallel to the longitudinal axis of the ulna.

Possible Substitutions. Scapular depression and upward rotation, trunk extension, elbow extension.

Note. In the supine position the humerus should be supported on a pad to place it in line with the acromion process. The measurement is the same as for internal rotation.[1]

Internal and External Rotation: Alternate Method

If shoulder limitation prevents positioning for the previously described method, the patient may be seated with humerus adducted to his side and elbow flexed to 90°. This method will be inaccurate in internal rotation if the patient has a large abdomen. (Internal rotation: 0° to 80°; external rotation: 0° to 60°).

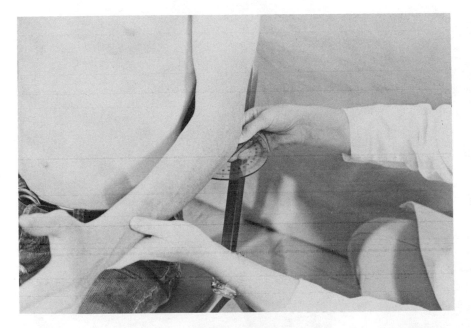

Figure 8.16 External rotation (alternate method): Start position.

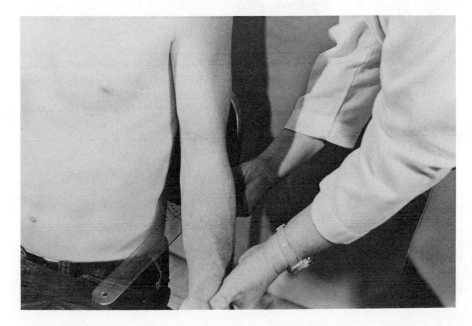

Figure 8.17 External rotation (alternate method): End position.

Elbow Flexion-Extension

Movement of the supinated forearm anteriorly in the sagittal plane (0° to 150°).

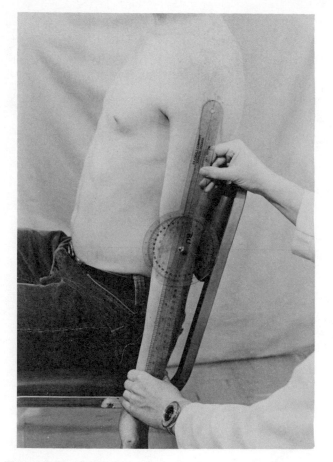

Figure 8.18 Starting position: Arm in anatomical position. This measurement is recorded as the limit of extension.

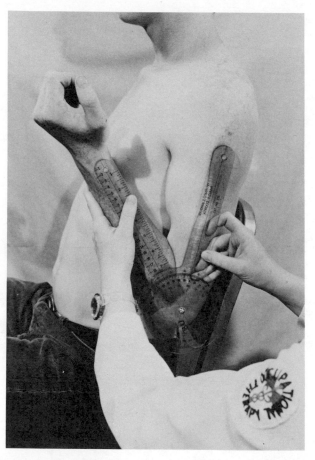

Figure 8.19 End position: Forearm has moved toward the humerus so that the hand approximates the shoulder to the limit of motion of elbow flexion.

Goniometer Placement

Axis. Lateral epicondyle of the humerus.
Stationary Arm. Parallel to the longitudinal axis of the humerus on the lateral aspect.

Movable Arm. Parallel to the longitudinal axis of the radius.

Forearm Supination

Rotation of the forearm laterally around its longitudinal axis from midposition (0° to 80°).

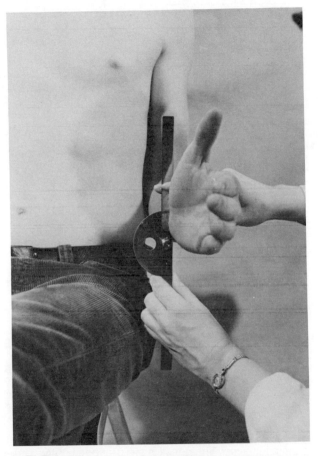

Figure 8.20 Starting position: Humerus adducted to the side and elbow flexed to 90° with the forearm in midposition.

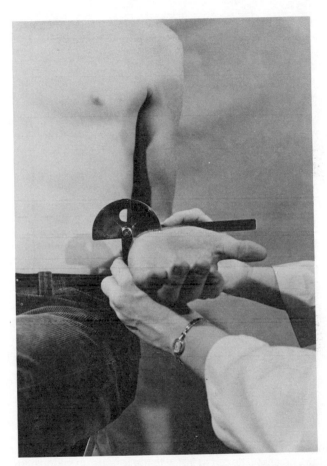

Figure 8.21 End position: Forearm rotated so that the palm faces up.

Goniometer Placement

Axis. Parallel to the longitudinal axis of the forearm displaced toward the ulna.

Stationary Arm. Perpendicular to the floor.

Movable Arm. Across the distal radius and ulna on the volar surface.

Possible Substitutions. Shoulder adduction and external rotation.

Forearm Supination: Alternate Method

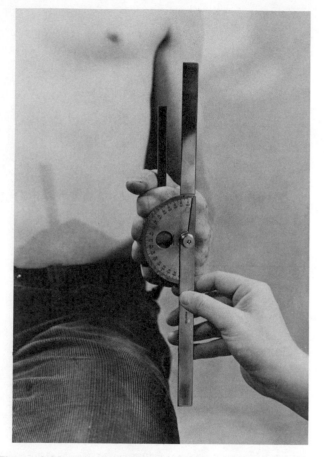

Figure 8.22 Starting position: Humerus adducted to the side and elbow flexed to 90° with the forearm in midposition. A pencil is held in the tightly closed fist with the pencil protruding from the radial side of the hand.

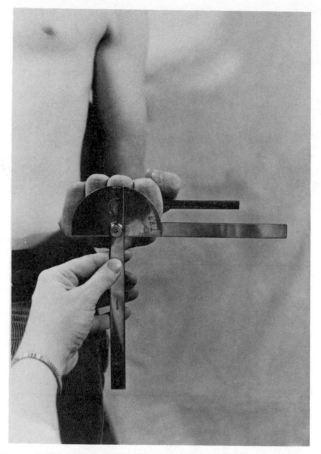

Figure 8.23 End position: The forearm is rotated so that the palm faces up. The pencil is still grasped tightly.

Goniometer Placement

Axis. Head of the third metacarpal, which coincides with the longitudinal axis of the forearm.
Stationary Arm. Perpendicular to the floor.
Movable Arm. Parallel to the pencil.

Possible Substitutions. Movement of pencil by release of grasp or by wrist extension and deviation, shoulder adduction, and external rotation.

Forearm Pronation

Rotation of the forearm medially around its longitudinal axis from midposition (0° to 80°).

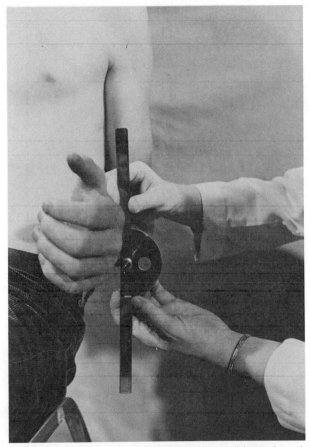

Figure 8.24 Starting position: Humerus adducted to the side and elbow flexed to 90° with the forearm in midposition.

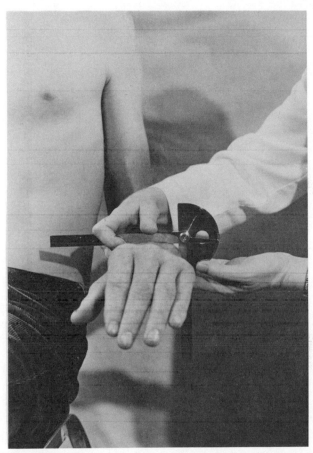

Figure 8.25 End position: Forearm rotated so that the palm faces down.

Goniometer Placement

Axis. Longitudinal axis of forearm displaced toward the ulnar side.

Stationary Arm. Perpendicular to the floor.

Movable Arm. Across the distal radius and ulna on the dorsal surface.

Possible Substitutions. Abduction and internal rotation of the shoulder.

Forearm Pronation: Alternate Method

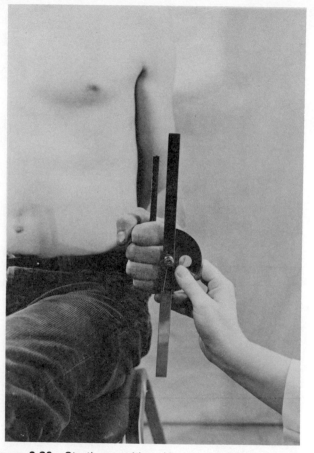

Figure 8.26 Starting position: Humerus adducted to the side and elbow flexed to 90° with the forearm in midposition. A pencil is held in the tightly closed fist, with the pencil protruding from the radial side of the hand.

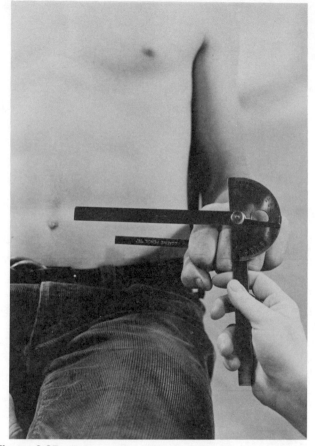

Figure 8.27 End position: The forearm is rotated so that the palm faces down. The pencil is still grasped tightly.

Goniometer Placement

Axis. Head of the third metacarpal, which coincides with the longitudinal axis of the forearm.

Stationary Arm. Perpendicular to the floor.

Movable Arm. Parallel to the pencil.

Possible Substitutions. Movement of pencil by release of grasp or by wrist flexion and deviation, or abduction and internal rotation of the shoulder.

Wrist Flexion (Volar Flexion)

Movement of the hand volarly in the sagittal plane (0° to 80°).

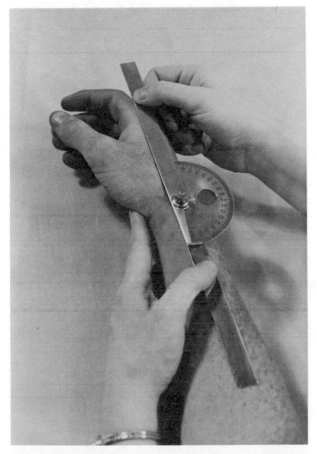

Figure 8.28 Starting position: Forearm rests on the table in midposition; wrist is in neutral position. The fingers are slightly extended or relaxed to eliminate the error that could occur due to tenodesis effect: the finger extensor tendons are too short to allow full wrist flexion with full finger flexion.

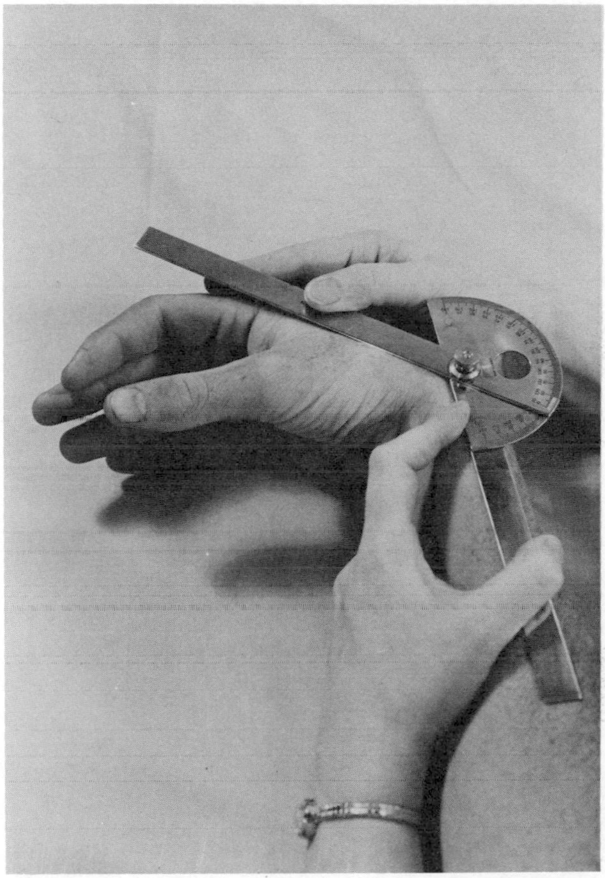

Figure 8.29 End position: The hand has moved toward the volar forearm to the limit of motion.

Axis is capitate
move arm a 3rd MC

Goniometer Placement

Axis. Over the styloid process of the radius, which is located on the lateral aspect of the wrist at the anatomical snuff box.

Stationary Arm. Parallel to the longitudinal axis of the radius.

Movable Arm. Parallel to the longitudinal axis of the second metacarpal.

Wrist Extension (Dorsiflexion)

Movement of the hand dorsally in the sagittal plane (0° to 70°).

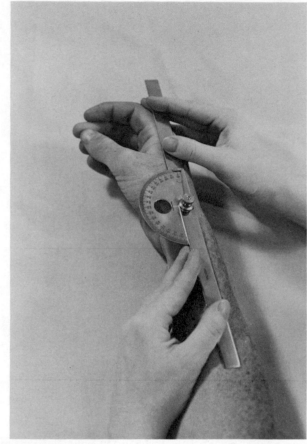

Figure 8.30 Starting position: The forearm rests on the table in midposition. The wrists is in neutral position. The fingers should be slightly flexed or relaxed to eliminate the error that could occur due to the finger flexor tendons being too short to allow full wrist extension with full finger extension.

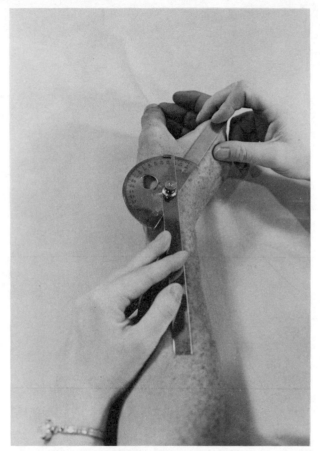

Figure 8.31 End position: The hand has moved toward the dorsal forearm to the limit of motion.

Goniometer Placement

Axis. Over the styloid process of the radius.
Stationary Arm. Parallel to the longitudinal axis of the radius.

Movable Arm. Parallel to the longitudinal axis of the second metacarpal.

Wrist Ulnar Deviation

Movement of the hand toward the ulnar side in a frontal plane (0° to 30°).

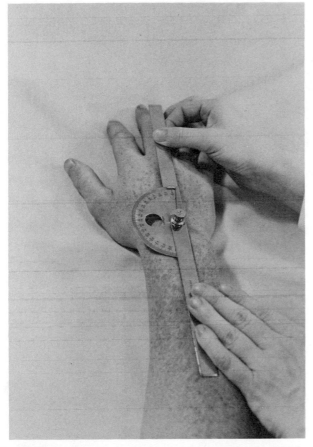

Figure 8.32 Starting position: The forearm is pronated with the volar surface of the forearm and palm resting lightly on the table. The wrist is in neutral position, with fingers relaxed.

line up w 3rd MC not 3rd digit

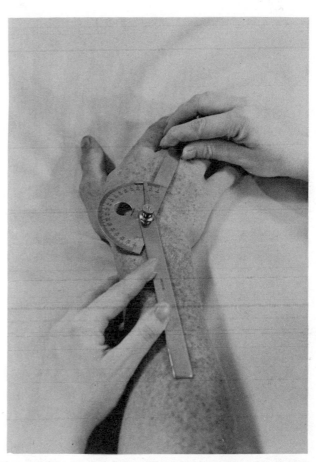

Figure 8.33 End position: The hand has moved so that the little finger approximates the ulna to the limit of motion.

Goniometer Placement

Axis. On the dorsal aspect of the wrist joint in line with the base of the third metacarpal.

Stationary Arm. Along the midline of the forearm on the dorsal surface.

Movable Arm. Along the midline of the third metacarpal.

Possible Substitutions. Wrist extension, wrist flexion.

Wrist Radial Deviation

Movement of the hand toward the radial side in a frontal plane (0° to 20°).

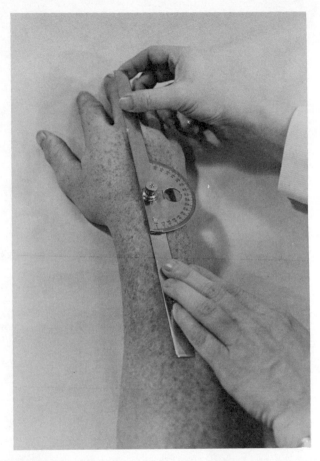

Figure 8.34 Starting position: The forearm is pronated, with the volar surface of the forearm and the palm resting lightly on the table. The wrist is in neutral position, fingers relaxed.

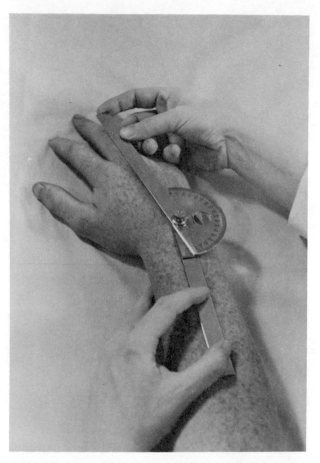

Figure 8.35 End position: The hand has moved so that the thumb approximates the radius to the limit of motion.

Goniometer Placement

Axis. On the dorsal aspect of the wrist joint in line with the base of the third metacarpal.

Stationary Arm. Along the midline of the forearm on the dorsal surface.

Movable Arm. Along the midline of the third metacarpal.

Possible Substitution. Wrist extension.

Thumb Carpometacarpal Flexion

Movement of the thumb across the palm in the frontal plane (0° to 15°).

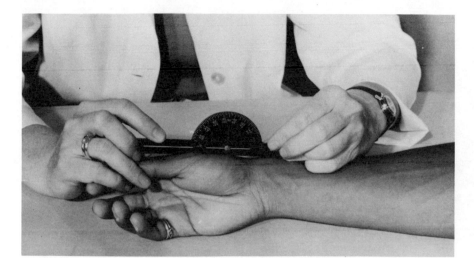

Figure 8.36 Starting position: The wrist is in neutral or slight ulnar deviation to align the second metacarpal and the radius. The carpometacarpal joint is in neutral, with the thumb next to the volar surface of the index finger.

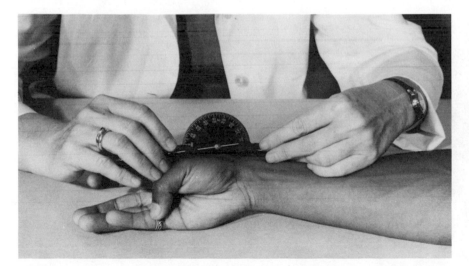

Figure 8.37 End position: The thumb has moved across the plane of the palm toward the ulnar side to the limit of motion in flexion.

Goniometer Placement

Axis. On the radial side of the wrist at the junction of the base of the first metacarpal and the trapezium.

Stationary Arm. Parallel to the longitudinal axis of the radius.

Movable Arm. Parallel to the longitudinal axis of the first metacarpal.

Note. For accuracy, the arms of the goniometer must remain in full contact with skin surfaces over the bones. However, excessive pressure with the edge of a half-circle goniometer must be avoided. These statements apply to all flexion–extension measurements of the thumb and fingers.

Thumb Carpometacarpal Extension

Movement of the thumb away from the palm in the frontal plane (0° to 20°).

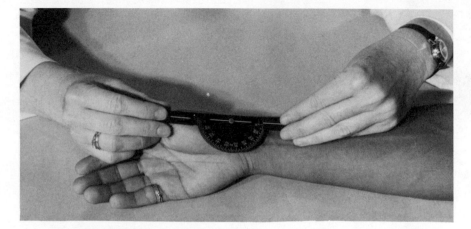

Figure 8.38 Starting position: The wrist is in neutral or slight ulnar deviation to align the second metacarpal and the radius. The carpometacarpal joint is in neutral with the thumb next to the volar surface of the index finger.

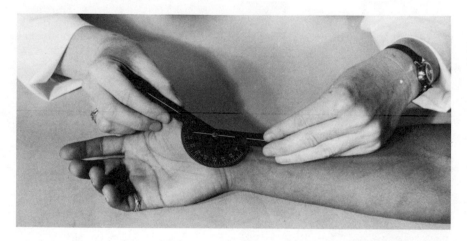

Figure 8.39 End position: The thumb has moved into full extension away from the palm toward the radial side to the limit of motion in extension.

Goniometer Placement

Axis. On the volar side of the wrist at the junction of the base of the first metacarpal and the trapezium.

Stationary Arm. Parallel to the longitudinal axis of the radius.

Movable Arm. Parallel to the longitudinal axis of the first metacarpal.

Thumb Metacarpophalangeal (MP) Flexion-Extension

Movement of the thumb across the palm in the frontal plane (0° to 50°).

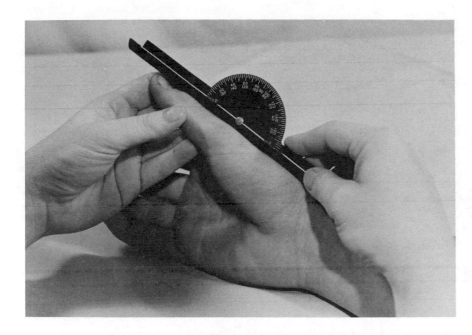

Figure 8.40 Starting position: The wrist is in neutral position or slight extension. The MP joint is in extension.

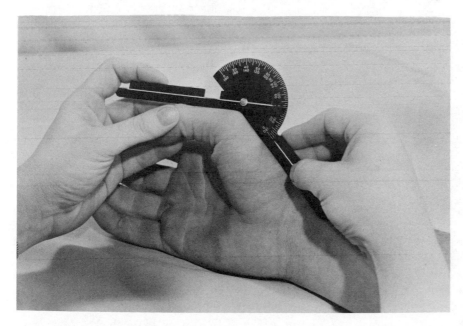

Figure 8.41 End position: The thumb has moved across the plane of the palm toward the ulnar side of the hand to the limit of motion in flexion.

Goniometer Placement

Axis. On the dorsal aspect of the MP joint.
Stationary Arm. On the dorsal surface, along the midline of the first metacarpal.

Movable Arm. On the dorsal surface, along the midline of the proximal phalanx of the thumb.

Thumb Interphalangeal (IP) Flexion-Extension

Movement of the distal phalanx of the thumb toward the volar surface of the proximal phalanx of the thumb (0° to 80°).

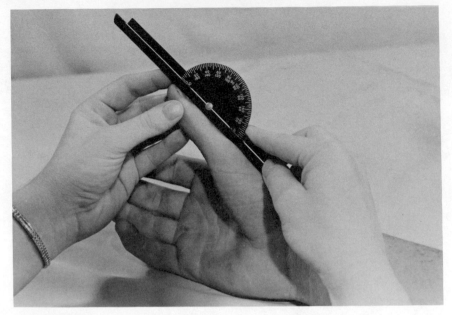

Figure 8.42 Starting position: The wrist is in neutral position or slight extension. The IP joint is in extension.

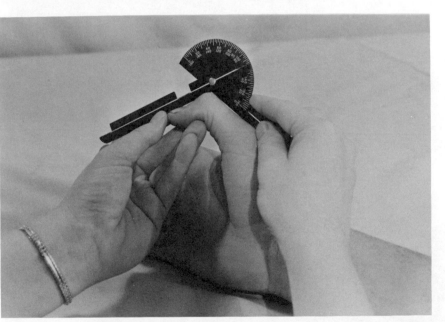

Figure 8.43 End position: The volar surface of the distal phalanx approximates the volar surface of the proximal phalanx to the limit of motion in flexion.

Goniometer Placement

Axis. On the dorsal aspect of the IP joint.

Stationary Arm. On the dorsal surface, along the proximal phalanx.

Movable Arm. On the dorsal surface, along the distal phalanx.

Note. If the thumbnail prevents full goniometer contact, shift the movable arm laterally to increase accuracy.

Alternate Goniometer Placement

Thumb MP and IP flexion-extension can be measured on the lateral aspect of the thumb using lateral aspects of the same landmarks.

Thumb Abduction

Movement of the thumb anteriorly in the sagittal plane, up away from the palm of the hand in line with the index finger (0° to 70°).

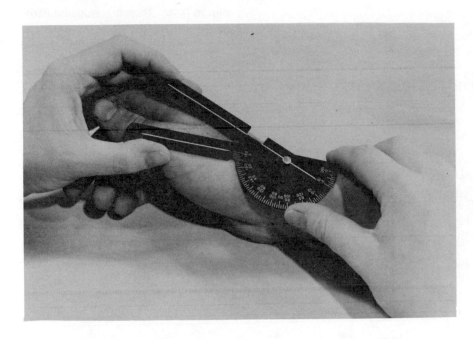

Figure 8.44 Starting position: The wrist is in neutral position and the thumb is touching the volar surface of the palm and index finger. *Note.* This is the zero starting position; although the goniometer may indicate 20° to 30° it is recorded as zero.

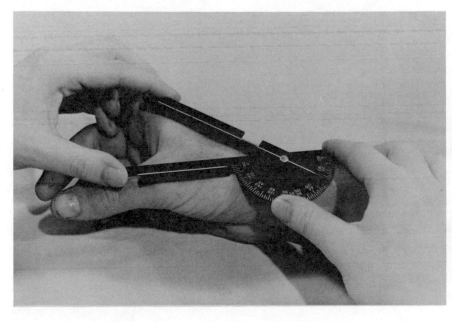

Figure 8.45 End position: The thumb has moved away from the palm in line with the index finger to the limit of motion.

Goniometer Placement

Axis. On the radial side of the wrist at the junction of the bases of the first and second metacarpals.

Stationary Arm. Along the second metacarpal on its lateral aspect.

Movable Arm. Along the first metacarpal on its dorsal surface.

Thumb Abduction and Opposition: Ruler Measurements

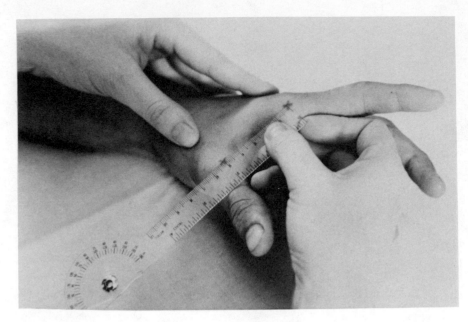

Figure 8.46 Thumb abduction: Ruler measurement of web space.

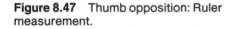

Figure 8.47 Thumb opposition: Ruler measurement.

Abduction. Take the measurement from the midpoint of the head of the first metacarpal to the midpoint of the head of the second metacarpal while the thumb is in full abduction.

Opposition. Rotary movement of the thumb to approximate the pad of the thumb to pads of the fingers.

Normally, a person can oppose to each of the fingers.

Measure the distance from the tip of the thumb (not the thumbnail) to the tip end of the little finger to record any deficit of opposition.

Finger Metacarpophalangeal Flexion

Movement of the finger at the MP joint in a sagittal plane (0° to 90°).

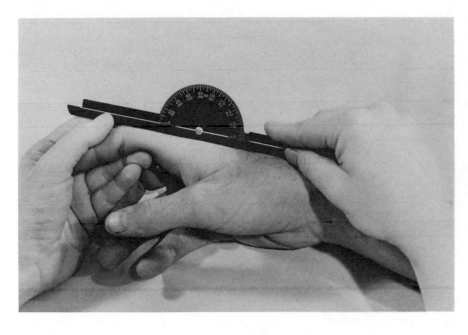

Figure 8.48 Starting position: The wrist is in neutral position or slight hyperextension. The MP joint is in extension.

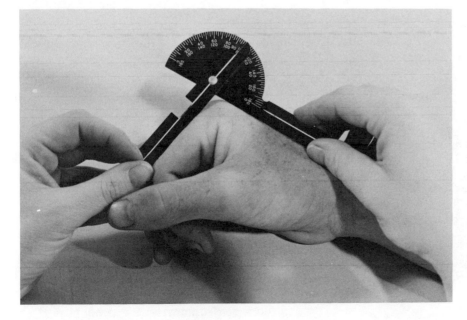

Figure 8.49 End position: The volar surface of the proximal phalanx approximates the palm to the limit of motion of flexion.

Goniometer Placement

Axis. On the dorsal aspect of the MP joint of the finger being measured.

Stationary Arm. On the dorsal surface along the midline of the metacarpal of the finger being measured.

Movable Arm. On the dorsal surface along the midline of the proximal phalanx of the finger being measured.

Finger Metacarpophalangeal Hyperextension

Movement of the finger at the MP joint dorsally in a sagittal plane (0° to 45°).

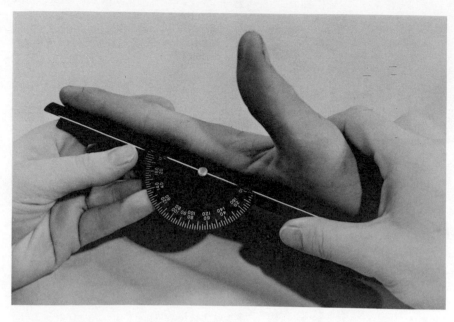

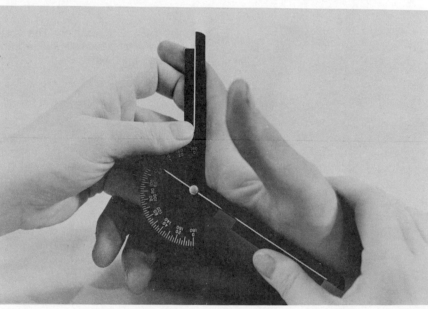

Figure 8.50 Starting position: The wrist is in neutral position or in slight flexion. The MP joint is in zero degrees (neutral position). The IP joints are relaxed.

Figure 8.51 End position: The dorsal surface of the proximal phalanx moves toward the dorsum of the hand to the limit of motion.

Goniometer Placement

Axis. On the volar aspect of the MP joint of the finger being measured.

Stationary Arm. Along the volar aspect of the midline of the metacarpal of the finger being measured.

Movable Arm. Along the volar aspect of the midline of the proximal phalanx of the finger being measured. Allow the PIP and DIP joints to flex.

Alternate Goniometer Placement

MP flexion and hyperextension can be measured from the lateral aspect of the index and little fingers by using the lateral aspects of the same landmarks noted here. The long finger and ring finger measurements are estimated by sighting in from the adjoining fingers. This alternate method may be more accurate in cases where there are enlarged joints or excess tissue on the patient's palm.

Finger Proximal Interphalangeal (PIP) Flexion-Extension

Movement of the middle phalanx toward the volar surface of the proximal phalanx in the sagittal plane (0° to 100°).

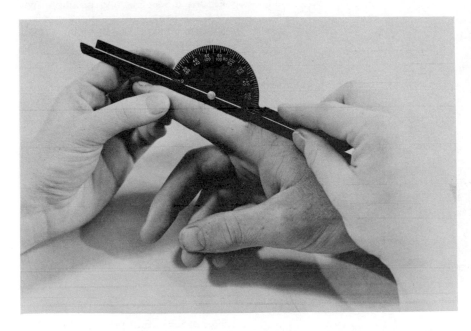

Figure 8.52 Starting position: The wrist is in neutral position or slight hyperextension. The PIP joint is in extension.

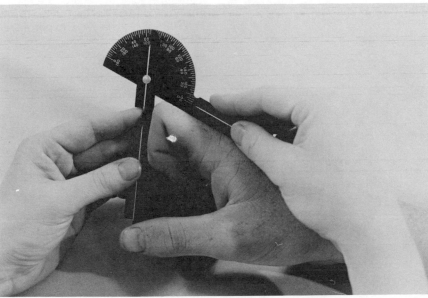

Figure 8.53 End position: The volar surface of the middle phalanx approximates the volar surface of the proximal phalanx to the limit of motion in flexion.

Goniometer Placement

Axis. On the dorsal aspect of the PIP joint of the finger being measured.

Stationary Arm. On the dorsal surface along the midline of the proximal phalanx of the finger being measured.

Movable Arm. On dorsal surface along the midline of the middle phalanx of the finger being measured.

Finger Distal Interphalangeal (DIP) Flexion-Extension

Movement of the distal phalanx toward the volar surface of the middle phalanx in a sagittal plane (0° to 90°).

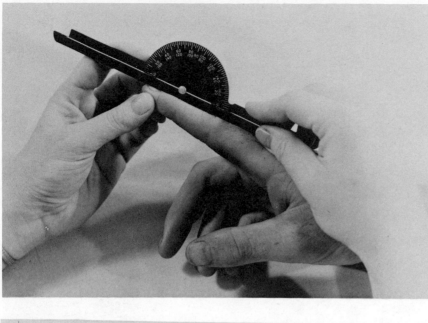

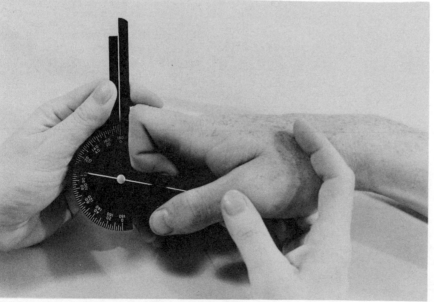

Figure 8.54 Starting position: The wrist is in neutral position or slight hyperextension. The DIP joint is in extension.

Figure 8.55 End position: The volar surface of the distal phalanx approximates the volar surface of the middle phalanx to the limit of motion in flexion. The PIP joint should flex to permit full DIP flexion.

Goniometer Placement

Axis. On the dorsal aspect of the DIP joint of the finger being measured.

Stationary Arm. On the dorsal surface along the midline of the middle phalanx of the finger being measured.

Movable Arm. On the dorsal surface along the midline of the distal phalanx of the finger being measured.

Note. If the fingernail prevents full goniometer contact, shift the movable arm laterally to increase accuracy.

Alternate Goniometer Placement

Finger PIP and DIP flexion-extension can be measured from the lateral aspect of each finger using the lateral aspect of the same landmarks. This method may be more accurate when joints are enlarged.

Finger Flexion: Ruler Measurements

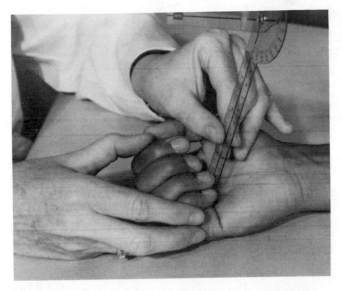

Figure 8.56 PIP and DIP flexion: Ruler measurement.

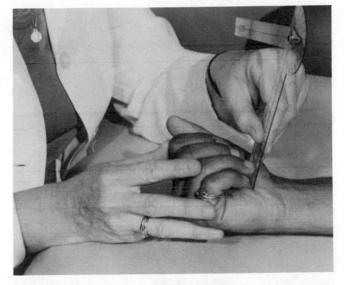

Figure 8.57 MP, PIP, and DIP flexion: Ruler measurement.

PIP and DIP Flexion

Measure from the tip of the finger to the distal palmar crease.

MP, PIP, and DIP Flexion

Measure from the tip of the finger to the base of the palm.[1]

Finger Abduction

Movement of the index, ring, and little fingers away from the midline of the hand in a frontal plane. The middle finger, which is the midline of the hand, abducts in both radial and ulnar directions.

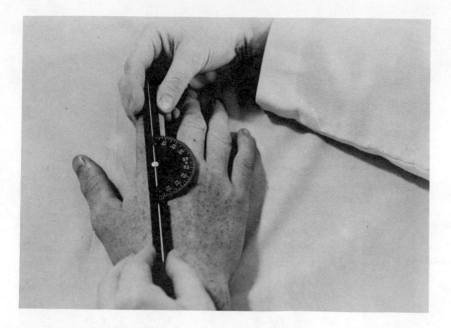

Figure 8.58 Starting position: The volar surface of the forearm and palm are resting lightly on a table. The metacarpal and the proximal phalanx of the finger being measured should be in a straight line.

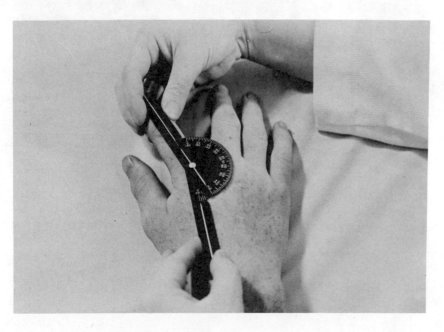

Figure 8.59 End position: The finger has moved away from the midposition to the limit of motion.

Goniometer Placement

Axis. On the dorsal aspect of the MP joint of the finger being measured.

Stationary Arm. Along the dorsal surface of the metacarpal of the finger being measured.

Movable Arm. Along the dorsal surface of the proximal phalanx of the finger being measured.

Alternate Measurement. Ruler measurements may be taken from the midpoint of the tip of each finger to the midpoint of the tip of the adjacent finger.

Finger Adduction

Movement of the index, ring, and little fingers toward the midline of the hand in a frontal plane.

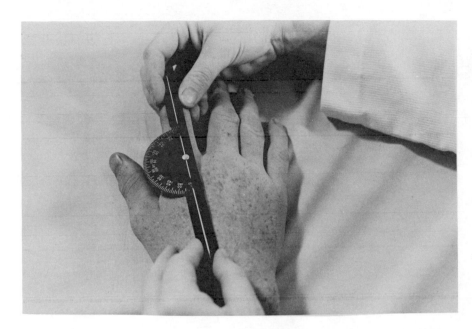

Figure 8.60 Starting position: The volar surface of the forearm and palm are resting lightly on a table. The metacarpal and the proximal phalanx of the finger being measured should be in a straight line.

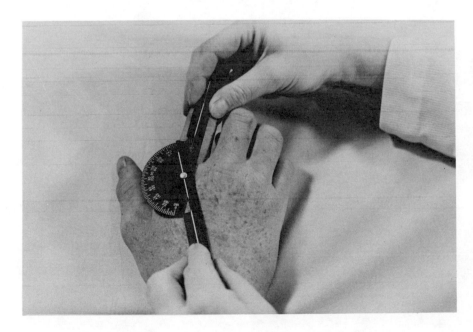

Figure 8.61 End position: The finger has moved toward the middle finger to the limit of motion. Move adjacent fingers out of the way if necessary to allow full excursion of movement.

Goniometer Placement

Axis. On the dorsal aspect of the MP joint of the finger being measured.

Stationary Arm. Along the dorsal surface of the metacarpal of the finger being measured. The middle finger is not measured.

Movable Arm. Along the dorsal surface of the proximal phalanx of the finger being measured.

MP Deviation Correction Measurement

In the case of ulnar deviation deformity of the metacarpophalangeal joints often seen in rheumatoid arthritis, this additional measurement is taken.

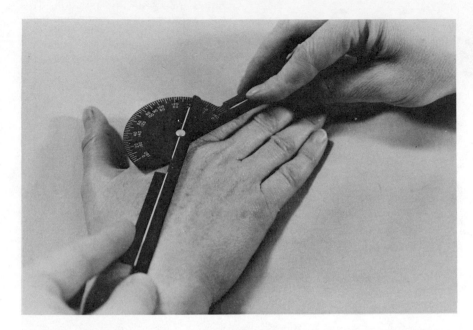

Figure 8.62 Starting position: The hand and forearm rest pronated on a flat surface. The finger is in the position of ulnar deviation in which the finger normally lies.

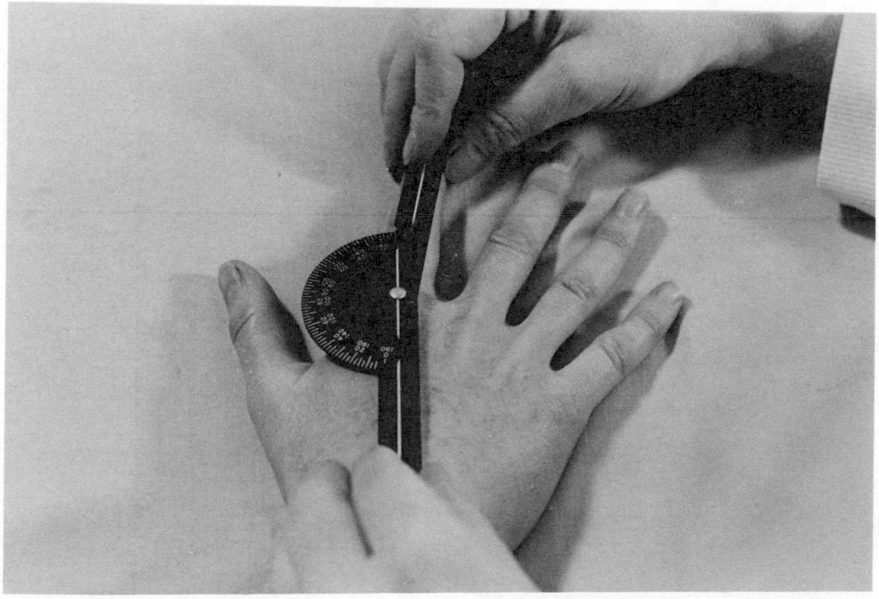

Figure 8.63 End position: Radial deviation of the finger.

Goniometer Placement

Axis. Over the MP joint of the finger being measured.

Stationary Arm. Placed along the dorsal midline of the metacarpal.

Movable Arm. Placed along the dorsal midline of the proximal phalanx.

The active range is compared to the passive range to determine if muscle weakness is present. Passive range of motion is compared to the norm of 0° deviation to determine if a fixed deformity exists.

MEASUREMENT OF THE LOWER EXTREMITY

Hip Flexion

Movement of the thigh anteriorly in a sagittal plane (0° to 120° with the knee flexed).

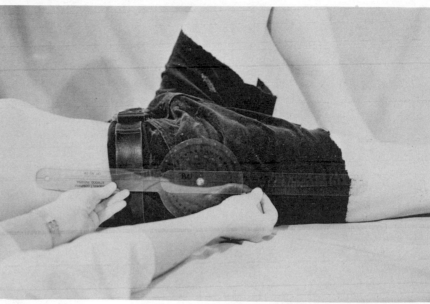

Figure 8.64 Starting position: Patient is supine. The leg being measured is fully extended. The opposite leg may be flexed or extended at the hip and knee.

Figure 8.65 End position: As the hip is flexed, the knee is allowed to flex. The anterior thigh approximates the anterior trunk to the limit of motion.

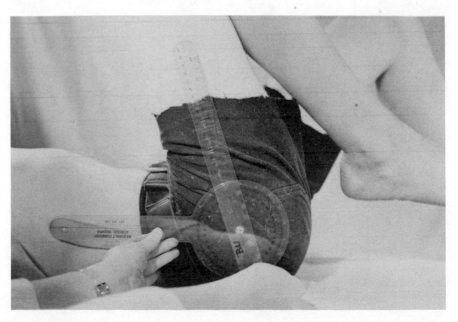

Goniometer Placement

Axis. On a point on the lateral aspect of the hip opposite the greater trochanter.

Stationary Arm. Perpendicular to a line drawn from the anterior superior iliac spine to the posterior superior iliac spine of the pelvis.

Movable Arm. Along the midline of the femur on the lateral aspect of the thigh, pointing toward the lateral epicondyle of the femur.

Hip Extension

Movement of the thigh posteriorly in a sagittal plane (0° to 30° with the knee extended).

This average range was determined by using the lateral trunk as a reference for placement of the stationary arm, a method that has been violated by others.[7,8]

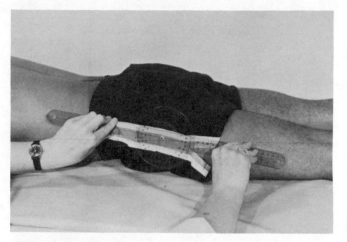

Figure 8.66 Starting position: The patient is prone with both legs fully extended.

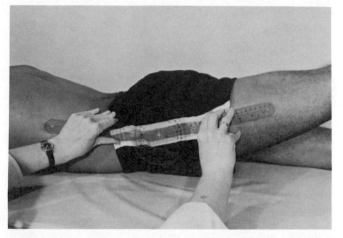

Figure 8.67 End position: The thigh is moved up off the table to the limit of motion. The knee remains extended.

Goniometer Placement

Axis. On a point on the lateral aspect of the hip opposite the greater trochanter.

Stationary Arm. Perpendicular to a line drawn from the anterior iliac spine to the posterior superior iliac spine of the pelvis.

Movable Arm. Along the midline of the femur on the lateral aspect of the thigh in line with the lateral epicondyle of the femur.

Note. Clayson et al.[9] described an adapted goniometer for measuring hip extension; one arm of the goniometer has a flexible metal band that can be secured to the anterior and posterior superior iliac spines to ensure accurate placement.

Hip Abduction ☆

Movement of the thigh laterally away from the midline
of the body in a frontal plane (0° to 45°).

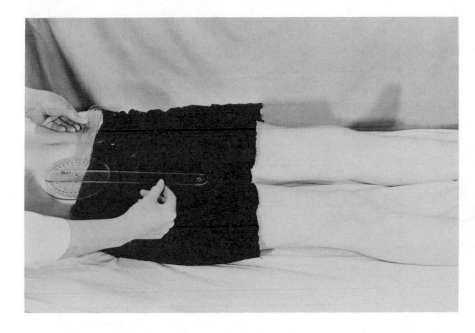

Figure 8.68 Starting position: Patient
is supine with legs extended.

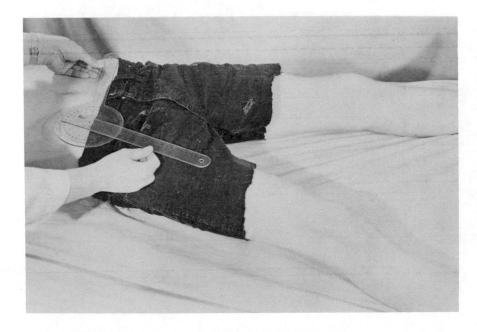

Figure 8.69 End position: The leg
being measured is moved laterally to
the limit of motion. Knee remains extended.

Goniometer Placement

Axis. The anterior superior iliac spine of the side
being measured.

Stationary Arm. On a line between the two anterior
superior iliac spines.

Movable Arm. Parallel to the midline of the femur on
the anterior surface of the thigh; it points toward the
patella.

Possible Substitution. Hip external rotation.

Hip Adduction

Movement of the thigh medially across the midline of the body in a frontal plane (0° to 30°).

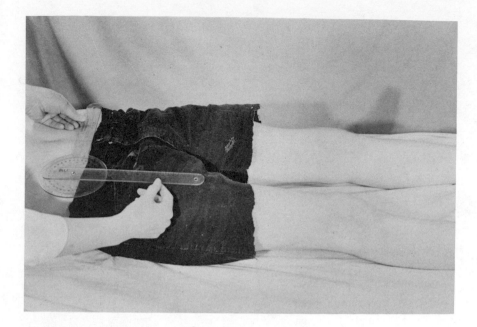

Figure 8.70 Starting position: The patient is supine with the legs extended.

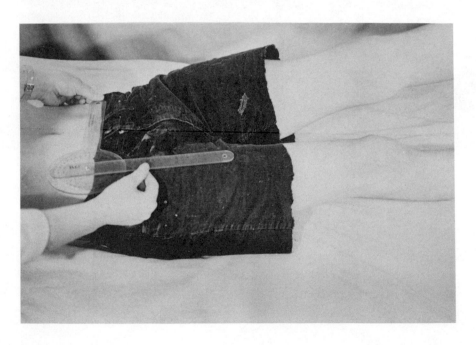

Figure 8.71 End position: The leg not being measured is flexed at the hip to move it out of the way. The leg being measured is moved medially across the midline of the body to the limit of motion.

Goniometer Placement

Axis. Anterior superior iliac spine of the side being measured.

Stationary Arm. On a line between the two anterior superior iliac spines.

Movable Arm. Parallel to the midline of the femur on the anterior surface of the thigh and pointing toward the patella.

Possible Substitution. Hip internal rotation.

Hip Internal Rotation

Movement of the femur medially around its longitudinal axis (0° to 45°).

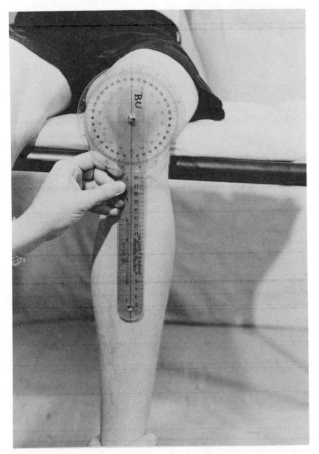

Figure 8.72 Starting position: The patient is seated with the hip flexed to 90°. The lower leg hangs over the edge of the plinth (treatment table).

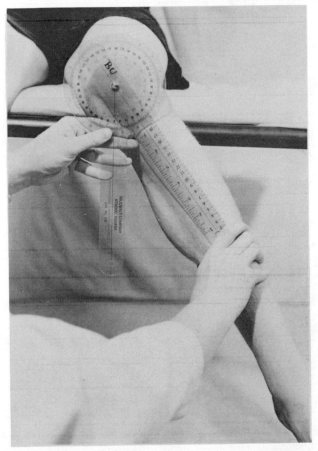

Figure 8.73 End position: The foot and lower leg are moved laterally while the thigh rotates medially but is not permitted to adduct or flex.

Goniometer Placement

Axis. Centered on the knee joint over the patella.
Stationary Arm. Perpendicular to the floor.

Movable Arm. Along the midline of the tibial shaft.

Hip External Rotation

Movement of the femur laterally around its longitudinal axis (0° to 45°).

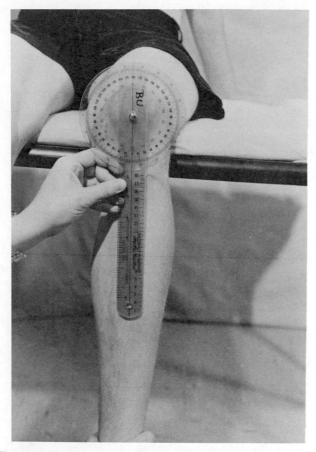

Figure 8.74 Starting position: The patient is seated with the hip and knee flexed to 90°. The lower leg hangs over the edge of the plinth (treatment table).

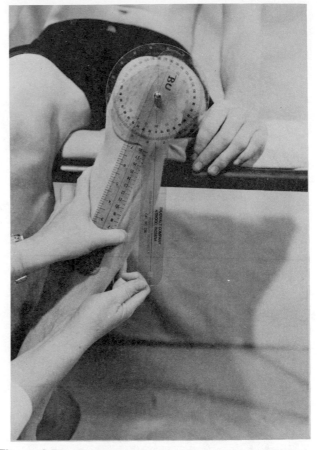

Figure 8.75 End position: The foot and lower leg are moved medially while the thigh rotates laterally but is not permitted to flex or abduct.

Goniometer Placement

Axis. Centered on the knee joint over the patella.
Stationary Arm. Perpendicular to the floor.

Movable Arm. Along the midline of the tibial shaft.

Hip Internal and External Rotation: Alternate Method

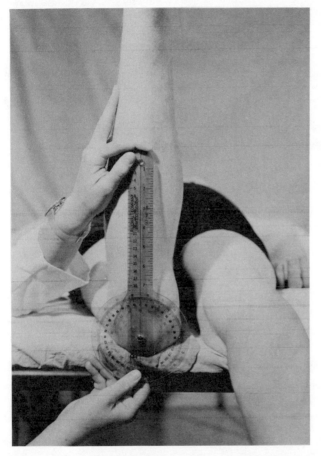

Figure 8.76 Starting position: Patient is prone with knee flexed to 90° and lower leg perpendicular to the plinth.

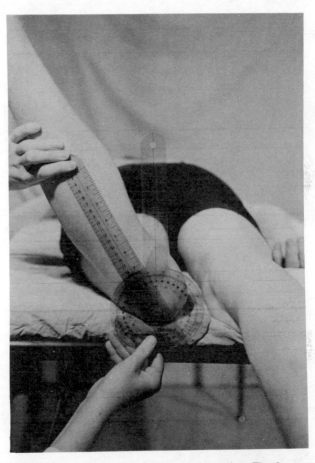

Figure 8.77 End position for internal rotation: The foot and lower leg are moved laterally to the limit of motion while the thigh rotates medially. No thigh adduction is permitted. For external rotation the foot and lower leg are moved medially while the thigh rotates laterally. No thigh abduction is permitted.

Goniometer Placement

Axis. Centered on the knee joint over the patella.
Stationary Arm. Perpendicular to the floor.

Movable Arm. Along the midline of the tibial shaft.

Knee Flexion-Extension

Movement of the lower leg posteriorly in a sagittal plane (0° to 135°).

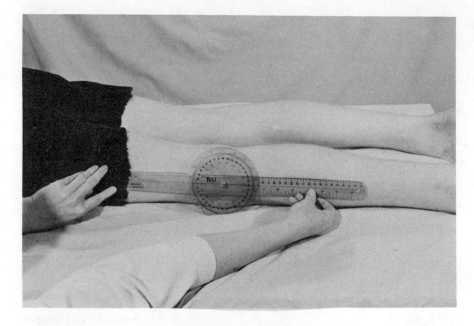

Figure 8.78 Starting position: Patient is prone with both legs fully extended and feet over the table edge. Alternate position: Patient sits with knees flexed and lower legs over the table edge.

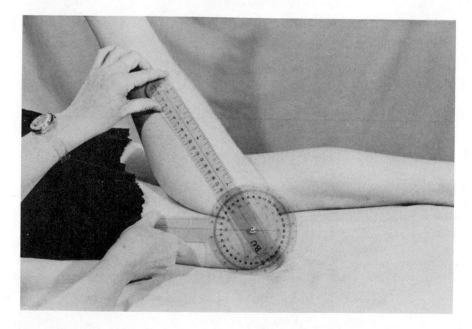

Figure 8.79 End position: The lower leg is moved so that the calf approximates the posterior thigh to the limit of flexion.

Goniometer Placement

Axis. The knee joint at the lateral tibial condyle.
Stationary Arm. Along the midline of the femur on the lateral aspect of the thigh.

Movable Arm. Along the lateral midline of the lower leg in line with the lateral malleolus.

Ankle Dorsiflexion-Plantar Flexion

Dorsiflexion is movement of the foot anteriorly in the sagittal plane (0° to 20°). Plantar flexion is movement of the foot posteriorly in a sagittal plane (0° to 50°).

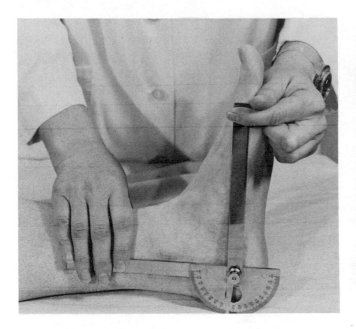

Figure 8.80 Starting position: The patient is sitting or supine with knee flexed. The foot is in neutral position (90°).

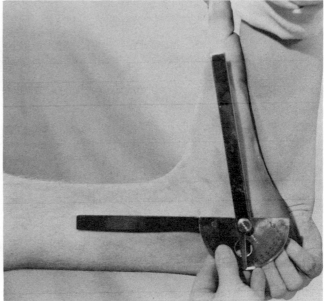

Figure 8.81 End position for dorsiflexion: The foot is moved so that the toes point up.

Goniometer Placement

Axis. On the medial aspect of the ankle joint approximately 1 inch below the medial malleolus.

Stationary Arm. Along the midline of the medial aspect of the lower leg.

Movable Arm. In line with the first metatarsal. The goniometer will read 90° at the start of the measurement, and this must be deducted when recording.

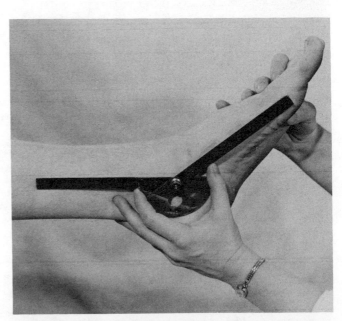

Figure 8.82 End position for plantar flexion: The foot is moved so that the toes point down.

Ankle Inversion

Inversion is movement of the forefoot to bring the sole of the foot to face medially (0° to 35°).

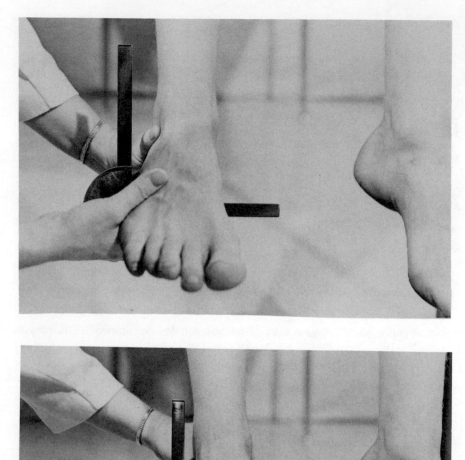

Figure 8.83 Starting position: The patient is supine or sitting with the knee flexed. The foot is in neutral position.

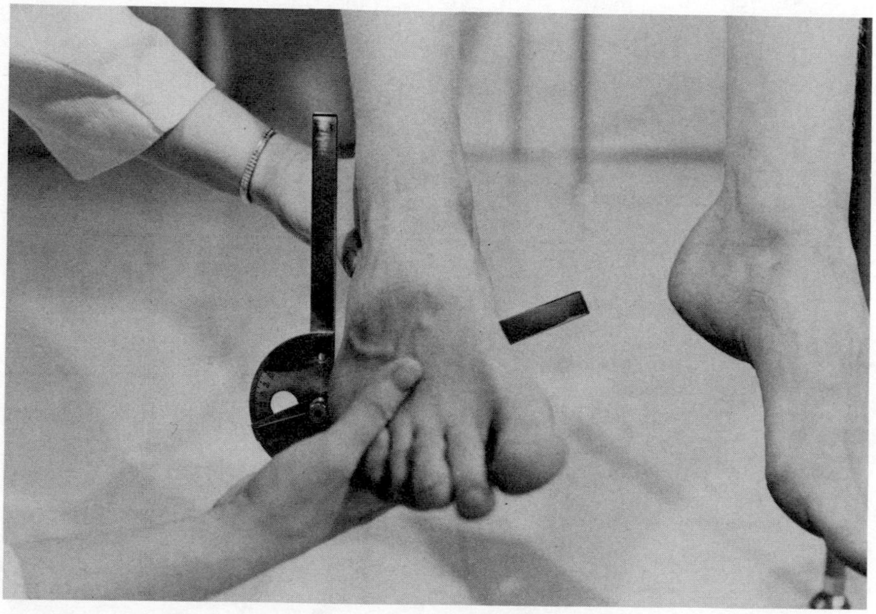

Figure 8.84 End position: The sole of the foot faces medially to the limit of motion. External rotation of the hip is prohibited.

Goniometer Placement

Axis. A point parallel to the longitudinal axis of the foot, displaced laterally.

Stationary Arm. Along the midline of the lateral aspect of the lower leg.

Movable Arm. Across the sole of the forefoot.

Note. The goniometer will read 90° at the start of the measurement and this must be deducted when recording.

Ankle Eversion

Eversion is movement of the forefoot to bring the sole of the foot to face laterally (0° to 15°).

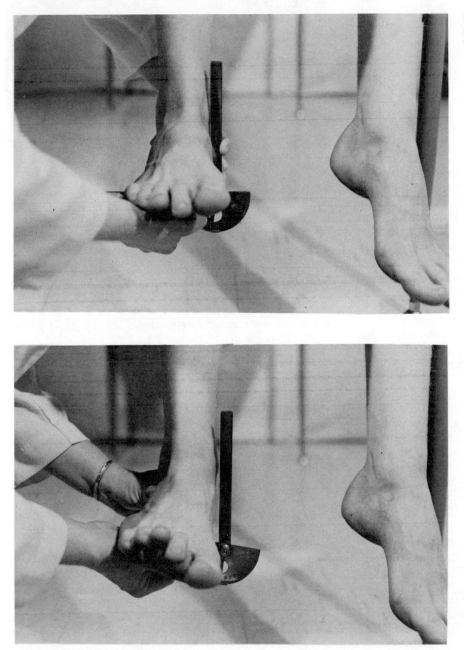

Figure 8.85 Starting position: The patient is supine or sitting with the knee flexed. The foot is in neutral position.

Figure 8.86 End position: The sole of the foot faces laterally to the limit of motion. Internal rotation of the hip is prohibited.

Goniometer Placement

Axis. A point parallel to the longitudinal axis of the foot displaced medially.

Stationary Arm. Along the midline of the lower leg on the medial aspect.

Movable Arm. Across the sole of the forefoot.

Note. The goniometer will read 90° at the start of motion, and this must be deducted when recording.

Palm Prints.[10,11] Imprints of the palm of the patient's whole hand are made on paper using either finger paint or a waterbased ink stamp pad. This presents a graphic record of deformities. Sequential palm prints indicate changes in these deformities over time. This method is frequently used to record the changes in deformities of the hands of rheumatoid arthritic patients.

Xerography.[12] Xerox photographs of the patient's whole hand are made for the same reasons that palm prints are made. Xerography, however, gives a clearer representation.

Outline. The hand is placed on a paper, and a tracing is made around the entire hand with the fingers in both an abducted and an adducted position. This is an alternative graphic representation of abduction and adduction of the fingers often used instead of, or as an adjunct to, goniometric measurement or ruler measurement.

Bubble Goniometer. This is a measuring tool that uses the principle of a carpenter's level in which a bubble of air within a column of liquid moves when the angle is changed. The bubble goniometer is designed like a watch in which the bubble rests at the highest point (equivalent to 12 o'clock), and the face is marked off in degrees rather than in minutes. It is currently most often used to measure the cervical spine.

Gravity Goniometer. This is a tool that resembles a round lollipop and is used to measure supination and pronation of the forearm. The round face of the instrument is marked off in degrees and has an indicator like a compass point that always points up due to the force of gravity. Its accuracy depends upon careful positioning as described for the alternate method of measuring supination and pronation using a pencil.

Electrogoniometer.[13] This is a device that electrically records the position of the joint or joints to which it is applied. A potentiometer whose resistance changes with changes in position is aligned with the joint to be measured. The electrical signal is recorded on paper as a graphic representation of the position of the joint. The degrees of change can be measured from the paper record, or the electronic signal can be digitized by computer. Electrogoniometers precisely measure change in exact limits of motion over the course of one treatment session if they remain in place; however, removal and replacement would decrease the accuracy of repeated measures of limits of motion. Changes in range of motion from treatment to treatment can be compared to document progress. Figure 8.87 shows one type of electrogoniometer, which measures movement of finger joints. Figure 12.2 shows one type of wrist electrogoniometer.

Measuring Cone for Thumb Abduction/Extension.[14] A yarn cone can be adapted to assess the first web space of burned hands. The measurement represents the diameter around which the thumb and index finger can be positioned passively. No norms exist; it

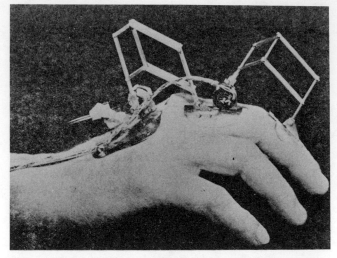

Figure 8.87 Electrogoniometer placed to measure MP and PIP flexion and extension of the long finger. (Reproduced with permission from Long, C., and Brown, M. E.: Electromyographic kinesiology of the hand: muscles moving the long finger. *Bone Joint Surg.*, 46-A(8):, 1683–1706, 1964.

is used to compare the patient's progress from time to time.

Functional. Range of motion is observed during the performance of activities to see if there are any limitations which interfere with function. This type of observation assists in determining if the patient's ROM limitations are significant.

Edema

Edema, one cause of limited range of motion, is quantified using volumetric measurements, which document changes in the mass of a body part via the technique of water displacement. A water vessel that is large enough to allow submersion of the whole hand up to a given point on the wrist is used. It has a spillover spout near the top of the water level. When the hand is placed in the volumeter, water is displaced and spills out of the vessel into a graduated beaker. An edematous hand will displace more water than a nonedematous hand so that a lower reading is considered an improvement. A study done to determine the ability of the therapist to consistently orient the extremity within the measuring device and to correctly measure the displaced water indicated high reliability over three repeated tests on 24 hands.[15]

Circumferential measurement using a centimeter tape measure is another way to measure edema and is preferred for body parts not easily submersed. Care must be taken to measure at exactly the same place from test to test.

The measurement of the affected part is compared to its contralateral counterpart to determine the extent of the edema. The short-term goal of treatment is stated, for example, "to decrease edema more than 5 milliliters," which is slightly more than the identified within-patient variance,[15] or "to reduce measurement by *x* number of millimeters."

Muscle Strength

Muscle strength has been defined "as the capacity of a muscle to produce the tension necessary for maintaining posture, initiating movement, or controlling movement during conditions of loading on the musculoskeletal system."[16] Weakness is defined as a lack or reduction of this tension-producing capacity of a muscle or muscle group.[16] When weakness limits function it is necessary to determine the degree and distribution of the weakness. In some cases, such as Landry-Guillain-Barré syndrome, weakness will be generalized, and therefore testing will be extensive. In other cases, such as a peripheral nerve injury, weakness will be limited to muscles innervated by the damaged nerve, and muscle testing will usually involve only these muscles. In other words the therapist tests those muscles that are involved and toward which treatment will be directed. If you treat it, measure it!

The commonly measured index to assess strength is maximum tension production under voluntary effort.[17] Strength of muscle contraction can be measured by means of spring scales, tensiometers, dynamometers, weights, or manual resistance.[18] Although the measurement of strength taken using apparatus is more exact, it is difficult and time-consuming to set up the apparatus as precisely as it must be in order to get accurate measurements of each muscle group. Therefore, clinicians use manual muscle testing, which they have found to be adequate for most clinical purposes. Since manual muscle testing is a measurement of maximum *voluntary* contraction of an isolated muscle or muscle group, strength testing is inappropriate for patients who lack the ability to contract one muscle or a muscle group in isolation, as is the case for patients with central nervous system damage.

Manual muscle testing can be performed as a break test or a make test.[16] In the "break" test, the limb is positioned so the muscle to be tested is at its greatest mechanical advantage and the patient is asked to hold the position as the tester imparts an external force to overcome the contractile force of the muscle or muscle group.[16] In other words, the therapist tries to "break" the patient's hold.

In the "make" test, the body segment imparts a force to some external object.[16] The object can be the therapist's hand or an instrument, e.g., a hand-held dynamometer, sometimes called a push scale. The object is stationed at the point where the muscle would be at greatest mechanical advantage. The patient presses the distal part of the limb against the object with as much an effort as he can generate, and the tension is estimated by the therapist or registered by the instrument. Changes in velocity of movement toward the object from test to test will affect the outcome.[16]

The term "mechanical advantage" refers to the length/tension relationship of a muscle. Total tension of a muscle is the sum of the passive tension exerted by the elastic components in the lengthened muscle and the active tension generated by the contractile elements of the contracting muscle.[19] Therefore, a muscle is able to generate its greatest total tension or sustain the heaviest load when positioned at an optimal length, which is usually slightly (10%) longer than resting length.[17,19] Developed (active) tension, which is total tension minus the elastic contribution, is greatest at resting length but decreases as the muscle is shortened; at less than 50% of resting length, the muscle cannot develop contractile tension.[19]

For those muscles or muscle groups too weak to resist an outside force, muscle strength is evaluated by isotonic contraction in which the muscle is required to move the mass of the body part against gravity but no applied resistance or with the effect of gravity eliminated.[20,21] Carlson[22] tested elbow flexion strength of 36 normal subjects comparing tests of isometric and isotonic strength and found that isometric strength was significantly greater than isotonic strength in these subjects, but there was a high positive relationship between the two types of contraction, indicating measurement of one is a good estimate of the other.

The evaluation of muscle strength presented here is the "break" test. Gravity as resistance is considered an important variable and is used for all motions where practical and possible, including supination and pronation, as well as motions of the fingers and toes. In our experience elimination of gravity has been observed to alter the performance ability of muscles of the fingers and is considered to be an important variable, even though the resistance offered by a small lever arm is, of course, less than that of a large lever. When standard procedures for evaluation against gravity and with gravity eliminated are given in the literature or are in general use, these are described. When a gravity-eliminated position is not described in the literature we applied the concepts to these muscles to describe a gravity-eliminated position. Tests of the upper and lower extremities described here are motion tests for the purpose of evaluating strength in terms of ability to perform functionally. Tests of individual muscles in the wrist and hand are given because of the clinical need for specific assessment to determine correct treatment procedures for hand rehabilitation and splinting.

TESTS OF ADDITIONAL MUSCLES

The movements of head, neck, trunk, and toes have not been included here. However, if the treatment program is to include strengthening of any of this musculature, then the therapist is responsible for the measurement and is referred to texts listed in the references for guidance in doing so.

MANUAL MUSCLE TESTING PROCEDURES

The therapist moves each of the patient's joints through passive range of motion to estimate what range of motion is available at each joint. The available range is considered to be "full range of motion" for the purposes of muscle testing. However, notation is made that a limitation exists if it does.

There are established procedures for muscle testing to make this evaluation as reliable as possible. The patient is *positioned* so that the direction of movement will be against gravity, or with gravity eliminated as appropriate to the strength of the muscle. As a consideration for the patient's comfort, all testing is done in one position before changing to another position. For efficient movement of the part distal to the joint and to ensure isolation of the muscle or muscle group being tested,[16] the proximal attachment must be *stabilized*. For weak patients, the therapist must provide this stability but must avoid placing hands over the muscles that are contracting. The supporting surface, e.g., plinth, may be used to provide stabilization for some muscles. The prime movers are *palpated* to ascertain that they are functioning during the motion. Palpation is, in fact, the basis for assigning a trace grade. The technique of palpation involves the therapist placing the finger pads firmly but lightly over the belly or tendon of the patient's muscle. It is sometimes necessary to have the patient try to do the motion, then relax, which causes the muscle to alternately contract and relax and allows verification that the correct muscle is being palpated. *Resistance* is applied on the distal end of the moving bone i.e., the bone into which the muscle inserts. If resistance is applied at any other point, the lever arm is lengthened or shortened and therefore the resistance is changed. For the break test, resistance is applied in a direction opposite to the motion after the patient has completed the motion.[16,21] The resistance should be applied as close to perpendicular as possible.[16] Gravity and/or muscles other than those being tested may *substitute* to cause the motion. Careful palpation and observation can identify these substitutions and the patient can be repositioned to eliminate them.

Reliability, that is, the reproducibility of scores when no change has occurred, is essential for meaningful evaluation. Of greatest importance to the reliability of the scores of repeated tests is the strict adherence to the exact procedures of muscle testing.

In addition, reliability of muscle testing scores is affected by the interest and cooperation of the patient, the experience of the tester, the temperature of the day and the limb, distractions to the patient or tester, and other environmental conditions.[23] Other factors known to affect outcome are ability to understand directions, posture, motivation, fatigue, and therapists' operational definitions of various grades. To increase reliability, these variables need to be controlled as much as possible from test to test. The test procedure should be clearly explained and each test motion described and demonstrated to the patient. Consistency of verbal instructions is very important.[16] The overall posture of head, neck, trunk, and other limbs during testing should be the same from test to test.[16] Motivation is affected by spectators during testing, fear of pain, noise, competition with self or others, or rewards, including therapist praise.[24]; these should be eliminated or kept the same from test to test. Fatigue differs for each person and each muscle[25]; in general, however,

a rest of 2 min between maximum effort of the same muscle is considered adequate.[24,25]

It is necessary for the therapist to develop a kinesthetic sense of what "normal" strength for each different muscle feels like. The number of fibers within a given muscle does not vary greatly among people but the size of fibers in a muscle varies and reflects strength[16]; the larger the fibers, the greater the potential strength of the muscle. To develop a kinesthetic sense of "normal," a student therapist must test many able-bodied people. Normal strength of each muscle varies according to a person's age, sex, size, body type, and occupation. When first beginning to test persons with muscle weakness, inexperienced therapists can learn the kinesthetic definition of minimal, moderate, and maximal resistance from experienced therapists by each testing the same patient and discussing the grade to be assigned.

The muscle or muscle group is assigned a grade according to the amount of resistance it can take. Two of the many grading systems that have evolved are presented here; Table 8.2 equates one numerical scale with the letter grading system. Each member of a particular department should learn and use one muscle grading system.

RECORDING MUSCLE STRENGTH

The grade for each motion or muscle, in the case of wrists and hands, is accurately recorded in the appropriate column on a form. The form should have columns to record the grades for the right and left sides of the body. The therapist must sign and date each test; if a test continues over several days, the dates should reflect that. A sample form is presented here (Table 8.3). The peripheral nerve and segmental levels are listed beside each muscle to assist the therapist in interpreting the results of the muscle test.

If the muscle test is a reevaluation, the scores are compared to the previous test to note changes. The frequency of reevaluation depends on the nature of the diagnosis. Where recovery is expected to be rapid, reevaluation is done frequently. If the repeated muscle test shows that the patient is making gains, the therapeutic program is considered beneficial. When repeated muscle tests show no gains despite programming adaptations, the patient is considered to have reached a plateau and may be considered to be no longer benefiting from restorative therapy. However, remember that the occupational therapist's goal is increased function. Therefore, she will be concerned with helping the patient to learn, by means of the rehabilitative approach, to compensate for his remaining disability before discharge.

Patients with degenerative diseases are expected to get weaker; therefore, therapy is aimed at maintaining their strength and function as long as possible. Repeated muscle tests are done to confirm that effect of therapy. A plateau for these patients is desirable and indicates that the therapy program is effective for maintaining strength and should be continued.

Table 8.2
MUSCLE TESTING GRADING SYSTEMS: NUMERICAL SCALE EQUATED WITH LETTER GRADING SYSTEM

Against Gravity	5	Normal	N	=	The part moves through full range of motion against maximum resistance and gravity. "Normal" differs for each muscle group and in persons of different ages, sex, and occupation.
	4	Good	G	=	The part moves through full range of motion against gravity and moderate resistance.
		Good minus	G–	=	The part moves through full range of motion against gravity and less than moderate resistance.
		Fair plus	F+	=	The part moves through full range of motion against gravity, takes minimal resistance, and then "breaks," i.e., relaxes suddenly.
	3	Fair	F	=	The part moves through full range of motion against gravity with no added resistance.
		Fair minus	F–	=	The part moves less than full range of motion against gravity.
Gravity Eliminated		Poor plus	P+	=	The part moves through full range of motion on a gravity-eliminated plane, takes minimal resistance, and then "breaks."
	2	Poor	P	=	The part moves through full range of motion on a gravity-eliminated plane, with no added resistance.
		Poor minus	P–	=	The part moves less than full range of motion on a gravity-eliminated plane.
	1	Trace	T	=	Tension is palpated in the muscle or the tendon but no motion occurs at the joint.
	0	Zero	0	=	No tension is palpated in the muscle or tendon.

Table 8.3
SAMPLE FORM FOR RECORDING MUSCLE STRENGTH

Patient's Name:_____

Diagnosis:_____

Patient's Case Number:_____ Date of Onset:_____

LEFT					RIGHT	
				Examiner		
				Date		

		S C A P U L A		**ELEVATION**
				    Upper Trapezius (accessory) CR XI, C_{3-4}
				    Levator Scapulae (dorsal scapular)C_5, C_{3-4}		

				DEPRESSION
				    Lower Trapezius (accessory) CR XI, C_{3-4}
				    Latissimus Dorsi (thoraco-dorsal) C_{6-8}		

				ADDUCTION
				    Middle Trapezius (accessory) CR XI, C_{3-4}
				    Rhomboids (dorsal scapular) C_5		

				ABDUCTION Serratus Anterior (long thoracic) C_{5-7}		

		S H O U L D E R		**FLEXION**
				    Anterior Deltoid (axillary) C_{5-6}
				    Coracobrachialis (musculocutaneous) C_{5-6}
				    Pectoralis Major-clavicular (pectoral) C_5-T_1
				    Biceps (musculocutaneous) C5-6		

				EXTENSION
				    Latissimus Dorsi (thoraco-dorsal) C_{6-8}
				    Teres Major (lower subscapular) C_{5-6}
				    Posterior Deltoid (axillary) C_{5-6}
				    Triceps-long head (radial) C_{7-8}		

				ABDUCTION
				    Supraspinatus (suprascapular) C_5
				    Middle Deltoid (axillary) C_{5-6}		

				ADDUCTION
				    Latissimus Dorsi (thoraco-dorsal) C_{6-8}
				    Teres Major (lower subscapular) C_{5-6}
				    Pectoralis Major (pectoral) C_5-T_1		

Table 8.3—_continued_

LEFT				RIGHT	
		Examiner			
		Date			

	SHOULDER Cont'd.	**INTERNAL ROTATION**
		    Subscapularis (upper & lower subscapular) C_{5-6}
		    Teres Major (lower subscapular) C_{5-6}
		    Latissimus Dorsi (thoraco-dorsal) C_{6-8}
		    Pectoralis Major (pectoral) $C_5\text{-}T_1$
		    Anterior Deltoid (axillary) C_{5-6}			

		EXTERNAL ROTATION
		    Infraspinatus (suprascapular) C_{5-6}
		    Teres Minor (axillary) C_{5-6}
		    Posterior Deltoid (axillary) C_{5-6}			

		HORIZONTAL ABDUCTION Posterior Deltoid (axillary) C_{5-6}			

		HORIZONTAL ADDUCTION
		    Pectoralis Major (pectoral) $C_5\text{-}T_1$
		    Anterior Deltoid (axillary) C_{5-6}			

	ELBOW	**FLEXION**
		    Biceps (musculocutaneous) C_{5-6}
		    Brachioradialis (radial) C_{5-6}
		    Brachialis (musculocutaneous) C_{5-6}			

		EXTENSION Triceps (radial) C_{7-8}			

	FOREARM	**SUPINATION**
		    Supinator (radial) C_6
		    Biceps (musculocutaneous) C_{5-6}			

		PRONATION
		    Pronator Teres (median) C_{6-7}
		    Pronator Quadratus (median) $C_8\text{-}T_1$			

	WRIST	**EXTENSION**
		    Ext. Carpi Radialis Longus (radial) C_{6-7}
		    Ext. Carpi Radialis Brevis (radial) C_{6-7}
		    Ext. Carpi Ulnaris (radial) C_{7-8}			

		FLEXION
		    Flexor Carpi Radialix (median) C_{6-7}
		    Palmaris Longus (median) C_8
		    Flexor Carpi Ulnaris (ulnar) C_{7-8}			

	FINGERS	P.I.P.	**FLEXION**
			    Flexor Superficialis 1st (median) $C_7\text{-}T_1$
			    Flexor Superficialis 2nd (median) $C_7\text{-}T_1$
			    Flexor Superficialis 3rd (median) $C_7\text{-}T_1$
			    Flexor Superficialis 4th (median) $C_7\text{-}T_1$		

Table 8.3—*continued*

LEFT						Examiner	RIGHT	
						Date		
			F	D.I.P.		Flexor Profundus 1st (median) C_8-T_1		
			I			Flexor Profundus 2nd (median) C_8-T_1		
			N			Flexor Profundus 3rd (ulnar) C_8-T_1		
			G			Flexor Profundus 4th (ulnar) C_8-T_1		
			E	5th MP		Flexor Digiti Minimi (ulnar) C_8-T_1		
			R			EXTENSION		
			S			Extensor Digitorum 1st (radial) C_{7-8}		
				M.P.		Extensor Digitorum 2nd (radial) C_{7-8}		
						Extensor Digitorum 3rd (radial) C_{7-8}		
						Extensor Digitorum 4th (radial) C_{7-8}		
						Extensor Digiti Minimi (radial) C_{7-8}		
						Lumbrical 1st (median) C_8-T_1		
						Lumbrical 2nd (median) C_8-T_1		
						Lumbrical 3rd (ulnar) C_8-T_1		
						Lumbrical 4th (ulnar) C_8-T_1		
			F			ABDUCTION		
			I			Dorsal Interosseus 1st (ulnar) C_8-T_1		
			N			Dorsal Interosseus 2nd (ulnar) C_8-T_1		
			G			Dorsal Interosseus 3rd (ulnar) C_8-T_1		
			E			Dorsal Interosseus 4th (ulnar) C_8-T_1		
			R			Abductor Digiti Minimi (ulnar) C_8-T_1		
			S			ADDUCTION		
						Palmar Interosseus 1st (ulnar) C_8-T_1		
						Palmar Interosseus 2nd (ulnar) C_8-T_1		
						Palmar Interosseus 3rd (ulnar) C_8-T_1		

Table 8.3—*continued*

LEFT				RIGHT	
			Examiner		
			Date		
			FLEXION		
		T H U M B	Flexor Pollicis Longus (median) C_8-T_1		
			Flexor Pollicis Brevis (median & ulnar) C_{6-8} & C_8-T_1		
			EXTENSION		
			Extensor Pollicis Longus (radial) C_{7-8}		
			Extensor Pollicis Brevis (radial) C_{7-8}		
			ABDUCTION		
			Abductor Pollicis Longus (radial) C7-8		
			Abductor Pollicis Brevis (median) C_8-T_1		
			ADDUCTION		
			Adductor Pollicis (ulnar) C_8-T_1		
			OPPOSITION		
			Opponens Pollicis (median) C_8-T_1		
		5th	Opponens Digiti Minimi (ulnar) C_8-T_1		
			FLEXION		
		H I P	Iliopsoas (femoral) L_{2-3}		
			EXTENSION		
			Gluteus Maximus (inf. gluteal) L_5-S_2		
			ABDUCTION		
			Gluteus Medius (sup. gluteal) L_4-S_1		
			Gluteus Minimus (sup. gluteal) L_4-S_1		

Table 8.3—*continued*

LEFT				RIGHT	
			Examiner		
			Date		
		HIP	ADDUCTION		
			Adductor Magnus (obturator)L3-4 (sciatic)L4-S3		
			Adductor Longus (obturator) L3-4		
			Adductor Brevis (obturator) L3-4		
			EXTERNAL ROTATION		
			Gluteus Maximus (inf. gluteal) L_5-S_2		
			Six small external rotators L_4-S_2		
			INTERNAL ROTATION		
			Gluteus Medius (sup. gluteal) L_4-S_1		
			Gluteus Minimus (sup. gluteal) L_4-S_1		
		KNEE	FLEXION		
			Hamstrings (sciatic) L_5-S_2		
			EXTENSION		
			Quadriceps (femoral) L_{2-4}		
		ANKLE	DORSIFLEXION		
			Tibialis Anterior (deep peroneal) L_4-S_1		
			Extensor Digitorum Longus (deep peroneal)L_4-S_1		
			Extensor Hallucis Longus (deep peroneal)L_4-S_1		
			PLANTAR FLEXION		
			Gastrocnemius (tibial) S1-2		
			Soleus (tibial) S_{-2}		
		FOOT	INVERSION		
			Tibialis Anterior (deep peroneal) L_4-S_1		
			Tibialis Posterior (tibial) L_5-S_1		
			EVERSION		
			Peroneus Longus (superficial peroneal)L_4-S_1		
			Peroneus Brevis (superficial peroneal)L_4-S_1		
			Peroneus Tertius (deep peroneal) L_4-S_1		

Innervations according to Lockhart, R. D., Hamilton, G. F., and Fyfe, F. W. *Anatomy of the Human Body.* Philadelphia: J. B. Lippincott, 1959.

MEASUREMENT OF THE UPPER EXTREMITY

The photograph of each against-gravity position shows the completed test motion and the application of resistance. The photograph of each gravity-eliminated position shows the support of the part during motion.

Scapular Elevation

Prime Movers
  Upper trapezius
  Levator scapulae

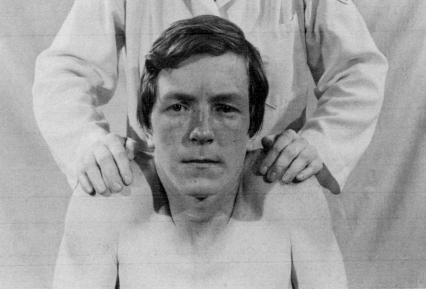

Figure 8.88 Resistance in the against-gravity position. Movement starts with patient sitting erect with arms at the side. Patient raises his shoulders toward his ears.

Figure 8.89 Gravity-eliminated position. With the patient prone, arms at the side, the therapist supports the shoulder as the patient attempts to move his shoulder toward his ear. The shoulder is lifted so the scapular motion will be on a gravity-eliminated plane. The therapist's left hand is palpating the upper trapezius.

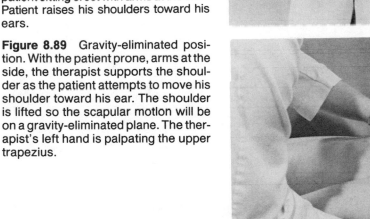

Stabilize. Trunk is stabilized against the plinth.

Palpation. Upper trapezius is palpated on the shoulder at the curve of the neck. The levator is palpated posteriorly to the sternocleidomastoid on the lateral side of the neck.

Resistance. The therapist's hand is placed over the acromion and pushes down toward scapular depression. A normal trapezius of an adult cannot be "broken" using the break test.

Substitution. Pushing on knees with hands.

Scapular Depression

Prime Movers
   Lower trapezius
   Latissimus dorsi

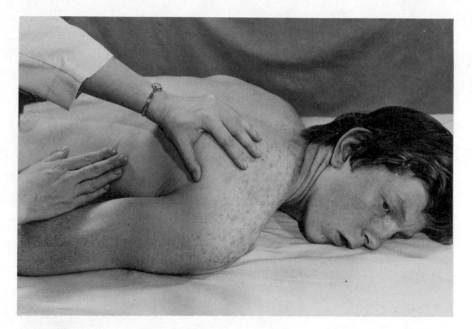

Figure 8.90 Resistance in the gravity-eliminated position. The patient is prone with the arm internally rotated and at the side. From resting position, patient moves the scapula caudally. The therapist's right hand is palpating the latissimus dorsi.

Against-gravity position. This is tested in the gravity-eliminated position, since the patient cannot be positioned to move against gravity.

Stabilize. Trunk is stabilized by the plinth.

Palpation. The lower trapezius is palpated lateral to the vertebral column as it passes diagonally from the lower thoracic vertebrae to the spine of the scapula. The latissimus dorsi is palpated along the posteriolateral rib cage or at its point of distal attachment in the posterior axilla.

Resistance. The therapist's hand is cupped over the inferior angle of the scapula and pushes upward toward scapular elevation. When the inferior angle is not easily accessible due to tissue bulk, resistance can be applied at the distal humerus *if* the shoulder joint is stable and pain-free.

Grading. Because of the positioning, it is not possible to accurately grade shoulder depressors for against-gravity grades. Experienced therapists estimate these grades and place a question mark (?) beside the grade.

Substitutions. In an upright position, gravity can substitute. In a prone position, the arm can be inched downward using the finger flexors.

Scapular Adduction

Prime Movers
  Middle trapezius
  Rhomboids

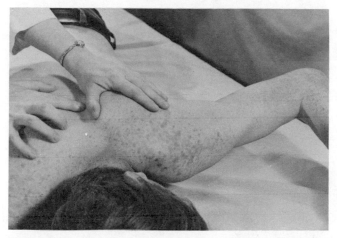

Figure 8.91 Test for middle trapezius against gravity and resistance. The shoulder is externally rotated. The patient lifts his arm up off the plinth to move the scapula toward the vertebral column. The theraplst's right index finger points to the middle trapezius.

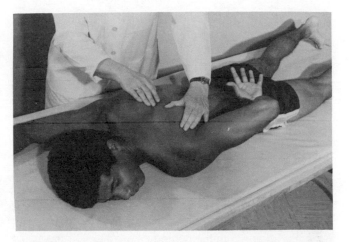

Figure 8.92 Test for rhomboids against gravity and resistance. The shoulder is internally rotated with the hand held over the lumbar region. The patient lifts his hand up off of the buttocks to move the scapula toward the vertebral column. The therapist's right hand palpates the rhomboids.

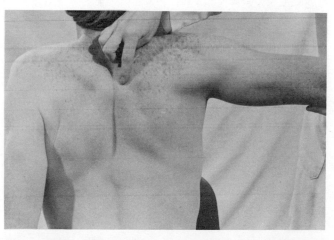

Figure 8.93 Gravity-eliminated position. The patient sits erect with the humerus abducted to 90° and supported. He attempts to move the scapula toward the vertebral column.

Stabilize. Trunk.

Palpation. Middle trapezius is palpated between the vertebral column and vertebral border of the scapula at the level of the spine of the scapula. With the arm in internal rotation and held over the back, the rhomboids are palpated along the vertebral border of the scapula, near the inferior angle.

Resistance. The whole length of the therapist's thumb is placed along the vertebral border of the scapula and the rest of the hand is placed on the dorsal surface of the scapula. The therapist pushes laterally.

Substitutions. None.

Scapular Abduction

Prime Mover
Serratus anterior

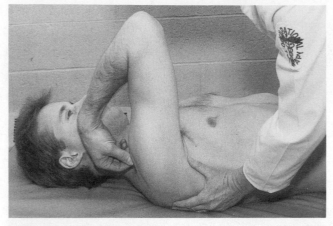

Figure 8.94 Resistance in the against-gravity position. The patient is supine with the humerus flexed to 90°; the elbow may be flexed or extended. The patient abducts the scapula so that the arm moves upward.

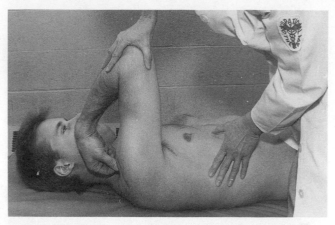

Figure 8.95 Alternative method of applying resistance in against-gravity position. The therapist's left hand palpates the digitations of the serratus anterior. See text for precautions.

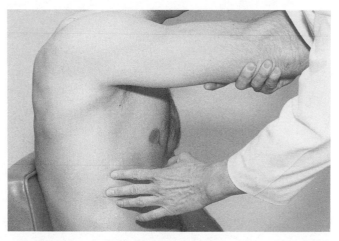

Figure 8.96 Gravity-eliminated position. The patient sits erect with the humerus flexed to 90° and supported; the elbow may be flexed or extended. He abducts the scapula so that the arm moves forward.

Stabilize. Trunk.

Palpation. Serratus anterior is palpated on the lateral ribs just lateral to the inferior angle of the scapula.

Resistance. According to the rule, resistance should be applied along the axillary border of the scapula (Fig. 8.94). Because it is difficult to apply resistance there, therapists often resist this motion either by grasping the distal humerus or by cupping the hand over the patient's elbow and pushing down or backward toward adduction (Fig. 8.95). Of course, this is an unsafe practice if the glenohumeral joint is unstable. Another reason for not testing in this way is that a normal serratus is very strong and normal shoulder flexors may "give" before the serratus does.[20]

Substitutions. In the gravity-eliminated position this motion can be achieved by inching the arm forward on the supportive surface using the finger flexors.

Shoulder Flexion

Prime Movers
  Anterior deltoid
  Coracobrachialis
  Pectoralis major—clavicular
  Biceps—both heads

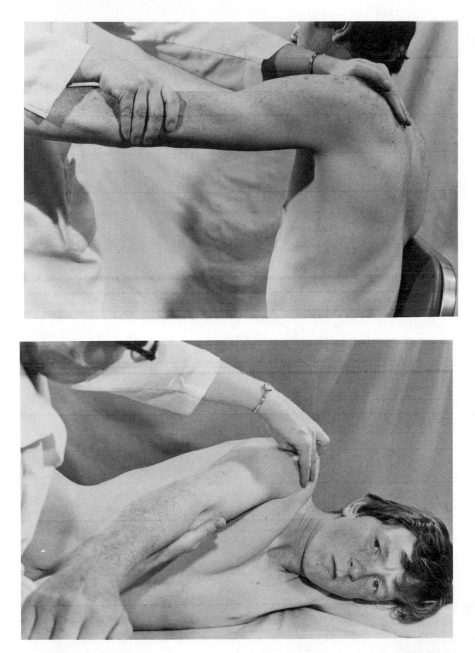

Figure 8.97 Resistance in the against-gravity position. The patient sits erect with the arm at the side in midposition. He flexes the humerus to 90° with the elbow extended.

Figure 8.98 Gravity-eliminated position. The patient is side-lying with arm in midposition along the side of the body. The arm is supported by the therapist or by a smooth testing board while the patient attempts to flex the humerus to 90° with the elbow extended. The therapist's left hand is palpating the anterior deltoid.

Stabilize. Scapula.

Palpation. Anterior deltoid is palpated immediately anterior to the glenohumeral joint. Coracobrachialis may be palpated medially to the biceps, which are palpated on the anterior aspect of the humerus. The clavicular head of the pectoralis major may be palpated below the clavicle on its way to insert on the humerus below the anterior deltoid.

Resistance. The therapist's hand is placed over the distal end of the humerus and pushes down toward extension. Movement above 90° involves scapular upward rotation; these motions are separated for muscle testing, although they are not separated for range of motion measurement.

Substitutions. Shoulder abductors; trunk extension.

Shoulder Extension

Prime Movers
    Latissimus dorsi
    Teres major
    Posterior deltoid
    Triceps—long head

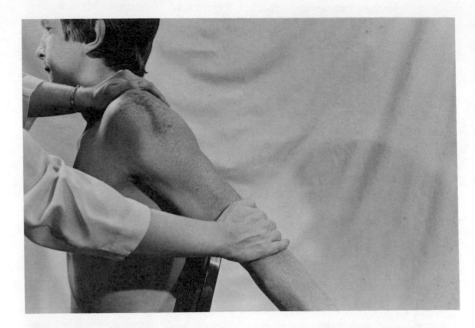

Figure 8.99 Resistance in the against-gravity position. Patient is sitting with the humerus internally rotated and the arm by the side. He extends the humerus. An alternate starting position is with the patient prone. *Note.* The therapist stands in front of the patient for safety to prevent the trunk from bending forward when resistance is applied.

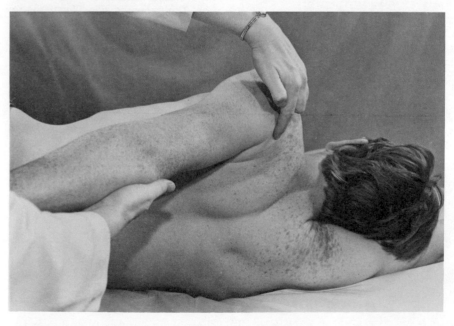

Figure 8.100 Gravity-eliminated position. The patient is side-lying with the humerus internally rotated and the arm supported with the elbow extended. Patient attempts to extend the humerus. The therapist is pointing to the posterior deltoid.

Stabilize. Scapula.

Palpation. The latissimus dorsi and the teres major form the posterior border of the axilla. The latissimus dorsi is located inferior to the teres major. The posterior deltoid is located immediately posterior to the glenohumeral joint. The triceps is palpated on the posterior aspect of the humerus.

Resistance. The therapist's hand is placed over the distal end of the humerus and pushes forward toward flexion.

Substitutions. Shoulder abductors; tipping the shoulder forward.

Shoulder Abduction

Prime Movers
   Supraspinatus
   Middle deltoid

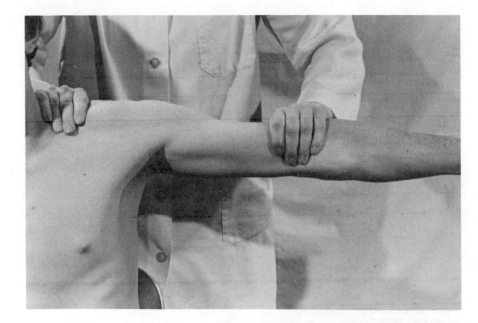

Figure 8.101 Resistance in the against-gravity position. The patient sits erect with the arm at the side in midposition. He abducts the humerus to 90° with the elbow extended.

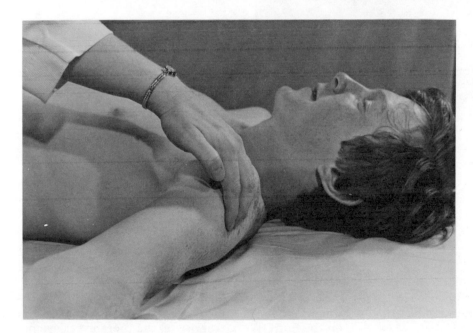

Figure 8.102 Gravity-eliminated position. The patient lies supine with the arm supported at the side in midposition. He attempts to abduct the arm to 90° with the elbow extended. The middle deltoid is palpated on top of the shoulder joint.

Stabilize. Scapula.

Palpation. The supraspinatus lies too deep for easy palpation. The middle deltoid is palpated below the acromion and lateral to the glenohumeral joint.

Resistance. The therapist's hand is placed over the distal end of the humerus and pushes the humerus down toward the body. Movement above 90° involves scapular upward rotation and is not measured.

Substitutions. The long head of the biceps can substitute if the humerus is allowed to be moved into external rotation; trunk lateral flexion.

Shoulder Adduction

Prime Movers
  Pectoralis major
  Teres major
  Latissimus dorsi

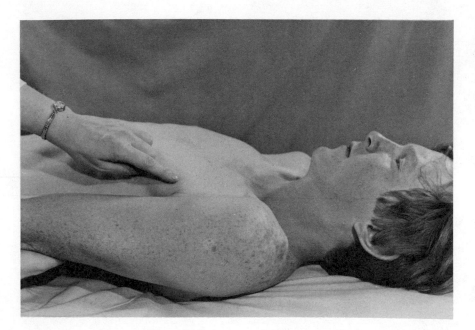

Figure 8.103 Resistance in the gravity-eliminated position. The patient is supine with the humerus abducted to 90° and in midposition. He adducts the humerus. The therapist is pointing to the sternal portion of the pectoralis major.

Test in the gravity-eliminated position since the patient cannot be positioned for this motion against gravity.

Stabilize. Trunk.

Palpation. The pectoralis major forms the anterior border of the axilla where it may be easily palpated. Palpation of the teres major and the latissimus dorsi has been previously described.

Resistance. The therapist's hand is placed on the medial side of the distal end of the humerus and pulls the humerus away from the patient's body.

Grading for antigravity grades again can only be estimated and a question mark entered beside the grade on the form. With experience, the therapist develops the skill to estimate reliably.

Substitutions. In an upright position gravity can substitute. On a supporting surface, the arm can be inched down using the finger flexors.

Shoulder Horizontal Abduction

Prime Mover
  Posterior deltoid

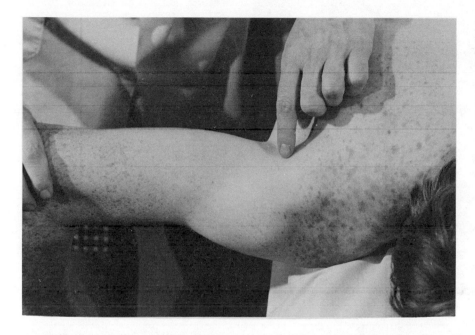

Figure 8.104 Resistance in the against-gravity position. The patient is positioned prone with the arm hanging in internal rotation over the edge of the table. He horizontally abducts the humerus, allowing the elbow to flex. The therapist is pointing to the posterior deltoid.

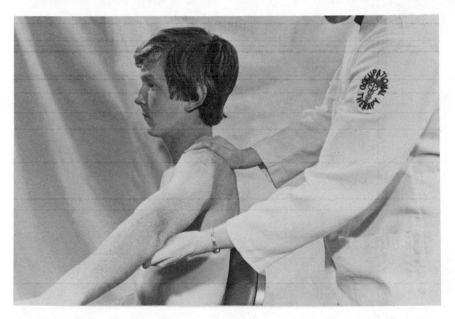

Figure 8.105 Gravity-eliminated position. The patient sits with the humerus flexed to 90° and the arm supported. He attempts to horizontally abduct the humerus.

Stabilize. Scapula. In the sitting position stabilize the trunk against the back of the chair.

Palpation. Posterior deltoid is palpated immediately posterior to the glenohumeral joint.

Resistance. Therapist's hand is placed on the posterior surface of the distal end of the humerus and pushes the arm downward or forward toward horizontal adduction.

Substitution. Trunk rotation in a sitting position.

Shoulder Horizontal Adduction

Prime Movers
  Pectoralis major
  Anterior deltoid

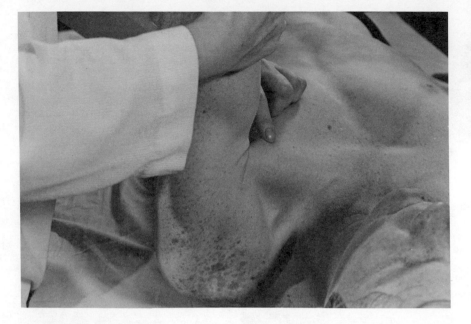

Figure 8.106 Resistance in the against-gravity position. The patient lies with the humerus abducted to 90°. The patient horizontally adducts the humerus to 90° of shoulder flexion. *Note*. In the supine position, if the triceps is weak, prevent the patient's hand from hitting his face. The therapist is pointing to the sternal portion of the pectoralis major. The clavicular portion can be seen to contract just caudal to the triangle formed by it, the clavicle, and the anterior deltoid.

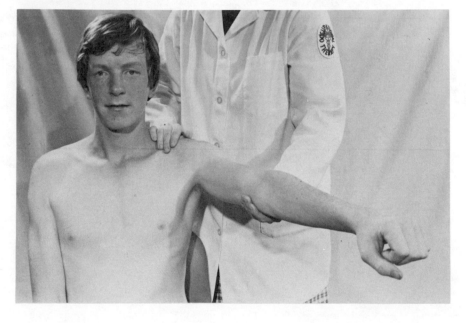

Figure 8.107 Gravity-eliminated position. The patient sits with the humerus abducted to 90° and attempts to horizontally adduct the humerus.

Stabilize. Scapula. In the sitting position stabilize the trunk against the back of the chair.

Palpation. The pectoralis major can be palpated along the anterior border of the axilla. The anterior deltoid is located immediately anterior to the glenohumeral joint below the acromion process.

Resistance. The therapist's hand is placed on the anterior surface of the distal end of the humerus and pushes the arm backward toward horizontal abduction.

Substitutions. In a sitting position, trunk rotation can substitute. The arm can be inched across the supporting surface using the finger flexors.

Shoulder External Rotation

Prime Movers
  Infraspinatus
  Teres minor
  Posterior deltoid

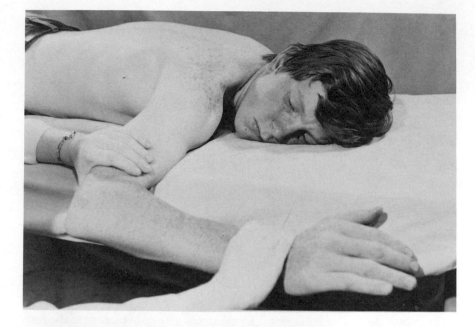

Figure 8.108 Resistance in the against-gravity position. The patient lies prone with the humerus abducted to 90° and supported on the table and the elbow flexed to 90° with the forearm dangling over the edge of the table. The patient externally rotates the humerus, bringing the dorsal surface of the hand toward the ceiling.

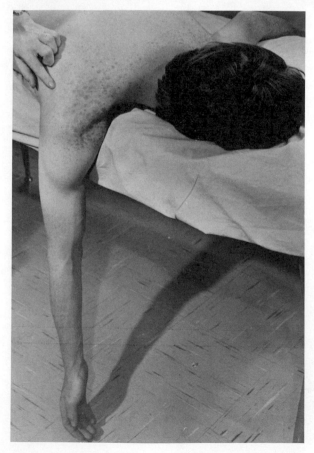

Figure 8.109 Gravity-eliminated position. The patient lies prone with the entire arm dangling over the edge of the table. He attempts to externally rotate the humerus.

Stabilize. Humerus at the elbow to allow only rotation.

Palpation. The infraspinatus is palpated inferiorly to the spine of the scapula. The teres minor is palpated between the posterior deltoid and the axillary border of the scapula; it is located superiorly to the teres major. Palpation of the posterior deltoid has been described.

Resistance. (1) Against gravity—the therapist's hand is placed on the dorsal surface of the distal end of the forearm and pushed toward the floor, keeping the patient's elbow supported and flexed to 90° to prevent supination. (2) Gravity-eliminated—the therapist's hand encircles the distal end of the humerus and turns the humerus toward internal rotation.

Alternate gravity-eliminated position: the therapist's hand is placed on the dorsal surface of the distal end of the forearm and pushes forward, keeping the elbow flexed to 90°.

Substitutions. Scapula adduction combined with downward rotation can substitute. The triceps may substitute when resistance is applied in an against gravity position or in the alternate gravity-eliminated position. Supination may be mistaken for external rotation in a gravity-eliminated position.

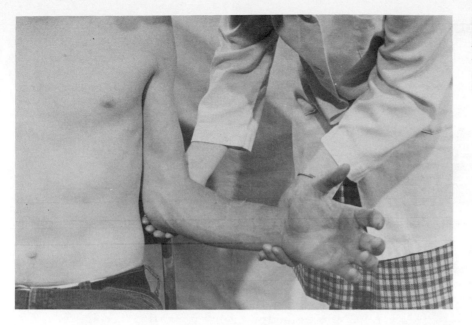

Figure 8.110 Alternate gravity-eliminated position. The patient sits with the humerus adducted and the elbow flexed to 90°. The hand moves laterally as the patient externally rotates the humerus.

Shoulder Internal Rotation

Prime Movers
    Subscapularis
    Teres major
    Latissimus dorsi
    Pectoralis major
    Anterior deltoid

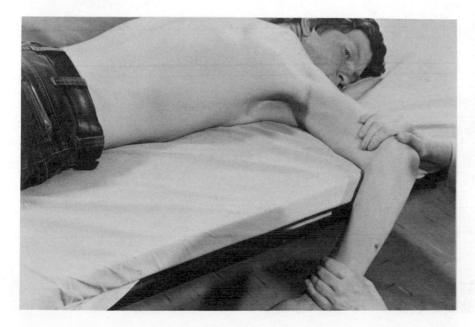

Figure 8.111 Resistance in the against-gravity position. The patient lies with the humerus abducted to 90° and supported on the table and the elbow flexed to 90° with the forearm dangling over the edge of the table. The patient internally rotates the humerus, bringing the palmar surface of the hand toward the ceiling.

Shoulder Internal Rotation *cont.*

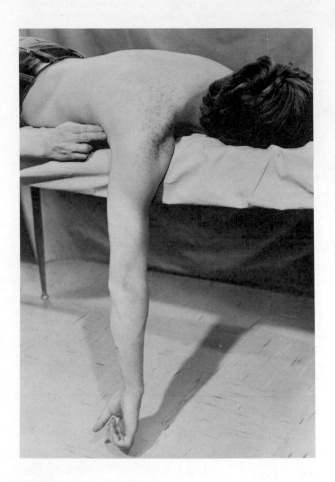

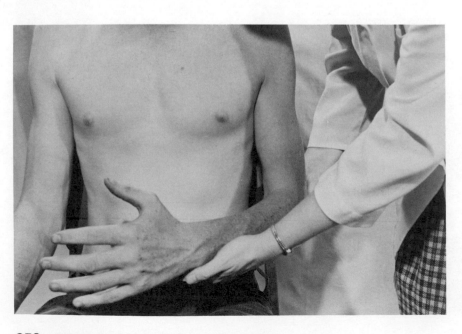

Figure 8.112 Gravity-eliminated position. The patient lies prone with the entire arm dangling over the edge of the table. He attempts to internally rotate the humerus. The therapist is palpating the teres major and latissimus dorsi.

Stabilize. Humerus at the elbow to allow only rotation.

Palpation. The subscapularis is not easily palpated but may be palpated in the posterior axilla. The teres major, latissimus dorsi, pectoralis major, and anterior deltoid are palpated as previously described.

Resistance. (1) Against gravity—the therapist's hand is placed on the volar surface of the distal end of the forearm and pushes toward the floor, keeping the elbow supported and flexed to 90°. (2) Gravity-eliminated—the therapist's hand encircles the distal end of the humerus and turns the humerus toward external rotation.

For alternate gravity-eliminated position: the therapist's hand is placed on the volar surface of the distal end of the forearm and pulls away from the abdomen, keeping the elbow flexed to 90°.

Substitutions. Scapula abduction combined with upward rotation can substitute. The triceps can substitute, as it did in external rotation. Pronation may be mistaken for internal rotation in a gravity-eliminated position.

Figure 8.113 Alternate gravity-eliminated position. The patient sits with the humerus adducted and the elbow flexed to 90°. Patient's hand moves toward the abdomen as he internally rotates the humerus.

Elbow Flexion

Prime Movers
  Biceps
  Brachialis
  Brachioradialis

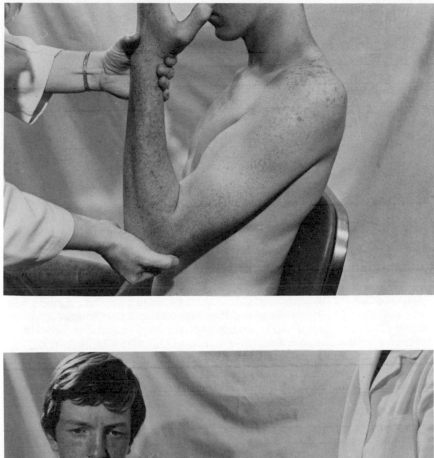

Figure 8.114 Resistance in the against-gravity position. The patient sits with his arm at the side in anatomical position. He raises his forearm so that the hand approximates the ipsilateral shoulder.

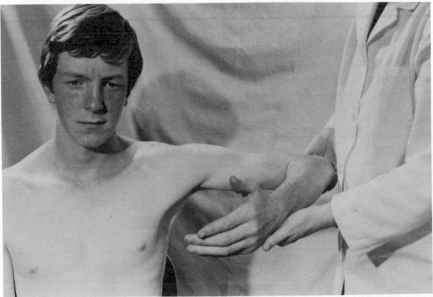

Figure 8.115 Gravity-eliminated position. The patient sits with the humerus abducted to 90° and the elbow extended, supported if necessary. The hand is relaxed. The patient attempts to flex the elbow.

Stabilize. Humerus.

Palpation. The biceps is easily palpated on the anterior surface of the humerus. With the biceps relaxed and the forearm pronated, the brachialis is palpated just medial to the distal biceps tendon. With the forearm in midposition the brachioradialis is palpated along the top of the proximal forearm.

Resistance. The therapist's hand is placed on the volar surface of the distal end of the forearm and pulls out toward extension.

Substitution. In a gravity-eliminated plane, the wrist flexors may substitute.

Elbow Extension

Prime Mover
Triceps

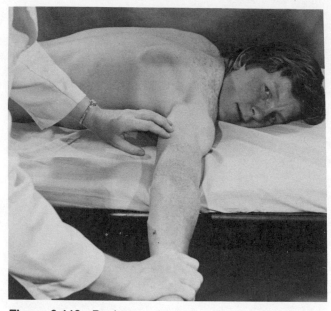

Figure 8.116 Resistance in the against-gravity position. The patient lies prone with the humerus abducted to 90° and supported on the table; the elbow is flexed and the forearm is hanging over the edge of the table. The patient extends the elbow. The therapist's left hand is palpating the long head of the triceps.

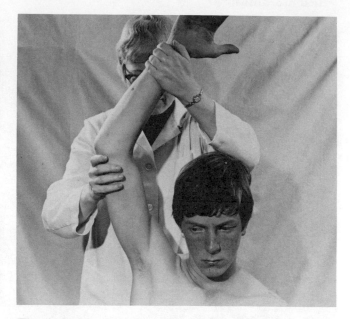

Figure 8.117 Alternate against-gravity position. The patient sits with the humerus flexed to 180° and the elbow fully flexed. He extends the elbow. *Note.* If the shoulder is flaccid, avoid shoulder abduction and external rotation when moving the arm into a position of full shoulder flexion. Without the protection of its cuff musculature, abduction and rotation may place stress on the joint capsule and may dislocate the head of the humerus.

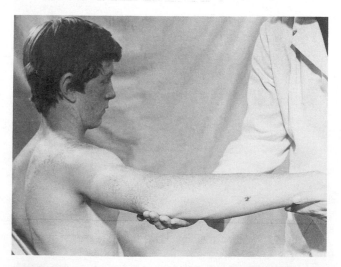

Figure 8.118 Gravity-eliminated position. The patient sits with the humerus abducted to 90° and supported if necessary; the elbow is fully flexed. The patient attempts to extend the elbow.

Stabilize. Humerus.

Palpation. The triceps is easily palpated on the posterior surface of the humerus.

Resistance. The therapist's hand is placed on the dorsal surface of the patient's forearm and pushes it toward flexion. Resistance is applied with the elbow in a position 10° to 15° less than full extension so that the elbow does not lock into position, which could unreliably indicate strength where none existed.

Substitutions. Gravity may substitute in a sitting position. In the gravity-eliminated position, no external rotation of the shoulder is permitted in order to avoid letting extension occur due to the assistance of gravity. On a supporting surface, finger flexion may be used to inch the forearm across the surface.

Pronation

Prime Movers
 Pronator teres
 Pronator quadratus

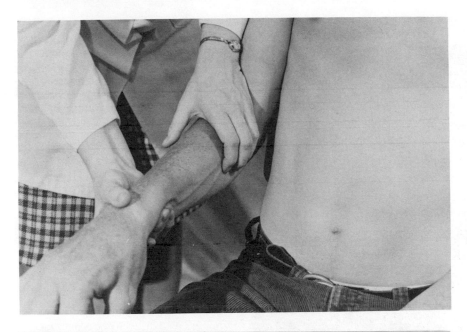

Figure 8.119 Resistance in the against-gravity position. The patient sits with the humerus adducted, the elbow flexed to 90°, the forearm supinated, and the wrist and fingers relaxed. The patient pronates to turn the palm down. *Note.* Gravity assists the motion beyond midposition. The therapist is palpating the pronator teres with her left hand.

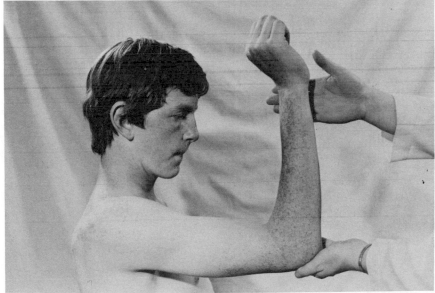

Figure 8.120 Gravity-eliminated position. The patient sits with the humerus flexed to 90° and supported, the elbow flexed to 90°, the forearm supinated, and the wrist and fingers relaxed. The patient pronates to turn the palm away from the face.

Stabilize. Humerus.

Palpation. The pronator teres is palpated medially to the distal attachment of the biceps tendon on the volar surface of the proximal forearm. Pronator quadratus is too deep to palpate.

Resistance. The therapist's hand encircles the patient's volar wrist with the therapist's index finger extended along the forearm. The forearm is turned in the direction of supination.

Alternate methods of applying resistance are: (1) The therapist encircles the distal forearm by cupping the forearm between his thenar eminence and four fingers to avoid hurting the patient by applying force through the tips of the fingers and thumb. (2) The therapist interlaces the fingers of both his hands, and the patient's distal forearm is cupped between the therapist's opposing palms.

Substitutions. The wrist and finger flexors may substitute.

Supination

Prime Movers
   Supinator
   Biceps

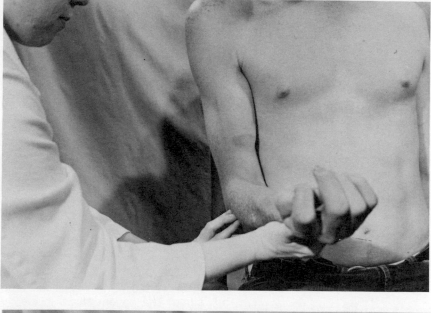

Figure 8.121 Resistance in the against-gravity position. The patient sits with the humerus adducted, the elbow flexed to 90°, the forearm pronated, and the wrist and fingers relaxed. The patient supinates to turn the palm up. *Note*. Gravity assists the motion beyond midposition. The therapist's left hand palpates the supinator.

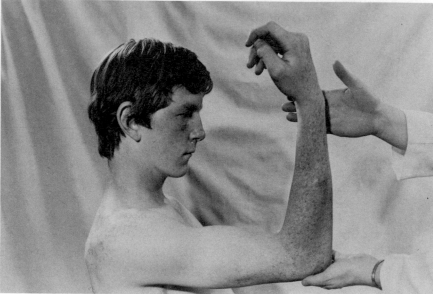

Figure 8.122 Gravity-eliminated position. The patient is positioned the same as for pronation, but with the forearm pronated. He attempts to turn the palm toward his face.

Note. To differentiate the supinator from the supination function of the biceps, test the supinator with elbow extended. The biceps does not supinate the extended arm unless resisted.[26]

Stabilize. Humerus.

Palpation. The supinator is palpated on the dorsal surface of the proximal forearm just distally to the head of the radius. Palpation of the biceps has been described.

Resistance. Same as for pronation except that the forearm is turned in the direction of pronation.

Substitutions. The wrist and finger extensors may substitute.

Muscles of the Wrist and Hand

Many tendons of wrist and hand muscles cross more than one joint. For this reason test positions for individual muscles must include ways to minimize the effect of other muscles crossing the joint. As a general rule, to minimize the effect of a muscle, place the part opposite to its prime action. For example, to minimize the effect of the extensor pollicis longus on extension of the proximal joint of the thumb, the distal joint is flexed.

Wrist Extension

1. Extensor carpi radialis longus (ECRL)

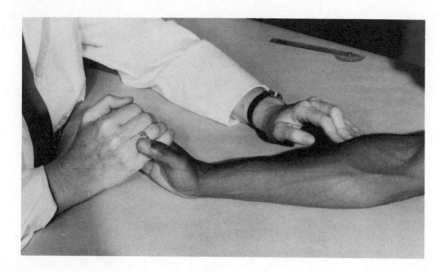

Figure 8.123 Resistance and palpation in the against-gravity position.

Position. (1) Against gravity—Forearm pronated to 45°, wrist flexed and ulnarly deviated, and the fingers and thumb relaxed. (2) Gravity-eliminated—Forearm in midposition, wrist flexed, fingers and thumb relaxed.

Stabilize. Forearm.

Test Motion. The patient extends the wrist toward the radial side.

Palpation. The tendon of the ECRL is palpated on the dorsal surface of the wrist at the base of the second metacarpal. The muscle belly is found on the dorsal proximal forearm adjacent to the brachioradialis.

Resistance. The therapist's palm is placed across the dorsum of the patient's hand on the radial side and pushes toward combined wrist flexion and ulnar deviation.

Substitutions. Extensor pollicis longus, extensor digitorum.

2. Extensor carpi radialis brevis (ECRB)

3. Extensor carpi ulnaris (ECU)

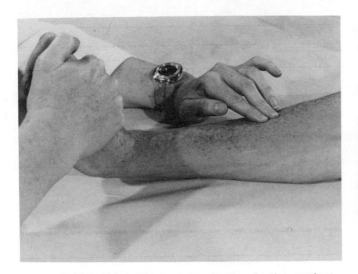

Figure 8.124 Resistance and palpation in the against-gravity position.

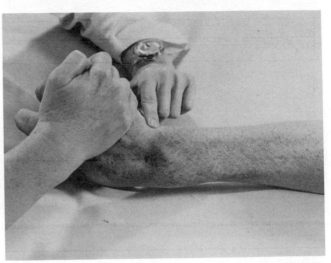

Figure 8.125 Resistance and palpation of the tendon in the against-gravity position.

Position. (1) Against gravity—Forearm is fully pronated, the wrist is flexed and undeviated, the fingers and thumb are relaxed. (2) Gravity-eliminated—Same as for ECRL.

Stabilize. Forearm.

Test Motion. The patient extends the wrist without deviation.

Palpation. The tendon of the ECRB is palpated on the dorsal surface of the wrist at the base of the third metacarpal adjacent to the ECRL. The muscle belly of ECRB is found distal to the belly of ECRL on the dorsal surface of the proximal forearm.

Resistance. The therapist's palm is placed across the dorsum of the patient's hand and pushes directly toward flexion.

Substitutions. Extensor pollicis longus; extensor digitorum.

Position. (1) Against gravity—Shoulder internally rotated, forearm fully pronated, wrist flexed and radially deviated, and fingers relaxed. (2) Gravity-eliminated—Forearm pronated to 45°, wrist flexed and radially deviated, fingers relaxed.

Stabilize. Forearm.

Test Motion. Patient extends the wrist toward the ulnar side.

Palpation. The ECU tendon is palpated on the dorsal surface of the wrist between the head of the ulna and the base of the fifth metacarpal. The muscle belly is found approximately 2 inches distal to the lateral epicondyle of the humerus.[27]

Resistance. The therapist's palm is placed across the dorsum of the patient's hand on the ulnar side and pushes toward combined wrist flexion and radial deviation.

Substitutions. Extensor digitorum.

Wrist Flexion

1. Flexor carpi radialis (FCR)

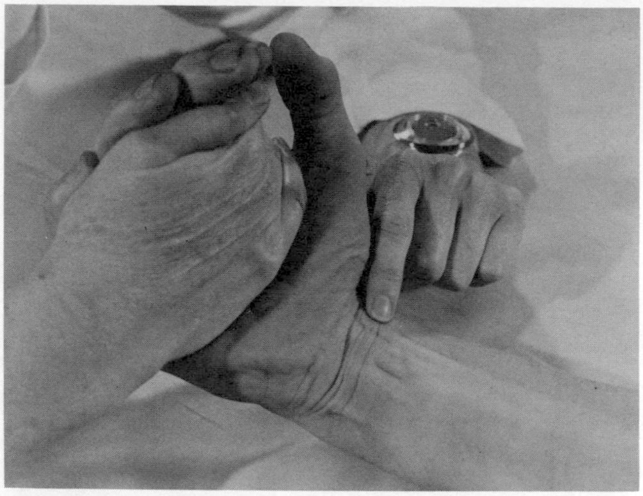

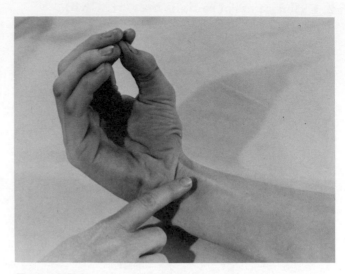

Figure 8.126 Resistance and palpation of the tendon in the against-gravity position.

Position. (1) Against gravity—Forearm supinated, wrist extended, and fingers and thumb relaxed. (2) Gravity-eliminated—Forearm in midposition, wrist extended, and fingers and thumb relaxed.

Stabilize. Forearm.

Test Motion. Patient flexes the wrist.

Palpation. The FCR tendon is palpated on the volar surface of the wrist in line with the second metacarpal and radial to the palmaris longus (if present).

Resistance. The therapist's fingers are placed across the patient's palm and pull toward wrist extension.

Substitutions. Abductor pollicis longus; flexor pollicis longus; flexor digitorum superficialis; and flexor digitorum profundus.

The palmaris longus is a weak wrist flexor that has a small muscle belly and long tendon. The tendon crosses the center of the volar surface of the wrist. If is not tested for strength and may not even be present. However, if it is present, it will stand out prominently in the middle of the wrist when wrist flexion is resisted or the palm cupped.

Position. (1) Against gravity—Shoulder adducted and externally rotated, forearm fully supinated, wrist extended, and fingers relaxed. (2) Gravity-eliminated—Forearm supinated to 45°, wrist extended, and fingers relaxed.

Stabilize. Forearm.

Test Motion. Patient flexes the wrist toward ulnar deviation.

2. Palmaris longus

Figure 8.127

3. Flexor carpi ulnaris (FCU)

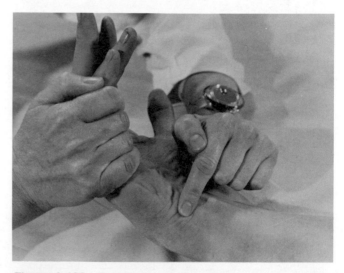

Figure 8.128 Resistance in the against-gravity position. The therapist's finger points to the tendon.

Palpation. The FCU tendon is palpated on the volar surface of the wrist just proximally to the pisiform bone.

Resistance. The therapist's fingers are placed across the patient's palm and pull toward wrist extension and radial deviation.

Substitutions. Flexor digitorum superficialis; flexor digitorum profundus.

Finger DIP Flexion

Flexor digitorum profundus (FDP)

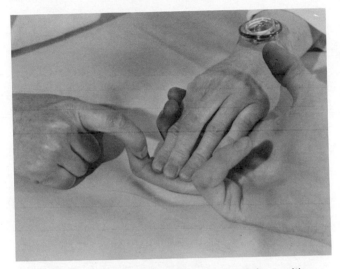

Figure 8.129 Resistance in the against-gravity position.

Finger PIP Flexion

Flexor digitorum superficialis (FDS)
Flexor digitorum profundus

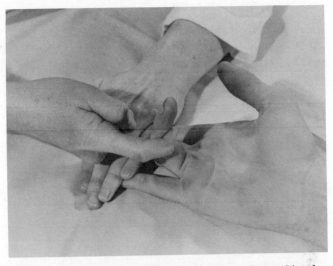

Figure 8.130 Resistance in the against-gravity position for flexor digitorum superficialis.

Position. (1) Against gravity—Forearm supinated and supported on a table; wrist and interphalangeal joints relaxed. (2) Gravity-eliminated—Forearm in midposition, resting on ulnar border on a table; wrist and interphalangeal joints relaxed in neutral position.

Stabilize. Middle phalanx of each finger as it is tested to prevent flexion of the proximal interphalangeal joint; wrist should remain in neutral position.

Test Motion. Flexion of the distal phalanx toward the middle phalanx.

Palpation. The belly of the FDP is palpated just volarly to the ulna in the proximal third of the forearm. The tendons are sometimes palpable on the volar surface of the middle phalanges.

Resistance. The therapist places one finger on the pad of the patient's finger and pulls toward extension.

Substitutions. Rebound effect of apparent flexion following contraction of extensors. Wrist extension causes tenodesis action.

Position (for flexor digitorum superficialis). (1) Against gravity—Forearm supinated and supported on the table; wrist and metacarpophalangeal joints relaxed. To rule out the influence of the profundus when testing the superficialis, hold all interphalangeal joints of the fingers not being tested into full extension. Because the profundus is essentially one muscle with four tendons, by preventing its action in three of the four fingers, it cannot work in the tested finger. In fact, the patient is unable to flex the distal joint of the tested finger at all! In some people the profundus slip to the index finger is such that this method cannot rule out its influence on the PIP joint of the index finger. This should be noted on the test form. (2) Gravity-eliminated—Forearm supported in midposition, with the wrist and MP joints relaxed in neutral position. Again rule out the influence of the FDP by holding all the joints of the nontested fingers in extension.

Stabilize. Proximal phalanx of the finger being tested and hold all joints of the other fingers into extension; the wrist should remain in neutral.

Test Motion. Patient flexes PIP joint.

Palpation. The superficialis is palpated on the volar surface of the proximal forearm toward the ulnar side. The tendons may be palpated at the wrist between the palmaris longus and the flexor carpi ulnaris.

Resistance. Using one finger, the therapist pulls the head of the middle phalanx toward extension.

Substitutions. Flexor digitorum profundus. Wrist extension causes tenodesis action.

Finger MP Flexion

Flexor digitorum profundus
Flexor digitorum superficialis
Dorsal interossei
Volar (Palmar) interossei
Flexor digiti minimi

The tests for the first four muscles have been or will be discussed under their alternate actions. The flexor of the little finger has no other action and is described here.

Finger Adduction

Volar (Palmar) interossei (3)

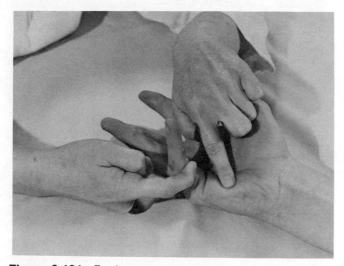

Figure 8.131 Resistance and palpation in the against-gravity position for flexor digiti minimi.

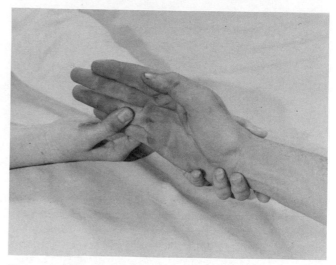

Figure 8.132 Resistance to palmar interossei 2 in the against-gravity position.

Position (for flexor digiti minimi). (1) Against gravity—Forearm supported in supination. (2) Gravity-eliminated—Forearm supported in midposition.

Stabilize. Other fingers in extension.

Test Motion. Patient flexes fifth finger at MP joint without flexing the interphalangeal joints.

Palpation. On the volar surface of the hypothenar eminence.

Resistance. Using one finger, the therapist pushes the head of the proximal phalanx toward extension. The therapist must be sure the interphalangeal joints remain extended.

Substitutions. Flexor digitorum profundus; flexor digitorum superficialis; third volar interosseus.

Position. (1) Against gravity—For palmar interossei 2 and 3, support the forearm on the ulnar border of the wrist with the fingers extended and abducted. For palmar interosseus 1, the arm is internally rotated, the forearm fully pronated so that the hand can be supported on the radial border, with the hand free and the fingers extended and abducted. (2) Gravity-eliminated—Forearm is supinated and supported.

Stabilize. Support the hand lightly.

Test Motion. As each is tested, the patient moves the index, ring, or little finger toward the middle finger.

Palpation. The palmar interossei are usually too deep to palpate with certainty. When these muscles are atrophied the areas between the metacarpals on the volar surface appear sunken.

Resistance. One by one, the therapist pulls the head of the proximal phalanx of each finger being tested away from the middle finger.

Substitutions. Extrinsic finger flexors; gravity, depending upon the position of the hand, most usually substitutes for the first palmar interosseus.

Finger Abduction

Dorsal interossei (4)
Abductor digiti minimi

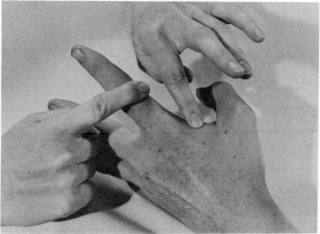

Figure 8.133 Resistance and palpation in the against-gravity position for dorsal interosseus 1.

Position. (1) Against gravity—For dorsal interossei 1 and 2, the forearm rests on the ulnar border on a supporting surface with the hand free and MPs adducted and slightly flexed. For dorsal interossei 3 and 4 and abductor digiti minimi, the arm is internally rotated, with the forearm fully pronated so that it can be supported on the radial border. The MPs are adducted and slightly flexed. Flexion of the MPs minimizes the abduction caused by the angle of pull of the extensor digitorum. (2) Gravity-eliminated—Forearm is pronated and supported with the hand free and MPs adducted and slightly flexed.

Stabilize. Support the hand lightly.

Test Motion. One by one, the patient moves the index finger away from the middle finger, the middle finger toward the index, the middle toward the ring finger, the ring finger toward the little finger, and the little finger away from the ring finger.

Palpation. The first dorsal interosseus fills the dorsal web space and can be easily palpated there. The abductor digiti minimi is palpated on the ulnar border of the fifth metacarpal. The other interossei lie between the metacarpals on the dorsal aspect of the hand where they may be palpated and on some people the tendons can be palpated as they enter the dorsal expansion near the heads of the metacarpals. When the dorsal interossei are atrophied, the spaces between the metacarpals appear sunken.

Resistance. The therapist pushes the head of the proximal phalanx of each finger, in turn, toward the direction opposite to its test motion.

Substitutions. Extensor digitorum; gravity, especially for dorsal interossei 3 and 4 and the abductor digiti minimi.

Finger MP Extension

Extensor digitorum (ED)
Extensor indicis proprius
Extensor digiti minimi

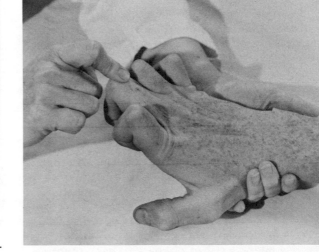

Figure 8.134 Resistance in the against-gravity position for extensor digitorum.

Position. (1) Against gravity—Forearm pronated and supported, wrist supported in neutral position, and fingers flexed at all joints. (2) Gravity-eliminated —Forearm supported in midposition, wrist in neutral, and fingers flexed.

Stabilize. Wrist and metacarpals.

Test Motion. Patient extends MP joints keeping the PIP and DIP joints flexed.

Palpation. The muscle belly of the ED is palpated on the dorsal-ulnar surface of the proximal forearm. Often the separate muscle bellies can be discerned. The tendons of this muscle are readily seen and palpated on the dorsum of the hand.

The extensor indicis tendon is located ulnarly to the extensor digitorum tendon. The belly of this muscle is palpated on the mid- to distal dorsal forearm between the radius and ulna.

The extensor digiti minimi tendon is palpated ulnarly to the ED. Actually, it is the tendon that looks as if it were the ED tendon to the little finger because the ED to the little finger is only a slip from the ED tendon to the ring finger.

Resistance. Using one finger, the therapist pushes the head of each proximal phalanx toward flexion, one at a time.

Substitution. Apparent extension of the fingers can occur due to the rebound effect of relaxation following finger flexion. Flexion of the wrist can cause finger extension through tenodesis action.

Finger Interphalangeal Extension

Lumbricales
Interossei
Extensor digitorum
Extensor indicis proprius
Extensor digiti minimi

According to electromyographical evidence, the intrinsics, especially the lumbricales, are the primary extensors of the interphalangeal joints.[28,29] Except for the lumbricales, the other muscles have been discussed. The lumbricales, arising as they do from the flexor profundus and inserting on the extensor digitorum, have a unique duty in regard to finger extension. Contracting against the noncontracting flexor profundus, the lumbricales pull the tendons of the profundus forward toward the fingertips. This slackens the profundus tendons distal to the insertion of the lumbricales, allowing the extensor digitorum to fully extend the interphalangeal joints, regardless of the position of the MP joints.[29,30] It has been electromyographically demonstrated that the profundus and the lumbricales operate out of phase with each other except during flexion of the metacarpophalangeal joints while the interphalangeal joints are extended or extending.[29] Electromyographic evidence exists which shows that the interossei flex the MP joints while extending the interphalangeal joints and, in fact, operate to extend only when the MP joints are flexed or flexing.[29]

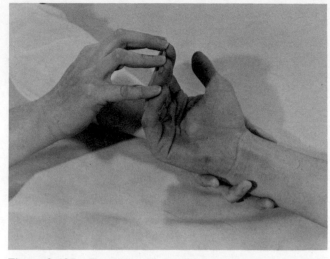

Figure 8.135 Resistance in the against-gravity position for testing lumbricales.

Position (lumbricales). There is no reliably good test for lumbrical function. Test 1 is the traditional test used. Test 2 is an hypothesized test. (1) Against gravity—Test 1: forearm supinated and supported. Wrist in neutral position, MPs extended, IPs flexed. Test 2: (alternate) MPs flexed and IPs extended. (2) Gravity-eliminated—same as above except that the forearm is supported in midposition.

Stabilize. Metacarpals.

Test Motion. Test 1—From the starting position, the patient simultaneously flexes his MP joints while extending his IP joints. The concept of this motion is difficult for patients to understand and will need practice.

Test 2—A perfectly adequate test, based on the electromyographical evidence, could be to have the patient maintain full IP extension while moving from a position of MP flexion to MP extension.

Palpation. Lumbricales lie too deeply to be palpated.

Resistance. Test 1—The therapist holds the tip of the finger being tested and pushes it toward starting position.

Test 2—The therapist places one finger on the patient's fingernail and pushes toward flexion.

Substitution. Nothing substitutes for DIP extension in the event of the loss of lumbrical function when the MP joint is extended. Other muscles of the dorsal expansion can substitute for DIP extension when the MP joint is flexed.

Thumb IP Extension

Extensor pollicis longus (EPL)

Thumb MP Extension

Extensor pollicis brevis (EPB)
Extensor pollicis longus

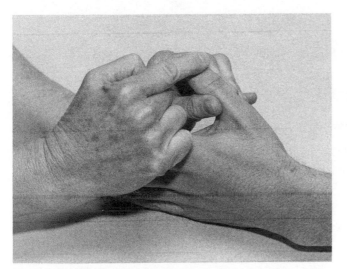

Figure 8.136 Resistance in the against-gravity position with stabilization of the proximal phalanx.

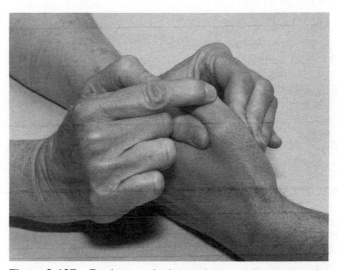

Figure 8.137 Resistance in the against-gravity position for extensor pollicis brevis with stabilization of the first metacarpal.

Position. (1) Against gravity—Forearm supported in midposition, thumb flexed. (2) Gravity-eliminated—Forearm pronated, thumb flexed.

Stabilize. Proximal phalanx.

Test Motion. Patient extends the IP joint of the thumb.

Palpation. The tendon of the EPL may be palpated on the ulnar border of the anatomical snuff box and also on the dorsal surface of the proximal phalanx of the thumb.

Resistance. The therapist places one finger over the dorsum of the distal phalanx (thumbnail) and pushes toward flexion.

Substitutions. Relaxation of the flexor pollicis longus will result in apparent extensor movement due to rebound effect.

Position (test for extensor pollicis brevis). (1) Against gravity—Forearm supported in midposition, MP joint flexed, IP joint flexed. (2) Gravity-eliminated—Forearm pronated, MP joint flexed, IP joint flexed.

Stabilize. First metacarpal in abduction.

Test Motion. The patient extends the MP joint, keeping the IP joint flexed to minimize the effect of the extensor pollicis longus. The EPB may not be present.

Palpation. The tendon of the EPB is palpated on the radial border of the anatomical snuff box medial to the tendon of the abductor pollicis longus.

Resistance. The therapist's index finger is placed on the dorsal surface of the head of the proximal phalanx and pushes toward flexion.

Substitution. Extensor pollicis longus.

Thumb Abduction

Abductor pollicis longus (APL)
Abductor pollicis brevis (APB)

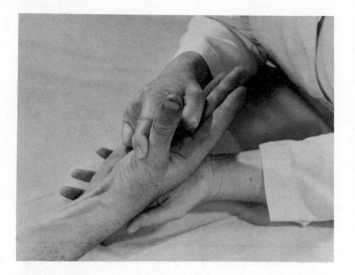

Figure 8.138 Resistance in the against-gravity position for abductor pollicis longus.

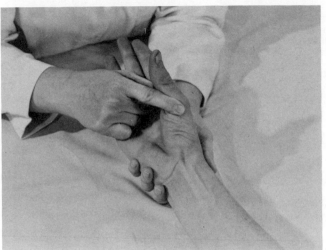

Figure 8.139 Resistance in the against-gravity position for abductor pollicis brevis.

Position (for abductor pollicis longus). (1) Against gravity—Forearm supinated to 45°, wrist in neutral, thumb adducted. (2) Gravity-eliminated—Forearm pronated to 45°, wrist in neutral, thumb adducted.

Stabilize. Support the wrist on the ulnar side and hold it in neutral position.

Test Motion. Patient abducts the thumb in a radial direction on a diagonal plane between extension and true abduction.

Palpation. The tendon of the APL is palpated at the wrist joint just distally to the radial styloid and laterally to the EPB.

Resistance. The therapist's finger presses the head of the first metacarpal toward adduction.

Substitutions. Abductor pollicis brevis; extensor pollicis brevis.

Position (for abductor pollicis brevis). (1) Against gravity—Forearm is supported in supination, wrist in neutral, thumb adducted. (2) Gravity-eliminated—Forearm is supported in midposition, wrist in neutral, thumb adducted.

Stabilize. Support the wrist in neutral position by holding it on the dorsal and ulnar side.

Test Motion. The patient abducts the thumb, bringing it straight up from the palm.

Palpation. APB is palpated over the center of the thenar eminence.

Resistance. The therapist's finger presses the head of the first metacarpal toward adduction.

Substitution. Abductor pollicis longus.

Thumb MP Flexion

Flexor pollicis brevis (FPB)
Flexor pollicis longus (FPL)

Thumb IP Flexion

Flexor pollicis longus

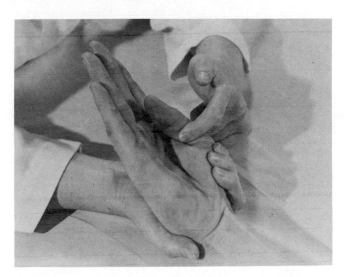

Figure 8.140 Resistance in the against-gravity position for flexor pollicis brevis with stabilization of the first metacarpal.

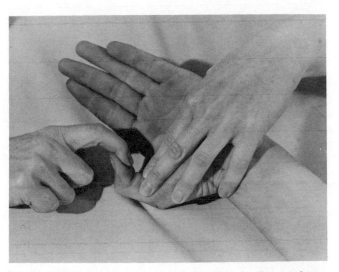

Figure 8.141 Resistance and palpation in the against-gravity position for flexor pollicis longus with stabilization of the proximal phalanx.

Position (for flexor pollicis brevis). (1) Against gravity—Elbow flexed and forearm supinated so that the palmar surface of the thumb faces the ceiling; thumb is extended at both the MP and IP joints. (2) Gravity-eliminated—Forearm supinated to 90° so that thumb can flex across the plane of the palm.

Stabilize. First metacarpal.

Test Motion. Patient flexes the MP joint but keeps the IP joint extended to minimize the influence of the flexor pollicis longus.

Palpation. The FPB is palpated on the thenar eminence just proximal to the MP joint, and medial to the abductor pollicis brevis.

Resistance. The therapist's finger pushes the head of the proximal phalanx toward extension.

Substitution. Flexor pollicis longus.

Position (for flexor pollicis longus). (1) Against gravity—Elbow flexed and forearm supinated so that the palmar surface of the thumb faces the ceiling; thumb extended at the MP and IP joints. (2) Gravity-eliminated—Forearm supinated to 90° so that the thumb can flex across the palm.

Stabilize. Proximal phalanx, holding MP joint in extension.

Test Motion. Patient flexes IP joint.

Palpation. The FPL tendon is palpated on the palmar surface of the proximal phalanx.

Resistance. The therapist's finger pushes the head of the distal phalanx toward extension.

Substitution. Relaxation of the extensor pollicis longus causes rebound movement.

Thumb Adduction

Adductor pollicis

Opposition

Opponens pollicis
Opponens digiti minimi

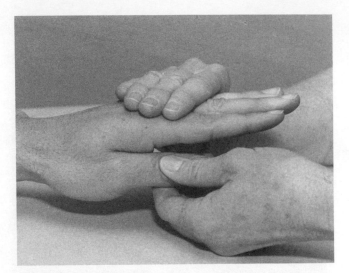

Figure 8.142 Resistance in the against-gravity position.

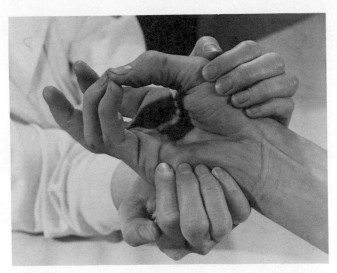

Figure 8.143 Resistance in the against-gravity position.

Position. (1) Against gravity—Forearm pronated, wrist and fingers in neutral, thumb abducted and MP and IP joints of the thumb in extension. (2) Gravity-eliminated—Same, except forearm in midposition.

Stabilize. Metacarpals of fingers, keeping the MP joints in neutral.

Test Motion. Patient brings the thumb toward the palm, without hyperextending the MP joint or flexing the MP or IP joints.

Palpation. Adductor pollicis is palpated on the palmar surface of the thumb web space.

Resistance. The therapist grasps the head of the proximal phalanx and pulls it away from the palm toward abduction.

Substitutions. Extensor pollicis longus, flexor pollicis longus; flexor pollicis brevis.

Position. (1) Against gravity—Forearm supinated and supported, wrist in neutral, thumb adducted and extended. (2) Gravity-eliminated—Elbow resting on the table with forearm perpendicular to the table, wrist in neutral, thumb adducted and extended.

Stabilize. Hold the wrist in a neutral position.

Test Motion. The patient brings the thumb away from and across the palm rotating it so that the pad of the thumb approximates the pad of the little finger. The little finger rotates around to meet the thumb.

Palpation. Place fingertips along the lateral side of the shaft of the first metacarpal where opponens pollicis may be palpated before it becomes deep to the abductor pollicis brevis. The opponens digit minimi can be palpated volarly along the shaft of the fifth metacarpal.

Resistance. The therapist holds along the first metacarpal and "derotates" the thumb or holds along the fifth metacarpal and "derotates" the little finger. These can be resisted simultaneously using both hands (see Fig. 8.143).

Substitutions. Abductor pollicis brevis; flexor pollicis brevis; flexor pollicis longus.

Hip Flexion

Prime Movers
   Iliopsoas
   Iliacus
   Psoas major

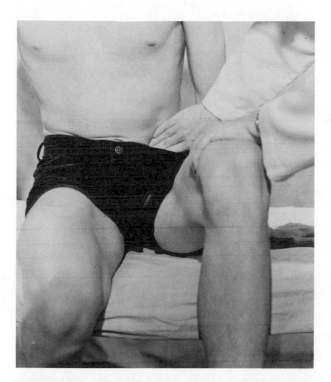

Figure 8.144 Resistance in the against-gravity position. The patient sits with his lower leg hanging over the edge of the sitting surface. He raises the thigh up from the surface; the knee remains flexed. The therapist's right hand is palpating the psoas major.

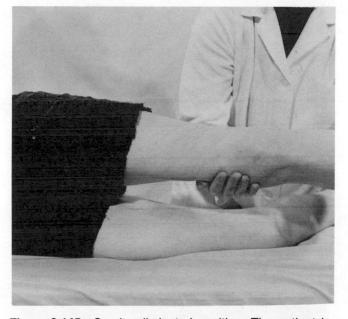

Figure 8.145 Gravity-eliminated position. The patient is side-lying on the side opposite the leg being tested. The leg to be tested is supported in extension at the hip and knee and in a position of 0° of abduction to align the leg and trunk. The patient flexes the hip as the therapist supports the leg in abduction; the knee may flex.

Stabilize. Pelvis.

Palpation. The iliacus is too deep to be palpated. In a sitting position the psoas major can be palpated with the patient bending forward to relax the abdominal muscles. The therapist's fingers are placed at the waist between the ribs and the iliac crest and pressure is applied posteriorly to feel the contraction of the psoas major as the hip flexes.[27]

Resistance. The therapist's hand is placed on the distal anterior thigh and presses downward toward extension.

Substitution. The abdominals can tilt the pelvis posteriorly to substitute for hip flexion in a gravity-eliminated position.

Hip Extension

Prime Movers
   Gluteus maximus
   Biceps femoris[26]

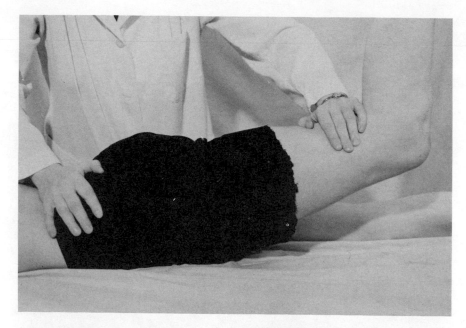

Figure 8.146 Resistance in the against-gravity position. The patient lies prone with knee flexed 90° or more[20,21] to test the gluteus maximus. The biceps femoris will be tested in its alternate function of knee flexion. The patient extends the hip keeping the knee flexed.

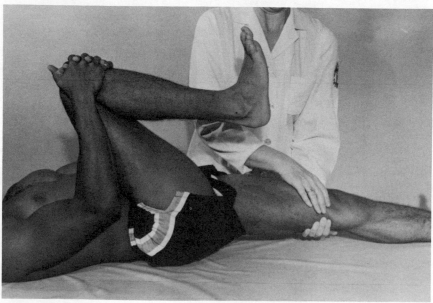

Figure 8.147 Alternate against-gravity position. Gluteus maximus and biceps femoris are tested together as hip extensors with the knee extended. The patient lies supine and holds the opposite leg in flexion at the hip and knee. The therapist holds the leg to be tested just above the knee and instructs the patient, "Do not let me raise your leg.[31] Grading: normal if trunk comes up from table; fair if the hip "gives" as the trunk begins to come up from the table.

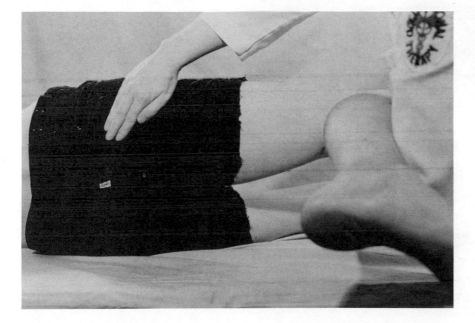

Figure 8.148 Gravity-eliminated position. The patient is side-lying with hip in neutral and knee flexed. The leg to be tested is on top. The patient extends the thigh. The therapist's hand indicates where to palpate the gluteus maximus.

Stabilize. Pelvis and lumbar spine.

Palpation. The gluteus maximus is the larger muscle of the buttock and can be easily palpated. The biceps femoris can be palpated on the posterior aspect of the thigh; its tendon bounds the popliteal fossa laterally.

Resistance. The therapist's hand is placed over the distal posterior thigh and presses downward or forward toward flexion.

Substitutions. Extension of the lumbar spine. The semimembranosus and semitendinosus assist resisted hip extension if the hip is abducted.[26]

Hip Abduction

Prime Movers
   Gluteus medius
   Gluteus minimus

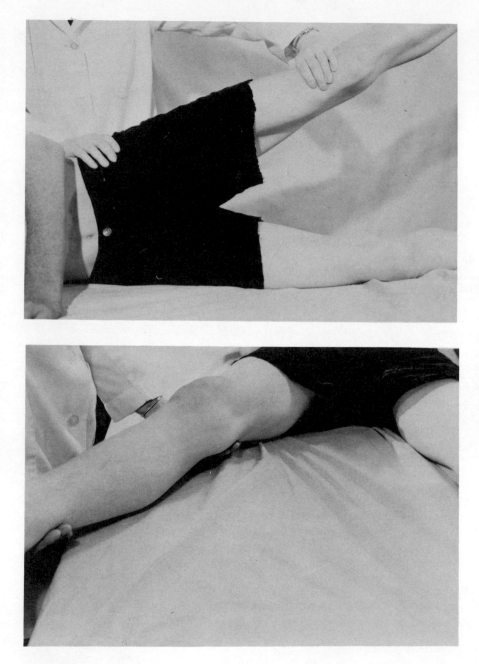

Figure 8.149 Resistance in the against-gravity position. The patient is side-lying on the side opposite the leg to be tested with that leg flexed at the hip and knee for balance. The leg to be tested is extended at the hip and knee and in alignment with the trunk. The patient moves the leg away from the midline of the body.

Figure 8.150 Gravity-eliminated position. The patient lies supine with hip and knee extended. He moves the leg away from midline.

Stabilize. Pelvis.

Palpation. The gluteus medius and minimus are palpated together laterally to the hip joint below the iliac crest.

Resistance. The therapist's hand is placed on the distal lateral thigh and pushes the leg toward the midline of the body.

Substitutions. Lateral flexion of the trunk; hip external rotation and flexion.

Hip Adduction

Prime Movers
   Adductor magnus
   Adductor longus
   Adductor brevis

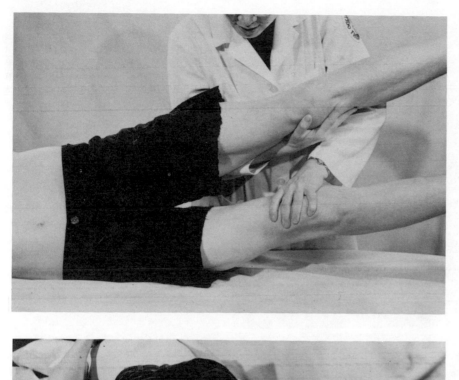

Figure 8.151 Resistance in the against-gravity position. The patient is side-lying on the leg to be tested with the other leg supported in abduction. Both legs are in extension at the hip and knee. The patient adducts the leg being tested, without rotating, to bring it toward the other leg and across the midline.

Figure 8.152 Gravity-eliminated position. The patient lies supine with both legs in abduction and extended at the hips and knees. The therapist supports the leg as the patient attempts to adduct across midline.

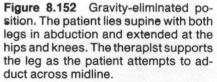

Stabilize. Pelvis.

Palpation. The adductors are palpated on the medial thigh.

Resistance. The therapist's hand is placed on the distal medial thigh and pushes the leg downward or outward toward abduction.

Substitutions. In the side-lying position hip internal rotation and flexion may substitute. In the supine position hip external rotation may substitute.

Hip Internal Rotation

Prime Movers
   Gluteus medius
   Gluteus minimus
   Tensor fasciae latae

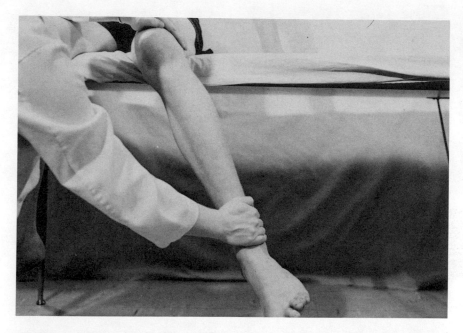

Figure 8.153 Resistance in the against-gravity position. The patient sits with the lower leg hanging over the edge of the sitting surface. The patient internally rotates the thigh, moving his foot laterally.

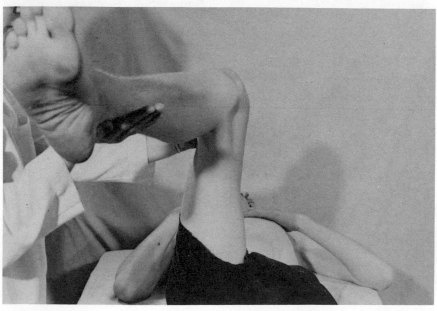

Figure 8.154 Gravity-eliminated position. The patient lies supine with hip flexed to 90°. The leg that is not being tested remains in extension. The patient internally rotates the thigh moving his foot laterally.

Stabilize. Femur above the knee to allow only rotation.

Palpation. Palpate the gluteus medius and minimus lateral to the hip joint. The tensor fasciae latae is located just anteriorly to the gluteus medius and below the anterior superior iliac spine.

Resistance. The therapist's hand is placed on the distal lateral part of the lower leg and pushes the foot medially, applying force toward external rotation.

Substitutions. Hip adduction and flexion.

Hip External Rotation

Prime Movers
  Gluteus maximus
  Obturator internus and externus
  Gemellus superior and inferior
  Piriformis
  Quadratus femoris

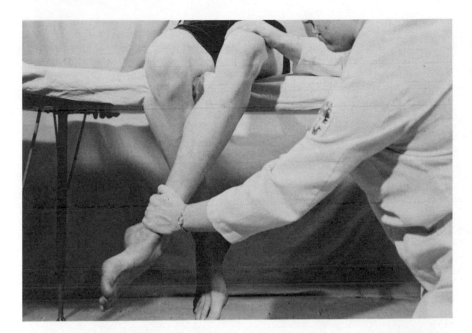

Figure 8.155 Resistance in the against-gravity position. The patient sits with the lower leg hanging over the edge of the sitting surface. The patient externally rotates the thigh, moving his foot medially.

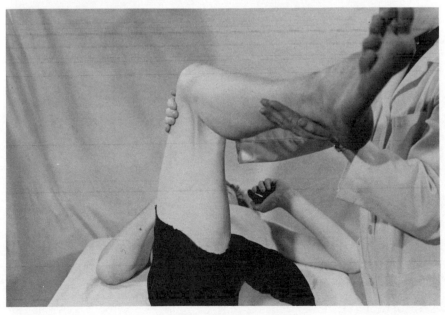

Figure 8.156 Gravity-eliminated position. The patient lies supine with the hip flexed to 90°. The leg not being tested remains in extension. The patient externally rotates the thigh, moving his foot medially.

Stabilize. Femur above the knee to allow only rotation.

Palpation. Palpation of the gluteus maximus has been described. The six small rotators are palpated as a group posterior to the greater trochanter of the femur.

Resistance. The therapist's hand is placed on the distal medial part of the lower leg and pulls the foot laterally toward internal rotation.

Substitutions. Hip abduction and flexion.

Knee Flexion

Prime Movers
  Hamstrings
    Semimembranosus
    Semitendinosus
    Biceps femoris

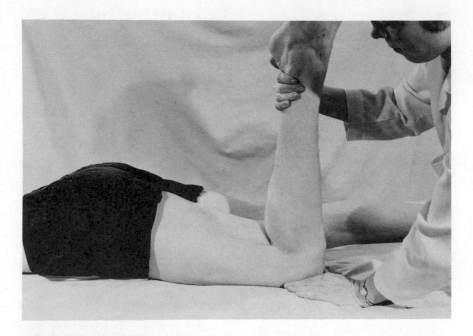

Figure 8.157 Resistance in the against-gravity position. The patient lies prone with both hips and knees extended, feet hanging free over the edge of the plinth. The patient moves the lower leg toward the back of the thigh. After the patient flexes his knee to 90° the motion becomes gravity-assisted. In deciding between a F– or F grade, the therapist must use clinical judgment or stand the patient up to have him flex to 120° against gravity.

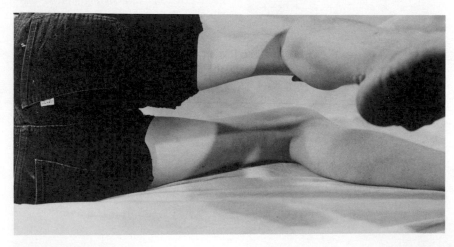

Figure 8.158 Gravity-eliminated position. The patient is side-lying on the side opposite the leg being tested. The leg to be tested is supported by the therapist. The patient moves the lower leg toward the back of the thigh.

Stabilize. Thigh against the plinth.

Palpation. These three muscles can be palpated on the posterior surface of the thigh. The tendon of the biceps femoris can be palpated on the lateral side of the popliteal space, and the tendon of the semitendinosus may be palpated on the medial side of the popliteal space. Both tendons become prominent when resistance is applied.[27] The biceps femoris can be isolated from the other muscles by rotating the lower leg externally with respect to the femur.[27] The semitendinosus will contract more prominently if the lower leg is rotated internally with respect to the femur.[27] The semimembranosus lies deep to the semitendinosus, but its lower portion may be palpated on both sides of the semitendinosus tendon.[27]

Resistance. The therapist's hand is placed on the distal end of the posterior surface of the tibia and pushes it toward extension. If resistance is applied off to one side, medially or laterally, either the lateral or medial hamstrings will contract more strongly.

Substitutions. When prone, gravity assists flexion beyond 90°. When sitting, gravity can flex the knee.

Knee Extension

Prime Movers
  Quadriceps
    Rectus femoris
    Vastus medialis
    Vastus intermedius
    Vastus lateralis

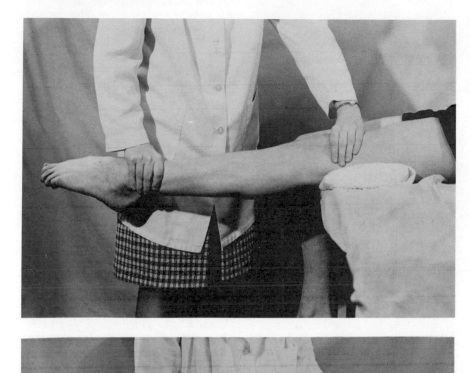

Figure 8.159 Resistance in the against-gravity position. The patient sits erect with the lower leg hanging free. A small pillow or rolled towel is placed between the edge of the plinth and the distal end of the thigh for the patient's comfort. Patient extends the knee.

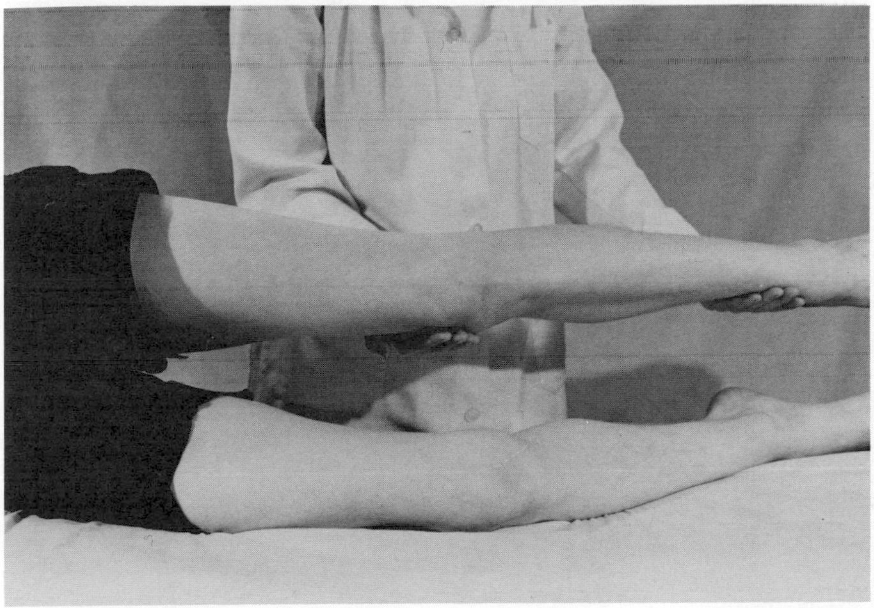

Figure 8.160 Gravity-eliminated position. Side-lying on the side opposite the leg being tested. The therapist supports the tested leg. The patient extends the knee from 90° of flexion.

Stabilize. Thigh.

Palpation. The tendon of the quadriceps may be palpated as it approaches the patella. Except for the vastus intermedius the muscle bellies can be palpated on the anterior surface of the thigh; the rectus is in the center and lies over the intermedius; the other vasti are palpated medially and laterally to the rectus.

Resistance. The therapist's hand is placed at the distal end of the anterior surface of the tibia. Resistance is applied slowly to build up to the patient's maximum in order to avoid injury to the knee which can result from applying sudden or excessive resistance. It is almost impossible to "break" a normal quadriceps.[32]

Substitutions. None.

Ankle Dorsiflexion

Prime Movers
Tibialis anterior
Extensor hallucis longus
Extensor digitorum longus

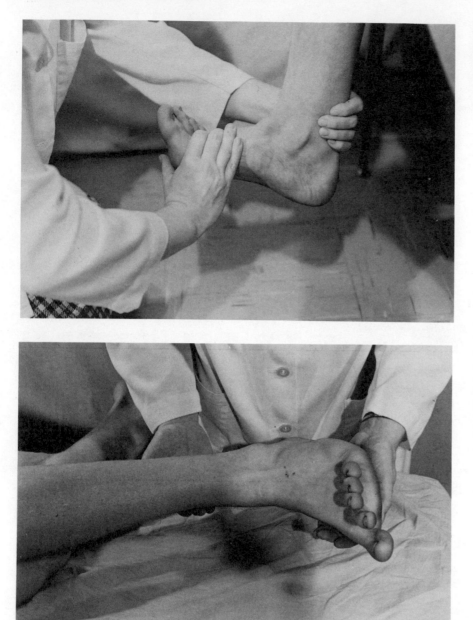

Figure 8.161 Resistance in the against-gravity position. The patient sits erect with the lower leg hanging free. The foot is in neutral position (perpendicular to lower leg). The patient moves the foot so that the dorsum of the foot approximates the anterior surface of the lower leg.

Figure 8.162 Gravity-eliminated position. The patient is side-lying on the side opposite the leg being tested. Tested leg is supported with knee flexed and foot in neutral position. The patient attempts to dorsiflex the ankle.

Stabilize. Lower leg.

Palpation. The belly of the tibialis anterior can be palpated immediately lateral to the shaft of the tibia. Its large tendon can be palpated on the anterior surface of the ankle, medial to the tendon of the extensor hallucis longus. The latter can be palpated in the middle of the anterior surface of the ankle. The extensor digitorum longus tendon is prominent on the lateral side of the anterior aspect of the ankle. The tendons of the hallucis and digitorum can be traced to their insertions on the toes.

Resistance. The therapist's hand is placed on the distal portion of the foot and pushes toward plantar flexion without allowing the foot to invert or evert.

Substitutions. None.

Ankle Plantar Flexion

Prime Movers
 Gastrocnemius
 Soleus

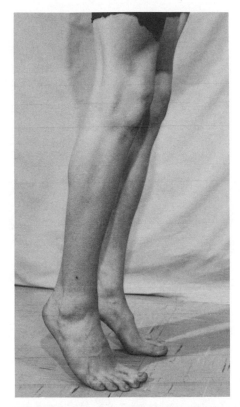

Figure 8.163 Test for plantar flexion to grade normal: standing on tip-toe.

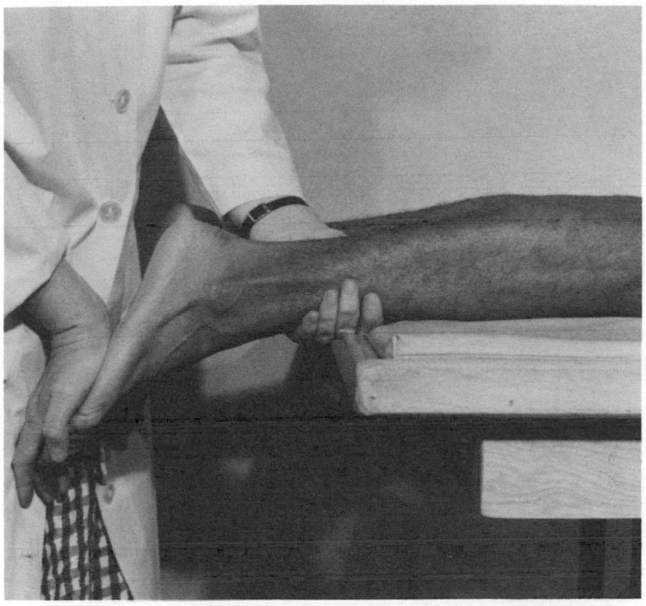

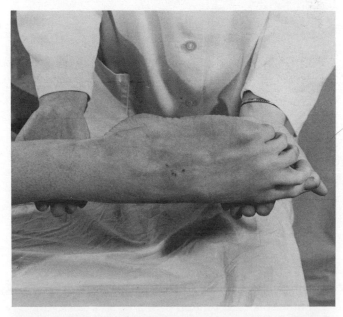

Figure 8.164 Resistance in the against-gravity position. The patient lies prone with the knee extended and the foot hanging free off the plinth. The foot is in neutral position (perpendicular to lower leg). The patient moves the foot so that the toes move away from the anterior surface of the lower leg.

Stabilize. Lower leg.

Palpation. The soleus is palpable at the distal portion of the lower leg. The gastrocnemius is the superficial muscle of the calf; the two heads can be palpated at their origin on either side of the posterior femur. The Achilles tendon is the insertion of both the soleus and gastrocnemius and is readily palpable. To separate the soleus from the gastrocnemius, the patient lies prone with his knee flexed to minimize the influence of the gastrocnemius and slight resistance is applied to plantar flexion.[27]

Resistance. When the patient rises on tip-toe the full body weight resists these muscles. To apply manual resistance, when the patient is unable to stand, the therapist's hand is placed at the distal portion of the foot and pushes the foot toward dorsiflexion.

Substitutions. Gravity substitutes when the person is lying supine or is sitting with feet off the supporting surface. The extrinsic toe flexors substitute weakly.

Figure 8.165 Gravity-eliminated position. The patient is side-lying on the side opposite to the leg being tested. The tested leg is supported. Foot is in neutral position. The patient attempts to plantar flex the ankle.

Ankle Inversion

Prime Movers
Tibialis posterior
Tibialis anterior

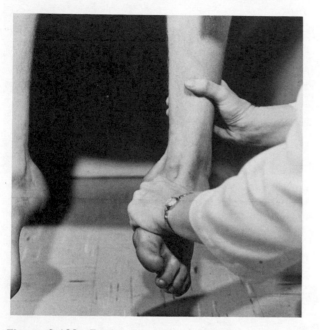

Figure 8.166 Resistance in the against-gravity position. The patient sits erect with the lower leg hanging free. Foot is in neutral position. The patient moves the foot so that the sole of the foot faces medially.

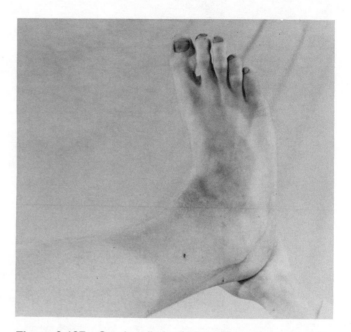

Figure 8.167 Gravity-eliminated position. The patient lies supine with the hip and knee flexed to 90°. Foot is in neutral position. The patient moves the foot so that the sole of the foot faces medially.

Stabilize. Distal part of the lower leg.

Palpation. The tendon of the tibialis posterior may be palpated on and above the medial malleolus. Palpation of the tibialis anterior has been described.

Resistance. The therapist places his hand on the medial surface of the forefoot and holds the first metatar-

sal between the heel of his hand and his fingers. He pulls the forefoot toward eversion.

Substitutions. Extrinsic toe flexors; external rotation of the hip when the patient is lying down with hips and knees extended.

Ankle Eversion

Prime Movers
   Peroneus longus
   Peroneus brevis
   Peroneus tertius

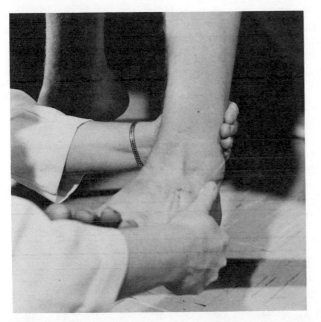

Figure 8.168 Resistance in the against-gravity position. The starting position is the same as for inversion; however, the patient moves the foot so that the sole of the foot faces laterally.

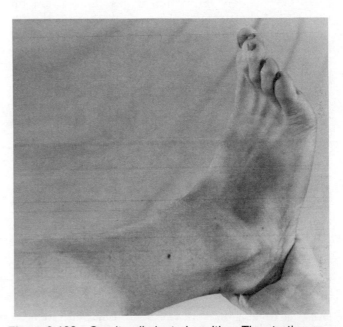

Figure 8.169 Gravity-eliminated position. The starting position is the same as for inversion; the patient moves the foot so that the sole of the foot faces laterally.

Stabilize. Distal lower leg.

Palpation. Peroneus longus is palpated just below the head of the fibula. The tendons of peroneus longus and brevis pass behind the lateral malleolus. The tendon of the peroneus brevis can be seen as it passes to its insertion on the fifth metatarsal. In some persons, the tendon of the longus may be distinguished from the brevis above the malleolus: the longus is adjacent but more posterior. Peroneus tertius is anterior to the lateral malleolus and is palpated lateral to the tendon to the fifth toe.[27]

Resistance. The therapist's hand is placed on the lateral surface of the forefoot and holds the fifth metatarsal between the heel of his hand and his fingers. He pulls the forefoot toward inversion.

Substitutions. Internal rotation of the hip when the patient is lying down with hips and knees extended; extensor digitorum longus.

DYNAMOMETRIC METHODS USED TO TEST MUSCLE STRENGTH

Therapists supplement manual strength testing with dynamometric measurements of grip and pinch for which norms have been established.[33] An abbreviated version of the norms are listed in Table 8.4. The standard method of measurement on which the norms are based reflects the recommendations of the American Society of Hand Therapists (ASHT) and is as follows.[34] The patient is seated with his shoulder adducted and neutrally rotated, elbow flexed at 90°, and the forearm and wrist in neutral position (Fig. 8.170). The handle of the Jamar dynamometer is set at the second position.[33,34] The task is demonstrated to the patient. After the dynamometer is positioned in the patient's hand, the therapist says, "ready? squeeze as hard as you can" and then urges the patient on throughout the attempt. The patient squeezes the dynamometer with as much force as he can, three separate times with a 2- to 3-min rest period between trials. The average of the three trials is recorded[34] and compared to that for the patient's uninvolved hand or norms for his age group to ascertain if he has a significant weakness. Test-retest reliability of this method is ≥0.88; interrater reliability is ≥0.99.[34] Some norms for the Jamar dynamometer used in different ways have also been published.[35,36]

The strength of pinch can be measured in pounds using a pinch meter. Norms for tip pinch, lateral pinch, and palmar pinch using the B & L pinch meter were established on the same sample as the grasp norms were established.[33] Some of the norms are included here (Table 8.5).

The standardized method of measuring used to derive these norms for the three types of pinch are as follows.

Tip Pinch

The patient pinches the ends of the pinch meter between the tips of his thumb and index finger, the norms for which are given here, or between the thumb and the index and middle fingers as pictured (Fig. 8.171) and for which norms are recorded elsewhere.[37] The test is administered by first giving the patient instructions and a demonstration. Then the therapist says, "ready? pinch as hard as you can." The patient is urged to pinch maximally as he attempts the pinch. He does three trials with a rest between each trial. The average of three trials is recorded. Test-retest reliability is reported as ≥0.69; interrater reliability is ≥0.99.[34]

Lateral Pinch

The patient pinches the meter between the pad of his thumb and the lateral surface of his index finger (Fig.

Table 8.4
GRASP DYNAMOMETER NORMS IN POUNDS
(MEAN OF THREE TRIALS)[a]

		20	30	40	50	60	70	75+
		Norms at Age (yr):						
Male	R	121	122	117	113	90	75	66
	L	104	110	113	102	77	65	55
Female	R	70	79	70	66	55	49	42
	L	61	68	62	57	46	41	37

[a]Adapted from Mathiowetz, V., et al. Grip and pinch strength: normative data for adults. *Arch. Phys. Med. Rehabil.* 66(2): 69–74, 1985. Based on a sample size of *n* = 628, aged 20–94 years. Average standard deviation: males, 28 R and 27 L; females, 17 R and 15 L.

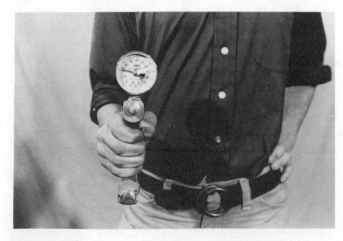

Figure 8.170 Grasp dynamometer.

Table 8.5
PINCH NORMS IN POUNDS
(MEAN OF THREE TRIALS)[a]

		Norms at Age (yr):						
		20	30	40	50	60	70	75+
Tip								
Male	R	18	17	18	18	16	14	14
	L	17	17	18	18	15	13	14
Female	R	11	12	11	12	10	10	9
	L	10	12	11	11	10	10	9

(average standard deviation: males, 4.0; females, 2.5)

Lateral								
Male	R	26	26	25	27	23	19	20
	L	26	26	25	26	22	19	19
Female	R	17	19	17	17	15	14	12
	L	16	18	16	16	14	14	11

(average standard deviation: males, 4.6; females, 3.7)

Palmar								
Male	R	26	25	24	24	22	18	19
	L	26	25	25	24	21	19	18
Female	R	17	19	17	17	15	14	12
	L	16	18	16	16	14	14	11

(average standard deviation: males, 5.0; females, 3.7)

[a]Adapted from Mathiowetz, V., et al. Grip and pinch strength: normative data for adults. *Arch. Phys. Med. Rehabil.,* 66(2): 69–74, 1985. Based on a sample size of *n* = 628, aged 20–94 years.

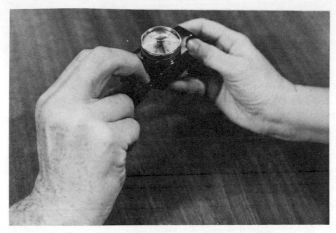

Figure 8.171 Pinch meter measuring tip pinch.

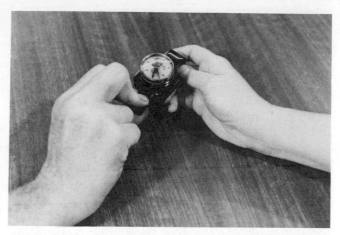

Figure 8.173 Pinch meter measuring palmar pinch.

8.172). The instructions and procedure are repeated as for tip pinch. Test-retest reliability is ≥0.74; interrater reliability is ≥0.98.[34]

Palmar Pinch (Three-Jaw-Chuck)

The patient pinches the pinch meter between the pad of his thumb and the pads of his index and middle fingers (Fig. 8.173). The instructions and procedure are the same as for tip pinch. Test-retest reliability is ≥0.97; interrater reliability is ≥0.74.[34]

As when using any instrument to measure, the instrument must be set at zero to start and it must be calibrated. Dynamometers and pinch meters can be calibrated using a calibrated push-type spring scale in which the number of pounds of push against the compression part of the meter are registered on the spring scale and should correspond to the reading on the face of the meter. Calibration can also be done by placing known weights on, or suspending them from, the compression part of the meter.[34,36]

Using these procedures, the Jamar dynamometer, designed by Bechtol,[38] was found to be accurate to within ± 3% and the B & L pinch meter to within ±

1%.[34,36] These instruments are preferred over other brands for documentation of industrial injury.[36]

However, a vigorometer has been found to be an acceptable alternative hand-strength measurement device for patients whose diagnoses contraindicate stress on joints and/or skin. It requires the patient to squeeze a rubber bulb rather than a steel handle. The vigorometer is a commercially available instrument for which norms have been published.[39]

To quantify strength of other muscle groups in a more objective way than manual muscle testing, a hand-held dynamometer can be used.[40] The force required to overcome the patient's maximal voluntary contraction in a "make" test is recorded. The patient pushes against the plate and piston of the dynamometer and the therapist offers the opposing force, which must be stronger than the patient's effort.[40,41] This method was found to have ≥0.84 test-retest reliability when done by an experienced therapist.[40] Stabilization and meeting muscle force may be particularly difficult for clinicians who are not physically strong,[40] a problem also encountered with manual muscle testing.

INTERPRETATION

After the muscle test scores have all been recorded, the therapist reviews the scores and looks for the muscles that are weak as well as the distribution and significance of the weakness. Any muscle which grades good minus (**G−**) or below is considered to be weak. Good plus (**G+**) muscles are functional and usually require no therapy. Good (**G**) muscles may or may not be functionally adequate for the patient, depending on his occupational tasks. The pattern of muscle weakness is important to notice. The pattern may be one of general weakness due to disuse secondary to immobilization. Or the pattern may reflect the level of spinal innervation in a patient after spinal cord injury or the distribution of a peripheral nerve in the case of peripheral nerve injury. A pattern of imbalance of forces in agonists and antagonists is potentially deforming; counterpositioning or splinting should be considered along with strengthening of the weak muscles. The

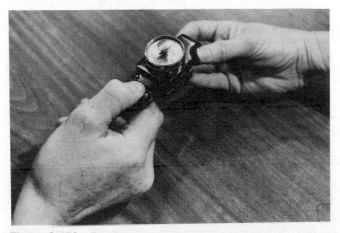

Figure 8.172 Pinch meter measuring lateral pinch.

pattern of significant strengths is also important to notice. For example, a muscle test of a spinal cord-injured patient that indicates some strength in a muscle innervated by a segment below the diagnosed level of injury is a hopeful sign for more recovery. Or, since muscles are reinnervated proximally to distally after peripheral nerve injury, muscle test results showing beginning return of strength in particular muscles help to trace the progress of nerve regeneration.

SHORT-TERM GOALS

Short-term goals are set to move the patient from the level of strength determined by testing to the next higher level, e.g., if a muscle grades **F**, the short-term goal is to improve strength to **F+**; if it grades **F+**, the goal is to increase strength to **G−** and so on. An example of this continuum is given in chapter 1.

Endurance

Endurance is the ability to sustain effort. Energy is needed for a person to produce the required intensity or rate of effort over a period of time necessary to complete a given exercise or activity. Length of time or duration of performance and the rate or intensity of the activity must both be considered when evaluating endurance. Factors influencing endurance may relate to muscle function, to oxygen supply from the cardiopulmonary system, or to combined impairment of muscle function and energy supply.[42] Anyone who suffers an illness or major trauma, and in fact anyone who is confined to bed for a few days, may experience generalized decrease of endurance. Friman[43] found that patients confined to bed with acute infectious diseases (i.e., influenza and pneumonia) had reduced endurance capacity that did not return to full capacity until more than 4 months after the acute disease. Decreased endurance is inevitable if decreased cardiac function or decreased respiratory efficiency is a major symptom of the patient's diagnosis. Endurance of one muscle or a muscle group may be decreased due to localized trauma or immobilization; the muscles tire more easily. Patients with decreased muscle strength may require increased energy output to sustain a level of activity and may consequently have decreased endurance.

Other factors influencing fatigue have been under investigation. Asmussen[44] studied muscle fatigue and found evidence to support a "central" component to muscle fatigue in addition to the "peripheral" factors. Subjects performed maximal dynamic muscle contractions to exhaustion using a finger or an arm ergograph. During 2-min rest periods between exercise bouts, complete rest of these muscles was compared with rests of diverting light activities using different muscle or mental activity, such as counting. More work could be done after the diverting rest than after the complete rest. In explanation of this effect, it was proposed that during complete rest the input from fatigued muscles causes the reticular formation to inhibit voluntary efforts, whereas during diverting activity impulses to the reticular formation from the other body parts influ-

ence the reticular formation to facilitate voluntary efforts. Two studies that support this idea have been published in the occupational therapy literature. In both studies the subjects were able to sustain effort significantly longer when doing an interesting activity as opposed to when they did comparable exercise.[45,46] The subjects in both these studies were normal young adults; research is needed to document a similar response in patients included in various diagnostic categories. Clamann and Broecker[47] recorded EMG activity of the triceps, biceps, adductor pollicis, and first dorsal interosseous muscles during maintained maximal voluntary contraction and repeated contractions of low and high force to distinguish between the effects of fatigue on type I (red tonic) and type II (pale phasic) muscle fibers. Triceps and biceps have predominantly type II fibers, adductor pollicis has type I fibers, and in the first dorsal interosseus the fibers are equal. Type II fibers were found to fatigue more quickly than type I fibers. Type II fibers fatigue during near-maximal effort, whereas type I fibers are difficult to fatigue at any level of force. Fiber type composition varies among individuals, accounting in part for differences in fatigue and endurance.

Endurance is measured by determining the amount of time or the number of repetitions that can be carried out before the point of fatigue occurs. Traditionally repetitive activities have been used by therapists to estimate muscular (peripheral) endurance.

Kottke[48] suggests the selection of a lightly resistive activity requiring 15% to 40% of maximal effort. If a low load is used it will take longer to reach the point of fatigue. Therefore, the resistance of the test activity must be kept constant from test to test to gauge improvement. The Box and Block Test, described in chapter 4, can be adapted to measure upper-extremity endurance in general by counting the number of blocks the patient can transfer before becoming fatigued. Endurance can also be evaluated by determining the amount of time a patient can actively hold or maintain a position or contraction.[25] Isometric holding, however, causes large increases in blood pressure and can stress the cardiopulmonary system.[49] Precautions regarding use of isometric exercise should be observed for cardiac patients and others for whom increased blood pressure is problematic. Time is also the measure of endurance for a splint or device. This type of endurance is often referred to as tolerance, e.g., wearing tolerance or sitting tolerance.

In addition to the fatigue of muscles, the ability to sustain effort is influenced by a person's cardiopulmonary status. Heart rate is an indicator of response to exercise that is easily evaluated by the therapist.[42] Heart rate reflects the intensity of activity and is a good indicator of work capacity for patients with decreased endurance and a sound cardiopulmonary system. A resting pulse is taken after 5 min of sitting quietly. Normal resting heart rate is between 65 and 85 beats/min. Then, after exercise, the pulse is taken again; an increase in direct proportion to the increase in work load is expected. Activities that produce a heart rate that is 60% to 75% of maximal heart rate will produce a training effect and are ideal for endurance training for the cardiopulmonary system for patients with no cardiac problem. The formula 220 − Age = Maximum Heart Rate is generally used, and 60% to 75% of the result is calculated to determine the desired heart rate during activity.

Testing of endurance for patients with cardiopulmonary deficits must be done in the presence of a physician or a cardiac nurse specialist because of the potential danger to the patient. Stress testing methods are explained in chapter 30.

For patients with decreased muscular endurance the short-term goal is to increase the endurance by a certain number of repetitions or over a more prolonged time, aiming at a level slightly higher than the results of the evaluation indicate the present capability of the patient to be.

STUDY QUESTIONS:

Evaluation

1. Describe the correct placement, in general, of a goniometer.
2. Define "limits of motion."
3. Why can you not accept a 4° increase in range of motion (ROM) measurement as indicative of patient improvement?
4. When is a detailed ROM measurement of a patient *not needed?*
5. What does it mean if active range of motion is less than passive range of motion?
6. ROM limitations can be caused by a number of underlying conditions. State the short-term goal for treatment of elbow flexion contracture found after removal of a cast used to immobilize a fractured humerus.
7. Why is manual muscle testing inappropriate for use with brain-injured patients?
8. What is the difference between a "break" test and a "make" test?
9. Of what importance is the length/tension relationship of a muscle in manual muscle testing?
10. Name the five procedures that must follow an established format in testing each muscle or motion.
11. For what muscle test grades is treatment to increase strength an appropriate goal?
12. How is endurance measured?

References

1. Moore, M. L. Clinical assessment of joint motion. In *Therapeutic Exercise*, 3rd edition. Edited by J. V. Basmajian. Baltimore: Williams & Wilkins. 1978.
2. Cole, T. M. Goniometry: the measurement of joint motion. In *Handbook of Physical Medicine and Rehabilitation*, 2nd edition. Edited by F. H. Krusen, F. J. Kottke and P. M. Ellwood. Philadelphia: W. B. Saunders, 1971.
3. Boone, D. C., et al. Reliability of goniometric measurements. *Phys. Ther., 58*(11): 1355–1360, 1978.
4. Rothstein, J. M., Miller, P. J., and Roettger, R. F. Goniometric reliability in a clinical setting: elbow and knee measurements. *Phys. Ther., 63*(10): 1611–1615, 1983.
5. Gerhardt, J. J., and Russe, O. A. *International SFTR Method of Measuring and Recording Joint Motion.* Bern, Switzerland: Hans Huber Publishers, 1975.
6. American Academy of Orthopaedic Surgeons. *Joint Motion: Method of Measuring and Recording.* Chicago, 1965.
7. Mundale, M. O., Hislop, H. J., Rabideau, R. J., and Kottke, F. J. Evaluation of extension of the hip. *Arch. Phys. Med. Rehabil., 37*: 75–80, 1956.
8. Kottke, F. J., and Kubicek, W. G. Relationship of the tilt of the pelvis to stable posture. *Arch. Phys. Med. Rehabil., 37*: 81–90, 1956.
9. Clayson, S. J., Mundale, M. O., and Kottke, F. J. Goniometer adaptation for measuring hip extension. *Arch. Phys. Med. Rehabil., 47*: 255–261, 1966.
10. Dworecka, F., et al. A practical approach to the evaluation of rheumatoid hand deformity. *Am. J. Orthop. Surg.*, 1968.
11. Brown, M. E. Rheumatoid arthritic hands: tactual visual approaches. *Am. J. Occup. Ther., 20*(1): 17–23, 1966.
12. Regenos, E., and Chyatte, S. Joint range and deformity recorded by xerography. *J. A. P. T. A., 50*(8): 190, 1970.
13. Wirta, R., and Taylor, D. Engineering Principles in Rehabilitation Medicine. In *Handbook of Physical Medicine and Rehabilitation*, 2nd edition. Edited by F. H. Krusen, F. J. Kottke, and P. M. Ellwood. Philadelphia: W. B. Saunders, 1971.
14. Schwanholt, C., and Stern, P. J. Brief or new: measuring cone for thumb abduction/extension. *Am. J. Occup. Ther., 38*(4): 263–264, 1984.
15. DeVore, G. L., and Hamilton, G. F. Volume measuring of the severely injured hand. *Am. J. Occup. Ther., 22*(1): 16–18, 1968.
16. Smidt, G. L., and Rogers, M. W. Factors contributing to the regulation and clinical assessment of muscular strength. *Phys. Ther., 62*(9): 1283–1290, 1983.
17. Darling, R. C. Exercise. In *Physiological Basis of Rehabilitation Medicine.* Edited by J. A. Downey and R. C. Darling. Philadelphia: W. B. Saunders, 1971.
18. Borden, R., and Colachis, S. Quantitative measurement of the good and normal ranges in muscle testing. *Phys. Ther., 48*(8): 839–843, 1968.
19. Gowitzke, B. A., and Milner, M. *Understanding the Scientific Bases of Human Movement.* 62nd edition. Baltimore: Williams & Wilkins, 1980.
20. Kendall, H. O., Kendall, F. P., and Wadsworth, G. E. *Muscles: Testing and Function.* Baltimore: Williams & Wilkins, 1971.
21. Daniels, L., and Worthingham, C. *Muscle Testing: Techniques of Manual Examination*, 3rd edition. Philadelphia: W. B. Saunders, 1972.
22. Carlson, B. R. Relationship between isometric and isotonic strength. *Arch. Phys. Med. Rehabil., 51*: 176–179, 1970.
23. Salter, N. Muscle and joint measurement. In *Therapeutic Exercise.* Edited by S. Licht. New Haven: Elizabeth Licht, 1958.
24. Caldwell, L. S., Chaffin, D. B., Dukes-Dobos, F. N., Kroemer, K. H. E., Laubach, L. L., Snook, S. H., and Wasserman, D. E. A proposed standard procedure for static muscle strength testing. *Am. Ind. Hyg. Assoc. J., 35*(4): 201–206, 1974.
25. Milner-Brown, H. S., Mellenthin, M., and Miller, R. G. Quantifying human muscle strength, endurance and fatigue. *Arch. Phys. Med. Rehabil., 67*(8): 530–535, 1986.
26. Basmajian, J. V., and DeLuca, C. J. *Muscles Alive: Their Functions Revealed by Electromyography*, 5th edition. Baltimore: Williams & Wilkins, 1985.
27. Lehmkuhl, L. D., and Smith, L. K. *Brunnstrom's Clinical Kinesiology*, 4th edition, Philadelphia: F. A. Davis, 1983.
28. Long, C., and Brown, M. E. EMG kinesiology of the hand. Part III. Lumbricales and flexor digitorum profundus to the long finger. *Arch. Phys. Med. Rehabil., 43*: 450–460, 1962.
29. Long, C. Intrinsic-extrinsic muscle control of the fingers. *J. Bone Joint Surg., 50A*(5): 973–984, 1968.
30. Landsmeer, J. M. F., and Long, C. The mechanism of finger control based on electromyograms and location analysis. *Acta Anat. (Basel), 60*: 330–347, 1965.
31. Diekmeyer, G. Altered test position for hip extensor muscles. *Phys. Ther., 58*(11): 1379, 1978.
32. Hines, T. Manual muscle examination. In *Therapeutic Exercise.* Edited by S. Licht. New Haven: Elizabeth Licht, 1958.
33. Mathiowetz, V., et al. Grip and pinch strength: normative data for adults. *Arch. Phys. Med. Rehabil., 66*(2): 69–74, 1985.
34. Mathiowetz, V., et al. Reliability and validity of grip and pinch strength evaluations. *Hand Surg., 9A*(2): 222–226, 1984.
35. Swanson, A. B., Matev, I. B., and DeGroot, G. The strength of the hand. *Inter-clinic Information Bulletin, 13*(10): 1–8, 1974.
36. Schmidt, R. T., and Toews, J. V. Grip strength as measured by the Jamar dynamometer. *Arch. Phys. Med. Rehabil., 51*(5): 321–327, 1970.
37. Kellor, M., Frost, J., Silverberg, N., Iverson, I., and Cummings, R. Hand strength and dexterity. *Am. J. Occup. Ther., 25*(2): 77–83, 1971.

38. Bechtol, C. O. Grip test: use of a dynamometer with adjustable handle spacing. *J. Bone Joint Surg., 36A*(7): 820–824, 832, 1954.
39. Fike, M. L., and Rousseau, E. Measurement of adult hand strength: a comparison of two instruments. *Occup. Ther. J. Res., 2*(1): 43–49, 1982.
40. Bohannon, R. W. Test-retest reliability of hand-held dynamometry during a single session of strength assessment. *Phys. Ther., 66*(2): 206–209, 1986.
41. Edwards, R. H. T., and Hyde, S. Methods of measuring muscle strength and fatigue. *Physiotherapy, 13*(2): 51–55, 1977.
42. Lunsford, B. R. Clinical indicators of endurance. *Phys. Ther., 58*(6): 704–709, 1978.
43. Friman, G. Effect of acute infectious disease on human isometric muscle endurance. *Upsala J. Med. Sci., 83*(2): 105–108, 1978.
44. Asmussen, E. Muscle fatigue. *Med. Sci. Sports, 11*(4): 313–321, 1979.
45. Kircher, M. A. Motivation as a factor of perceived exertion in purposeful versus nonpurposeful activity. *Am. J. Occup. Ther., 38*(3): 165–170, 1984.
46. Steinbeck, T. M. Purposeful activity and performance. *Am. J. Occup. Ther., 40*(8): 529–534, 1986.
47. Clamann, H. P., and Broecker, K. T. Relation between force and fatigability of red and pale skeletal muscles in man. *Am. J. Phys. Med., 58*(2): 70–85, 1979.
48. Kottke, F. Therapeutic exercise. In *Handbook of Physical Medicine and Rehabilitation*, 2nd edition. Edited by F. H. Krusen, F. J. Kottke, and P. M. Ellwood. Philadelphia: W. B. Saunders, 1971.
49. Whipp, B. J., and Phillips, E. E., Jr. Cardiopulmonary and metabolic responses to sustained isometric exercise. *Arch. Phys. Med. Rehabil. 51*: 398–402, 1970.
50. Zimmerman, M. E. The functional motion test as an evaluation tool for patients with lower motor neuron disturbances. *Am. J. Occup. Ther., 23*(1): 49–56, 1969.

Supplementary Reading

Bohannon, R. W. Manual muscle test scores and dynamometer test scores of knee extension strength. *Phys. Ther., 67*(6): 390–392, 1986.
Bonder, B. Standardized assessments: ethical principles for use. *Am. J. Occup. Ther., 39*(7): 473–474, 1985.
Fish, D. R., and Wingate, L. Sources of goniometric error at the elbow. *Phys. Ther., 65*(11): 1666–1670, 1985.
Handler, M. Standardized tests in hand rehabilitation. *American Occupational Therapy Association Physical Disabilities Special Interest Section Newsletter, 6*(4): 3, 1983.
Loessin Grohmann, J. E. Comparison of two methods of goniometry. *Phys. Ther., 63*(6): 922–925, 1983.
Mayerson, N. H., and Milano, R. A. Goniometric measurement reliability in physical medicine. *Arch. Phys. Med. Rehabil., 65*(2): 92–94, 1984.
Reddon, J. R. et al. Hand dynamometer: effects of trials and sessions. *Percept. Mot. Skills, 61*: 1195–1198, 1985.
Smith, J. R., and Walker, J. M. Knee and elbow range of motion in healthy older individuals. *Physical & Occupational Therapy in Geriatrics, 2*(4): 31–38, 1983.
Walker, P. S., Davidson, W., and Erkman, M. J. An apparatus to assess function of the hand. *Hand Surg. 3*(2): 189–193, 1978.
Yack, H. J. Techniques for clinical assessment of human movement. *Phys. Ther., 64*(12): 1821–1830, 1984.

chapter
9

Treatment

Catherine A. Trombly

The goal of occupational therapy is to enable patients to be independent in their activities of daily living. When patients are prevented from accomplishing their daily tasks because of limited range of motion (ROM), strength, or endurance, preventative or restorative treatment is required. The biomechanical approach is used to treat deficits secondary to sudden or cumulative trauma or disease affecting the musculoskeletal system, spinal cord, or peripheral nervous system, integumentary (skin) system, or cardiopulmonary system. Based on evaluation findings, problems are identified and treatment goals are established.

Goal: To Prevent Limitation of Range of Motion

Many range of motion limitations *can and should be prevented*. Patients who are unable to move their own joints, and for whom motion is not contraindicated, should receive passive range of motion exercises and the part should be properly positioned between treatments.

If edema exists, range of motion will be limited and contractures, due to both the lack of movement and to the developing viscosity of the fluid, are a possibility. A subgoal would be to reduce edema using principles of dynamic muscle contraction, positioning, and compression.

PRINCIPLE: MOVEMENT THROUGH FULL RANGE OF MOTION

The *methods* used for ranging (movement through full range of motion) include teaching the patient to actively move the joints that are involved or adjacent to an injury or passively moving the joints if the patient is paralyzed. In the case of edema, active ranging is preferred because the contraction of the muscles will help pump the fluid out of the extremity. However, if active range of motion (AROM) is not possible, passive range of motion (PROM) must be done.

For AROM and PROM the ranging technique is the same. Each involved joint is slowly and gently moved three times, twice daily[1] from one limit of motion to the other.[2] Exception: The hands of quadriplegic persons who will rely on tenodesis action for grasp must be ranged in the following manner to allow finger flexor tendons to develop necessary tightness for function. When flexing the fingers, the wrist must be fully extended, and when extending the fingers, the wrist must be fully flexed.

Battery-operated continuous passive motion (CPM) machines are commercially available orthoses used to maintain ROM and prevent postoperative swelling by continually moving the part from one limit of motion to the other. CPM is a well tolerated painless procedure that stimulates healing and remodeling of tissue.[3,4] There are CPM units for large joints as well as hands. In the hand units, one to five digits can be exercised simultaneously. The limits of motion are adjustable to fit the patient's requirements and the speed of each full cycle can be set. CPM used postoperatively is prescribed by the physician, who should specify the safe limits of motion and duration of daily treatment. CPM is contraindicated in cases of unstable fractures or joints or lacerations of nerves or arteries. Continuous passive motion instituted immediately postoperatively and continued for at least 1 week has been found to prevent loss of increased range of joint motion obtained at surgery.[3] It has also been found to be successful in correcting knee flexion contractures in one patient who continued to worsen despite treatment with manual passive ranging and stretching.[5]

PRINCIPLE: POSITIONING

Positioning of joints to avoid development of deformities is essential. All potentially nonfunctional positions are avoided throughout the day and night. Positioning can be accomplished by the use of orthoses, pillows, rolled towels, positioning boards, etc. For example, when the patient is in bed, footboards may be used to prevent foot drop, and sandbags or trochanter rolls can be placed along the lateral aspect of the thigh to prevent hip external rotation.[6,7] Elevating a patient's edematous hand by use of a suspension sling will allow the fluid to drain back to the body.

Sometimes contractures and subsequent ankylosis are unavoidable due to the disease process. In these instances positioning, splinting, and bracing are used to ensure that ankylosis occurs in as nearly a functional position as possible. Functional positions are those that if fixed will still allow the person to manage his self-care and other functional tasks. For example, the functional position of the hand and wrist is slight (10° to 30°) extension of the wrist, opposition and abduction of the thumb, and semiflexion of the finger joints. If the hand contracted in that position, the person would be able to use it to hold objects. If, however, the hand were to contract in a fully flexed position, it would not only be useless but would also present a hygiene problem. If it contracted in full extension, it would have no holding capability and be equally useless. When positioning a patient using props or orthoses, the occupational therapist must be vigilant in anticipating eventual outcomes of prolonged immobilization that could compromise function.

PRINCIPLE: COMPRESSION

Edema can be controlled by compression with elastic strip bandages or tubular bandages. Care must be exercised so that these are applied correctly and do not constrict circulation in the more distal part of the extremity. Skin color is observed regularly to confirm that circulation is preserved. Coban® (3M Co., St. Paul, MN) a self-adherent elastic wrap bandage, is wrapped around the part spirally in a distal to proximal direction[8] and by overlapping the edge by at least 25% of the width of the material so that the fluid can flow evenly back toward the body and not be trapped in pockets of unwrapped tissues. Tubigrip® (Mark One Health Care Products, Inc., Philadelphia, PA) is a tubular elastic support bandage that provides graduated constant pressure support when the correct size is applied.

Goal: To Increase Passive Range of Motion

If the results of evaluation of PROM indicate that limitations in joint motions are significant, i.e., if they impair the patient's ability to function independently in life tasks or are likely to lead to deformity, then treatment may be indicated. Whereas some significant limitations of ROM can be ameliorated or corrected by activity or exercise, some cannot. Problems that can be changed include contractures of soft tissue, i.e., skin, muscle, tendon, and ligament. Problems that cannot be changed include bony ankylosis or arthrodesis, long-standing contractures in which there are extensive fibrotic changes in soft tissue, and severe joint destruction with subluxation. Occupational therapy for limited ROM problems that cannot be treated restoratively is rehabilitative in nature and focuses on providing techniques and/or equipment to compensate for the problems of limited range of motion, and is described in Part Five.

PRINCIPLE: STRETCH

It is important that stretch be done to the point of maximal stretch, defined as a few degrees beyond the point of discomfort, and held there for a few seconds. The stretching may be active or passive.

The patient controls the amount of stretch and force in active stretching, while the setup of the activity or exercise equipment controls the direction of force. By using activities that combine active stretch and minimal resistance to the contracting muscle, the patient can make instantaneous adjustments in the force of the stretch in response to pain by relaxing the contraction and moving away from the stretched position. Passive stretch, on the other hand, does not have the luxury of an internal feedback system, so that the force applied by an external source cannot be immediately adjusted by the patient or therapist to accommodate to small pain signals experienced by the patient. Nonetheless, passive stretch is usually more effective than active stretch because the therapist carefully ensures that each limited joint is stretched to the point of maximal stretch. When precautions are in effect, however, passive stretch must be done with extreme caution, and active stretch is preferable. Precautions are noted below.

Use of an electrogoniometer that provides feedback to the patient when he has achieved the desired limit of motion may increase the effectiveness of active stretching. A simple electrogoniometer that can be constructed by an occupational therapist has been described by Brown et al.[9] When feedback units are used in combination with activity, effectiveness of treatment may be enhanced.

Active Stretching

At the limited joint, the patient contracts the muscles antagonistic to the contracture in order to stretch the contracture. For example, if there is a flexion contracture, the extensors must contract to pull against it. The patient controls the force, speed, extent, and direction of the stretch within his own tolerance for pain. It is the therapist's role to instruct the patient and to encourage him to frequently stretch the part correctly throughout the day, as well as during a treatment session.

Passive Stretching

An external force stretches the contracture at the limited joint. It is used when the patient does not have sufficient strength in the antagonist to do active stretching.

Methods to provide passive stretching include orthoses that provide traction, manual stretching, joint mobilization techniques, exercise, and/or activities. All methods stretch the tissue beyond its customary limit of motion. Different tissues tolerate stretch differently; tight muscles can be stretched more vigorously than tight joints.[1] The force, speed, direction, and extent of stretch must be controlled. The *force* must be enough to put tension on the tissue, but not enough to rupture it. The *speed* should be slow to allow the tissue to gradually adjust. The *direction* of stretch is exactly opposite to the tightness. The *extent* of stretch is to the point of maximal stretch, defined above. Precautions are to be observed.

Orthotic devices that provide a continuous, gentle stretch (traction) are used to supplement gains made by means of exercise or activity as well as to provide a form of controlled, continuous, passive stretching. One such device is the glove flexion mitt used to put a constant stretch on extensor contractures of the metacarpophalangeal and interphalangeal joints. To make the mitt, an ordinary workman's glove is adapted by adding rubber bands to the fingertips, which are anchored to the wrist.[10] Other orthoses are described in chapter 13.

Manual stretching, a form of passive stretching, is done by the therapist. Ideally, the environment and the therapist are quiet and relaxed to encourage relaxation of the patient. The patient is informed about the process of manual stretching and that it involves tolerable pain. He is instructed that he is responsible for indicating when discomfort occurs in order for the procedure to be done properly. For stoic patients, the importance of this must be emphasized. Real pain would defeat the results of stretching, since it would interfere with relaxation of the tissue being stretched, which is required for an adequate result. The therapist holds the extremity in such a way that the part proximal to the joint is stabilized and the part distal to the joint is moved in the exact plane of movement opposite to the tightness. The motions used in stretching are identical to the motions described in chapter 8 for range of motion evaluation. The patient is encouraged to move the part with the therapist if he can, because during active motion the tight antagonistic muscles are reflexly programmed to relax, and therefore more motion may consequently be obtained. The therapist moves the part smoothly, slowly, and gently to the point of mild discomfort,[11] which the patient indicates verbally or by facial expression. The therapist then moves the part to the point of maximal stretch. There should be relief of discomfort immediately following release of stretch. Residual pain after stretching indicates that the stretch was too forceful and caused tearing of soft tissues or blood vessels.[1]

Gentle stretching that achieves small increments of gain over a period of time is more effective than vigorous stretching aimed at large gains quickly. As a protective mechanism, connective tissue resists quick, vigorous stretching, which is therefore ineffective or injurious.[1] The method of moving gently to the point of maximal stretch and holding this position allows connective tissue, having the property of plasticity, to adjust its length gradually over time. The duration of the stretch when applied manually is usually only several seconds to a minute. It is clinically recognized that continuous stretching is most effective; however, gains are also noted using briefly held stretch. There are no research studies that specify the minimal amount of time required for effective stretching. Twenty seconds has been recommended for athletes who stretch their muscles before strenuous activity.[11]

During each treatment session, each joint with limitation of PROM is gently stretched in the described manner several times to ensure achieving maximal stretch at least once. In order to maximize gains achieved by stretching it is necessary to stretch daily, because it has been determined by microscopic examination of connective tissue that the process involved in contracture formation begins in 1 day.[1]

In ligament or tendon tightness resulting from weakness of the shoulder musculature, it has been clinically demonstrated that pain, caused by the weight of the arm pulling on the rotator cuff muscles, can be reduced by approximating the head of the humerus into the glenoid fossa, while simultaneously ranging or stretching this joint. In ligament, muscle, or tendon tightness of the wrist, thumb, and fingers it has been clinically demonstrated that pain associated with stretching can be reduced by traction applied to each joint to separate the articular surfaces during stretching.[1]

Joint mobilization techniques are primarily used in physical therapy; however, the occupational therapist may find the techniques useful to increase range of motion in stiff hands and wrists.

Maitland[12] has described methods of joint manipulation and joint mobilization. Manipulation is defined as either a sudden thrusting movement of small amplitude or as a steady controlled stretch strong enough to break adhesions. Manipulation is often done under anesthesia and is never used without extensive special training. Mobilization is defined as passive movements done at such a speed that the patient could prevent them if he chose. Two types of movement are included: (1) oscillatory movement (two to three per sec) of small or large amplitude applied anywhere within the range of motion or (2) sustained stretching with tiny amplitude oscillations done at the limit of range. The oscillatory movements may be of the physiologic movements or accessory movements (also called "joint play," i.e., movement possible within a joint but not under voluntary control).

Grades of movement have been defined to aid prescribing mobilization treatment and recording progress.

Grade I: Small-amplitude movement performed at the beginning of the range.

Grade II: Large-amplitude movement performed within the range but not reaching the limit of the range. If the movement is performed near the beginning of the range it is expressed as II−; if it is taken deeply into range yet not to the limit, it is expressed as II+.

Grade III: Large-amplitude movement performed up to the limit of range. III− indicates a gentle approach to the limit, whereas III+ indicates movement that pushes vigorously into the limit.

Grade IV: Small-amplitude movement performed at the limit of range. IV— and IV+ can be used to describe the vigor of the movement, as in the case of grade III.

Treatment of stiff joints recommended by Maitland[12] includes small-amplitude oscillatory movements done for approximately 2 min at the limit of range of the functionally limited physiologic movement. This is followed by small-amplitude, strong stretching oscillatory movements of the accessory movements of the joint. These two types of movements are alternated until progress is achieved. If soreness develops, movement is changed to grade II type. The reader is referred to Maitland's manual, *Peripheral Manipulation*,[12] for the details of this treatment method.

An exercise that has been found to be effective in increasing the PROM of shortened tissue is the proprioceptive neuromuscular facilitation (PNF) technique called "hold/relax."[13] The "hold/relax" procedure involves a brief (4 to 6 sec[14]) and maximal isometric contraction performed at the point of limitation. The tight muscle is contracted maximally and then relaxed for 2 sec.[14] During the relaxation phase, the therapist moves the part in the direction opposite to the contraction into the new maximal range and holds it for 8 sec.[14] The effect in the lower extremities has been found to last up to 90 min.[14] The "hold/relax" procedure may be repeated at each succeeding limit of range until a large gain in range is made. Example: if there were a contracture of elbow flexors, the elbow would be extended to its limit. The patient would be instructed to isometrically contract his flexors maximally, then relax, at which moment the therapist would smoothly extend the elbow into greater range until resistance was felt. The "hold/relax" procedure is repeated until increments of gain are achieved. The technique is neurophysiologically based on the hypothesis that after a motor unit is maximally activated, it is inhibited (relaxes) due to Golgi tendon organ (GTO) influence. When a muscle contracts maximally, most or all motor units fire simultaneously, therefore stimulating all or most of the GTOs of that muscle with the effect of inhibiting all the active motor units, enabling the part to be gently moved to greater range.

The comparative effectiveness of passive stretch and "hold/relax" (isometric exercise) has been studied on young adult normal males. One study[13] found "hold/relax" to be the more effective procedure, and the other study[15] found no statistically significant difference between isometric contraction and passive stretch. Both treatments produced improved range of motion as compared to no treatment.[13,15] In a study of 30 young adult females, "contract/relax," an isotonic contraction against maximal resistance, was found superior to "hold/relax" in increasing ROM; both improved ROM as compared to no treatment.[16]

Activity used for increasing PROM must provide a gentle active stretch by use of slow, repetitive isotonic contraction of the muscles opposite the contracture or by use of a prolonged passive stretched position of the tissue producing limitation. In both types of activity, the requirement is that the range be increased slightly beyond the patient's limitation. The use of activity for stretching is empirically based on the idea that a person involved in an interesting and purposeful activity will gain greater range because he is relaxed, not anticipating pain, is motivated to complete the task, and will be more likely to move as the activity demands. The ROM Dance Program, devised by Harlowe and Yu as a home program for rheumatoid arthritic patients, is an example of use of purposeful, meaningful activity to achieve physical goals. The program is comprised of expressive dance techniques as well as relaxation techniques for use during rest periods.[17,18] The 7-min dance, modeled after T'ai-Chi Ch'uan, incorporates joint motion in all ranges recommended for patients with rheumatoid arthritis. The dance is done while listening to or reciting a poem that is meant to evoke pleasurable images of warmth and friendship.[17,18] An outcome study indicated that significant gains in ROM were made by the experimental subjects as compared to control subjects who did a "traditional home program."[18] Compliance was not significantly different between the groups; however, this conclusion may be contaminated by measurement error.[18]

The selected activity must be interesting to the patient and must intrinsically demand the correct motion. This means that the performance of the activity as it is set up for the patient must involve the desired motion, without unreasonable contrivance or the necessity for the patient to concentrate on the movement itself rather than the goal of the activity. Reasonable adaptations, however, are permissible and, in fact, may be necessary in order to elicit the desired motion. Creativity on the part of the therapist to devise appropriate adaptations is desirable, as long as the adaptation does not change the nature of the activity, put the patient in an awkward position, or cause him to perform unnatural movements. An example of an adaptation of an activity to provide active stretch of an elbow flexion contracture of a jigsaw puzzle enthusiast could be to position the puzzle pieces just beyond his comfortable range, requiring him to extend his elbow to reach for them. One point to remember, though, is that if the contracture existed when the limb was not immobilized in some way, then active stretch will not be effective; if he was free to move and did not during his daily activities then it is unlikely gains will be made using activity to correct the contracture.

Adaptations to activity can be made through the tools or equipment used in doing the activity. Equipment used in activities can provide traction (passive stretch) if resistance is provided by means of springs, weights, elastic material, or the weight of the tool. An example of how weights are used to adapt an activity can be seen in woodworking (sanding long boards such as used to make a book case). Each of the shelf boards are attached in turn to an inclined sanding frame. The patient tries to push the sander to the end of the board. Weights are attached to the sander by suspending

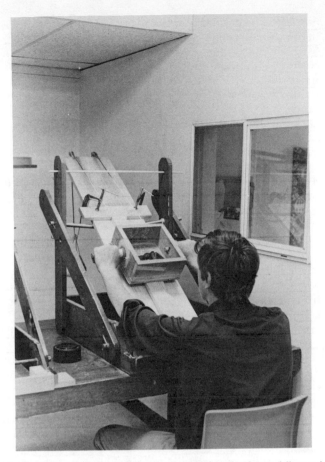

Figure 9.1 Sanding on an inclined plane using a bilateral sander with pulleys and weights attached.

them from a rope through a pulley at the top of the incline, creating an upward force that stretches the shoulder extensors and elbow flexors (Fig. 9.1).

Adaptations made to adjust the size or location of handles of craft or recreational equipment can require the patient to move further into range actively. The size or location is gradually changed by the therapist as the patient improves.[19]

One cannot prescribe activity for specific purposes similar to the way a physician prescribes medication because each person moves in his own characteristic ways. The therapist must carefully monitor the patient's method of doing an activity and not assume that the activity, *per se*, will evoke the desired result in all persons. Two examples illustrate this. Pressing the weft of finger weaving using a passive hand and the force of shoulder extensors provides stretch to the finger flexors. Actively pressing the weft into place using finger flexion, on the other hand, stretches the finger extensors because the flexors contract. Both methods accomplish the same activity goal. The other example is similar: Pressing clay into a mold has been used successfully, in combination with other exercises, to stretch finger flexor tightness.[20] However, if the patient had actually pressed the clay into the mold using finger flexion instead of a passively held hand, then ex-

tensors would have been stretched. It is best to avoid the use of an activity that requires a motion that is habitual for the patient, but if done in this habitual manner, does not meet the therapy goal. Otherwise, the patient must concentrate on the new movement and will often revert back to the habitual method.

Precautions

Inflammation, sensory loss, or consequences of immobilization preclude stretching or require modifications of procedure.

Inflammation weakens the structure of collagen tissues,[21] which include bone, cartilage, tendon, ligament, artery, fascia, dermis, and other connective tissues. Care must be taken not to stretch inflamed tissue.[1] If steroids are used to treat the inflammation, they may cause side effects such as osteoporosis that would also require modified procedures.

Sensory loss prevents the patient from monitoring pain, thus permitting overstretching to occur unless the therapist pays particular attention to the tension of the tissues being stretched. Overstretching causes internal bleeding with subsequent scar formation that may eventually ossify.[1] An unfortunate common example of such calcification, heterotropic ossification, occurs in hip and elbow flexor musculature of spinal cord-injured patients[1] because of the cumulative effects of overstretching inherent in daily life tasks.

Stretching tissue after it has been immobilized must be done carefully because prolonged immobilization or bed rest produces many side effects. One is osteoporosis. Bone loses calcium because there has been no compression forces on the bone to maintain its integrity,[21] and it can be more easily fractured by tension or shear forces. Tendons and ligaments also change biochemically and lose tensile strength in the absence of motion and stress.[21] Muscle filaments, which must slide during muscle contraction, have not been sliding during immobilization; therefore, they lose that ability. The resultant adhesions may be torn when stretched. Bed rest causes a decrease in blood pressure in the extremities, which reduces the stress necessary for maintaining the strength of the collagen fibers of the vessel walls; consequently, blood vessels are weakened.[21] To reduce the effects of immobilization and bed rest, the physician may prescribe weight bearing, isometric muscle contraction, or CPM.

Goal: To Increase Strength

If evaluation of the patient's strength reveals a significant limitation, one that prevents the person from carrying out his life tasks or that may lead to deformity, then treatment is aimed at gradually increasing the patient's strength. Weakness is potentially deforming if muscles on one side of a joint are weak in comparison to their antagonists.

Strength of contraction is gained when more motor units are recruited, which occurs when a muscle is stressed by increasing the load or speed requirements of a movement or when the muscle begins to tire. Muscle fibers of repeatedly recruited motor units hypertrophy in response to increased resistance[21-23] or load, thereby increasing strength.

PRINCIPLE: INCREASE STRESS TO MUSCLE

Stress is applied to the muscle or muscle group to the point of fatigue.[24] Parameters that may be manipulated to alter the stress on a muscle include *type of exercise, intensity* or load (resistance), *duration* of a held contraction or exercise period, *rate* or velocity of contraction (repetitions per period of time), and the *frequency of exercise* (exercise periods/day). Each parameter may be manipulated independently of one another. There may be precautionary reasons, for example, why the load should not be increased for a given patient. In that case, the therapist has the option of increasing one of the other parameters, for example, frequency (treatment twice daily), to thereby stress the muscle which will result in a strength gain.

The intensity of exercise refers to the amount of resistance offered. Although research is limited, intensities as low as 50% to 67% of maximum capability appear to increase strength.[25,26] Resistance is graded by the type of exercise chosen, by adding a load to the extremity, by changing the length of the lever arm or changing the point where the load is applied to the limb, or by changing the plane of movement. It must be remembered that the weight of the extremity itself is a load as are the weights of tools and the resistiveness of work materials.

Increasing the duration of a contraction causes fatigue of the active muscles. As fatigue progresses more motor units are recruited to maintain the goal posture. The muscle fibers in these later recruited units, therefore, have the opportunity to hypertrophy, which would not occur if they had not been activated. Also, it should be noted that a weak muscle activates more motor units to exert a given force than a strong muscle does.[27,28]

By choosing a certain type of exercise, intensity can be graded low to high, from full assistance to full resistance. The choice, based on the measured strength of the muscle(s), should require effort. The appropriate level of exercise for a patient who cannot move at all is *passive exercise* to maintain range of motion. If the patient is able to contract the contralateral muscle or muscle group, it should be exercised since 30–50% increases in strength of the nonexercised muscle group have been demonstrated as a result of cross-education.[22,29,30] Grading along the continuum of increasing resistance, *active assistive exercise* is selected for muscles that grade poor minus (P−) and fair minus (F−). Gravity is eliminated during exercise of the P− muscle, but the F− muscle works against gravity by definition. Active assistive exercise means that the patient moves the part as much as he can for strengthening and is then assisted to complete the motion in order to maintain mobility. The motion may be completed by the therapist or by the force of therapeutic equipment. The next increment in the gradation of resistance is *active*

exercise. The patient moves the part through full range of motion without assistance or outside resistance. Muscles that grade poor (P) or fair (F) would be exercised in this manner. Again, gravity would be eliminated for the P muscle, but not for the F muscle.

Finally, exercise becomes *active resistive*. Muscles that grade poor plus (P+), fair plus (F+), and good (G−, G, G+) are exercised in this manner. Gravity is eliminated when exercising the P+ muscle. The amount of resistance applied increases with increasing strength.

The plane of movement alters the force of gravity. Tools or utensils of some sort are usually required in order to use activity in therapy. Therefore, muscles must be able to take the resistance of the tool and the material being worked on. A fair-graded muscle operating against gravity cannot take resistance. However, if this muscle were changed to a gravity-eliminated plane, a tool could be used.

Another factor that should be considered in designing a strengthening program is the type of muscle contraction to be required. Exercise to increase muscle strength can be accomplished by means of isotonic or isometric contraction. An isotonic concentric contraction is one in which the internal force produced by the muscle exceeds the external force of the resistance and the muscle shortens.[31] An isotonic eccentric contraction is a lengthening contraction that occurs when an external force greater than the internal force is added to an already shortened muscle.[31] In an isometric (static) contraction the internal and external forces are in equilibrium and the external length of the muscle remains the same.[31] The effectiveness of concentric[32-34] and isometric[26,35-38] exercise to increase strength has been documented. The three types of contraction are illustrated in these examples. Raising a mug of coffee to your mouth requires concentric contraction of the elbow flexors, whereas carefully lowering the mug requires eccentric contraction of the same muscle group. In operating a hand printing press (Fig. 9.2), concentric contraction of the shoulder extensors is used to pull the handle down and eccentric contraction of the same muscle group allows the handle to return gently to its starting position. Maintaining the grasp on the handle of the printing press and on the mug are examples of isometric contraction.

If a person is required to use isotonic contraction in his important daily life tasks, then treatment should utilize isotonic contraction because transfer of the effects of training is poor between isometric and isotonic training programs.[24,25,35,39] Ability gained in isometric training has been found to transfer after several days of further isotonic training; however, ability gained in isotonic training did not transfer to the isometric task.[24]

When no movement of the joint is permitted or possible because of a cast, isometric contraction is the only choice.

When hypertension or cardiovascular conditions are problems for the patient, then isometric contraction should be avoided, since it has been found that isomet-

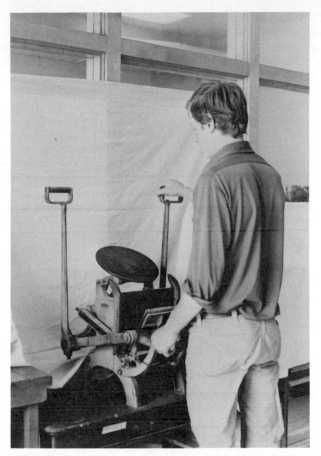

Figure 9.2 Hand printing press adapted with bilateral handles.

ric contraction of either small or large muscles increases the systolic and diastolic blood pressure and heart rate.[40,41] Grasp and pinch, grasp in combination with pushing using total body force, and manual muscle testing of upper extremity musculature were studied in 40 normal subjects aged 19 to 30.[41] Significant increases in systolic and diastolic blood pressure and heart rate were found, which increased with duration of contraction. Approximately 25% of the subjects had to be eliminated from the study when their values exceeded safe limits.[41]

More weight can be lowered by a given muscle during an eccentric contraction than can be lifted concentrically or held at any one point. A corollary is that less effort is exerted during lowering a given weight than is required to lift it. In comparing the relative effects of eccentric and concentric contractions, Mannheimer[42] reasoned that since more force is generated during eccentric contraction, strength gain should be greater using eccentric contraction. In his study of 26 normal male subjects, strength was gained faster by use of eccentric contractions, but there was no significant difference in the amount of strength gain after 1 month. When an agonist muscle is significantly weaker than its antagonist, then an exercise or activity that requires the weaker muscle to contract concentrically and then eccentrically for the return motion may be more effective than one that requires reciprocal contraction of the agonist and antagonist.

Lawrence[43] found isotonic extension of the knee more effective than isometric exercise for increasing strength of the quadriceps; however, the method of measuring gains (amount of weight that could be lifted through range once) was an isotonic measure and may have biased the outcome. Another study that compared isotonic and isometric exercise of the quadriceps found equal strengthening potential of the two types of exercise even with less than maximal resistance, as long as the muscle worked to the point of fatigue.[24]

In terms of work (work = force × distance), a muscle doing an eccentric contraction is doing negative work and one doing concentric contraction is doing positive work. Since negative work (meaning that work is being done to the muscle) is easier to do, i.e., less tension is required for the same load, it may be advantageous to start very weak muscles doing eccentric contraction.[39] The eccentric contraction should be a slow, *controlled,* lengthening in the direction of the pull of gravity. No research was found to support this hypothesis. Eccentric contraction is less stressful cardiovascularly[21,31,39] and thus would be a factor in choosing exercise for patients with cardiac or pulmonary conditions.

Isokinetic exercise has also been found effective to increase strength. Isokinetic exercise is dynamic concentric exercise to agonist and antagonist in which the rate of movement is controlled, that is, the same for each repetition.[1] Physical therapists use machines that deliver the correct rate of motion to the patient undergoing treatment. Some machines also vary the resistance to the motion to accommodate the differing tensions of the muscle at its different lengths throughout the motion. In this way, isokinetic exercise using such machines is similar to PNF in that both use the concept of accommodating maximal resistance throughout range. DeLateur et al[34] found the same relative effectiveness of isokinetic and isotonic exercise and transfer of training was positive between them.

Great intra- and intersubject differences have been seen electromyographically in the patterns of muscle contraction people use to accomplish the same goal.[28,44] In order for a particular treatment program to be effective for a particular person, careful monitoring, preferably using electromyographic biofeedback (see chapter 12), should be done.

Methods by which strengthening can be achieved include exercise, activity, or a combination of both. The use of non-product-related exercise in occupational therapy is a source of continuing controversy.[45,46] Exercise allows greater control over the intensity, rate, and duration. The therapist can grade any or all of the parameters more exactly. Improvement can be graphed and understood easily by the patient and others. Activity, on the other hand, provides interest, a motivator for some patients to endure the stress necessary to make gains. Those activities that can be adapted to provide some control over the parameters are chosen.

Isotonic activity should be characterized by repetition, movement to full range, and a means to gradually increase resistance (weight of tool, change in materials, etc.). Isometric activity should be characterized by a requirement to hold the contraction for increased periods of time and/or against increased loads. Improvement is noted in the amount of work accomplished each work period. Calculation of work can be done using these formulae: Static work = force × duration. Dynamic work = force × distance load lifted × number of repetitions.

Weakness rarely exists in only one motion. If one activity involving several motions provided the correct amount of resistance for each of the motions needing strengthening, this activity would be ideal. Usually, however, the therapist must plan different activities within a given treatment period to provide exercise to all the weak muscles of a patient. The therapist should plan several activities that would provide exercise to each motion to be strengthened and then allow the patient to select the activities of interest.

Isometric Exercise and Activity

For muscles graded trace (T) strength, isometric contraction to increase the strength and passive exercise to maintain range of motion are most appropriate. Lawrence[47] reports successful case outcomes using two kinds of isometric exercise programs: *Progressive Prolonged Isometric Tension Method* and *Progressive Weighted Isometric Exercise Method*. The Prolonged Method is defined as holding the isometric contraction, at whatever level the patient is capable, for the longest period of time. This is repeated 10 times. The duration of maximal contraction is determined by trial and error during the 1st treatment day. The time is increased as the patient improves so that maximal effort is exerted to hold the contraction for 10 repetitions with rest periods between. The Weighted Method requires the patient to hold a contraction against weight determined by the DeLorme method, described below, for a given period of time (30 or 45 sec), with 15-sec rest periods interspersed between the 10 repetitions.

Brief Maximal Isometric Exercise.[36] A maximal isometric contraction held for 6 sec once per day has been found to be effective in increasing strength. Unfortunately it is difficult to detect without instrumentation whether the patient is exerting his maximal effort. Hislop[26] found that holding the contraction for 15 sec twice per day was more effective than for lesser amounts of time.

Isometric contraction is achieved in activity by grasp of handles (the amount of grasp increases with increasingly resistive material that the tool is used against), stabilization of materials being worked on, or by positioning projects so that the limbs must maintain antigravity positions during the work.

Isotonic Assistive Exercise and Activity

Active assistive exercise can be accomplished manually. The patient moves the part as far as he can, and the therapist completes the motion. This is the method of choice for movements not easily exercised using equipment or activity. In progressive assistive exercise (PAE), equipment is used to provide the minimal amount of weight required to complete the motion after the patient has moved as far as he can by means of muscle contraction. As the strength increases, the task is made more difficult by reducing the amount of weight, i.e., the amount of assistance.[32]

The schedule for weight reduction is based on the repetition minimum, which is determined by trial and error on the 1st day of treatment. The repetition minimum is the least amount of weight necessary to assist the limb to full range, 10 times. On the second treatment day, the program begins using this schedule:

10 repetitions with 200% of repetition minimum, rest 2 to 4 min
10 repetitions with 150% of repetition minimum, rest 2 to 4 min
10 repetitions with 100% of repetition minimum

In other words, if 12 pounds are required to assist the patient to flex the shoulder through full range 10 times, the program would start out using 24 pounds, then 18, then 12.

The assistance is offered the muscle through the use of apparatus, such as a counterbalanced sling or skate with weights and pulley attached. The antagonistic muscles must be strong enough to work against any weight used to assist the completion of motion by the weak muscles in order to return the apparatus to starting position. The therapeutic skate has free-moving ball bearings on the bottom of the skate to assist the patient to move more easily on a flat, smooth surface in a gravity-eliminated plane. The motions that can best be exercised by using this apparatus are shoulder-horizontal abduction and adduction and elbow flexion and extension. Assistance is achieved by use of weights hanging on a rope that passes through a pulley. Location of the pulley on the board provides guidance for the correct direction of movement (Fig. 9.3). The overhead counterbalanced sling suspension suspends (Fig. 9.4) the extremity from ropes that extend from the elbow and wrist cuffs to the overhead bar and finally to weights at the back of the apparatus. Antigravity motions of the proximal extremity, such as shoulder abduction, flexion, and external rotation, can be assisted.

Dynamic orthoses that assist motions provide active assistive exercise (see chapter 13).

Few opportunities exist to provide assistive exercise by use of activity. Although a strong extremity can assist a weak one to do the gross, repetitious motions of an activity, the resistance offered by the activity itself must be low. Rolling dough or sanding using a bilateral sander would be too resistive for muscles requiring active assistive exercise, whereas polishing a smooth surface would be possible, but limited in scope. The beater

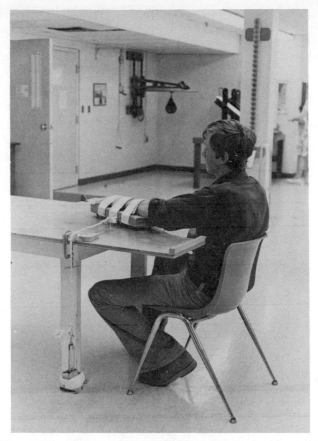

Figure 9.3 Skate with pulley and weight attached to resist horizontal adduction or assist horizontal abduction.

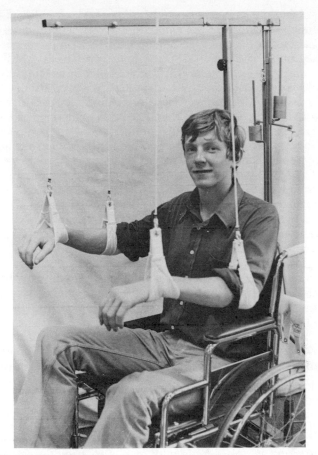

Figure 9.4 Deltoid Aid counterbalanced sling.

of a floor loom can be weighted to provide progressively less assistance in the direction of weakness. If the elbow extensors are weak, the beater can be modified using weights and pulleys or springs to assist the return motion. These can be changed to be less assistive as the patient progresses.

Isotonic Active Exercise and Activity

Active exercise requires the patient to complete the range of motion without assistance or resistance. Activities are selected that allow these criteria to be met. For example, eating finger food offers no appreciable resistance and the active motion can be done by F elbow flexors. Contraction of the biceps in this case is alternately concentric and eccentric: the force against which the muscle works in both cases is that offered by the force of gravity on the lever arm (forearm and hand). An activity that demands contraction of the same muscle during both phases of a movement offers greater exercise potential than one in which return motion is accomplished by the antagonist muscles or by an outside force.

Since most activities require the use of a tool or object that offers resistance, it is easier to find ways to strengthen F muscles if they are put on a gravity-eliminated plane where they can take resistance. For example, an F biceps on a gravity-eliminated plane

could take enough resistance to function in a game of chess. In this example, when moving in a gravity-eliminated plane, the type of contraction of the biceps is concentric. Grading of this type of exercise could be accomplished by changing the rate of contraction, the duration, and/or frequency of exercise bouts.

Isotonic Active Resistive Exercise and Activity

Progressive Resistive Exercise (PRE). DeLorme organized an elaborate system of gradation of resistance to achieve maximal strength quickly.[48] The rationale for PRE was to provide a warm-up exercise period so that a greater maximal strength could be achieved. Studies compared the effectiveness of DeLorme's original technique to modified, less time-consuming versions and found them equally effective in attaining the same final outcome of increased strength. In the original technique the resistance was increased in increments of 10% of maximal resistance (repetition maximum or RM) up to 100% at 10 repetitions of each increment. Between each set of repetitions the patient rested 2 to 4 min. This was a time-consuming process. Two of the modifications found to be equally effective are presented here. The amount of weight the patient can carry 10 times through range of motion using his maximal effort is designated the 10 RM. Determination of 10 RM is done by trial and error: a load is selected that is anticipated to be maximal, and then weight is added or subtracted until 10 RM is established.[1] Jones[49] found that the trial and error method of determining the 10 RM is extremely reliable, even if the subject must lift a load 70 times to determine the 10 RM.

The DeLorme and Watkins modification[32] consists of 10 repetitions at 50% of 10 RM; 10 repetitions at 75% of 10 RM; and 10 repetitions at 100% of 10 RM. In other words, if the 10 RM is 12 pounds, then the patient does 10 repetitions using 6 pounds followed by a rest. Ten repetitions of 9 and 12 pounds each would then be done with rest periods between change of resistance. The McGovern and Luscombe modification[33] requires five repetitions at 50% of 10 RM and 10 repetitions at 100% of 10 RM. In either modification, between each set of repetitions, the patient rests for 2 to 4 min. This sequence is repeated once daily, 5 days per week. The weight is increased as strength improves.

Regressive Resistive Exercise (RRE). McGovern and Luscombe[33] reported a modified sequence of the original work of Zinovieff (Oxford technique) in which strength was increased as effectively using RRE as using PRE. The modification is: 10 repetitions at 100% of 10 RM; 10 repetitions at 75% of 10 RM; and 10 repetitions at 50% of 10 RM. The 10 RM is determined as described above for PRE. These researchers based this plan of RRE on the rationale that resistance should decrease as the muscle fatigues and contracts less effectively.

The overhead counterbalanced sling suspension was previously pictured (Fig. 9.4) and described as a means of providing active assistive exercise for antigravity motions of the shoulder. It can also provide active resistive exercise to motions working against the pull of the weights. The motions that can be resisted by this device are scapular depression, shoulder adduction, shoulder extension, and shoulder internal rotation. The overhead suspension can be positioned for use with patients in a semireclined position and is consequently often selected in the initial strengthening program for patients with quadriplegia and other conditions with proximal weakness for whom treatment begins before the patient has gained full sitting tolerance. The counterbalanced weights provide direct and easily gradable resistance through a large range of motion. Springs can be used instead of the weights but can be graded only by knowing the force of each spring and by selecting the appropriate number of springs. The skate, described above, can be set up to provide resistance to horizontal abduction or adduction or elbow flexion or extension through weights on a pulley or by use of a motor that puts a preselected amount of tension on the cable attached to the skate.[50]

Exercise of the wrist extensors of a C_6 quadriplegic person who will rely on tenodesis grasp may be done by supporting the forearm on an inclined board set at the edge of the table. The hand and wrist are free. A cuff is placed on the hand around the metacarpals to hold the weights (Fig. 9.5). In another example, exercise for a weak extensor digitorum may be accomplished with the forearm and hand supported on a table with the fingers free. Finger loops, to which weights are at-

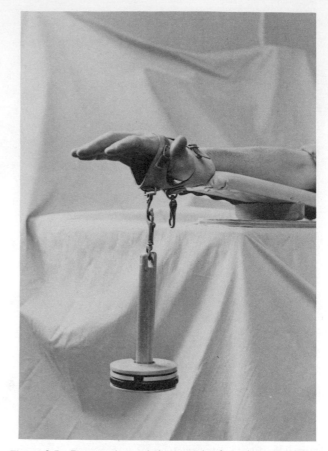

Figure 9.5 Progressive resistive exercise for wrist extension.

tached, are placed on each finger over the proximal phalanx (Fig. 9.6).

In occupational therapy, activities that involve repetitious movements and whose resistance can be graded in small increments can be used to provide active resistive exercise. One example is woodworking, in which the weight of the sanding block or other tools can be graded (Fig. 9.7). Another example is a game in which the equipment or playing pieces can be changed to increase the resistance, such as grading balls from balloons to medicine balls or grading checkers from foam rubber pieces to lead pieces. A third example is weaving on a loom whose beater and/or harnesses can be weighted or otherwise adapted. A method of adapting a floor loom to provide PRE to shoulder depressor muscles has been devised. Although successful in increasing strength, the quality of the project suffered.[51] Some patients would not tolerate that and would therefore prefer to first do strengthening exercise and then do the weaving normally to increase endurance by using the newly acquired strength functionally.

Goal: To Increase Endurance

PRINCIPLE: INCREASED DURATION AT LESS THAN 50% MAXIMAL INTENSITY AND RATE

Fatigue develops in a muscle fiber if insufficient recovery time is allowed for reabsorption of lactic acid. A

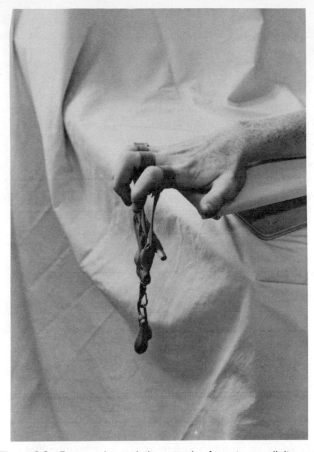

Figure 9.6 Progressive resistive exercise for extensor digitorum.

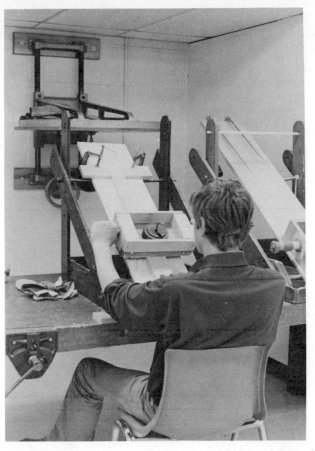

Figure 9.7 Standing on an inclined plane using a bilateral sander with weights for resistance.

person can sustain isometric contraction equivalent to 50% of maximum voluntary contraction (MVC) up to 1 min.[52] The static contraction required in postural activity is generally below 10% MVC; exhaustion of muscle engaged in static activity at more than 20% MVC is mainly due to ischemia created within the muscle due to the constriction forces.[52] In normal subjects, contraction time and percentage of MVC are inversely related. As percentage of MVC increases, time to fatigue decreases. If isometric contractions (up to 75%) are intermittent, allowing better circulation within the muscle, total contraction time increases before fatigue ensues.[52]

In ordinary daily activities that are lightly resistive, motor units are activated asynchronously; after a motor unit ceases activity, the muscle fibers recover to some degree while fellow units take their turn. Fatigue occurs slowly as contrasted to the rapidity of fatigue that occurs after maximal contraction in which many more units must contract simultaneously and do not have the opportunity to recover during the period of the contraction. Exercise to increase endurance, therefore, utilizes moderately fatiguing activity for progressively longer periods of time with intervals of rest to allow metabolic recovery.[1]

Activity or exercise used to increase endurance is graded by increasing the duration of the exercise period, which means increasing the number of repetitions of an isotonic contraction or length of time an isometric contraction is held. An interim method of upgrading the work output of the patient who is not ready to increase the duration is to increase the frequency of exercise or activity per day or per week.

Occupational therapy provides the patient with interest-sustaining activities that are gradable along the dimensions of time or repetition. In normal subjects activity has been documented to significantly increase effort and time to fatigue over that achieved with comparable exercises.[53,54] As an example, a patient can operate a bicycle jigsaw, rather than a stationary bicycle, to increase both general endurance and specific endurance of lower-extremity musculature while sawing a woodworking project of his choice (Fig. 9.8). As another example, a patient with severely low endurance can do light activities, such as mosaic tiles or turkish knotting (Fig. 9.9). The pieces completed each day can be counted, and progress can be easily measured by the therapist and the patient.

With the current emphasis on physical fitness in the United States, some persons prefer exercise to crafts. In that case, the person will want to continue beyond the PRE or RRE regime required to increase strength. The resistance can be reduced to less than 50% of 10

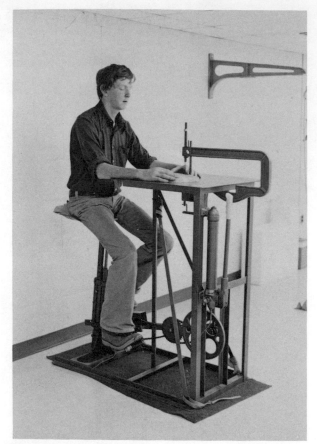

Figure 9.8 Bicycle jigsaw.

RM and the activity continued for a longer period of time.[1] A record of the time the patient can engage in the activity to the point of fatigue indicates changes in endurance. As the muscle increases in strength, the amount of resistance that can be used in endurance activities will also increase.

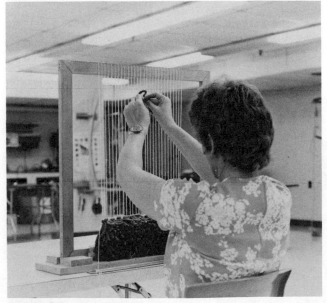

Figure 9.9 Turkish knot weaving.

Recalling that DeLateur et al.[24] found that strengthening occurred even with less than maximal resistance if a muscle worked to the point of fatigue, and recognizing that the ability to sustain effort requires less than maximal effort in order for metabolic recovery to occur, the relationship between activity to increase strength and activity to increase endurance can be clarified. When the objective of treatment is to increase endurance, less than maximal effort is required, but strengthening will also occur if the activity is repeated to the point of fatigue.

Programming for increasing endurance in patients with cardiopulmonary problems is discussed in chapter 24.

STUDY QUESTIONS
Treatment

1. For whom is treatment using the biomechanical approach appropriate?
2. What treatments can be appropriately used to prevent development of range of motion limitations?
3. Describe the functional position of the hand.
4. What treatments can be appropriately used to correct range of motion limitations?
5. Name the four parameters that must be controlled during passive stretching.
6. How should passive stretching treatment be modified if the patient acknowledges residual pain after treatment?
7. What are the two mechanisms by which strength of contraction increases?
8. What are the five parameters that can be manipulated to alter stress on muscle to increase strength?
9. Define concentric, eccentric, and isometric contractions and give examples of each.
10. What are the characteristics that isotonic activity should have to promote strengthening? Isometric?
11. Compare and contrast progressive assistive exercise with progressive resistive exercise in terms of goal, method, and level of strength for which each is appropriate.
12. What are the necessary characteristics of exercise, or activity, used to increase endurance?

References

1. Kottke, F. Therapeutic Exercise. In *Handbook of Physical Medicine and Rehabilitation,* 2nd edition. Edited by F. H. Krusen, F. J. Kottke, and P. M. Ellwood. Philadelphia: W. B. Saunders, 1971.
2. Tookey, P., and Larson, *C. Range of Motion Exercise: Key to Joint Mobility.* Minneapolis: American Rehabilitation Foundation, 1968.
3. Salter, R. B. *Textbook of Disorders and Injuries of the Musculoskeletal System,* 2nd edition. Baltimore: Williams & Wilkins, 1983.
4. Salter, R. B., et al. Clinical application of basic research on continuous passive motion for disorders and injuries of synovial joints: a preliminary report of a feasibility study. *J. Orthop. Res.,* 1:325–342, 1984.
5. Stap, L. J., and Woodfin, P. M. Continuous passive motion in the treatment of knee flexion contracture. *Phys. Ther.,* 66(11): 1720–1722, 1986.
6. Bergstrom, D., and Coles, C. *Basic Positioning Procedures.* Minneapolis: Kenny Rehabilitation Institute, 1971.
7. Feinberg, J., and Andree, M. Dynamic foot splint for the Hoffman apparatus. *Am. J. Occup. Ther.,* 34(1): 45, 1980.
8. Enos, L., Lane, R., and MacDougal, B. A. Brief or new: the use of self-adherent wrap in hand rehabilitation. *Am. J. Occup. Ther.,* 38(4): 265–266, 1984.
9. Brown, D. M., DeBacher, G., and Basmajian, J. V. Feedback goniometers for hand rehabilitation. *Am. J. Occup. Ther.,* 33(7): 458–463, 1979.

10. Heurich, M., and Polansky, S. An adaptation of the glove flexion mitt. *Am. J. Occup. Ther.*, 32(2): 110–111, 1978.
11. Agre, J. C. Static stretching for athletes. *Arch. Phys. Med. Rehabil.*, 59(11): 561, 1978.
12. Maitland, G. D. *Peripheral Manipulation,* 2nd edition. Boston: Butterworths, 1977.
13. Tanigawa, M. Comparison of the hold-relax procedure and passive mobilization on increasing muscle length. *Phys. Ther.*, 52(7): 725–735, 1972.
14. Moller, M., Ekstrand, J., Oberg, B., and Gillquist, J. Duration of stretching effect on range of motion in lower extremities. *Arch. Phys. Med. Rehabil.*, 66(3): 171–173, 1985.
15. Medeiros, J. M., et. al. The influence of isometric exercise and passive stretch on hip joint motion. *Phys. Ther.*, 57(5): 518–523, 1977.
16. Markos, P. Comparison of hold-relax and contract-relax and contralateral effects. Unpublished master's thesis, Boston University, 1977.
17. Harlowe, D. The ROM Dance Program. *American Occupational Therapy Association Physical Disabilities Special Interest Section Newsletter,* 5(4): 1, 4, 1982.
18. Van Deusen, J., and Harlowe, D. The efficacy of the ROM Dance Program for adults with rheumatoid arthritis. *Am. J. Occup. Ther.*, 41(2): 90–95, 1987.
19. Maughan, I. V. Graduated supination-pronation attachments for table and floor looms. *Am. J. Occup. Ther.*, 16(6): 285–286, 1962.
20. Eyler, R. Treatment of flexion contractures in occupational therapy. *Am. J. Occup. Ther.*, 19(2): 86–88, 1965.
21. Downey, J., and Darling, R. *Physiological Basis of Rehabilitation Medicine.* Philadelphia: W. B. Saunders, 1971.
22. Moritani, T., and DeVries, H. A. Neural factors versus hypertrophy in the time course of muscle strength gain. *Am. J. Phys. Med.* 58(3): 115–130, 1979.
23. MacDougall, J. D., et al. Biochemical adaptation of human skeletal muscle to heavy resistance training and immobilization. *J. Appl. Physiol.*, 43(4): 700–703, 1977.
24. DeLateur, B., et al., Isotonic versus isometric exercises: a double-shift transfer-of-training study. *Arch. Phys. Med. Rehabil.*, 53(5): 212–216, 1972.
25. Dons, B., Bollerup, K., Bonde-Petersen, F., and Hancke, S. The effect of weight-lifting exercise related to muscle fiber composition and muscle cross-sectional area in humans. *Eur. J. Appl. Physiol.*, 40: 95–106, 1979.
26. Hislop, H. Quantitative changes in human muscular strength during isometric exercise. *Phys. Ther.*, 43(1): 21–38, 1963.
27. Fuglsang-Frederiksen, A. Electrical activity and force during voluntary contraction of normal and diseased muscle. *Acta Neurol. Scand.* 63 (Suppl. 83): 22–23, 1981.
28. Trombly, C. A., and Quintana, L. A. Activity analysis: electromyographic and electrogoniometric verification. *Occup. Ther. J. Res.*, 3(2): 104–120, 1983.
29. Hellebrandt, F. A., and Waterland, J. C. Indirect learning. The influence of unimanual exercise on related muscle groups of the same and opposite side. *Am. J. Phys. Med.*, 41: 45–55, 1962.
30. Stromberg, B. V. Contralateral therapy in upper extremity rehabilitation. *Am. J. Phys. Med.* 65(3): 135–143, 1986.
31. Gowitzke, B. A., and Milner, M. *Understanding the Scientific Bases of Human Movement,* 2nd edition. Baltimore: Williams & Wilkins, 1980.
32. DeLorme, T. L., and Watkins, A. L. Technics of progressive resistance exercise. *Arch. Phys. Med. Rehabil.*, 29: 263–273, 1948.
33. McGovern, R. E., and Luscombe, H. B. Useful modifications of progressive resistive exercise technique. *Arch. Phys. Med. Rehabil.*, 34: 475–477, 1953.
34. DeLateur, B., et al. Comparison of effectiveness of isokinetic and isotonic exercise in quadriceps strengthening. *Arch. Phys. Med. Rehabil.*, 53: 60–64, 1972.
35. Carlson, B. R. Relationship between isometric and isotonic strength. *Arch. Phys. Med. Rehabil.*, 51(3): 176–179, 1970.
36. Rose, D. L., et al. Effects of brief maximal exercise on the strength of the quadriceps femoris. *Arch. Phys. Med. Rehabil.*, 38: 157–164, 1957.
37. Lawrence, M. S. Strengthening the quadriceps femoris: progressive weighted isometric exercise method. *Phys. Ther. Rev.*, 40(8): 577–584, 1960.
38. Hislop, H. Response of immobilized muscle to isometric exercise. *Phys. Ther.*, 44(5): 339–347, 1964.
39. Rasch, P. J. The present status of negative (eccentric) exercise: A review. *Am. Correct. Ther. J.*, 28(3): 77–94, 1974.
40. Riendl, A. M., et al. Cardiovascular response of human subjects to isometric contraction of large and small muscle groups. *Proc. Soc. Exp. Biol. Med.*, 154: 171–174, 1977.
41. Smith, D. A., and Lukens, S. A. Stress effects of isometric contraction in occupational therapy. *Occup. Ther. J. Res.*, 3(4): 222–239, 1983.
42. Mannheimer, J. A., comparison of strength gain between concentric and eccentric contraction. *Phys. Ther.*, 49(11): 1201–1207, 1969.
43. Lawrence, M. S. Comparative increase in muscle strength in the quadriceps femoris by isometric and isotonic exercise and effects on the contralateral muscle. *Phys. Ther.*, 42(1): 15–20, 1962.
44. Hinson, M., and Rosentswieg, J. Comparative electromyographic values of isometric, isotonic, and isokinetic contraction. *Res. Q.*, 44(1): 71-78, 1973.
45. Trombly, C. A. Letters to the editor: include exercise in purposeful activity. *Am. J. Occup. Ther.*, 36(7): 467–468, 1982.
46. Hollis, L. I. Identifying occupational therapy: the use of purposeful activities. *American Occupational Therapy Association Physical Disabilities Special Interest Section Newsletter,* 9(4): 2–3, 1986.
47. Lawrence, M. S. Strengthening the quadriceps. Progressively prolonged isometric tension method. *Phys. Ther. Rev.*, 36(10): 658–661, 1956.
48. DeLorme, T. Restoration of muscle power by heavy resistance exercises. *J. Bone Joint Surg.*, 27: 645–667, 1945.
49. Jones, R. E. Reliability of the ten repetition maximum for assessing progressive resistance exercise. *J.A.P.T.A.* 42(10): 661–662, 1962.
50. Roemer, R. B., Culler, M. A., and Swartt, T. Automated upper extremity progressive resistance exercise system, *Am. J. Occup. Ther.*, 32(2): 105–108, 1978.
51. Hultkrans, R., and Sandeen, A. Application of progressive resistive exercise to occupational therapy. *Am. J. Occup. Ther.*, 11(4): 238–240, 1957.
52. Monod, H. Contractility of muscle during prolonged static and repetitive dynamic activity, *Ergonomics*, 28(1): 81–89, 1985.
53. Kircher, M. A. Motivation as a factor of perceived exertion in purposeful versus nonpurposeful activity. *Am. J. Occup. Ther.*, 38(3): 165–170, 1984.
54. Steinbeck, T. M. Purposeful activity and performance. *Am. J. Occup. Ther.*, 40(8): 529–534, 1986.

Supplementary Reading

Arem, A. J., and Madden, J. W. Effects of stress on healing wounds. I. Intermittent noncyclical tension. *J. Surg. Res.*, 20: 93–102, 1976.
Bell, C. C. Endurance, strength, and coordination exercise without cardiovascular or respiratory distress. *J. N. Natl. Med. Assoc.*, 71(3): 265–270, 1979.
Chapman, E. A., deVries, H. A., and Swezey, R. Joint stiffness: effects of exercise on young and old men. *J. Gerontol.*, 27(2): 218–221, 1972.
Goldberg, R. The rationale for early motion in fracture management. *American Occupational Therapy Association Physical Disabilities Special Interest Section Newsletter,* 6(3): 3, 1983.
Hellebrandt, F. A., and Houtz, S. J. Mechanisms of muscle training in man: experimental demonstration of the overload principle. *Phys. Ther. Rev.*, 36(6): 371–383, 1956.
Lesser, M. The effects of rhythmic exercise on the range of motion in older adults. *Am. Correct. Ther. J.*, 32(4): 118–122, 1978.
Melvin, J. L. Roles and functions of occupational therapy in hand rehabilitation. *Am. J. Occup. Ther.*, 39(12): 795–798, 1985.
McGourty, L. K., Givens, A., and Fader, P. B. Roles and functions of occupational therapy in burn care delivery. *Am. J. Occup. Ther.*, 39(12): 791–794, 1985.
Moritani, T., and deVries, H. A. Potential for gross muscle hypertrophy in older men. *J. Gerontol.*, 35(5): 672–682, 1980.
Petrofsky, J. S., et al. Comparison of physiological responses of women and men to isometric exercise. *J. Appl. Physiol.*, 38(5): 863–868, 1975.
Phelps, P. E., and Weeks, P. M. Management of the thumb-index web space contracture. *Am. J. Occup. Ther.*, 30(9): 543–550, 1976.
Rodgers, M. M. and Cavanagh, P. R. Glossary of biomechanical terms, concepts, and units. *Phys. Ther.*, 64(12): 1886–1902, 1984.
Rose, D. L., and Page, P. B. Conscious proprioception and increase in muscle strength. *Arch. Phys. Med. Rehabil.*, 50(1): 6–10, 1969.
Vasudevan, S. V., and Melvin, J. L. Upper extremity edema control: rationale of the techniques. *Am. J. Occup. Ther.*, 33(8): 520–523, 1979.
Weeks, P. M., Wray, R. C., and Kuxhaus, M. The results of nonoperative management of stiff joints in the hand. *Plast. Reconstr. Surg.*, 61(1): 58–63, 1978.
Zinovieff, A. N. Heavy-resistance exercises: the "Oxford technique." *Br. J. Phys. Med.*, 14: 129–132, 1951.

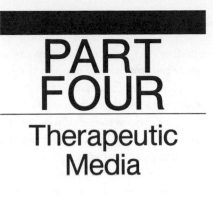

PART
FOUR
Therapeutic
Media

Purposeful activity is the unique medium of occupational therapy. Occupational therapists are concerned with occupation or purposeful activity from two standpoints. One is a concern with occupational performance tasks, defined as those life tasks of self-care, work, and play/leisure that individuals must perform to meet their own needs and to be contributing members of the community.[1] Therapists are interested in the balance among work, self-maintenance, and play/leisure within the person's life and the patient's ability to function successfully within these spheres. The other standpoint is the use of purposeful activity to evaluate, facilitate, restore, and maintain function[2] consistent with a person's roles in life. Occupational therapists believe that a person develops cognitive, perceptual, psychosocial, and motor skills through engagement in activity of interest and purpose. Although this is a basic tenet of occupational therapy, there has been less consensus concerning what constitutes purposeful activity.

The AOTA Commission on Practice[2] has officially defined purposeful activities as "tasks or experiences in which the person actively participates." It further states that activities are purposeful when they "assist and build upon the individual's abilities and lead to achievement of personal goals."[2]

Chapters 5, 6, and 9 of this text include suggestions for exercises as well as the more traditionally used games or craft activities to implement the therapeutic principles believed appropriate to restore performance components. Performance components are the skills a person needs to carry out his self-care, work, and play/leisure tasks in life.[1] The reason exercise was included along with more traditional activities was that it is the opinion of the editor of this textbook that any activity that requires mental processing of information and/or movement to achieve a goal, as exercise does, meets the official definition of purposeful activity just as goal-directed physical manipulation of objects does.[3] The patient is "actively participating" while exercising and exercises "build upon individual abilities and lead to achievement of personal goals." Both exercise and activity are endeavors that involve goal setting, and therefore the central nervous system would view them as purposeful, a requirement to activate the neural circuits needed to accomplish the task.[4] Although exercise is considered here as a legitimate treatment medium for occupational therapists engaged in treating physically disabled patients when the patient prefers it, activities that relate to a person's value system while providing the therapeutic benefit being sought are to be preferred not only because of their documented motivational value[5,6] but also their ability to elicit multifaceted outcomes more representative of life situations.

Activities used for therapy must have intrinsic and/or potential therapeutic value. The therapist analyzes activities to determine their intrinsic value to meet certain goals. Based on these analyses, the therapist selects an activity expected to implement the immediate treatment goal for the particular patient or may need to adapt an activity to develop its potential value to meet the goal. Guidelines for activity selection, analysis, and adaptation to remediate physical problems are presented in the first two chapters of this section. Persons with physical disabilities will not only need to develop motor skills, but may also need to develop skills in other areas. Any one activity used in therapy may offer opportunity for skill development in cognition, perception, psychosocial function, and/or movement. Because a thorough presentation of occupational therapy rationale for treatment of cognitive, perceptual, or psychosocial problems is beyond the scope of this text, activity selection, analysis, and adaptation for these problems are not included here. The reader is referred to the references cited at the end of chapters 2 and 7 for in-depth study of these areas.

Therapists who treat patients with physical disabilities do not limit the modalities of their practice to occupation.[7] They believe that the therapeutic process requires use of adjunctive media to enable the patient to participate or gain maximum benefit from participation in purposeful activity. There are no clear guidelines at this time as to which modalities are or are not legitimate components of occupational therapy practice for the physically disabled,[1,8] although there is considerable discussion within the profession.[7-11] Biofeedback, orthoses, and wheelchair adaptations are frequently used adjuncts to engagement of the patient in functional, purposeful activity or to achieve biomechanical, neurodevelopmental, and rehabilitative goals that therapists may have for patients. Chapters in this section describe these adjunctive therapies.

References

1. Shriver, D. J., and Foto, M. AOTA Commission on Practice: standards of practice for occupational therapy. *Am. J. Occup. Ther., 37*(12): 802–804, 1983.
2. Hinojosa, J., and Shapiro, D. AOTA Commission on Practice position paper: purposeful activities. *Am. J. Occup. Ther., 37*(12): 805–806, 1983.
3. Trombly, C. A. Letters to the editor: include exercise in purposeful activity. *Am. J. Occup. Ther., 36*(7): 467–468, 1982.
4. Granit, R. *The Purposive Brain.* Cambridge, MA: MIT Press, 1977.
5. Kircher, M. A. Motivation as a factor of perceived exertion in purposeful versus nonpurposeful activity. *Am. J. Occup. Ther., 38*(3): 165–170, 1984.
6. Steinbeck, T. M. Purposeful activity and performance. *Am. J. Occup. Ther., 40*(8): 529–534, 1986.
7. English, C., et al. The Issue Is: on the role of the occupational therapist in physical dysfunction. *Am. J. Occup. Ther., 36*(3): 1990–202, 1982.
8. American Occupational Therapy Association, Inc. Association policy: occupational therapists and modalities. *Am. J. Occup. Ther., 37*(12): 816, 1983.
9. Huss, A. J. From kinesiology to adaptation. *Am. J. Occup. Ther., 35*(9): 574–580, 1981.
10. Bissell, J. C., and Mailloux, Z. The use of crafts in occupational therapy for the physically disabled. *Am. J. Occup. Ther., 35*(6): 369–374, 1981.
11. West, W. L. A reaffirmed philosophy and practice of occupational therapy for the 1980s. *Am. J. Occup. Ther., 38*(1): 15–23, 1984.

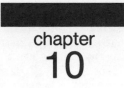

chapter
10

Activity Selection and Analysis

Catherine A. Trombly

Occupational therapists use activity as an enabling force toward wellness. Activity is defined as a process involving mental function and action,[1] implying active involvement with the environment.[2] Activity is the means by which basic needs are fulfilled and a sense of mastery and competence is achieved.

The occupational therapist designs activity experiences to translate therapeutic theories and principles that apply to the particular patient's source of dysfunction into concrete tasks which will promote movement and behavior away from dysfunction toward function.[3] Activities are selected for their inherent therapeutic properties and also for their meaningfulness to the patient. Engagement in meaningful, purposeful activity makes the patient his own cotherapist.

In this text, activities are defined as arts, crafts, sports and exercise, games, and daily life tasks including vocational tasks. Because activities used in therapy may be fun, familiar, or appear ordinary, the therapeutic purpose of the activity may not be readily apparent to the patient. Therefore, the therapist must clearly explain to him, his family, and other health care providers the relationship between the selected activity and the process of restoration of particular function(s).

Activity Selection

In treatment situations, after interpreting evaluation data and listing problems, goals are stated. Each goal represents the next level of progress for the patient. The occupational therapist selects the best activity to meet each goal of the patient's program. The best activity is one that intrinsically demands the exact response that has been determined to need improvement. Contrived methods of doing an ordinary activity in order to make it therapeutic may diminish the value of the activity in the eyes of the patient. Contrived methods also require the patient to constantly focus his attention directly on his movements rather than the end purpose of the activity. This, at the least, di-

minishes satisfaction and may even interfere with developing coordinated, smooth voluntary motion.

Although the therapist may determine what seems to be the ideal therapeutic activity to accomplish a particular goal, it would be inappropriate to assign that activity to the patient. He should be allowed to choose an activity from several that can be equally effective. If he chooses the activity, he is more likely to be committed to doing it as prescribed. Several activities may be required during one treatment session in order to work on all current therapeutic goals.

Generally, activities used to increase physical function should be within the patient's capabilities, should allow gradation of response to progress the patient to the next higher level of function, and should be as repetitive as required to evoke the therapeutic benefit. Repeating well-learned responses is not therapeutic. The choice must also take the person's cognitive and perceptual abilities, emotional status, and interests into consideration. Some cognitive aspects of the activity to be considered include the number and complexity of the steps involved in doing the activity, the requirements for organization and sequencing of the steps or stimuli, and the amount of concentration and memory required. Some perceptual factors to be considered are whether the activity requires the patient to distinguish figure from ground, position in space, construct a two- or three-dimensional object, or follow verbal or spatial directions. Other cognitive/perceptual considerations are found in chapter 7. Some psychosocial aspects of an activity that may be important to patients include whether the activity must be done alone or in a group; the length of time required to complete the activity; whether fine, detailed work or large, expansive movements are involved; how easily errors can be corrected; and how much skill is required to produce a satisfying outcome.

The selected activity should have a reasonable end goal or product. If the therapist suggests the use of sanding to strengthen the anterior deltoid, then the patient should sand pieces of something that become a product. If the patient is not interested in producing a product, the selection of sanding as the activity is inappropriate. It is poor practice to require the outward appearance of productive activity when no product is involved. Sanding a board not intended to be used, riding a bicycle jigsaw without sawing, and screwing "millions" of screws into a board for no decorative or other purpose are all examples of poor activity selection. Sports, games, or exercise may be better choices for this patient.

In addition to the general characteristics listed above, activities must have specific characteristics related to the intended goal. The therapist needs to know these characteristics, which stem from basic treatment principles used to achieve the goal. For example, if the goal is to increase strength of the elbow extensors without increasing strength of the elbow flexors, the principle is to increase resistance to the triceps. Therefore the activity must call the triceps into action, must offer the correct amount of resistance, and must involve a return motion that does not strengthen the biceps (eccentric contraction of the triceps or return by use of springs, etc.).

For the goals commonly addressed by occupational therapists some specific characteristics are listed here in simplistic form. The therapist's thinking process and subsequent activity choices will become more refined as she becomes skilled in synthesizing all therapeutic principles applicable to a particular patient. The dimensions along which the activity needs to be graded also are listed; when more than one dimension is listed, the therapist should be careful to grade the changes in one dimension at a time so that the patient has more of a chance at success.

ACTIVITY CHARACTERISTICS

To Retrain Sensory Awareness and/or Discrimination

The activity must provide components that offer a variety of textures, shapes, and sizes, graded from large, distinct, common shapes to small, less common shapes with less distinct differences between them. The texture of the various objects needs to be graded from diverse, coarse materials to similar, smooth materials. The patient and the therapist must also involve themselves in a teaching/relearning interactive experience in which the characteristics of the objects are discussed and correct identification by touch rewarded.

To Decrease Hypersensitivity

The activity should involve objects or media whose textures can be graded from soft to hard to rough and the contact with the objects can be graded from touching them to rubbing them to tapping them.

To Normalize Tone

The activity must involve controlled (location, intensity, duration) sensory experiences.

To increase tone, appropriate tactile, proprioceptive, thermal, and/or vestibular facilitatory stimuli offered to the particular muscle group(s) should be a prominent feature of the activity. It is important that if a particular type of response (tonic or phasic) is sought, stimuli known to elicit that type of response be offered.

To decrease tone, the activity should offer inhibitory sensory stimulation to the target muscle group(s) or to the patient as a whole.

To Reacquire Maturationally Based Postural and Movement Patterns

The activity must elicit the appropriate level of postural adjustment. One activity or a series of activities must progress the patient along the continuum of righting reactions in developmental sequence and/or increasingly challenge equilibrium reactions within a developmental posture.

To Recapitulate Ontogenetic Sequence

To develop stability (or decrease mobility), the activity should involve developmentally correct postures; offer resistance to axial or proximal limb musculature and/or demand weight bearing for a period of time to develop cocontraction; and be gradable to require increased duration of the holding response and then allow increasing amounts of controlled movement of the stabilized joints after stability responses are learned.

To develop mobility, the activity should involve developmentally correct movement patterns; offer little or no resistance; and be gradable to demand increasing control of gross movement and movement of specific joints in developmental order as the patient gains control of gross movement.

To Reacquire Skilled Voluntary Movement

The activity must demand responses that build on the patient's present abilities; it should offer opportunity to self-monitor successful movements; and it should provide for vast amounts of varied practice to enable learning to occur.

To Increase Coordination and Dexterity

The activity should allow as much range of motion as the patient can control and allow grading from slow, gross motions at the point where the patient is able to function to more precise, faster movements.

To Increase Active Range of Motion

The activity must require that the part of the body being treated move to its limit repeatedly and be gradable, naturally or through adaptations, to demand greater amounts of movement as the patient's limit changes.

To Increase Passive Range of Motion

The activity must provide controlled stretch or traction to the part being treated for a defined period of time. See chapter 9 for precautions.

To Increase Strength

Stress can be graded by increasing the velocity and/or resistance needed to complete the task and by increasing the number of repetitions of an isotonic contraction or the amount of time an isometric contraction is held.

To Increase Cardiopulmonary Endurance

The activity should be slightly more demanding metabolically than the patient's current status. The demand can be graded by increasing the frequency of doing a particular task, by changing the muscles used in the task (see chapter 30), by increasing the duration a task is done, or by increasing the intensity. The metabolic intensities of some activities have been measured; some of these are listed in chapter 30.

To Increase Muscular Endurance

The activity must be repetitious over a controlled number of times or period of time. It should be resistive to 50% or less of maximal strength.

To Decrease Edema

The activity should involve repetitive isotonic contractions of the muscles in the edematous part. An activity that requires repeated movement of the extremity into an elevated position would be beneficial in helping to drain the fluid out of the extremity.

Activity Analysis

The occupational therapist's job begins where the theoretical bases for improved movement leave off; the therapist must translate these theories into activities appropriate for the individual client. Activity analysis is the process used to do that translation.

Activity analysis is one of the key process skills of the occupational therapist by which activities are closely examined to determine their components and what level of capability is demanded to enable a person to do the activity. When selecting an activity, the therapist matches the particular patient's capabilities to the demand level of the activity. The match involves either challenging the patient's present level (activity used restoratively) or ensuring success at his present level (activity involved in daily occupational performance tasks). If an activity or task is part of the patient's daily life, then the comparison between task demands and patient capabilities determines whether the patient will be able to do the activity independently, with adaptation, or not at all. If an activity is to be used to restore one or more abilities found significantly deficient during evaluation, then the activity must challenge that patient's present level of ability so that through effort and/or practice the patient improves. For example, if a patient has **P**− triceps—can actively extend his elbow less than full range with gravity eliminated—the therapist selects an activity that requires him to reach a few degrees beyond his present limit so that his effort is challenged. As soon as he is repeatedly successful in reaching to that location, the activity must be modified to require him to move a few more degrees and so on.

The therapist who is skilled in analysis can more easily select the most appropriate activity from those that are available and are of interest to the patient. The therapist's ability to select activities to meet the needs of the patient comes from her fund of knowledge of the demands of various activities, which she has developed by constant practice of analyzing activity observed throughout the course of a day. Activity analysis skill should become second nature to an occupational therapist.

Students often ask why isn't there a book published with all activities analyzed and cross-referenced with disabilities so that activity prescription can be more like drug prescription. Perhaps that can be done in the decades to come when electromyographic and kinematic analyses and computers will be used routinely. Right now it can't be done validly because any differences in the position or size of the patient, the relative position of the work to the patient, the tools, the materials, or the patient's manner of working change the outcome of the analysis.

Motor analysis of activities may be done from a neurodevelopmental and/or biomechanical point of view. The biomechanical analysis of each activity is the basis of all analysis. The nervous system utilizes the least amount of muscle contraction required to meet the goal.[4] Therefore, the therapist has to be aware of the biomechanical demands, or lack of them, offered by activities used for restoration of neuromotor control. The extent of movement required, the length of the lever arms, the effects of gravity, and the postural requirements all influence the motor response governed by the central nervous system.

Traditionally analysis has been done by observing others or by doing the activity oneself while attending to what muscles should contract and relax, based on anatomical studies of muscles, joints, and bony levers. That method is used here, as it is still the most universal one. However, electromyographic kinesiological analyses of some exercises and activities have been done.

Some of the conclusions are contrary to our expectations based on anatomical studies or simplified application of neurophysiological data to movement.

BIOMECHANICAL ANALYSIS

The components of analysis of activity for remediation of physical disabilities were first put forth by Licht.[5] His "kinetic" analysis was a reaction to "craft" analysis, which focused on the craft rather than the process, which is the therapeutic aspect of activity as treatment medium.[5]

The therapist begins the biomechanical analysis of the activity by establishing the exact placement of the selected tools and equipment in relation to the patient. Changes in the equipment, supplies, or placement change the demands of the activity. Only analysis of a specific activity under specific circumstances is valid.[5] The *steps of an activity are identified.* For example, the steps of hammering a nail are: (1) reach for and pick up the hammer; (2) carry the hammer to the start position; (3) pick up the nail; (4) place the nail; (5) hit the nail; and (6) return the hammer to the start position.

Each step is then subdivided into motions. For example, hitting the nail involves elbow flexion and extension if the person is standing and the nail is located in front of him waist high or below. Hitting the nail could use other motions, such as shoulder internal and external rotation, depending on the location of the nail in relation to the person. Wrist stabilization (cocontraction) in extension and cylindrical grasp are also "motions" associated with that step. The potential *repetitions* of each motion are noted. Only steps 3, 4, and 5 would be analyzed because they are the repetitive, therapeutic aspects of this activity. Steps 1, 2, and 6 occur too infrequently to be therapeutic. The *range of each of the motions is estimated* by observation of the patient, another person, or the therapist herself, preferably in a mirror, while the activity is performed. Each motion is further analyzed to *determine which muscle(s) are required* based on anatomical, kinesiological, and electromyographical knowledge. By examining the *effect of gravity,* the *minimal strength necessary* to do the motion can be estimated. The *kind of contraction* demanded for each muscle group in each motion involved in the activity is established by definition, i.e., concentric, eccentric, isometric. Table 10.1 facilitates the analysis of activities using a biomechanical approach by structuring the components to be examined.

NEURODEVELOPMENTAL ANALYSIS

Neurodevelopmental analysis includes consideration of the developmental and neurophysiological aspects of activity. Patients with brain damage will be treated using activities based on development of voluntary motor skill. The sensory stimulation that an activity offers affects the neurophysiological response.

Analysis involves repeated observation of normal persons doing the activity to determine the characteristics of it. Table 10.2 will guide the therapist in this analysis. The position in which the activity is done and/or the movements involved are noted for their developmental level according to known sequences. Movements and positions involved in the activity are observed to determine what automatic postural reactions (righting and equilibrium) are required or are being encouraged and whether primitive reflexes are being reinforced. For example, if a patient were to reach out to the side to place or pick up an object while watching his hand, the asymmetric tonic neck reflex would be reinforced. A game of catch while sitting unsupported would encourage equilibrium reactions as the patient reached for or threw the ball.

Another characteristic to be observed is whether the activity demands stability and/or mobility responses and at which joints. For example, throwing a ball requires stability of the neck, trunk, scapula, and lower extremities and mobility of the throwing arm. Batting a baseball is an example of stability of hands and wrists and mobility of the shoulder and scapula.

The amount of attention required in the performance of an activity and whether attention is directed toward the movement itself or toward the end goal is

Table 10.1
BIOMECHANICAL ACTIVITY ANALYSIS

1. Name of the activity:
2. Describe how the person and the materials are positioned, especially in relation to one another:
3. What precautions must be considered when using this activity?
4. Analyze the activity:

Steps/Motions	Repetition	ROM	Primary Muscles	Gravity Assists/ Resists/ No Effect	Minimal Strength Required	Type of Contraction
Step 1: Motions:						
Step 2: Motions:						

5. How can this activity be graded to increase:
   a. strength?
   b. active range of motion?
   c. passive range of motion?
   d. coordination?
   e. endurance?
   f. or reduce edema?
6. For which short-term goal(s) would this activity be appropriate?
7. What must be stabilized to enable certain patients to do this activity and how will that stabilization be provided?

Table 10.2
NEURODEVELOPMENTAL ACTIVITY ANALYSIS

1. Name of the activity:

2. Describe how the person and materials are positioned, especially in relation to one another:

3. What precautions must be considered when using this activity?

4. Which *automatic postural reactions* must be intact for successful completion of the goal of the activity? Which are elicited by the activity?

5. What *developmental posture* is demanded by the activity?

6. Does this activity demand a *stability or mobility* response or a combination of the two? In which joints?

7. What *pattern of motion* is demanded by this activity? Is this pattern opposite to primitive reflex patterns or limb synergies or does the activity reinforce these unwanted patterns?

8. Does the activity demand movement of the *whole limb or isolated control* of single joints? Which ones?

9. Does this activity require *unilateral or bilateral* responses? Are the bilateral responses *symmetrical, asymmetrical, or reciprocal?*

10. What *muscle groups* are required to contract?

11. Does this activity demand *attention* to the movement (closed-loop control) or does movement proceed automatically towards a goal (open-loop control)?

12. What *controlled sensory stimulation* is offered by the activity? What is the nature of the stimulation? To which muscle groups?

Stimulus	Facilitatory or Inhibitory?	Muscle Group

12. What is the next level of motor control? How can this activity be graded to progress the patient to that level?

13. In summary, for treatment of which short-term goal(s) can this activity be used?

---

noted. Cortical control is directed toward the focus of attention.

The kinds of sensation that the activity offers are noted. It should not offer a type of sensory stimulation improper for the needs of the patient. Correct stimulation can be applied as adjunctive treatment if the activity itself does not offer it.

ELECTROMYOGRAPHIC ANALYSIS

Electromyography (EMG) is the process of recording the electrical activity produced by a contracting muscle. When a muscle is at rest, no activity is recorded. As the muscle contracts to maximum, the electrical activity increases proportionately.

A tremendous amount of research on activity must be done. Not only do activities used in therapy need to be electromyographically analyzed to provide basic knowledge concerning patterns and degree of muscle usage, but some premises also need to be confirmed. For instance, one premise is that an activity inherently demands that certain muscles or motions will be used and can therefore be prescribed based on the demands determined through traditional activity analysis. However, evidence indicates that persons will do the activity using various muscle patterns or combinations of other abilities that affect strategy,[6,7] which ultimately changes patterns of muscle contraction. That is how

the central nervous system works—it sees the goal within an environmental context, assesses the resources in relation to the demand (muscles of a given strength needed to provide the necessary forces etc.), and activates what is necessary to achieve the goal, given the resources. So the idea that doing a certain activity will always exercise a certain weak muscle may be too naive.

Some studies have been done to document the pattern, amplitude, and timing of electrical activity of muscles under controlled conditions. The reader is referred to *Muscles Alive: Their Functions Revealed by Electromyography*[4] for a compilation of studies. A few studies will be presented here because of their unique interest to occupational therapists, especially related to restoration of hand function.

A series of studies of intrinsic and extrinsic hand muscles made under loaded (resisted)[8] and unloaded[9] conditions led Long to conclude that in power grip, the extrinsic muscles provide the major gripping force. All extrinsics (agonists and antagonists) are used in proportion to the force used against the object grasped. The flexor superficialis, which is rarely seen to be active in the unloaded hand except when the wrist is flexed, becomes active in the loaded hand in proportion to the loading. The major intrinsic muscles of power grip are the interossei, active as phalangeal rotators and metacarpophalangeal (MP) flexors. Spherical grip evoked more intrinsic activity than any other test grip. The lumbricals are not significantly used in power grip.

In pinch, compression is provided by the extrinsic muscles, assisted by the MP flexion force of the interossei and the flexor pollicis brevis and the adducting force of the adductor pollicis. The opponens is acting to rotate and position the thumb[8].

In precision handling, specific extrinsic muscles provide gross motion and compressive forces. In rotation motions, the interossei are important contributors. The lumbricals are interphalangeal (IP) joint extensors as well as abductors-adductors and rotators of the first phalanges. Thenar muscles active in precision handling are the triad of flexor pollicis brevis, opponens pollicis, and abductor pollicis brevis. The adductor pollicis brevis is least active[8,9].

In another study[10] of 52 normal subjects the finger extrinsics (flexor profundus [FP], extensor digitorum [ED] and flexor superficialis [FS]) were monitored during five types of basic movement components of activity: resisted grasp, resisted finger extension, fast extension, slow extension, and unresisted grasp and release. The results, similar to those reported by Long,[8] indicated that rapid and resisted movement generated a high percentage of maximum voluntary contraction (MVC) of all three extrinsic finger muscles whether they were agonist or antagonist. Unresisted slow movement generated a low percentage of MVC. A reciprocal relationship between agonist and antagonist was the most common pattern seen, although no muscle was totally silent as antagonist. True cocontraction pattern was seen only in the most resistive exercise—grasp.

Study[11] of 10 post-cerebrovascular-accident (CVA) subjects with active grasp but little to no active finger extension, using the same basic exercises listed above and monitoring the same three extrinsic muscles under the same conditions, led to these conclusions: during resisted grasp, the FP and ED contracted maximally. Following grasp, extension motion was unchanged indicating that the FP was not inhibited since range of motion (ROM) did not increase nor was extensor motion jeopardized. The flexor muscles were seen to act independently and can therefore not be considered as a unit when doing activity analyses. Changes in movement as a result of these exercises that had been hypothesized from neurophysiological analyses did not occur consistently in all subjects, indicating need for case-by-case review of the data and further study of more subjects.

In comparison to normal subjects,[12] the post-CVA subjects recruited a lower percentage of MVC during rapid or resisted exercise and a higher percentage of MVC during slow unresisted exercise. Because of reduced innervation to motor units, the patients seemed to need to use proportionately more of their available motor units to accomplish the unresisted tasks, a finding similar to that seen in quadriplegics.[13] Patterns of muscle usage, although similar between groups, were not identical; therefore, EMG analyses of muscle usage by normal subjects cannot be extrapolated to activity analyses for persons with brain damage. The intersubject variability was also greater among patients than among normal subjects, as would be expected as each stroke results in different losses.

In another study of particular interest to occupational therapists, muscles of nine subjects were monitored during resisted and unresisted bilateral sanding on an inclined plane set at different angles.[13] It was concluded that this activity primarily required output of the anterior and middle deltoid during both the upstroke and downstroke under the resisted and unresisted conditions. The amount of muscle output increased as the upward incline of the board increased and as the resistance increased. The triceps was mildly active in the upward stroke in subjects with normal upper extremities and excessively active in three quadriplegic subjects (up to 320% MVC). Biceps and pectoralis major did not substantially contribute in any subject or under different conditions of angle or load.

A study of 16 activities used in therapy was done using 15 normal subjects[14]. The FP, the ED and the dorsal interossei I, and the abductor pollicis brevis/opponens (ABD/OPP) were monitored. Similar to previous reports, the FP and ED increased their output as resistance increased. Each was more active as an antagonist during resisted activity than during unresisted activity when each was a prime mover. For instance, the ED recruited 58% MVC during resisted grasp but only 19% MVC or less during unresisted opening of the hand. There was simultaneous contraction of agonist and antagonist even in low-resistance activities in which skill or precision was involved. The size of the object grasped and released (marble versus tennis ball) did not affect the level of muscle contraction. There was increasing variability among subjects in the amount of output of the muscles as resistance increased probably because each person uses his own strategies to overcome resistance and accomplish the goal. The activities in which each muscle was most active ($>$ 50% MVC) in 50% or more of 15 normal subjects are listed in Table 10.3. Activities which evoked 25% or less MVC of all four muscles in 50% or more of the subjects were grasp and release of tennis balls or marbles, Hindu puzzle, and mosaic tiles. These would be suitable to use for developing coordination and dexterity rather than increasing strength.

EMG studies have shown variability among subjects doing the same exercise or activity[4,10,13-15]; therefore, even with EMG information incorporated into activity analysis, the analysis will not be perfect for a particular patient because of individual differences in muscle action and differences in movement strategies. If it is essential that a particular muscle of a particular patient

Table 10.3
ACTIVITIES THAT CALLED FORTH MORE THAN 50% OUTPUT IN FOUR HAND MUSCLES OF AT LEAST 50% OF THE 15 NORMAL SUBJECTS

Muscles	Activities
Extensor digitorum	Extension game (lift Velcro checker off of Velcro board using finger extension); Theraplast donut (extend fingers and abduct thumb to spread a donut-shaped piece of Theraplast).
Flexor profundus	Closing the lid of a large jar; Theraplast grasp (grasp of a 2.5-cm cylinder of Theraplast and squeeze maximally); Theraplast donut and extension game.
Dorsal interosseous	Theraplast grasp and Theraplast pinch (pinch a 2.5-cm ball of Theraplast between the pads of the thumb and index finger).
Abductor pollicis brevis/opponens	Opening and closing of a large jar lid; Theraplast pinch; Theraplast grasp; tip pinch game (lift Velcro checker off of Velcro board using tip pinch).

be contracting to a certain level of activity, as may be the case in tendon transfer rehabilitation, then it is best to monitor the muscle directly using EMG biofeedback while the patient does the activity. EMG analyses performed on normal subjects cannot be applied to patients with dysfunctional nervous systems.[11,12]

STUDY QUESTIONS:

Activity Selection and Analysis

1. Why is activity used in occupational therapy?
2. What are the general characteristics required of an activity to be used to treat physical dysfunction?
3. How do goals and treatment principles relate to selection of activity for therapy?
4. How does activity analysis relate to activity selection?
5. Name the seven components of biomechanical activity analysis.
6. What 10 factors are considered in neurodevelopmental activity analysis?
7. What is electromyography and why is it useful?
8. According to electromyographic studies of grasp and pinch, what muscles provide the major compression forces?
9. What activities have been shown to activate a high percentage of maximum voluntary contraction (MVC) of the flexor profundus in normal subjects?
10. Do weak patients seem to use more or less of total percent of MVC available to them as compared to normal subjects?

References

1. Mish, F. C., editor. *Webster's Ninth New Collegiate Dictionary.* Springfield, MA: Merriam-Webster, Publishers, 1984.
2. West, W. L. A reaffirmed philosophy and practice of occupational therapy for the 1980s. *Am. J. Occup. Ther., 38*(1): 15–23, 1984.
3. Cynkin, S. *Occupational Therapy: Toward Health Through Activity.* Boston: Little, Brown & Company, 1979.
4. Basmajian, J. V., and DeLuca, C. J. *Muscles Alive: Their Functions Revealed by Electromyography, 5th edition.* Baltimore: Williams & Wilkins, 1985.
5. Licht, S. Kinetic analysis of crafts and occupations. *Occupational Therapy and Rehabilitation, 26:* 75–78, 1947.
6. Fleishman, E. A. On the relation between abilities, learning, and human performance. *Am. Psychol. 27*(Nov): 1017–1032, 1972.
7. Beltel, P. A. Multivariate relationships among visual-perceptual attributes and gross-motor tasks with different environmental demands. *J. Motor Behavior, 12*(1): 29–40, 1980.
8. Long, C., et al. Intrinsic-extrinsic muscle control of the hand in power grip and precision handling. *J. Bone Joint Surg., 52-A*(5): 853–867, 1970.
9. Long, C. Intrinsic-extrinsic muscle control of the fingers. *J. Bone Joint Surg., 50-A:* 973–984, 1968.
10. Trombly, C. A., and Quintana, L. A. Activity analysis: electromyographic and electrogonimetric verification. *Occup. Ther. J. Res., 3*(2): 104–120, 1983.
11. Trombly, C. A., and Quintana, L. A. The effects of exercise on finger extension of CVA patients. *Am. J. Occup. Ther., 37*(3): 195–202, 495, 1983.
12. Trombly, C. A., and Quintana, L. A. Differences in response to exercise by post-CVA and normal subjects. *Occup. Ther. J. Res., 5*(1): 39–58, 1985.
13. Spaulding, S. J., and Robinson, K. L. Electromyographic study of the upper extremity during bilateral sanding: unresisted and resisted conditions. *Am. J. Occup. Ther., 38*(4): 258–262, 1984.
14. Trombly, C. A., and Cole, J. M. Electromyographic study of four hand muscles during selected activities. *Am. J. Occup. Ther., 33*(7): 440–449, 1979.
15. Bagg, S. D., and Forrest, W. J. Electromyographic study of the scapular rotators during arm abduction in the scapular plane. *Am. J. Phys. Med., 65*(3): 111–123, 1986.

Supplementary Reading

Ayres, A. J. Occupational therapy for motor disorders resulting from impairment of the central nervous system. *Rehabilitation Literature, 21*(10): 302–310, 1960.
Barris, R., Cordero, J., and Christiaansen, R. Occupational therapists' use of media. *Am. J. Occup. Ther., 40*(10): 679–684, 1986.
Bissell, J. C., and Mailloux, Z. The use of crafts in occupational therapy for the physically disabled. *Am. J. Occup. Ther., 35*(6): 369–374, 1981.
Breines, E. The issue is: An attempt to define purposeful activity. *Am. J. Occup. Ther., 38*(8): 543–544, 1984.
Fidler, G. From crafts to competence. *Am. J. Occup. Ther., 35*(9): 567–573, 1981.
Hollis, L. I. Identifying occupational therapy: the use of purposeful activities. *American Occupational Therapy Association Physical Disabilities Special Interest Section Newsletter, 9*(4): 2–3, 1986.
Kielhofner, G., editor. *A Model of Human Occupation: Theory and Application.* Baltimore: Williams & Wilkins, 1985.
Kircher, M. A. Motivation as a factor of perceived exertion in purposeful versus nonpurposeful activity. *Am. J. Occup. Ther., 38*(3): 165–170, 1984.
Levine, R. E. The influence of the arts-and-crafts movement on the professional status of occupational therapy. *Am. J. Occup. Ther., 41*(4): 248–254, 1987.
Llorens, L. A. Activity analysis for cognitive-perceptual-motor dysfunction. *Am. J. Occup. Ther., 27*(8): 453–456, 1973.
Llorens, L. A. Activity analysis: agreement among factors in a sensory processing model. *Am. J. Occup. Ther., 40*(2): 103–110, 1986.
Marteniuk, R. G. Motor skill performance and learning: considerations for rehabilitation. *Physiother. Can. 31*(4): 187–202, 1979.
Matsutsuyu, J. S. The interest check list. *Am. J. Occup. Ther., 23*(4): 323–328, 1969.

Newall, A. R., Robinson, K. L., and Spaulding, S. J. An electromyographic study of shoulder muscles during bilateral sanding: a pilot study. *Can. J. Occup. Ther., 48*(4): 163–168, 1981.

Peganoff, S. A. The use of aquatics with cerebral palsied adults. *Am. J. Occup. Ther., 38*(7): 469–473, 1984.

Project Magic. Can magic work miracles? *Accent on Living, 30*(2): 52–55, 1985.

Reed, E. S. An outline of a theory of action systems. *J. Motor Behavior, 14:* 98–134, 1982.

Rogers, J. C. Why study occupation? *Am. J. Occup. Ther., 38*(1): 47–49, 1984.

Rogers, J. C., Weinstein, J. M., and Figone, J. J. The interest checklist: an empirical assessment. *Am. J. Occup. Ther., 32*(10): 628–636, 1978.

Smedley, R. R., et al. Slot machines: their use in rehabilitation after stroke. *Arch. Phys. Med. Rehabil., 67*(8): 546–549, 1986.

Steinbeck, T. M. Purposeful activity and performance. *Am. J. Occup. Ther., 40*(8): 529–534, 1986.

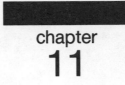

chapter
11

Activity Adaptation

Catherine A. Trombly and Anna Deane Scott

Activity adaptation is the process of modifying a familiar craft/game/sport or other activity to accomplish a therapeutic goal. There are two reasons to adapt an activity in the treatment of the physically disabled. One is to modify the activity to make it therapeutic when ordinarily it would not be so in the unadapted form. Many examples of this can be seen in occupational therapy clinics. Some such examples are floor loom adaptations to provide exercise to muscles not usually involved in weaving[1]; wall checkers in which the board is painted on the wall and has pegs at each square to hold the enlarged checkers; and biofeedback units electronically coupled to switches to turn appliances on and off.

The other reason for adaptation is to graduate the exercise offered by the activity along therapeutic continua to accomplish goals. Although the same amount of assistance or resistance may be offered manually by the therapist while the patient performs an unadapted activity, adaptation is preferred because the resistance or assistance will be consistent over time; the patient can work independently and thereby have feelings of competence and satisfaction; and, in cases where the patient is learning a new pattern of motion, the therapist would be an interference. One instance of adapting for exercise gradation is to change the size of the implements of the activity. To increase coordination, the activity must be graded along a continuum from gross, coarse movement to fine, accurate movement. Checkers and other board games lend themselves easily to such gradations; the board and pieces can be changed from large to small. The person who is a checker aficionado can continue a favorite game while continuing to benefit therapeutically.

The characteristics of a good adaptation are the following: The adaptation accomplishes the specific goal. The adaptation does not encourage or require odd movements or postures. Positioning must be reasonable for the activity involved. The adaptation is soundly constructed and is not potentially dangerous to the patient. The adaptation does not require the patient to think in terms of the movement, per se. Adaptations must be such that they intrinsically demand a certain response by the patient, one that he does not have to concentrate on performing. Finally, it does not demean the patient; some contrived adaptations seem ridiculous to the patient, and therefore he is embarrassed to use them.

When adapting activities, as with all therapeutic techniques, it is vital for the patient to understand the reason that an activity will be done in an adapted manner.

Principles of adaptation correspond to the treatment principles given in chapters 5 and 9. Activity adaptations that implement these principles are described here.

Positioning the Task Relative to the Person

The position of the person relative to the work to be done dictates the movement demanded by the activity, and therefore which muscle groups are likely to be used and how much the muscles must work.[2] Adaptation by positioning refers to changes in incline of work surface, height of work surface, or placement of pieces to be added to the project (Fig. 11.1-11.3).

Activities that are usually done on a flat surface, such as finger painting, board games, sanding wood, or using the exercise skate, can be made more or less resistive by changing the incline of the surface. For example, if the surface is inclined down, forward, and away from the patient, resistance is given to shoulder extension and elbow flexion. If the incline is up, resistance is given to shoulder flexion and elbow extension.

The standard horizontal work surface itself can be raised or lowered to make demands on certain muscle groups or to alter the effect of gravity. For example, a table raised to axilla height allows flexion and extension of the elbow on a gravity-eliminated plane. Another example is to lower the table surface to elbow height so that supination/pronation movements are evoked while eliminating shoulder rotation by allowing the upper arm to remain adducted during the process of moving items around on the table surface. Using a

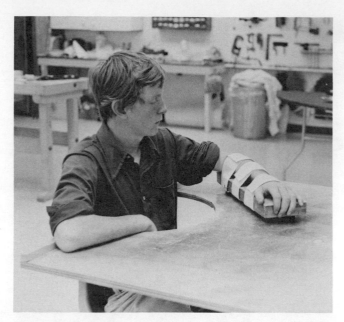

Figure 11.1 Skate and skateboard positioned at midchest level.

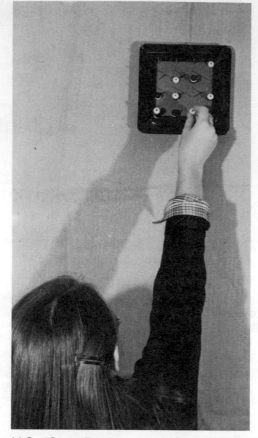

Figure 11.2 "Score Four" game mounted on the wall to require shoulder flexion and elbow extension.

skate, if the skateboard is adjusted to axilla height, shoulder horizontal abduction or adduction can be resisted. If the table is adjusted waist high, shoulder external or internal rotation can be resisted.

Placing items such as mosaic tiles, pieces of yarn, beads, darts, bean bags, etc., in various locations changes the motion required to reach them when performing an activity in an otherwise standard manner. Placement may be high enough to encourage shoulder flexion or abduction; lateral to encourage shoulder rotation, trunk rotation, or horizontal motion; or low to encourage trunk flexion, or lateral trunk flexion.

Positioning can evoke responses within developmental patterns. For example, in sitting or side-sitting, placement of the pieces of an activity to one side will require that the person reach with one arm, stabilize with the other arm, and rotate the trunk to reach them. Activities requiring reaching for objects will evoke equilibrium responses.

Adding Weights

The addition of weights adapts an activity to meet such goals as increase of strength, promotion of cocontraction, and increase of passive range of motion by stretch.

Some nonresistive activities can be made resistive by adding weights to the apparatus, directly or by use of pulleys, while others may be made resistive by adding weights to the person himself. For example, to resist shoulder extension and elbow flexion, weights can be suspended from pulleys attached across from the person on a flat or inclined surface with the weight lines running from each handle of a bilateral sanding block.

The line of pull can be reversed to resist shoulder flexion and elbow extension by attaching the pulleys behind the person.

Resistance can be changed on all looms[3]; however, the floor looms lend themselves to more versatility in the application of the resistance. Weights can be added directly to the harnesses, treadles, or beater or can be added indirectly to the beater by the use of a pulley system (Fig. 11.4).

Weights can be attached directly to the person by means of weighted cuffs, as well as by pulley line attachments. For example, when using a weighted wrist cuff, leather lacing can become resistive to external rotation and elbow flexion. As another example, braid weaving can be made resistive to shoulder flexion by means of weights and pulleys attached over the back of the person's chair with the lines running to a cuff fastened around the person's humerus.

Tools also are weights and can be selected or adjusted to offer graded resistance. Some of the possibilities include the following. Hammers can be graded from lightweight tack hammers to heavy ball-peen or claw hammers. Weaving can be done on table looms, and as the patient gains range and/or strength, larger, heavier floor looms may be used.

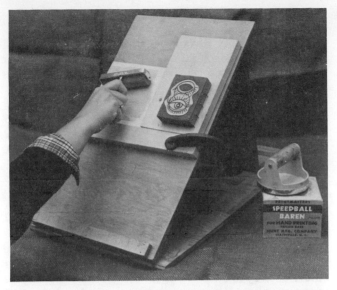

Figure 11.3 Block printing repositioned. Block is held in place by resting on nails below and to the right of the block. Height can be changed by moving the board C-clamped to the incline board.

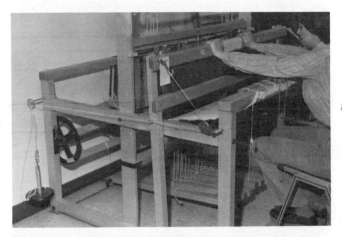

Figure 11.4 Floor loom adapted with weights and pulleys to resist elbow extension.

Adding Springs and Rubber Bands

Springs and rubber bands are means of adapting activity to increase strength or the cocontraction response through resistance, to assist a weak muscle, or to stretch muscle and other soft tissue to increase passive range of motion. When offering resistance, the spring or rubber band is positioned so that its pull is opposite to the pull of motion of the target muscle group, whereas if used for assistance, they are set to pull in the same direction as the contracting muscle. Springs or rubber bands applied for the purpose of stretching are placed so the pull is against the tissue to be stretched (see chapter 9 for precautions).

Springs of graduated tensions may be applied directly to the equipment. A beater of a floor loom can be made resistive to elbow extension or flexion by attaching springs either from the breast beam to the beater to resist elbow extension or from the beater to the castle, the center upright of the loom, to resist elbow flexion. A grip sander, which has springs in the handle, will resist finger flexion when the person squeezes to use it.[2]

Rubber bands can be added to smaller pieces of equipment and can be graded from thin and light tension to thick and heavy tension. For example, a rubber band can be wrapped around the pincer end of a spring-type clothespin to add resistance while it is used in games involving picking up small pieces.

When rubber bands or springs are used to create a force of resistance in one direction the return motion can involve passive stretch of the same muscle group during motion in the opposite direction, unless the person does an eccentric contraction of the resisted muscles to prevent the stretching pull. For example, if a spring is attached to a loom's beater to resist elbow flexion when the beater is pulled toward the person, on the return motion, the spring will pull into extension, thereby stretching the flexors unless the patient eccentrically contracts the flexors. Eccentric contraction would be desired as it would also exercise the weak flexors.

Change of Length of Lever Arm

The amount of work a muscle or muscle group is doing depends on the resistance. Resistance is determined by the pull of gravity on the limb and the implements the patient is using which together act as the resistance lever arm. The effect of a given amount of resistance can be altered by lengthening or shortening the resistance lever arm. The longer the lever arm, the greater the force required to counterbalance it. The lever arm can be lengthened or shortened by changing the location of the resistance on the limb; for example, applying a weight at the end of the humerus rather than at the wrist reduces the amount of force that the shoulder flexors must generate to lift the weight. The lever arm can also be altered by "shortening or lengthening" the limb; for example, by flexing the knee, which shortens the limb, less resistance is offered to hip extension than if the knee were extended. Another example is carrying an object close to the body, which requires less activity of back muscles than if the object were carried at arm's length. Use of a reacher to pick up an object increases the resistance, and therefore the muscle output required, than if the object were picked up directly. Use of a large paint brush to paint a picture on the wall increases the resistance over using finger paint to make the picture.

On the other hand, increasing the length of the force lever arm decreases the muscle output needed to accomplish a task. For example, in Figure 11.5, if the clothespin were adapted to have longer handles, less pinch force would be required to open the end of it the same distance.

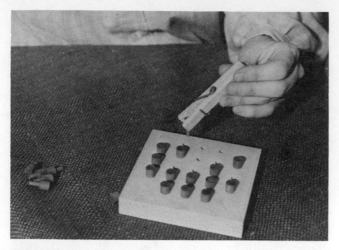

Figure 11.5 Game is played using a clothespin to move the pieces to strengthen pinch.

Attention to lengths of lever arms is important not only in adapting activity to make it more therapeutic but also in adapting utensils and tools used in daily life tasks to enable weak persons to be able to use them and in guiding workers in methods of lifting and handling on their jobs to avoid musculoskeletal injuries.

Change of Materials or Texture of Materials

Gradation along the strengthening continuum may be accomplished by selection of material by type and also by variations of texture or density to change resistance. Coordination can be challenged by changing the material used to that of a finer, more delicate nature. Cutaneous stimulation changes as objects or surfaces that the person uses are more or less textured and has the effect of facilitating or inhibiting the muscles associated with the skin surface stimulated. Padding handles with textured material offers sensory stimulation to the finger flexors.

Resistance can be changed, for example, by starting a cutting project with tissue paper and then progressing to heavier materials, such as construction paper, cloth, or leather. Metal tooling can be graded for resistance by choosing materials in grades from thin aluminum to thick copper. Sandpaper is graded from extra fine to coarse, and resistance increases with the coarser grade. Mixing can be graded from making jello to scrambled eggs to biscuit batter, etc. If materials are graded in the opposite direction, that is, from heavy to light, then the activity will demand increased coordination from the patient. Weaving may begin using rug roving and be graded toward fine linen threads as the patient progresses in coordination. By making balls from yarn or terry toweling, carpeting surfaces the person works on, etc., the therapist adapts the activity to increase sensory stimulation.

Change of the Size or Shape of Objects

Playing pieces of board games can be made a different size (Figure 11.6) or shape than they standardly are

and can therefore offer a therapeutic benefit that the standard objects would not. For example, checkers, which are usually flat pieces approximately 2.5 cm in diameter, can be made cylindrical, square, cubes, or spheres and can range in size from tiny to as large as a person's reach permits.

By reducing the size or changing the shape of the pieces being worked on, the goal of increased dexterity and fine coordination is facilitated. Therapists creatively change sizes of craft materials, such as weaving thread, tiles, paint-by-number guidelines, ceramic pieces, etc., and recreational materials, such as puzzle pieces, chess men, target games, etc., to increase coordination. Tools are adapted by changing the size or shape of their handles or adding handles to tools that do not normally have them. Plans for an adapted cone-handled sander have been published.[4] The actual size of the tool used can be changed in which case tools offer more or less resistance. For example, saws range in size from small coping saws or hack saws to large crosscut or rip saws. Resistance of saws can also be graded by the number of teeth per inch on the blade; the lesser the number of teeth, the greater the resistance. Woodworking planes vary in size, and the amount of exposed blade can be adjusted to provide resistance. Scissors also vary in size, and the resistance can be increased by tightening the screw.

Change of Method of Doing the Activity

Bowling, basketball, and many other sports can be done from a seated position as opposed to the normal standing position. Change of rules adapts some sports, such as track and field events, to certain requirements of the physically disabled. Sewing and needlework, normally bilateral activities, can be made unilateral by adaptations that hold the material steady for the working hand. (See Figure 19.1.) Holes can be punched in leather or packs of paper by use of a drill press in lieu of regular leather or paper punches. Block printing can be done in a hand- or foot-operated printing press rather than in a block printing press. Instead of foot races, crawling races can be done. Instead of rolling over on a therapy mat, rolling can be done on a shag rug to provide greater sensory stimulation.

Change of method is used both for exercise (Fig. 11.6 and 11.7) and for compensation (Fig. 11.8). By changing the method an activity is made possible when under ordinary circumstances it would not be possible because of the person's disability. This compensatory adaptation allows the therapist to offer activity of interest to the patient while at the same time accomplishing certain therapeutic goals.

Sometimes therapists must devise new games or activities to provide therapy to a particular muscle group at an intensity greater than would be available in everyday activities. The finger extensors are such a muscle group for which a game has been devised and the instructions published.[5]

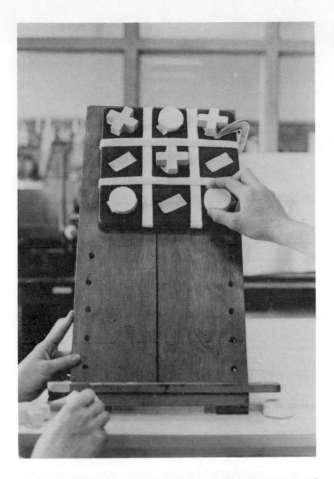

Figure 11.6 Adapted tic-tac-toe repositioned to require shoulder motions and size changed to accommodate poor coordination. The pieces are held in place with Velcro.

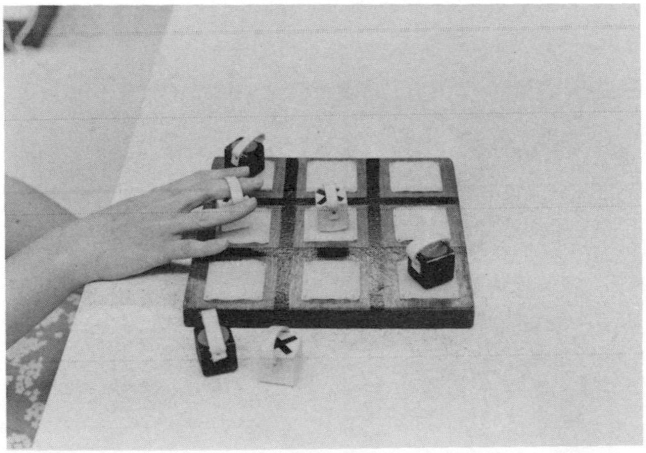

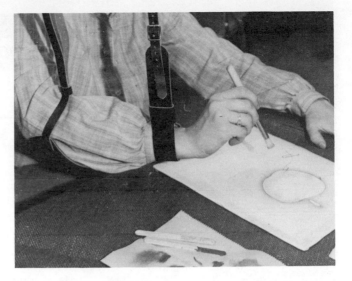

Figure 11.8 Stenciling is made possible by use of a suspension sling. Exercise to wrist extensors is obtained.

STUDY QUESTIONS:

Activity Adaptation

1. What are the two reasons given for adapting an activity for use in therapy?
2. What are the five characteristics of good adaptations?
3. What therapeutic goals can be accomplished by:
   a. changing the position of the task relative to the person?
   b. adding weights to tools or game pieces?
   c. adding springs or rubber bands to craft equipment or tools?
   d. changing the length of lever arms of tools, equipment, or the limb itself?
   e. changing the material to be used in a project?
   f. changing the method of doing an activity?

References

1. Hultkrans, R., and Sandeen, A. Application of progressive resistive exercise to occupational therapy. *Am. J. Occup. Ther., 11*(4): 238–240, 1957.
2. McGrain, P. and Hague, M. A. An electromyographic study of the middle deltoid and middle trapezius muscles during warping. *Occup. Ther. J. Res., 7*(4): 225–233, 1987.
3. Bellman, J. B., Myers, C., and Norton, C. G. *Therapeutic Devices 1956–1976 American Journal of Occupational Therapy.* Rockville, MD: The American Occupational Therapy Association, 1977.
4. Gans, S. O., and Braband, N. Brief or new: adapted cone-handled sander. *Am. J. Occup. Ther., 39*(1): 49–51, 1985.
5. Gesior, C., and Mann, D. Finger extension game. *Am. J. Occup. Ther., 40*(1): 44–48, 1986.

Supplementary Reading

Brunyate, R. W. A study of the use of magnetic toys in the treatment of cerebral palsied children. *Am. J. Occup. Ther., 8*(4): 151–155, 1954.
Hollis, L. I. Identifying occupational therapy: the use of purposeful activities. *American Occupational Therapy Association Physical Disabilities Special Interest Section Newsletter, 9*(4): 2–3, 1986.

Figure 11.7 Adapted tic-tac-toe to exercise finger extensors; pieces are held by Velcro and require force to lift them.

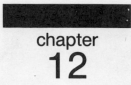
Biofeedback as an Adjunct to Therapy

Catherine A. Trombly

Feedback is necessary for motor learning.[1] Augmented feedback is regularly offered by therapists who verbally call the patient's attention to outcome of actions (accuracy of placement, speed of task completion, number of repetitions completed, etc.) or by use of videotapes[2] or mirrors.

Biofeedback, a coined term meaning biological feedback,[3] refers to the process of using instrumentation to feed back to the patient sensory information not usually in conscious awareness. By receiving and processing such information, the person can learn to control the monitored function because he knows the effects of his efforts, i.e., has knowledge of results. The use of biofeedback by occupational therapists is a natural extension of their use of feedback[4] to motivate and inform the patient about his success and progress.

General feedback, of the type given verbally by therapists, is characterized as motivational, whereas artificial sensory feedback, such as offered by biofeedback instruments, is informational.[1] The advantages of electronic feedback over that offered by the therapist are fourfold[1,5]: Electronic feedback offers information quantitatively (the signal is in proportion to patient output) rather than qualitatively ("OK, good!"). Information is given objectively and consistently and does not rely on the alertness of the therapist, which may waver and cause the patient to receive unstable feedback. The therapist can only give information about what she sees, which is on a gross, external level, whereas the instrument can convey information on a minute, internal level (motor unit activity, imperceptible degrees of motion, change in weight distribution or force, etc). Electronic feedback is continuous, immediate, and offered during performance, which enhances neuromuscular reeducation; feedback from the therapist is given after the response has occurred, which can disrupt learning. A basic tenet of motor learning is that learning or relearning increases as feedback becomes more specific and immediate.[5]

Biofeedback instruments can make a person aware of the state of contraction of voluntary or involuntary muscles, blood pressure level, skin temperature, heart rate, or brain activity. Other devices are available to provide information concerning joint position and small changes in joint motion, smoothness of movement, weight distribution,[5] pressure exerted on a tool or object, or posture. These instruments and devices are being incorporated into therapeutic programs by occupational therapists, as well as other health professionals.

This chapter will focus on electromyographic (EMG) and electrogoniometric biofeedback. EMG biofeedback is used to make the patient aware of the state of contraction of his muscles (Fig. 12.1). Electrogoniometric biofeedback is used to inform the patient of joint position or small increments of movement he may not notice (Fig. 12.2). Other types of biofeedback used in therapy will be described briefly.

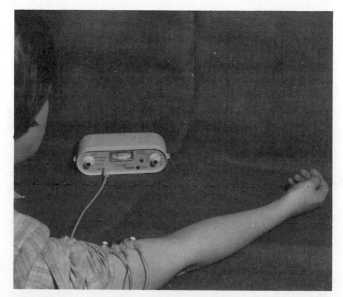

Figure 12.1 Electromyographic biofeedback using Cyborg J33 instrument.

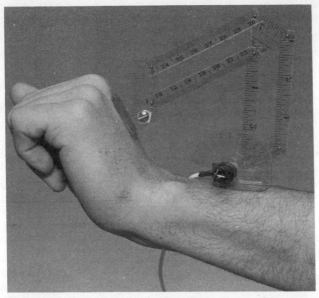

Figure 12.2 Electrogoniometric biofeedback. Elgon was designed and built by Gary de Bacher, Ph.D., Assistant Professor of Rehabilitation Medicine at Emory University and Rehabilitation Engineer at Center for Rehabilitation Medicine, Atlanta, Georgia.

Patients with motor dysfunction need to relearn voluntary control over impaired muscles or how to disrupt synergistic motor patterns,[6] or they must redevelop a motor program or develop a compensatory plan for action.

For those patients who are able to perform some action, biofeedback can be used as an adjunct to ongoing therapy[7] to inform both the patient and the therapist of the effects of treatment procedures chosen to improve the person's motor control, the results of which may surprise the therapist who has chosen the procedure based on common beliefs.[3] When the goal is to increase or decrease muscle participation in a movement, EMG biofeedback validates contraction of a particular muscle at a particular level during activity or exercise.[5] When the goal is to increase active range of motion (AROM), electrogoniometric biofeedback can be used to validate limits of motion.

Sometimes biofeedback itself is the treatment. As treatment, the focus is on manipulating the signal under voluntary effort. For example, the patient monitors the effect of his effort to contract or relax a muscle or to move a joint a certain amount. If the patient is paralyzed and cannot move, biofeedback becomes the therapeutic modality of choice to inform the patient that his efforts are having an effect.[1,3] Since he cannot move, he cannot gain knowledge of results by observing his own movements, and so neither the patient nor therapist can know whether the adopted strategy is useful or useless in reorganizing the motor system.[1] Motor unit recruitment in the target muscle has been shown to be significantly greater under conditions of biofeedback versus no biofeedback, all other variables

held constant.[8] Likewise, if the patient is spastic and trying to learn to relax muscle contraction, biofeedback gives him information concerning the effectiveness of his strategies and rewards his efforts.

Biofeedback Equipment

All biofeedback instruments have three major components: the transducer, the processing unit, and the output display.

The transducer is what detects the change in the parameter being measured. Different transducers are used to pick up different types of signals. In general, there are two types of signals monitored for biofeedback purposes. One type is the actual electrical signals produced by neural electrochemical changes in the body. Muscle fiber depolarization or brain cell depolarization are examples of this type. EMG, electroencephalographic (EEG), and electrocardiographic (EEG) biofeedback are of this type. The AC (alternating current) processing circuit amplifies the tiny biological signal that the body generates. This type probably can be considered true biofeedback or feedback of a biological signal.

The other type of signal used for biofeedback purposes is the result of a mechanical or chemical change of the transducer secondary to the change in the body. The change in the transducer causes a change in the resistance of the DC (direct current) processing circuit. When the resistance in the circuit changes, more or less electricity flows through the circuit, making the signal greater or lesser.

EMG and ECG transducers are electrodes, that is, small pieces of metal that convert ionic bioelectric current to electronic current.[3,9] The electrodes are taped to the patient's skin to detect the tiny electrical signals that skeletal or heart muscle generates during contraction and to transmit these signals to the amplifier for processing and display. The signal that is processed is the difference of potential (voltage) detected by the two electrodes.

The electrogoniometric transducer, the potentiometer, is a type of variable resistor that changes resistance when rotated. One arm of the potentiometer is connected to the moveable arm of the goniometer and the other to the stationary arm. When the positions of the arms of the goniometer change in relation to each other, the potentiometer changes the amount of resistance it offers to the flow of electricity in the circuit. The electrical signal that is spoken of in this case comes from a battery or other voltage source outside of the patient. It is processed through a special circuit called a Wheatstone Bridge. The bridge circuit has four resistors connected in a parallel circuit. Each of the two branches of this parallel circuit has a fixed-value and a variable resistor. Of the two variable ones, one is the potentiometer and the other is a resistor that can be set by the calibrating knob on the instrument. When one branch (AB) of the Wheatstone Bridge circuit matches the other branch (CD), no electricity flows to the display because there is no potential difference in the two branches.[10,11] Electrons have negative charges and tend to move toward a more positive, or less negative, place in the circuit. There has to be a difference in potential (or charge) for the electrons to flow. When the resistance of the CD branch changes because the elgon moves and changes the resistance of the potentiometer, then there is a difference in potential between the two branches of the bridge and electricity flows and the display indicates this.[10,11] In the process of calibrating the elgon, the arms of the elgon (and hence the potentiometer) are placed in given positions and baseline is established by balancing the bridge circuit (AB = CD) so no electricity flows. This corresponds to "zero" or one limit of joint motion. The moveable arm of the elgon is then moved to the other limit of motion, which changes the potentiometer so that less resistance is offered to the flow of electricity in the CD branch, causing a potential difference between branch AB and branch CD. The electrical signal that corresponds to the amount of motion away from baseline to the other limit of joint motion is displayed on the output device.

As long as the elgon is placed correctly and secured so it does not move on the patient's skin, the signal fed back to the patient is a valid representation of his movement. If the elgon is replaced exactly each day and calibrated properly, the signal is reliable; that is, it stays the same from day to day except in response to true patient changes in movement.

The processing unit contains electrical circuits that amplify (enlarge), rectify (make all positive polarity), filter (smooth), and integrate (collect, store, or sum)[12] the signal in preparation for its display. There are two types of processing circuits. In an AC circuit, the polarity of the signal reverses periodically and its magnitude changes over time.[10-12] In a DC circuit neither the polarity nor the magnitude of the signal changes over time. Although some biofeedback instruments are simple on-off types (signal reaches criteria and display comes on), most have a level detector that requires the signal to reach a certain level or threshold before the display is activated. This is an important feature that allows shaping of the patient's response by requiring improvement to obtain the reward of the display. According to operant conditioning methodology, a response that in any way approximates the final performance is rewarded at first, then, as that is learned, only a better response is rewarded, and so on until the final level of performance is achieved.

Preferably, the output of the feedback display changes in proportion to the effort, which gives the patient information on the quality of his response. However, some simple feedback devices that simply turn on and off indicating the response to be correct or incorrect may be adequate for a particular use.

The biofeedback signal can be thought of as a switch to turn a display device on or off. The type of display can take many forms. One type is an oscilloscope on which the direct picture of the raw (nonintegrated) EMG signal can be displayed. Another is a computer monitor on which an analogue of the raw EMG signal can be plotted over time.[13] Output of both of these display devices can be fed to computers and recorded on paper for record keeping or research. Another type of display is the sound of the EMG signal broadcast over a speaker. Other types of displays include buzzers of various types, lights, or meters. One particularly motivating type of display for children or adolescents to reward maintained response is the use of a switching unit that turns some electrical appliance on and keeps it running as long as the desired level of signal indicates maintained effort. The switching unit can be reversed to keep the equipment running as long as no unwanted signal is detected, for example, in the case of control of spasticity or maintained upright posture. Any type of appliance can be attached to the switching unit: radio, television, electronic toys, tape player, etc. The signal can also be displayed on a computer monitor, and when it reaches correct levels can be rewarded by whatever the computer is programmed to offer.

The selection of type of display is usually limited in any occupational therapy department but there is always a choice between audio or visual displays. Some patients may know which type of feedback would be most helpful to them; others may need to discover it by trial and error. If the patient is confused by one, another can be tried. Perhaps in the future there will be clearer, research-based, guidelines for choice. One study on persons with intact proprioception indicated that use of augmented visual feedback decreased reliance on proprioceptive feedback.[14] Differences in outcome of eventual gains in motor relearning between choice of visual or auditory feedback needs study in a clinical population with defective proprioception.

There may be times when two channels of information are of interest, for example, output of both agonist and antagonist. If the display devices are meters or lights, visual monitoring of both channels simultaneously is too difficult, but monitoring one visual display (agonist) and one auditory display (antagonist) or monitoring one display that relates the two visual signals to each other may be possible. Some patients are unable to do this, however.[15,16] Another way to monitor dual outputs is to use a unit that permits linking the outputs so that only when both conditions (for example, contraction of agonist and relaxation of antagonist, or contraction of two synergistic muscles) are above threshold will the display reward the effort. However, neither the patient nor therapist will know which of the two conditions is at fault if the reward fails to appear. New multichannel instruments[13] that provide graphic visual feedback via computer monitor enable simultaneous visual monitoring of several outputs because the signals are processed and chunked into meaningful bits of displayed information.

Electromyographic Biofeedback

Each motor unit is composed of many muscle fibers, which depolarize (fire) more or less simultaneously when the neuron belonging to that unit activates them.

If many motor units fire at the same time, their signals add together and the amplitude of the resultant signal is larger as an indication of that summation. When no contraction of extrafusal muscle is occurring (when the muscle is at rest), no signal is generated. Physicians have studied these signals for many years, using a process called clinical electromyography, to detect and/or diagnose neuromuscular diseases. Marinacci and Horande[17] very cleverly figured that viewing this information could be therapeutic to persons relearning to control their muscles.

When a muscle fiber depolarizes in response to a neural impulse, a small electrical charge or voltage is generated. In Figure 12.3, an attempt is made to conceptually relate the EMG signal to the physiologic changes it represents. The circular "scope" to the right of the figure shows what the electrodes are "seeing." In the top drawing, the representative muscle fiber of a motor unit is in a resting state with positive K+ charges outside and negative Na- charges within.[18] As depolarization occurs, in the second drawing, the left electrode is seeing a negative charge in relation to what the right one sees; therefore, the tracing dips negatively. In the third drawing, both electrodes are seeing a negative charge as the wave of depolarization moves along and since there is no difference in potential detected, the tracing returns to zero. In the fourth drawing, the left electrode is positive in relation to the right as repolarization begins; therefore, the tracing deflects to the positive side of the recording. Finally in the last drawing, as the repolarization wave progresses, again there is no difference detected and the tracing returns to zero, completing the EMG action potential for that motor unit. The EMG signal is an AC signal.

ELECTRODE SELECTION

Two electrodes are used to transmit the signal of each muscle being monitored. Surface electrodes are small metal discs. Any type of metal may be used. However, because the electrical conductivity differs among metals, both electrodes should be of the same material. If they are not, then the signal is contaminated by differences in ionic interchange between the gel and the different metals. Most surface electrodes used today are the silver-silver chloride type. The chloriding provides a stable ionic transmission[3] between the electrode and the electrolyte (gel). The size of electrodes affects validity of the signal because the pickup area is circumferential around the electrode configuration on the skin and conical in depth (Fig. 12.4). Large electrodes, which have more metal surface, offer less resistance than small ones and enable the electrons to flow easier. Small electrodes allow more specific monitoring than large ones and should absolutely be used to monitor muscles of the hand or the closely packed muscles of the forearm. Even then the signal may contain output from both the extensor digitorum (ED) and the extensor carpi radialis, rather than just the ED, for example.

SPECIFICATIONS FOR EMG BIOFEEDBACK INSTRUMENTS

For biofeedback to be effective for learning, it must be valid; that is, the signal must actually represent the monitored change. For that reason it is important to know how the signal is processed and what factors associated with the processing can affect validity. The EMG signal that is to be processed is characterized by its amplitude (size), measured in microvolts, and fre-

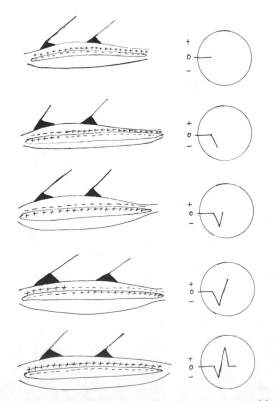

Figure 12.3 Schematic of how the electromyographic signal is generated by the muscle.

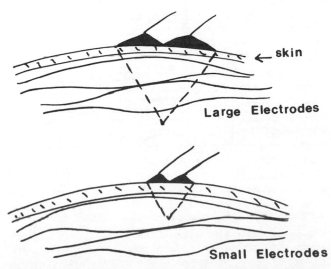

Figure 12.4 Schematic denoting the pickup area of different-sized electrodes.

quency (shape), measured in hertz (Hz) or cycles per second. The processing unit needs to be sensitive enough to process the tiny signal and linear in its representation of the input signal in the displayed output signal. Additionally, the amplifier must have certain specifications that should be considered when purchasing EMG biofeedback instruments. They are described below.

Range

This specification refers to all the levels of amplitude and frequency over which the device is expected to operate.[12] The specification sheet will state the amplitude range in terms of microvolts ($\mu V = 1/1,000,000$ V). The signal of one motor unit has an amplitude of 0 at rest to approximately 250 μV[19] for a large motor unit; many motor units firing simultaneously results in voltages of 1000 μV or higher. Frequency range is specified under terms such as "filters," "bandwidth," or simply "frequency range" and is described below.

Frequency Range. Frequency in the specifications of biofeedback instruments does not refer to the repetition rate of motor unit firing but rather to the mathematical description (harmonics) of the waveform. If you were to visualize the output of one motor unit, it would have a characteristic shape that is composed of many frequencies of waveforms. Figure 12.5 schematically illustrates this concept. Near the baseline are low-frequency waves and near the peak are high-frequency waves. To present the shape of that motor unit, waveforms of various frequencies are represented and their electrical values summate.[9,20]

The frequency range must be adequate to accommodate the major portion of the EMG signal. A range of 10 Hz to 10 kHz (kHz = 1000 Hz) will give a good representation of the shape of the EMG signal. Although the frequency components of the waveform of the EMG signal can approximate 10,000 Hz, an instrument that processes less than 1000 Hz will produce a good signal

for biofeedback. For diagnostic EMG, a true picture of the signal is necessary; therefore, the physician uses an oscilloscope with a very high frequency capability that faithfully reproduces the shape of the signal.[9] The biofeedback instrument with its limited frequency range still gives accurate information about whether the muscle is or is not contracting and whether it is contracting more or less than previously. Even though the frequencies of the EMG signal do go as low as 1 Hz, the low-frequency filter switch is usually set above that to eliminate from the processed signal slowly fluctuating DC signals generated at the electrode-electrolyte interface, called movement artifact.

Figure 12.6 illustrates the effect of use of a 200-Hz low band-pass filter and a 20 Hz high band-pass filter. Frequencies less than 200 Hz but more than 20 Hz are passed, but those above or below those frequencies are not so that the resultant electrical signal for that motor unit is reduced and the shape is changed (imagine that the peak is lost). When the filters cut out frequency components of the wave form of the signal below and above the values set by the high-pass and low-pass filters, respectively, the amplitude of the signal is attenuated[12] because less electrical energy is permitted to pass. Therefore, if the setting of the filter switch of the biofeedback instrument is changed, the output signal will be affected independent of the patient's effort. For reliable recording from treatment to treatment, these settings should be constant across sessions.

Signal-to-Noise Ratio

This specifies the ratio of amplification of the signal in relationship to the amount of electronic noise that exists within the machine itself and is processed into the output. The signal-to-noise ratio should be at least 1000:1,[12] which means that the EMG signal is processed 1000 times more than the noise. This specification may be listed as a given amount of noise at a

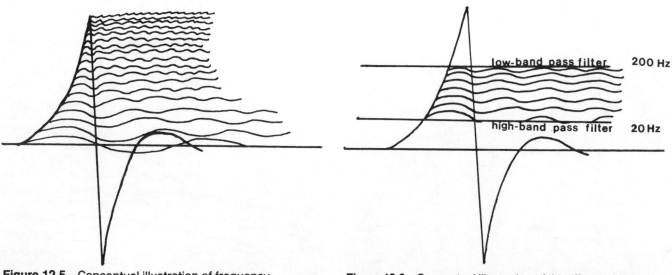

Figure 12.5 Conceptual illustration of frequency.

Figure 12.6 Conceptual illustration of the effects of filters.

certain frequency range, e.g., 5 µV when set at 2 Hz to 10 kHz. Since the patient has no control over this noise signal he can be frustrated by false feedback if it is allowed to be a large part of the processed signal.

Common Mode Rejection Ratio

Amplifiers used for electromyography are differential amplifiers; that is, they process that part of the signal that is different from the signal held in common. This type of amplifier is used because the bioelectric signal is so small in relation to the ambient, non-EMG electrical signals produced by house current. When monitoring one muscle, three electrodes are used: two are placed on the skin over the muscle. They pick up not only the muscle signal but also ambient signals that the antenna-like body has captured from the atmosphere. The other electrode is placed anyplace else on the body. That single electrode also picks up the ambient signals, but not the muscle signals. The differential amplifier then processes that part of the signal that is different among the three electrodes—the muscle signal.[9,19]

Common mode rejection ratio (CMRR) refers to how efficiently the differential amplifier amplifies the wanted muscle signal over the unwanted common signal. The higher the CMRR, the better, because the wanted signal is that much more likely to be processed over the unwanted one. For example, a CMRR rating of 100,000:1 means that the wanted signal is processed 100,000 times more than the common signal.

If the electrodes are different in size or composition or the resistances are different due to incomplete skin preparation or a dirty electrode, then instead of the differential amplifier receiving a common level of interference signal from each electrode, it receives different levels from each. Therefore, the interference is not all cancelled out. What happens then is that this artifact become part of the signal and gives false information to the patient.

Input Impedance

Each measuring instrument has a certain internal resistance that appears across the input leads.[10] Resistance within an AC circuit is called impedance, which includes reactance in addition to resistance.[11] The resistance offered by the reactive element is frequency-dependent.

In a series-type circuit, the total voltage (electromotive force) is dropped (used up) as it pushes the electrons over the resistors in the circuit. If there are two resistors, the voltage will be divided between the two resistors. If one resistor is larger than the other, then more force will be used up in pushing the electrons over the large resistor and less force dropped over the other. If the voltage were recorded over the large resistor, the voltage reading would be large; whereas if it were recorded over the smaller resistor, the signal would be less. Two impedances connected in series will also behave as a voltage divider.[10] In a conceptual way, we can think of the electrode-electrolyte interface as one resistor in series with the instrument, the other resistor.

Since the output signal is taken over the instrument "resistor", it is desirable that it have a larger value than the electrode "resistor." If the case were vice versa, then the output signal would be diminished because there would be a large voltage drop over the electrode "resistor" and less available to drop over the instrument "resistor." High impedance of the electrode-skin combination, in relation to the input impedance of the amplifier, results in attenuated EMG signals and increased noise levels.[12,21] The therapist has some control over this by reducing the electrode-skin resistance through proper care of electrodes and skin preparation to be discussed below. Surface electrodes, properly applied, may have impedances of up to 10 kilohms.[12] The input impedance of the amplifier is specified by the manufacturer. It should be high (> 100 times the expected electrode impedance.[10] The high input impedance of the biofeedback unit will allow the CMRR to account for the inevitable small differences in electrode impedances.

PATIENT SELECTION

Cognitive processing abilities have not been studied in relation to the effectiveness of biofeedback.[22] Obviously, the patient must be able to understand the relationship between his effort and the feedback. Characteristics reported to be associated with success include greater AROM at the start of treatment and less spasticity.[23,24] Variables *not associated* with successful use of biofeedback include age,[8,25-27] sex, and side affected by stroke,[25,27] type of injury (peripheral or central nervous system,[8] amount of previous rehabilitation or duration of injury,[8,26-27] or number of biofeedback treatments. Proprioceptive loss has been found to greatly impair functional success and receptive aphasia to slightly reduce it in patients treated with biofeedback.[25]

There is much variability in electromyographic output for patients with central nervous system dysfunction; therefore, if a patient fails to benefit on the first try, another try is justified.

ELECTRODE PLACEMENT

The muscle to be trained is carefully palpated to determine its margins so that the electrodes can be located over the belly of the muscle. They are aligned parallel to its line of pull. The reason for this is that since the signal is a difference between what each electrode "sees" and since theoretically the wave of depolarization passes down the parallel muscle fibers equally, then if the electrodes were placed perpendicular to the line of pull, little potential difference would be seen and the signal would be miniscule or absent. Even though the wave of depolarization does not actually proceed in such an orderly way, the signal is still better when electrodes are placed in line with the muscle fibers than it would be if the electrodes were placed across the muscle fibers.

The spacing of the electrodes affects the size and specificity of the signal. Closely placed electrodes pick up signals more superficially and from a more circumscribed area than do widely spaced electrodes (Fig. 12.7). Spacing the electrodes apart during early sessions to reeducate a weak muscle, as long as the electrodes are still within the margins of the muscle belly, will pick up whatever signals may be generated by this muscle and its synergists and give the patient positive reinforcement. On the other hand, to relax spasticity, close spacing will reduce the pickup area, making it more specific, and consequently increase the likelihood of success.

The ground or common electrode can be located anywhere on the body, preferably over a bony prominence or on the earlobe, where no muscle is actively contracting. This is the electrode that tells the differential amplifier to cancel out all signals picked up by the other two electrodes that are seen in common with this electrode. This electrode does not "ground" the person to prevent shock. It should be mentioned, as an aside, that all medical instrumentation should meet safety standards and should be periodically checked for electrical leakage.

ELECTRODE APPLICATION

Knowing how the signal is transmitted from muscle to amplifier will help the therapist understand that careful application of the electrodes is essential for obtaining a valid signal. The electrical signal generated by ionic exchange during depolarization of muscle fibers moves away from the muscle, through the saline of the tissues, and toward the surface of the body (as well as deeper into the body). The body is a volume conductor; that is, electrical signals are conducted throughout its volume as opposed to a wire, which conducts electricity along its length. At the surface, the skin has a dead, horny layer that is in effect a resistor. This layer needs

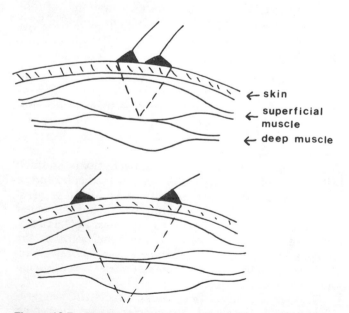

← skin

← superficial muscle

← deep muscle

Figure 12.7 Electrode placement affects pickup of signals.

to be removed or its resistance reduced to allow valid conduction of the signal via electrodes. One way to reduce the resistance is to rub the skin with rough material (gauze pad) and then rub a little electrode gel into the skin. The electrode gel is also put into the cup of the electrode housing. When the electrode is placed over the skin where the gel was rubbed in, the electrical signal continues its journey from body saline to gel to electrode and up the wires to the amplifier. At the point where the gel and electrode meet (the electrode-electrolyte interface) an ionic exchange occurs which results in a DC voltage.[12] The amplifier has a component called a capacitor that does not conduct DC signals; therefore, they are stopped before they enter the processing section. As long as the electrode remains stationary on the skin, this voltage does not get processed and does not contaminate the bioelectric signal, which is AC voltage. However, if the electrode moves because it is touched or isn't taped down well, then the DC signal begins fluctuating and the capacitor sees it as an AC signal, accepts it, and sends it on for processing, causing artifact or a false signal.

Procedure for Applying Electrodes

Of course the electrodes must be in good condition. If there is a break in the wire or in the connection of the wire to the electrode, the circuit will be open and therefore a 60-Hz artifact signal (ambient noise) may be all that is processed. To test the integrity of an electrode, place one lead of an ohm meter on the metal electrode (not the plastic housing) and the other lead on the metal plug of the electrode. If the electrode is intact, no resistance (0 ohms) will be measured on the ohm meter.[9]

Disposable electrodes, some pregelled, are available; therapists should follow the manufacturer's directions for application. The following process applies to cup-type commercially available electrodes, which are commonly used.

1. If the patient is hairy, the hair is shaved off.

2. The skin is rubbed with gauze and alcohol to remove body oil and the layer of dead skin cells. When the site is reddened, it is ready. Do not cause an abrasion. Some gel can be rubbed into the skin in distinct areas. It cannot be allowed to communicate between the sites because it will short-circuit (stop) the signal.

3. While the alcohol is drying, the electrode is prepared. An adhesive electrode collar with its protective ring is peeled off the backing and placed exactly around the bottom of the plastic rim of the electrode. The cup of the electrode is filled with electrolyte, and a straight-edge paper is used to level the gel in the cup. The remaining gel is inspected for bubbles and, if found, these are broken. Bubbles cause artifact due to the disturbance of the electrode-electrolyte interface. The electrode with its leveled amount of gel is attached to the skin after removing the protective ring from the collar. The periphery of the electrode is pressed into place before the center is pressed to prevent oozing of the gel. Oozing causes short circuiting and/or poor attachment.

4. It is useful to tape the lead (wire) near the electrode to the skin. Also if the patient is going to move during the treatment, the leads should be taped in place to prevent them from swinging, which causes artifact.

Electrodes should be carefully handled because breaks can easily occur in the leads, which of course makes them inoperative. Obviously each time the electrodes are removed and reapplied, a different population of motor units is being sampled, which affects the reliability of day-to-day recordings. The more exactly they are replaced, the more reliable the signal.

In summary, to ensure valid processing of the EMG signal for biofeedback purposes:

1. The electrodes should be of the same material and be clean.
2. The electrodes should be properly applied, including reducing the skin resistance and filling the wells of the electrode properly with electrolyte.
3. The electrodes should be of the correct size for the size of the muscle being monitored and should be taped down securely.
4. The electrodes should be placed exactly over the belly of the muscle and in a longitudinal configuration. Palpation, not simply a chart of electrode placement sites, should be used to locate the electrodes.
5. The electrodes should be spaced for valid recording of the monitored muscle: close together for small or superficial muscles and at a distance for large muscles.
6. The amplifier should have proper frequency range, signal-to-noise ratio, common mode rejection ratio, and input impedance, and the filter switches should be set properly.

TRAINING

Although there is no universally correct method, some procedures used in training persons using electromyographic biofeedback are:

1. The patient is oriented to the apparatus and procedure. A trial, using a nondysfunctional limb, allows the patient to understand the treatment and begin to determine strategies for achieving the goal with the impaired limb.

2. Baseline level of activity of the monitored muscle is determined. This level is found by adjusting the settings until no signal is produced but would be if the dial were turned the slightest amount.

3. The threshold goal is set by the therapist so that the patient must reach the goal to gain correct feedback. If the muscle is being reeducated, the baseline level is low; the goal is to get greater output, and therefore the threshold is set a small increment greater than baseline in order to get feedback. If the muscle is being inhibited, the baseline is high; the goal is to decrease output; therefore, the threshold is set a small amount below baseline. Feedback in this case occurs when the

signal turns off (unless the machine is equipped with a special arrangement by which absence of signal turns the feedback display on). This example may clarify:

Goal	Baseline	Threshold	Feedback
Reeducate	10μV	15μV	Display "on"
Decrease spasticity	20μV	15μV	Display "off"

4. For brief (10- to 15-min) treatment periods, the patient follows a treatment protocol appropriate for the goal. These are described here:

Goal: Reeducation of Muscle Contraction

These techniques are appropriate for weak (O or T) or flaccid muscles. To start, the electrodes are large and are spaced apart but within the muscle's limits. As the patient improves, the electrode spacing and size are reduced.[28] The target threshold is set above baseline level.

The patient is encouraged to contract the muscle and facilitation techniques are used. Especially useful techniques are the tonic reflexes, muscle and tendon tapping, and vibration. Vibration, unfortunately, introduces an artifact similar to 60-Hz artifact into the output due to the electromagnetic forces generated by the available vibrators. This is a time when an oscilloscope could help distinguish between artifact and signal.

As the patient achieves success, the threshold is raised. The performance is improved and shaped by increasing the threshold as success occurs at each previous level. When success consistently occurs at the maximum threshold level for that patient the patient is gradually weaned from EMG feedback. Weaning is done by preventing the patient from receiving the feedback while the therapist continues to monitor the output. As his performance deteriorates, then feedback is allowed so that he might regain control. Once control is regained, feedback is removed again. The weaning process continues until the patient is successful without the feedback.

Kelley et al.[28] have outlined specific procedures for use with hemiplegic patients to reeducate muscle contraction.

Goal: Reduction of Spasticity[29,30]

The atmosphere should be relaxing, and the therapist should use a soothing voice. The electrodes should be closely spaced. The best position for achieving relaxation is determined. The target baseline is set below baseline level. The patient is encouraged to relax and shut off the signal. Relaxation methods such as imagery (imagining soothing scenes), Jacobson's relaxation techniques,[31] and contract/relax are some techniques used.

The patient seeks to maintain silence of the signal for as long as possible. Then he tries to keep the muscle relaxed despite contraction of muscles of the opposite extremity, arousal, or mental effort (counting backward for example). When relaxation can be achieved in various positions under these conditions, relaxation during elicitation of the stretch reflex is the next goal. The patient's limb is moved slowly at first while he tries to maintain relaxation. As he succeeds, the speed of passive movement is increased. After this is achieved fairly well, relaxation during unresisted contraction of the antagonist is aimed for.

Once the patient is consistently successful in learning to relax his spastic muscles, he needs to be weaned from the instrument. Weaning involves making the feedback unavailable to him but still monitored by the therapist for as long as he can maintain an acceptable level of inhibition. It is helpful if the therapist has access to an oscilloscope to monitor EMG signals at least from time to time in order to know what exactly is happening. The information from a feedback display is not specific; it does not differentiate between a signal from many small and moderately sized motor units and one from one or two huge units firing repeatedly, nor between EMG and artifact.[29,32]

Electrogoniometric Biofeedback

Devices, such as electrogoniometers, that combine information into a single entity that is easily codable and relates in a more straightforward way to movement[33] should result in greater success than has been reported for EMG biofeedback. Electrogoniometric biofeedback is more useful than EMG when increased range of motion is the goal.[34] EMG biofeedback is not relevant to goal-directed actions,[35] probably because the same movement patterns can be performed using different muscles.[1] Also, many variables other than muscle contraction are reflected in the EMG signal.[19] The EMG output does not mathematically relate to force generated nor linearly relate to joint angle; therefore it may be more helpful in learning specific muscle contraction[29,36] or relaxation than in learning movement per se. EMG does not relate to joint angle for two reasons: (1) different amounts of tension are required in a muscle depending on the limb's relation to gravity, e.g., more tension is needed in the biceps to hold a position of 90° of elbow flexion than 120°. (2) Tension is a composite of motor unit recruitment and viscoelastic properties of muscle and tendon tissue. The more tension generated because of stretch of the viscoelastic components of muscle, the less motor unit recruitment is needed to maintain the same tension.[37]

The electrogoniometer is a device that measures joint angle electronically. It is fastened over the bones adjacent to the joint being monitored using straps, tape, electrode collars,[29] or rubber contact cement. It is important that the axis of the potentiometer be aligned with the axis of joint motion similar to a manual goniometer used to measure ROM (chapter 8). In the case of a parallel linkage electrogoniometer (Fig. 12.2), the device needs to be aligned so that the hinge in the linkages nearest the joint is located directly above the joint when the joint is in neutral position.

The signal that is being picked up for processing is a voltage signal, the amplitude of which varies depending on the position of the arms of the goniometer. The voltage is DC, which means the magnitude and polarity remain fixed with relation to time.[12] The signal can be displayed on a meter, by switching on a light, over a speaker, on a paper record,[38] on a computer monitor,[13] or by turning equipment off and on.

TRAINING TO INCREASE MOVEMENT

The procedures found useful in training persons using electrogoniometric biofeedback are the following:[34]

1. The patient's AROM and passive range of motion (PROM) are measured using a standard goniometer, and these baseline measurements are recorded. The patient must have some pain-free AROM to use the electrogoniometric feedback to advantage.

2. The dysfunctional joint, or a key joint if many are dysfunctional, is selected, and the electrogoniometer is carefully positioned over it as described above.

3. The target angle or threshold is set by the therapist. For the first session, this should be an easily attainable angle that the patient can successfully achieve. Concentration and voluntary effort are used by the patient. The therapist encourages. Facilitation techniques may be useful to increase muscle contraction. The session should last no more than 10 to 15 min, as tolerated, with the person working at his own pace and with ample rest periods. Using biofeedback to achieve certain goals takes full concentration and is tiring.

4. Later sessions can increase in duration and frequency, as tolerated. The target angle is changed in small increments so that the goal is always achieved at each session.

5. As the range of motion increases, the feedback can be used in combination with therapeutic activities to maintain motivation.

Measuring Success

The transducers must be placed absolutely exactly each time they are used with a certain patient if comparison of progress is to be made with any degree of reliability.

To measure the success of EMG biofeedback, the microvolt level recorded by the instrument can be used from day to day, but *only* if the same, cleaned electrodes are replaced exactly as previously and if the skin is prepared as well as before[29] so that the skin resistance is the same. This can be measured using an electrode impedance meter. Then differences will still be seen, which are measurement error, because replaced electrodes are possibly sampling a different population of motor units and the electrode/electrolyte interface is different, which could potentially change the processing of the signal by the differential amplifier.

Measurement of the difference from the beginning to the end of a treatment period is an accurate reflection of the gains made at that session. Gains so noted can be compared validly and reliably from day to day.

The gains achieved during electrogoniometric biofeedback can be determined by comparing the degrees of ROM gained within one treatment session to those gained in another. The absolute improvement in range cannot accurately be determined from one treatment period to the next, unless the electrogoniometer is reapplied and calibrated exactly the same each time.

Effectiveness

In controlled, counterbalanced studies of EMG biofeedback versus no biofeedback, it has been found that significant improvement resulted from the use of EMG biofeedback in normal subjects and those with hemiparesis and peripheral nerve lesions.[8,39]

By far the most commonly reported use of biofeedback for recovery of motor control has been with stroke patients. This probably reflects the belief that function of these patients would improve if motor unit recruitment were increased and/or spasticity reduced. Wolf et al.[27] reported that success, in terms of function, was achieved in 19 of 28 upper extremities and 20 of 36 lower extremities by use of biofeedback and was maintained 1 year later. On the other hand, in another study, significant improvement in numerous neuromuscular measures was found in 22 stroke patients given 60 EMG biofeedback treatments as compared to 9 control (no treatment) patients. However, no significant improvements related to function were found.[23] Another study reported that after an average of 50 therapy sessions, 5 chronic cerebrovascular accident patients with impaired expressive aphasia and auditory comprehension were successfully retrained to use their right upper extremities at the gross assist level and that self-esteem improved and depression was alleviated.[40] Another study, which looked at the effects on 12 hemiparetic patients, of EMG biofeedback combined with neurodevelopmental treatment versus neurodevelopmental treatment alone, concluded that there was no significant difference between groups.[35] Only very large treatment effects could be expected to be discerned in a study with such a small sample.

In one review of 32 papers that have been published during the last quarter century on the use of EMG biofeedback for stroke patients, it was concluded that no solid scientific evidence exists for or against the use of EMG biofeedback with stroke patients.[41]

The placebo effects of biofeedback cannot be underestimated. In a study in which actual EMG biofeedback, simulated EMG (therapist muscle activity was being fed to the patient), and no feedback were compared in a group of 24 hemiparetic patients, the two feedback conditions were found to result in significant increases in muscle function (increased EMG amplitude and ROM) as compared to control.[42]

Electrogoniometry has been found effective in decreasing the amount of genu recurvatum, hyperextension of knee, during stance phase of gait, in 13 subjects who underwent three weeks of daily training.[43]

Other Biofeedback Devices

MERCURY SWITCH TRANSDUCERS

There are other types of biofeedback that you may use depending on the types of diagnoses seen in a particular clinic.

In stress reduction therapy, one parameter monitored could be blood pressure; the patient would be trying to learn strategies to decrease it. Blood pressure can be monitored using a pressure transducer or strain guage to detect force displacements or volume changes.[10,11] Changes in the volume of blood in the body part, such as a finger, cause the transducer to be activated, which in turn causes proportional changes in resistance in the circuit. When resistance changes in the circuit, the voltage output changes. This voltage signal is then displayed to the patient so that he can learn to control his response to stress.

Skin temperature is measured using a thermistor transducer, which is very sensitive to small changes in temperature.[10,11] Use of it allows the patient to learn to control peripheral vascular dilation (sensed as warmth) and constriction (sensed as cool). Skin temperature monitoring is an indirect method of monitoring blood pressure. If the peripheral blood vessels dilate, the blood pressure decreases. The increased peripheral blood flow warms the distal body parts. The thermistor reacts to this change in temperature by reducing the resistance to the flow of electrons in the circuit. Patients with Raynaud's disease or migrane headaches use skin temperature feedback to learn to control vasodilation. The thermistor transducer is very sensitive to small changes of temperature.

Heart rate can be measured using a mercury strain guage transducer, which detects beats per minute.[10,11] The mercury strain guage is an elastic tube filled with mercury (Hg). Wire contacts are made with the Hg at each end of the tube so that resistance can be measured between the two ends. As each beat occurs, the force stretches the tube. The resistance in the circuit changes because when the column of Hg is made longer and thinner, it offers more resistance to the flow of electrons in the circuit than a short, fat column does. This idea of resistance to electron flow can be compared to differences in water flow seen when a pipe with a 1-inch diameter is used versus one with a 5-inch diameter. Heart rate also can be measured using a reflected light photoelectric transducer—plethysmyography.[10,11] Variation in light reflected from transluscent tissue illuminated by a small lamp is measured. As the amount of blood perfusing the tissue changes, so does the amount of light reflected to the photocell. The photocell changes its resistance to electron flow as a result of the brightening or dimming of light impinging on it. Heart rate is monitored during exercise and activity to make the patient aware of his cardiac responses under different circumstances.

Brain activity, or EEG, is measured using electrodes that sense the electrical charges in the brain cells. The frequency of these charges changes when the area of the brain being monitored is active compared with when it is at rest. Professionals who monitor brain activity are interested in teaching patients to relax, and the patient's efforts are rewarded by an increase in the appearance of delta (slowest) waves. EEG biofeedback is not frequently used because other, simpler ways can be used to teach the patient to relax and because artifact, or false signals, can easily spoil the feedback.

The transducers that measure galvanic skin response or GSR are electrodes like those used for muscle feedback. The electrodes detect a change in skin resistance caused by the change in the sweat level on the skin. As anxiety increases, sweating increases, and resistance decreases because sweat is salt water, which is a good ionic conductor. Dry skin acts more like an insulator that resists the ionic or electronic flow.[10]

Other devices are used to monitor smoothness of movement (accelerometers), pressure exerted on a tool, force exerted on the floor,[20] etc. These devices use strain guages as the sensing transducer. The strain guage is made of fine wire mounted on a stiff backing. When pressure or force is applied to the strain guage, the backing bends, stretching the wire. When a wire is stretched, it gets thinner and longer so its resistance increases. In the case of force or pressure detection, the strain guage is directly deformed and the wire stretched when the pressure or force is exerted. The accelerometer, on the other hand, has the strain guage mounted on a blade of steel with a small weight placed at the other end of the blade. Movement results in bending the blade, which in turn stretches the wire of the strain guage, changing the resistance. The jerkier the movement, the greater the change in resistance, which is reflected in the output.[10,11]

ACCELEROMETER

This transducer provides a voltage signal proportional to changes in velocity. The greater the variability in velocity, the greater the output.[5] One use is to monitor angular deflection of head position[44] in which the accelerometer is used to switch a feedback display on and off. It also can be used to decrease intention tremor or to improve smoothness of motion. A smooth movement would be characterized by a fairly uniform velocity and reduced output of the accelerometer.

Still other devices are simple on/off switches that let a person know if something has or has not happened. For example, to monitor bilaterally equal weight bearing, foot switches can be placed in the patient's shoes. Only when both switches are closed (have full weight) will the circuit be activated. Or if the therapist is interested in making sure that heel strike occurs in walking, a heel switch can be used in each shoe that closes the circuit when stepped on and activates the signal. Or to ensure that the patient is maintaining an upright posture,[45,46] or a neglected limb is not being forgotten,[47] a mercury switch can be used. A mercury switch is a glass vial that contains some Hg and has the two wires of the circuit protruding into it. The circuit is open (no electrical flow) when the vial is tipped so that the Hg flows away from the wires, and it is closed when the Hg flows around the wires and completes the circuit, activating the display. If the goal were for a patient to maintain upright posture, this type of switch could be used with a radio as the display device so that the radio program would switch off if the patient moved away from upright position.

Another clever device is an on/off switch to detect joint position to ensure that a patient is exercising or stretching to full range.[48] It uses a travel-type burglar alarm that has a string attached to the alarm. When the string is pulled beyond a certain point, the alarm sounds. The string can be threaded through a flexible drinking straw to keep it in place over the joint.

To develop coordination, an infrared light "magic pen" can be used to trace a design. If the pen strays off the black line, the light is reflected back to the pen and activates a beep—a form of negative reinforcement.[49] To make the reinforcement positive, the patient has to trace a white line on a dark background and a pleasant, continuous sound has to be the feedback signal to indicate that the patient stays on the line.

Directions for building other simple feedback systems have been published.[29,50]

Future Developments

The idea of using EMG templates of performance to improve sports performance in athletes is being explored and tested.[51] The templates are patterns of the amplitude and timing of EMG activity from strategic muscles during a best performance. Other practice efforts are compared to this template for correctness, and the athlete seeks to decrease the discrepancies between template and practice performance. This idea could be useful in retraining motor patterns in patients.

Another way to use normative data is to train patients to produce muscle activity similar to that produced by normal subjects doing the same activities. One study reports use of EMG biofeedback to train a patient with low back pain to reduce output of back muscles during movement to levels found in normal subjects matched by age and sex.[52]

The growing use of computers, which can chunk complex information that results from functional actions into usable feedback signals, will increase the use of augmented sensory feedback in therapy in the future. Perhaps even further into the future, computers will examine the patient's performance, compare it to a template of correct performance, and tell the patient, in language he can understand, what to do to correct the performance. The technology is here; the motor control strategies are not yet completely known nor do "templates of correctness" exist. Only recently have invariant characteristics of movement, the programmed aspects, begun to be discovered.[53,54] These characteristics, rather than EMG amplitude, which varies from trial to trial, may be more appropriately monitored. Clinical instrumentation and protocols have not yet been developed.

STUDY QUESTIONS:

BIOFEEDBACK

1. Define a) biofeedback; b) electromyographic (EMG) biofeedback; c) electrogoniometric biofeedback.
2. Name five functions that the patient can be made aware of through biofeedback.
3. What is the major reason an occupational therapist would use biofeedback?
4. What does the EMG signal represent?
5. What two factors are important to consider
   a. in selecting electrodes for EMG biofeedback?
   b. in placing electrodes for EMG biofeedback?
6. Explain what effect changing the frequency filter switch(es) on the EMG biofeedback instrument will have.
7. Define artifact. What will cause artifact to appear in the processed signal?
8. What is the function of the third (common) electrode used in EMG biofeedback?
9. Describe an EMG biofeedback procedure used to reeducate a weak muscle.
10. Describe the procedure to increase movement.

References

1. Mulder, T., and Hulstyn, W. Sensory feedback therapy and theoretical knowledge of motor control and learning. *Am. J. Phys. Med., 63*(5): 226–244, 1984.
2. Holm, M. B. Video as a medium in occupational therapy. *Am. J. Occup. Ther., 37*(8): 531–534, 1983.
3. DeWeerdt, W., and Harrison, M. A. Electromyographic biofeedback for stroke patients: some practical considerations. *Physiotherapy, 72*(2): 106–108, 1986.
4. Weiss-Lambrou, R. To whom does biofeedback belong? *Am. J. Occup. Ther., 36*(1): 49, 1982.
5. Wolf, S. L. Biofeedback applications in rehabilitation medicine: implications for performance in sports. In *Biofeedback and Sports Science*. Edited by J. H. Sandweiss and S. L. Wolf. New York: Plenum Press, 1985.
6. Honer, J., Mohr, T., and Roth, R. Electromyographic biofeedback to dissociate an upper extremity synergy pattern. *Phys. Ther., 62*(3): 299–303, 1982.
7. Runck, B. *Biofeedback: Issues in Treatment and Assessment*. Publication No. (ADM)80-1032. Washington, DC: National Institute of Mental Health, Department of Health and Human Services, 1980.
8. Middaugh, S. J., and Miller, M. C. Electromyographic biofeedback: effect on voluntary muscle contractions in paretic subjects. *Arch. Phys. Med. Rehabil., 61*(1): 24–29, 1980.
9. Reiner, S. and Rogoff, J. B. Instrumentation. In *Practical Electromyography*. Edited by E. W. Johnson. Baltimore: Williams & Wilkins, 1980.
10. Bergveld, P. *Electromedical Instrumentation: A Guide for Medical Personnel*. New York: Cambridge University Press, 1980.
11. Yanoff, H. M. *Biomedical Electronics*, 2nd edition. Philadelphia: F. A. Davis, 1972.
12. Cohen, B. A. Basic biofeedback electronics for the clinician. In *Biofeedback—Principles and Practice for Clinicians*. Edited by J. V. Basmajian. Baltimore: Williams & Wilkins, 1979.
13. Self Regulation Systems, 14770 N.E. 95th St., Redmond, WA 98052.
14. Adams, J. A., Gopher, D., and Lintern, G. Effects of visual and proprioceptive feedback on motor learning. *J. Motor Behavior, 9*(11): 11–22, 1977.
15. Burnside, I. G., Tobias, H. S., and Bursill, D. Electromyographic feedback in the remobilization of stroke patients: a controlled trial. *Arch. Phys. Med. Rehabil., 63*(5): 217–222, 1982.
16. Weiss-Lambrou, R., and Dutil, E. The effect of differing feedback conditions on grip strength: a pilot study. *Occup. Ther. J. Res., 6*(2): 93–103, 1986.
17. Marinacci, A. A. and Horande, M. Electromyogram in neuromuscular re-education. *Bull. Los Angeles Neurol. Soc., 25*: 57–71, 1960.
18. Eyzaguirre, C., and Fidone, S. J. *Physiology of the Nervous System*, 2nd edition. Chicago: Year Book Medical Publishers, 1975.
19. Basmajian, J. V., and De Luca. C. J. *Muscles Alive: Their Functions Revealed by Electromyography*, 5th edition. Baltimore: Williams & Wilkins, 1985.
20. Yack, H. J. Techniques for clinical assessment of human movement. *Phys. Ther., 64*(12): 1821–1830, 1984.
21. Baker, M. P., and Wolf, S. L. Biofeedback strategies in the physical therapy clinic. In *Biofeedback—Principles and Practice for Clinicians*. Edited by J. V. Basmajian. Baltimore: Williams & Wilkins, 1979.
22. Wolf, S. L. Electromyographic biofeedback applications to stroke patients. *Phys. Ther., 63*(9): 1448–1459, 1983.
23. Wolf, S. L., and Binder-Macleod, S.A. Electromyographic biofeedback applications to the hemiplegic patient: changes in upper extremity neuromuscular and functional status. *Phys. Ther., 63*(9): 1393–1403, 1983.
24. Basmajian, J. V., et al. EMG feedback treatment of upper limb in hemiplegic stroke patients: a pilot study. *Arch. Phys. Med. Rehabil., 63*(12): 613–616, 1982.
25. Wolf, S. L., Baker, M. P., and Kelly, J. L. EMG biofeedback in stroke: effect of patient characteristics. *Arch. Phys. Med. Rehabil., 60*: 96–102, 1979.
26. Greenberg, S., and Fowler, R. S. Kinesthetic biofeedback: a treatment modality for elbow range of motion in hemiplegia. *Am. J. Occup. Ther., 34*(11): 738–743, 1980.
27. Wolf, S. L., Baker, M. P., and Kelly, J. L. EMG biofeedback in stroke: a 1-year follow-up on the effect of patient characteristics. *Arch. Phys. Med. Rehabil., 61*(8): 351–355, 1980.
28. Kelly, J. L., Baker, M. P., and Wolf, S. L. Procedures for EMG biofeedback training in involved upper extremities of hemiplegic patients. *Phys. Ther., 59*(12): 1500–1507, 1979.
29. De Bacher, G. Biofeedback in spasticity control. In *Biofeedback—Principles and Practice for Clinicians*. Edited by J. V. Basmajian. Baltimore: Williams & Wilkins, 1979.
30. Brown, D. M., and Nahai, F. Biofeedback strategies of the occupational therapist in total hand rehabilitation. In *Biofeedback—Principles and Practice for Clinicians*. Edited by J. V. Basmajian. Baltimore: Williams & Wilkins, 1979.
31. Jacobson, E. Electrical measurements concerning muscular contraction (tonus) and the cultivation of relaxation in man: studies on arm flexors. *Am. J. Physiol., 107*: 230, 1933.
32. Regenos, E, M., and Wolf, S. L. Involuntary single motor unit discharges in spastic muscles during EMG biofeedback training. *Arch. Phys. Med. Rehabil., 60*(2): 72–73, 1979.
33. Newell, K. M., and Walter, C. B. Kinematic and kinetic parameters as information feedback in motor skill acquisition. *J. Human Movement Studies, 7*: 235–254, 1981.
34. Brown, D. M., DeBacher, G., and Basmajian, J. V. Feedback goniometers for hand rehabilitation. *Am. J. Occup. Ther., 33*: 458–463, 1979.
35. Mulder, T., Hulstijn, W., and Van Der Meer, J. EMG feedback and the restoration of motor control: a controlled group study of 12 hemiparetic patients. *Am. J. Phys. Med., 65*(4): 173–188, 1986.
36. Harris, F. A. Exteroceptive feedback of position and movement in remediation for disorders of coordination. In *Behavioral Psychology in Rehabilitation Medicine: Clinical Applications*. Edited by L. P. Ince, Baltimore: Williams & Wilkins, 1980.
37. Long, C., Thomas D., and Crochetiere, W. J. Viscoelastic factors in hand control. *Excerpta Med. Int. Congr. Ser.* Proceedings of the IVth International Congress of Physical Medicine, Paris, September 6–11. No. 107: 440–445, 1964.
38. Morris, A. F., and Brown, M. Electronic training devices for hand rehabilitation. *Am. J. Occup. Ther., 30*(6): 376–379, 1976.
39. Middaugh, S. J. EMG feedback as muscle reeducation technique: A controlled study. *Phys. Ther., 58*: 15–22, 1978.
40. Balliet, R., Levy, B., and Blood, K. M. T. Upper extremity sensory feedback therapy in chronic cerebrovascular accident patients with impaired expressive aphasia and auditory comprehension. *Arch. Phys. Med. Rehabil., 67*(5): 304–310, 1986.
41. DeWeerdt, W., and Harrison, M. A. The efficacy of electromyographic feedback for stroke patients: a critical review of the main literature. *Physiotherapy, 72*(2): 108–118, 1986.
42. Hurd, W. W., Pegram, V., and Nepomuceno, C. Comparison of actual and simulated EMG biofeedback in the treatment of hemiplegic patients. *Am. J. Phys. Med., 59*(2): 73–82, 1980.
43. Hogue, R. E., and McCandless, S. Genu recurvatum: auditory biofeedback treatment for adult patients with stroke or head injuries. *Arch. Phys. Med. Rehabil., 64*(8): 368–370, 1983.

44. Leiper, C. I., et al. Sensory feedback for head control in cerebral palsy. *Phys. Ther.*, 61(4): 512–518, 1981.
45. O'Brien, M., and Tsurumi, K. The effect of two body positions on head righting in severely disabled individuals with cerebral palsy. *Am. J. Occup. Ther.*, 37(10): 673–680, 1983.
46. Bjork, L., and Wetzel, A. A positional biofeedback device for sitting balance. *Phys. Ther.*, 63(9): 1460–1461, 1983.
47. Gruskin, A. K., Abitante, S. M., and Gorski, A. T. Auditory feedback device in a patient with left-sided neglect. *Arch. Phys. Med. Rehabil.*, 64: 606–607, 1983.
48. Bohannon, R. W., and Short, D. Compact device for positional biofeedback. *Phys. Ther.*, 64: 1692, 1984.
49. Talbot, M. L., and Junkala, J. The effects of auditorally augmented feedback on the eye-hand coordination of students with cerebral palsy. *Am. J. Occup. Ther.*, 35(8): 525–528, 1981.
50. Hallum, A. How to build simple inexpensive biofeedback systems. *Phys. Ther.*, 64(8): 1235–1239, 1984.
51. Sandweiss, J. H. Biofeedback and sports medicine. In *Biofeedback and Sports Science*. Edited by J. H. Sandweiss and S. L. Wolf. New York: Plenum Press, 1985.
52. Jones, A. L., and Wolf, S. L. Treating chronic low back pain: EMG biofeedback training during movement. *Phys. Ther.*, 60(1): 58–63, 1980.
53. Schmidt, R. A. The search for invariance in skilled movement behavior. *Res. Q. Exerc. Sport*, 56(2): 188–200, 1985.
54. Schmidt, R. A. *Motor Control and Learning: A Behavioral Emphasis.* 2nd ed. Champaign, IL: Human Kinetics Publishers, Inc., 1988.

Supplementary Reading

Abildness, A. H. *Biofeedback Strategies.* Rockville, MD: The American Occupational Therapy Association, 1982.

Basmajian, J. V., and Blumenstein, R. *Electrode Placement in EMG Biofeedback.* Baltimore: Williams & Wilkins, 1980.

Binder-Macleod, S. A. Biofeedback in stroke rehabilitation. In *Biofeedback: Principles and Practice for Clinicians,* 2nd edition. Edited by J. V. Basmajian. Baltimore: Williams & Wilkins, 1983.

Bowman, B. R., Baker, L. L. and Waters, R. L. Positional feedback and electrical stimulation: an automated treatment for the heimplegic wrist. *Arch. Phys. Med. Rehabil.,* 60(11): 497–502, 1979.

Delp, H. L., and Newton, R. A. Effects of brief cold exposure on finger dexterity and sensibility in subjects with Raynaud's phenomenon. *Phys. Ther.,* 66(4): 503–507, 1986.

Ince, L. P., and Leon, M. S. Biofeedback treatment of upper extremity dysfunction in Guillian-Barre Syndrome. *Arch. Phys. Med. Rehabil.,* 67(1): 30–33, 1986.

Knutzen, K. M., Bates, B. T., and Hamill, J. Electrogoniometry of postsurgical knee bracing in running. *Am. J. Phys. Med.,* 62(4): 172–181, 1983.

McWilliams, P. A. *Personal Computers and the Disabled.* Garden City, NY: Doubleday & Co., 1984.

Thomas, D., and Long, C. Electrogoniometer for the fingers: kinesiologic tracking device. *Am. J. Med. Electronics, 3:* 96–100, 1964.

Thompson, S. B. N., Hards, B., and Bate, R. Computer-assisted visual feedback for new hand and arm therapy apparatus. *Br. J. Occup. Ther.,* 49(1): 19–21, 1986.

Orthoses: Purposes and Types

Catherine A. Trombly

Orthotic rehabilitation involves the prescription, design, fabrication, checkout, and training in the use of special devices applied to patients to substitute for lost function. Several rehabilitation professionals bring their special expertise to different aspects of the orthotic rehabilitation process. The physician is responsible for prescribing the device. The certified orthotist is an expert in design and fabrication of all types of permanent orthoses, especially complicated spinal and lower-extremity orthoses and upper-extremity orthoses used to restore function. The occupational therapist is an expert in the adaptive use of the upper extremities in occupational performance tasks and has taken major responsibility for the checkout and training in the use of permanent orthoses for the upper extremities, as well as design and fabrication of thermoplastic splints. The physical therapist is an expert in movement and mobility, especially locomotion and gait, and is responsible for the checkout and training in the use of trunk and lower-extremity orthoses. The rehabilitation engineer is an expert in technical problem solving involving mechanical and/or electrical solutions to unique problems of particular patients. Occupational therapists and rehabilitation engineers often collaborate to solve problems encountered by patients in performing their tasks of daily life. The therapist presents the parameters of the problem to the engineer in terms of patient abilities and disabilities and the functional and psychological goals that the device needs to meet or allow. The engineer then proposes technical solutions, and together they apply them to the patient and evaluate the outcome.

An orthosis is a device added to a person's body to support, position, or immobilize a part; to correct deformities; to assist weak muscles and restore function; or to modify tone. Orthoses are classified descriptively according to the part they include. For example, a wrist cock-up splint is a wrist-hand orthosis (WHO)[1] and a long leg brace is a knee-ankle-foot orthosis (KAFO).

Within that classification, there may be several types. For example, a wrist cock-up splint and a flexor hinge hand splint are both WHOs. In this chapter, traditional names, which communicate exactly which splint is meant, will be used. Orthoses for the hands are often called splints.

There are two basic classifications of splints: static and dynamic (also known as lively.)[1] Static splints, which have no moving parts, prevent motion and are used to rest[2] or rigidly support[1] the splinted part. Because immobilization causes such unwanted effects as atrophy and stiffness, a static splint should never be used longer than physiologically required and should never include joints other than those being treated.[2] A dynamic splint is preferable if it is equally effective. Dynamic splints have moving parts to permit, control, or restore movement.[2,3] The movement in dynamic splints may be intrinsically powered by another body part[1] or electrical stimulation of the patient's muscles. Extrinsic power can be provided by elastics, springs, gas-operated devices, or motors.[1]

Orthoses are categorized here by the most common goal for which they are used; however, it is not meant that that goal is their only goal. The same orthosis may fulfill several functions. For example, a dynamic splint that provides prehension function also provides static positioning of the thumb in a functional position. The therapist should clearly have the goal(s) and precautions in mind when selecting a splint for a particular patient. The representative sampling of orthoses in this chapter is not meant to be exhaustive. The reader is referred to the references for additional information.

To Support or Immobilize a Painful Joint; To Position To Prevent Deformities or Enhance Function

When a patient lacks the ability to keep the joint aligned or to hold a part in a functional position, such as in the case of weakness of the extensor pollicis brevis, or has suffered soft tissue injury that may result in deformities as healing progresses, such as in the case of burns, orthoses to maintain a functional position are needed. During acute episodes of rheumatoid arthritis or other instances when rest of a joint is required to relieve pain or to protect joint integrity, supportive types of splints are used.

These types of splints are often worn all day, all night, or both, to provide the best benefit. *However,* in every case, the splint is removed several times a day for gentle passive range of motion exercises to maintain the patient's mobility.

Some common examples of these kinds of orthoses are as follows.

PROXIMAL SUPPORTS

The *suspension sling* is a device that supports the upper extremity with cuffs that fit under the elbow and wrist. These cuffs are suspended from a spring attached overhead. Suspension slings can be used unilaterally or bilaterally. Some are designed for suspension from a rod that attaches to the wheelchair (Fig. 13.1), some are mounted on floor stands, and others are suspended directly from the ceiling. Regardless of how the sling is suspended, the distance between the point of suspension and the cuffs should be as far as is practical, because the longer the pendulum, the wider the arc of motion and, consequently, the longer the relatively flat section of the arc.[1] Movement is easier for the patient in the flatter area of the arc because the resistance offered by the inclined ends of the arc is eliminated or minimized.[1]

Arm slings have been developed to prevent shoulder subluxation in patients with brachial plexus injuries,[4] polymyositis,[5] and hemiplegia.[6] Some slings support and immobilize the whole arm[4] (Fig. 13.2), whereas

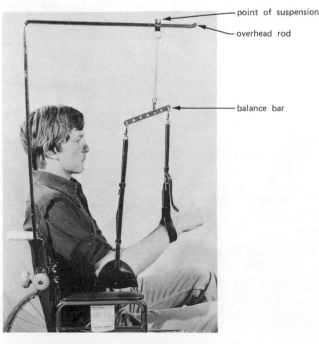

point of suspension
overhead rod
balance bar

Figure 13.1 Suspension sling.

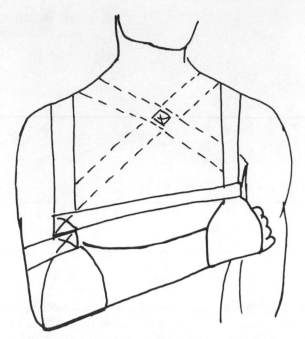

Figure 13.2 Double trough arm sling to support a flaccid shoulder. Dotted lines indicate placement of the straps on the back.

others support only the shoulder and leave the rest of the arm free for function[5,6] (Fig. 13.3). There are at least 25 styles and no consensus as to which type is best for a particular goal, nor as to whether a sling should be used at all for hemiplegic shoulders. A survey of Canadian physical and occupational therapists determined that the most frequently used slings for the hemiplegic shoulder were the Cuff Type Arm Sling (76%) and the Bobath Axilla Roll (62%).[7] The Cuff Type Arm Sling has an elbow cuff attached to the strap that goes across the patient's back, over the unaffected shoulder, and ends in a wrist cuff so that the patient's hand is positioned about waist high.[7] The Bobath Axilla Roll is described below. One study has documented by x-ray that a sling designed to support both the shoulder and forearm during ambulation, but only the shoulder when the patient is seated and using a lapboard, does in fact reduce subluxation; patients also reported reduced pain.[8] The sling is complicated and difficult to don, however.[8]

Some slings are commercially available. In using these, or any sling, the therapist must not only check them for size and comfort, but must also be sure the sling does not prevent function the patient has and should be using, nor create new problems for the patient such as edema in the dependent hand, nor increase disability by positioning in patterns of spasticity or pulling the head of the humerus out of the glenoid fossa. A checklist of 19 desirable and 4 undesirable characteristics of slings has been published to aid in selection of a sling for a particular patient.[9]

Occupational therapists make some slings. Instructions for the sling pictured in Fig. 13.2, called the Double Trough Arm Sling by Boyd and Gaylard,[7] are as

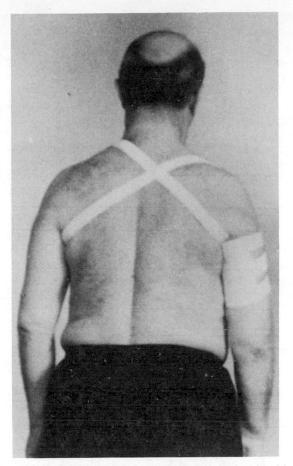

Figure 13.3 Arm sling to support hemiplegic shoulder. (Reproduced with permission from Bobath, B, *Adult Hemiplegia: Evaluation and Treatment,* 2nd edition. London: Heinemann Medical Books, 1978.)

follows. Elbow and wrist cuffs are connected by 2-inch webbing that extends from the elbow cuff, up the front of the chest, over the affected shoulder, across the back, around the unaffected side to the wrist cuff, around the wrist cuff, up the front of the chest, and over the unaffected shoulder, across the back to the elbow cuff under the affected arm. The webbing makes a figure-of-eight on the patient's back. The crossed areas are permanently sewn, as is the webbing to the cuffs. Stabilizing pieces are added behind the elbow and between the elbow and wrist straps in front. Needless to say, the nursing staff and the patient need careful instruction in applying this sling correctly. The Bobath Axilla Roll holds the humerus slightly abducted, which orients the humeral head more directly into the glenoid fossa while supporting the joint.[6] The patient wears the sling when he is ambulating or in his wheelchair. It is constructed by rolling up an 8- to 10-inch-wide piece of soft foam rubber jelly roll fashion to fit under the axilla. The roll is secured in place with a figure-of-eight harness, similar to that used for upper-extremity prostheses, made from an ace bandage or webbing. An alternative strapping procedure uses a chest strap that passes through the roll; the chest strap

is suspended by two straps over the affected shoulder, one directly attached and the other diagonally attached.[10] When using this axilla roll sling care must be taken that the humerus is not displaced laterally[6] and the radial nerve is not compressed. The addition of a distal support component could help prevent these risks while still encouraging arm swinging during ambulation.[11]

The use of a humeral cuff (Fig. 13.3) suspended by a figure-of-eight harness to support the humerus while allowing use of the extremity is also suggested by the Bobaths[6] and is now commercially available.[12]

Wheelchair arm boards are often preferred to the use of slings for a wheelchair-bound patient because they allow the humeral head to approximate the glenoid fossa at an angle, its more natural position, and they support the hand so that edema is less likely to occur (Fig. 13.4). Ideally the board supports the wrist and fingers in a functional position. Sixty-four percent of therapists in one study[7] chose arm boards to protect the hemiplegic shoulder. The sling would be preferred while patients were ambulating, of course.

Arm boards are now commercially available although the occupational therapist may need to custom-make one to suit a particular patient's problem. Various designs have been published.[6,13-16] The arm board is approximately 10 to 12 cm wide, padded, and may have straps to hold the arm in place. It attaches over the regular wheelchair armrest.

An alternative to an arm board is the use of a *wheelchair lapboard.* It was used by 81% of the therapists responding to a survey about support devices for the hemiplegic shoulder.[7] The lapboard provides all the advantages of the arm board plus allowing the arm to be positioned forward to pull the scapula forward, a position of choice for hemiplegic patients.[6] In the opinion of some, the lapboard seems "more natural and less a badge of disability" than a sling or arm board.[17] Clear plexiglass lapboards allow the patient to see his whole body. Lapboards do make independent wheelchair propulsion difficult, however.

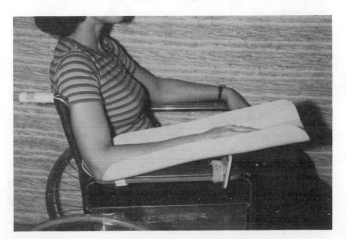

Figure 13.4 One type of wheelchair arm board.

DISTAL SUPPORTS: HAND SPLINTS

Volar wrist cock-up splints (Fig. 13.5 and 13.6) support the wrist in a position of 20–30° of dorsiflexion. The person for whom a wrist cock-up splint would be appropriate would have use of the fingers. This splint can be made of plaster of Paris bandage, thermoplastics, or metal. It is a simple splint that extends from the distal palmar crease, over the wrist, to approximately two-thirds the length of the forearm. Small hands do not require such a long splint because that amount of leverage offered by the forearm piece is not needed for the light weight of the small hand. The palmar piece is trimmed to avoid interfering with the thenar eminence and is molded to the palm to support the arches of the hand.

Other wrist support splints, available commercially, are elasticized cuffs with metal stays to support the wrist. Such a splint may be worn while working or engaging in sports. One study[18] found that although immobilization is not complete with this style of splint, working speed on hand tasks is subtly slower, a factor to be weighed for the working patient.

A *resting pan splint* (Fig. 13.7 and 13.8) is chosen for patients who need to have the wrist, fingers, and thumb supported in functional position. A resting splint may be of volar or dorsal design, depending on patient needs and preferences. The commercially available splints may be adjusted somewhat, but some changes cannot be made, e.g., the pictured splints are too short for these persons. However, it saves time to have a stock of these splints already made for use with average-sized persons, especially in the case of burn patients where time is of the essence and a splint cannot be formed directly on the newly burned skin anyway.

A variation of the resting pan has been devised to splint the burned hand after primary excision and early skin grafting.[19,20] The splint is made prior to surgery. A large circular piece of splint material is added to the finger part of the splint to act as an outrigger. Dress hooks are cemented to the fingernails of the patient and rubber bands attached to them and stretched to the perimeter of the circular piece to hold the fingers abducted and partially flexed at the metacarpophalangeal (MP) joints, and extended at the proximal

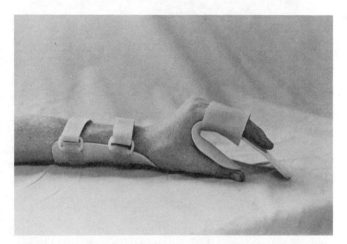

Figure 13.7 One type of commercially available volar resting pan splint. The fit is not ideal for this person: the arches of the hand are not maintained and the forearm piece is too short.

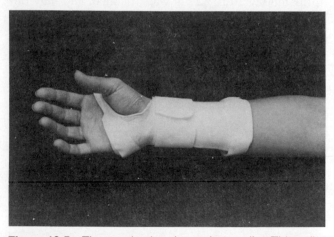

Figure 13.5 Thermoplastic volar cock-up splint. This splint would be improved if the palmar edge were rolled along the distal crease to prevent pressure on the skin during hand use.

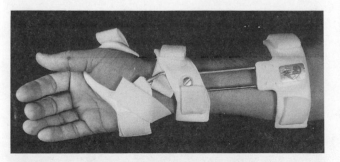

Figure 13.6 Wire-Foam™ wrist-hand orthosis: volar wrist splint. (Courtesy of LMB Hand Rehab Products, Inc., San Luis Obispo, CA 93406.)

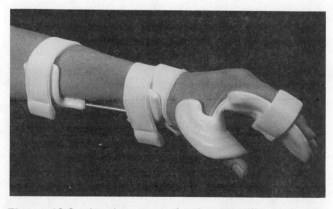

Figure 13.8 Another type of volar wrist-finger-thumb-orthosis: resting splint. (Courtesy of LMB Hand Rehab Products, Inc., San Luis Obispo, CA 93406.)

interphalangeal (PIP) and distal interphalangeal (DIP) joints.

Long and short opponens splints (Fig. 13.9–13.13) are designed to support the thumb in an abducted and opposed position. The long opponens hand splint also supports the wrist and has been used effectively for positioning the quadriplegic hand and/or resting the hand following trauma, deQuervain's syndrome, or thumb tendon repair.[22] These splints would be used for patients with finger function; however, either splint can be modified by adding a platform to support nonfunctioning fingers.

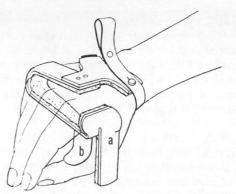

Figure 13.11 Schematic of short opponens splint. **a,** opponens bar; **b,** C-bar. The modifications noted for Figure 13.9 would apply here also. (Reproduced with permission from Long, C., and Schutt, A. Upper limb orthotics. In *Orthotics Etcetera,* 3rd edition. Edited by J. B. Redford. Baltimore: Williams & Wilkins, 1986.)

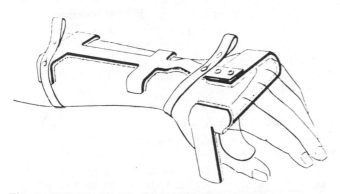

Figure 13.9 Schematic of long opponens splint; when fabricated, the palmar bar would be flared to conform to the distal transverse arch, and the ulnar edge of the hand piece would be lowered to follow the oblique line of the metacarpals during grasp. The forearm piece would extend two-thirds the length of the volar forearm. (Reproduced with permission from Long, C. Upper limb bracing. In *Orthotics Etcetera,* 1st edition. Edited by S. Licht and H. Kamenetz. Baltimore: Waverly Press, 1966.)

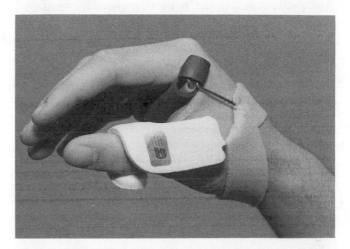

Figure 13.12 Wire-Foam™ thumb palmar abduction support. (With permission from LMB Hand Rehab Products, Inc., San Luis Obispo, CA 93406.)

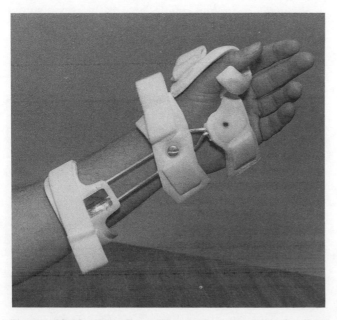

Figure 13.10 Wire-Foam™ wrist/thumb orthosis. With permission from LMB Hand Rehab Products, Inc., San Luis Obispo, CA 93406.)

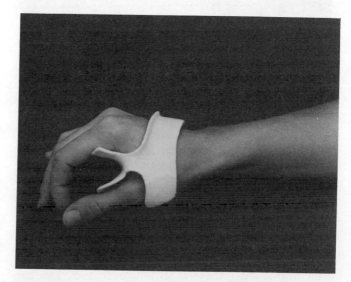

Figure 13.13 Short opponens splint made from Orthoplast.

CHAPTER 13 Orthoses: Purposes and Types **333**

Thumb carpometacarpal (CMC) stabilization splint[23,24] is a short, static splint that slips over the first metacarpal to relieve pain and increase hand function. The thumb CMC stabilization splint restricts motion of the thumb CMC and MP joints but allows motion of the IP joint and wrist. It is indicated for patients with degenerative joint disease who experience pain during activities.

Finger deviation support splint (Fig. 13.14), a static variation of the Rancho finger deviation dynamic splint (see reference 1), is used to support the MP joints of rheumatoid arthritic patients in semiextension and good alignment during hand use[22] to counteract the normal tendency for the MP joints to sublux and deviate ulnarly during grasp, which is believed to stress the already disease-weakened ligaments.

Finger stabilizer splint (Fig. 13.15) is the name given to a variety of splints designed to stabilize one or more joints of a finger in flexion or extension. These splints are easily constructed from thermoplastic materials and are also commercially available.

To Correct Deformities

Static and dynamic orthoses are used to provide prolonged stretch to correct contractures or to provide prolonged pressure to reduce scarring. Orthoses to stretch out contractures are adjusted to provide stretch of the tissue to the point at which the patient indicates discomfort rather than at the point of maximal stretch, which would result in intolerable pain if prolonged. As in manual stretching, gentle pressure over a long time is preferred to rapid, forceful stretching. Adjustments to static splints are required as the tissue adjusts to each new position. It is advantageous

if the orthosis is adjustable, rather than requiring refabrication to the new position.

Wearing time of the orthosis is gradually increased as the patient is able to tolerate the device. The importance of wearing the splint for the designated time must be emphasized to the patient. After wearing tolerance has increased to several hours it might be preferable for the patient to wear the device at night when he is asleep, freeing the part for active use during the day. If sleep is interrupted due to discomfort from the splint, the force is too great.[1]

Splints designed to correct or prevent scarring secondary to burns must provide firm, even pressure over the entire surface. These splints are worn constantly except for the brief period needed for hygiene.

The following orthoses were selected to illustrate the principles involved in increasing range of motion or preventing scarring. Others are available, or the therapist may need to design one to suit a particular patient's unique problem.

PROXIMAL CORRECTION

Neck extension splint (Fig. 29.1), also called the conformer neck splint, is used for patients whose neck has been burned to hold the neck extended and to prevent the fusion of the chin to the chest during the healing process.[25,26] It can also be used to reduce the thickness of scar tissue through the constant, uniform pressure offered against the developing scar tissue.

The transparent face mask has been used successfully to prevent hypertrophic scarring of facial tissue after deep, partial, or full thickness thermal injury.[27] The mask is made of cellulose acetate butyrate (Uvex), a high-temperature plastic. Directions for making the negative and positive molds and the mask are published.

Shoulder abduction splint, also called an airplane splint, (Fig. 13.16) is designed to maintain or increase range of motion in shoulder abduction and can be fabricated to place the shoulder in internal or external ro-

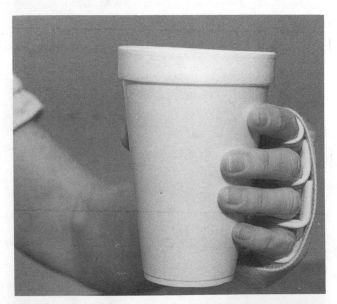

Figure 13.14 Wire-Foam™ proximal phalangeal splint (ulnar deviation splint) for the arthritic patient. (With permission from LMB Hand Rehab Products, Inc., San Luis Obispo, CA 93406.)

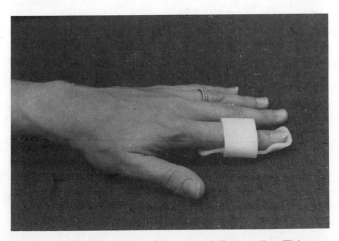

Figure 13.15 One type of finger stabilizer splint. This one immobilizes the proximal interphalangeal and distal interphalangeal joints.

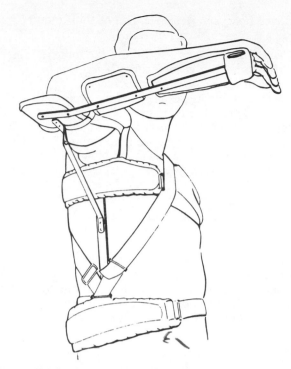

Figure 13.16 Shoulder abduction or airplane splint. (Reproduced with permission from Long, C., and Schutt, A. Upper limb orthotics. In *Orthotics Etcetera,* 3rd edition. Edited by J. B. Redford. Baltimore: Williams & Wilkins, 1986.)

tation, as well as any degree of abduction. The *Axillary spacer,*[28] used in the treatment of rotator cuff tears, places the shoulder in approximately 60° abduction, 30° horizontal abduction, and 15° external rotation.

Elbow flexion contractures can be corrected by use of a *turnbuckle splint* (Fig. 13.17), *Wire-Foam™ elbow extension spring* (Fig. 13.18),[22] or a *Dynasplint®*

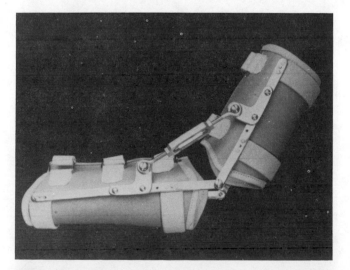

Figure 13.17 Turnbuckle splint for elbow flexion contractures. (Reproduced with permission from Green, D. P., and McCoy, H. Turnbuckle orthotic correction of elbow-flexion contractures after acute injuries. *J. Bone Joint Surg., 61A*(7): 1092–1095, 1979.)

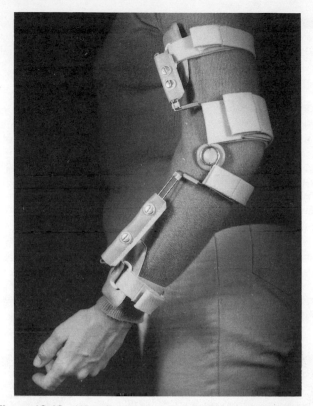

Figure 13.18 Wire-Foam™ extension spring splint. (Courtesy of LMB Hand Rehab Products, Inc., San Luis Obispo, CA, 93406.)

(Dynasplint Systems, Inc.). The turnbuckle splint utilizes a turnbuckle on the lateral aspect of a hinged elbow brace to exert force towards extension. It can be adjusted in fine gradations and has been used successfully to stretch contractures in 12 of 15 patients (80%) on whom it was researched.[29] The average increase in range of motion was 43°; the average reduction of deformity was 37°. The Wire-Foam™ elbow extension spring splint, designed by Charles Brown, O.T.R., exerts continual gentle force via two coiled springs located at the axis of elbow motion.[22] The Dynasplint® is a precisely adjustable splint composed of two stainless steel struts placed laterally and medially, upper arm and forearm cuffs, and compression-coil springs that can be adjusted with a screwdriver.[30]

Elbow extension contractures are rare. To increase range toward elbow flexion, a splint can be made that incorporates upper-arm and forearm cuffs with springs or elastic traction for continual stretch. Alternatively, turnbuckles or Klenzak or Lehrman fracture brace joints[31] can be used to provide the adjustable traction. The splint would be similar to that shown in Fig. 13.17 but the direction of force would be reversed.

DISTAL CORRECTION

Volar cock-up splints (Fig. 13.5 and 13.6) can be used to provide a gentle force toward wrist hyperextension to stretch the wrist flexors while permitting active finger flexion. If the wrist contracture is secondary to spasticity, the resting pan type splints (Fig. 13.7 and 13.8), or similarly styled splints, must be used to exert traction not only on the wrist flexors but also the extrinsic finger flexors.

Metacarpophalangeal flexion splint with outrigger (Fig. 13.19) can be easily constructed using thermoplastics.[20] Finger loops are placed over the proximal phalanges and attach via rubber bands to a volar outrigger to force the MP joints into flexion. For the angle of pull of the rubber bands to be perpendicular, the outrigger must extend the correct distance from the surface of the splint and be changed as the patient improves. If the patient can actively maintain wrist extension; a "knuckle bender" type splint (Fig. 13.20) can be used to provide the force toward MP flexion. This splint is commercially available from several manufacturers. All fingers are forced into the same degree of flexion, whereas the MP flexion splint with outrigger can be used when some of the fingers need a force different from what others need. The reverse knuckle bender (Fig. 13.21) forces the MP joints into extension.

Glove flexion mitt is a splint used to force the fingers into flexion.[32] It has sometimes been used as exercise equipment to resist finger extension. The splint is made from a cotton gardener's glove. Rubber bands are attached from the fingertips to a button secured at the wrist. Directions for construction of an adaptation of the mitt for a patient whose impairment is limited to less than all fingers has been published.[33]

Interphalangeal extension splint with lumbrical bar[34] (Fig. 13.22) prohibits MP joint hyperextension while a dorsal outrigger provides attachment for finger loops and rubber bands set at an angle of 90°, which exert a rotary force to pull the interphalangeal joints into extension.

Finger knuckle bender[35] is a commercially available splint that works on the same principle as the knuckle bender for MP joints, except that this one forces flexion of one PIP joint only. Reverse finger knuckle benders (Fig. 13.23) are also available for extension of the PIP joints.

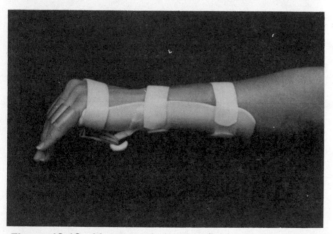

Figure 13.19 Metacarophalangeal flexion splint with outrigger.

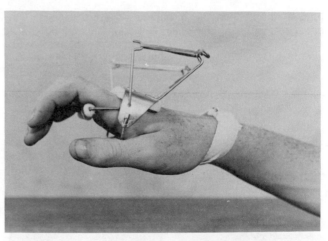

Figure 13.21 Bunnell reverse knuckle bender.

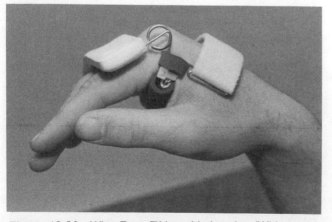

Figure 13.20 Wire-Foam™ knuckle bender. (With permission from LMB Hand Rehab Products, Inc., San Luis Obispo, CA 93406.)

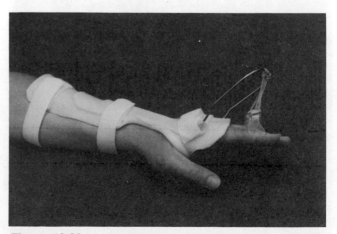

Figure 13.22 Interphalangeal extension splint with lumbrical bar.

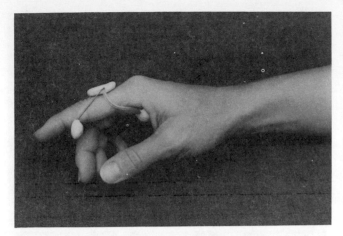

Figure 13.23 Reverse finger knuckle bender.

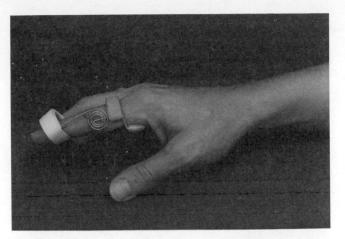

Figure 13.24 Spring safety pin splint, See text for other names for this splint.

Fingernail splint utilizes dress hooks that are cemented to the dorsal surfaces of the fingernails. Rubber bands extend from these hooks to an outrigger to pull all joints of the fingers into flexion or extension.[36] The length and location of the outrigger controls the direction and extent of pull. This type of splint may be used for burn patients and others for whom skin contact is contraindicated.

Spring safety pin splint[35] or **spring coil finger extension** assist ("Capener"; **spring coil finger extension** assist ("Capener"; "Wynn-Parry splint")[22] (Fig. 13.24 and 13.25) is commercially available and uses spring steel wires to stretch out a PIP joint contracture and/or to assist the joint into extension, while permitting active finger flexion. To correct a flexion contracture of both PIP and DIP joints, a spring coil long finger extension assist splint can be used. To stretch a PIP joint extension contracture or to assist flexion, a spring coil finger flexion assist can be used (Fig. 13.26).[22] For DIP or PIP joints, finger flexion spring splints (Fig. 13.27) and extension finger spring splints (Fig. 13.28) are available.

Static PIP extension block splints, designed by Hollis[37] (Fig. 13.29), are easily constructed from bits of thermoplastic splinting material to prevent or correct swan neck deformity since the splint will prevent PIP hyperextension.

Foot-drop splint (Fig. 13.30) is used when a person is confined to bed and lacks the ability to keep his feet dorsiflexed; plantar flexion contractures often develop. Foot-drop splints are made to hold the foot perpendicular to the leg, as if the patient were standing up straight. The newer thermoplastic materials lend themselves nicely to this application.

Orthoses To Restore Function

Orthoses that assist weak muscles or substitute for absent motor power may enable functional activities to be performed more easily by the patient.

DISTAL FUNCTION: HAND SPLINTS

The following dynamic splints were selected to illustrate orthoses used to assist weakness and to increase

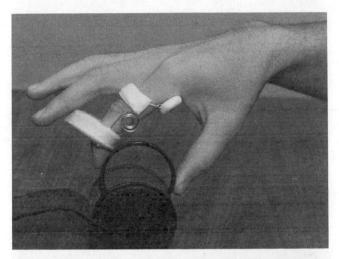

Figure 13.25 Pinching with Wire-Foam™ spring coil finger extension assist in place. The distal strap appears large here, but simply was not trimmed prior to the photo.

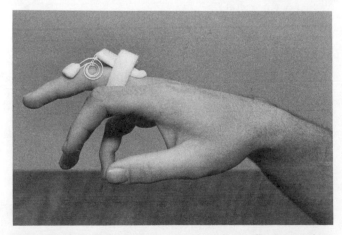

Figure 13.26 Wire-Foam™ spring coil finger flexion assist. (With permission from LMB Hand Rehab Products, Inc., San Luis Obispo, CA 93406.)

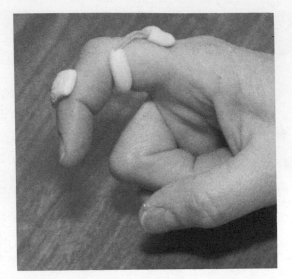

Figure 13.27 Finger flexion spring splint. (With permission from LMB Hand Rehab Products, Inc., San Luis Obispo, CA 93406.)

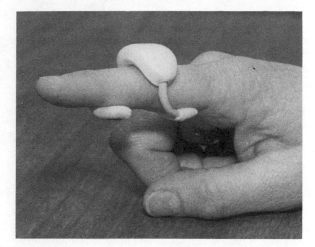

Figure 13.28 Finger extension spring splint. (With permission from LMB Hand Rehab Products, Inc., San Luis Obispo, CA 93406.)

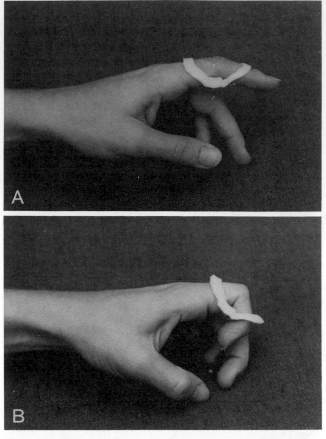

Figure 13.29 Finger splint for swan neck deformity. **A.** Prevents hyperextension of proximal interphalangeal joint. **B.** Allows flexion.

strength. Assistance may be given to a motion by use of rubber bands that are adjusted so that after the patient has moved as far as he can, the rubber band completes the motion. Assistance can also be provided by use of springs or coiled wire. The weak muscle is strengthened by actively moving the part as far as it can before the assisting mechanism completes the motion. The opposing muscles may also be strengthened if they are required to work against the elastic, wires, or springs. Corrective splints may be used alternatively to assist weak muscles. For example, a spring safety pin splint, described above to correct a PIP flexion contracture, can also assist weak extensor movement.

Long Opponens Hand Splint with Action Wrist and Dorsiflexion Assist (Fig. 13.31)

This is a dorsal splint that supports the thumb and assists the weak wrist extensors by way of the rubber

band that extends from the proximal band of the splint to the hand piece.

Wrist-Hand Orthosis With Metacarpophalangeal Extension Assist (Fig. 13.32)

This splint is used for radial nerve injuries; it supports the wrist in extension and the thumb in abduction and extension, and assists MP extension while allowing finger flexion. The MP extension assist is a dorsal outrigger from which cuffs are suspended by way of rubber bands that support the fingers individually to assist weak MP extension. The pull of the rubber bands must be perpendicular to the proximal phalanx for the full benefit of the pull to be applied in moving the finger around the axis of the joint, rather than applying traction or compression forces on the joint. The tension of the rubber bands is adjusted to complete the extension motion while allowing the patient to actively extend and flex to his limits. This orthotic design may also be used to increase range of motion of the fingers when there is a flexor contracture by increasing the tension of the rubber bands to stretch the fingers into extension.

Low-Profile Dorsal Dynamic Splint

This splint is designed to support the wrist and assist the weak finger extensors of patients with radial nerve

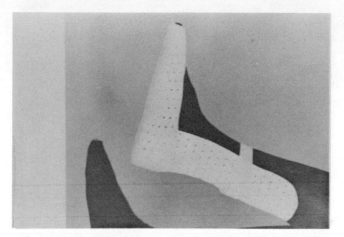

Figure 13.30 Orthoplast splint to prevent foot-drop. (Reproduced with permission from Johnson & Johnson, New Brunswick, NJ 08903.)

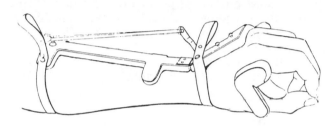

Figure 13.31 Long opponens hand splint with action wrist and dorsiflexion assist. (Reproduced with permission from Long, C., and Schutt, A. Upper limb orthotics. In *Orthotics Etcetera,* 3rd edition. Edited by J. B. Redford. Baltimore: Williams & Wilkins, 1986.

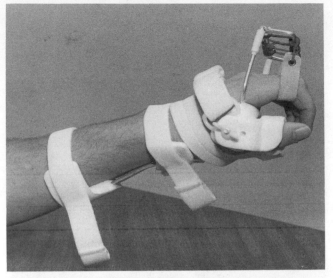

Figure 13.32 Wire-Foam™ wrist orthosis with metacarpophalangeal extension assist. (With permission from LMB Hand Rehab Products, Inc., San Luis Obispo, CA 93406.)

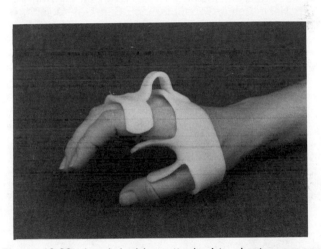

Figure 13.33 Lumbrical bar attached to short opponens splint.

injuries. The fingers are supported by elastic slings attached to wire prongs that lie close to the extended fingers. The splint allows active finger flexion. This splint has the advantage of being less cumbersome than splints with outriggers. Directions for construction are published by Sellers[38] and Colditz.[39]

Thumb Abduction Assist (Fig. 13.12)

This splint dynamically extends and abducts the thumb.[22]

Metacarpophalangeal Stop or Lumbrical Bar (Fig. 13.33)

The bar is attached to a hand splint dorsally and exerts a force over the proximal phalanges to hold the MP joints into slight flexion. The force of the extensor digitorum is thereby transferred to the interphalangeal joints. For these reasons this bar prevents the development of claw hand deformity ("intrinsic-minus hand") that results due to absent interossei and lumbricales. The bar can be constructed to exert the force against all or selected fingers. It may be used in conjunction with DIP extension outriggers (Fig. 13.34) and/or thumb abduction-extension assist (Fig. 13.35).

MP extension assist with thumb abduction and extension assist (Fig. 13.36) is used for a low radial nerve in-

jury, one in which the patient still has control of wrist extension. It allows active grasp of objects and assists release.

PERMANENT FUNCTIONAL ORTHOSES

Residual weakness of the upper extremity that results in an inability to move the limb effectively to orient the hand to objects or an inability to pinch or grasp an object can be partially compensated for by the use of permanent orthoses. For a permanent orthosis to be useful to the patient, he must accept it, value it, and incorporate it into his body image. A prime prerequisite to acceptance is that the device allow the patient to do something *he wants to do* that he cannot do without the orthosis.[1,40,41] Other factors that influence the acceptance are mechanical reliability, cosmesis, ease of application and control, and thorough training to the point of automaticity of control.

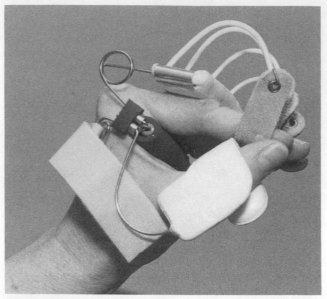

Figure 13.34 Wire-Foam™ metacarpophalangeal flexion spring with thumb palmar abduction support and finger interphalangeal extension assists. (With permission from LMB Hand Rehab Products, Inc., San Luis Obispo, CA 93406.)

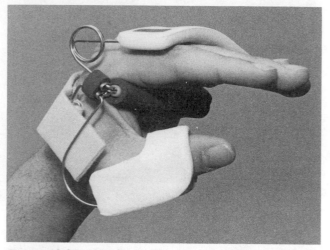

Figure 13.35 Wire-Foam™ metacarpophalangeal flexion spring with thumb palmar abduction support. (With permission from LMB Hand Rehab Products, Inc., San Luis Obispo, CA 93406.)

The principles of orthotic training are borrowed from the field of prosthetics and include checkout of the fit and mechanical aspects of the orthosis; instruction in the names of the parts, the care of the orthosis, and how to put it on and remove it; controls training; and use training. Intensive practice under various conditions is an essential aspect of the training.

Flexor Hinge Hand Splints

Palmar prehension, or three-jaw chuck prehension, is provided by flexor hinge hand splints by these three factors: (a) the thumb is posted into a position of ab-

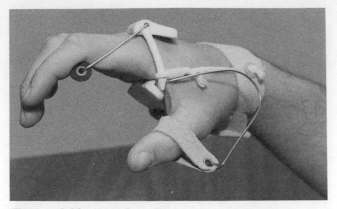

Figure 13.36 Wire-Foam™ metacarpophalangeal extension spring with thumb abduction extension assist. (With permission from MB Hand Rehab Products, Inc., San Luis Obispo, CA 93406.)

duction and partial opposition; (b) the MP and interphalangeal joints of the thumb are posted into extension; and (c) the index and middle fingers are splinted into a semiflexed position so that when the mechanical joint at the MP joint flexes, the pads of the fingers meet the pad of the thumb (Fig. 13.37). If the wrist is included in the splint, it is usually held in about 15° of dorsiflexion.

The power for the pinching motion of the fingers is supplied by power from the person's remaining musculature that is mechanically harnessed or, if that is not possible, by an external power source, such as a motor, carbon dioxide, or electric stimulation.

Finger-Driven Flexor Hinge Hand Splint. For the patient who has active flexion of the ring and/or little fingers, prehension is powered by these fingers. Prehension is accomplished by the force obtained when the patient presses down on a rod that extends from the middle and index fingers to under the ring and little fingers. When the patient wants to pinch, he flexes the ulnar fingers, and the bar transfers this power to the radial fingers. If the patient lacks active extension, a spring can be added to pull the fingers away from the thumb. This splint may be a hand splint only or may also incorporate the wrist to which it would give static support.

Checkout involves inspection of the splint both on and off the patient for proper construction and fit. The criteria of fit outlined in chapter 14 apply to these hand splints. In addition, the mechanism must operate smoothly and allow pinch of thin flat objects as well as large objects. The joint of the splint must *exactly* coincide with the axis of the patient's second MP joint. Straps and fastenings must facilitate independent application and removal.

The patient will probably be able to apply and remove his own hand splint and should practice this until he is able to do so in less than 1 min. Speed is important because the splint impedes some tasks, such as propelling a wheelchair, and unless it can be quickly put on and off as needed, it will be discarded as just one more hindrance.[41]

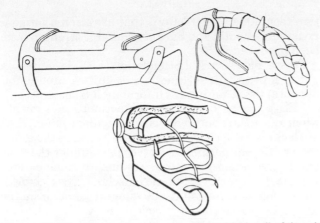

Figure 13.37 Flexor hinge hand splint with detail of thumb post and finger piece. (Reproduced with permission from Long, C. Upper limb bracing. In *Orthotics Etcetera*, 1st edition. Edited by S. Licht and H. Kamenetz. Baltimore: Waverly Press, 1966.)

Controls training teaches the patient to pick up, move, and release objects of different sizes, textures, weights, and crushability. Firm objects of about 1 inch (2.5 cm) in circumference and with semirough texture are easiest to handle. As the patient's skill increases, objects are graded in size, smoothness, flatness, and fragility. Marshmallows, paper cups, fresh jelly donuts, playing cards, coins, pencils, and metal or glass objects are all challenges. In order for a person with a posted thumb to pick up flat objects, the objects must be pushed so that they partially overhang the table or must be placed on a soft surface, such as a sheet of foam rubber, to allow the thumb to get under the object. Tip prehension, which the splint does not provide, is normally used to pick up these types of things. The absence of active wrist motion in a splint requires that the patient compensatorily abduct and internally rotate at the shoulder in order to pick something up. If the patient has proprioceptive feedback along with the fine control of the extrinsic hand muscles, controls training will be rapidly accomplished.

Use training involves a systematic trial of occupational performance tasks to discover which require the splint, how these tasks may best be accomplished, and if metal or glass objects need to be coated or covered to provide friction. If slipping of objects is a frequent problem it is preferable to have the patient wear a large-size secretary's rubber finger cover over the thumb post to provide friction. The maximal weight of any object that can be lifted will depend both on the strength of pinch and the strength of the proximal extremity. A pinch meter that records in ounces (grams) is used to measure amount of pinch possible when using a prehension splint.

Wrist-Driven Flexor Hinge Hand Splint (Tenodesis). The thumb is posted and the radial fingers are splinted as described above. In addition to the joint located at the patient's second MP joint to allow finger flexion, there is also a joint located at the exact axis of the wrist on the radial side to allow wrist movement.

The C_6 quadriplegic patient who has active wrist extension can pinch using this splint because the power of wrist extension is transferred to prehension through a power transfer bar (Fig. 13.38). This splint augments the natural tenodesis grasp the patient has and enlarges his scope of abilities. In a properly adjusted splint, the wrist to pinch strength ratio is 2:1.

Using the tenodesis splint the patient must abduct and internally rotate his shoulder to approach an object on a table properly. Ratchet-type mechanisms[42] are available that lock the splint into position to relieve the patient of the necessity of maintaining active wrist extension during holding. The ratchet mechanism is released by pressure. Some C_4, C_5 quadriplegic patients, who cannot actively use a wrist driven flexor hinge hand splint because they lack active wrist extension, use a ratchet splint in preference to an externally powered splint.[42] They passively engage the mechanism by pushing their wrist into extension against their body, wheelchair, or a table. The mechanism remains locked in that position until the release pushbutton is depressed.

The *checkout* procedure for a wrist-driven flexor hinge hand splint is the same as described above for the finger-driven flexor hinge hand splint, with the addition of checking the exactness of the location of the wrist joint axis. The strength of pinch is also measured because the length of the transfer bar can be changed by the orthotist if this is necessary to increase the strength of pinch.[43]

The patient must learn to put on and remove this hand splint rapidly for the same reasons as stated for the finger-driven flexor hinge hand splint.

Controls and use training are also the same as described above, although patients using this type of splint will require more practice because usually the patient who uses this splint lacks sensory feedback from the fingers. Also, the patient must learn how to orient the splint to approach objects of different shapes and must practice until this becomes automatic.

Externally Powered Flexor Hinge Hand Splint. The basic splint is the same as that used for the wrist-driven flexor hinge hand splint with these exceptions: The wrist joint is fixed at about 15° to 20° of dorsiflexion; there is no transfer bar; a short bar extends from the finger piece to allow distal attachment of the external power mechanism; and a spring provides mo-

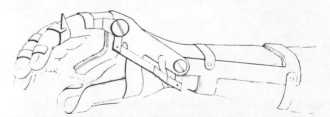

Figure 13.38 Wrist-driven flexor hinge hand splint. (Reproduced with permission from Long, C., and Schutt, A. Upper limb orthotics. In *Orthotics Etcetera*, 3rd edition. Edited by J. B. Redford. Baltimore: Williams & Wilkins, 1986.)

tion of the radial fingers in one direction, usually extension. The name implies that the power source is located outside the patient's body. This complicates the learning process for the patient because he must learn to control switches, valves, or other transducers to operate the power source.

Power to drive hand splints can be obtained from any of the following:

1. A small rotary motor that runs forward, backward, and holds when stopped. One end of a cable is attached to the motor and the other end of the cable is attached to the bar that extends from the finger piece of the splint (Fig. 13.39). As the cable is pulled in by the motor, the fingers are flexed and pinch against the thumb. As the cable is reeled out, the spring pulls the fingers into extension. The patient can control the extent of the opening by turning the motor on and off more or less quickly. Some motors are proportional and operate fast or slow, depending upon the force the patient exerts on the control switch.

2. Electrical stimulation of one of a patient's muscles over which he has no control.[44] When the electrical stimulation is on, the muscle contracts, and when the stimulation ceases the muscle relaxes. The opposite motion, usually flexion, is accomplished by a spring. Originally, this type of splint seemed to have limited value for quadriplegics because the stimulated muscle rapidly fatigued. This fatigue phenomenon occurred when the finger extensor muscles were repetitively stimulated with enough voltage to overcome the strong pull of the spring that is needed for the pinch used in daily tasks (3 to 4 pounds) and these muscles lost their ability to continue to contract. Stimulating the flexor muscles instead of the extensor was not a satisfactory solution; fatigue developed due to the prolonged tetany needed for maintained holding. This problem seems to have been overcome by using a program of electrically induced exercise and by utilizing a sequential stimula-

tion technique. Contractions that are strong, fatigue-resistant, smooth, and have controllable strength have been produced.[45]

Functional Electrical Stimulation (FES) is defined as a neural prosthetic technique that utilizes stimulation of neural tissue for inward information transfer.[46]

FES provides or improves functional movements when, due to an abnormal neuromuscular system, they are lacking.[47] Electrical pulses are applied to the efferent or afferent peripheral nerve fibers under the control of the patient, who thus regains, to some extent, voluntary control over paretic muscles.[47] The electrical pulses can be delivered to the efferent nerve or motor end plate to activate the muscle directly. They also can be applied afferently via stimulation of cutaneous nerves and low-threshold afferent nerve fibers to produce complex reflex patterns of movement by activating central efferent pathways.[47] No exoskeletal support, i.e., flexor hinge hand splint or brace, is used with FES. Afferent FES has been used successfully to enable paraplegics to walk[47-49] and to provide correct walking patterns in children with cerebral palsy and in adult hemiparetics. After many repetitions, the walking pattern seems to be relearned. FES is also used to attempt to restore finger extension in hemiparetic patients; however, carryover of function after a period of FES training has not been as successful to date.[50,51] This is probably because for learning to occur, the afferent-central-efferent loop must be completed, which it is for stepping motions since they are probably organized subcortically. However, finger extension is cortically directed, and the afferent input stops at the level of the lesion, never to reach the central-efferent part of the loop.[51]

Seeking other upper-extremity movement via FES is not seen as a viable research direction since the movement of the upper extremity is too complex, involving a variety of possible responses to a given goal situation requiring complex control of each joint simultaneously. Conscious control of such a system is beyond human capability and no automatic control systems exist that enable anything except robot-like preprogrammed compound movements.[47]

3. An "artificial muscle" (Fig. 13.40) is made of a tubular, helically woven nylon sleeve covering a leakproof rubber bladder. When gas (carbon dioxide) is allowed to flow into the bladder it enlarges as a balloon would; however, the constraint of the helical weave of the sleeve causes the ends of the "muscle" to move closer together as the circumference increases. When the gas is released, the "muscle" gets thin and long again. A Chinese finger trap operates on the same principle. The end of the "muscle" is attached to the finger piece and causes the fingers to flex when it is distended, while a spring causes extension when the tension in the "muscle" is reduced.

The *control transducer* of the externally powered splint is operated by a part of the patient's body over which he has voluntary control, where he has normal sensation, and which does not activate the transducer

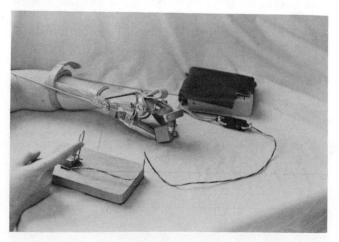

Figure 13.39 Demonstration of microswitch control of externally powered (motor) flexor hinge hand splint. A fingertip's pressure is sufficient to activate the switch, which would be mounted where the patient could voluntarily control it.

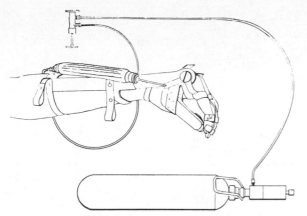

Figure 13.40 "Artificial muscle" driven flexor hinge hand splint. (Reproduced with permission from Long, C., and Schutt, A. Upper limb orthotics. In *Orthotics Etcetera*, 3rd edition. Edited by J. B. Redford. Baltimore: Williams & Wilkins, 1986.)

accidentally during habitual motions. For a C_4, C_5 quadriplegic this means upper trapezius-, tongue-, or chin-operated controls. If shoulder elevation is to be used, the opposite shoulder is usually chosen to reduce the likelihood of associated unintentional activation. Spotty muscle weakness such as occurs in polio may preserve control sites in the lower extremities if none exist in the upper body.

The motor can be controlled by microswitches that require about 1 ounce of pressure to activate (Fig. 13.39). These microswitches may be mounted over the patient's shoulder so he can elevate or retract the shoulder to touch and activate them (Fig. 13.41), or near his face so his tongue can press them, or in a joystick arrangement that can be controlled by the chin pushing on the stick, or in a figure-of-eight harness configuration so that scapular protraction activates it,[1] or in any other position where the patient can exert voluntary pressure. The microswitches must be mounted so that the patient can activate two switches —forward and reverse—for each motor.

The motor also can be controlled by myoelectric signals that when amplified can electronically switch the motor.[52,53] The electrical activity of the voluntarily contracting control muscle is picked up using surface electrodes. Forward and reverse directions of the motor are achieved by using a low-amplitude signal to switch forward and a high-amplitude signal to switch backward or vice versa instead of using two muscles as with the two switches mentioned above. A protocol for determination of suitable controller muscles has been published.[54]

Voice activation of the motor is a possible, but as yet unreliable, method of control because extraneous noise also activates the motor.

In electrical stimulation splints, the flow of electrical stimulation can be controlled by myoelectric signals or by a potentiometer, which is an electrical component that increases or decreases the resistance to the flow of electricity as the armature is moved, or by a switch. The switch or potentiometer can be arranged so it can be controlled by shoulder elevation or any other movement the patient can control.

The "artificial muscle" (also known as the McKibben muscle after the physicist who invented it) is controlled by a three-position valve: when the stem of the valve is pushed all the way in, the gas flows to activate the "muscle"; when released, the valve holds the gas in place, and the fingers remain in whatever position they were (Fig. 13.42). When the stem of the valve is pushed halfway in, the gas is allowed to escape, which deflates the "muscle." The gas can be allowed to escape in short, quick spurts, thus opening the fingers a little at a time; this is called feathering the valve.

Checkout of Externally Powered Hand Splints. The checkout involves all that has been cited for the two other flexor hinge hand splints above. In addition, the reliability of the control mechanism must be carefully checked: the signal used to close the splint must always close the splint and always work with the same amount of pressure of the control site. If the cable is too short or the spring too forceful, pinching thin objects (paper) will be prevented and the cable or spring will need adjustment. Adjustments would need to be made also if large (2-inch) items could not be grasped. A stop can be

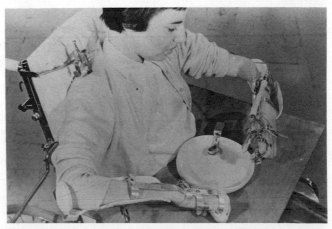

Figure 13.42 Patient using an artificial muscle-powered flexor hinge hand splint on the left hand with control valve mounted over right shoulder, activated by scapular elevation. (Photograph used with permission of Doris Brennan.)

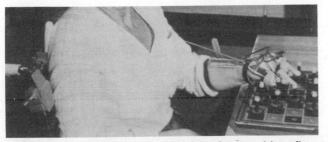

Figure 13.41 Microswitch activation of motor-driven flexor hinge hand splint via retraction of the opposite shoulder.

incorporated into this splint to prevent excessive pressure on the fingertips in the closed position; however, it should still allow holding paper or playing cards if the patient needs to do this.

Rarely will a patient who needs this type of splint be able to put it on and off by himself. However, he should be able to clearly instruct another and should receive supervised practice in giving this instruction. He must also instruct others in the care and recharging of the power unit. Battery-powered splints (motor, electrical stimulation) can be charged overnight using the charger that comes with the unit. The CO_2 gas bottle refill may need to be obtained from the orthotist; fire station supply houses or bottling plants have CO_2 and often are willing to fill the empty bottle, but the proper adapter must be obtained from an orthotist. A full 12-inch bottle of CO_2 lasts about 3 weeks if the splint is opened and closed once every 5 min, 8 hours per day. This amount of use is rare since the splint is opened and closed once to grasp something which is then usually held; no gas is used during the holding phase.

All hand splints should be treated like fine jewelry: washed, polished, and stored where they cannot be bent or misaligned. An out-of-kilter hand splint is dangerous; at the very least it exerts pressure that can cause decubiti and at worst can exert undesired forces on the joints.

Controls training must be thoroughly completed before use training is attempted to decrease the inevitable frustration. Controls training begins with observation of the effect of the control motion on the hand splint.[55,56] The hand splint may be on the patient's hand, but if it cannot be seen easily, the splint is best mounted some other place so the patient can watch it while simultaneously feeling his controlling movement. Electronic feedback devices are helpful adjuncts to training.[57] Once the effect of the control motion is learned, the patient begins the same practice of picking up, moving, and releasing various objects as described above for the other flexor hinge hand splints. A good test of the patient's automaticity of control of the splint is to have him pick up, on signal, a cube that has been placed on a premarked spot and to release it into a small box placed 6 to 8 inches away. The time in tenths of seconds is recorded. This is repeated 20 or so times during each training session. The mean and the standard deviation are computed (see Table 14.1). A low standard deviation indicates consistency of operation, a sign of skill. Tasks attempted during use training will be limited by the patient's disability. Adaptations beyond the orthosis will probably be necessary to accomplish these, and the reader is referred to the chapter on spinal cord injury for specifics.

PROXIMAL FUNCTION

The *suspension sling* (Fig. 13.1) can be adjusted to assist certain movements of the upper extremities. Remember that whenever a motion is assisted, its opposite is resisted. For example, the patient must have relatively strong shoulder horizontal abductor muscles if the suspension sling is adjusted to assist weak shoulder horizontal adductors. Motions that can be assisted using an overhead suspension sling are shoulder horizontal abduction and adduction, shoulder external and internal rotation, shoulder abduction, and elbow flexion and extension. Adjustments to assist weak muscles are made to parts of the suspension sling as follows:

Motion Assisted by Suspension Sling	Adjustment
Shoulder motions:	
Horizontal abduction	The overhead rod is rotated laterally; that is, the top part of the rod is turned out away from the patient, which carries the suspended arm out toward horizontal abduction.
Horizontal adduction	The overhead rod is rotated medially; that is, the top part of the rod is turned in toward the patient. The suspended arm is thereby carried in toward horizontal adduction.
Abduction	The distance between the spring and the overhead rod is shortened to pull the arm into abduction.

Some adjustments are made by moving the position of the cuffs on the balance bar.

External rotation	The cuffs are moved back on the bar to shift the weight toward the elbow.
Internal rotation	The cuffs are moved forward on the balance bar to shift the weight toward the hand.
Elbow motions:	
Flexion	The point of suspension is moved backward on the overhead rod, which puts the hand back toward the patient's face.
Extension	The point of suspension is moved forward on the overhead rod, which puts the hand out away from the patient's face.

Each adjustment is made in as small an increment as is just necessary to assist the patient's motion.

Mobile Arm Supports (MAS)

This term, once inclusive of suspension arm slings and feeders, now refers only to feeders. Their former name was ball-bearing forearm orthoses (BFO). MAS are frictionless arm supports that are usually mounted on a wheelchair but also may extend from a waist belt for ambulatory patients. They utilize the principle of the inclined plane in which gravity causes movement when something is inclined away from horizontal. They assist weak shoulder and elbow muscles to place the hand

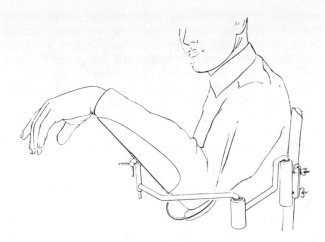

Figure 13.43 Georgia Warm Springs feeder (mobile arm support). (Reproduced with permission from Long, C., and Schutt, A. Upper limb orthotics. In *Orthotics Etcetera*, 3rd edition. Edited by J. B. Redford. Baltimore: Williams & Wilkins, 1986.)

in space as needed. Adjustments are made to individually tailor the assistance of the MAS for each person's disability.

The neutral set up and adjustments for a Rancho Los Amigos type mobile arm support are described here. The Georgia Warm Springs feeder (Fig. 13.43) is very similar to the Rancho one (Fig. 13.44) with two exceptions, the proximal ball-bearing wheelchair bracket assembly and the rocker arm assembly. The bracket of the Georgia Warm Springs feeder is adjustable and the rocker arm assembly is offset which allows unimpeded vertical motions. The Michigan feeder (see Fig. 13.45) allows more precise adjustment of the position of the proximal ball-bearing and the rocker assembly. The Michigan rocker assembly allows adjustment in the Z coordinate of movement (up and down), which allows the therapist to match the axis of the motion of the forearm trough to the exact axis of the bulk of the forearm, thereby enabling a weaker patient to use the feeder effectively.

Adjustment of Mobile Arm Supports. The principles of setup and balancing described below generally apply to all designs of mobile arm supports, although the exact methods of adjusting the pieces are slightly different.

Neutral setup of the MAS is sufficient for the patient who has generalized, balanced weakness throughout the upper extremity. Modifications of this neutral setup must be made for patients with other patterns of weakness. Many therapists prefer to adjust the MAS initially into neutral position before proceeding to make modifications in the balance as required by the patient's pattern of weakness.

A properly balanced MAS will hold, without any effort on the patient's part, the forearm in a position of 45° from the horizontal and the upper arm in approximately 45° of combined shoulder abduction and flexion.

In order for MAS to be fitted to the patient, he ought to be able to sit for 1 hour. The Rancho assembly requires that the patient sit upright, whereas the Georgia Warm Springs or Michigan types allow 5° to 10° of recline of the wheelchair back. He must have good lateral trunk stability, which may be provided by corsets, seat adaptations, braces, or restraints if he does not have it actively. MAS cannot be used in bed or when the patient is semireclined in his wheelchair. He can use suspension slings in these positions, however.

The patient must have some source of power to operate the MAS, although some external power can be added for very weak patients. If the patient is too weak to operate a MAS, the alternative is use of environmental control units.[1,58]

Passive range of motion (PROM) must be within normal limits in order to obtain the most benefit from the MAS. Limited range of motion combined with very limited strength precludes the use of feeders in most cases.[40] Incoordination or poor head or trunk control are contraindications for the use of MAS.

If the patient wears a hand splint, this is put on *before* beginning to balance the feeders. MAS are applied bilaterally, one at a time.

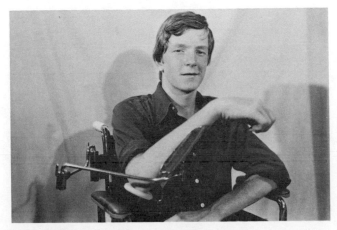

Figure 13.44 Rancho mobile arm support.

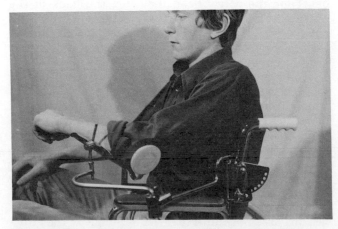

Figure 13.45 Michigan feeder (mobile arm support).

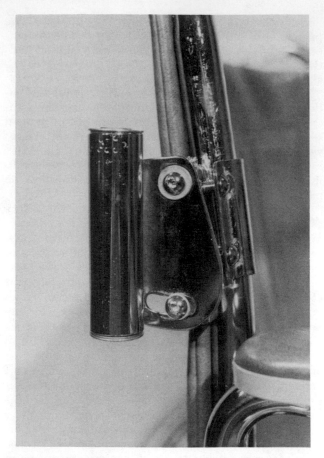

Figure 13.46 Ball-bearing feeder bracket assembly (Rancho type).

assembly also determines the horizontal motion at the shoulder. Neutral = set the ball bearing perpendicular to the floor so that the proximal arm, when inserted, falls neither forward nor backward. Move the bracket out (posteriorly around the wheelchair upright) to assist horizontal abduction; move it in (anteriorly around the upright) to assist horizontal adduction.

PROXIMAL SWIVEL ARM (FIG. 13.47).   This piece permits humeral motion. The distal ball bearing is located at the end of the proximal swivel arm to hold the distal swivel arm. The distal ball bearing may be angled down to assist elbow extension or upward to assist elbow flexion. The patient's permanent feeders will be angled by the orthotist; there is an adjustable proximal arm available for trial purposes (Fig. 13.48). The proximal arms are interchangeable unless adapted, in which case the right and left ones must be marked.

ELEVATING PROXIMAL ARM (FIG. 13.49).   The elevating proximal arm is a component that may be selected in lieu of the standard proximal arm. This component is used to assist a weak (F-) deltoid. A strong rubber band assists the weak deltoid muscle to abduct and flex the shoulder, thus allowing the hand to be brought toward the head.

DISTAL SWIVEL ARM (FIG. 13.50).   This piece corresponds to the forearm; it permits elbow motion in the horizontal plane. It supports the rocker arm assembly and feeder trough. Right and left distal swivel arms differ; to distinguish them, hold the solid end in your hand, the arm should angle in toward you in both cases (R or L). The hollow post at the distal end of the arm may need to be cut lower if the patient is having trouble inwardly rotating. The curvature of the distal arm occasionally may need to be different than standard for a particular pa-

All screws, nuts, etc., *must be secured* to prevent slipping of the MAS while the patient is attempting to use it, even during fitting.

Parts, Functions, and Adjustments of Mobile Arm Supports. BALL-BEARING FEEDER BRACKET ASSEMBLY (FIG. 13.46). The bracket is the piece that attaches to the wheelchair upright. The ball-bearing assembly is the piece that fits into the bracket and holds the proximal ball-bearing rings. There is a right and left assembly: the bevel for the screw head indicates the back of the bracket. It may be necessary to put tape on the wheelchair upright before applying the bracket to prevent the bracket from slipping down the smooth wheelchair upright under the weight of the patient's arm.

This assembly determines the height of the feeder in relation to the patient's body. Neutral = set at a height equal to midhumerus. Raise to enable the patient to get his hand to his mouth or for the elbow dial of the trough to clear the lapboard. Lower the bracket if the patient's shoulders are pushed into elevation. The height of the patient's seat cushion affects this setting. This assembly holds the proximal swivel arm. To prevent pushing the bottom ball bearing out, be sure that the proximal arm is pushed all the way down through the ball-bearing assembly until the first 90° angle of the proximal arm rests against the top of the assembly. This

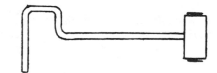

Figure 13.47 Proximal swivel arm.

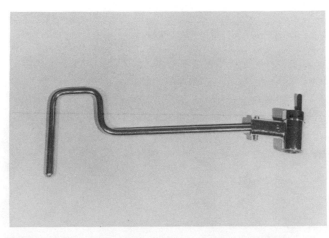

Figure 13.48 Adjustable type proximal swivel arm.

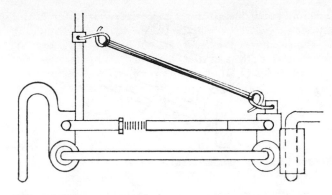

Figure 13.49 Elevating proximal arm for a mobile arm support. (Reproduced with permission from Long, C., and Schutt, A. Upper limb orthotics. In *Orthotics Etcetera*, 3rd edition. Edited by J. B. Redford. Baltimore: Williams & Wilkins, 1986.)

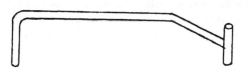

Figure 13.50 Distal swivel arm.

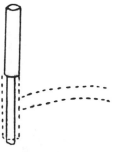

Figure 13.51 The post.

tient to allow the elbow dial of the trough to clear the distal arm during vertical motion. The orthotist will do this. Be sure the patient is using a proper motion pattern before you take the problem to the orthotist. The length of the distal arm, like the proximal arm, is standard; however, an unusually small or large patient may need special length arms. To fit correctly, the distal ball bearing should be located directly opposite the patient's elbow; not behind the elbow nor in front of it.

POST (FIG. 13.51). The post provides added height at the distal end of the distal arm for specific activities. This part must be added by another person whenever it is needed; therefore, an effort should be made to balance the feeders without using this. If one must be used permanently, the orthotist can make the permanent post of the distal arm higher to alleviate the need for this piece.

HORIZONTAL STOP (FIG. 13.52). The horizontal stop limits horizontal motion to within the patient's controllable limits. The horizontal stop can also be used to transfer

motion from the shoulder to the elbow by applying it at the proximal ball bearing to prevent horizontal abduction; this will result in elbow extension when the patient attempts horizontal abduction. If the patient lacks shoulder power, it can be used to transfer power proximally by applying it at the distal ball bearing. The horizontal stop is usually applied to the ball bearing on the outside to limit horizontal abduction or extension rather than inside to limit adduction or flexion. Neutral setup is no stop used.

ROCKER ARM ASSEMBLIES. Five will be described here; any one of these may be used on any MAS setup.

1. Rancho type (Fig. 13.53) permits vertical motion of the feeder trough. It swivels to produce added horizontal motion at the elbow. Right and left are indistinguishable. The trough is attached to this part, which is inserted into the distal end of the distal swivel arm.

2. Georgia Warm Springs type (Fig. 13.54) provides an offset that permits the elbow dial of the trough to

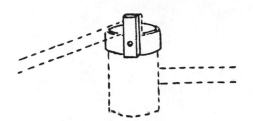

Figure 13.52 The horizontal stop.

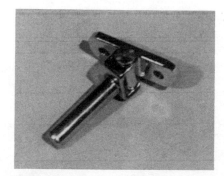

Figure 13.53 Rancho type rocker arm assembly.

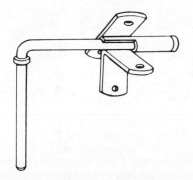

Figure 13.54 Georgia Warm Springs type offset rocker arm assembly.

clear the distal arm. The functions listed above for the Rancho type are also offered. The right and left differ; when inserted into the distal arm, the assembly should angle toward the patient.

3. Michigan type (Fig. 13.55) allows, in addition to the features of the two assemblies noted above, adjustment in the Z axis (vertical) and thereby allows the pivot point to be located directly opposite the center of gravity of the forearm. A weak patient is more easily able to use this type.

4. Modular adjustment mechanism (Fig. 13.56) improves on the Rancho type assembly by alleviating the need for unscrewing the assembly when making proximal/distal adjustments on the trough.[59]

5. Supinator assist (Fig. 13.57) is a special rocker arm assembly that provides mechanical supination, actually humeral external rotation, during flexion and reciprocal pronation during internal rotation. The amount of supination-pronation can be controlled by

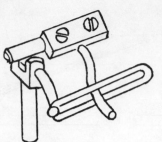

Figure 13.57 Supinator assist.

limiting the length of the wire loop. The supinator assist can be mounted onto a Rancho or offset rocker assembly. Right and left differ: the wire loop is on the side toward the patient.

VERTICAL STOP (FIG. 13.58). The vertical stop is attached to the offset rocker assembly to limit vertical motion. It keeps the motion within the controllable limits of the patient. It may be used to limit both up and down motions or only one or the other by adjusting the screws. Neutral setup = no stop.

TROUGHS. Two types will be described. (1) Trough with elbow dial (Fig. 13.59). The length of the trough is 2 inches less than the distance from the olecranon to the head of the ulna. The distal end is flared. The motion of the wrist should not be impeded. The distal lip of the trough should not limit circulation in the patient's hand. The trough supports the forearm. It is possible to adjust the location of the trough on the rocker assembly to assist either internal rotation (hand heavy—move the trough forward on the rocker assembly) or external rotation (elbow heavy—move the trough backward on the rocker assembly). For neutral setting, set the trough on the rocker assembly so that the forearm rests at an angle of 45° in relation to the lapboard. The elbow dial can be bent forward or backward to provide fine adjustment to assist internal or external rotation. The dial offers good, stable elbow support, although it restricts some elbow extension in the process. However, this does not limit function significantly. In neutral setup, the elbow dial is in line

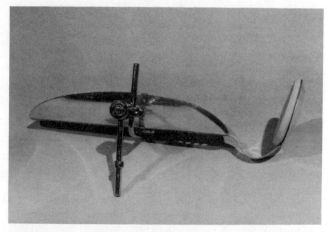

Figure 13.55 Michigan type rocker arm assembly attached to trough.

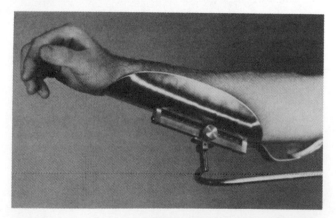

Figure 13.56 Modular adjustment mechanism attached to Rancho type rocker arm assembly. In this photograph the trough is too long for the person; see section on troughs in the text. (Reproduced with permission from Drew, W. E., and Stern, P. H. Modular adjustment mechanism for the balanced forearm orthosis. *Arch. Phys. Med. Rehabil.*, 60*(2):* 81, 1979.)

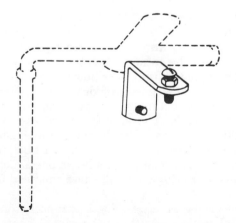

Figure 13.58 Vertical stop.

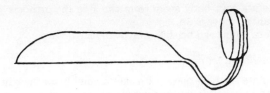

Figure 13.59 Forearm trough with elbow dial.

with the center line of the trough; to accommodate right or left arms, the dial is angled in slightly toward the patient.

(2) The "flying saucer" feeder trough (Fig. 13.60) supports the forearm. It is used in cases where the patient has active elbow flexion and external rotation of the humerus and does not need the vertical motion. This part supplants both the trough and the rocker arm assembly.

Once the MAS is assembled, always mark the location of pieces in relation to one another before making changes during the balancing so that it is easy to return to the previous position, which may prove to be the better adjustment after all. When the MAS is finally balanced, erase all extraneous marks and remark all final positions in case the MAS are knocked out of adjustment and need to be rebalanced. Be sure all screws are *tight.*

Movement Patterns and Equipment Adjustments to Achieve Motion in Mobile Arm Supports. It is preferable to instruct the patient in movement patterns to achieve certain motions in the neutrally adjusted mobile arm supports. However, as is frequently the case, the patient may be too weak to be able to do these motions. In that case the equipment can be adjusted to assist the motions that are weakest. It is not advisable to require the patient to practice the motions a long time before making the equipment adjustments because he will become discouraged and may reject the orthosis. The movement patterns and the equipment adjustments are not listed here in any order of preference. One motion, or one adjustment, may be all that is necessary; or for greater effect a combination of two or more motions, two or more adjustments, or a combination of a motion plus an adjustment may be necessary for the extremely weak patient. Use only the movement patterns and adjustments that are completely safe for the patient, use the least energy, most nearly approximate normal or acceptable movement, and that are most effective. The process of discovery of the correct combination is one of trial and error. The pa-

tient should not be allowed to become fatigued in the process, however, because fatigue invalidates the adjustments. The movement patterns listed below are adapted from a manual once available from Georgia Warm Springs Rehabilitation Center.

DESIRED MOTION: HAND TO MOUTH

Instructions for Movement Patterns.

1. Depress your shoulder while adducting your humerus.
2. Externally rotate your shoulder.
3. Bend laterally toward the same side that the MAS you want to move is on.
4. Shift your body weight toward the side that the MAS you want to move is on (only if enough strength to regain balance).
5. Straighten up or lean back in the chair.
6. Rotate your trunk toward the side the MAS that you want to move is on.
7. Tilt or turn your head toward the MAS that you want to move.
8. Press the elbow dial against a friction pad placed on the lapboard near the waist by depressing your scapula. This may cause enough supination to aim the eating utensil toward your mouth.

Equipment Adjustment

1. Move rocker assembly forward on trough. (Make "elbow heavy.")
2. Turn ball-bearing bracket assembly toward individual.
3. Adjust the proximal swivel arm up.
4. Position the anterior vertical stop to decrease internal rotation.
5. Raise the ball-bearing bracket assembly on the wheelchair upright.
6. Adapt the utensil's length or angle.
7. Raise the trough by use of a post.
8. Lower the posterior vertical stop under the trough to permit additional shoulder external rotation.

DESIRED MOTION: HAND TO TABLE

Instructions for Movement Patterns

1. *Elevate and internally rotate your shoulder to lower the hand.*
2. *Roll the shoulder forward, which encourages horizontal adduction with shoulder flexion, internal rotation, and elbow extension.*
3. *Laterally bend toward the side opposite from the MAS that you want to move.*
4. *Shift your body weight to the side opposite from the MAS that you want to move if your balance can be regained.*
5. *Rotate your trunk toward the side opposite from the MAS that you want to move.*
6. *Tilt or turn your head away from the MAS that you want to move.*

Equipment Adjustment

1. Move the rocker assembly further back on the trough ("hand heavy").
2. Turn the ball-bearing bracket assembly backward, away from individual.
3. Adjust the proximal swivel arm down.
4. Position the anterior vertical stop under the trough to allow more elbow extension (internal rotation).

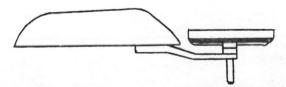

Figure 13.60 "Flying saucer" forearm trough for feeder; this replaces the distal arm as well as the trough and rocker arm assembly.

5. Lower the ball-bearing feeder bracket assembly on the wheelchair upright.
6. Lower the trough by removing the post or cutting down the distal channel into which the rocker arm assembly fits.

DESIRED MOTION: HORIZONTAL ABDUCTION

Instructions for Movement Patterns

1. Shift your body weight toward the side that the orthosis you want to move is on.
2. Rotate your trunk toward the side that the orthosis you want to move is on.
3. Turn your head briskly toward the orthosis.

Equipment Adjustment

1. Rotate the ball-bearing bracket assembly on the wheelchair upright backward, away from the individual.
2. Shorten the proximal swivel arm.

DESIRED MOTION: HORIZONTAL ADDUCTION

Instructions for Movement Pattern

1. Shift your body weight away from the side the orthosis you want to move is on.

2. Rotate your body away from the side the orthosis you want to move is on.
3. Turn your head briskly away from the orthosis.

Equipment Adjustment

1. Rotate the ball-bearing bracket assembly on the wheelchair upright forward, toward the individual.
2. Lengthen the proximal swivel arm.

Checkout and Training for Mobile Arm Supports. Checkout of the mobile arm support may be done using the form shown in Table 13.1

The patient will not be able to put on his MAS independently but must instruct others in their proper application. Patients can remove the MAS by lifting their arms slightly, causing the MAS to move away. The MAS, except for the ball-bearing bracket assembly, is removed when the wheelchair is stored. Care must be taken that the bracket assembly does not get knocked out of alignment when the chair is put into the car or when the patient is wheeled through doorways because this will change the entire balance of the MAS.

Controls training involves having the patient move the MAS as far as he can *horizontally* from side to side and then from front to back. If the patient needs much

Table 13.1
CHECKOUT SHEET FOR MOBILE ARM SUPPORTS[a]

Patient's Name_____ Type Feeder (R)_____

Date Fitted_____ (L)_____

I. Patient's position in wheel chair

Yes	No	Is patient able to sit up straight?
Yes	No	Are hips well back in chair?
Yes	No	Is spine in good vertical alignment?
Yes	No	Does patient have lateral trunk stability?
Yes	No	Is chair seat adequate for comfort and stability?
Yes	No	If patient wears hand splints, does he have them on?
Yes	No	Does patient meet requirements for passive ROM and coordination?

II. Mechanical Checkout

Yes	No	Are all screws tight?
Yes	No	Is bracket tight on wheelchair?
Yes	No	Are all joints freely movable?
Yes	No	Is proximal arm all the way down into the bracket?
Yes	No	Is bracket at proper height so shoulders are not forced into elevation?
Yes	No	Does elbow dial clear lapboard when trough is in "up" position?
Yes	No	Is patient's hand (in "up" position) as close to mouth as possible?
Yes	No	Can patient obtain maximal active reach?
Yes	No	Is feeder trough short enough to allow wrist flexion or to prevent pressure on blood vessels?
Yes	No	Are trough edges rolled so that they do not contact forearm?
Yes	No	Is elbow secure and comfortable in elbow support?
Yes	No	In vertical motion, does the dial clear the distal arm?

III. Control checkout

Yes	No	Can patient control motion of proximal arm from either extreme?
Yes	No	Can patient control motion of distal arm from either extreme?
Yes	No	Can patient control vertical motion from either extreme?
Yes	No	Have stops been applied to limit range within controllable limits if necessary?

[a] Devised by staff at Rancho Los Amigos Hospital, Downey, CA.

practice to do these motions effortlessly, then activities requiring horizontal motions, such as drawing with felt-tipped pens, turning large-sized magazine pages, playing board games, etc., offer some stimulation to the exercise. The patient learns to control first one feeder, then the other. Both are usually worn for balance, but if the patient is tall and has lateral instability he may be more stable if his non-training arm is out of the feeder and resting on the lapboard. Next, *vertical* motions are learned, first out to the side, which is easiest, then in front of the face, and then at any point within his horizontal range. Games that require picking up playing pieces and movement in space are interesting exercises for the patient.

Use training is not initiated before the patient has excellent control of the feeders *and* his hand splint if he has one. Use training activities will include feeding, grooming, use of telephone, typewriter, calculators, computers, and other electronic devices, page turning, games, and possibly writing and drawing.

Pronator Lively Splint for C₅ Tetraplegic Arm (Fig. 13.61)

This splint provides active elbow extension through the use of coiled springs mounted at the elbow joint and pronation through the use of specially designed springs. The assisted arm movement enables the C₅ spinal cord-injured patient to use a prehension splint functionally and is an alternative to MAS for those patients with good shoulder musculature.[60]

Often the use of orthoses that enable the otherwise paralyzed patient to move results in increased strength and endurance. The need for the orthosis or need for modification of it should be reevaluated over time. Patients with degenerating diseases should be reevaluated regularly so that their orthotic prescription can be current with their level of function to allow as much independence as possible. The need for increased orthoses is a psychologically critical time for the patient, and attention should be given to the mourning process.

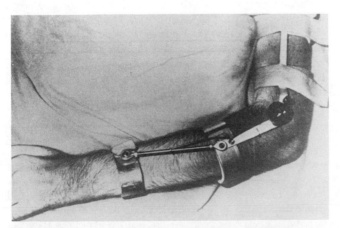

Figure 13.61 "Lively" pronator splint for C₅ tetraplegic arm. (Reproduced with permission from Abraham, D., Shrosbree, M. B., and Key, A. G. A functional splint for the C₅ tetraplegic arm. *Paraplegia, 17:* 198–203, 1979–80.)

Orthoses To Modify Tone

Through splinting, therapists have implemented the principle of prolonged stretch to reduce spasticity. According to that principle, when a muscle is held in an elongated position, the muscle spindles will be rebiased to a longer length, making them less likely to become activated by small movements. Other treatment principles incorporated into some splinting designs for the spastic patient include neutral warmth or grasp of a hard cone to inhibit spasticity, positioning opposite to patterns of spasticity to inhibit or prevent development of spasticity, tactile stimulation of antagonists to facilitate them and reciprocally inhibit the spastic muscles, and quick stretch to facilitate hypotonic muscles.

Splinting of the spastic hand is controversial. A poll of 100 registered therapists concerning their practice of splinting the hemiplegic hand resulted in no clear direction or rationale for whether or not splinting should be used or what type should be used at various stages of recovery.[62] Some therapists choose volar splints; others choose dorsal splints, fearing the effects of sensory stimulation of the flexor surface and hoping to use the sensory stimulation of the dorsal surface to facilitate extension. One pilot study found that volar splinting did tend to increase spasticity, whereas dorsal splinting tended to decrease it in hemiplegic patients.[63] Zislis[64] compared the effects of dorsal and ventral splints in one hemiplegic patient. The fingers were abducted in the ventral splint and adducted in the dorsal splint, which clouds the comparison. Electromyography demonstrated a decrease in motor unit output of the spastic flexors using the ventral splint and an increase using the dorsal splint. Another study of three hemiparetic subjects[65] found that none of three splints (volar resting pan, finger spreader, hard cone) immediately reduced electromyographic activity. The volar resting pan splint actually increased the electromyographic activity as compared to no splint. In a study of 10 subjects with hypertonic wrist flexors, half of whom were assigned to use of a volar resting pan with finger separators and half to a spasticity-reduction splint with dorsal forearm piece, static splinting reduced the viscoelastic components of hypertonicity.[66] No measure was taken of the neural component. No significant differences were found between the splint styles.[66] Age was found to be an intervening variable in that subjects 35 years of age and younger showed more of a change than those 65 years of age and older.[66] This study points out that some of the controversy about splinting may reflect differential effects of splinting on the two components of spasticity. Successful reduction of the viscoelastic component has been reported,[66,67] whereas the neural component remained unchanged[67] or increased or decreased in other studies seemingly without clear reasons. Inhibitory splinting can be considered a neurorehabilitation treatment when aimed at the neural component of spasticity. Like other such treatments, it is successful for some and not others. Until the controlling variables are identified to guide treatment planning, therapists must use knowledge and judgment in applying splints and in monitoring the outcome.

A spastic patient, or potentially spastic patient, if splinted at all, must have a splint that incorporates both the wrist and the fingers because the effect of splinting one part of the spastic hand in extension is to cause flexion contractures of the unsplinted part.

Splint designs for the hemiplegic hand include the dorsal or volar resting pans (Fig. 13.7), the orthokinetic splint, and the finger abduction splints (Fig. 13.62 and 13.63).

Spasticity reduction splint (Fig. 13.62) is a variation of the resting pan.[68] The splint is molded to provide 30° of wrist hyperextension, 45° of MP flexion, full interphalangeal extension, finger abduction, and thumb extension and abduction. This position duplicates a suggested reflex-inhibiting pattern of Bobath. No data on the effectiveness of this splint in reducing spasticity have been published.

In a study of 10 hemiplegic patients, Kaplan[69] reported increased free range of motion (decreased

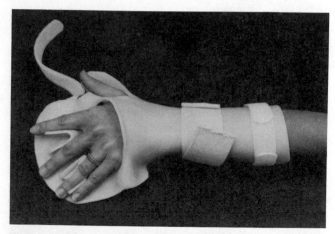

Figure 13.62 Spasticity reduction splint.

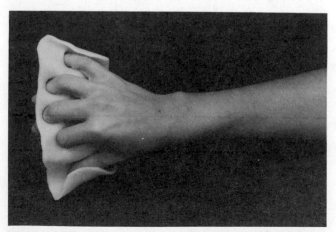

Figure 13.63 Finger abduction splint for the spastic hand.

spasticity) at the wrist and fingers following splinting of the affected arm into maximal extension.[69] The wrist was hyperextended to approximately 90° and the fingers and thumb to 0°. The fingers were adducted. This dorsal splint, with textured lining for sensory stimulation, was worn at least 8 hours per day as tolerated by the patient.

Finger abduction splint for the spastic hand (Fig. 13.63) utilizes Bobath's reflex-inhibiting pattern theory. Originally, the splint was constructed of a block of foam with holes punched through the foam to allow insertion of the fingers and thumb in an abducted position.[6] A more permanent splint has been designed for the same purpose using low-temperature splinting materials.[70]

Zislis[64] demonstrated electromyographically on one poststroke patient a decrease in finger flexor activity when a volar splint that held the fingers extended and abducted was used as compared to a dorsal splint that maintained the fingers extended and adducted. The thumb was not included in either splint; the wrist was held in neutral position in both.

Orthokinetic splint for the spastic hemiplegic was developed by A. Joy Huss and uses ideas from Rood as its theoretical base: a firm surface in the palm of the hand will inhibit the extrinsic flexor muscles, and tactile stimulation of the extensor surface of the forearm will facilitate extensor tone. The hand and forearm pieces are made of low-temperature plastics. The hand piece is shaped into a cone; the larger end of the cone is ulnar-directed. The forearm shell extends two-thirds of the length of the forearm from approximately 3 cm from the wrist crease. The cone is attached to the forearm piece by two side supports that are bent to follow the contour of the hand laterally. The side supports are attached loosely, using rivets, so that the wrist is free to move. The forearm piece is secured to the patient using elastic bandage for straps[71] to simulate the benefits of an orthokinetic cuff. No data on the effectiveness have been published.

Inflatable splint is a double plastic cuff long enough to envelop the part to be splinted. It was originally designed as an emergency immobilizer splint for the limbs, but has been adopted for use with spastic patients. It provides deep pressure therapy[72] and warmth. It is worn for 15 to 20 min before movement therapy begins[73] and then continues to be worn in conjunction with simulated weight-bearing exercise to correctly position the intermediate joints of the arm and to provide sensory stimulation to reduce spastic tone during exercise.[72]

Serial casting of spastic limbs is developing as a treatment choice for brain-injured[67] and stroke[74,75] patients. The casts are replaced as the limb is stretched more and more away from the contracted spastic posture with each cast change, so that greater free ROM is obtained over time. There is some evidence that prolonged immobilization of the limb (3 months with removal for washing and free movement twice daily) in a position of full stretch will decrease the spasticity, increase the range of free movement, and increase the tone of the antagonists (except in cases of wrist and finger extensors).[75] Pain and skin damage may occur during prolonged immobilization unless the device is well constructed and the condition of the limb is frequently monitored.[75] Plaster of paris was found to erode the skin,[75] and the newer plastic materials may be preferable.

Another study in which immobilization was followed by night casting in a half-shell cast for a total of 16 days was beneficial to one patient with severe elbow flexor spasticity.[74] In this study plaster cast was preferred to plastic splints.

Guidelines and results of chart review of 201 head trauma patients who were serially casted for lower-extremity spasticity have been published.[67]

A *dynamic sling,* designed by Mary Jo Winsinky, R.P.T., has been used to facilitate the elbow extensors via stretch and resistance offered by a surgical tubing strap as the patient walks. It also is believed to inhibit finger flexion, and possibly the whole flexor pattern, by use of the cone held in the hand. To construct this sling, the plastic cone is placed on a length of rubber tubing or strapping long enough to loop over the patient's shoulder while he holds the cone and has his elbow flexed to 90° or less. A knot is made in the tubing and pushed inside the cone out of view. The large end of the cone is worn ulnarward, and the tubing crosses under the axilla if the sling is applied correctly (Fig. 13.64). It may be necessary to fasten the tubing onto the shoulder and to strap the hand onto the cone.[76]

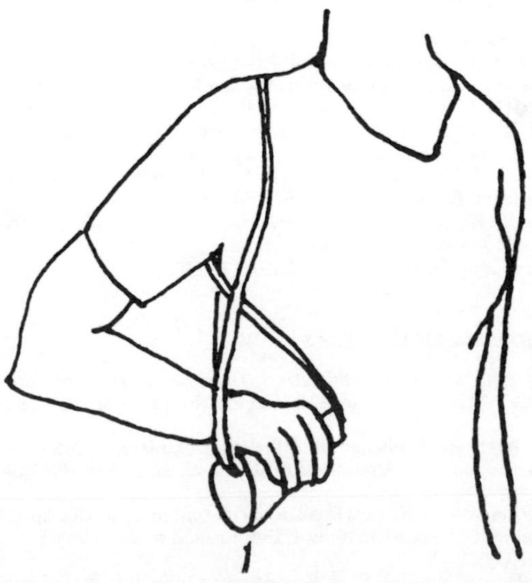

Figure 13.64 Dynamic sling to facilitate hypotonic elbow extensor muscles of a hemiparetic patient.

STUDY QUESTIONS:

Orthoses: Purposes and Types

1. What are the roles of various rehabilitation professionals in orthotic rehabilitation?
2. Define orthosis.
3. Name the goals for which splinting may be used.
4. Discuss why a static splint might be chosen and the precautions related to such splints.
5. What are the pros and cons of the various orthoses that can be used to support the shoulder of a hemiplegic patient?
6. Discuss when a wrist orthosis with MP extension assists and thumb abduction-extension assist would be selected for a patient as opposed to a resting pan splint.
7. Select a splint for a patient with a combined ulnar and median nerve injury.
8. Define wearing tolerance.
9. Select two splints that could be used for swan neck deformity of one finger and discuss the reasons for choosing one over the other for a particular patient.
10. Select correct styles of all parts of a mobile arm support for a weak patient with particular weakness of the internal rotators and absent triceps. State how each part will be adjusted for this patient.
11. Describe a therapy session to improve a patient's horizontal control of a mobile arm support.
12. Select a splint to reduce excessive flexor tone of the wrist, discuss reasons for the choice, and state the principle(s) that it implements.

References

1. Long, C., and Schutt, A. Upper limb orthotics. In *Orthotics Etcetera, 3rd* edition. Edited by J. B. Redford. Baltimore: Williams & Wilkins, 1986.
2. Cailliet, R. *Hand Pain and Impairment, 3rd* edition. Philadelphia: F. A. Davis, 1982.
3. Shafer, A. A. *Common Problems, Useful Solutions in Hand Rehabilitation.* Dedham, MA: AliMed,® Inc., 1986.
4. DeVore, G. L. A sling to prevent a subluxed shoulder. *Am. J. Occup. Ther., 24*(5): 580–581, 1970.
5. Neal, M. R., and Williamson, J. Collar sling for bilateral shoulder subluxation. *Am. J. Occup. Ther., 34*(6): 400–401, 1980.
6. Bobath, B. *Adult Hemiplegia: Evaluation and Treatment,* 2nd edition. London: Heinemann Medical Books, 1978.
7. Boyd, E., and Gaylard, A. Shoulder supports with stroke patients: a Canadian survey. *Can. J. Occup. Ther., 53*(2): 61–67, 1986.
8. Rajaram, V., and Holtz, M. Shoulder forearm support for the subluxed shoulder. *Arch. Phys. Med. Rehabil., 66*(3): 191–192, 1985.
9. Smith, R. O., and Okamoto, G. A. Checklist for the prescription of slings for the hemiplegic patient. *Am. J. Occup. Ther., 35*(2): 91–95, 1981.
10. Walker, J. Modified strapping of roll sling. *Am. J. Occup. Ther., 37*(2): 110–111, 1983.
11. Claus, B. S., and Godfrey, K. J. Brief or new: a distal support sling for the hemiplegic patient. *Am. J. Occup. Ther., 39*(8): 536–537, 1985.
12. *Catalogue.* Smith & Nephew Roylan, Menomonee Falls, WI 53051, 1987.
13. Ferreri, J., and Tumminelli, J. A swivel cock-up splint-type armtrough. *Am. J. Occup. Ther., 28*(6): 359, 1974.
14. Iveson, E., Phillips, M., and Ream, W. D. A removable armtrough for wheelchair patients. *Am. J. Occup. Ther., 26*(5): 269, 1972.
15. Goold, N. J. A versatile wheelchair armrest attachment. *Am. J. Occup. Ther., 30*(8): 502–504, 1976.
16. Salo, R. E. A hammock wheelchair armrest. *Am. J. Occup. Ther., 32*(8): 525, 1978.
17. Enstrom, J., and Davies, J. Lapboard modifications to help support a flaccid upper extremity. *Phys. Ther., 60*(6): 795–796, 1980.
18. Carlson, J. D., and Trombly, C. A. The effect of wrist immobilization on performance of the Jebsen Hand Function Test. *Am. J. Occup. Ther., 37*(3): 167–175, 1983.
19. Fishwick, G. M., and Tobin, D. G. Splinting the burned hand with pri-

mary excision and early grafting. *Am. J. Occup. Ther.,32*(3): 182–183, 1978.

20. Tenney, C. G., and Lisak, J. M. *Atlas of Hand Splinting*. Boston: Little, Brown & Company, 1986.
21. Long, C. Upper limb bracing. In *Orthotics Etcetera, 1st* edition. Edited by S. Licht and H. Kamenetz. Baltimore: Waverly Press, 1966.
22. *Catalogue*. LMB Hand Rehab Products, Inc., San Luis Obispo, CA 93406, 1986.
23. Melvin, J. L. *Rheumatic Disease: Occupational Therapy and Rehabilitation, 2nd* edition. Philadelphia: F. A. Davis, 1982.
24. Parks, B. J., Barrett, K. P., and Voss, K. The use of Hexcelite in splinting the thumb. *Am. J. Occup. Ther., 37*(4): 266–267, 1983.
25. Making the least of burn scars. *Emerg Med., 4:* 24–45, 1972.
26. Larson, D. *The Prevention and Correction of Burn Scar Contracture and Hypertrophy*. Galveston, TX: Shriner's Burn Institute, University of Texas Medical Branch, 1973.
27. Rivers, E. A., Strate, R. G., and Salem, L. D. The transparent face mask. *Am. J. Occup. Ther., 33*(2): 108–113, 1979.
28. Jardine, J., Lee, H., and Simons, A. Rotator cuff treatment protocol. *The American Occupational Therapy Association Physical Disabilities Special Interest Section Newsletter, 6*(3): 1, 3, 4, 1983.
29. Green, D. P., and McCoy, H. Turnbuckle orthotic correction of elbow-flexion contractures after acute injuries. *J. Bone Joint Surg., 61A*(7): 1092-1095, 1979.
30. Hepburn, G. R., and Crivelli, K. J. Use of elbow Dynasplint for reduction of elbow flexion contractures: a case study. *The Journal of Orthopaedic and Sports Physical Therapy, 5*(5): 269–274, 1984.
31. Collins, K., et al Customized adjustable orthoses: their use in spasticity. *Arch. Phys. Med. Rehabil., 66*(6): 397–398, 1985.
32. Malick, M. H. *Manual on Dynamic Hand Splinting with Thermoplastic Materials*. New York: ABC Inc., 1974.
33. Heurich, M., and Polansky, S. An adaptation of the glove flexion mitt. *Am. J. Occup. Ther., 32*(2): 110–111, 1978.
34. Anderson, M. *Upper Extremity Orthotics*. Springfield, IL: Charles C Thomas, 1965.
35. Bunnell, S. *Surgery of the Hand,* 3rd edition. Philadelphia: J. B. Lippincott, 1956.
36. Von Prince, K., Cureri, W., and Pruitt, B. Application of fingernail hooks in splinting burned hands. *Am. J. Occup. Ther., 24*(8): 556–559, 1970.
37. Fess, E. E., Gettle, K. S., and Strickland, J. W. *Hand Splinting: Principles and Methods*. St. Louis: C. V. Mosby Company, 1981.
38. Sellers, J. A low-profile dorsal dynamic splint. *Am. J. Occup. Ther., 34*(3): 213, 1980.
39. Colditz, J. C. Low profile dynamic splinting of the injured hand. *Am. J. Occup. Ther., 37*(3): 182–188, 1983.
40. Yasuda, Y. L., Bowman, K., and Hsu, J. D. Mobile arm supports: criteria for successful use in muscle disease patients. *Arch. Phys. Med. Rehabil., 67*(4): 253–256, 1986.
41. Nichols, P. J. R., et al. The value of flexor hinge hand splints. *Prosthet. Orthot. Int., 2*(2): 86–94, 1978.
42. McKenzie, M. The ratchet handsplint. *Am. J. Occup. Ther., 27*(8): 477–479, 1973.
43. Stenehjem, J., Swenson, J., and Sprague, C. Wrist driven flexor hinge orthosis: linkage design improvements. *Arch. Phys. Med. Rehabil., 64*(11): 566–568, 1983.
44. Long, C., and Masciarelli, V. An electrophysiological splint for the hand. *Arch. Phys. Med. Rehabil., 44*(9): 499–503, 1963.
45. Peckham, P. H., and Mortimer, J. T. Restoration of hand function in the quadriplegic through electrical stimulation. In *Functional Electrical Stimulation*. Edited by F. T. Hambrecht and J. B. Reswick. New York: Marcel Dekker, 1977.
46. Hambrecht, F. T., and Reswick, J. B., editors. *Functional Electrical Stimulation*. New York: Marcel Dekker, 1977.
47. Vodovnik, L., Kralj, A., and Bajd, T. Modification of abnormal motor control with functional electrical stimulation of peripheral nerves. In *Recent Achievements in Restorative Neurology 1: Upper Motor Neuron Functions and Dysfunctions*. Edited by J. Eccles and N. Dimitrijevic. Basel: S. Karger Publishers, 1985.
48. Vodovnik, L., and Grobelnik, S. Multichannel functional electrical stimulation—facts and expectations. *Prosthet. Orthot. Int., 1:* 43–46, 1977.
49. Kralj, A., Bajd, T., and Turk, R. Electrical stimulation providing functional use of paraplegic patient muscles. *Med. Prog. Technol., 7:*3–9, 1980.
50. Gracanin, F. Functional electrical stimulation in control of motor output and movements. In *Contemporary Clinical Neurophysiology*. Edited by W. A. Cobb and H. Van Duijn. Amsterdam: Elsevier, 1978.
51. Vodovnik, L., Kralj, A., Stanic, U., Acimovic, R., and Gros, N. Recent applications of functional electrical stimulation to stroke patients in Ljubljana. *Clin. Orthop., 131:* 64–70, 1978.

52. Trombly, C., Prentke, E., and Long, C. Myoelectrically controlled electric torque motor for the flexor hinge hand splint. *Orthop. Prosthet. Appl. J., 21:* 39–43, 1967.
53. Silverstein, F., French J., and Siebens, A. A myoelectric hand splint. *Am. J. Occup. Ther., 28*(2):99–101, 1974.
54. Rudin, N. J., Gilmore, L. D., Roy, S. H., and DeLuca, C. J. New motor control assessment techniques for evaluating individuals with severe handicaps: a case study. *J. Rehabil. Res. Dev., 24*(3): 57–74, 1987.
55. Trombly, C. Principles of operant conditioning related to orthotic training of quadriplegic patients. *Am. J. Occup. Ther., 20*(5): 217–220, 1966.
56. Trombly, C. Myoelectric control of orthotic devices for the severely paralyzed. *Am. J. Occup. Ther., 22*(5): 385–389, 1968.
57. Seeger, B. R., Caudrey, D. J., and McAllister, G. M. Skill evaluator and trainer for electrically operated devices: An evaluation of the SET. *Arch. Phys. Med. Rehabil., 66*(6): 387–390, 1985.
58. Warren, C. G., and Enders, A. Introduction to systems and devices for the disabled. In *Orthotics Etcetera, 3rd* edition. Edited by J. B. Redford. Baltimore: Williams & Wilkins, 1986.
59. Drew, W. E., and Stern, P. H. Modular adjustment mechanism for the balanced forearm orthosis. *Arch. Phys. Med. Rehabil., 60*(2): 81, 1979.
60. Abraham, D., Shrosbree, M. B., and Key, A. G. A functional splint for the C₅ tetraplegic arm. *Paraplegia, 17:*198–203, 1979–80.
61. Herman, R., and Schaumberg, H. Alterations in dynamic and static properties of the stretch reflex in patients with spastic hemiplegia. *Arch. Phys. Med. Rehabil., 49*(4): 199–204, 1968.
62. Neuhaus, B. E., et al. A survey of rationales for and against hand splinting in hemiplegia. *Am. J. Occup. Ther., 35*(2): 83–90, 1981.
63. Charait, S. A comparison of volar and dorsal splinting of the hemiplegic hand. *Am. J. Occup. Ther., 22*(4): 319–321, 1968.
64. Zislis, J. Splinting of the hand in a spastic hemiplegic. *Arch. Phys. Med. Rehabil., 45*(1): 41–43, 1964.
65. Mathiowetz, V., Bolding, D. J., and Trombly, C. A. Immediate effects of positioning devices on the normal and spastic hand measured by electromyography. *Am. J. Occup. Ther., 37*(4): 247–254, 1983.
66. McPherson, J. J., et al. A comparison of dorsal and volar resting hand splints in the reduction of hypertonus. *Am. J. Occup. Ther., 36*(10): 664–670, 1982.
67. Booth, B. J., Doyle, M., and Montgomery, J. Serial casting for the management of spasticity in the head-injured adult. *Phys. Ther., 63*(12): 1960–1966, 1983.
68. Snook, J. H. Spasticity reduction splint. *Am. J. Occup. Ther., 33*(10): 648–651, 1979.
69. Kaplan, N. Effect of splinting on reflex inhibition and sensorimotor stimulation in treatment of spasticity. *Arch. Phys. Med. Rehabil., 43*(11): 565–569, 1962.
70. Doubilet, L., and Polkow, L. S. Theory and design of a finger abduction splint for the spastic hand. *Am. J. Occup. Ther., 31*(5): 320–322, 1977.
71. Kiel, J. L. Making the dynamic orthokinetic wrist splint for flexor spasticity in hand and wrist. In *Sensorimotor Evaluation and Treatment Procedures for Allied Health Personnel,* 2nd edition. Edited by S. D. Farber and A. J. Huss. Indianapolis: Indiana University Foundation, 1974.
72. Johnstone, M. *Restoration of Motor Function in the Stroke Patient, 2nd* edition. London: Churchill Livingstone, 1983.
73. Johnstone, M. Inflatable splint for the hemiplegic arm. *Physiotherapy, 61*(12): 377, 1975.
74. King, T. I. Plaster splinting as a means of reducing elbow flexor spasticity: a case study. *Am. J. Occup. Ther., 36*(10): 671–673, 1982.
75. Brennan, J. B. Response to stretch of hypertonic muscle groups in hemiplegia. *Br. Med. J., 1*(5136): 1504–1507, 1959.
76. Farber, S. D., and Huss, A. J. *Sensorimotor Evaluation and Treatment Methods for Allied Health Personnel, second edition*. Indianapolis: The Indiana University Foundation, 1974.

Supplementary Reading

Adaptive Equipment Rehabilitation Technology: Information Packet. Rockville, MD: The American Occupational Therapy Association, 1986.

Callahan, A. D., and McEntee, P. Splinting proximal interphalangeal joint flexion contractures: A new design. *Am. J. Occup. Ther., 40*(6): 408–411, 1986.

Dovelle, S., Heeter, P. K., and Phillips, D. A dynamic traction splint for the management of extrinsic tendon tightness. *Am. J. Occup. Ther., 41*(2): 123–125, 1987.

Exner, C. E., and Bonder, B. R. Comparative effects of three hand splints on bilateral hand use, grasp, and arm-hand posture in hemiplegic children: a pilot study. *Occup. Ther. J. Res., 3*(2): 75–92, 1983.

Hooper, R. M., and North, E. R. Dynamic interphalangeal extension splint design. *Am. J. Occup. Ther., 36*(4): 257–262, 1982.

Huddleston, O. L., Henderson, W., and Campbell, J. The static night splint. *Am. J. Occup. Ther., 12*(5): 245–246, 1958.

Jamison, S. L., and Dayhoff, N. E. A hard hand positioning device to decrease wrist and finger hypertonicity: a sensorimotor approach for the patient with nonprogressive brain damage. *Nurs. Res., 29*(5):285–289, 1980.

Johnson, B. M., Flynn, M. J. G., and Beckenbaugh, R. D. A dynamic splint for use after total wrist arthroplasty. *Am. J. Occup. Ther., 35*(3): 179–184, 1981.

Lopez, M. S., and Hanley, K. F. Splint modification for flexor tendon repairs. *Am. J. Occup. Ther., 38*(6): 398–403, 1984.

McPherson, J. J. Objective evaluation of a splint designed to reduce hypertonicity. *Am. J. Occup. Ther., 35*(3): 189–194, 1981.

McPherson, J. J., Becker, A. H., and Franszczak, N. Dynamic splint to reduce the passive component of hypertonicity. *Arch. Phys. Med. Rehabil., 66*(4): 249–252, 1985.

Pollock, D., and Sell, H. Myoelectric control sites in the high-level quadriplegic patient. *Arch. Phys. Med. Rehabil., 59*(5): 217–220, 1978.

Smith, D. G., and Siegars, J. B. Engineering student design projects in a rehabilitation setting. *Am. J. Occup. Ther., 36*(6): 396–397, 1982.

Woodson, A. M. Proposal for splinting the adult hemiplegic hand to promote function. *Occup. Ther. Health Care,* 4(3/4): 85–95, 1987.

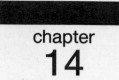

chapter
14

Materials and Methods of Construction of Temporary Orthoses

Catherine A. Trombly

Orthoses used in treatment to position or immobilize for protection of a joint or relief of pain, to increase range of motion, or to decrease spasticity are often considered temporary. They are typically purchased commercially or made by an occupational therapist from thermoplastic materials. Orthoses used to restore function are usually needed on a permanent basis and are machined from metals by a certified orthotist. Unfortunately, the supply of certified orthotists does not yet meet the demand, and the therapist may find it necessary to make the intricate metal splints that substitute for function. Anderson[1] graphically demonstrates this process; however, it is recommended that if the therapist is to have this duty, he or she should enroll in a postgraduate course for advanced training in the fitting and fabrication of permanent orthoses.

Hand Splint Construction by the Occupational Therapist

SELECTING THE SPLINT DESIGN

To decide whether a hand splint is needed and what type is required, the therapist examines the patient's hand to determine the position of pain, or why the hand is not operating functionally to provide grasp and prehension, or why it is not being held in a functional position at rest. The functional position of the hand is 15° to 30° of wrist dorsiflexion, neutral to slight ulnar deviation of the wrist, partial flexion of the metacarpophalangeal and interphalangeal joints of the fingers and thumb, and thumb abduction and opposition. At rest, the normal hand assumes this position due to the balance of biomechanical forces that is brought about by the shape of the joints and the viscoelastic properties of the ligaments, tendons, skin, and innervated muscles. Changes in any of these factors will result in a hand problem that may require a hand splint.

The ideal goal of hand splinting is to restore or preserve normal hand function. To determine what splint design will be necessary to achieve the desired result, the therapist applies corrective forces manually to the patient's hand. While applying these forces the therapist notes how much and where force is needed to put the hand into a functional position or to assist it to move in functional grasp and prehension patterns. The therapist must remember that a relationship exists between the position of the wrist and the position and operation of the fingers due to tenodesis effect. This is an important fact to remember when deciding whether to make a short hand splint or one that crosses and supports the wrist. Both grasp and release should be at least potentially permitted by the position of the wrist in the splint. It should be remembered that by splinting only the wrist or only the fingers of a patient with flexor spasticity, increased flexion of the unsplinted joint will occur.

Mechanical principles must be considered in the decision about splint design.[2] One principle is the relationship between the total force exerted and the area over which that force is applied: the smaller the area, the greater the force applied. To prevent pressure sores, especially over bony areas, the force should be distributed over as large an area as possible. This principle would therefore be important in selecting the correct width of the splint itself, of the straps and the finger loops. By fabricating the splint so that the edges that contact the skin are rolled is another application of this principle. The principle of mechanical advantage refers to the relationship between the length of the force arm and that of the resistance arm of a lever system. A volar splint represents a class I lever in which the axis is located at the wrist joint, the weight of the hand is the resistance, and the weight of the forearm is the force.[2] Remembering from kinesiology that $F \times FA = RA \times R$ or $F = RA \times R/FA$, it can be seen that if the resistance and resistance arm (palmar support) remain unchanged, the force exerted on the forearm skin can be reduced by increasing the length of the force arm (forearm piece). These two principles, which relate to forces applied in parallel, support the clinical experience that long, wide splints are more comfortable and more durable than short, narrow ones.[2]

A third principle especially relates to outrigger design and placement. Force has both rotational and translational components. The rotational component provides motion that brings the part in a circular arc around the joint axis. The translational, or linear, component compresses or distracts the joint surfaces. If the force to stretch out a joint is applied perpendicularly, i.e., 90°, the force is entirely rotational. As the angle of application moves away from perpendicular, the translational component increases. If the force is applied at greater than 90°, it tends to compress the joint, whereas at angles less than 90°, it tends to distract the joint. Rarely are these situations wanted in a splint. Therefore, in a dynamic splint designed to stretch out a contracture, the outrigger must be continually corrected to keep pace with the patient's new position so that the traction is always applied perpendicularly.[3]

The torque of rotational force at the joint is equal to the product of the force and the length of the lever arm on which it acts. The longer the lever arm, the greater the torque. A finger cuff placed at the distal interphalangeal joint to apply stretch may exert too great a torque for the comfort of the patient and may therefore initially need to be placed more proximally to be within the pain tolerance of the patient.[2] The exact placement of cuffs, and stabilizers to provide a counterbalancing force if necessary, depends on the relative degree of passive mobility of successive joints.[2] If all joints within a finger are immobile, the cuff can be applied distally to exert force across all joints. If an intermediate joint has normal range of motion, a stabilizer will need to be added to direct the pull toward the impaired joint.

Friction, of course, should not be and is not a factor in the well-fitted and well-designed splint. Friction occurs when one surface (splint) moves in relation to the surface it contacts (skin); damage occurs to the softer surface.[2]

Once the therapist has the design parameters of the hand splint in mind, she can use a standard splint design for which patterns exist,[4–8] adapt a standard design to fit the particular problem, or design a new splint and make the pattern for the patient's unique problem.

FITTING THE PATTERN (FIG. 14.1–14.4)

For each splint made, the pattern will have to be fitted to the particular person. Standard patterns almost never fit perfectly. There are two stages to the fitting process: gross adaptation of the pattern to the particular hand and final adjustment. Gross adaptation, or sizing, of the pattern is done directly on the hand or on the nonaffected hand.

If the hand splint is simple, the method of sizing the pattern is to trace the outline of the patient's hand onto a flat piece of paper. The locations of the patient's joints are indicated on this drawing. Then the outline of the splint pattern is drawn over the drawing of the hand, meeting the landmarks of the hand as it should.

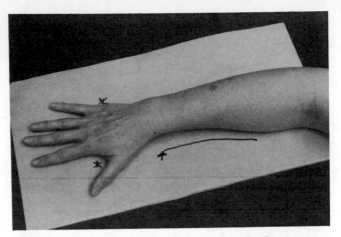

Figure 14.1 Important points of fit are marked onto paper pattern.

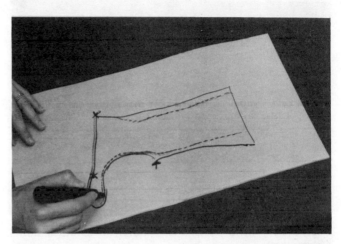

Figure 14.2 The pattern is drawn onto the paper to fit the tracing of the patient's hand.

This is a two-dimensional process, and extra length must be allowed in parts that wrap around to accommodate the thickness of both the material and the hand. Final sizing is done by cutting the pattern out of paper toweling, dampening it, and smoothing it onto the patient's hand. An alternative method is to draw the pattern on a paper towel that is placed over the entire surface of the hand and arm that the splint is meant to cover. The pattern is drawn freehand to fit the contour of the hand, which is palpated beneath the paper towel. If the therapist finds it difficult to draw the contour of the splint freehand, she may use the too small or too large patterns available in the books cited as references to this chapter and change the size by adding to or trimming away the pattern until it fits without altering the basic shape of the pattern.

Final adjustment of the pattern is done by dampening the paper towel pattern to help it conform to the hand and by carefully checking the fit at every point both with the hand stationary and when the fingers and wrist are gently moved if movement is meant to

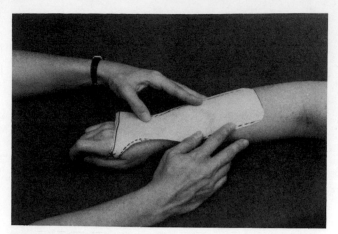

Figure 14.3 Paper pattern is fitted to the patient's hand.

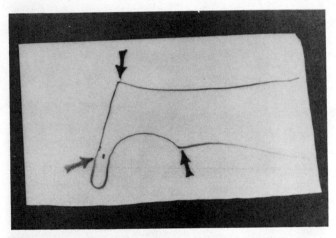

Figure 14.4 The pattern is transferred to the material (Aquaplast).

take place. Extra material is snipped away or tucks made, and lacking material is added until the final pattern is perfected. The thickness of the splinting material to be used must be allowed for in the paper pattern; any part that wraps around must be longer by twice the thickness of the material.

Recommended Criteria of Fit of a Hand Splint

Because of the need to apply correct forces and to make the orthosis comfortable and safe, certain recommendations for fitting hand splints have evolved. These criteria of fit are also used during the checkout process to be described later.

1. Any splint follows the contour of the hand and forearm as closely as possible to prevent pressure points and/or friction.

2. The longitudinal and distal transverse arches are maintained to preserve the ability to grasp various-shaped objects.[2] The distal transverse arch consists of the relatively immobile radial metacarpals around which the mobile thumb and ulnar metacarpals ro-

tate.[2] If viewed in the transverse plane, the metacarpal heads of the normal fisted hand describe an oblique line that descends from high to low from the radial to ulnar side.[2] The splint will accommodate this obliquity by being higher on the radial side than the ulnar side. The longitudinal arch includes the carpals, metacarpals, and phalanges and allows approximately 280° of total active flexion of each finger.[2]

3. The fingers are in functional position: semiflexion.

4. The thumb is in functional position: abduction and opposition.

5. The wrist is in neutral position or in 15° to 30° of dorsiflexion, depending on the patient's condition and the purpose of the splint.

6. A wrist splint extends two-thirds the length of the forearm for proper leverage. It does not extend so far as to interfere with elbow motion.

7. Except in special circumstances, volar hand splints must allow 90° of metacarpophalangeal flexion and therefore not extend beyond the distal palmar crease. This crease also guides the correct oblique angle the splint should have to accommodate the decreased length of the metacarpals from radial to ulnar fingers.[2]

8. Because a splint should not unnecessarily restrict motion that the patient has, the ideal length of a short hand splint is that it extend on the dorsum of the hand from the most distal wrist crease to a diagonal line drawn over the dorsum of the hand proximal to the metacarpophalangeal joints and connecting the ends of the volar palmar creases. This length will prevent restriction of motion at the wrist and at the metacarpophalangeal joints.

9. Finger and thumb pieces are long enough to give adequate support but not so long as to interfere with pinch or cause pressure on opposing fingertips.

10. The splint does not impinge on the thenar eminence, which would restrict motion.

11. For stability and comfort, the width of the forearm piece extends from the lateral to the medial midline of the forearm.

12. Bony prominences are kept free from pressure either by not covering them or by pushing out space above them.

13. Allowance is made in dorsal hand splints for padding over the metacarpal area because of the need to protect superficial bones and tendons.

14. The straps are wide to distribute the pressure; tight, narrow, encircling parts and straps are avoided.

15. Outriggers are positioned so that the rotational force is applied perpendicularly to the bone to which it attaches.[3]

16. The dynamic force exerted by elastics is not so strong as to distort the joint.

17. Splints that have joints fit so that the axis of joint motion and the axis of splint motion are aligned.

18. There is no indication of excessive pressure (reddened skin areas 20 min after removal of the hand splint) after the splint has been worn for ½ hour.

SELECTION OF MATERIAL

Materials commonly used by occupational therapists include plaster of paris bandage and thermoplastics. A representative sampling of thermoplastics will be discussed; the advantages and disadvantages of each can be judged by the reader on the basis of the properties of each and the methods required to work with each. This is not a comprehensive list of available materials. The reader is referred to rehabilitation supply house catalogues and conference displays for the latest materials as they are developed.

High-temperature plastics become soft and can be formed when they are heated in the oven to about 300° to 350°F[5] (149° to 177°C). Because they are so hot when malleable, these plastics must be formed on a mold. These materials are strong and rigid when cooled; therefore, splint designs having more delicate parts can be used. Royalite, Plastazote, and Kydex are examples of this type of material. Royalite comes in a variety of colors. Preformed resting hand and wrist splints made of this material are commercially available. Plastazote is a lightweight, strong, but soft, material that looks foamy but is actually a closed cell material and therefore water-resistant. Plastazote (foamed cross-linked polyethylene) comes in various densities and colors. Kydex is similar to Royalite except that it stays malleable for a longer period when heated and is available in colors of flesh beige to parchment.[8]

Low-temperature plastics are heated to 140° to 170°F (60° to 77°C) in hot water before forming directly onto the patient after a momentary pause to allow some air-cooling.[5] They can be reheated and adjusted if an error is made. Orthoplast, Aquaplast, Polyform, and Hexcelite are examples of these plastics. Orthoplast is a white, waxy, smooth or perforated material that is elastic when hot. It fuses to itself when hot, which is desirable when adding pieces but which ruins the splint if it happens accidentally. Polyform[8] is a whitish-beige, waxy surfaced material that is self-adhering when hot, rigid when cool, nontoxic, and biodegradable. It has a critical working temperature range of 140° to 167°F; below 140°F it will not soften enough to be workable and above 167°F it will become too pliable, sticky, and stretched out.[7] Aquaplast is an off-white material that molds easily—"drapes onto the skin"—when warm. A less pliable version is available, called Green Stripe Aquaplast. Both types are equally rigid when cool.[9] Aquaplast is transparent when warm, which allows immediate correction of pressure areas. It fuses to itself and other materials unless they are lubricated or wet and cool. Hexcelite is a white mesh material that is both lightweight and highly ventilated. It permits evaporation of perspiration, which reduces risk of skin maceration.[10] It is rigid enough to be used for casting and fracture bracing and flexible enough for orthotic uses. The open weave allows observation of the skin during molding to aid in precise fitting.[11] It bonds to itself. Polyform and Aquaplast are more stretchy than Orthoplast, and therefore some therapists prefer them for molding outriggers and other intricate parts or small finger splints.

Splints made of low-temperature plastics lose their shape if left in hot cars, submerged in hot water, or left near radiators. In time, the cumulative effects of body heat may also loosen the fit.

Plaster of paris does not require heating to form it, but in the process of curing, heat is generated; therefore, the patient's skin must be protected. Splints are made from plaster of paris bandage, a gauze material impregnated with plaster of paris. It requires 2 to 12 hours of drying time. It is not washable as the other materials are unless the splint has been treated by painting it with varnish or enamel. It is comparably very inexpensive, so plaster bandage is often chosen when a splint needs frequent modification. Wires for outriggers and reinforcement are easily added.

SPLINTMAKING PROCEDURES (FIG. 14.5–14.14)

After the splint design has been selected, the pattern fitted to the patient, and the material selected to best suit both the purpose of the splint and the skill of the therapist, the procedures listed below for the material selected are followed for the actual construction of the splint.

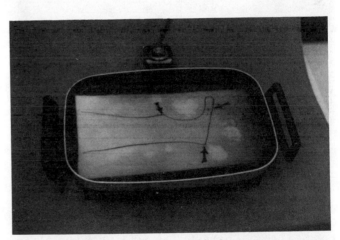

Figure 14.5 Aquaplast is warmed before cutting.

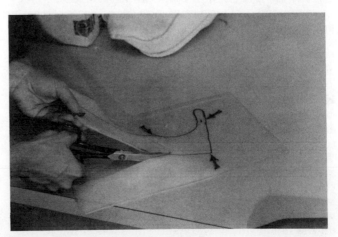

Figure 14.6 The splint is cut out.

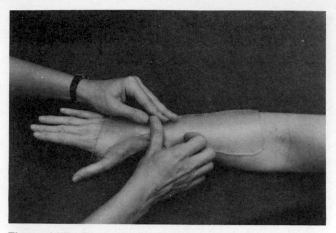

Figure 14.7 The splint is fitted to conform to the contours of the forearm.

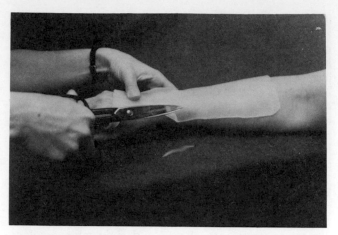

Figure 14.9 Adjustments are made as necessary by snipping off excess material.

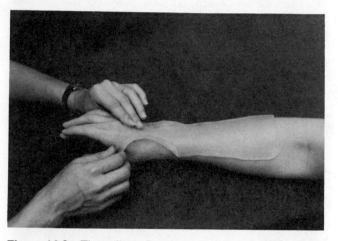

Figure 14.8 The splint is fitted to the contours of the hand.

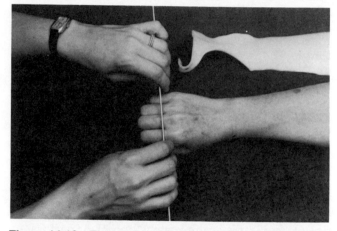

Figure 14.10 The width of the outrigger is measured.

Royalite® (Uniroyal, Inc.) and Kydex® (Rohm & Haas). *Marking the Pattern onto the Material.* Any writing instrument may be used. Sharp curves must be notched because Royalite does not stretch and Kydex has only a limited stretch characteristic when heated.

Cutting. A jig saw or band saw may be used.

Reinforcing. This is not necessary because these are very strong and rigid materials.

Finishing Edges. Sand or file the edges using a power sander, sandpaper, or a wood file. The edges may also be buffed using a machine buffer.

Adding Straps. Prior to shaping the Royalite or Kydex, holes are drilled for the rivets that will hold the straps on. Straps are made from 1-inch (2.5-cm) wide cotton webbing and fastened with a Velcro closure. A 1- to 2-inch (2.5- to 5-cm) strip of the hook part of the Velcro is glued or riveted to the outside of the splint after the splint is shaped, and a similar-sized strip of the soft part of the Velcro is glued and sewn to the strap. In this way only the soft part comes into contact with the patient's skin. The closure is usually located on the radial side of the splint since it is easier for the patient to fasten. Attach the straps using rivets after

the splint is shaped. A rounded anvil may be necessary to use as a striking surface if the strap is added to a curved area: the rivet must be applied so that it is smooth on the inside of the splint to prevent irritation to the patient's skin. Straps may also be added using contact cement or self-adhesive Velcro.

Adding Outriggers. Outriggers are extensions added to splints. They are used to suspend rubber bands with finger cuffs attached to them to support or stretch the fingers or thumb into certain positions. The outrigger must be angled in such a way as to allow the rubber band to approach the finger at a 90° angle (Fig. 14.11). Outriggers of Royalite, Kydex, or aluminum may be added using rivets. The holes for the rivets are drilled prior to shaping.

Shaping. Place the cut-out splint on a flat surface such as a board or a cookie sheet. Heat the Royalite in a 300°F oven (149°C) or the Kydex in a 350°F (177°C) oven for several minutes to soften the material in preparation for shaping; bubbling indicates overheating. Use potholder mitts while forming the hot material over a wooden or a plaster of paris mold of the patient's hand. These materials set into shape as they cool,

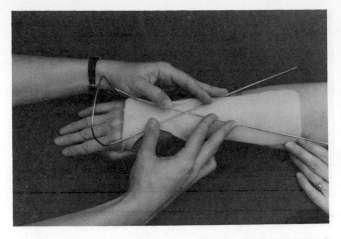

Figure 14.11 After shaping, the length of the outrigger is measured.

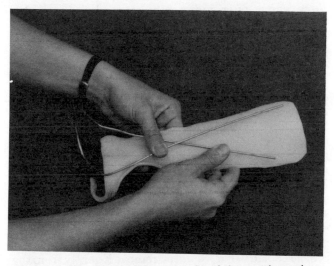

Figure 14.12 After cutting, the fit of the outrigger is re-checked.

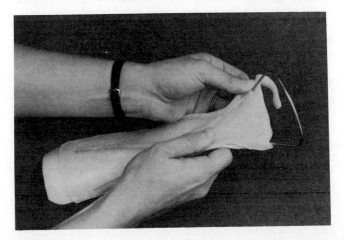

Figure 14.13 The reinforcement piece of Aquaplast is added to hold the outrigger in place.

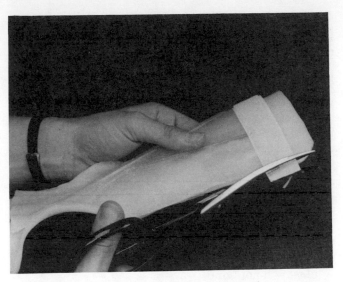

Figure 14.14 Straps are added and trimmed.

which happens very quickly for Royalite and a little less quickly for Kydex.

Plastazote® (Smith & Nephew Rolyan, Inc.)[12,13]
Marking the Pattern onto the Material. Use a pencil to mark the pattern. Plastazote comes in 2- to 30-mm thicknesses. The usual thickness chosen for neck collars and arm splints is 9 mm. This thickness need not be taken into consideration when preparing the paper pattern because the material expands approximately 25 to 30 mm when heated.

Cutting. A sharp knife or scissors may be used to cut the cold material.

Reinforcing. Two sheets of Plastazote placed one on top of the other in a 140°C (284°F) oven will laminate. A piece of solid, low-density polyethylene sheeting can be inserted between the layers before fusion for added strength.

Finishing Edges. A very sharp knife is used for trimming; an emery wheel or no. 1 glass paper is used for smoothing. Warm water and detergent wash marks off.

Adding Straps. Rivets or double-sided tape are used to attach the straps.

Shaping. A layer of closely fitting stockinet is placed on the patient. The splint is placed on a board covered with the easy-release paper provided with the material or dusted with French chalk and put into a 140°C oven (284°F) for a period of time that is twelve times (in seconds) the thickness (in millimeters). It must not be heated above 160°C (320°F). The material cools quickly. The surface temperature is checked before applying it to the patient. Mold it directly on the patient, who has been protected with stockinet, by gently stretching it to fit the contours. Plastazote sets in the same amount of time it takes to heat it and may be removed from the patient after 2 to 3 min. It is cooled thoroughly before finishing.

Orthoplast® (Johnson & Johnson).[14] *Marking the Pattern onto the Material.* Use a grease crayon. Ball point pen ink cannot be removed and a pencil will not mark. The pattern must not have slender, delicate parts because such parts will require excessive reinforcement to be strong enough, which will make the splint unacceptably bulky.

Cutting. Scissors are used to cut the material after it is heated for a few moments in hot water. Long strokes are made with the scissors to get as smooth an edge as possible.

Reinforcing. Several methods may be used:

1. A strip of Orthoplast can be fused to the as-yet unformed splint by heating both pieces and firmly pressing them together at exactly the place where the reinforcement is desired. You cannot separate fused Orthoplast. On the other hand, dirty Orthoplast will not bond.
2. For added strength, an aluminum strip or wire may be embedded between the two pieces of Orthoplast before they are fused.
3. A soda straw may be placed between the two pieces of Orthoplast before they are fused so that the reinforcing Orthoplast piece becomes semitubular and therefore stronger than a flat piece.
4. Edges can be "hemmed," that is, folded over to add strength. This method gives a finished look if done very neatly.

Finishing Edges. Soften the Orthoplast edges with a bonding iron and smooth the edges with the iron or with a finger. Folded edges need no further finishing.

Adding Straps. There are several methods by which straps can be added to an Orthoplast splint. One way is to use contact cement to hold the strap and the hook part of Velcro on. Self-adhesive Velcro may also be used. Another way is to use a leather punch to punch holes in the splint where rivets will be used to hold on the straps. A third way is unique to Orthoplast, Polyform, and Hexcelite because of their self-bonding characteristic: the straps are attached using strips or buttons of Orthoplast in the following manner (Fig. 14.15). A narrow (approximately 3-mm or ⅛-inch) strip of Orthoplast is cut one and a half times as long as the strap is wide. For example, if the strap is 1 inch wide, the little Orthoplast strip will be about 1½ inches long. Two large holes are punched in the webbing strap, and it is aligned onto the splint in the desired location. A bonding iron is used to heat a small area adjacent to the edge of the strap, then one end of the little strip of Orthoplast is heated and bonded there next to the strap. In the same manner, the little strip is bonded to the underlying Orthoplast first in one hole of the strap, then in the other, then on the far edge.

Adding Outriggers. Wire, aluminum, or Royalite outriggers can be added to Orthoplast by embedding the ends between layers of Orthoplast and fusing them there. This must be done before the splint is actually shaped. The outrigger may be also riveted for strength.

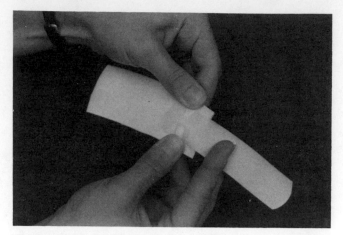

Figure 14.15 Orthoplast strap applied to a scrap piece using self-bonding method.

Very short outriggers can be made of doubled Orthoplast fused together and can be attached by fusion. Orthoplast is too weak to be used for longer outriggers. If the splint is already formed, the small Orthoplast outrigger may be attached by spot heating the splint at the desired location and fusing the hot outrigger to it, or the outrigger can be added using rivets.

Shaping. Heat the Orthoplast in 140° to 170°F (60° to 77°C) water. Remove the Orthoplast from the hot water by using tongs. Dry it or expose it to the air momentarily to cool it to a reasonable temperature before forming it directly on the patient. Smooth and hold the entire splint until it cools and hardens, which may be speeded up by immersing the splinted hand in cool water or ice water. Immersion in ice water produces physiological effects in a person; therefore, if the splint is to be cooled using ice water, remove it gently from the patient after a few moments when it has begun to firm up, then put it in the ice water. A large splint should be loosely wrapped in ace bandage or should have a piece of close-fitting stockinet placed over it to help hold it in proper contour during the cooling and hardening process. Orthoplast is very elastic and molds very well in convex and concave curves if repeatedly smoothed over curved areas.

Polyform® (Smith & Nephew Rolyan, Inc.).[7] *Marking the Pattern onto the Material.* A pen or scratch awl may be used on cold Polyform. A fingernail will mark soft Polyform.

Cutting. Scissors are used to cut the material after it has been warmed for 20 to 25 sec in water that is 150° to 160°F (66° to 71°C). Care must be taken to prevent this highly self-adhering material from fusing during the cutting process. Rose pruners or a saw can be used to cut unheated Polyform.

Reinforcing. Press together two dry pieces of properly heated Polyform and they will fuse. Aluminum or wire strips may be added between the fused layers for added support, although this may be rarely necessary due to the rigidity of the cooled material. The edges can be "hemmed" or rolled over for reinforcement and for a finished look.

Finishing Edges. Heated edges can be smoothed with the finger, the edges can be rolled, or cold Polyform can be filed, sanded, or buffed.

Adding Straps. This can be done in the same ways as described for Orthoplast.

Adding Outriggers. Aluminum outriggers can be added by riveting them or embedding them between layers of Polyform from which the clear coating is scraped off and which are then fused together. Outriggers made of doubled-over and fused Polyform are probably rigid enough to be used to support weak digits. The Polyform outrigger adheres to a Polyform splint best if both it and the part to which it is being attached are dry and hot. Polyform will not stick to Orthoplast, polyethylene, polypropylene, wax paper, human skin, or hair.

Shaping. The best method for softening Polyform for shaping is to use heated water. The recommended temperature range for ⅛-inch Polyform is 150° to 160°F (66° to 71°C). Do not lay it on the bottom of a pan because if it overheats, it will stick. A heat gun can be used to heat small areas. Overheating causes the material to become sticky. If this should happen, lay it on a flat surface to cool slightly. The material can be formed directly on the patient. It stretches and follows concave and convex contours easily. This property makes it a useful material to use to make adapted handles on utensils or tools. Scrap pieces can be used for this purpose.

Aquaplast® (WFR/Aquaplast Corp.).[4,9] Use regular Aquaplast for small splints and Green Stripe for large ones. The therapist's hands must be wet at all times when working on warm Aquaplast.

Marking the Pattern onto the Material. The wet pattern is simply placed under the transparent material, and the splint is cut out according to the pattern. Or a grease pencil can be used to trace the pattern onto the material.

Cutting. The splint design can be cut using long-bladed shears when the material is warm, but hazy and no longer sticky. A piece the size of the splint should be cut from the stock when the material is cold by using a razor-blade knife to score the material and then breaking off the piece. A band saw or heavy shears can also be used when the material is cold.

Reinforcing. Regular Aquaplast can be used for reinforcement. It instantly self-bonds in a softened state. Heat the reinforcement in water until it is transparent; spot heat the splint where the attachment is to be made; apply the reinforcement piece and feather the edges with a wet finger. A bond will not occur if there is grease on the material.

Finishing Edges. Use a potato peeler or leather edger to bevel the edges. Then, dip the edge into hot water and polish it with the heel of the hand. Quench in cold water to set the new, smooth edge. Edges can also be hemmed over within the first minute after being removed from the hot water.

Adding Straps. To attach a patch of hook Velcro, spot heat the splint where the patch is to be applied, while at the same time softening a thin strip of Aquaplast. Place the patch of Velcro over the heated spot, wet your fingers, and stretch the thin strip of Aquaplast around the Velcro, overlapping the edge all around, and press it down firmly. To attach a strap, cut notches on both edges of the strap near the end to be attached to the splint. Spot heat the splint where the strap is to go, while warming a patch of Aquaplast of a size large enough to cover the end of the strap. With a wet finger, press the soft patch around the end of the strap and into the notches to bond the strap to the splint. Self-adhesive Velcro can also be used.

Adding Outriggers. Outriggers are attached in the same manner that reinforcements are. Both surfaces must be hot; dry heat forms the most secure bonds. Rivets may also be used.

Shaping. Heat in 140°F (60°C) water just until the material becomes transparent. An Aquaplast Frypan Guard *must* be used to prevent the Aquaplast from sticking to the pan when hot. When soft, lift the Aquaplast out of the hot water on the Frypan Guard mesh. Place it, mesh side down, on a terry towel. Wet your hands to handle the material. The patient's arm must also be wet with water and then the slightly cooled (about 30 sec) Aquaplast can be molded directly. Mold into and around concave and convex surfaces. It will cling to the limb when stretched. Aquaplast shrinks 2% as it cools and will become too tight around bony prominences unless spread slightly as it cools. As Aquaplast cools, the splint will lift from the skin, signifying it is rigid enough to remove without deforming. Hasten cooling by immersing in cold water or by using an ice pack or cold spray.

Hinges. Hinges can be formed between two pieces of Aquaplast (or other splinting material) using rivets by making the holes slightly larger than the rivet post. The rivet is hammered until it is secure, but not tight, and the pieces may still move freely.

Hexcelite® (Hexcel Medical, Ltd.).[10,15] *Marking the Pattern onto the Material.* The pattern is not marked on the material, but rather the paper pattern is laid atop the required layers of Hexcelite and cut out, allowing 1 cm excess all around to be used for a turned-over edge.

Cutting. Hexcelite is easily cut hot or cold.

Reinforcing. Several layers may be used together to provide the amount of rigidity required. Holding the layers together, the splint is heated for 10 sec. After the excess water is blotted away, the splint is rolled out on a flat, hard surface using a rolling pin to ensure good bonding between the layers. The tools, work surface, and therapist's hands must all be wet to avoid bonding. Rolling the 1-cm edge over also provides some stability while avoiding the rough edges of the cut material.

Finishing Edges. While the material is still soft, and after the edges have been rolled over, they are smoothed by rubbing them with a flat metal edge.

Adding Straps. A hole is cut in the strap. Small double patches of Hexcelite are cut approximately 1 cm larger than the end of the strap. Hot water is poured onto the sites of the splint where the straps will be attached (bonding occurs only if both Hexcelite surfaces are hot). The heated patches are secured atop the strap, making sure a good bond is achieved through the cutout.

D-rings may be attached to the splint by cutting lengths of Hexcelite slightly wider than the D-ring. The Hexcelite is then softened, stretched diagonally, and threaded through the D-ring. The material is folded and pressed together into a fan shape. The ring must be pivoted while the Hexcelite is setting up to ensure free movement. When it is set, the ends of the Hexcelite are softened and attached to the splint as described for attaching straps. The top of the ring should be located just below the edge of the splint to prevent pinching the patient's skin when cinching the strap.

Adding Outriggers. This step is not mentioned in the technical literature; however, it seems plausible that this could be done similarly to the way it is done using plaster of paris. Finger spreaders are added by bonding the parts as described above.

Shaping. Heat the Hexcelite in 160°F (71°C) water. A thin film of lanolin should be applied to the patient's limb. Blot the excess water off the splint and apply the softened splint directly to the limb and gently mold according to the criteria of good fit listed above while avoiding pressure points. Hold in position for about 1 min until the splint is firm enough to remove it. The splint can be reheated if remolding is necessary.

Plaster of Paris Bandage. To make a slab-type splint from plaster of paris bandage, cut strips equal to the length of the pattern. Enough strips are cut to make 8 to 10 layers. The number of layers needed depends on the amount of support required. The pattern is drawn on the bandage using a pencil and may be cut out with large scissors. Any outriggers or straps should then be made because they will be embedded in the plaster as the splint is formed. Outriggers can be made from coat hangers or from brass welding rods that will not rust. The part of the outrigger that will be embedded in the splint must conform to the shape of the part to be splinted. If the outrigger rod is round rather than flat, the part to be embedded should be flattened or serpentined so that it will not rotate between the layers of plaster bandage.

Allowing extra length, place a close-fitting tubular stockinet bandage over the part of the patient's limb to be splinted. Then dip half of the plaster layers in lukewarm water one at a time; cooler water slows down setting time and warmer water speeds up setting time. Gently squeeze out the bandage until it just stops dripping; more water slows down setting time and less water speeds up setting time. Next, place the bandage over the part to be splinted, for example, the anterior wrist, palm, and forearm when making a cock-up splint, making sure the pattern of the strip conforms as it should. Smooth it with the fingers to spread the plaster particles into the gauze bandage. Apply several layers in this manner.

The stockinet should be trimmed to within ½ to ¾ inch from the edge of the plaster and folded up onto the plaster bandage to form a "hem." Wetting the stockinet will hold it to the plaster as it is turned up. If outriggers or reinforcing aluminum strips are to be added to the basic splint, these should now be added by attaching the outrigger with small strips of wet plaster bandage that are looped over the metal rod and pressed onto the plaster; small squares of plaster bandage also help reinforce and secure the outrigger. Next, lay the straps across the splint at the proper locations. Now wet, squeeze, and smooth the remaining plaster layers and place them on the splint to cover the stockinet edges, outriggers, and straps. Additional plaster strips should be placed near strap edges and to cover any edges which are uneven. Sprinkle talcum powder and rub it into the splint surface to obtain a smooth, shiny surface.

Note. The curing process of plaster produces heat and causes slight shrinking. If the patient is sensitive to heat, several layers of stockinet must be used. The splint may be carefully removed from the patient for the curing and drying process as soon as the shape has been set.

Making a Mold of Patient's Hand. To make a mold that can be used to form a splint made of the high-temperature materials, it is necessary to make a negative mold first, then a positive mold. The process of making a palmar mold of the hand and forearm will be described. This type of mold can be used to form a resting pan, wrist cock-up, or other volar splints that do not have circumferential parts. The same process may be used to make a dorsal mold, of course. The process for making a mold of the entire hand or forearm, that is, one that encircles these parts, is complicated and will not be included here. The reader is referred to Malick.[5,8]

NEGATIVE PLASTER OF PARIS PALMAR MOLD.[5] Cut three or four pieces of plaster of paris bandage long enough to extend from the patient's fingertips to approximately 1 inch (2.5 cm) below the elbow. Cut a 4- to 5-inch (10 to 12.5-cm) slit in the end of each piece of the bandage approximately 1½ inches (3.7 cm) from the side edge of the bandage; this will allow the thumb to be positioned in abduction. Apply mineral oil or petroleum jelly to the entire area to be covered by the plaster bandage. Loosely roll up the first piece of plaster bandage and dip it into a bowl of lukewarm water. Holding the rolled bandage by two ends, gently squeeze excess water out but do not wring it so hard that much of the plaster is squeezed out. Unroll the bandage strip, place it over the forearm and hand of the patient, and smooth it carefully to eliminate wrinkles and to work the plaster into the bandage. The patient's limb must be held in a functional position while this mold is being made.

Repeat with the remaining pieces of bandage, making certain to smooth each carefully so that the layers of bandage will adhere to each other.

The limb is held in the functional position until the plaster hardens. Fast-setting plaster bandage sets in about 5 min.

Mark vertical lines on each side of the cast using a rule and indelible pencil and indicate the width that the cast edges should be separated at these points; these lines and measurements are used to realign the cast should it become distorted in the process of removing it from the patient or pouring the positive mold.

Slide the patient's hand out of the mold. Realign the mold according to the markings and maintain this position by using narrow strips of plaster bandage to bridge the open side of the mold.

An alternative way to construct a negative mold, when exact fit over contoured areas is important, is to use a silicone elastomer. Directions for use of Alginate Dental Impression Material have been published.[16] Apply petroleum jelly over the entire area to be molded. The Alginate (Jeltrate) is prepared in a flexible bowl using cold water by quickly spatulating the mixture against the sides of the bowl to eliminate bubbles. It is poured over the part to be molded. It would be helpful to place the hand and arm in a small plastic dishpan that has one end cut out to accommodate the arm that must be held flat in position. The excess material could then be easily discarded. After the Alginate sets, it is reinforced with at least four layers of plaster bandage, which are smoothed into the impression contours. After the plaster bandage begins to set, the patient is asked to move or contract his muscles to help break the vacuum to remove the mold. The ends are covered with plaster bandage to form a "bowl" shape to receive the plaster of paris that will be used to make the positive mold.

POSITIVE MOLD.   Place strips of plaster bandage over the finger, thumb, and elbow edges of the negative mold to make the mold a container that will hold the plaster when poured. Use a brush to coat the inside of the negative mold with a substance such as liquid green soap, which will allow the positive mold to eventually be separated from the negative mold.

Mix plaster of paris in a flexible bowl or in a waxed milk carton by placing about 2 cups of water into the bowl and slowly adding and mixing plaster until it is of the consistency of cake batter.

Pour the plaster into the negative mold, gently shaking and tapping the negative mold to eliminate air bubbles. Add more plaster to fill the mold and tap again. Insert a metal rod lengthwise into the thumb section to reinforce it and a larger rod or dowel into the length of the whole mold. These rods protrude from the mold and allow it to be held securely in a vise when later using the positive mold for shaping the high-temperature plastics.

Allow the plaster to set. *Do not pour excess plaster into a sink drain; it will harden there.* When the excess plaster has set up in the bowl, that is the clue that the mold is also ready for the next step. Remove the excess plaster from the bowl by flexing the sides of the bowl and dispose of it in the trash.

Gently remove the positive mold from the negative one by removing the narrow strips of bandage that were used to bridge the width of the negative mold and by spreading the sides of the negative mold as you extract the positive. Be careful not to damage the more delicate thumb part.

Smooth any ridges by using a file, sandpaper, or a piece of wire mesh screening. After the plaster has dried for about ½ hour, sand it smooth. Allow to dry overnight before using it.

Checkout of the Splint

It is the responsibility of the occupational therapist to check out the fit of any upper-extremity orthosis or any splint which he or she has made. The checkout is the process of examining the fit, function, and reliability of the orthosis. The checkout is done before establishing a wearing schedule and before either controls or use training. Periodic recheck of the orthosis may be necessary for those patients who wear the orthosis on a permanent or long-term basis.

The checkout considers the following points:

1. Does the orthosis actually accomplish the purpose for which it was intended? If not, it must be remade or redesigned.

2. Are the insides, edges, rivets, etc., padded and/or smooth to prevent skin abrasions? If not, they must be smoothed or padded. Many manufacturers of orthotic materials also manufacture self-adhesive padding material that can be cut with scissors and quickly applied. The size of the splint must allow for the extra room needed for adding padding.

3. Are there red areas on the patient's skin, indicating pressure, which remain for 20 min after the splint has been removed following wear for ½ hour? If so, pressure must be relieved by spot heating the thermoplastic splint and pushing the material out away from the patient. *Do not add padding;* this increases the pressure. A plaster splint will need to be remade.

4. Does the splint conform to the recommended criteria of good fit stated previously? If not, it must be corrected by cutting, reshaping, or even rebuilding.

The forms in Tables 14.1 and 14.2 are examples of ones that may be used for orthotic check-out.

Establishing the Wearing Schedule

A patient adjusts to his new splint over time by following a wearing schedule that designates the amount of time the splint is to be worn and the amount of time the splint should remain off. The wearing schedule for a splint designed to correct deformity will start with a very brief wearing period, whereas a supporting splint will start with a wearing schedule of ½ hour or longer on and ½ hour off. When the splint is off, the patient will exercise the part or do his hygiene or other tasks

Table 14.1
CHECKOUT FOR HAND SPLINTS

		General Considerations
Yes	No	Is the splint on the patient correctly?
Yes	No	Does this splint needlessly immobilize a joint?
Yes	No	If the splint, or parts of it, immobilizes a joint, is the splint removed periodically and the joints moved through passive range of motion?
Yes	No	Does this splint actually accomplish the function for which it was intended?
Yes	No	Does this splint cover the least amount of skin area to permit tactile sensation, but also provide good distribution of force over sufficiently large areas?
Yes	No	After wearing the splint for ½ hour does the patient have reddened areas?
Yes	No	Do these disappear within 15 to 20 minutes?
Yes	No	Is the splint cosmetically acceptable to the patient?
		Traction Splints
Yes	No	If elastics are used, do they pull perpendicularly to the part as they should?
Yes	No	Is the tension in the elastics exactly right (just enough to provide a small force beyond that needed to pull the part to the limit of range of motion)?
Yes	No	If this is a static traction splint, is the force just enough to push slightly beyond the limit of range of motion?
Yes	No	Is the traction force distributed over as large an area as possible?
Yes	No	Is the force adjusted periodically to keep up with the changes in the patient's limits of range of motion?
Yes	No	Has a wearing schedule been established?
		Externally Powered Hand Splints
Yes	No	Is the splint mechanism reliable? If not, what seems to be the problem?
Yes	No	Is the control located at a site over which the patient has voluntary control, has sensation, and which does not trigger the control accidentally during habitual movements?
Yes	No	Does the control work reliably, i.e., the same signal repeatedly causes same response?
Yes	No	Can the patient operate the controls with the splint held in any position?
Yes	No	Can the patient put it on by himself or clearly instruct another in its application?
Yes	No	Is the power source ready for use? When does it get refilled or recharged?_____ By whom?_____ How?_____
Yes	No	Does the splint prevent the patient from doing any functional activity he can otherwise do? What?_____ Why?_____
		Can the patient pick up correctly:
Yes	No	Squashable things (paper cup, marshmallow, cotton, etc.)
Yes	No	Glass or metal objects
Yes	No	Thin things (cards, paper, checkers)
Yes	No	Small things (pencil, dice)
Yes	No	Eating utensils
Yes	No	Large things (beer can, cup, razor)

As an indication of the patient's level of learning to control an externally powered orthosis, evaluate the variability of performance over time.

Each day, measure the time, in tenths of seconds, of 20 trials of picking up and releasing a 1-inch cube on command. Be sure that the cube is placed at the same place each time and that the patient starts from the same position each time. The cube is released into a small box that is consistently positioned. The variability of one 20-trial session can be estimated by noting the range of scores and measured by calculating the standard deviation. The more consistent the perfomance, the lower the deviation, indicating that learning has occurred. Graphing each day's standard deviation will allow the patient to track his progress and the therapist to know when learning levels off.

One formula for standard deviation is:

$$ SD = \sqrt{\frac{\Sigma x^2}{n-1}} $$

Where Σ = sum, x = difference between each score and the mean of all trials, and n = number of trials.

permitted by the physician. No splint remains on for 24 hours without being removed to permit exercise and hygiene.

The wearing period is gradually increased to the full amount of time prescribed. The time is increased as the discomfort subsides or the patient learns to tolerate the strangeness of a device attached to him. A reasonable tolerance to a splint that is meant to be used at night is developed during the day so that the patient's sleep will not be repeatedly interrupted by discomfort or the handling of the splint by the nurse as it is removed and reapplied.

The wearing schedule is established by the physician who ordered the orthosis, by the therapist who made or checked it out, or preferably by these two professionals in collaboration with each other.

Table 14.2

FACTORS TO EVALUATE IN CHECKING OUT A HAND SPLINT[a]

A. Fit:
  1. Are all bony prominences, such as the head of the ulna, free from pressure?
  2. Is available passive range of motion permitted at wrist and metacarpophalangeal and interphalangeal joints if desired?
  3. Does the palmar piece conform to the contour of the palmar arch?
  4. Does the forearm piece conform to the contour of the forearm?
  5. If the splint has an action wrist, does the forearm piece stay in position during wrist extension, so that the joint of the splint remains aligned with the wrist joint?
  6. Do all splint joints approximate their corresponding anatomical joints?
  7. Is the lumbrical bar or metacarpophalangeal flexion control placed so that it lies just proximally to the proximal interphalangeal joints?
  8. Does the C-bar extend just proximally to the interphalangeal joint of the thumb so that it does not restrict motion of this joint?
  9. Does the opponens bar hold the first metacarpal opposed, that is, in front of the palm and under the second metacarpal?
  10. If the thumb is posted, does the thumb post hold the interphalangeal joint of the thumb extended, the thumb opposed and in full abduction, or as close to that position as the patient's passive range of motion will allow?
  11. Is splint construction sturdy enough to hold the wrist in functional position as the patient moves his fingers?
B. Comfort (applies to patients who have sensation):
  1. Is the splint comfortable? If not, can it be made comfortable by:
    a. easing the corrective forces?
    b. improving the fit?
    c. adjusting the tension or angles of pull of elastics or springs?
  2. How long can the patient wear the splint without discomfort?
C. Function:
  1. When relaxed, is the hand as near the functional position as the passive range of motion will permit?
  2. Does the splint restrict full forearm pronation, thereby interfering with effective prehension?
  3. In a prehension splint, do the index and middle finger pads have maximal contact with the thumb pad?
  4. During pinching, are thumb and finger pads free of metal?
  5. Does the splint permit functional grasp of small and large objects?
  6. Is release of grasp adequate for function?
  7. With a flexor hinge splint, are ulnar fingers positioned so that they do not interfere with pinch or grasp?
  8. Is the wrist of a flexor hinge splint positioned so that the patient can pick up objects from flat surfaces?
  9. Is the splint made for ease of application and removal by patient?
  10. Do corrective parts obtain maximal correction within the patient's tolerance?
  11. In a wrist-driven splint, does the amount of pinch force represent an effective relationship to wrist extensor power?
  12. Is release of pinch adequate for function?
  13. Do extension assists restrict maximal pinch?
D. Information that might be recorded to help evaluate function:
  1. What is the force of the muscle power driving the splint?
  2. What is the lateral prehension force without the splint?
  3. What is the palmar prehension force without the splint?
  4. What is the prehension force in the splint?
  5. How many inches is the finger opening of the splint with the patient's hand in it? Measure from the tip of thumb to tip of index finger.

[a]Revised and adapted from a form developed by the Occupational Therapy Department of Rancho Los Amigos Hospital, Downey, CA.

Handle Adaptations

Three materials are pliable enough to be fashioned into adapted handles. Hexcelite[17] and Polyform[18] bond to themselves so that they can be rolled into a tube to lengthen a handle of a tool or utensil. Keys or other small knobs can be enlarged by pressing pieces of the material, cut to extend beyond the edges of the object, together to enclose the piece to be enlarged.

Adapt-It[19] is a low-temperature thermoplastic pellet material. It can be softened using boiling water in any hot water container, including a styrofoam cup. As the pellets melt they form a transparent ball around the stirrer (tongue depressor, etc.). The ball of resin is removed from the cup and blotted dry. When cooled to the touch, it is pulled from the stirrer, kneaded, and formed into whatever shape desired. It hardens as it cools; cooling can be speeded up by use of cold water or ice.

STUDY QUESTIONS:

Materials and Methods of Construction of Temporary Orthoses

1. What is the goal of hand splinting?
2. Explain the mechanical principles that support the clinical observation that long, wide splints cause fewer secondary problems than do short, narrow ones.

3. Why are outriggers mounted so the line of pull is perpendicular to the part?
4. How would you know if a splint was exerting too much pressure on a patient's skin?
5. What points are considered during checkout of a splint?
6. Which of the splinting materials described here would you choose to make a thumb carpometacarpal stabilization splint for a 50-year-old female gardener with degenerative joint disease? On what factors is your choice based?
7. Describe how you could enlarge the handles of wooden cooking spoons for a patient with arthritis.
8. A quadriplegic patient is learning to operate his externally powered flexor hinge hand splint by picking up and releasing a 1-inch block into a box 20 times a day. On one day he achieved the following scores (recorded in sec.):

4.2	5.4	4.3	2.7
6.8	9.0	3.1	3.0
3.4	2.6	3.5	1.5
2.1	8.7	5.3	1.0
7.2	3.6	4.1	2.2
rest	rest	rest	end

How variable is his performance for the whole session? Calculate standard deviation. How can you determine whether his performance improved (learning) or deteriorated (fatigue) over time?

References

1. Anderson, M. *Upper Extremity Orthotics*, 3rd edition. Springfield, IL: Charles C Thomas, 1974.
2. Fess, E. E., Gettle, K. S., and Strickland, J. W. *Hand Splinting: Principles and Methods*. St. Louis: C. V. Mosby, 1981.
3. Colditz, J. C. Low profile dynamic splinting of the injured hand. *Am. J. Occup. Ther.*, 37(3): 182–188, 1983.
4. Wasserman, J. *Splinting with Aquaplast*, 2nd revision. Ramsey, NJ: WFR/Aquaplast Corp., 1983.
5. Malick, M. *Manual on Static Hand Splinting*. Pittsburgh: Harmarville Rehabilitation Center, 1972.
6. Tenney, C. G., and Lisak, J. M. *Atlas of Hand Splinting*. Boston: Little, Brown & Company, 1986.
7. Peterson, T. *Making Polyform Splints*. Technical Bulletins 4-105R-2, 4-123, 4-124, 4-125. Menomonee Falls, WI: Smith & Nephew Rolyan Inc. (out of print).
8. Malick, M. *Manual on Dynamic Hand Splinting with Thermoplastic Materials*. Pittsburgh: Harmarville Rehabilitation Center, 1974.
9. *Technical Bulletin 10/06/77*. WFR/Aquaplast Corporation, P.O. Box 327, Ramsey, NJ 07746.
10. *Technical Bulletin TC-486-5M*. Kirschner Medical, 10 West Aylesbury Rd., Timonium, MD 21093.
11. Parks, B. J., Barrett, K. P., and Voss, K. The use of hexcelite in splinting the thumb. *Am. J. Occup. Ther.*, 37(4): 266-267, 1983.
12. *Technical Information Manual: Plastazote*. Menomonee Falls, WI: Smith & Nephew Rolyan Inc., 1974.
13. *The Basic Principles of Evazote and Plastazote Moulding and Thermoforming*. Technical Information # ERP114. Croydon Surrey, Great Britain: Bakelite Xylonite, 1978.
14. *Orthoplast Splints: Instructions for Use*. New Brunswick: Johnson & Johnson.
15. Hicks, S., and McFetridge, L. Hand and wrist resting splint: suggested procedures. In *Hexcelite: Splinting and Seating Techniques*. Hexcel Ltd., Catherine House, 63 Guilford Rd., Lightwater, Surrey GU 18 5SA, England.
16. Rivers, E. A., Strate, R. G., and Solem, L. D. The transparent face mask. *Am. J. Occup. Ther.*, 33(2): 108–113, 1979.
17. Hicks, S., and Wathen, G. An aid to independence: suggested procedure. In *Hexcelite: Splinting and Seating Techniques*. Hexcel, Ltd., Catherine House, 63 Guilford Rd., Lightwater, Surrey GU 18 5SA, England.
18. Hansen, A. M. W. *Making Adaptive Equipment with Polyform*. Technical Bulletin 2-128-R1. Menomonee Falls, WI: Smith & Nephew Rolyan, Inc. (out of print).
19. *Adapt-It*. *Technical Bulletin*. WFR/Aquaplast Corp., P.O. Box 327, Ramsey, NJ 07446.

Supplementary Reading

Couchman, P. J. The use of Hexcelite as a splinting material for the acutely burned hand. *American Occupational Therapy Association Physical Disabilities Special Interest Newsletter*, 4(3): 3, 1981.
Mildenberger, L. A., Amadio, P. C., and An, K.-N. Dynamic splinting: a systemic approach to the selection of elastic traction. *Arch. Phys. Med. Rehabil.*, 67(4): 241–244, 1986.
Williams, M., and Lissner, H. R. *Biomechanics of Human Motion*. Philadelphia: W. B. Saunders, 1962.
Ziegler, E. A problem-solving approach to orthotic design. *The American Occupational Therapy Association Physical Disabilities Special Interest Section Newsletter*, 9(2): 4–5, 1986.

chapter
15

Wheelchair Measurement and Prescription

Catherine A. Trombly and Anna Deane Scott

It is essential that a wheelchair be correctly prescribed to meet the needs of the patient. It must be the type that offers the support required, is the correct size for comfort and prevention of decubiti, and has the features and accessories needed for safety and maximal independence.

Guidelines have been developed and validated for wheelchair selection for an elderly population in order to efficiently and correctly prescribe wheelchairs to meet the needs and capabilities of that population.[1] Guidelines for others have not been published; however, the catalogues of the many manufacturers of wheelchairs can be consulted to help in selecting the best wheelchair to suit each particular person. Complicating the choice will be whether the patient's eventual physical status is expected to be different from his current status. The choice needs to anticipate any change by either compromising between immediate and future needs or by being modifiable in the future while meeting the needs of the present.[2]

It may or may not be the occupational therapist's duty to measure the patient and prescribe the wheelchair, depending on the customary division of labor between occupational and physical therapy at a particular facility. Ideally this should be a collaborative decision among the occupational therapist, physical therapist, and the patient. The patient needs to develop a sense of ownership and control over this major orthosis and therefore should have opportunity to ensure that the choice fits his life-style and sense of style. The ordering of a person's permanent wheelchair is one of the psychological crises spoken of in chapter 2. The therapists, especially the occupational therapist, should be particularly attuned to the patient's emotional status at this time. Both therapists should be involved in the decision because each has certain functional goals in mind that the wheelchair should facilitate, or at least not prohibit. The therapists may also plan use of other orthotic equipment or adapted equipment for which the wheelchair must be compatible.

The occupational therapist will be responsible for ensuring that the patient learns how to use the wheelchair and its features in all expected situations of daily living. The occupational therapist is also the professional who usually does the checkout and controls training—driving skills—if the patient has an electric wheelchair. If the patient has a manually operated chair, he must learn mobility skills (chapter 17) for which either the occupational or physical therapist may take responsibility.

The therapist who takes major responsibility for teaching the patient how to use the wheelchair should also teach the patient and his family how to care for it. Care includes keeping the wheelchair clean and lubricated and, if electric, the battery charged. Care instruction also includes providing information about how to inspect the chair and do routine preventative and corrective maintenance[3] as well as where to get repair or replacement service.

Patients who use a wheelchair permanently will need a seat cushion for comfort; those with sensory loss will also require one to assist in prevention of decubiti (see chapter 3). Many cushions are commercially available, and all types relieve some pressure on the ischial tuberosities and distribute it over the buttocks and thighs. A high-density foam cushion may be used initially, but may be replaced with another type (flotation or air filled) for permanent use.[4] See chapter 3 for a discussion of cushion types. A bed pillow or low-density foam rubber cushion will not do as a cushion, even if only used for comfort, because these "bottom out," that is, collapse under the weight of the person and then no longer provide any cushioning.

Type

ELECTRIC WHEELCHAIR

An electric wheelchair allows independent access to the community[5] to high-level quadriplegic individuals and to others who are unable to propel a standard wheelchair or would need to use excessive energy to do so. Some models are small and maneuverable with a molded or cushioned seat and a center bar control stick. Others are similar to a standard wheelchair with a power drive control box located on the left or right side near the arm rest (Fig. 15.1). The joystick, when pushed in the direction the patient wishes to move, activates microswitches that control one or both motors. The speed (2.4 to 5 miles per hour[6]) can be proportional to the pressure applied to the joystick or preselected for the user who would have difficulty controlling proportional speed. Methods of adapting the joystick using PVC pipe to allow patients with varying grip abilities to use it have been published.[7] For persons unable to use hand or finger control, a power-driven chair can be operated by puff and sip (expiration and inspiration) mouth controls or by microswitch controls mounted so that the foot, chin, or other body part can activate them. The choice depends on the patient's remaining function; for example, puff and sip controls can be used by a patient with good vital capacity and mouth control; chin control can be used by a patient with good neck and head control. The choice also depends on whether the control function interferes with performance of other daily life tasks that would need to be done simultaneously. Another consideration is that the control device be constructed and mounted so that it does not hamper other life tasks by its presence; for example, an unadapted sip and puff controller might be in the way during eating or telephoning.

In prescribing the electric wheelchair, a choice about battery type must be made. The best battery for a wheelchair is the deep cycling type[8] such as designed for powering fishing motors, golf carts, etc., rather than the starting-lighting-ignition type used in automobiles.[9] The latter is not meant to be deep cycled (discharged so that it cannot deliver the voltage needed and recharged) repeatedly, as is required for wheelchair use.[9] Because the deep cycling battery will be damaged if not fully and properly charged every time, a

very accurate charger designed for this type of battery must be used. Other types of batteries require other chargers.[10]

MANUALLY OPERATED WHEELCHAIR (FIG. 15.2)

This type of wheelchair is selected if a person is able to propel the wheelchair independently. There are three frame types to consider. The outdoor frame, which has the large wheels in the back and casters in front, is most frequently prescribed because it is the most maneuverable, easiest to propel, and allows the tilt needed for curbs.[11] An amputee frame is designed for the bilateral lower extremity amputee; the rear axle is offset behind the large rear wheels. This design, accommodating to the fact that the person's weight is concentrated further back in the wheelchair, prevents the chair from tipping over backwards. The amputee frame can be ordered with or without footrests, depending on whether or not artificial limbs are worn.[11] An indoor frame is least often selected; it has the large wheels in the front with back casters. Occasionally people prefer or need this chair for indoor use if reaching rear wheels is difficult due to limited range of motion. It rolls over door sills and rug edges more easily but is impractical for curbs and restricts access for transfers.[11]

Frame construction is selected to suit the expected activity level of the user. Heavy-duty construction is for rugged use by heavy or overweight people. A lightweight chair is half the weight of a standard chair and requires less energy to propel or to lift in and out of a car; it is for moderately active people.[11] An active-duty lightweight chair combines heavy-duty bracing and durability with lightweight metals to provide a chair for very active people when rugged use and maneuverability are both desirable.[11] There are also frame constructions for special uses. The sportsman model has a lower back and safety features for active use in competitive sports.[12] A lightweight outdoor frame is available with a lower seat height for the hemiplegic patient who uses one leg to propel the chair.[13] A one-arm drive chair has both handrims on the same side so that the two wheels can be controlled simultaneously or individually by a person who operates the chair with one arm.[11] This option is excellent for some patients but rarely for a stroke patient with cognitive and/or perceptual dysfunction.

Postural Supports

For patients who cannot assume an upright posture in a wheelchair or who need the back reclined at times to change position, a semireclining or fully reclining wheelchair with an extension for head support may be needed (Fig. 15.3).[11]

There are inserts and attachments for wheelchairs as well as chairs of unique design available for special posture problems. Postura® (Everest & Jennings) is one such support system; it has components that provide adjustable postural support for persons with severe disabilities. The modular postural support system consists of a removable firm seat that can be adjusted in depth and/or inclined to shift the weight toward the back of the chair.[11,14] Both the seat and the back are

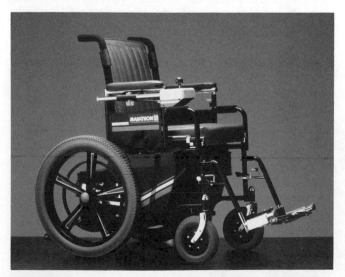

Figure 15.1 Electric wheelchair. (Reproduced with permission from Everest & Jennings, Inc., Los Angeles, CA.)

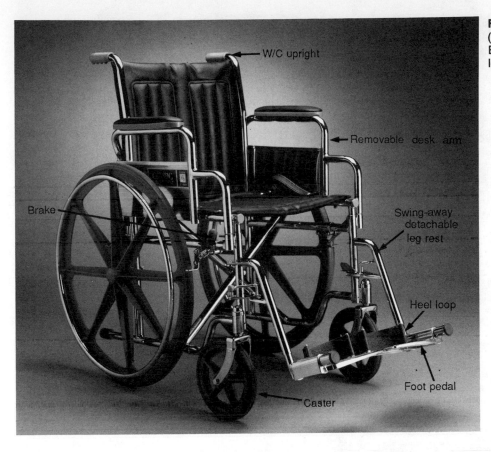

Figure 15.2 Standard wheelchair. (Reproduced with permission from Everest & Jennings, Inc., Los Angeles, CA.)

W/C upright

Removable desk arm

Brake

Swing-away detachable leg rest

Heel loop

Foot pedal

Caster

covered with foam and vinyl. Optional additions to the system include a headrest, lateral trunk supports, side cushions, and abduction wedge (a triangular cushion to keep the legs separated), and a leg rest cradle for full support of both legs.

When postural supports are required, wheelchairs with semireclining or fully reclining backs are most often selected, although the components can also be used on a wheelchair with a fixed back and detachable arms.[14] The Postura system is compatible with many Everest & Jennings standard wheelchairs.[14] For the severely deformed patient, custom molded support systems are available.[14]

Size

The wheelchair size is determined by measuring the seated patient with a tape measure and then selecting a wheelchair that will fit.

SEAT WIDTH

This measurement is taken across the hips or thighs at the widest part and should include the width of braces if worn. Then 5 cm (2 inches) are added to allow for a 2.5-cm (1 inch) clearance on each side.[15] This width will prevent rubbing against the side panels and allow for ease of transfers, while keeping the chair as narrow as possible for ease of propulsion and accessibility through doorways.

SEAT DEPTH

This measurement is taken from the most posterior part of the buttocks along the thigh to the bend behind the knee. Then 5 cm to 7.5 cm (2 to 3 inches) are subtracted to avoid having the seat upholstery press into the popliteal area while still having enough depth to support the thighs and distribute the weight.[15]

SEAT HEIGHT

Leg length is measured from under the distal thigh to the heel of the shoe. The seat height needed is determined by adding 5 cm (2 inches) to the leg length measurement. This will allow a 5-cm (2-inch) clearance from the footrests to the floor so the footrests will clear thresholds, inclines, and uneven surfaces.[15] If a seat cushion is to be used, it will raise the height of the seat, and for many people it is all that is needed to raise the seat height enough for the footrests to be adjusted for adequate clearance. Special seat heights are available for unusually tall individuals. In addition to having a 5-cm (2-inch) minimal floor clearance, the footrests should be adjusted so that the patient's distal thigh is approximately 2.5 cm (1 inch) above the front of the seat upholstery or cushion to avoid pressure under the distal thigh. It is important that the footrests be no higher than necessary to achieve this distal thigh clearance or the patient's weight will no longer be distributed over the large area of the thighs but be placed over the ischial tuberosities, a prime site of decubiti (pressure sores).

ARMREST HEIGHT

Arm height is measured from the seat to the elbow which is flexed to 90°. Then 2.5 cm (1 inch) is added to determine the height of the armrest.[15] This height sup-

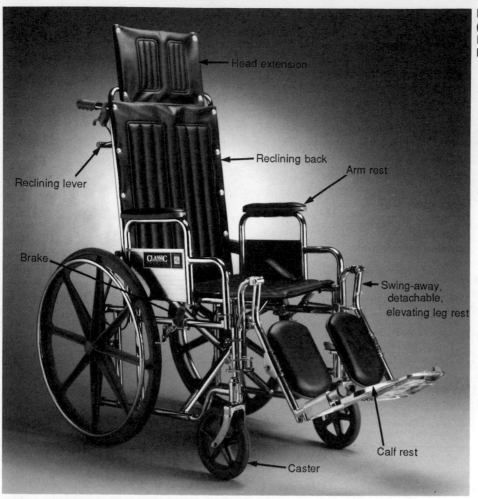

Figure 15.3 Reclining wheelchair. (Reproduced with permission from Everest & Jennings, Inc., Los Angeles, CA.)

Head extension

Reclining back

Reclining lever

Arm rest

Reclining lever

Brake

CLASSIC

Swing-away, detachable, elevating leg rest

Calf rest

Caster

ports the arms comfortably without encouraging slouching if too low or elevation of the scapulae if too high. Use of a seat cushion would also affect this measurement.

BACK HEIGHT

Measurement is taken from the seat to the axilla. Then at least 10 cm (4 inches) are subtracted from this measurement to determine the height of the back upholstery. The current trend is to lower the back height even more than that to increase arm freedom and functional capabilities when trunk strength is sufficient to permit reduced back support.[15]

These measurements are then compared to the sizes of standard models designed to meet the needs of the majority of people, and a wheelchair of the correct size for the individual patient is selected. Universal standards do not yet exist. Table 15.1 lists the standard dimensions used by one manufacturer; see catalogues of other manufacturers for their standard dimensions. If custom modifications are required for any dimension these can be specified but are expensive.[11]

Features and Accessories

Many features and accessories can be selected for a standard wheelchair according to the needs of the pa-

tient. Consideration should be given to the choice of types of casters, arm styles, footrests or leg rests, and accessories for safety or special needs.

CASTERS

Casters are the small wheels located in front on the outdoor frame wheelchair; there is a choice of 5-inch or 8-inch diameter. Casters that are 8 inches in diameter are most frequently selected because they are stable and roll more easily over a variety of surfaces. Caster locks are available for the 8-inch casters to prevent rotation of the casters during transfers. Casters that are set forward are available for increased stability. Rubber bumpers can be ordered to cover the axle of the 8-inch casters for ankle protection if one or both legs are used to propel the chair.

ARMRESTS

Wheelchair arms may be fixed as a permanent part of the chair or may be detachable, so that the arms may be removed for transfers. The wheelchair with fixed arms is lighter and narrower than the detachable-arm wheelchair but requires front transfers from the chair. An offset fixed arm, chosen when patient's seat width exceeds the standard dimension, is constructed so that the arm comes up just beside the seat frame rather

Table 15.1
STANDARD DIMENSIONS USED BY ONE MANUFACTURER[a] (in inches)

Standard Dimensions	Seat Width	Seat Depth	Seat Height	Arm Height	Back Height
Adult	18	16	20	10	16½
Designed for full-grown adults of average size and build.					
Narrow Adult	16	16	20	10	16½
For relatively slender full-grown adults. Combines dimensions of both Adult and Junior models.					
Slim Adult	14	16	20	10	16½
Designed for the thin, tall adult or youth.					
Junior	16	16	18½	10	16½
For full-grown adults with smaller-than-average body size.					
Low Seat	18	16	17½	10	16½
For shorter persons who desire a lower seat height or for persons who propel chair with foot.					

[a]Reproduced with permission from *Measuring the Patient*. Los Angeles, CA: Everest & Jennings, Inc., 1979.

than straight up from the seat edge and consequently adds 4.4 cm (1¾ inches) to the seat width without adding to the width of the wheelchair, thus keeping it within the limits of doorways. Detachable arms are necessary for depression or sliding board transfers. They add 3.75 cm (1½ inches) to the width of the wheelchair. Wraparound detachable arms are constructed to avoid adding to the width of the wheelchair, but the ability to exchange or reverse the arms is sacrificed. A desk-arm style (Fig. 15.2) is available in the offset fixed or detachable styles; the arm is low in front with a smaller padded area at the back for an armrest. The low part allows the wheelchair to be rolled under the edge of a table or desk to enable the person to move closer to these surfaces. Locks for the detachable armrests prevent them from being inadvertently detached when used for leverage by the patient, who may pull on the armrest to assist in changing position or when the wheelchair is lifted in and out of the car. An adjustable-height feature is available in all detachable arm styles. This is particularly useful when a variety of cushions may be used or for severe disabilities when the height of the arms may need to be adjusted as trunk stability changes.

FOOTRESTS

Footrests may be nondetachable or detachable. Swinging detachable footrests (Fig. 15.2 and 15.3) can be moved off to the side without detaching them, which permits closer access to the bed, toilet, or other surfaces. Detachable footrests are essential for a forward transfer into the tub or for other transfers where a side approach is not possible and the footrest would prevent getting close to the transfer surface. Elevating leg rests are needed if the chair is a reclining one, implying that the patient will rest part of the day without the need to transfer back to bed, or if the patient's disability requires elevation of one or both legs. The leg rest

has a padded support for the leg in addition to the foot plate so that the leg is supported when the height of elevation is adjusted. Elevating leg rests may be ordered detachable or nondetachable.

TIRE TYPES

Wheels and casters are available in solid, semipneumatic, or pneumatic types. Pneumatic tires are air filled, similar to a bicycle tire; they give a cushioned ride for outdoor use over rough ground. Pneumatic tires, however, make the wheelchair difficult to push and they are subject to flats. Semipneumatic tires also soften the ride and increase the difficulty of chair propulsion, but the tires are not inflated and will not go flat. If the wheelchair is primarily used indoors or on paved surfaces standard solid tires are adequate.

FOOTPLATES

Footplates are standard on all wheelchairs, but additional features or accessories may be selected. Size variations are available to extend the width of the pedal forward or backward. Plastic-coated footplates, heel loops, or metal heel rests are ordered if the person's feet have a tendency to slide off of the pedals. Toe loops or ankle straps may be needed for patients with excessive clonus, spasms, or involuntary movements in order to keep their feet on the pedals. Pop-up footplates have a spring action that offers an assist to tipping up the pedals. Footplates can be ordered with an angle adjustment for providing foot support when the angle of the ankle is a problem. Several styles of heel straps or a leg rest panel may be attached across the footrest uprights behind both heels or calves to assist in keeping the legs in position on the footrests.

SPECIALIZED ACCESSORIES

Other accessories may be needed for safety, convenience, or special needs. A *Grade-Aid*[11] is an accessory that attaches under the brake for use going up inclines. It releases when the chair is pushed forward and stops against the wheel between pushes to prevent the wheelchair from losing ground by rolling backwards as the patient propels the wheelchair forward up a ramp or incline. The *Grade-Aid* is disengaged when the chair is on a level or downhill surface. *Brake lever extensions* permit locking and unlocking the brakes when the patient cannot reach down to the standard-sized levers or when the patient is too weak to use standard brakes; the increased lever arm length reduces the force required. An extension for the brake on the involved side is often ordered for a hemiplegic patient for ease in reaching the opposite brake with the noninvolved hand. If tipping the wheelchair forward is a likely hazard, a *forward stabilizer* can be attached in front of the caster to stop against the floor if the chair tips forward. Also *antitipping devices* can be attached to the projections at the rear of the wheelchair frame to extend and angle them toward the floor to prevent the wheelchair from tipping backwards. These are generally used with persons who are unable to do a wheelie (see chapter 17) and in situations such as going uphill with a lightweight wheelchair. A *cane or crutch holder* is available for the back of the wheelchair so that canes or crutches may be carried conveniently when using the chair. A *"Quad" release* ("Lever-Ease" or "Cam Ease") for swinging detachable footrests or leg rests has an easier release mechanism than the standard and is for quadriplegic patients or others with limited hand use. *Reduce-a-Width*[11] is a crank-handled device that attaches to one side of the wheelchair arm and seat; the handle can be turned to reduce the wheelchair width temporarily for passage through a narrow doorway. Special *handrims* may be needed by a patient with weak or absent grasp. Friction to assist weak grasp is provided by plastic-coated handrims or rubber handrim covers. If grasp is very weak or absent, the wheelchair can be propelled by pushing the palms against projections on the handrims; these include knobs spaced around the rim or rubber-tipped projections extending vertically or obliquely from the handrim. Choice of the type of projections should take into consideration the fact that some projections add up to 10 cm (4 inches) to the wheelchair width. A *seat belt* is advisable for patients with excessive involuntary movement, severe spasms, or any problem that would make falling out of the wheelchair a possible hazard during functional activities or if the chair stopped suddenly. Items available for special posture or positioning needs are a *solid seat*, a *solid* or *padded back*, and a *body positioner* for lateral trunk support. A *zippered* or *detachable back* is available when a transfer in and out of the back of the wheelchair is required. A *carrying pocket* fits across the back of the wheelchair and is useful for books or other items. *Antifolding devices* are available for theft prevention; they prevent the wheelchair from folding and thus make it difficult to transport the chair.

STUDY QUESTIONS:
WHEELCHAIR MEASUREMENT AND PRESCRIPTION

1. Discuss the occupational therapist's role in wheelchair prescription.
2. How can a severely paralyzed person control an electric wheelchair?
3. What information contributes to choice of frame construction of a manually operated wheelchair?
4. Can a patient with poor trunk control use a wheelchair? What is used to make this possible?
5. What are the five dimensions measured to guide wheelchair selection?
6. Under what circumstances would detachable, desk-arm style armrests be prescribed?
7. Under what circumstances would detachable, swing-away footrests be prescribed?
8. What precautionary equipment can be added to the wheelchair to prevent tipping over in forward or backward directions?

References

1. Bradey, E., et al. A validity study of guidelines for wheelchair selection. *Can. J. Occup. Ther.,* 53(1): 19–24, 1986.
2. Kamenetz, H. L. Wheelchairs and other indoor vehicles for the disabled. In *Orthotic Etcetera,* 3rd edition. Edited by J. B. Redford. Baltimore: Williams & Wilkins, 1986.
3. *Care & Service.* Camarillo, CA: Everest & Jennings, Inc., 1983.
4. Garber, S. L. Wheelchair cushions: a historical view. *Am. J. Occup. Ther.,* 39(7): 453–459, 1985.
5. Breed, A. L., and Ibler, I. The motorized wheelchair: new freedom, new responsibility and new problems. *Dev. Med. Child Neurol.,* 24: 366–371, 1982.
6. *The Power Rolls® IV Catalogue.* Elyria, OH: Invacare, 1981.
7. Kozole, K. P., and Hedman, G. E. Modular hand tiller system for joystick operation of powered wheelchairs. *Arch. Phys. Med. Rehabil.,* 66(3): 193–194, 1985.
8. Border, V. Wheelchair batteries: which is best? *Accent on Living,* 30(3): 28–30, 1985.
9. Wise, E. H. The best battery for your wheelchair or for your van lift. *Accent on Living,* 23(3): 98–103, 1978.
10. Border, V. Battery chargers. *Accent on Living,* 30(3): 32–35, 1985.
11. *Wheelchair Selection.* Camarillo, CA: Everest & Jennings, Inc., 1979.
12. Quadra Wheelchairs, Inc. 31117 Via Colinas, Westlake Village, CA, 91362.
13. *Premier 2 Catalogue.* Camarillo, CA: Everest & Jennings, Inc., 1987.
14. Medhat, M. A., and Trautman, P. Seating devices for the disabled. In *Orthotic Etcetera,* 3rd edition. Edited by J. B. Redford. Baltimore: Williams & Wilkins, 1986.
15. *Measuring the Patient.* Camarillo, CA: Everest & Jennings, Inc., 1979.

Supplementary Reading

Fried, P., and Balick, J. Sip and puff control evaluator and trainer. *Am. J. Occup. Ther.,* 32(6): 398, 1978.
Garee, B., editor. *Wheelchairs and Accessories, An Accent Guide.* Bloomington, IL: Accent Special Publications, Cheever Publishing, Inc., 1981.
Glaser, R. M., et al. An exercise test to evaluate fitness for wheelchair activity. *Paraplegia,* 16(4): 341–349, 1978–79.
Mildenberger, L. A. Brief or new: disk hand [w/c] control for persons with high-level spinal cord injuries. *Am. J. Occup. Ther.,* 39(3): 200–201, 1985.
Practice Division, American Occupational Therapy Association. *Adaptive Equipment Rehabilitation Technology: Information Packet.* Rockville, MD: The American Occupational Therapy Association, 1986.
Safety and Handling. Camarillo, CA: Everest & Jennings, Inc., 1983.

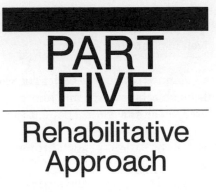

PART FIVE
Rehabilitative Approach

The rehabilitative approach is a compensatory approach appropriate for patients who will need to live with a disability on a temporary or permanent basis. The goal of this approach is the essence of occupational therapy—to enable patients to live as independently and in the most satisfying way that their residual disability allows. In this approach, the therapist focuses on developing the patient's competence in his occupational performance tasks. Anything a person does related to his duties, roles, or life satisfactions is an occupational performance task. The ability to do these tasks depends on a person's basic capacities (i.e., strength, perception, motor control, etc.). When the basic capacities are normal, occupational therapy is not needed. It is when one or more of the basic capacities is lacking and cannot be restored that the occupational therapist is called upon to help the person adapt his methods, tools, and/or environment to enable development of abilities of daily life and, through practice, to relearn the skills, habits, and roles needed for independence. Independence is an attitude as much as a fact. Independent living is defined as the ability to set a life's direction, control it, and take responsibility for it.[1] Occupational therapy is concerned with instilling that attitude, in addition to teaching physical compensation. One way that the occupational therapist promotes the patient's attitude of independence is by fostering his sense of competency; that is, she offers opportunities that allow him to reaffirm his capacity to interact effectively with his environment.[2]

The physical compensation aspect of the rehabilitative approach is an educational process.[3] The therapist teaches the patient to use his remaining abilities in adapted methods of independent living and also teaches him the principles and concepts of those methods so that he may become an independent problem solver. A successful educational process requires that the learning objectives be defined (goals set) and that the teacher know the material and present it so that the learner can understand. Teaching methods will need to be adapted to accommodate persons who have information reception or processing deficits, such as those who are blind or deaf, or have other sensory losses; those who have perceptual deficits or information organizing or retention deficits; or those with retrieval (memory) deficits.[3] Suggestions for environmental support and teaching techniques that apply to all, especially the elderly, have been published.[3] They include:

1. The environment should be organized and familiar, especially during early stages of learning.
2. The therapist facilitates and motivates learning through a calm, confident, patient, enthusiastic, and interested manner.
3. Positive reinforcement should be given in the early stages of learning for good effort as well as successful performance.

4. Relevant information should be presented, visually or verbally, in a well-organized way at a rate consistent with the patient's capacity to understand.

5. Instructions should be given in clear, simple, concrete, age-relevant language, one step at a time.

6. Demonstrations should be planned so that the patient can see the process and relate to the spatial orientation of the objects involved and himself in relation to the objects.

7. Choice of task should relate to goals that reflect patient values and preferences, and the patient should be helped to see the connection.

8. Tasks chosen should be within the patient's capability but challenge his current level of performance.

9. Adequate time to practice should be allowed, and feedback should be given after or during each trial to guide knowledge of correctness of response.

Principles of adaptation of teaching methods are included in the chapters on sensory and cognitive/perceptual evaluation and treatment as well as in the application chapters.

When a person with a disability is unable to accomplish daily life tasks in the usual way, adapted techniques or equipment may enable him to be independent. Adapted techniques are preferred to equipment because they make the person's life more flexible and independent and have less handicapping status. If independence is not possible without equipment, a decision on how to implement adaptation must be made. Many assistive devices are commercially available from rehabilitation supply companies or from gadget catalogues sent in the mail to the general public. Equipment supplied by these sources is preferred because it is economical (compared to a therapist's time) and the quality of workmanship is usually good. However, therapy does not become a process of simply selecting the solution from a catalogue. That piece of equipment may or may not solve the person's problem. The therapist must analyze what specific abilities the patient has and what the piece of equipment requires and can offer to determine if there is a satisfactory match. She then must evaluate its effectiveness and train the patient in its use.

When equipment is needed but is unique and cannot be commercially manufactured, the therapist must use ingenuity to devise specialized adaptations. Adapted equipment needs to be sturdy for daily use by a disabled person, who may stress it more than a normal person would. The quality of workmanship needs to be excellent: smooth edges, finished joints, polished, and permanent looking. "Rube Goldberg" type adaptations are unacceptable. These are poorly designed, excessive, put together with "rubber bands and bubblegum," and are less effective than they should be for the extent of the adaptation.

Part Five deals with evaluation and treatment related to occupational performance tasks and access to the environment. Principles of compensation for each type of problem are stated and will serve as a basis for the therapist's and/or patient's creative problem solving when procedures or pieces of equipment listed are inadequate for a particular patient. Some patients present several disability problems at once; e.g., the rheumatoid arthritic patient may be limited in both range of motion and strength. When more than one problem exists, the therapist needs to consult those sections of the chapters applicable to each problem of a particular patient and combine the principles in the solution. When no technique or equipment can compensate for a problem, the patient will need help and support in deciding whether to eliminate the task from his daily life or to be dependent on someone else for performance of that task.

References

1. Services for Independent Living. 25100 Euclid Ave., Euclid, OH 44117.
2. White, R. Motivation reconsidered: the concept of competence. *Psychol. Rev.,* 56: 297–333, 1959.
3. Ager, C. L. Teaching strategies for the elderly. *Physical & Occupational Therapy in Geriatrics,* 4(4): 3–14, 1986.

Supplementary Reading

Hurff, J. McC. Gaming technique: an assessment and training tool for individuals with learning deficits. *Am. J. Occup. Ther.,* 35(11): 728–735, 1981.

Creighton, C. Therapeutic activities study shows free time unfulfilling for many. *O. T. Week,* 2 (April 28): 4, 31, 1988.

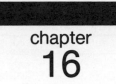

chapter
16

Evaluation of Occupational Performance Tasks

Catherine A. Trombly

Independence in occupational performance tasks is the goal of rehabilitation in general and occupational therapy in particular. Whenever a person suffers a trauma or disease that results in a physical impairment, independence in these tasks is jeopardized. The occupational therapist must determine the patient's abilities and limitations. Evaluation of occupational performance tasks consists of systematic observation and/or interview to determine what tasks cannot be performed and what the limiting factors are. If the limiting factors can be improved or eliminated by direct restorative treatment, the therapist chooses one of the other two treatment approaches that is appropriate to the problem. If, however, the limiting factors are not amenable to change, the therapist teaches the patient to compensate for these limitations.

The format of the evaluation instrument is usually a checklist on which the therapist indicates whether each item can be done independently, with equipment, with supervision, with assistance, or not at all. Items that are not applicable to that person are marked NA. See Table 16.1. The level of measurement of most evaluations of occupational performance tasks is ordinal; that is, the score can be located on a ranking from dependent/is unable to independent/is able. Space is available on forms for periodic reevaluation. It is important to at least record the level of performance at admission and at discharge, since these records may be used for program evaluation, to justify service to third-party payers, in legal actions, and in determining whether a patient will be discharged home or to an extended-care facility.[1]

Evaluation instruments should be valid, reliable, and sensitive enough to detect important changes. A valid test is one that measures what it purports to measure. Most evaluations of functional performance are valid on their face, i.e., have logical validity.[2] The evaluation instrument should weight each item that defines the activity fairly in order to have content validity. The items are samples of a universe of behavior,

but some are more important than others[2], e.g., "can use the stove safely" is a more important item than "can stir batter" in the universe of "meal preparation." If each were weighted equally, then the score would not accurately define the patient's "meal preparation" ability. A reliable test is one that measures the parameter under study consistently no matter who is scoring (interrater reliability) or when the scoring occurs (test-retest reliability). Reliability has rarely been established for the evaluations of occupational performance tasks in use. The tasks listed in departmentally composed tests are rarely even operationally defined, the initial step in establishing reliability. To operationally define something is to describe it so that another person could duplicate the process and arrive at the same conclusion or score. Sensitivity, the third characteristic of a good test, refers to the ability to detect the smallest increment of change that would be considered a significant change for the purpose of the test. As an example, for a therapist working on a day-to-day basis with a patient to increase ability to dress, the test should be sensitive enough to allow progress to be noted when different areas of the body can be dressed or different articles of clothing applied. However, for program evaluation the crucial piece of information is whether or not the patient is or is not independent in dressing, and therefore the tool used to measure is preferably less discriminating.

Observation is the most direct method of assessing functional ability[1] and is preferred for accuracy, detection of faulty or unsafe methods, and for determination of the underlying reason that a particular task cannot be performed. It is, however, time consuming and costly.[1] Self-report through interview is the easiest, fastest, and most inexpensive direct method of assessing functional abilities.[1] There is a concern, however, that the interview may not accurately reflect the patient's abilities. If a patient reports questionable data and does not permit observation, the therapist should verify the report with others who have knowl-

Table 16.1
EVALUATION OF INDEPENDENT LIVING/DAILY LIVING SKILLS[a]

Name: _____ Diagnosis: _____

Key to Grading:
    Independence Grades:
        4 Normal performance
        3 Adequate performance, but dependent on special apparatus or environmental condition (specify in comment section)
    Dependence Grades:
        2 Supervision needed to complete
        1 Assistance needed to complete
        0 Activity impossible
        X Not indicated for testing at present time
        NA Not applicable

Date:						
Rater:						
Functional Mobility						
Turn over in bed						
Sit up in bed						
Procure object from table beside bed						
Transfer from bed to w/c						
Transfer from w/c to toilet						
Transfer from w/c to tub/shower						
Get in and out of chairs						
Get in and out of car						
Wheelchair turning						
Wheelchair forward 30 ft						
Wheelchair up ramp						
Wheelchair down ramp						
Wheelchair forward 100 ft						
Get down and up from floor						
Move on floor not in upright position						
Retrieve object from floor						
Operate automatic elevator						
Open and go through door with sills						
Do 7-inch steps with rails						
Do 7-inch steps without rails						
Cross street with traffic light						
Get wheelchair in and out of car						
Walk forward 30 ft						
Walk backward 10 ft						
Walk sidewards						
Walk carrying object						
Walk forward 100 ft						
Do bus steps						
Drive automobile						
Feeding/Eating						
Swallow liquids and solids						
Chew foods						
Eat with fingers						
Eat with fork						
Eat with spoon						
Cut with knife						
Drink from glass/cup						

edge of the patient's actual performance. False information is not a conscious intent to deceive but may reflect denial of the problem, carryover of the premorbid self-concept, or a strong wish to be independent that seems real. A study that compared results of self-report with observation of functional performance of 47 elderly patients with hip fractures found high agreement between the two, especially for self-care tasks performed daily.[1]

Evaluation of all occupational performance tasks is not done at the same time. Ability to do self-care, personal mobility, and to do leisure time activities within the current limits of the disability are usually done early and form the basis for the whole occupational therapy treatment plan that includes restorative therapy to enable independence. As recovery plateaus and discharge planning decisions are being considered, evaluations concerned with access to home and community, transportation, care of the home and children, hobbies, sports and family recreation, and job/educational abilities are done as applicable. In addition to the physical requirements of these tasks, soundness of judgment and perceptual/cognitive skills must be assessed to determine if these tasks can be safely and effectively accomplished.

Independent Living/Daily Living Skills

In the area of daily living skills, which includes self-care, mobility, and communication, observation of the various activities should be done at the time of day when these activities are normally done and in the location where the patient usually performs the tasks. Remember that people may have strong feelings of modesty regarding personal care that should be respected. The entire self-care evaluation is not done at one time because it is fatiguing. The therapist should discontinue the evaluation if fatigue occurs. Items that would be unsafe or obviously unsuccessful are postponed until the patient's physical status improves; these are marked X (not indicated for testing at present) or some equivalent designation.

If the patient is not independent in some required task at the time of discharge, plans must be developed to ensure that this task is done by others or that additional training is received.

Most standardized self-care evaluations were designed for program evaluation to document the level of independence achieved by patients because of a particular program. The most frequently cited standardized self-care tests are the Katz Index,[3] the Revised Kenny Self-Care Evaluation,[4] and the Barthel Index.[5] The Barthel Index and the Kenny Evaluation are more sensitive to change of a particular patient than the Katz Index.[6] The Barthel Index is more inclusive than the Kenny Evaluation or the Katz Index.[6]

The Katz Index evaluates six functions; scoring is based on ontogenetic development of self-care skills.[3,6] The Barthel Index looks at 10 functions. Total score can range from 0 to 100 (total independence) in increments of 5. Functions are weighted according to impor-

tance to independence.[5,6] A score of 60 seems to be the transition point from dependency to assisted independence.[7] The Revised Kenny Self-Care Evaluation, a more sensitive instrument, looks at seven categories of self-care, each of which are broken down into specific tasks that define the activity. The patient scores either independent (I), dependent (D), needs assistance (A), or needs supervision (S) on each task. The activity is given a number score depending on the number of I's, D's, A's, or S's earned. The category score is an average of the activity scores. The total self-care score is a total of the category scores.[4]

The Klein-Bell Activities of Daily Living Scale© is even more sensitive to small changes than the Revised Kenny Self-Care Evaluation. It documents basic activities of daily living (BADL) skills. The areas tested include dressing, elimination, mobility, bathing and hygiene, eating, and emergency telephone communications.[8] Each area is broken down into tasks, and each task is broken down into step-by-step simple behavioral items. There are 170 such items on the scale, which are scored "achieved" (no physical or verbal assistance) or "failed" (assistance needed). If the person can do the item with adapted equipment, he scores "achieved." Interrater agreement of 92% has been determined from scoring of 30 patients by three pairs of occupational therapists and three pairs of registered nurses, even without extensive training.[9] Validity was established on 14 patients by comparing the total score at discharge against the hours of assistance required. A correlation of $r = -0.86$ was obtained, indicating that the amount of assistance decreases as the Klein-Bell score increases. This appears to be a very useful test because it is as sensitive as a therapist needs to document daily gains and because the validity and reliability have been determined to some degree. Unfortunately, the Klein-Bell Activities of Daily Living Scale has not yet been published and must be obtained directly from the authors.

The Additive Activities Profile Test (ADAPT)© Quality of Life Scale evaluates activities of daily living in relation to the degree of physical fitness or maximal oxygen consumption ($\dot{V}O_2$ max); a correlation of $r = 0.83$ was found between maximal oxygen uptake level and score on this test in a study of 39 pulmonary patients aged 40 to 73.[10] ADAPT is a self-administered paper and pencil test that orders 105 activities according to the $\dot{V}O_2$ required for each.[10]

An example of a nonstandardized activities of daily living (ADL) evaluation form is included here (Table 16.1).

Work

Work, including homemaking, child care, and employment, is another area of concern to occupational therapists,[11] although measures of independent living usually reflect only basic self-care and not other important aspects of the patient's life-style.

A five-item screening test based on instrumental activities of daily living (IADL) needed for community residence—as opposed to BADL such as feeding, grooming, or dressing—has been devised for the community-living elderly to identify those in need of more extensive assessment, assistance, or protected placement.[12] IADL assessments are culture specific; this one was devised for the urban United States. The five items included in this assessment were the ability to do housework, to travel in the community, to shop for food and clothing, to prepare meals, and to handle personal finances.[12] An Activity Index, by which domestic chores, work, and leisure tasks are evaluated and scored as to the frequency and recency of performance, has been developed to aid in goal setting and to document changes in life-style due to disability.[13]

These tests are not sensitive enough for day-to-day treatment planning, nor are they standardized. Except for self-care and prevocational tests, no standardized evaluations of occupational performance tasks exist.

Homemaking includes meal planning, preparation, service and clean up, marketing for food and clothing, and routine and seasonal care of the home and one's clothing. Yardwork and other maintenance tasks may have been the responsibility of the patient and may be considered homemaking tasks. There are no standardized scales of functional performance for homemakers. An example of a nonstandardized evaluation form is included here (Table 16.2).

Child Care/Parenting includes, but is not limited to, the physical care of children and use of age-appropriate activities, communication, and behavior to facilitate child development.[11] Since no standard evaluations exist, the therapist must analyze the tasks, taking the age(s) and personalities of the children into account to determine what assistance the patient may need in this area.

Employment evaluation includes determination of whether the patient has the ability to perform the necessary job skills and is otherwise prepared for employment in terms of work habits, work product quality, ability to learn or acquire new skills, and ability to work with others as team member, supervisor, or supervisee. Many prevocational evaluations exist, some of which are described in chapter 21.

Play/Leisure refers to skill and performance in choosing, performing, or engaging in activities for amusement, relaxation, spontaneous enjoyment, and/or self-expression.[11] An interest scale has been developed,[14,15] but there are no scales to evaluate performance of the many types of recreational activities patients may want to engage in. The occupational therapist will need to analyze the activity of the patient's choice (chapter 10) to determine its basic steps and then evaluate the patient's capability to perform it independently or with adaptation.

STUDY QUESTIONS:

Evaluation of Occupational Performance Tasks

1. What are the methods used to evaluate occupational performance tasks?
2. What are the pros and cons of each method?

3. What are the necessary three characteristics of standardized evaluation instruments? Define each.
4. Define operational definition.
5. What is the relationship of evaluation of occupational performance tasks to development of the occupational therapy treatment plan?
6. Choose one of the mentioned self-care evaluations, describe it, and state its strengths and weaknesses.
7. Define instrumental activities of daily living and basic activities of daily living.
8. What procedure does the occupational therapist use when there is no test for the particular occupational performance task domain she is interested in evaluating?

References

1. Harris, B. A., et al. Validity of self-report measures of functional disability. *Topics in Geriatric Rehabilitation, 1*(3): 31–41, 1986.
2. Hasselkus, B. R., and Safrit, M. J. Measurements in occupational therapy. *Am. J. Occup. Ther., 30*(7): 429–436, 1976.
3. Katz, S., et al. Studies of illness in the aged. The index of ADL: a standardized measure of biological and psychosocial function. *J.A.M.A., 185*(12): 914–919, 1963.
4. Iversen, I. A., et al. *The Revised Kenny Self Care Evaluation.* Publication 722, Sister Kenny Institute. Minneapolis: Abbott-Northwestern Hospital, 1973.
5. Mahoney, F. I., and Barthel, D. W. Functional evaluation: the Barthel index. *Md. State Med. J., 14*(2): 61–65, 1965.
6. Gresham, G. E., Phillips, T. F., and Labi, M. L. C. ADL status in stroke: relative merits of three standard indexes. *Arch. Phys. Med. Rehabil., 61*(8): 355–358, 1980.
7. Granger, C. V., et al. Stroke rehabilitation: analysis of repeated Barthel index measures. *Arch. Phys. Med. Rehabil., 60*(1): 14—17, 1979.
8. Klein, R. M., and Bell, B. J. *Manual: Klein-Bell Activities of Daily Living Scale.* Seattle: School of Medicine, University of Washington, 1979.
9. Klein, R. M., and Bell, B. Self-care skills: behavioral measurement with Klein-Bell ADL Scale. *Arch. Phys. Med. Rehabil., 63*(7): 335–338, 1982.
10. Daughton, D. M., et al. Maximum oxygen consumption and the ADAPT Quality-of-Life Scale. *Arch. Phys. Med. Rehabil., 63*(12): 620–622, 1982.
11. *AOTA Uniform Terminology System for Reporting Occupational Therapy Services.* Rockville, MD: The American Occupational Therapy Association, 1979.
12. Fillenbaum, G. G. Screening the elderly: a brief instrumental activities of daily living measure. *J. Am. Geriatr. Soc., 33*(10): 698–706, 1985.
13. Holbrook, M., and Skilbeck, C. E. An activities index for use with stroke patients. *Age Aging, 12*: 166–170, 1983.
14. Matsutsuyu, J. S. Interest checklist. *Am. J. Occup. Ther., 23*(4): 323–328, 1969.
15. Rogers, J. C., Weinstein, J. M., and Figone, J. J. The interest checklist: an empirical assessment. *Am. J. Occup. Ther., 32*(10): 628–630, 1978.

Supplementary Readings

Casanova, J. S., and Ferber, J. Comprehensive evaluation of basic living skills. *Am. J. Occup. Ther., 30*(2): 101–105, 1976.
Harvey, R. F., and Jellinek, H. M. Functional performance assessment: a program approach. *Arch. Phys. Med. Rehabil., 62*(9): 456–461, 1981.
Jacobson, N. S. Uses versus abuses of observational measures. *Behavioral Assessment, 7*: 323–330, 1985.
Kirchman, M. M. Measuring the quality of life. *Occup. Ther. J. Res., 6*(1): 21–32, 1986.
Klein-Parris, C., Clermont-Michel, T., and O'Neill, J. Effectiveness and efficiency of criterion testing versus interviewing for collecting functional assessment information. *Am. J. Occup. Ther., 40*(7): 486–491, 1986.
Law, M. C., and Polatajko, H. J. Diagnostic tests in occupational therapy: a model for evaluation. *Occup. Ther. J. Res., 7*(2): 111–122, 1987.
Lawton, E. B. Activities of daily living test: geriatric considerations. *Physical & Occupational Therapy in Geriatrics, 1*(1): 11–20, 1980.
Smith, R. O., et al. The effects of introducing the Klein-Bell ADL Scale in a rehabilitation service. *Am. J. Occup. Ther., 40*(6): 420–424, 1986.
Stratton, M. Behavioral assessment scale of oral functions in feeding. *Am. J. Occup. Ther., 35*(11): 719–721, 1981.

Table 16.1—continued

Grooming and Hygiene						
Use handkerchief						
Wash hands						
Wash face						
Brush teeth						
Comb hair						
Care for nails						
Shave or make-up						
Arrange clothes at toilet						
Use toilet paper						
Bathe self						
Shampoo hair						
Care for menstrual period						
Manage catheter						
Dressing						
Choose appropriate clothing						
Put on/remove cardigan garment						
Put on/remove slipover garment						
Put on/remove outer coat						
Put on/remove trousers						
Put on/remove socks						
Put on/remove shoes						
Put on/remove underwear						
Tie shoes						
Tie bow or tie						
Lock and unlock lower-extremity orthoses						
Put on/remove lower-extremity orthoses						
Put on/remove slings, MAS, or prostheses						
Put on/remove handsplints						
Object Manipulation						
Operate switches (all types)						
Operate faucets (all types)						
Flush toilet						
Operate locks						
Plug in cord						
Wind watch or clock						
Open and close drawers						
Open and close windows						
Use scissors						
Handle Money						
Functional Communication						
Write name						
Handle own mail						
Use phone						
Use typewriter/computer						
Use artificial vocalization systems						
Use communication boards, etc.						

[a]Evaluation adapted from: University of Illinois, College of Medicine, School of Associated Medical Sciences, Curriculum in Occupational Therapy.

Table 16.2
HOMEMAKING EVALUATION[a]

Name _____

Diagnosis _____ Onset _____

Disability _____

Precautions _____

Expected ambulation _____ Present level _____ Dominant hand _____

Visual limitations _____ Type of diet _____

Expected homemaker status: Assistive _____ Full-time _____

Description of home: Owned _____ Rented _____ Steps _____ Elevator _____

    Floors _____ No. of rooms _____ Special problems _____

_____

Diagram house interior (use reverse side of sheet)

Patient's expected responsibilities:

    Meal preparation_____Meal service_____Washing dishes_____Marketing _____

    Clothes washing: machine_____by hand_____. Drying clothes: _____

    machine_____hanging_____. Ironing_____Mending_____Washing windows _____

    Floor care: sweep_____, vacuum_____, wash_____. Cleaning: dusting _____,

    tidy up_____, heavy cleaning (walls, closets, cupboard, oven, refrigerator) _____.

Does the patient appear motivated toward homemaking activities? _____

Available help for household chores: _____

Available equipment

    *Range:*_____microwave_____electric_____gas_____automatic pilot _____

       Location of controls_____location of oven_____self-cleaning? _____

       Description:

    Food preparation tools: Can opener: electric or manual _____.

       Knives: electric_____standard_____. Are knives sharp? _____

       Coffeepot: percolator or drip?_____electric_____standard _____.

       Fry pan: electric_____standard _____.

    Refrigerator: Door opens: right_____left_____Freezer location: _____

       Shelves: rotary_____pullout_____stable _____

       Self-defrosting? yes_____no_____partially_____Description: _____

    Sink: one well_____two well_____drainboard on right_____left _____

       height_____standard_____deep_____shallow_____space under sink? _____

    Garbage disposal: yes_____no_____switch located? _____

    Dishwasher: top loading _____ front loading _____ location of controls: front_____back_____

       description _____

    Washer: automatic_____top loading_____front loading _____

       Location:_____ Controls: front_____back_____

    Dryer: electric_____gas_____. Location: _____.

       Controls: front_____back_____clothesline location _____

       Height_____. Can it be lowered? _____ Method of transporting

       clothes and pins: _____

    Ironing board: Adjustable?_____Location:_____Iron: standard _____

       steam_____Location of table or rack for finished clothes? _____

    Vacuum cleaner: upright_____tank_____built-in attachments _____

_____

    Method of emptying _____

Electric mixer: portable _____ standard _____ *Blender:* _____

Electric roaster: _____ *Hot plate:* _____ *Tea cart:* _____

Knife sharpener: _____ *Toaster:* _____ *Toaster oven:* _____

Kitchen chair: _____

Cookbook: shortcut recipes _____ special diet _____

Table 16.2—*continued*

Scoring key: 0 = unable,   1 = with physical assistance,   2 = with verbal assistance or supervision,
3 = with adapted equipment,   4 = independent.

Homemaking Tasks	Initial	Discharge	Methods or person to be responsible for:
Cleaning activities			
Pick up objects from floor			
Wipe up spills (counter/floor)			
Make beds			
Change bed linens			
Use dust mop/shake			
Use broom			
Use dust pan			
Dust high and low surfaces			
Use vacuum cleaner			
Tidy up			
Transport cleaning materials			
Use wet mop/wring out			
Meal preparation			
Turn on water			
Light match and gas oven or burner			
Pour hot liquids			
Serve hot foods			
Open packaged foods			
Open ½ gallon milk carton			
Pour from milk carton			
Carry hot foods or pans			
Open screw top jars			
Use can opener			
Remove food from refrigerator			
Remove articles from cupboards			
Peel vegetables			
Use knives safely			
Break an egg			
Stir batter			
Use measuring spoons			
Use egg beater			
Pour batter			
Grease pan			
Open oven safely			
Use oven mitts			
Put pan in oven			
Use electric mixer/blender			
Use scissors			
Butter bread			
Baste meat			

Table 16.2—_continued_

Use microwave oven			
Plan week's menu			
Meal service			
Set table			
Carry food to table			
Serve food at table			
Fold napkins			
Put on and remove table covering			
Sweep crumbs			
Scrape dishes			
Clear table			
Wash dishes and/or load dishwasher			
Dry dishes			
Dry silverware			
Scrub pots			
Wipe stove and table			
Laundry			
Sort clothes			
Hand laundry			
Use clothes pins			
Use clothesline/rack			
Plug in cord			
Iron shirt or dress			
Fold ironed clothes			
Set up ironing board			
Use washer			
Use dryer			
Fold clothes			
Sewing			
Thread needle			
Tie knot			
Sew on button			
Cut thread			
Mend rips			
Use sewing machine			
Heavy cleaning			
Cleaning stove/oven			
Clean and defrost refrigerator			
Wax floors			
Washing windows			
Cleaning tub			
Turn mattress			
Change storm windows/screens			

Table 16.2—*continued*

Marketing			
In person			
Order by phone			
Receive and put away			

Summarize patient's capabilities following initial evaluation:
Summarize patient's capabilities following training/at discharge:
Special equipment needed: (describe, list source and estimated cost.)
Summarize plans for tasks not within patient's capability:

[a]Adapted from a form devised by the Occupational Therapy Department of Highland View Cuyahoga County Hospital, Cleveland, OH 44122.

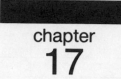

chapter
17

Activities of Daily Living

Catherine A. Trombly and Lee Ann Quintana

Activities of daily living (ADL) are those occupational performance tasks that a person does each day to prepare for, or as an adjunct to, role tasks. The term activities of daily living is not exactly synonymous with self-care. Self-care is a more limited term that refers to the ability to dress, feed, toilet, bathe, and groom oneself, as well as miscellaneous common skills, such as using the telephone, communicating by writing, and handling mail, paper money, coins, books, or newspapers. ADL also includes mobility, which refers to being able to turn over in bed, come to a sitting position, move, and transfer from place to place. Driving is included in this chapter since it is considered an adjunctive daily task. Procedures to be used in cases of emergency (fire,[1,2] tornado warning, automobile breakdown, etc.) should be discussed and supplemented with written instructions for those who may encounter such eventualities when they are alone.

The occupational therapist is the rehabilitation specialist responsible for increasing the patient's independence in ADL. All other therapy is supportive of that goal. Using the biomechanical or neurodevelopmental approaches, the therapist attempts to increase the patient's capabilities. If restorative therapy is able to return the patient to normalcy, no special therapy will be needed to increase independence in ADL; the patient will be doing the tasks as he is able. However, in many cases restorative therapy improves the patient's capabilities, but these remain less than normal. In these cases, the occupational therapist teaches the person new methods of doing these tasks or introduces or devises adapted equipment that will enable the person to be independent of another person for the task. Teaching the adapted method is preferred to using equipment so that the person can become truly independent. Issuing adapted equipment to make the person partially independent is sometimes justified, but depends on the investment the patient has and the sense of satisfaction he receives in doing that particular task for himself.

The actual process of teaching the person the new techniques or how to use the adapted device depends on the patient's capacity for learning. For those patients without brain damage and of average intelligence, the teaching methods can be discussion, demonstration, or simply describing methods that others have found helpful. The patient may have suggestions about how a task might be accomplished, and his ideas should be respected and encouraged. Many techniques commonly in use have been developed by therapist-patient collaboration. Non-brain-damaged persons should be taught in such a way that they become independent problem solvers. They need to learn to identify the problem, to understand the principle involved, and to be able to match a solution from a repertoire of solutions that have been found helpful in the past or that others have used. Practice will improve speed and ease of performance.

Patients with brain damage require more attention to the actual teaching process, which will be guided by the patient's particular learning problem. If the patient is unable to automatically do the task using old habit programs, he will be relearning a skill; therefore, much repetition is necessary. The learning may or may not transfer to other familiar tasks; therefore, he may need to practice each task until it is learned. Brain-damaged patients may not become problem solvers, and their prognosis for independence outside of a sheltered or familiar environment may be limited. Some ADL tasks are not even attempted if judgment is impaired.

Patients who suffer damage to their dominant hemispheres usually have difficulty processing verbal or written language but are able to benefit from demonstrated or pictorial instruction. Those who suffer damage to their nondominant hemispheres may have difficulty with spatial relationships; therefore, step-by-step verbal instruction is usually processed better than demonstration. Brain-damaged patients often have difficulty processing abstract information or large "chunks" of information at a time and need the instructions reduced to one- or two-word concrete cues. Given consistently over the course of practice sessions, these key word cues help the patient chain the task from beginning to end. It may be necessary to practice one step at a time; steps may be combined as learning progresses. Some patients, however, can only do the task if the whole chain is completed.[3]

Some profoundly brain-damaged, yet teachable, patients benefit from backward chaining. Backward chaining is an adaptation of Skinner's Law of Chaining, which he describes in this way: "The response of one reflex may produce the eliciting or discriminative stimulus of another."[4] In backward chaining of dressing skills, for example, assistance is given to do the task until the last step of the process is reached; the patient performs this one step independently with the satisfaction of having completed the task. Once the patient has mastered the final step, the therapist assists only to the next to the last step and the patient completes the two remaining steps. This process continues until the patient can do the entire task from start to finish independently.

There are some patients who are unable to learn, and their therapy must be deferred until their mental condition clears. Learning is prevented by loss of recent (or short-term) memory, severe receptive aphasia, disorientation to person or place, or ideational apraxia, the inability to identify or know the use of common objects. High anxiety also blocks learning, and therapy to reduce anxiety would be necessary if the patient exhibits this condition.

Since the rehabilitation approach involves teaching as its method of implementation, those patients who speak a language not known to the therapist and who do not understand demonstration will need to be taught through the help of an interpreter.

To plan treatment, results of the ADL evaluation must be considered with knowledge of the disability and with the results of sensorimotor evaluations so that reasonable expectations concerning the level of independence to be achieved can be estimated. To ensure success, the patient must have the prerequisite strength, mobility, endurance, balance, and coordination required for each task before it is attempted. Lack of sensation must be compensated for. Initially, if the patient lacks some of these prerequisite capabilities for a task, adapted methods or equipment may make completion of the task possible. These methods and/or use of equipment will be modified and/or withdrawn as the patient progresses.

LEVEL OF INDEPENDENCE

It is important that the occupational therapist accurately document the patient's level of independence. When evaluating the patient's ability to perform a task, note must be made of: (1) how much physical assistance is required (e.g., patient requires assistance pulling up pants), (2) the amount of verbal cues required (e.g., patient may require verbal cues for correctly sequencing the task), (3) what position the task is completed in (e.g., in bed, up in the wheelchair, at the sink, etc.), (4) what type of adaptive equipment is used, and (5) how much time or amount of energy/endurance is required (e.g., a quadriplegic patient who takes two hours to dress is not functionally independent). From this information, the patient's level of independence is rated from independent to dependent (Table 17.1). For example, if donning a button-down shirt were broken down into five steps [i.e., (1) setting up and positioning

Table 17.1
LEVELS OF INDEPENDENCE

Independent	Patient is able to complete the task including setup, with or without adaptive equipment. Note should be made of adaptive equipment used.
Independent with setup	Patient is able to complete the task once someone sets it up for him (e.g., able to dress but unable to get clothes out of the closet; able to feed self once someone applies his adaptive equipment).
Supervision	Patient is able to perform the task but cannot be left alone due to cognitive deficits, poor balance, etc.
Minimal assistance	Patient requires minimal physical assistance or verbal cues to complete the task; assistance with 25% of the task.
Moderate assistance	Patient requires moderate physical assistance or verbal cues to complete the task; assistance with 50% of the task.
Maximum assistance	Patient requires maximum physical assistance or verbal cues to complete the task; assistance with 75% of the task.
Dependent	Patient is unable to do any part of the task.

the shirt, (2) putting the arms in the correct armholes, (3) putting the shirt over the head, (4) pulling the shirt down in back, and (5) buttoning the shirt], the patient requiring minimal assist would need help with only one of these steps. The patient who needed help with two or three of these steps would require moderate assist, while patients needing help with four steps would need maximum assist. Description of the amount of verbal cues required is generally used with brain-damaged patients with cognitive/perceptual deficits. They can be used in combination with the amount of physical assistance required (e.g., the patient requires minimal assistance and moderate verbal cues to don a pullover shirt).

The therapist must then set realistic goals with the patient. They must take into account the patient's attitude and desires as well as the discharge situation. If the task takes a long time or a lot of energy and the patient would rather have someone else do the task for him, his wishes must be respected. In this case, the goal may be related to the patient directing his own care. The discharge situation is important as well. The patient may be able to dress independently in the hospital using the electric bed, but if the plan is to discharge the patient home without a hospital bed, then the discharge goal must accurately reflect this (i.e., independent in dressing without use of electric bed).

Mobility and Transfers

Mobility refers to movements on one surface involving change of position or location. Bed mobility (e.g., rolling side to side, going from supine to sit, etc.), wheelchair mobility (propelling the wheelchair and managing its parts), and driving are examples of mobility that the occupational therapist may be responsible for teaching. In addition, while responsibility for teaching ambulation belongs with the physical therapist, the occupational therapist is responsible for teaching functional ambulation skills (e.g., if the patient now ambulates with a cane, how does he manage to move his coffee cup from the counter to the table? Is he able to reach up/down into cabinets safely? etc.).

Transfers refer to movement from one surface to another. For example, movements from the bed to the wheelchair or from the wheelchair to the car seat are transfers. The type of transfer used depends on the degree of disability. If the patient is unable to move at all, a lift is required to carry him from one surface to another. If the patient is unable to bear weight on his lower extremities, and has weak upper extremities, an assisted or independent sliding transfer is taught. If the patient is unable to bear weight on his lower extremities but has strong upper extremities enabling him to depress his scapulae to lift his buttocks off of the surface, a depression transfer is the appropriate choice. If weight bearing on the lower extremities is possible and permitted, a pivot transfer is used. When standing balance is a problem, this transfer is assisted.

Transfers will be described going in one direction. Reversing the process will accomplish the transfer in the other direction. **Note that the wheelchair must be locked for all transfers.** Transfers are most easily accomplished when the heights of the two surfaces involved in the transfer are the same.

When lifting or assisting a patient to transfer, the therapist must protect her own back by using proper body mechanics. The stronger leg muscles are used by keeping the back straight and bending the knees whenever the patient is lifted up or lowered. The therapist evaluates her size and strength relative to the size and weight of the patient. The therapist should not attempt a lift that seems unmanageable. If the therapist should overestimate her strength or underestimate the weight of the patient and feels the patient slipping from her support, she should ease him to the floor and cushion the fall as well as she can.

Again, it is important that the occupational therapist accurately document the patient's level of independence in mobility and transfer skills. The levels noted in Table 17.1 are used as well as the following: (1) contact guard—the therapist maintains physical contact with the patient but does not help, the contact is used in case of sudden loss of balance; (2) close supervision—the therapist is within reach of the patient, but not in continual contact; this is generally used when there are still occasional losses of balance; and (3) distant supervision—the therapist is in the same area as the patient; generally the patient is able to do the task but requires supervision due to cognitive/perceptual deficits.

LIMITED RANGE OF MOTION

Mobility and transfers can be done by persons with limited range of motion. The important factor in these activities is the correct use of joints and avoidance of deforming forces (see chapter 27). Correct joint use includes avoidance of moving on twisted joints and use of the larger, stronger joints of the arms and legs instead of the small joints of the wrists and fingers whenever possible. Deforming forces are those that require the joints to forcefully assume positions that are typical deformities (e.g., ulnar deviation of the metacarpophalangeal joints). Some special devices to protect certain joints during crutch ambulation are crutches with forearm platforms or troughs to protect the distal upper-extremity joints of rheumatoid arthritics from the joint-deforming stresses of resisted grasp and weight bearing on the hands and wrists. Enlarged or padded hand grips on crutches or canes can be used for patients with limited grasp or to protect joints of the rheumatoid arthritic hand. Rubber or foam rubber hand grips are commercially available, or a customized hand grip can be fabricated using thermoplastics.

For those with limited range of motion of the hips and knees combined with muscle weakness, coming to a standing position is facilitated by use of raised seating. Some examples are: (1) a raised toilet seat that can be attached to the rim of the toilet; (2) high or adjustable-height chairs such as executive office chairs; (3) a portable or electric or spring-loaded lift for existing chairs that tilts the chair seat forward to assist standing; (4) an additional cushion placed in existing chairs to raise the seat height to the required level; (5) a wheelchair fitted with an hydraulically controlled elevating seat that raises the seat when the patient is preparing to transfer.

A mobility aid for home and office use, available for those with weakness combined with the limited range of hip motion, is a glider chair that has casters on each leg. The chair is propelled by the feet. It can also be used for locomotion by patients limited by pain. The patient's ability to transfer to this type of chair must be carefully considered; since the wheels generally do not lock, the patient will be transferring to/from an unstable surface.

If the person is unable to bear weight on the legs and has weak arms, a sliding depression transfer is chosen. This transfer can be assisted or independent, depending on the extent of the person's disability.

Assisted Sliding Transfer

A sliding or transfer board is used to bridge the space between the transfer surfaces. A plastic sliding board is commercially available that has a very slippery surface. Wooden sliding boards are available as well. These come in various lengths, depending on the needs of the patient. A longer sliding board may be necessary for bridging the space between a wheelchair and the car, whereas a shorter board would be more appropriate for toilet transfers. The sliding board is positioned with one end well under the patient's hips and the other end on the surface to which the patient is transferring. Assistance is provided by holding the patient around the rib cage, waist, or waistband of trousers and sliding him along the board. The patient can place his arms around the therapist's neck or waist during the transfer. After the patient is safely onto the new surface, the legs are carried into place by the patient if possible or by the therapist if necessary.

Independent Sliding Transfer

A sliding transfer is done independently by the person doing a series of mini-depression transfers as he slides along the sliding board from one surface to the next (Fig. 17.1). A board may not be needed if the surfaces are contiguous.

DECREASED STRENGTH

The ability to roll over and the ability to sit up in bed are necessary prerequisites to being able to dress and transfer. To roll over, the person with decreased strength in all four extremities holds the bedside rail or the arm of the wheelchair, which has been placed beside the bed and locked. He holds by grasping with the hand closest to that side of the bed or, if he lacks grasp, by hooking the distal forearm or extended wrist around

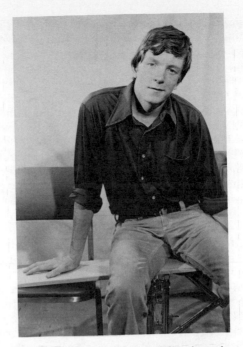

Figure 17.1 Transferring using a sliding board.

the rail or the wheelchair handle. To gain the momentum necessary for rolling the upper trunk over, he then flings the other arm across the body using proximal musculature. He may then need to reach down and hook his extended wrist under his distal thigh to pull the leg over.

There are several methods a weak person can use to sit up. One is to use the vertical bars on the bedside rail to pull up using first a near bar and then each next bar to pull up to sitting. A sitting position beyond 90° of hip flexion must be achieved to maintain balance. Another method is to use a rope ladder, which is tied to the foot of the bed. It has webbing bars attached between two webbing strips to form the ladder. The process is the same as used with the bedside rail: the arms are looped through successive bars to progressively achieve a sitting position.

To avoid the necessity for equipment, the patient can learn to come to a sitting position as follows: (1) roll to one side, for example, the right; (2) fling the top arm (left) backward to rest the elbow on the bed; (3) roll onto the left elbow and quickly fling the right arm back to rest the palm of the hand or fist on the bed; (4) roll to the right and quickly move the left arm to rest the hand on the bed; (5) having achieved a semisitting position resting on both hands, with the elbows extended or locked, the hands are "walked" forward to come to a forward-leaning position of greater than 90° of hip flexion to maintain balance.

Dependent Transfers

If the person is so weak that he is unable to roll over and come to a sitting position in bed, he is transferred by lifting.

A **three-person carry** is used to transfer a person who is lying down and must remain in a supported recumbent position. The three lifters position themselves on the same side of the individual to be transferred. They bend their knees and keep their backs straight. The person near the head puts one hand under the patient's neck and the other hand under the patient's scapulae; the person in the middle puts one hand under the patient's scapulae and the other hand under the patient's hips; the third person puts one hand under the patient's hips and the other hand under the patient's knees. On signal from the person supporting the head, all three lifters pull and roll the patient toward themselves to hold him against their chests as they rise to a standing position using their legs to lift. The person at the head continues to direct the transfer by leading the turn toward the transfer surface.

A **two-person carry** is used to transfer a person who can be placed in a sitting position. One lifter is positioned at the patient's head. After pulling the patient toward the edge of the bed and into a partial sitting position, the lifter flexes the patient's elbows so that the patient's forearms rest across his body. The lifter pushes his hands in under the axillae from back to front to grasp both of the patient's forearms just distal to the elbows. The other lifter assists by moving the patient's hips over to the edge of the bed by holding the patient securely under the knees. On signal from the person supporting the upper body, both lifters move the patient from the bed.

A **log roll transfer** can be done by one person. The wheelchair is locked in position, facing the foot of the bed, with the seat near the patient's hips, detachable arm removed, and a pillow over the wheel. The patient is rolled onto his side with his back toward the chair, his hips toward the chair seat at the edge of the bed, and with arms and legs flexed, which distributes the weight to prevent rolling out of bed. The hips are moved onto the chair seat while the upper trunk and legs remain on the bed. Then the upper trunk is moved to an upright position in the chair and, finally, the feet are moved from the bed to the footrests of the wheelchair.

Mechanically Assisted Transfer. If the person who is to do the lift is weak compared to the size of the patient, and the patient is allowed to sit, a **mechanical lifter** can be used. One device (Hoyer lift)[5] has a seat and back support made of nylon material that is positioned under the patient. This support is then hooked to the hydraulic lifting mechanism, which, when pumped, will lift the patient off the surface. The device is wheeled to the other surface, and slow release of the hydraulic mechanism lowers the patient to the surface. Similarly, devices have been adapted from a garage door opener[6] and a battery-operated winch[7] that allow independent "dependent" transfer from one specific place to the other, e.g., bed or wheelchair to commode. The use of a mechanical lift may mean the difference between discharge home or discharge to nursing home.[6]

Assisted Transfers

Several styles of assisted transfer are available. The **assisted sliding transfer** has already been described. Other types are listed here.

A **swivel trapeze bar** attached to an orthopedic frame at the head of the bed can be used to help lift the patient if he has upper-extremity strength equal to lifting half his body weight. The wheelchair is positioned next to the bed, with the armrest removed and the brakes locked. The patient holds onto the trapeze by hooking his extended wrists around the bar to pull to sitting and then puts both forearms across the bar, assisted, if needed. The patient then contracts his elbow flexors to support the weight of his upper trunk. The therapist holds the patient's legs and pulls him off of the bed surface toward the foot of the bed and swings his lower body over to the chair. The trapeze swivels with the motions. Once seated, the patient releases his arms from the trapeze and positions his trunk in the chair.

A patient may also need assistance positioning himself in the wheelchair. A position change may be accomplished by one person standing behind the wheelchair. The wheelchair is locked and tipped backwards to its point of balance on the large back wheels. Shaking the chair assists gravity in sliding the patient's hips back into the chair. **Caution: Do not shake the chair if the patient has spasticity.** If the patient needs more assistance than this, his elbows are flexed so that his forearms rest across his body. The therapist pushes her arms in between the patient's arms and chest wall under the axillae to grasp each forearm just distal to the elbow. Force is applied upward to pull the patient into an upright posture. While lifting, the therapist guards the balance of the wheelchair with one knee to prevent it from toppling over backward.

Independent Transfers

Patients with weak upper and lower extremities may be able to do an **independent sliding transfer** (see Fig. 17.1), described previously. The **swivel trapeze bar transfer**, also previously described, can be done independently if upper extremity strength permits. The patient would lift his legs from the bed to the wheelchair foot rests himself after he was in the wheelchair.

Independent Depression Transfer. For patients with paralyzed lower extremities but strong scapular depression and elbow extension, an independent depression transfer is done in this way: the wheelchair is positioned as close to the surface being transferred to as possible, and the brakes are locked. The feet are lifted off the footrests and placed on the floor one by one. Each footrest is raised out of the way. If the patient has poor trunk balance, he can hook one of his arms around the wheelchair upright while leaning to pull up the footrests with the other. The arm of the wheelchair on the side to which the transfer is to be done is removed. The patient slides forward on the seat of the wheelchair. He places one hand at a distance onto the surface he is transferring to and the other under his hip. He pushes down using scapular depression and elbow extension to lift the buttocks clear of the wheelchair and swings over to the other surface in one quick, smooth action.

Sometimes, it is not possible to get the wheelchair close enough to the transfer surface. This most often occurs in toilet or bathtub transfers. In this case, a sturdy straight-backed chair can be used to bridge the gap between the wheelchair and the toilet or tub seat.[8] A zipper back on the wheelchair may be needed to allow the patient to transfer directly backward when space near the toilet is severely limited or due to a particular patient's limitations.

Wheelchair Mobility

An electric wheelchair is required for persons too weak to propel a standard wheelchair (see chapter 15). For the patient who is confined to a wheelchair but has adequate upper-extremity strength to propel a standard wheelchair, mobility training is important. A graded program toward independent wheelchair mobility proceeds as follows: from level, smooth surfaces to inclined, rough surfaces, which are very difficult to manage in a wheelchair.

The patient also needs to learn to conquer curbs. At first the therapist assists. She first explains the procedure, as tipping the wheelchair unexpectedly could scare the patient. To assist a wheelchair up a curb, the therapist approaches the curb with the front of the wheelchair and depresses the foot projection on the back of the wheelchair frame while pulling back on the handles to put the casters over the curb. To assist a wheelchair down a curb, the therapist approaches the curb backwards, letting the large back wheels down first and then the casters. An alternative method of assisting a wheelchair down a curb uses a forward approach: tip the wheelchair back onto the large back wheels to the point of balance where the center of gravity is over the rear axle and then let the large wheels gently down the curb.

Good upper-extremity strength and the ability to do a "wheelie" are needed to maneuver curbs independently. A wheelie is done by giving a quick forward push on the handrims while simultaneously throwing the trunk back against the seat back[9]; this tips the chair backward and raises the casters off the floor. The patient then has to balance the wheelchair on its point of balance over the rear axle. Learning to do a wheelie takes much practice and some courage. A Wheelie Training Aid has been developed to allow the patient to practice without the need for a staff member present to guard.[9] Two nylon webbing straps are suspended from the ceiling and attached by way of pipe clamps to the handles of the wheelchair. The straps catch the patient and prevent him from going over backward when he fails to catch the balance point.[9]

To go up a curb the patient approaches the curb forwards. As the casters near the curb, he does a wheelie or pulls back quickly on the handrims to raise the front of the chair, which lifts the casters onto the curb. Then, while leaning forward, he propels the large back wheels onto the curb. To go down a curb the patient approaches the curb backwards, leans forward in the chair, and rolls down the curb. An alternative method for going down a curb uses a forward approach; the patient does a wheelie and rolls off the curb. (Fig. 17.2).

Ascending and descending several stairs requires the assistance of two people. To take a person in a wheelchair up a flight of stairs, approach the stairs backwards. One person stands behind the chair and tips it backwards into its balanced position. The second person stands in front of the chair and holds onto the leg rest upright (making sure they are holding onto part of the frame of the chair, not a detachable part). While maintaining the chair at its point of balance on the back wheel, the person behind the chair pulls it up each step in succession while the person at the foot assists in lifting and maintains the point of balance. To take a person in a wheelchair down a flight of stairs, approach the stairs forward and with the wheelchair in a balanced position. The two people reverse the process for ascending stairs to lower the chair down each step in succession. If the person can do an independent floor to wheelchair transfer, it would be possible for him to "bump" himself up and down the stairs in an emergency and pull his wheelchair after him.

INCOORDINATION

No special techniques are used to enable persons with incoordination to move in bed or to transfer. Unless they have concomitant weakness, in which case the techniques listed under the previous section would be used, they are able to do these activities. The problem of safety arises, and these patients must pay particular attention to safety factors. If judgment is poor, the patient will be dependent on others for supervision during transfer.

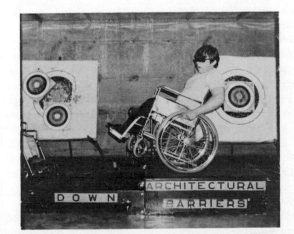

Figure 17.2 A "wheelie" demonstrated by a student at the University of Illinois.

Some incoordinated persons find it easier to propel a standard wheelchair by using their feet. Pushing backwards is easiest, but a rear view mirror is needed to prevent accidents!

LOSS OF THE USE OF ONE SIDE OF THE BODY

The person who has suffered a stroke and lost the use of one side of the body must relearn how to roll over and come to a sitting position in bed. The hemiplegic patient is generally able to roll toward the affected side, but experiences difficulty rolling toward the unaffected side. In one method of rolling to the unaffected side from a supine position, the hemiplegic patient puts his unaffected foot under the affected ankle, carries his affected arm across his body, and then pulls himself over onto his unaffected side by holding the side of the bed. Another method is for the patient to clasp his hands, extend his elbows, and flex his shoulders above 90° so that he is reaching upward. Then he quickly swings his arms from one side to the other side, building momentum. Finally, the momentum carries him onto his side.[10]

One method of coming to sitting on the edge of the bed is to put the unaffected foot under the affected ankle and carry the legs to the edge of the bed. Next, the affected arm is carried across the body, while the head is simultaneously pulled forward and the uninvolved arm pushes against the bed to come to a sitting position. The patient continues the upward thrust of his upper body while swinging his legs over the side of the bed. The important thing to remember is that he should roll all the way onto his side before pushing to sit up. This puts the arm in a better position to push up and puts less strain on the back. He should be guarded until the therapist is satisfied that he can do this procedure independently and safely. A hard mattress reduces the danger of falling. If the mattress at home is soft, a bed board can be suggested.

Another method of coming to sitting is advocated by Bobath.[10] At first the patient starts by clasping his hands and rolling over into the sound side as described. With the arms still clasped together, he bends his sound elbow and pushes it against the bed to lift the upper trunk off the bed. He brings his sound leg over the edge of the bed, which brings him to a semisitting position. He then pushes with both arms (still clasped), while flexing the head toward the affected side, to bring himself upright. The affected leg is simultaneously lowered as he pushes upright. The therapist may need to assist with the head lateral flexion and swinging the affected leg off the bed until the patient learns the technique and gains sufficient strength.

Assisted Transfers

The hemiplegic person is able to accept weight on one or both lower extremities and is therefore a candidate for a pivot transfer. Initially, the patient always transfers with his strong side leading, or toward the non-

involved side, but the patient must learn to transfer in both directions if he is to be independent.

Assisted 90° Pivot Transfer. For a pivot transfer from wheelchair to chair, the locked wheelchair is positioned at an acute angle to the side of the chair placed on the patient's noninvolved side. The therapist faces the patient, who is sitting with his feet on the floor, approximately 20 to 30 cm apart. The patient must first scoot forward in the chair. The therapist assists by having the patient lean to one side and then gently pulls the opposite hip forward in the chair; the patient leans to the other side and the other hip is pulled forward. This is repeated until the patient is near the front edge of the chair. The therapist bends her knees to meet and support the patient's knees. She reaches under the patient's arm to position her hands on the scapula of the involved side or takes hold of the waistband of the patient's trousers. As the patient leans forward and pushes down on the wheelchair armrest with the noninvolved arm to assist standing, the therapist supports one of the patient's knees and assists it into extension while lifting from the scapula or trousers (Fig. 17.3). The important thing is to get the patient to lean forward enough to get his center of gravity over the feet when coming to standing. Patients are

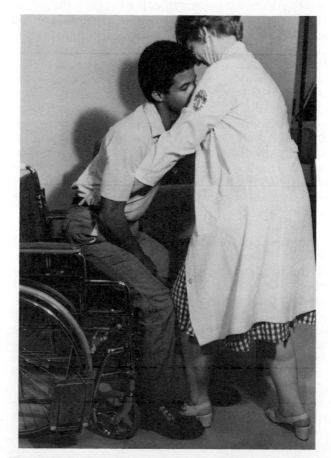

Figure 17.3 Assisted pivot transfer: rising from one surface.

often afraid to lean forward enough, but if they don't the therapist ends up doing more work than she needs to do. The therapist may place one hand on the patient's upper back/neck area to assist and guide the patient to bend forward enough.

After the patient is standing and balanced, the therapist pivots with the patient to turn so that the patient now stands in front of the chair. The therapist helps to lower the patient into the chair slowly by bending her knees as the patient sits. The patient puts his noninvolved hand on the armrest to assist in lowering himself slowly into the chair (Fig. 17.4). The patient must bend forward during sitting to keep the center of gravity over the feet; if he doesn't, sitting will be uncontrolled and he'll "flop" down into the chair. Before the student therapist does the transfer with a patient, she needs to experiment and practice to determine how to place her feet in relation to the patient's feet to offer the best stability to the patient's knee and to prevent tripping each other.

Independent Transfer

Independent 90° Pivot Transfer. In this transfer, the process is the same as noted above, except that it is done without help. To review, the wheelchair is

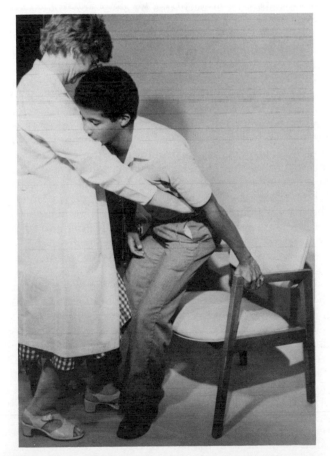

Figure 17.4 Assisted pivot transfer: lowering onto the other surface.

locked in position next to the surface to be transferred to, which is located on the patient's noninvolved side. The front of the wheelchair seat should be perpendicular to, or at an acute angle to, the front of the seating surface to be transferred to. The patient lifts the footrests and slides forward in the wheelchair. The feet are flat and slightly apart on the floor.

Using a rocking motion to gain momentum, the patient then presses with the noninvolved foot to extend that leg while pushing down on the arm of the wheelchair with the noninvolved arm to come to a standing position. Once balanced in a fully standing position, the patient reaches to the surface to which he is transferring, pivots, and lowers himself to the surface.

A modified pivot transfer is sometimes used when the patient's standing balance is poor. In this case, the same procedure would be followed as above, except the patient would not come to a fully standing position. As soon as he had come to a partial stand, he would reach for the surface he is transferring to and pivot. If transferring toward the involved side, the noninvolved arm would maintain contact with the armrest throughout the pivot: the noninvolved arm would push down on the arm of the chair, the patient would raise the buttocks off of the chair and pivot to the new surface while the noninvolved arm maintained contact to assist with balance.

Independent 180° Pivot Transfer. The 180° independent pivot transfer is done similarly to the 90° pivot but requires the patient to turn much more after standing to reach the surface to which he is transferring. This transfer is chosen when required by the circumstances such as in a bathroom or other areas where the wheelchair cannot be positioned for the 90° pivot. Grab bars assist in doing a 180° pivot safely.

Wheelchair Mobility

If the patient is confined to a wheelchair either temporarily or permanently, he can learn to propel a standard wheelchair. To do so, the hemiplegic patient uses both the unaffected arm and leg. The leg provides both power and compensatory steering. A one-arm drive wheelchair, which is commercially available, is confusing to hemiplegics but would be appropriate for patients who have a disability that leaves one arm as the only functional extremity and who have the cognitive and perceptual abilities to learn to operate the chair.

BLINDNESS

This disability of course does not interfere with bed mobility or transfers. Ambulatory mobility is limited, however.

Mobility is taught by a peripatologist, a specialist in blind mobility. Through extensive special training, a blind person can become independently mobile. The long cane method is preferred. The technique of using a guide dog requires specialized training for the person and the dog. Seeing eye dogs, in harness, are working and should never be diverted by someone else or petted without permission of the owner. When a blind person is being led, in lieu of independent mobility, the blind person holds the leader's upper arm and walks about one-half step behind the leader. The leader holds his arm close to his body so that the blind person gets sensory input from the leader's arm and body. In that way, the blind person can sense unevenness in the terrain, steps, turning corners, etc. Verbal cautioning is unnecessary unless there is an overhanging object, such as a branch of a tree, in the path.

Self-Care

In studies of independence in self-care, Katz et al.[11] found that patients with chronic illness regained independence in the following order: feeding, continence, transferring, going to toilet (social and cultural aspects), dressing, and bathing. They hypothesized from observations that loss of these functions would occur in reverse order. Comparison of their conclusions concerning the sequence of the development of self-care independence with child developmental and anthropological observations revealed an ontogenetic consistency. Based on their findings it would seem appropriate for treatment planning to follow this sequence. Some additions can be made, such as the insertion of grooming after feeding, and undressing before dressing. Conversely, some diagnostic conditions may require modifications of this sequence. For example, a spinal cord-injured patient may transfer before he develops continence and, in fact, may never regain continence. A study of the recovery of functional skills in head-injured adults concluded that development of gross hand functions (grasp and pinches) precedes basic and personal ADLs. These are followed by social and community skills, and the last to recover in this population are tasks requiring fine finger dexterity.[12]

Not all patients achieve total independence in self-care. It may be necessary for the occupational therapist to train family members in proper methods of supervising or assisting the patient to perform tasks in the most efficient and safe manner for both patient and family member. In some cases independence is a matter of teaching the patient to direct his own care.

All tasks that the patient will be required to perform independently once discharged must be practiced in a manner similar to the way they will be done. For example, if a patient will bathe in a tub at home, it is inadequate to only practice sponge bathing while hospitalized. It is also inadequate to eliminate from practice the details of self-care such as nail care, ear care, menstrual care, handling catheter, hair setting, contact lens care and use, etc., or to assume that all self-care tasks that a particular person may need to learn are listed on the evaluation checklist.

As each task is taught, all potentially needed equipment should be close at hand. For early training in dressing, clothing that is a size too large should be used since it can be managed more easily. Attention should also be placed on the design details of clothing as some designs are more easily donned by persons with certain disabilities. The details to be considered are the cut of the garment, the sleeve style, type of closure or fasteners, and fabric.[13] Clothing design for the handicapped is just beginning to be attended to by designers and pattern makers. Methods to adapt clothing for wheelchair users, and other disabled persons, have been published by the Sister Kenny Institute.[14] Wishes and preferences of the patient must be respected; common use and fashion may influence what the patient will wear rather than ease.[15]

If the patient must learn to feed himself using adapted utensils, one training sequence is to start with sticky foods that will not easily slide off of the spoon. Skill and endurance in the use of the equipment is sought through practice. Once skilled in basic use of the utensil, the patient is ready to feed himself an entire meal. The therapist should ensure that the meal will be easy to eat, i.e., not spaghetti for dinner and sliced peaches for dessert! The first independent meal should be a pleasant, successful experience, not one spent adjusting the equipment.

Communication devices have burgeoned with the development of rehabilitation engineering. There are three types of devices: (1) direct selection devices that print, out of a fairly large array, the one item that the person points to or activates by some control transducer; (2) scanning devices in which the device points to the item or groups of items in an array one at a time and may or may not print it; and (3) encoding devices that accept codes (e.g., Morse code) and translate them into whole messages.[16,17] These devices are used by those too incoordinated to speak clearly or by those too paralyzed to write or use a standard typewriter for written communication. It is necessary to evaluate the patient and choose the best type of equipment for him.[16,17] The cost may be prohibitive[17] for the ideal solution, but less sophisticated devices, such as language boards that simply have the alphabet or phrases written on them to which the patient points, may increase the person's abilities. Because the more sophisticated instruments may enable an otherwise unemployable person to be employed, the cost may be justified, and financial help may be available from the Vocational Rehabilitation Services.

Techniques and equipment for self-care presented in this chapter are not the only methods of accomplishing these particular tasks. This presentation is not meant to be exhaustive but rather to provide the student therapist with a repertoire of basic skills with which she can approach her patient with confidence. The principles of solutions for each problem are key pieces of information allowing the student to evaluate other techniques or equipment to meet the needs of the patient. Many tasks not mentioned here either do not require adaptation, or the adaptation can be extrapolated from the examples cited. Sources of equipment are rehabilitation supply stores and catalog mail order businesses. The annual *Accent on Living Buyer's Guide* lists sources for all types of equipment.[18] Although there are many pieces of adaptive equipment available for purchase, the occupational therapist needs to know and evaluate each piece of equipment before recommending it to her patient.

LIMITED RANGE OF MOTION

The principles of compensation for limited or restricted range of motion are to increase the person's reach by means of extending handles and to substitute for limited range by use of adaptations.

Feeding

The problem may be one of inability to close the hand enough to grasp the utensil or the inability to bring the hand to the mouth.

Enlarged or elongated handles can be added to spoons or forks. The elongated handle may need to be angled to enable the patient to reach his mouth. Remember that the longer the handle, the heavier and less stable is the device; therefore, the handle should be only as long as is absolutely necessary. Handles may be temporarily enlarged by wrapping a washcloth, foam rubber, or other material around the handle and securing it with a rubber band. Commercially available utensils with handles of plastic or adjustable aluminum can be used more permanently. Also, thermoplastics can be used to mold and enlarge handles for permanent use (see chapter 13).

A universal cuff, or utensil holder, can be used when grasp is not possible. This cuff fits around the palm and has a pocket for insertion of the handle of a utensil (Fig. 17.5).

Grooming

The problems are the same as for feeding. Enlarged or extended handles can be attached to a comb (Fig. 17.6), brush, toothbrush, shampoo brush, lipstick tube, or safety razor.

Aerosol deodorant, hair spray, powder, and perfume can be used by those with limited range.

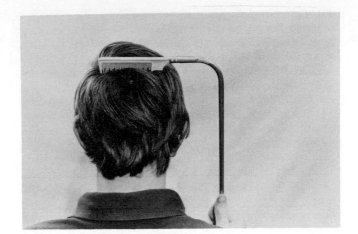

Figure 17.6 Long-handled comb.

Another person may be needed to thoroughly wash and curl a woman's hair; a simple hair style is recommended.

Toileting

The problem is the inability to reach. The patient may not be able to sit on a low commode; therefore, a raised toilet seat would be necessary. The toilet tissue dispenser should be located within reach.

Gravity will assist in pulling clothes down; larger clothes slide off more easily. A dressing stick (a long rod with a hook attached to one end) can be used to pull up the clothing. Wiping tongs can extend reach when using toilet tissue. If grasp is poor, the tissue can be wrapped around the hand to eliminate the need for grasping it. A bidet eliminates the need for wiping by hand. Sanitary napkins with adhesive strips can be used more easily than tampons; the protective paper can be removed using the teeth.

Dressing

Lack of reach and grasp and the inability to raise the arms at the shoulders or to bend the legs at the hips or knees are possible problems encountered in dressing by arthritic patients. For 3 months following hip replacement, patients are restricted from flexing the hip past 90°, adducting the leg past midline, externally rotating the leg, or bearing full weight on the leg.[19]

A dressing stick can be used to pull clothing over the feet or to reach hangers in the closet. Reaching tongs can be used to remove clothes from shelves, to start clothes over parts of the body, or to pick up objects from the floor (Fig. 17.7).

Putting on socks or stockings is a major problem for people who are unable to reach their feet or not allowed to flex the hip. For them, a sock or stocking aid (Fig. 17.8) is a valuable piece of adapted equipment.[19] This may be purchased or made from x-ray film or thermoplastic splinting material by cutting a triangle with rounded corners out of the material, and attaching three straps or strings to the base of the triangle. To use, the triangular material is made into a cone shape,

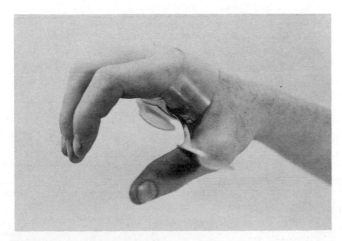

Figure 17.5 Universal cuff.

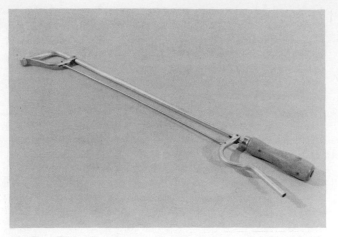

Figure 17.7 Voluntary opening reacher that remains closed to hold objects without exertion of the patient.

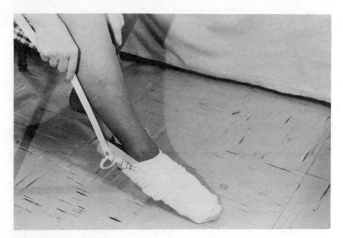

Figure 17.8 One type of stocking aid.

and the cone is inserted into the foot of the stocking; the top of the stocking is pushed down below the top edge of the cone. While the strings are held, the stocking aid with stocking in place is tossed over the toes, and the person's foot is moved into the foot of the stocking. The cone is then removed by pulling the strings, bringing it out of the stocking behind the heel. The stocking will now be within reach and can be pulled up onto the leg.

An alternative method is to place a piece of foam rubber on the floor to help get the stocking onto the foot after it is placed on the toe with a reacher. This method consists of pushing the foot forward across the foam rubber, which provides friction and holds the stocking as the foot slides into the stocking.[8] As this method can be done standing up or sitting on a high stool, it may be particularly helpful to post-hip replacement patients who are not allowed to flex the hip.

Another solution is to sew a garter to each end of a long piece of webbing. The garters are attached to either side of a sock or stocking to pull them up to a point on the leg where they may be reached.

A long shoe horn assists in putting on shoes when the feet cannot be reached.[19] Some long shoe horns have a hook on the opposite end that may be used as a dressing stick. Loafer-style shoes or elastic shoelaces avoid the need to tie shoelaces.

Garters attached to webbing straps may be used to pull up slacks. Cardigan shirts are used instead of slip-over garments. The dressing stick or reacher is used to bring the garment around the shoulders.

Zippers, especially easy sliding, large-toothed plastic ones, were found to be the easiest clothing fastener for 97 arthritic women.[15] Snaps and buttons were rated as difficult, although vertical buttonholes made buttoning easier.[15] Velcro tabs can replace buttons, snaps, or hooks if limited mobility in the fingers prevents buttoning or fastening, although few clothes come with this type of fastener, and therefore the patient's clothing must be adapted. To preserve the look of a buttoned garment, the buttonhole is sewn closed, and the button is attached over the hole. The hook and pile Velcro tabs are sewn to replace the button.[20]

Bathing

The transfer into the tub is facilitated by grab bars **securely** mounted to the studs in the wall beside the bathtub or attached to the side of the bathtub. A securely fastened rubber mat should be placed in the tub, even if the tub has a nonskid surface, and one outside the tub, unless the bathroom is carpeted.

A tub seat is used when the patient is unable, or not allowed, to get down into or up from the bottom of the tub.[19] Different heights and styles are available and need to be evaluated for each patient in terms of stability and ease of transfer. A hand-held shower hose is used for rinsing if a tub seat is required.

The same problems of reach and grasp encountered in dressing are seen to interfere with bathing. Flat handles on faucets do not require grasp and allow better leverage for turning them on. It is helpful if the soap is on a string. It can be purchased that way or made by drilling a hole through a cake of soap and attaching a cord. The soap is either worn around the neck or hung within easy reach. When grasp is limited, a sponge or terrycloth bath mitt may be preferred. A long-handled bath sponge can be used to reach the feet or back[19]; some are designed to hold the soap inside of the sponge. A terrycloth bathrobe is effective for drying.

Miscellaneous

Writing and telephoning may be problem areas. If pinch is limited, the size of the writing instrument can be increased by using sponge rubber or a foam rubber hair curler,[8] or the pencil can be passed through the holes in a practice golf ball. If the person cannot raise the telephone receiver to the ear and hold it there, an extended arm that clamps on the table permanently holds the receiver at a convenient height. If the extended arm is of the gooseneck type, the receiver can be put in different positions. A lever is attached to the phone to depress the activator buttons, and the phone is answered by raising this lever.

DECREASED STRENGTH

The principles of compensation for weakness or decreased strength are to use gravity to assist, to change body mechanics or leverage, to use lightweight devices, and to use electrical appliances. When muscle weakness involves all four extremities, the techniques and devices are extensive; therefore, this section will focus on compensation for involvement of all four extremities. If the patient is weak in his lower extremities with normal upper extremities, many of the techniques or devices will be unnecessary. Other equipment suggestions have been listed in the chapter on spinal cord injury.

Feeding

The problem is the inability to grasp and/or bring the hand to the mouth.

Mobile arm supports or suspension slings (see chapter 13) may be required for proximal weakness, or a table or lapboard at axilla height may be used to offer support for the arm and to eliminate gravity. As strength increases, the surface can be lowered.

A universal cuff can be used to hold the utensil if grasp is absent. A "spork," a utensil that combines the bowl of a spoon with the tines of a fork, is used with the cuff to eliminate the need to change utensils. Some of these have a swivel feature to substitute for the inability to supinate. Gravity and weight of the food keep the bowl level on the way to the mouth; sporks with enlarged handles can be purchased (Fig. 17.9). Some splints provide pinch to hold the utensils. Lightweight utensils are used. If the patient has weak grasp without a splint, lightweight, enlarged handles can be used. For cutting, a sharp, serrated knife is used since less force is needed and it is less likely to slip.

Sandwich holders that hold a sandwich in a trough and have a handle that the patient can manage are available.

An attachable, open-bottomed handle can be added to a glass or soda can to permit picking them up in the absence of grasp. A mug with a T-shaped handle or a handle that allows all four fingers to be inserted provides leverage and stabilizes the fingers around the mug, allowing pick up when only tenodesis grasp is present. A stretch terrycloth coaster placed around a glass can provide friction to assist a weak grasp.[8]

Grooming

The inability to grasp and pinch needs to be dealt with to enable the patient to groom himself. A universal cuff or a splint can be used to hold a rattail comb, toothbrush, lipstick tube, or safety razor if grasp is absent. If grasp is weak, lightweight, enlarged handles may be enough. Electric razor holders that have a handcuff provide a safer method of shaving than use of a safety razor. If the patient wants to use a safety razor, those with a floating head, which will follow the curves of the face are best. A small, plastic brush with or without a cuff attachment may be used to assist in shampooing hair.[8]

Toileting

Transfers, the handling of the body to lower and raise the clothing, and the lack of pinch and grasp are problems.

Pants can be generally pushed down while in the wheelchair by the patient leaning to one side and then the other. If the patient has precarious balance, it may be necessary to transfer back to the wheelchair before raising the clothing. If the patient uses an indwelling catheter or external drainage device, the collection bag can be emptied into the toilet without the need to transfer or remove clothing.

A raised toilet seat is used by quadriplegic individuals to create a space between the seat and toilet bowl rim to allow for insertion of a suppository.

Digit stimulators and suppository inserters are commercially available for those with weak or absent pinch. They are attached to handcuffs for use by quadriplegic patients and the suppository inserter has a spring ejector that releases the suppository after it is properly positioned in the rectum. An inspection mirror is needed if the patient lacks anal sensation.

For those patients with weak grasp and pinch, toilet tissue can be wrapped around the hand for use. Menstrual needs can be met by adaptations to positioning, pants, pad versus tampon, and aids such as mirrors or knee spreaders.[21]

Dressing

Dressing problems include the need to learn new ways of using the stronger limbs to move the paralyzed limbs to dress them, as well as the need to compensate for the lack of pinch and grasp.

While in bed and by using the wrist extensors and elbow flexors, patients with spinal cord injuries at C_6 and below can pull the knees up to dress the lower extremities.

A dressing stick with a loop attached to the end opposite the hook can help quadriplegics. They pull against the loop, using wrist extension, to stabilize tenodesis grasp of the stick.

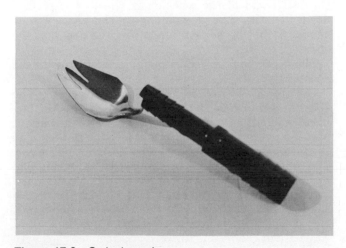

Figure 17.9 Swivel spork.

The sock aid and long-handled shoehorn previously mentioned may be useful. Loops of twill tape can be added to the cuffs of socks to facilitate pulling them on by hooking the thumb in the loop.

The buttonhook, attached to a cuff or with a built-up handle, is used when fingers are unable to manipulate buttons. The hook is inserted through the buttonhole to hook the button and pull it through the buttonhole. The other hand is used to hold the garment near the buttonhole (Fig. 17.10).

A loop of string or leather lacing may be attached to the zipper pull of trousers or other garments, so that in the absence of pinch, the thumb can be hooked in the loop to close the zipper. A hook can also be used.

Primarily, the following methods of quadriplegic dressing were described by Margaret Runge, O.T.R., in an article, "Self Dressing Techniques for Patients with Spinal Cord Injury" in the *American Journal of Occupational Therapy*.[22]

Trousers (and Undershorts).
While the patient is sitting in bed with side rails up, the trousers are positioned with the front up and legs over the bottom of the bed. The trousers are positioned by tossing them or using a dressing stick with a wrist loop.

One leg is lifted by hooking the opposite wrist or forearm under the knee, and the foot is put into the pants leg. The thumb of the other hand hooks a belt loop or pocket to hold the trousers open. Working in a cross-body position aids stability for those with poor balance. The other foot is inserted. The palms of the hands are used to pat and slide the trousers onto the calves, attempting to get the trouser cuffs over the feet. The wrist(s) is hooked under the waistband or in the pockets to pull the trousers up over the knees. The patient continues to pull on the waistband or pockets while returning to supine position to pull the trousers up onto the thighs. This may need to be repeated. Hooking the wrist or thumbs in the crotch helps pull up the trousers. In a side-lying position, the thumb of the top arm is hooked in the back belt loop, and the pants are pulled over the buttocks. Then the patient rolls to

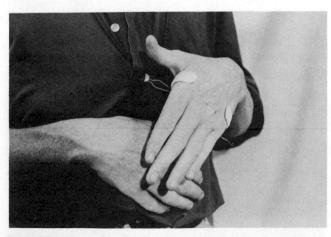

Figure 17.10 Buttonhook on a cuff. Note zipper pull hook on other end.

the other side and repeats the process until the trousers are on. In a supine position, the trousers can be fastened using a zipper pull loop and Velcro tab closing or buttonhook. Removing the trousers is accomplished essentially by reversing the procedures and pushing the pants off.

Socks.
While sitting in the wheelchair, the patient crosses one leg over the other and uses tenodesis pinch to put on the sock and the palms of the hands to help pull it on. If the patient is unable to cross his legs, the foot can be placed on a stool or chair. If trunk balance is poor, one arm can be hooked around the wheelchair upright while reaching with the other hand, or the socks can be put on in a sitting position in bed by crossing first one leg and then the other. A sock cone or aid may be helpful in getting the sock over the toes if the patient is unable to reach his feet. Socks are removed by pushing them off with a dressing stick, long shoehorn, or the thumb hooked in the sock edge.

Long Leg Braces (KAFO; Knee-Ankle-Foot Orthosis) for Paraplegics.
While the patient is sitting in bed, the brace is positioned beside the leg, and then the patient lifts his leg over into the brace. If the shoe is attached to the brace, the foot is first put into the shoe. It is helpful to unlock and flex the knee of the brace to press the shoe against the bed and pull on the uprights to get the heel into the shoe. Then, with the knee still flexed, the shoe can be tied. Next, the knee is straightened, the knee pad is fastened, and then the thigh band is fastened.

For a brace to be worn under trousers, the brace must be attached to the shoe with removable calipers. In this instance, the patient first puts on his socks, the brace, his trousers, then his shoes, and finally attaches the brace to the shoe.

Once the patient is in the wheelchair, other garments are put on.

Shoes.
Loafer-type shoes are most practical for nonambulatory patients. Shoes are put on by crossing one leg at a time as for putting on socks. The shoe is pulled onto the foot by holding the sole of the shoe in the palm of the hand. With the foot on the floor, or on the foot pedal of the wheelchair, the foot is pushed down into the shoe by pushing on the knee. A long shoehorn may be helpful for getting the heel into the shoe.

Shoes can be removed by pushing them off with the shoehorn.

Cardigan Garments (Shirts or Blouses).
The shirt is positioned with the brand label of the shirt facing down and the collar toward the knees. The patient puts his arms under the shirt and into the sleeves. The shirt is pushed on until the sleeves are over the elbows. The shirt is gathered up by using wrist extension and by hooking the thumbs under the shirt back. Then the shirt is placed over the head. The patient shrugs his shoulders to get the shirt down across the shoulders. He hooks his wrists into the sleeves to free the axillae. The patient then leans forward and reaches back with one hand to rub on the shirt back in order to pull it

down. The shirt fronts are lined up, and buttoning begins from the bottom button up, using a buttonhook.

A cardigan garment is removed by pushing first one side and then the other off the shoulders and then alternately elevating and depressing the shoulders to allow gravity to assist in lowering the shirt down the arms. Then one thumb is hooked into the opposite sleeve to pull the shirt over the elbow, and the arm is removed from the shirt.

With the exception of buttons, an overhead garment is put on in a similar manner and removed by hooking one thumb in the back of the neckline and pulling the shirt over the head. The sleeves are then pushed off each arm.

Bra. Either a front- or back-closure style can be used. Velcro can replace hooks for fastening, but many patients can manage the standard hook fastener if it is hooked in front at waist level. After the bra is hooked, it is positioned with the cups in front, and the arms are placed through the shoulder straps. Then, by hooking the opposite thumb under a strap, one strap at a time is pulled over the shoulder.

Bathing

The problems include the transfer,[23] sitting equilibrium,[23] lack of lower-extremity movement, and lack of pinch and grasp.

A padded board placed across one end of the tub provides a level transfer surface. The padding helps to prevent decubiti. The back of the wall of the tub enclosure can be used for trunk support. A padded straight chair can be used either in the tub or in a shower stall. Suction cups or "skis" on the bottom of the chair provide stability for transfers. Other bath seats are available with and without back support or padding. Transfer tub seats, which have two legs in the tub and two legs outside the tub, allow for easier transfers from the wheelchair. Each patient's requirements need to be evaluated and a seat selected to fit them.

Grab bars secured to the studs of the wall help during the transfer and while seated. A suction cup-backed bath mat is used in the bottom of the tub.

The faucets must be placed within reach and must have flat handles for ease in tapping them off and on using the fist. A hand-held shower is used. If the shower does not have a mixer valve, water temperature is adjusted by turning on the cold water first and then adding the hot to prevent scalding desensitized skin. Soap on a string or dispenser soap is helpful. A bath mitt is used if grasp is weak or absent. A large towel is used for drying off before transferring back to the wheelchair. Bathing and drying the feet and legs is a particular problem for patients with poor trunk balance, and they may prefer to do foot hygiene while in bed.[23]

A custom-made shower stall installed in a person's home provides the best solution for a patient confined to a wheelchair. The shower area has a raised slope to prevent the water from running out, but allows the passage of a special shower wheelchair. Such a chair is meant to be wet without being damaged. Plans for such bath enclosures have been published in the popular press.

Miscellaneous

The quadriplegic patient will encounter problems with holding a book and turning the pages, with writing or recording notes in business or school, and possibly in telephoning.

If a person is unable to hold a book, bookholders are available. Some support a book on a table, whereas others are designed to hold a book overhead for reading supine in bed. If a person is reading supine, prism glasses are needed to direct the vision to a 90° angle so that the book may be seen.

If page turning is difficult, some of the following ways of increasing friction might be of assistance: (1) Tacky Fingers, which is a sticky substance available in stationery stores, can be applied to a patient's weak fingers; (2) a rubber thimble or finger cot can be put on a posted thumb when the patient wears a splint; (3) a pencil with the eraser end down can be used in a universal cuff or hand splint; and (4) a mouthstick with a friction tip end can be used. Electric page turners, which automatically turn pages when activated by microswitch or other means of control, are available for the severely disabled.

An alternative for the severely paralyzed is "talking books." These are records that were originally only made available to the blind, but are now by law available to the physically handicapped. The Library of Congress has a large collection of records, including many current issues of magazines. The records are free and can be ordered by mail or through the hospitals division of the local library. Particular books needed by students or professionals will be recorded on request. With the advent of cassette tape players, many popular books have been recorded and are available for purchase at bookstores or on loan at public libraries. A special mouthstick has been devised to assist independent use of a cassette tape player by severely paralyzed persons.[24]

Splints that provide pinch can be used to hold a writing instrument. If pinch is absent, and the patient does not use a splint, a pencil holder (Fig. 17.11) that encircles the pencil as well as the thumb and index finger can be made of thermoplastic materials.[25] Felt-tip pens mark with little pressure and are therefore easier to use when writing.

If the arms cannot be used, a mouthstick with pencil attached can, with practice, become an effective writing tool.

If writing is not possible or speed of recording is important, as in taking notes in the classroom, a tape recorder can be used. If necessary, the mechanical controls can be adapted.[20] If the recorder has electronic controls, it can be adapted by use of microswitches or other transducers.

Electric typewriters with automatic carriage return can be used by paralyzed persons who type using either typing sticks or a mouthstick. A mouthstick is prefera-

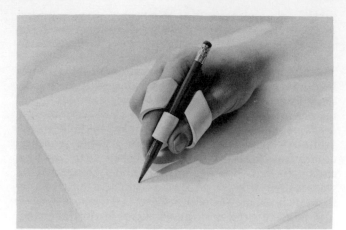

Figure 17.11 An Orthoplast pencil holder.

bly made by a dentist, who molds a mouthpiece of dental acrylic to conform to the patient's dentition; to the mouthpiece is added a lightweight wooden, plastic, or aluminum rod with an eraser or other type of end piece. Mouthsticks can be purchased commercially that have various interchangeable tips such as pencil, pen, brush, etc. Self-correcting ribbon may be useful, depending on the manner in which it is activated by the particular typewriter. The IBM machine can be fitted with a paper roll dispenser that feeds 20-cm (8-inch) paper into the typewriter for persons unable to pick up sheets of paper and start them into the machine. Personal computers with printers and word processing software are ideal for the patient who must do a lot of writing.

Severely disabled quadriplegics unable to use mechanical controls of a typewriter keyboard have been successful in using a newly developed voice-controlled computer terminal that types out the spoken message. Further development and study of this device for use in providing employment opportunities for the severely disabled are ongoing.[26]

C_6 level quadriplegics can pick up the telephone receiver and bring it to the ear. An executive shoulder rest attached to the receiver holds it there until the conversation is finished. Push-button phones are easiest to manage and are readily available, even for use in areas that do not have Touch-Tone® service. The push buttons can be depressed using a mouthstick or typing stick. Phone service is available that requires the patient to press one code number to initiate automatic dialing. For patients with greater paralysis, automatic telephone dialers are available.[16,27] An operator's headset can be used instead of the handset.

INCOORDINATION

The principles of compensation for problems of incoordination are to provide stability and to substitute for lack of fine skill. The patient is taught to use his body in as stable a posture as is possible, to sit when possible, and to stabilize the upper extremities by bearing weight on them against a surface or by holding the upper arms close to the body, or both. Stabilizing the

head may improve a person's ability to control his upper extremities. Friction surfaces, weighted utensils, or weighted cuffs added to the distal segments of the extremities, and the use of larger and/or less precise fasteners, all contribute to increasing independence by lessening the effects of the incoordination.

Feeding

The plate is stabilized on a friction surface (wet towel, wet sponge cloth, nonskid mat, etc.). A plate guard or scoop dish can be used to prevent the food from being pushed off the plate. The utensil may be weighted for stability, may have an enlarged handle to facilitate grasp, and may be plastisol-coated to protect the person's teeth. Sharp utensils are to be avoided. A weight cuff on the wrist is often chosen rather than a weighted utensil because the cuff can be heavier; also the cuff makes it unnecessary to weight each item that the patient will use (Fig. 17.12). The person may successfully drink from a covered glass or cup that has a sipping spout. A cup can be so adapted by using plastic food wrap as a cover, with a straw poked through it.[8] Some may use a long plastic straw that is held in place by a straw holder attachment; the patient moves his head to the straw, but he does not touch it with his hand. A severely incoordinated person with good strength and endurance may use an upper-extremity control brace, or friction feeder,[28] which supports the arm and dampens the patient's motion through the use of friction disks at each joint. The amount of friction can be adjusted.

Grooming

Weighted cuffs on the wrists may help some patients gain greater accuracy while grooming. Large lipstick tubes are easier to use than small ones. The arms will

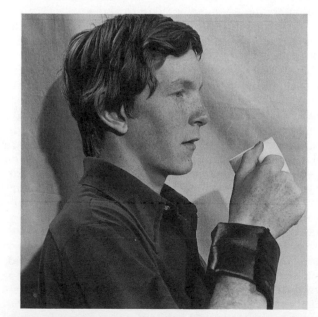

Figure 17.12 Weight cuff used to damp intention tremor or other incoordinated movements.

need to be stabilized to use lipstick. A simple hairstyle that does not need setting or arrangement is the best choice. For a patient who has difficulty holding a large comb, a military-style brush with a strap can be used.

Roll-on or stick deodorant is preferred to aerosol since these types eliminate the risk of accidentally spraying the substance into the eyes. An electric razor is preferred to a safety razor both because it is more easily held and because a safety razor can cause a cut if it is involuntarily moved sideways over the skin. Patients with fairly good head control improve their accuracy by holding the electric razor steady and moving their face over the cutting surface. An electric toothbrush is also useful both because it is heavier and because it can he held steady while the head is moved. This same principle can be employed when filing the nails: fasten the emery board to a flat surface and move each nail over the emery board. Cutting the nails may be an unsafe procedure for incoordinated patients; therefore, filing is recommended. Sanitary napkins with adhesive strips to hold them in place are preferred to tampons.

Dressing

Clothes that facilitate independent dressing are front-opening, loosely fitting garments with large buttons, Velcro tape closures, or zippers. The wrinkle-resistant and stain-shedding materials enable the person to look well groomed throughout the day. To overcome difficulty with buttoning, a buttonhook with an enlarged and/or weighted handle, if necessary, can be used. A loop of ribbon, leather, or metal chain can be attached to the zipper pull so that the person can hook it with a finger instead of pinching the zipper pull. To eliminate the need to fasten hooks on a bra, these can be replaced with Velcro. To don the bra, it is easier for the patient to put it around her waist, which is thinner and puts less tension on the garment, then fasten it in front where she can see what she is doing, turn it around, put her arms in, and pull it up into place. Elastic straps make this a relatively easy procedure. Some persons prefer to use an all elastic slipover-type bra with no hooks. Shoes can be of the loafer style or can have flip closures to eliminate tying. Many shoes are now available with Velcro closures. Patients who ambulate may need to wear tie shoes for stability and support. Tie shoes can be adapted using zipper shoelaces or elastic shoelaces. If a man wears a tie, he may choose to slide the knot down and pull the tie off over his head without undoing the knot or to use clip ties if his degree of coordination allows that.

Bathing

The patient may independently bathe, but must adhere closely to safety precautions. A bath mat with rubber suction cups is placed outside the tub to stand on while transferring and another is placed in the tub. It is important to be certain that the mats are securely stuck before trusting one's safety to them. Safety grab bars should be placed where they would be most useful to the particular person's needs: one mounted into the studs of the wall at the side of the tub and one mounted on the rim of the tub may be necessary. A bath chair or seat can eliminate the difficulty of trying to stand up from a sitting position at the bottom of the tub and provide a stable position for the patient when trying to wash his feet. If a seat is used, a hand-held shower spray needs to be available. If the patient chooses to shower instead of bathe, the mats, safety bars, and seat also must be provided. In either case, the water should be drawn once the patient has transferred in and is seated; a mixer tap is ideal, but if unavailable, the cool water should be turned on first and the hot water added to prevent scalding.

Soap on a string keeps the soap retrievable, or a bath mitt with a pocket to hold the soap can be used. The water should be drained before the person attempts to stand to transfer out of the tub. An extra large towel or large terry wraparound robe facilitates the drying process.

Miscellaneous

Communication is a problem to some incoordinated persons. For typing, a shield that covers the keyboard and has holes cut out over the keys prevents misstrikes. These shields are available for computer keyboards as well as for typewriters. If a shield is not available for a particular keyboard, one can easily be made from acrylic. A board placed in front of the typewriter on which the forearms can be stabilized would offer support for the arms while typing. IBM distributes a wooden armrest that attaches to the front of the keyboard.

For the severely incoordinated person, computer-operated typing (or communication) systems have been developed. One such is the **Auto Com**, developed at the University of Wisconsin in Madison. It has a large board with the letters alphabetically arranged and numbers and other characters similar to a typewriter. The letters selected are transferred to a TV monitor. Corrections are more easily made than on a conventional typewriter. The unit has been reported as an aid to classroom communication for a severely involved cerebral-palsied child at Kennedy Memorial Hospital in Boston.[29]

Communications systems can be accessed in a variety of ways including touch, activation by a light that is worn on a head band, strategically placed switches, and voice. Today, the attempt is made to use existing hardware and develop software that can be used by the disabled. An important job for the occupational therapist and rehabilitation engineer is to determine the interface, or means of access to the system for the patient. It is the interface that will often determine the outcome of a user/device relationship.[30]

Manual Communications Module, which is a portable, frequency-selective communication device, has been used successfully by severely involved cerebral-palsied adults to substitute for verbal communication in social situations.[31] It is operated by a keyboard and has a LED (light-emitting diode) display. It can also be used to communicate over the telephone to someone who has a compatible unit for decoding and was, in fact, originally designed for that purpose for the deaf.[31]

LOSS OF THE USE OF ONE UPPER EXTREMITY OR ONE SIDE OF THE BODY

The methods described below pertain to the hemiplegic patient who has lost the use of one side of his body. The methods and equipment may also be used by the unilateral upper-extremity amputee if necessary. However, the amputee will need less adaptation because he has normal trunk and lower-extremity function, as well as normal perception and cognition. Persons with temporary casts or restrictions of use of one upper extremity can also benefit from these ideas.

The principles of compensation for loss of use of one upper extremity or one side of the body are to provide substitution for the stabilizing or holding function of the involved upper extremity and to adapt the few truly bilateral activities so they can be done unilaterally.

Feeding

This is essentially a one-handed task, except for cutting meat and spreading bread. These tasks can be done by use of adapted equipment.

Meat can be simultaneously stabilized and cut by use of a rocker knife, a knife with a sharp curved blade that cuts when rocked over the meat (Fig. 17.13). The tool that combines a rocker knife and fork is dangerous and is to be avoided.

Bread can be spread if stabilized on a nonslip surface or trapped in the corner of a spikeboard and spread toward the corner (Fig. 17.14). Soft spreads facilitate this process.

Grooming

The problem here is the need to attend to the unaffected extremity and to find substitutions for two-handed activities.

Applying deodorant to the unaffected arm is more easily done using an aerosol spray unless the person has excellent range and can reach the axilla and

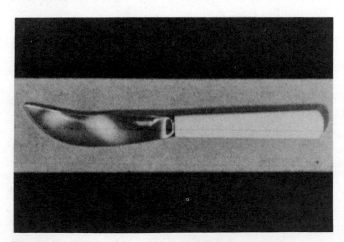

Figure 17.13 Rocker knife for one-handed cutting.

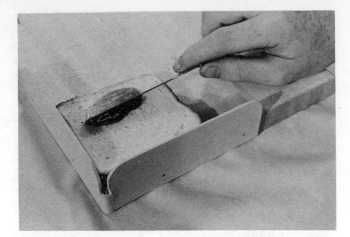

Figure 17.14 Spreading one handed by trapping bread in the corner of a spike board.

thereby use other types of applicators. To allow application of deodorant to the affected axilla, that arm is passively placed away from the body.

Fingernails of the unaffected hand are cleaned by rubbing them on a small suction cup brush attached to the basin; they are filed by rubbing the nails over an emery board secured to a table or other flat surface. The nails of the affected hand can be cleaned and trimmed using the person's habitual methods.

Using a suction denture brush, the person can scrub his dentures by rubbing them over the brush, which is fastened to the inside of the basin. Partially filling the basin with water and laying a facecloth in the bottom cushions the dentures if they are dropped accidentally.

An electric razor is recommended if judgment is impaired; accidents are possible with a safety razor.

Toileting

The problem is arranging the clothing, which is normally a two-handed activity.

There should be a grab bar mounted on the wall beside the toilet or a Versa Frame mounted on the toilet to assist transfers. Once standing, anyone wearing trousers unfastens them, and gravity takes them down. If the patient's balance is precarious and will interfere with retrieving them after using the toilet, the person can put the affected hand in the pocket, which prevents the trousers from sliding below the knees. A woman can lean her affected side against the adjacent wall, if available, for balance; she can then raise her dress on the affected side and tuck it between her body and the affected arm. Then she lowers her underpants to knee level and pulls the dress up on the unaffected side. A dress or skirt that wraps around facilitates this process by allowing the woman to reach across the front of herself and pull the material forward to anchor it between her body and the affected arm; then she lowers her underpants and holds the remaining material aside while seating herself using the grab bar. The toilet tissue should be mounted conveniently to the unaffected side. The patient will be able to manage menstrual needs by use of tampons or adhesive-type sanitary napkins.

Dressing

The following methods are taken from material prepared by the occupational therapy staff of Highland View Cuyahoga County Hospital in Cleveland, Ohio, and from an article in the *American Journal of Occupational Therapy* by Gladys Brett, O.T.R.[32] As a general rule, the affected limb is dressed first and undressed last.

Shirt or Cardigan Garment. *A. Overhead Method to Put on and Remove.* This method is least confusing for a patient with sensory and perceptual impairment, but is cumbersome for dresses and is not used for coats.

1. To keep the shirt from twisting, hold the collar and shake.
2. Put the shirt on the lap, label facing up, and the collar next to the abdomen; drape the shirttail over the knees.
3. Open the sleeve for the affected arm from the armhole to the cuff.
4. Pick up the affected hand and put it into the sleeve.
5. Pull the sleeve up over the elbow; if not pulled past the elbow, the hand will fall out when continuing.
6. Put the unaffected hand into the armhole. Raise the arm out and push it through the sleeve.
7. Gather the back of the shirt from tail to collar.
8. Hold the gathered shirt up, lean forward, duck the head, and put the shirt over the head.
9. To straighten the shirt, lean forward, work the shirt down over the shoulders (often the shirt gets caught on the affected shoulder and must first be pushed back over the shoulder), and reach back and pull the tail down.
10. To button, line up the shirt fronts and match each button with the correct buttonhole, starting with the bottom button.

To remove the shirt, the patient unbuttons it, leans forward, and uses the unaffected hand to gather the shirt up in back of the neck. He ducks the head, pulls the shirt over the head, then takes the shirt off the unaffected arm first.

B. Over-the-Shoulder Method to Put on and Remove. The more aware patient may prefer this method, especially if he has some voluntary control of his affected extremity and can place his extremity into the garment, because it is similar to the customary method. This method is also used for coats.

1. To keep the shirt from twisting, hold the collar and shake.
2. Put the shirt on the lap, label facing up, and the collar next to the abdomen, with the shirttail draped over the knees.
3. Put the affected hand into one sleeve.
4. Pull the sleeve up over the elbow.

5. Grasp the collar at the point closest to the unaffected side.
6. Hold tightly to the collar, lean forward, and bring the collar and shirt around the affected side and behind the neck to the unaffected side.
7. Put the unaffected hand into the other armhole. Raise the arm out and up to push it through the sleeve.
8. To straighten the shirt, lean forward, work the shirt down over the shoulders, reach back and pull the tail down, and then straighten the sleeve under the affected axilla.
9. To button, line up shirt fronts and match each button with the correct buttonhole, starting with the bottom button.

To remove the shirt, unbutton it and use the unaffected hand to throw the shirt back off the unaffected shoulder. Work the shirt sleeve off the unaffected arm. Press the shirt cuff against the leg and pull the arm out. Lean forward. Use the unaffected hand to pull the shirt across the back. Take the shirt off of the affected arm.

Pullover Garment. *Putting on:*

1. Garment is positioned on the lap, bottom toward chest and label facing down.
2. Using the unaffected hand, roll up the bottom edge of the shirt back, all the way up to the sleeve on the affected side.
3. Spread the armhole opening as large as possible. Using the unaffected hand, place the affected arm into the armhole and pull the sleeve up onto the arm *past the elbow.*
4. Insert the unaffected arm into the other sleeve.
5. Gather the shirt back from bottom edge to neck, lean forward, duck the head, and pass the shirt over the head.
6. Adjust the shirt on the involved side up and onto the shoulder and remove twists.

Removing:

1. Starting at top back, gather the shirt up, lean forward, duck the head, and pull the shirt forward over the head.
2. Remove the unaffected arm, then the affected arm.

Trousers. Modifications of these methods are used for men's and women's underclothing and pantyhose.

Putting on Trousers:

1. Sit. **Note:** If wheelchair is used, brakes should be locked and footrests should be in "up" position and/or swung out of the way. Move the unaffected leg beyond the midline of the body for balance.
2. Grasp the ankle or calf of the affected leg. Lift and cross the affected leg over the unaffected leg.
3. Pull the trousers onto the affected leg up to, but not above, the knee.

4. Uncross the legs.
5. Put the unaffected leg into the other pant leg.
6. Remain sitting. Pull the pants up above the knees.
7. To prevent the pants from dropping when standing, put the affected hand into the pant pocket, or the thumb into a belt loop.
8. Stand up. Pull the pants up over the hips; button and zip pants while standing. Persons with **poor balance**: remain seated and pull the pants up over the hips by shifting from side to side; button and zip pants from a seated position.

Removing Trousers. Sit. **Note**: If sitting in wheelchair, be sure wheelchair is locked. Unfasten the pants. Work the trousers down on the hips as far as possible. Stand. Let the trousers drop past the knees. Sit. Remove the trousers from the unaffected leg. Cross the affected leg over the unaffected leg. Remove the trousers from the affected leg. Uncross the legs.

Alternate method for persons with **poor balance**: place locked wheelchair or chair against a wall. Sit. Unfasten the trousers. Work the trousers down on the hips as far as possible. Put the wheelchair foot rests in "up" position and/or swing them out of the way. Lean back against the chair and press down with the unaffected leg to raise the buttocks slightly. Lean from side to side in the chair. Use the noninvolved arm to work the trousers down past the hips. Remove the trousers from the unaffected leg. Cross the affected leg over the unaffected leg. Remove the trousers from the affected leg. Uncross the legs.

Socks or Stockings. *Putting on:*

1. The person sits in a straight chair (with arms if balance is questionable) or in a locked wheelchair with foot pedals in "up" position.
2. The unaffected leg is placed slightly beyond midline of body toward the affected side, and the affected leg is crossed over it by grasping the ankle. If the person has difficulty in maintaining the leg in this position, a small stool under the unaffected leg will increase hip flexion angle and hold the affected leg more securely. If the patient cannot cross his legs, the heel is rested on a small stool, and a reacher is used to put the sock onto the toe and pull it up.
3. The top of the sock is opened by inserting the fist into the cuff area and then opening the fist and spreading the fingers.
4. The sock is put on the foot by slipping the toes into the cuff opening made under the spread hand. The sock is then pulled into place, and wrinkles are eliminated.

Removing. The leg is positioned as it is when putting the sock on. The sock is then pushed off with the unaffected hand.

Shoes. A loafer-type shoe is put on the affected foot with the shoe on the floor. The foot is started into the shoe, and a shoehorn is used to help ease the foot into the shoe. A tie shoe is put onto the affected foot after the leg is crossed over the unaffected one to bring the foot closer. If the laces have been thoroughly loosened, the person is often able to work the shoe on while the leg is crossed over by grasping the heel of the shoe with the unaffected hand and working it back and forth over the heel until it goes on completely. Sometimes, it is necessary to insert a shoehorn while the leg is crossed over and then carefully lower the foot with the shoe half on and finish getting the shoe on the foot by repeatedly pushing down on the knee and adjusting the shoehorn.

Tying the shoes is a problem. It is possible to tie a conventional bow one-handed, but it requires fine dexterity and normal perception. The amputee may prefer to do this or use loafer-style shoes. The hemiplegic patient can use flip-, zipper-, or Velcro-closure shoes. The person may use adaptations such as Know-bows, Wrap-a-laces, or elastic laces. Or he can learn a simplified, effective one-handed shoe tie as illustrated (Fig. 17.15). By putting the lace through the last hole from the outside of the shoe toward the tongue of the shoe, the tension of the foot against the shoe will hold the lace tight while the bow is being tied. One-hand shoe tying is especially difficult for patients with cognitive/perceptual deficits.

Short Leg Brace (AFO: Ankle-Foot Orthosis). If the patient uses a metal brace, it is usually designed so that the fastener is on the side toward the unaffected hand. Velcro closures are used primarily.

Putting on:

1. Pull the tongue of the shoe up through the laces so it does not push down into the shoe as the brace is put on.
2. Sit. Use a straight chair with arms or a locked wheelchair with the footrests up and/or swung out of the way. Bring the unaffected leg past midline in front of the body. Cross the affected leg over the unaffected leg.
3. Use the unaffected hand to hold the brace by the calf band. Swing the brace back and then forward so that the heel is between the side bars and the leg is in front of the calf band. Continue to swing the shoe forward until the toes are at the shoe opening.
4. Turn the shoe inward and insert the toes at a slight angle. This keeps the toes from catching at the sides of the shoe.
5. Pull the brace on as far as possible. Hold the brace in place by pressing on the calf band with the unaffected leg.
6. Use a shoehorn; insert it flat and directly under the heel of the foot in the back.
7. Leave the shoehorn in place. Grasp the calf band.
8. Pulling up on the calf band, uncross the leg.
9. Position the affected foot on the floor so that the heel is at a point just ahead of the knee. Push the heel forward while moving the shoehorn into an upright position with the unaffected hand.

1. Tie a knot in one end of the shoelace.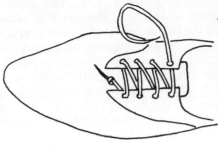

   Thread the unknotted end up through the hole nearest the toe of the shoe, on the left side.

2. Take the lace across the tongue of the shoe and up under the flap on the opposite side of the shoe.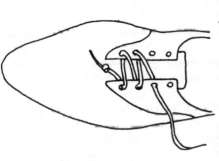

3. Continue to go across the tongue and up under the flap on the next highest hole on the opposite side until you reach the top (or go down through the last hole so the tension will be maintained for tying.)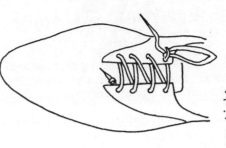

4. Circle around toward the toe of the shoe and go under the part of the lace that is going across the tongue to the last hole.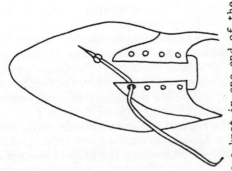

5. Circle around toward the top of the shoe. Pull free lace through the loop down toward the ankle and out to the left side.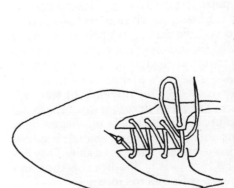

6. Pull loop tight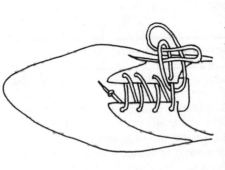

From: Highland View Cuyahoga County Hospital, Cleveland, Ohio 44122 (with permission)

Figure 17.15 One-handed shoe tie—left hemiplegic.

10. Work the foot into the shoe by pushing downward on the knee and moving the shoehorn back and forth. If the shoelaces are loose enough, a shoehorn may not be necessary.
11. Grasp the brace upright and pull up until the foot slips into place in the shoe. Remove the shoehorn.
12. Fasten the strap, being careful not to snag stockings. Fasten the shoes.

Removing. Sit. Cross the affected leg over the unaffected leg. Unfasten the straps and the laces. Push down on the calf band of the brace until the shoe is off the foot.

If the patient uses a posterior shell or molded AFO, the brace is put on the leg and the strap is fastened before the shoe is put on. It may be necessary to add another strap near the ankle to hold the brace onto the foot while attempting to put on the shoe. The shoe is put on as mentioned above for the unaffected foot. It is difficult to put the shoe on with the posterior shell in place. If all else fails (as this method could bend/break the brace—check with your orthotist first), the plastic AFO can be placed into the shoe first and then the patient puts his foot in in a method similar to that described for putting on a metal brace. The important thing to remember is to have the laces very, very loose to allow the maximum room possible for getting the foot into the brace and shoe.

Bra. To put on a bra, it is placed around the back at waist level and turned to hook in front where the patient can see what she is doing. It is then rotated to proper position, the affected arm is placed through the shoulder strap, and then the unaffected arm is placed through the other shoulder strap. The bra is pulled up into place. It is removed by reversing the process.

In some cases the patient is able to leave the bra closures hooked and don the bra by putting it over her head in a manner similar to donning a pullover garment. A plump patient may need an adapted front-closing bra if she cannot approximate the two edges of the bra to fasten it. Two flat metal belt keepers are sewn on the side of the bra opening that is on the involved side. Two cotton twill straps are sewn opposite these keepers on the other side of the bra opening. The hook Velcro is sewn as tabs on the ends of the twill straps near the bra. The pile Velcro is sewn at the distal ends of these straps. After the bra is on, fastening is done by threading these straps from the noninvolved side through the keepers on the involved side. They are pulled to bring the two ends of the bra together, and then they are secured with Velcro closures.

Bathing

The bathing arrangements described for patients with incoordination apply to hemiplegic persons also. In addition, these patients find a long-handled bath sponge that has a pocket to hold the soap useful to allow bathing of the unaffected upper arm and the back. The lower arm of the unaffected side is bathed by putting the soapy washcloth across the knees and rubbing the arm back and forth over it, unless the patient has some return of function and can use a bath mitt on the affected hand.

If sensory impairment exists, extra precautions should be taken to be certain of water temperature.

The hemiplegic patient should dry himself as much as possible while still seated on the bath chair before transferring out of the tub. The water is completely drained from the tub before the transfer is attempted. The patient may need assistance with the transfer if there is not enough room near the tub to position the wheelchair so that his noninvolved side leads.

A unilateral amputee can bathe as usual, but a rubber mat or nonskid strips in the tub, a grab bar, and letting the water drain before exiting are worthwhile safety measures.

Miscellaneous

A one-handed typing method has been developed for persons with the use of only one upper extremity.[8] Persons with only one functional arm need to stabilize the paper when writing in longhand. The paper can be secured using masking tape, a clipboard, a weight, the affected extremity acting as a weight, or other similar means.

BLINDNESS

Organization and consistency in the placement of objects is necessary for the blind person to be able to efficiently locate things. Memory training may be necessary for the newly blinded individual. He will need to develop increased awareness of the information that he receives from his senses of smell, touch, hearing, and taste. This awareness does not automatically occur but must be developed through training. Orientation to the environment is achieved through these senses, although a verbal description of the surroundings by someone else is extremely valuable. The American Foundation of the Blind is a major source of obtaining information and adapted devices for blind persons.

Feeding

The patient explores the placement of dishes, glasses, and utensils at his place. If dining alone, he explores the location and identifies the food by feel, using fork and taste. If dining with a companion, he can be instructed verbally using a clock method of description, e.g., meat is located at 3 o'clock. When pouring liquid, the correct amount is determined by the weight of the cup when it is full. Salt is distinguished from pepper by taste or use of differently shaped shakers. Food is cut by finding the edge of the food with the fork, moving the fork by a bite-sized amount onto the meat, and then cutting the food, keeping the knife in contact with the fork.

Grooming

A major problem is identification of objects. This can be done through the use of taste, touch (size, shape, texture), location, or braille labels. The application of cosmetics or toiletries is another problem; fingers of the assistive hand can be guides, e.g., when shaving sideburns or applying eyebrow pencil. Aerosol sprays may not be preferred because the blind person cannot determine the extent of the spray, although in some cases, such as with perfume, this does not matter.

Dressing

The blind person has no difficulty with the physical aspects of dressing. The only problems that arise relate to appearance. The blind person needs a system to coordinate colors of clothes and compatibility of style. One system of identification is to use French knots in certain patterns to designate color or identify all components of a total costume. Another system is to store clothes of like color together. Hems, buttons, seams, and socks should be checked for mending. Colorless wax polishes can be used to shine shoes. Clothes should always be hung properly to prevent wrinkles. Wrinkle-free, stain-resistant, no-iron fabrics are preferred. Listening to the weather report guides the person's selection of appropriate clothing, as for anyone. Clothing selection should be done with the assistance of a sighted person who can describe colors and style. Purchase of garments of the same style in different colors should be avoided because color identification is often done by remembering which style is a certain color.

Miscellaneous

The blind person can use a signature or writing guide to stay within boundaries while writing in longhand. Braille can be written by hand using a stylus and plate or on a machine similar to a courtroom stenotype. Braille writing is done mirror image to the way it is read.

Besides braille and talking books, new technological advances are providing new means for the blind to "read" regular print. One such device is the **Optacon**.[33] The Telesensory Systems' **Optacon** converts printed letters into direct tactual representations of the letters for use by the blind. The Optacon measures $2 \times 6 \times 8$ inches and can be carried around for use in reading posted messages, signs, or library materials not available in braille. A miniature camera, attached to the device by a cord, receives the printed word, and phototransistors send signals that are converted by the Optacon into a pattern on vibrating reeds where the fingers interpret the pattern. Speed of reading is slower than with braille, but when braille translations or readers are unavailable or impractical, it is a valuable tool. Its price limits general use.

Other computer devices change the printed word into spoken language.

Telephoning is no problem for the blind person as soon as he memorizes the dial or touch buttons.

The person can tell time using a braille watch. Sounds of the day, the radio, or TV can provide a general orientation to time. Clocks that announce the time are sold in gadget catalogues.

Tactile discrimination enables the person to identify coins; paper money is discriminated by the way it is folded after its denomination has been identified previously by someone else. Consistency is important here as in all aspects of the blind person's life. Some countries use paper money of different sizes for different denominations, but unfortunately that is not so in the United States yet. A machine is available that announces the value of paper money fed into it and would be helpful in a business, but is too cumbersome to be carried around for use by shoppers.

REDUCED CARDIOPULMONARY ENDURANCE

Patients with cardiopulmonary diseases have reduced ability to use oxygen needed for muscle (including cardiac muscle) and brain functions. If oxygen deprivation is severe enough, neuropsychological changes involving memory, perception, and information processing occur. These would affect the effectiveness of the teaching/learning process as well as the performance of the patient.

Principles used with these patients include conservation of energy, pacing and rest during activity, matching activity demands to patient ability, and avoidance of stressful positions and environmental stressors.

Energy conservation techniques are elaborated on in chapter 18. They include elimination of unnecessary tasks, working when seated if possible, planning ahead to have all required equipment present before starting a task, combining tasks to eliminate extra work, using electrical appliances to conserve personal energy, use of lightweight utensils and tools, and working with gravity assisting, not resisting.

Cardiac patients are cautioned to stop activity when they experience angina or shortness of breath (SOB). Chronic obstructive pulmonary disease (COPD) patients are taught to work slowly and to pace themselves and take "resting pauses"[34] during tasks. Both types of patients are taught to intersperse rest periods throughout the day.

Some activities require higher levels of metabolism than do others. One way to guide activity selection is to monitor the patient's breathing or heart rate. Dyspnea (SOB) signals the COPD patient that the activity he is doing is beyond the level of exertion. Angina or excessive increase in heart rate (20 beats over resting rate) signals the myocardial infarct patient that he has reached his limit. Another way to decide on appropriate level of activities for patients is to use metabolic equivalent tables (MET) (see chapter 30) or to use a task analysis system that rates activities according to six characteristics: rate, resistance, muscle groups used, involvement of trunk muscles, arm position, and isometric work or straining involved.[35] Most self-care activities require less than three METs; however, showering, tub bathing, toileting, and washing and setting hair require higher levels.[36] It should be remembered that MET charts are averages and do not account for particular circumstances and can therefore not be used without also monitoring the patient.

Stressful positions to be avoided include bending over [34,37,38] (slip-on shoes, sock aid, reacher, and long-handled sponge can be used to assist ADL independence); reaching overhead[34,38,39] (store clothes and utensils within easy reach, or rest arms on something or repeatedly lower them to rest if reaching is necessary); and isometric contractions including pushing, pulling, and maintained grasp. Patients are taught to exhale[37,38] or count if they do these tasks.

A hot, humid environment increases SOB and reduces the patient's ability to do activity. A COPD patient can feel "suffocated" in a shower.[34]

Driving

The ability to drive provides the greatest freedom of mobility for the physically disabled. In those cases that do not involve brain damage, the potential for driving is good. Those with limited range of motion may require special seating, but may otherwise be able to drive. Those with severely limited lower-extremity range can use hand-controlled automobiles as developed for spinal cord-injured patients.

Many persons with decreased strength can be safe drivers with the proper selection of the car, necessary adaptations, and training in the use of hand or foot controls as appropriate to the disability. Quadriplegic patients with a level of injury at C_6 or below are considered potential candidates for driver training.

CAR SELECTION

If a wheelchair-bound person is to use a sedan-type car independently, it must be a two-door sedan that is large enough to allow access for the wheelchair to be stored behind the front seat, with a high enough door opening space to accommodate the wheelchair handles, and with a large enough door to allow space in front for ease of transfer. The person may choose to remain in his wheelchair and use a van with a ramp or hydraulic lift, in which case wheelchair tie downs will be required to stabilize the wheelchair.

Hand controls can be attached to the brake and accelerator. There are many different types of hand controls. Most require at least moderate strength (4 to 6 kg) to push or pull the levers, but some "less effort" or "zero effort" models that require about 1 kg for acceleration, braking, and steering are now being produced.[40] However, they are very expensive since they must have an emergency backup system to keep the controls "less effort" in the event of engine failure.[40]

In an effort to control for equipment-dependent accidents, the Veterans Administration (VA) now requires that driving controls meet quality requirements before they are purchased by the VA for disabled veterans.[41,42] Governmental standards setting minimal levels of acceptable safety and quality for automobile driving aids have been published in the *Federal Register* (40[65]:15,017, Apr. 3, 1975). When choosing hand controls, all disabled drivers would be wise to adhere to the VA requirements.

Foot controls can be used to steer by those with no upper-extremity function.[43] Finger controls are similar to hand controls but are more sensitive to smaller movements and can be operated by finger motion only.

An automatic transmission is needed if hand or foot controls are used. Power seats, power steering, power brakes, and power windows may be recommended. The car may have a hand-operated dimmer switch on the turn signal, or one can be added.

Other adapted equipment needed include the following:

1. A swivel steering wheel knob or cuff allows the steering wheel to be operated with one hand while the other controls the hand-operated accelerator and brake.
2. A handle can be attached to the windshield wiper knob to give leverage for operating the windshield washer.
3. A piece of wood secured to the keys for the door and ignition provides leverage for turning the key.
4. A seat belt and shoulder harness are essential.
5. A two-way radio receiver is useful to call for assistance if needed.

One method the person could use to transfer into a two-door car and bring the wheelchair in is as follows. He would approach the car on the passenger side, move the power seat all the way back, and transfer into the car using either a depression transfer, a sliding board transfer, or a gutter hook-assisted transfer. This latter transfer uses a loop suspended from a flat wide metal hook that fits in the rain gutter of the car above the door. The loop is used to pull against, similarly to using a trapeze when transferring from the bed. Once transferred into the car, the person secures his trunk balance, and then leans to remove the wheelchair cushion. He folds the chair and puts the casters on the edge of the car near the entrance to the back seat. He moves to the driver's seat and then moves the entire seat forward. He tips the seat back on the passenger side forward and leans to reach the front casters of the wheelchair to pull it into the space behind the passenger seat. A board that levels the back floor makes transfer of the wheelchair easier. Then he tips the passenger seat back into place and adjusts the entire seat to a comfortable driving position. He reaches across to close the passenger door. A stick with a hook may be helpful to extend the reach. If spasm is a problem or a possibility, the legs are positioned so that spasm would not send the feet against the brake or accelerator.

If it is not possible for the patient to get the wheelchair into the car independently, hydraulic lifts are available that attach across the roof of the car and lift the wheelchair up and into the car.[8]

When parking the car, it is important to remember that a 1.3-meter (4 foot) space on the passenger side is required for transfer. It is wisest to park on a flat area and at the right of a line of cars. Parking spaces designated for handicapped drivers are marked to allow for transfer space.

Incoordinated persons may or may not be able to drive safely, depending on the severity of their disability.

A driving simulator (e.g., Doron Driver Evaluation and Training System[44]) can be used before driver training to evaluate defensive driving skills, hazard perception, and emergency procedures.[45] The patient sits in a mock-up car module with standard (or adapted) driving devices mounted as in a car. He watches a movie, steers, and reacts to the driving situations as they appear on the screen. His timing and responses are electronically recorded. If these aspects of driving are all right, a driver-training course for handicapped persons is then appropriate for the disabled driver. Such a course is similar to the training course for all new drivers, except that it teaches the person to use necessary adapted equipment safely. Occupational therapists often direct these programs. Most states require disabled drivers to be reeducated before examining them for a license.

Persons with the loss of use of one side of the body due to stroke may, with medical clearance, drive with few adaptations. Medical clearance is needed not so much for physical health problems, but rather the sequelae of the stroke. Whether or not the patient has hemianopsia; impaired perception, thought processes, or judgment; or slow automatic reactions must be taken into account before the patient is cleared for driving training. The driver-training simulator provides the opportunity to test whether these deficits exist without actually jeopardizing others by testing the patient in traffic. An evaluation with a simulator is recommended for all patients with brain damage or probable brain damage, such as COPD patients, because judgment deficits and slow reactions are sometimes not apparent during other evaluations but would definitely interfere with safe driving abilities. If the patient passes this simulated test, driving retraining or license tests are allowed.

The car of a person with loss of one upper extremity ought to have automatic transmission and power steering. A swivel steering wheel knob is needed to steer safely. If the patient has lost the use of his right arm, the gear shift lever and turn indicator will need to be remounted on the left of the steering column. A left-foot accelerator may also be indicated; these can be ordered as accessories on a new car.

STUDY QUESTIONS:

Activities of Daily Living

1. What conditions interfere with the patient's ability to benefit from instruction concerning ADL methods?
2. Define transfer, in rehabilitation terms.
3. How is the type of transfer to be used for a particular patient decided on?
4. State the steps of an independent depression transfer.
5. How and why is a "wheelie" done?
6. State the steps of an assisted 90° pivot transfer.
7. What principle of compensation is being implemented when a patient with limited or restricted range of motion uses a stocking aid?
8. What device is used to enable use of utensils when a patient lacks grasp?
9. Describe the steps a C_6 quadriplegic will use to put on his trousers.
10. Describe how a C_6 quadriplegic college student will be able to do tasks required of his role.
11. What are the principles of compensation used for problems of incoordination?
12. What principle of compensation is being used by an above-elbow amputee who uses a nail file taped to the counter to trim his fingernails?
13. State the steps a stroke patient can use to put on and remove a cardigan-type garment.
14. Name five energy conservation techniques and give an example of each that could be used by a cardiac patient.
15. What automobile adaptations will be required to enable a right below-elbow amputee to drive safely?

References

1. Coleman R. J. Fire—an alarming situation. *Accent on Living, 29*(1): 66–71, 1984.
2. Schroeder, C., and Benedict, P. Egress during fire—wheelchair exiting in an emergency. *Am. J. Occup. Ther., 38*: 541–542, 1984.
3. Brodal, A. Self-observations and neuro-anatomical considerations after a stroke. *Brain, 96*: 675–694, 1973.
4. Skinner, B. F. *The Behavior of Organisms*. New York: Appleton-Century-Crofts, 1938.
5. Ted Hoyer & Company, Inc., 2222 Minnesota Avenue, Oshkosh, WI 54901.
6. Alexander, L. Bed to commode lift increases independence. *Accent on Living, 23*(4): 108–109, 1979.
7. Petersen, R. Electric lift. *Accent on Living, 28*(4): 100–102, 1984.
8. Lowman, E., and Klinger, J. *Aids to Independent Living*. New York: McGraw-Hill (Blakiston Division), 1969.
9. Dutton, N., Davis, K., Lupo, S., and Wepman, S. "Wheelie" aide. *Phys. Ther., 59*(1): 35–36, 1979.
10. Bobath, B. *Adult Hemiplegia: Evaluation and Treatment*, 2nd edition. London: William Heinemann Medical Books, 1978.
11. Katz, S., et al. Studies of illness in the aged. The index of ADL: a standardized measure of biological and psychosocial function. *J.A.M.A., 185*(12): 914–919, 1963.
12. Panikoff, L. B. Recovery trends in functional skills in the head-injured adult. *Am. J. Occup. Ther., 37*(11): 735–743, 1983.
13. Levitan-Rheingold, N., Hotte, E. B., and Mandel, D. R. Learning to dress: a fundamental skill toward independence for the disabled. *Rehabil. Lit., 41*(3–4): 72–75, 1980.
14. Bower, M. T. *Clothing for the Handicapped: Fashion Adaptations for Adults and Children*. Minneapolis: Sister Kenny Institute, 1978.
15. Dallas, M. J., and White, L. W. Clothing fasteners for women with arthritis. *Am. J. Occup. Ther., 36*: 515–518, 1982.
16. Vanderheiden, G. C. Augmentative modes of communication for severely speech- and motor-impaired. *Clin. Orthop., 148*: 70–86, 1980.
17. Communication devices available but are out of reach to many. *Accent on Living, 25*(4): 26–35, 1981.
18. Garee, B., editor. *Accent on Living: Buyer's Guide*, P.O. Box 700, Bloomington, IL 61710.
19. Sieger, M. S., and Fisher, L. A. Adaptive equipment used in the rehabilitation of hip arthroplasty patients. *Am. J. Occup. Ther., 36*: 515–518, 1982.
20. Reich, N., and Otten, P. Are buttons and zippers confidence trippers? *Accent on Living, 25*(3): 98–99, 1980.
21. Duckworth, B. Overview of menstrual management for disabled women. *Can. J. Occup. Ther., 53*: 25–29, 1986.
22. Runge, M. Self dressing techniques for patients with spinal cord injury. *Am. J. Occup. Ther., 21*: 367–375, 1967.
23. Shillam, L. L., Beeman, C., and Loshin, P. M. Effect of occupational therapy intervention on bathing independence of disabled persons. *Am. J. Occup. Ther., 37*: 766–768, 1983.
24. Kelly, S. N. Adaptations for independent use of cassette tape recorder/radio by high-level quadriplegic patients. *Am. J. Occup. Ther., 37*: 766–768, 1983.
25. Barsamian, P. *More Splinting with Aquaplast*. WRF/Aquaplast Corp., P.O. Box 635, Wycoff, NJ 07481, 1983.
26. Glenn, J. W., Miller, K. H., and Broman, M. T. Voice terminal: may offer opportunities for employment to the disabled. *Am. J. Occup. Ther., 30*: 308–312, 1976.

27. Gadgets galore: Buy 'em or make 'em cheap. *Accent on Living, 25*(4): 37, 1981.
28. Holser, P., Jones, M., and Ilanit, T. A study of the upper extremity control brace. *Am. J. Occup. Ther., 16*: 170–175, 1962.
29. Bullock, A., et al. Communication and the nonverbal multihandicapped child. *Am. J. Occup. Ther., 29*: 150–152, 1975.
30. Levy, R. Interface modalities of technical aids used by people with disability. *Am. J. Occup. Ther., 37*: 761–765, 1983.
31. Workman, A. A. Communication system for the nonverbal severely disabled. *Am. J. Occup. Ther., 33*: 194–195, 1979.
32. Brett, G. Dressing techniques for the severely involved hemiplegic patient. *Am. J. Occup. Ther., 14*: 262–264, 1960.
33. Goldish, L., and Taylor, H. The Optacon: a valuable device for blind persons. *The New Outlook for the Blind, 68*: 49–56, 1974.
34. Barstow, R. E. Coping with emphysema. *Nurs. Clin. North Am., 9*(1): 137–145, 1974.
35. Ogden, L. D. Guidelines for analysis and testing of activities of daily living with cardiac patients. *American Occupational Therapy Association Physical Disabilities Special Interest Section Newsletter, 3*(4): 1, 3, 1980.
36. Huntley, N., and Mullivan, M. A., editors. *Basics of Cardiac Rehabilitation.* Minneapolis, MN: The Minnesota Occupational Therapy Association, 1978.
37. Pomerantz, P., Flannery, E. L., and Findling, P. K. Occupational therapy for chronic obstructive lung disease. *Am. J. Occup. Ther., 29*: 407–411, 1975.
38. Berzins, G. F. An occupational therapy program for the chronic obstructive pulmonary disease patient. *Am. J. Occup. Ther., 24*: 181–186, 1970.
39. Ogden, L. D. Activity guidelines for early subacute and high-risk cardiac patients. *Am. J. Occup. Ther., 33*: 291–298, 1979.
40. Risk, H. F. Pros and cons of the "less effort" steering and braking systems for the severely handicapped driver. *Am. Corr. Ther. J., 34*(5): 154–155, 1980.
41. VA evaluates car hand controls. *Accent on Living, 21*(2): 46, 1976.
42. Alarming statistics? Disabled drivers have more accidents. N.Y. study. *Accent on Living, 23*(4): 44–45, 1979.
43. Rosenkoetter, R. Valerie drives with her bare feet. *Accent on Living, 25*(1): 100–102, 1980.
44. Doron Precision Industries, P.O. Box 400, Binghampton, NY 13902.
45. Quigley, F. L., and DeLise, J. A. Assessing the driving potential of cerebral vascular accident patients. *Am. J. Occup. Ther., 37*: 474–478, 1983.

Supplementary Reading

Communication

Andrews, B., Miller, S., Horrocks, D., Jibowu, M. O. N., and Chawla, J. C. Electronic communications and environmental control systems for the severely disabled. *Paraplegia, 17*: 153–156, 1979–1980.

Beukelman, D. R., and Yorkston, K. N. Nonvocal communication: performance evaluation. *Arch. Phys. Med. Rehabil., 61*: 272–275, 1980.

Joubert, A. F. Fingercom—an electronic communicator for the disabled. *Med. Biol. Eng. Comput., 17*(4): 489–491, 1979.

Ross, J. A. A study of the application of Blissymbolics as a means of communication for a young brain damaged adult. *Br. J. Disord. Commun., 14*(2): 103–109, 1980.

Steadman, J. W., Ferris, C. D., and Rhodine, C. N. Prosthetic communication device. *Arch. Phys. Med. Rehabil., 62*(2): 93–97, 1980.

Mobility

Flaherty, P., and Jurkovich, S. *Transfer for Patients with Acute and Chronic Conditions.* Minneapolis, MN: American Rehabilitation Foundation, 1970.

Hinrichsen, L. C., Nordstrom, C., and Law, D. F. Device to assist training in balancing on the rear wheels of a wheelchair. *Phys. Ther., 64*(5): 672–673, 1984.

McGee, M., and Hertling, D. Equipment and transfer techniques used by C_6 quadriplegic patients. *Phys. Ther., 61*(2): 1372–1375, 1977.

Self-Care

Arthritis Foundation. *Self-help Manual for Patients with Arthritis.* 3400 Peachtree Road NE, Atlanta, GA 30326. 1980.

Asenjo, A. A. *Step-by-Step Guide to Personal Management for Blind Persons.* New York: American Foundation for Blind, 1970.

Ford, J. R., and Duckworth, B. *Physical Management for the Quadriplegic Patient.* Philadelphia: F. A. Davis, 1974.

Lawton, E. B. *Activities of Daily Living for Physical Rehabilitation.* New York: McGraw-Hill (Blakiston Division), 1963.

Newton, A. Clothing: a positive part of the rehabilitation process. *J. Rehabil., 42*(5): 18–22, 1976.

Occupational Therapy and Nursing Education Staff at Kenney Rehabilitation Institute. *Self-Care for the Hemiplegic.* Minneapolis, MN: American Rehabilitation Foundation, 1970.

Paralyzed Veterans of America. *Wheeling to Fire Safety.* 25100 Euclid Ave., Suite 109, Euclid, OH 44117.

Pendleton, H. McH., and Sommerville, N. J. Project Threshold: an approach to using assistive devices. *American Occupational Therapy Association Physical Disabilities Special Interest Section Newsletter, 5*(1): 1, 4, 1982.

Poole, J., and Parkinson, M. M. Bilateral shoulder disarticulation: equipment used to facilitate independence. *Am. J. Occup. Ther., 34*: 379–399, 1980.

Rogers, J. C., and Snow, T. An assessment of the feeding behaviors of the institutionalized elderly. *Am. J. Occup. Ther., 36*: 375–380, 1982.

Strub, N., and Levine, R. E. Self care: a comparison of patients' institutional and home performance. *Occup. Ther. J. Res., 7*(1): 53–56, 1987.

Yep, J. O. Tools for aiding physically disabled individuals to increase independence in dressing. *J. Rehabil., 43*(5): 39–41, 1977.

Driving

Jones, R., Giddens, H., and Croft, D. Assessment and training of brain-damaged drivers. *Am. J. Occup. Ther., 37*: 754–760, 1983.

Kent, H. Automobile modifications for the disabled. In *Orthotics Etcetera*, 3rd edition. Edited by J. B. Redford. Baltimore: Williams & Wilkins, 1986.

Sivak, M., et al. Improved driving performance following perceptual training in persons with brain damage. *Arch. Phys. Med. Rehabil., 65*(4): 163–167, 1984.

Resources

Communication

Adaptive Communication Systems, Box 12440, Pittsburgh, PA 15231.
Prentke Romich Company, 1022 Heyl Road, Wooster, OH 44691.
Zygo Industries, Box 1008, Portland, OR 97207.

Self-Care

ABLEDATA. National Rehabilitation Information System Center, 4407 Eighth St., NE, Washington, DC 20017 (202/635-6090). A computer data base of rehabilitation products accessed via brokers or directly via computer terminal.

American Foundation for the Blind, 15 W. 16th St. New York, NY 10011.
Comfortably Yours: Aids for Easier Living, catalogue. 52 West Hunter Ave., Maywood, NJ 07607.
FashionABLE, 5 Crescent Ave., Box S, Rocky Hill, NJ 08553.

Fred Sammons, Inc. *Professional Health Care Catalog, Enrichments: Helping Hands for Special Needs*, and *Orthopedic Catalog*, Box 32, Brookfield, IL 60513.

J. A. Preston Corporation, catalogue. 60 Page Rd., Clifton, NJ 07012.
The Left Hand, catalogue. 140 W. 22nd Street, New York, NY 10011.

Maddak, Inc., catalogue. 6 Industrial Rd., Pequannock, NJ 07440.
Rehab Aids, catalogue. Box 612, Tamiami Station, Miami, FL 33144.

Sears, Roebuck & Co. *Home Health Care Catalogue.* Sears Tower, Chicago, IL 60684.

Susquehanna Rehab Products, Rd. 2, Box 41, 9 Overlook Drive, Wrightsville, PA 17368.
Techni-Flair, adapted clothing catalogue. P.O. Box 40, Cotter, AR 72626.
Technology for Independent Living, resource guide, includes section on equipment for adapted driving and advice on car selection. RESNA, 4405 EastWest Highway, Bethesda, MD 20814.

chapter
18

Homemaking and Child Care

Catherine A. Trombly

Training in adapted methods of homemaking and child care begins when the patient's function has been restored to the expected near-maximal level. This training, therefore, usually takes place close to the time of discharge. Some homemaking activities may appropriately be used as therapeutic media in restorative therapy.

Work Simplification

Homemaking and child care are energy consuming for anyone, but for disabled persons who must use adapted methods these activities require an even greater expenditure of energy and, unless modified, may consume a disproportionate amount of the person's remaining energy.[1] Techniques to conserve personal energy become indispensable for these individuals. The principles and some suggestions are listed here. Other suggestions that can be used are frequently being published these days in magazine and newspaper columns aimed at the able-bodied working wife and mother who also needs to conserve energy.

The principles of energy conservation or work simplification listed here apply in general to all the disability categories presented and to all aspects of occupational performance tasks.

LIMIT THE AMOUNT OF WORK

Eliminate steps of a job or whole jobs that are not essential to one's life-style. The patient should determine for herself what is necessary by asking herself why it is necessary, if the job is worth the expenditure of energy required, and what would happen if the job were left undone.

Some short cuts to suggest include the following. Permanent-press and jersey materials to eliminate the need for ironing. Making a bed entirely from undersheet to spread at one corner before moving to do the same at the next corners to eliminate walking. Teaching family members to put their belongings and laundry in the proper place to eliminate the need to tidy-up the house. Soaking dishes to eliminate the need to scrub them. Allowing the dishes to air dry to eliminate drying. The step of returning clean dishes to the cupboard can be eliminated by reusing them directly from the dish drainer or dishwasher. The use of plastic tablecloths or paper placemats instead of cloth ones eliminates laundry. The use of casserole dishes for cooking and serving eliminates an extra set of dishes to wash. Frozen entrees and other prepared foods eliminate preparation and the need to wash the cooking dishes. Shopping by telephone and by mail order eliminates a task that requires tremendous amounts of energy; this method of shopping may be the only way the person can do this task. The use of the freezer eliminates the need to do frequent marketing. The use of paper diapers eliminates this aspect of laundering.

PLAN AHEAD

Plan the week's activities so that heavy tasks can be distributed over the days. The full day's activities should be carefully planned to incorporate periods of rest between bouts of work and to alternate active jobs with quiet ones. A flexible, written plan improves the homemaker's efficiency. The tasks should be prioritized so that those that must be done are done before the person runs out of time and energy. If a task doesn't seem to be getting done day after day because of its low priority, perhaps it is not important and can be eliminated. Each activity should be thought out ahead of time and all necessary supplies and equipment gathered prior to doing the job. The equipment should be put away before starting the next task so that if energy fails, the home is still tidy. A plan for the family's contribution to running the household is needed also.

ORGANIZE STORAGE

Supplies and equipment should be stored where first used and within easy reach. Duplicate sets of equipment in different locations are useful: for example, floor care equipment located on both the first and second floors of a two-story house. Extraneous, seldom-used equipment should be stored out of the way. If possible, things should not be stored behind other things nor under other things because of the energy consumed in trying to reach them. Vertical storage of dishes, baking pans, etc., is ideal. Narrow shelf storage or easily gliding pull-out shelves solve some storage problems; peg boards, lazy susans, and back of the counter or under the cabinet storage solve others.

SIT TO WORK

Sitting requires less energy than standing. Arrange work areas so that implements are within easy reach of the posture normally assumed for each task. Reaching is also energy consuming.

USE CORRECT EQUIPMENT

Energy is conserved if the tools fit the job and are in good condition. Lightweight equipment and utensils also conserve energy. Personal energy is also conserved if electrically powered equipment is used and indeed such equipment may be the only method by which a disabled person can accomplish a task. A dishwasher that does not require prior rinsing of the dishes, a self-cleaning electric stove, a self-defrosting refrigerator with an easily accessible freezer, a garbage disposal, a microwave oven (not for patients with pacemakers), crock pot, toaster oven, and an electric can opener are valuable energy-saving tools and are recommended for the disabled homemaker. As many of these as can be afforded should be purchased according to the priority established by each homemaker's needs and requirements. The specific features that each appliance should have in order to be used by a person with a particular disability should be discussed with the patient so that these features can be sought when shopping for equipment.

USE EFFICIENT METHODS

The patient should be taught to use the two arms in symmetrical, smooth motions when possible; to use the force available from muscles at proximal joints rather than the smaller, more distal joints and muscles; to use leverage; and to work with gravity assisting rather than resisting. Objects should be slid, not lifted. Contiguous counter space, especially between the sink, stove, and refrigerator, is very important. Use a wheeled service cart and laundry basket when possible to transport items. Avoid prolonged holding by using stabilization when possible. Suction cup bases, heavy pots and pans, nonskid mats, wet towels, and wet sponge cloths are all ways to stabilize. Locate switches and controls within easy, safe reach; appliance controls ought to be located in the front for accessibility. Be sure lighting is good.

REST

Fatigue leads to poor body mechanics and decreased safety awareness. Regular rest periods should be incorporated into the day's work plan. Mothers of young children are advised to rest when the child sleeps, even though it is tempting to use that time for doing a task uninterrupted.

It is strongly recommended, to conserve the energy of disabled homemakers, that they assign to other family members, to temporary hired household help, or to a commercial cleaning service such heavy tasks as cleaning the oven, defrosting the refrigerator, vacuuming wall to wall carpet, washing walls, floors, curtains, etc.

USE CORRECT BODY MECHANICS

Use of correct body mechanics is absolutely necessary for those with chronic low back pain, but it is also recommended for all persons engaged in physical work inside or outside of the home. The principles of good body mechanics elaborate on the ideas of joint alignment, use of large muscles instead of small, and working in harmony with gravity. Specifically, the principles are keep the head aligned with the trunk (tuck the chin); keep the shoulders and hips parallel (don't twist the trunk); maintain pelvic tilt (tuck the buttocks or keep one foot raised on a low stool while standing); maintain good balance (position the feet shoulder-distance apart, one foot forward); keep the back straight (bend at the hips and knees simultaneously rather than bend over at the waist); and push before pulling and pull before lifting.[2] If the person must lift and carry, he should keep the object close to the body to reduce the length of the resistance lever arm and subsequently the strain on trunk muscles and spinal ligaments.

Homemaker Training

Homemaking takes place on two levels: managerial and participative performance of tasks. The severely disabled homemaker may be an effective home manager, directing the efforts of other family members or paid household help. She can manage the finances and oversee the shopping. Training for this level may not be necessary for the experienced homemaker; some discussions about how this could be done might suffice. An inexperienced homemaker may need practice in hypothetical financial management and in directing others effectively by words alone.

Homemaker services, Home Health Aides, and Meals-on-Wheels are all programs available in many communities that enable a patient with limited abilities to remain in her home by providing essential services that the homemaker is unable to do. Each program offers different types and levels of services. For the homemaker who can afford it, commercial housekeeping services are increasing in availability and can be hired for weekly or seasonal cleaning chores.

The activities that the homemaker can reasonably expect to do should be discussed in detail and practiced. The therapist should suggest adapted methods or adapted equipment that will make the task possible if the homemaker is unable to do it in a standard way. To train the participative homemaker in tasks for which she needs to learn new methods, the therapist should be skilled in demonstrating the technique in a way that is as close as possible to the manner in which the disabled person will be expected to do it. The therapist should sit or stand beside the person while demonstrating to eliminate right-left confusion. The patient performs the activity in imitation of the therapist while the therapist cues the patient about the key points. Practice increases skill and should not be bypassed.

For mothers of infants, a flexible baby doll that is life-sized and weighted to simulate a baby may be used for practice of child care methods. To be realistic, the weight must be distributed throughout the doll, not just in the hollow head and limbs. A mother who is questionably safe in caring for the lifeless doll would be advised to have help in the care of her lively youngster.

Child care is complicated by the nature of the disability, the particular demands of children at various developmental stages, and by environmental conditions.[3] The child aged 8 months to 2½ years is the greatest challenge because he is mobile and can't be reasoned with.[3] He needs to be contained in a safe area.[3] All the energy-saving suggestions that put controls of appliances, supplies, and equipment within reach of the mother do so for the child also!

The handicapped mother will need to be a consistent disciplinarian insofar as she must rely on the child's obedience for his own safety. A toddler must come when called and must stop doing things when told. A disabled mother must teach her child to accommodate to her disability.[4] Even a toddler is helpful in picking things up off the floor for mother and in running to get something. The toddler can also be taught to climb safely in and out of his crib and can learn to assist in dressing himself. Children will learn to accommodate to the mother's disability as they grow older. Older children can be very helpful; the mother can learn to direct their activities verbally for the benefit of all and in such a way that increases their self-esteem and does not make them feel imposed upon. The children learn important personal skills and values in the process of helping mother.[4]

Mothering involves more than physical care of the child, and the disabled mother is encouraged to allow time in her daily routine to play with and counsel her child.

In addition to the suggestions listed above that apply generally to homemakers, the following sections note some other specific suggestions for types of disability. Given the principles, and learning some examples of applying the principle, the clever housewife will devise methods that suit her best to solve household problems. Training must emphasize the problem-solving method so that the housewife develops true independence in devising new methods for herself and purchasing useful household equipment. Manufacturers are increasing the availability of labor-saving household equipment, supplies, and packaging to cater to the working woman; this trend is a boon to the knowledgeable disabled homemaker.

COMPENSATION FOR LIMITED RANGE OF MOTION

The principles are to extend the person's reach via extended handles and to confine the work to a compact area.

Marketing

Since the patient may need assistance because many items are placed out of reach, marketing by phone or mail is recommended.

Food Preparation, Service, and Cleanup

Reacher tongs can be used to get lightweight objects from high or low places. A wall oven or countertop microwave oven eliminates bending. Small electrical appliances can be placed within easy reach. If ambulatory aids are used, a wheeled cart may be needed, unless dishes can be slid along a counter to a point near the table. A sponge cloth mitt, commercially available, or one made from terry cloth[5] will be useful for arthritic persons for washing dishes. Joint protection methods specific to persons with rheumatoid arthritis can be found in chapter 27.

Housecleaning

Articles that extend the person's reach such as reacher tongs for picking up objects from the floor or holding a dust rag to reach distant places, a feather duster, a long-handled sponge to clean the bathtub, and a long-handled dustpan are often necessary. A child's broom and mop are handy for wiping up spills.[6] Vacuum cleaner wand attachments can be used for cleaning out-of-reach places. The duster attachment of the vacuum cleaner is also helpful. Beds should be placed so the patient can work from both sides without leaning while making them. A self-wringing sponge mop and a flexible-handled dry mop are useful for patients with limited range of motion.

Laundry

If the patient is ambulatory, a top-loading automatic washer and raised dryer would eliminate bending; however, if the patient is wheelchair bound, a front-loading washer and dryer would be best. If the patient is wheelchair bound and must use a top-loading machine, a mirror mounted over it at an angle to enable the person to see into the tub and a reacher stick or tongs will be necessary. Maytag washer and dryer controls can be optionally fitted with larger four-pronged knobs.[7]

Mending would be best accomplished with a sewing machine. The patient may need assistance with threading the needle or need to use a needle-threading device.

Child Care

To eliminate the need for bending, a raised playpen could be used, and the crib mattress could be raised. A crib that accommodates the mother's wheelchair and has storage and a sliding railing to allow access to the baby was designed for a wheelchair-bound mother (Fig. 18.1).[4] The baby could be bathed in the kitchen sink or a bathinet.

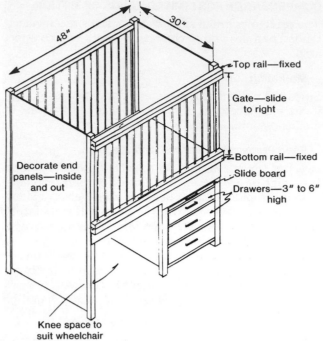

Figure 18.1 Crib with knee space to accommodate a wheelchair, handy storage, and sliding gate side rails. Designed by Lee and Gordon Heintzman. (Reproduced with permission from Dunn, V.M. Tips on raising children from a wheelchair. *Accent on Living* 22(4):78–83, 1978.)

PREVENTION OF CHRONIC BACK PAIN

The body mechanics principles listed above especially apply to patients with back pain.

Marketing

The problems are lifting low-placed items, prolonged standing, and carrying parcels. To reach low-placed items, the person should kneel on one knee (simultaneously bending the hip and knee, keeping the back straight); then holding the item close to the body, he should stand to lift. Lifting the item to an intermediate position before standing is also useful if the item does not have to be held at arm's length to do so. If prolonged standing is a necessity, the person should place one foot on a low object such as the bottom of a market food carriage; this causes the pelvis to tilt anteriorly into proper alignment. Bagged parcels should be as lightweight as they reasonably can be, or a wheeled cart should be used. If the bags must be carried, they should be carried close to the body either at waist height or one on each side if they have handles.[2]

Food Preparation, Service, and Cleanup

The problems are reaching and lifting low-placed utensils or ingredients, putting heavy dishes in and out of the oven, using a front-loading dishwasher, prolonged standing, and carrying heavy objects. Again, good body mechanics must be used to avoid bending at the waist. The person should sit during food preparation or alter-

natively put one foot on a low stool. Carrying should be eliminated as much as possible by sliding things on countertops between appliances or by use of a wheeled cart.

Housecleaning

This activity with all its required bending and reaching is a major problem for patients with chronic low back pain. As many of these tasks as possible should be assigned to others. Adaptations that eliminate the need to bend should be used (Fig. 18.2 is an example).

All principles of body mechanics apply. As with changing any habit, much practice with feedback is needed to unlearn bad habits and relearn the task using good habits of posture and movement. The therapist should work with the patient to not only solve the problems that the homemaker is expected to face but also to provide the opportunity to actually practice using equipment and situations similar to those that the patient will encounter at home. Verbal feedback is helpful, but videotaping the person's performance and discussing the good and poor aspects of it may be more beneficial. The person also needs to learn what types of tasks he or she can and cannot do and how long a task can be engaged in before it produces pain. In this way, the person can be in control of his or her disability by stopping the activity before pain is experienced.

Laundry

Problems include carrying baskets of laundry, bending over to remove clothes from a top-loading washer or to use front-loading appliances, bending to hang clothes

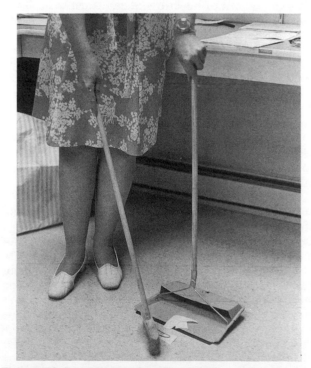

Figure 18.2 Extended-handle cleaning utensils assist reach and alleviate bending.

on a clothesline, and standing to iron. The same principles apply: wheeled carts instead of carrying or carry light loads near the body; sit to work; place objects at waist height to avoid the need to bend repeatedly; tilt the pelvis by elevating one foot.

Child Care

Carrying an infant and bending over to care for infants and small children are major sources of low back pain. Carrying a child in an infant seat is particularly stressful. Children should be carried close to the trunk. Prolonged carrying is probably best done in a carrier. Choice of front or back pack carrier depends on the person's particular back problem. A front-style carrier requires the back muscles to contract against the load, whereas a back style compresses the vertebrae.

Working with the child on a surface that does not require bending means that the mother either lowers herself to bed or floor level or raises the child to her waist level.

COMPENSATION FOR WEAKNESS

The principles are to use lightweight and/or powered equipment and to allow gravity to assist. These principles, along with strict adherence to energy conservation techniques, are also applicable to patients with low endurance.

Marketing

It is advisable to purchase small containers and pieces of meat because they are more easily handled and are lightweight. Forethought concerning opening of the packages should direct the patient toward zipper-pull boxes and plastic bags that can be cut with scissors, etc. Groceries should be bagged in more rather than fewer bags to reduce the energy required to carry each.[8]

Food Preparation, Service, and Cleanup

Lightweight utensils, pots, and pans, stored within easy reach, are necessary. Electric equipment, such as a can opener, countertop mixer, knife, small broiler oven, microwave oven, fry pan, and blender with a lightweight container conserve energy and/or allow the seated patient to work at convenient tabletop height. Knives and peelers should be very sharp so the tool does its job easily. A French chef's knife allows the patient to use leverage rather than a back-and-forth sawing motion for chopping. Built-up handles on cooking utensils may be needed for patients who use splints. A spike board to stabilize the vegetable or meat being cut may be necessary (Fig. 18.3). A spike board is a hardwood cutting board that has three aluminum, or preferably stainless steel, nails hammered through the middle of the board so that the pointed ends protrude about 2 inches to hold the food. It usually has suction cup legs to stabilize the board on the counter. The spike board should be finished using vegetable oil, not varnish. When not in use, the spikes on the board should be covered by wedges of cork.

Loop handles of various types can be added to cooking utensils, such as spatulas,[9] or to dishes to be used in

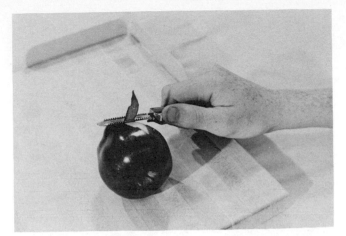

Figure 18.3 One-handed peeling of an apple stabilized on stainless steel nails of a spike board.

microwave ovens[10] to aid a patient with little or no grasp to use them. It is important to remember when building adapted equipment for use in microwave ovens that metal or glue may not be used.

Scissors, if they can be used, are useful to open packages or to cut vegetables and some meats. Resting the side of the container that a person is pouring from onto the edge of the container that is being poured to (which must be stabilized) utilizes leverage rather than energy. An egg can be cracked by someone with weak hands, such as a C_6 quadriplegic, by grossly grasping it and throwing it sharply into the bottom of an empty bowl where it will split in two and the shell can be removed. If the egg must be separated, it can be poured into a commercial egg separator.

The stove should have push-button controls located in the front. If the patient is confined to a wheelchair, a mirror mounted over the back of the stove and angled to reflect what is cooking in the pots may be necessary.

An automatic ice maker in the refrigerator alleviates the dependency on someone else to get ice or the need to warm the ice tray to release the ice. If the patient is confined to a wheelchair, the freezer of the refrigerator is best located beside the cold storage area rather than on the top or bottom.

The wheelchair homemaker will need to have a convenient work area that accommodates the wheelchair and allows her to be comfortable while working. Suggestions have been published in the popular press.[11] The sink and at least one countertop should be modified so that the wheelchair can fit under. Use of a "sink escalator," which is two boards joined by hinges that fits onto the countertop and over the edge of the sink, enables a weak person to slide heavy pots and pans into and out of the sink.[12] A lap apron is useful for the wheelchair homemaker because it provides a firm surface to place things on and has a lip to prevent their being knocked off in transit (Fig. 18.4). It does not interfere with pushing the wheelchair. However, it is dangerous to carry hot items, especially liquids, using this.

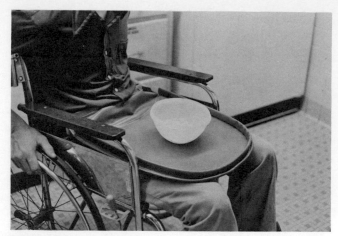

Figure 18.4 Lap apron.

Housecleaning

The use of a self-propelled vacuum cleaner allows some weak persons to do this job; maintenance of balance against the pull of the vacuum cleaner is a consideration, however. Use of lightweight tools, such as dry mops, brooms, sponge mops, etc., may enable floor care. Aerosol cleanser for tub and basin dissolves grime with little rubbing.

Patients with cardiopulmonary disorders should not do tasks that exceed their safe level as determined by exercise testing. They should alternate light and heavy tasks and be careful to rest for one hour after meals since energy is being used in digestion.

If fitted sheets are used on a bed, they should be loose fitting. Fitted sheets can be adapted by opening the two fitted corners at the bottom edge and sewing Velcro strips, so that when the bed is made the corners can be snugged up using the Velcro.[13] When making a bed, weak patients usually do not tuck the bed clothing in. Lightweight blankets and spreads are used. The idea of enclosing blankets or a quilt inside of a large pillowcase-like covering that is common in Europe makes a neat bed without the need to tuck sheets in. The covering acts like the sheet and spread and is laundered as frequently as sheets would be. These cases open entirely on one side which aids in putting the quilt inside. They can be purchased in specialty stores or made by sewing together sheets cut to the correct size. Velcro would be a better fastener than buttons.

If the patient works from a wheelchair, the bed must be placed so the wheelchair can get around it. The patient completes the bedmaking at each corner before moving to the next.

Laundry

Choice of a front- or top-loading washer depends on whether the patient is wheelchair bound or ambulatory. If wheelchair bound, the patient can transport the clothes by putting them in a drawstring duffel bag, hooking the string over a wheelchair handle,[14] and dragging the bag.

Push-button controls on the washer and dryer are easier to use than knobs. If knobs are used, they may need to be adapted to allow the patient to use them. Premeasured packages of soap and bleach avoid the need to handle large containers. It would be economical if these supplies were purchased in larger containers and then measured into individual packets by someone able to do it. A table for folding clothes should be convenient to the dryer and of the correct height. Hangers should be nearby for immediate hanging of permanent-press items as they are removed from the dryer. If the patient chooses to iron, the iron should be set so that it is a little cooler than usual. An asbestos pad can be used on the end of the ironing board so the iron can be placed there to eliminate the need of standing the iron up each time while preparing the clothes for the next ironing stroke.

Child Care

A weak mother may not be able to participate fully in the care of her child; she should reserve the most fun things for herself if possible and delegate the more mechanical tasks to the helper. The safest place for a weak mother to handle her baby is on the floor, if she is able to get up and down from the floor. The baby can be sponge-bathed, dressed, fed, and played with there. Of course, the floor should be clean, carpeted, and draft-free. If the mother is unable to get to the floor, a crib with a swing-open side (Fig. 18.1) will allow the mother to wheel her wheelchair close to the baby or allow the ambulatory mother to sit on the crib mattress while with the baby. Crib mattress heights are adjustable.

Feeding the baby can best be done with the child in an infant seat or propped up on pillows. Premeasured formula is ideal but expensive. Formula prepared by another family member can be stored in the refrigerator for the day; the nipple covers should be on loosely. Breast feeding eliminates the work of formula preparation and bottle sterilization. An electric baby dish that warms the solid food can be placed in a convenient position and keeps the food warm throughout the mealtime.

Clothing for baby should be large, made of stretchy material, and have closures the mother can handle. Commercially available disposable diapers with tape tab closures eliminate pins, plastic pants, and laundry.

Emergency help should be easily, quickly, and consistently available.

COMPENSATION FOR INCOORDINATION

Principles involve the use of techniques to stabilize the proximal segments of the limbs, to damp the movement of distal segments using weight, and to provide an environment in which the person feels safe and competent. Unless severely disabled, the incoordinated homemaker is likely to be independent.

Marketing

Depending upon the severity of the disability, the patient may need help taking items from the shelves and putting things away at home.

Food Preparation, Service, and Cleanup

The major problem facing the incoordinated person in the kitchen is the need for stability to prevent spillage, breakage, or accidents with sharp utensils or hot equipment, food, or beverages. In addition to the stabilizing methods mentioned in the chapter on self-care, heavy equipment or utensils offer stability. Cast iron pots, ironstone dishes, and heavy bowls serve these patients best because they aid in stabilizing the distal part of the extremities. Casseroles and pots and pans with double handles offer greater stability by anchoring the distal parts of both upper extremities. Weighted wrist cuffs may also be used to dampen tremors or provide anchoring.

Nonslip mats and sponge cloths can be used under most items to provide friction and stability. A spike board to anchor meat, fruit, and vegetables while cutting them is useful (Fig. 18.3). A serrated knife is less likely to slip than a straight-edged one.[15] When cutting or peeling, the patient must stabilize her arms proximally and direct the stroke away from herself. A French fry basket may be placed in a saucepan before vegetables are put in for cooking; this allows draining the vegetables by lifting out the basket to lessen the chance for scald burns. Prepared foods are especially useful for this homemaker.

A countertop mixer should be used rather than a hand-held mixer. An electric skillet used at the table eliminates the need for transferring items from the oven or stove. A milk carton holder with a handle helps in pouring milk.

The stove should have front controls. The patient must avoid reaching over hot pots to the back of the stove. Starting the oven after the food has been placed in seems safest. Lighting a gas stove would be unsafe.

Sliding the food and dishes along contiguous counter surfaces is safest. A wheeled cart that is weighted at its base may also be used safely with training. Double-handled or large-handled serving dishes are best.

When washing dishes, a dish towel or sponge cloth could be put on the bottom of the sink to cushion the fall of dishes and glassware and/or the sink could be filled with water before putting in the dishes. Dishes of chip-resistant material will look best the longest. Soaking dishes, rinsing by hand spray, and drip drying eliminate some handling when breakage could occur.

Disposable nonslip place mats would be helpful in table setting.

Housecleaning

Heavier work tools provide stability. A duster mitten may be more useful than trying to maintain grasp of a duster. Bric-a-brac ought to be eliminated or stored where dusting will be unnecessary. Fitted sheets for the bed are helpful.

Laundry

Premeasured soap and bleach packages avoid measuring-type spills. Ironing should be eliminated by the use of no-iron materials.

Child Care

A mildly incoordinate person can care for an infant using such stabilizing measures as holding her proximal extremities close to her body and sitting to work. She can hold the baby safely in the tub by using a bath seat (Fig.18.5). She can use a wide safety strap on the dressing table. It is also safer for this mother to work with her child on the floor. Disposable, tape-tab diapers and Velcro-closing clothing are recommended. Feeding an infant with a spoon may not be safe unless the incoordination is truly minimal.

A more severely incoordinate mother would be unsafe in the care of an infant, but may be able to assist her toddler to dress if clothing is selected properly. *Suggestions for Physically Handicapped Mothers on Clothing for Pre-School Children* by Eleanor Boettke[16] is an old reference (1957) but the principles apply. Ideas from *Self-Help Clothing for Handicapped Children*[17] can be adapted to enable the child to dress independently.

COMPENSATION FOR THE LOSS OF USE OF ONE UPPER EXTREMITY OR ONE SIDE OF THE BODY

The two problems for the one-handed homemaker are to find a way to stabilize the object being worked on, which is usually done by a person's assistor hand, and to accomplish the few truly bilateral activities.

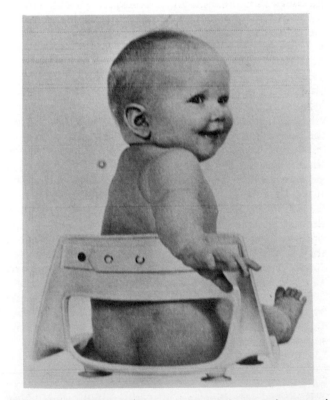

Figure 18.5 Infant bath seat with suction cup base and waist strap. (Reproduced with permission from Lowman, E., and Klinger, J. *Aids to Independent Living: Self Help for the Handicapped.* New York: McGraw-Hill (Blakiston Division), 1969.)

The principles that apply here are to find methods or equipment to substitute for the lost functions.

Marketing

A heavy marketing cart may be used for support by an ambulatory independent hemiplegic person while walking in the supermarket, but he must not rely on it for support when bending to reach items. A lightweight cart is unsafe to lean on while walking. The hemiplegic person should give a light cart a push, then use his cane or walker to walk to meet the cart. Some hemiplegic persons have visual perceptual problems that may interfere with the efficiency of their shopping, e.g., hemianopsia, impairment of figure-ground discrimination, and discrimination of depth perception. A wheelchair-bound hemiplegic person may find phone and mail shopping more suitable; actual visits to the shops will require assistance.

The upper-extremity unilateral amputee will rarely need assistance while shopping. The bilateral amputee may need assistance, depending on his skill with his prostheses.

Food Preparation, Service, and Cleanup

The unilateral upper-extremity amputee can be totally independent using methods and equipment outlined below and in other references. The hemiplegic patient may be less independent due to lower-extremity involvement and concomitant cognitive and perceptual disabilities. Compensatory techniques for minimizing the effects of the cognitive and perceptual deficits are mentioned in chapter 22.

To stabilize dishes, bowls, pots, etc., a suction cup base, a wet towel or sponge cloth, a nonslip rubber pad, or placemat can be placed under them. For holding a bowl securely, a slide-out cutting board can be adapted by cutting out a circular hole to fit the size of bowls usually used. A pattern for a portable cut-out bowl holder that also allows easy emptying of a bowl has been published.[12] Heavy pans will stay in place during stirring. An anchoring device is commercially available; it holds the handle of the pot in one place while the pot is on the stove. Directions for construction are also published.[12] A spike board holds meat, vegetables, and fruit while cutting or peeling. Some spike boards have metal lips at two edges to form a raised corner against which a slice of bread can be snugged while spreading butter etc. on it (see Fig. 17.14). A jar, box, or flip-top can can be opened by stabilizing the item between the knees, holding it against the counter edge with the patient's body, or putting it in a shallow drawer that is held as closed as possible by the person's body. A jar opener is a solution for screw-on lids (see Fig. 27.2). Items can be "cornered" to stabilize them when working on them; for example, a dish can be cornered in the sink while washing it.

Bilateral activities can be made unilateral by use of adaptations. Beating batter or eggs can be done using one-handed egg beaters, which are commercially available, or an electric mixer. Cans can be opened using a one-handed can opener[18] (Fig. 18.6) or by placing the

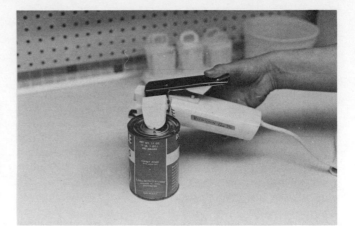

Figure 18.6 Ronson electric can opener that can be used one handed.

can on sponges stacked high enough to put the can in contact with the cutting teeth of a regular electric can opener (Fig. 18.7). Zip-open packages are easiest to open and should be purchased when possible. Other packages can be opened by stabilizing the package on its long edge and cutting the top with a sharp knife. Scissors, especially lightweight cushioned grip scissors, are very useful for many tasks in the kitchen, such as opening plastic or cellophane bags. Milk bottles with caps are easier to open than milk cartons, although the latter are possible by prying the edges apart with a table knife. The carton must be stabilized, of course. To drain vegetables, a slotted spoon can be used, or a French fry basket, put in the pot before the vegetables, will drain them when it is lifted.

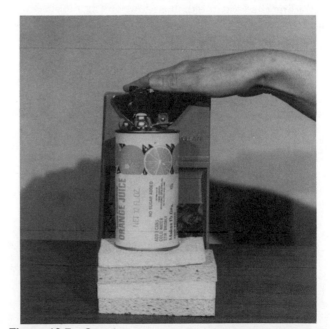

Figure 18.7 Opening a can one handed by supporting the can on sponges while activating a standard electric can opener.

Putting casseroles in the oven is very difficult; lightweight ones with one handle long enough so the patient can grasp it safely or ones with two swing-over-the-top handles that can be held by one hand are possibilities. Sliding the casserole from a pushcart to the pulled-out oven shelf is safest but possible only if the heights of these are equal. To pull out the oven shelf, a device can be made from an 1/2-inch thick slat of wood about 15 inches long. It has a notch at one end to push the oven shelf back into the oven and a hooked notch on one side edge to pull the shelf out.[12,19]

To sift flour, one-handed sifters are available. To roll dough, hold the rolling pin in the center. To crack and separate an egg, use the chef's egg crack: hold the egg in the palm using the four fingers and thumb. There should be a separation between the index and middle fingers. Crack the egg sharply on the side of the bowl at the point between the index and middle fingers, then, as in one motion, pull the two halves of the egg apart by further separating the fingers. Commercial egg separators are available to separate the yolk from the white.

The pans, dishes, etc., should be stored vertically to alleviate the need to lift off items stored on top of other items, put them down, get the needed one, and then put the others back.

For cutting, a sharp knife can be used on a stabilized object. A rocker knife or meat-cutting wheel (wallpaper casing wheel)[20] can be used on nonstabilized objects because the push force is downward. To meet specific needs, there are many gadgets available, such as an egg slicer, grapefruit sectioner, garlic press, one-handed food chopper, etc. Serving salad can be done using commercially available "salad scissors" in which two salad servers are joined with a scissor grip.

Transporting items can be done by using a wheeled cart, a basket, an apron with large pockets, or similar solutions.

Dishwashing is facilitated by soaking and air drying the dishes. For loss of use of one hand, the soiled dishes should all be placed on one side of the sink and the dish drainer on the other side, so the flow of work is energy conserving. A hand-held spray is helpful for rinsing. A restaurant-style suction-based brush is used for glassware. A sponge cloth or rubber mat in the bottom of the sink reduces breakage and provides a friction surface to hold the utensil against for scrubbing. Cleaning up as one prepares meals reduces the likelihood of stuck-on soil. If spills do become stuck on the stove or counter, a wet sponge can be put on the spills and eventually they will soften and wipe off.

Housecleaning

Bedmaking is facilitated for the hemiplegic person with figure-ground deficit if the top sheet is a contrasting color to the bottom sheet. Again, the bed could be made completely at each corner before going on to the next to conserve energy.

A long-handled dustpan that balances open when placed on the floor is useful. Floor spills must be cleaned up immediately to prevent falls. There are sponge mops that can be squeezed one handed by sliding the squeezer mechanism up the handle. A string mop can be wrung by the use of a self-wringing pail by which the water is extracted when a lever is pushed. An electric floor scrubber may be useful. The new no-wax floors are easiest to maintain.

A tank-type vacuum cleaner permits the patient to sit and reach areas to be cleaned using the long hose.

Sewing

The one-handed homemaker can sew by using an electric machine with foot or knee controls or sew by hand by stabilizing the material with weights or in an embroidery hoop mounted in a convenient place. The needle can be threaded while it is held in a pin cushion or a bar of soap. Material can be cut if it is weighted to prevent slipping.

Child Care

For feeding, the infant should be propped up on pillows, rested against the arm of an upholstered chair, or be in an infant seat. There are highchairs with one-handed tray release mechanisms. The screw-top nursing bottles are easier to manage than the plastic liner type. An electric baby dish heats the food in a safe manner and keeps the food warm during the meal. Tongs could be used to take hot baby food jars out of the warming water if this method is used.

To bathe the baby, before drawing the water into the tub or kitchen sink, strap the baby into a suction-based bath seat (see Fig. 18.5) to secure him. Turn the cold water on before the hot. Let the water out and dry the baby as well as possible before lifting him out onto another dry towel.

For dressing the baby, disposable diapers with tab closures are easiest. It is not impossible to use regular pinned diapers but requires much practice. Zippers are difficult to fasten unless the mother can devise a method to hold the bottom taut. Dressing the baby on a dressing table that has a wide Velcro closure strap to secure the baby is convenient because it reduces the amount of squirming possible, but dressing can be done most safely on the floor. To put the baby on the floor, the mother can first sit on a chair and then slide the baby gently down her legs to the floor. Playing with the baby on the floor is more worry free.

COMPENSATION FOR BLINDNESS

The principles are to substitute senses of smell, touch, and hearing, to adhere to an established routine and order, and to pay careful attention to the task at hand.[21]

There are many books written on the details of methods used by blind persons. A few of the more common methods are mentioned here.

Marketing

A companion is needed for shopping in the store, although the person may shop independently by telephone. Help will be needed to label nondistinguishable items with braille tags[21,22] when the order is delivered.

The blind person must organize storage in a consistent, noncluttered manner because she relies on her memory to find things.

Food Preparation, Service, and Cleanup

Frozen dinners are useful. Learning to use the stove is a terrifying experience for the newly blinded person. It is recommended that the person become very familiar with the contours and controls of the stove before attempting to use it with the power on.[21] Push-button controls are easiest, but braille markings can be used for the dial type. The timer or accessory timer also needs to be marked in braille. Some manufacturers offer braille overlays for the control panels of their microwave ovens and instructions for the care and use of the oven on audio cassette.[23] Long oven mitts should be used when using the oven. The patient should learn emergency measures for cooking fires, some of which may be caused by failure to remember putting a pot holder on a burner or leaving it on the oven door while basting and then shutting the door with it still there.

The organization of the refrigerator must be consistent; pull-out shelves reduce the likelihood of knocking over items and spills. Contiguous counter space also reduces accidental dropping and spilling.

Catalogues of useful items for the blind have been published and include a dispenser for sugar in one-teaspoon amounts (cubes or packages are an alternative), a pot for pouring off water without removing the lid (the French fry basket idea already mentioned is an alternative), a knife with a thickness guide for slicing meats, cheese, tomatoes, etc.[24,25]

The blind person relies heavily on his memory and senses of hearing, smell, and touch to work in the kitchen. Hot and cold water, in some houses, sound differently running from the tap; macaroni and ziti sound different when the box is shaken[21]; boiling water makes noise; spices and foods smell differently; ripe fruit and vegetables smell and feel differently from unripe. The fingertips of the assistive hand guide the working hand when peeling, slicing, etc.

Cookbooks are available in braille or on cassette.

Housecleaning

Bedmaking is no problem after the bedclothing is centered on the bed by matching the centerfold to the center of the bedframe and discriminating the top from the bottom of the sheets by feeling the hems. Dusting is facilitated by getting rid of clutter. Spray waxes are less desirable than liquids because the person cannot see the extent of the sprayed liquids. Liquid cleansers should be applied to the cloth, not directly to the furniture. Tidying and cleaning the bathroom as it is used keeps the room ready for use of visitors as well as reducing the need for frequent all-over cleaning. Vacuuming, mopping, etc., are done systematically by devising a system to remember what has and has not been done. Furniture is placed consistently. Animals should be taught to lie in out-of-the-way places.

Laundry

Fasten paired items together when they are taken off, using sock holders, pins, etc. Prepacked, individual measures of detergent and/or bleach are convenient. Ironing, if not eliminated, can be done by using a cooler iron (Braille markings) than usual for the fabric type (determined by touch) and by smoothing the material with one hand while ironing with the other. If a person lacks skill in this bilateral activity, the smoothing hand can wear an oven mitt or glove.

STUDY QUESTIONS:

Homemaking and Child Care

1. What are the principles of energy conservation?
2. Give examples of each as they apply to a homemaker.
3. What are the principles of body mechanics?
4. Analyze the task of cleaning the bathroom and state how the principles of body mechanics can be applied to this task.
5. Plan a therapy session to train a participative homemaker with rheumatoid arthritis to prepare a simple meal.
6. What are the principles of compensation used for quadriplegic homemakers?
7. What are the problems encountered by persons with loss of the use of one upper extremity and how do they compensate?
8. What are the compensation principles for persons with blindness or limited vision?

References

1. Gilbert, D.W. Energy expenditures for the disabled homemaker: Review of studies. *Am. J. Occup. Ther.* 19(6): 321–328, 1965.
2. Frederick, B.B., et al. *Body Mechanics Instruction Manual: A Guide for Therapists.* Redmond, WA: Express Publications, 1979.
3. Chamberlain, M.A. Social implications of rheumatoid arthritis in young mothers. *Rheumatol. Rehabil.* (Suppl): 70–73, 1979.
4. Dunn, V.M. Tips on raising children from a wheelchair. *Accent on Living,* 22(4):78–83, 1978.
5. Vorburger, L. Wash up. *Accent on Living,* 25(2): 125, 1980.
6. Lunsk, A.S. Clean sweep. *Accent on Living,* 25(1): 62, 1980.
7. New Products and Services. *Accent on Living,* 22(4): 93–98, 1978.
8. Barstow, R.E. Coping with emphysema. *Nurs. Clin. North Am.* 9(1): 137–145, 1974.
9. Burkhardt, B. Loop-handled utensils. *Am. J. Occup. Ther.,* 29(7): 423, 1975.
10. Collins, A.D. Adapted plate for use in a microwave oven. *Am. J. Occup. Ther.,* 32(9): 586–587, 1978.
11. Cala, M. House retrofits that make it easier for the handicapped. *Home Mechanix,* 81(683): 90–96, 1985.
12. Strebel, M.B. *Adaptations and Techniques for the Disabled Homemaker,* 5th edition. Minneapolis, MN: Sister Kenny Institute, 1980.
13. Fastow, K. Adapted fitted bed sheets. *Am. J. Occup. Ther.,* 31(6): 393, 1977.
14. Compton, A.E. Handy tote bag. *Accent on Living,* 25(1): 63, 1980.
15. Klinger, J., Frieden, F., and Sullivan, R. *Mealtime Manual for the Aged and Handicapped.* New York: Simon & Schuster (Essandess Special Edition), 1970.
16. Boettke, E.M. *Suggestions for Physically Handicapped Mothers on Clothing for Pre-School Children.* Storrs, CT: School of Home Economics, University of Connecticut, 1957.
17. Bare, C., Boettke, E., and Waggoner, N. *Self-Help Clothing for Handicapped Children.* Chicago: National Society for Crippled Children and Adults, 1962.
18. Lowman, E., and Klinger, J. *Aids to Independent Living: Self Help for the Handicapped.* New York: McGraw-Hill, (Blakiston Division), 1969.
19. Mulberry, O.L. Tips, tools & techniques. *Better Homes and Gardens,* November 1983, p. 200.

20. Souga, C. Meat cutting wheel for one-handed patients. *Am. J. Occup. Ther., 22*(3): 211, 1968.
21. Caldwell, J. Her special touch. *The Boston Globe,* January 12, 1983, pp. 25, 38.
22. (AID) for blind seen in new alphabet. *Accent on Living, 19*(4): 42–44, 1975.
23. Microcooking by braille. *Better Homes and Gardens,* March 1984, p. 16.
24. *Aids and Appliances.* American Foundation for the Blind, Inc., 15 West 16th St., New York, NY 10011.
25. National Federation for the Blind, 1800 Johnson St., Baltimore, MD 21230.

Supplementary Reading

Bingham, B. *Cooking with Fragile Hands.* Naples, FL: Creative Cuisine, 1985.
Oppliger, H.R., and Brunner, E. Electronic measuring cup for the blind. *IEEE Trans. Biomed. Eng., 24*(4):386–388, 1977.
Patricelli, J., and Eckroth, J. Adapted knife for partial hand amputation patients. *Am. J. Occup. Ther., 36*(3):193–194, 1982.

Payne, K. Doing the impossible—it's all in learning how. *Accent on Living,* Spring 1980, pp. 38–49.
Sarno, M.T., and Buonaguro, A. Factors associated with independent meal preparation in aphasic females: a pilot study. *Occup. Ther. J. Res.* 3(1):23–34, 1983.
Schafer, R. Occupational therapy for lower extremity problems. *Am. J. Occup. Ther., 27*(3):132–137, 1973.
Wright, S.B. Being independent—mobility aids can help. *Accent on Living, 24*(3):46–48, 1979.

Selected Resources

Aids Unlimited, 1101 North Calvert St., Suite 1901, Baltimore, MD 21202.
Appliance Information Service, Administrative Center, Benton Harbor, MI 49022.
Buyer's Guide (yearly publication) *Accent on Living,* P.O. Box 700, Bloomington, IL 61701.
Frederiksborg Køkkenet Ap.S., »»Tvinnemosegård««, Hillerødvej, 3540 Lynge, Denmark.

chapter
19

Leisure Time Activities for the Physically Disabled

Catherine A. Trombly

Leisure time activities can add zest to the life of physically disabled persons, just as they do to the life of the nondisabled. In a survey of 3000 men and women aged 30, 50, and 70 years, the following activities were ranked fourth through eighth as important contributors to the overall quality of their lives: participation in active recreation, such as sports, travel, dramatics, games, and playing musical instruments; learning, that is, acquiring desired knowledge or solving problems; a close relationship with a person of the opposite sex; socialization and participation in clubs; and creative expression through music, art, writing, or collecting.[1] Material comforts, interesting and worthwhile work, and health and personal safety ranked first through third.[1] The results of this study not only indicate the importance of leisure pursuits in a person's life but also give a clue to therapists that until a person's medical condition is stabilized or the outcome predictable to him and until his work and financial and living situations are under control, expectations that he pursue leisure time activities may be premature.

Play is intrinsically motivated and self-regulated by the individual[2] and thereby contributes to a person's feeling of being in control of his own life. Recreational activities can provide opportunities to redevelop social relationships,[3] to redevelop competency and self-esteem, and to maintain or increase strength and endurance and other physical gains made in the rehabilitation program.[4,5] For these reasons, development of avocational interests and skills should be included as part of the rehabilitation process. The patient who had no hobbies or interests other than work prior to disability can be encouraged to develop hobbies by experiencing their benefits while in a rehabilitation program.

The newly disabled person may need guidance in choosing and initiating activities that are both interesting and useful to his growth and development as a person as well as possible within his capabilities. One

study indicated that the depression following a major disabling accident (spinal cord injury) reduced the person's motivation to participate or be interested in recreational interests previously enjoyed.[4] Another study tested and found support for the hypothesis that increasing the level of physical fitness of poststroke patients would also improve their self-concept.[6] Too often the all-consuming interest becomes the disability and the limitations it imposes; interest in recreational activities can put the focus on achievement.

The occupational therapist's role in this aspect of the patient's life is based on the assumption that "play is a need-fulfilling and appropriate occupation in the life of every person."[2] Knowledge of motor and psychosocial activity analyses enables the occupational therapist to suggest recreational pursuits that are within the capabilities of the person and that will contribute to the goals the disabled person has for his life. The occupational therapist can devise or suggest adapted methods or specialized equipment needed by the disabled person to accomplish the particular activity of his choice. The adaptations are made using the same principles as cited in the chapters on self-care and homemaking. Sometimes, the specific solution needs to be collaboratively worked out by an expert in the sport or activity, the patient, and the occupational therapist, all contributing their knowledge of the particular situation. As with any adapted method or device, it must be evaluated for function and reliability and the patient must be thoroughly trained in its use.

If a therapeutic recreation specialist is part of the rehabilitation team, the occupational therapist may be less involved in selecting and adapting activities to meet the patient's goals, but may be more active in helping the patient discover what physical and mental abilities he has to capitalize on and what life goals and values may be met through avocational pursuits.

Some examples of activities and suggestions for adaptations of equipment or method are included here. This is by no means an exhaustive survey; the reader is referred to the literature and to special societies cited in the references.

referred to the literature and to special societies cited in the references.

Arts and Crafts

Involvement in the arts can be passive or active. Music, art, drama, literature, and dance or rhythmic movement can all be enjoyed on several levels. They offer the participant refreshment from daily work and a sense of achievement if participation is active.

Musical instruments can be adapted to enable some disabled musicians to continue their interest. For example, a person with weak forearms and elbows can use a piano if a smooth wooden shelf is attached to the piano in front of the keys to rest the arms on while playing.[7] An adaptation has been devised to enable a bilateral upper-extremity amputee to play the guitar.[8] Computerized musical instruments that are switch operated enable severely disabled persons to continue their interests in creating music. Some instruments are more suitable than others for persons with certain remaining capacities; an analysis has been published for various levels of upper-extremity amputation that could be applied to persons with other disabilities also.[9]

Paintbrush handles can be enlarged for easier grasp or adapted to be held in the mouth.[7] Paint cups can be secured in a cutout board to stabilize them to prevent spilling for a person with incoordination. Easels can be readily adjusted to a suitable angle.[7]

Wheelchair square dancing is an organized recreation in a number of communities.

Involvement in crafts not only gives one a sense of accomplishment, but also may help maintain physical gains of the rehabilitation process and may even result in limited earnings if the product is clever and the workmanship good. One popular craft is needlework. Sewing aids are available to hold, mark, or cut material. Self-threading needles allow threading by pushing the thread into the eye of the needle while the needle is held in a cake of soap, beeswax, a pin cushion, etc. Needlework can be held in place on a pillow or on hoops or other frames that attach to the table (Fig. 19.1) or clamp on a person's knee to allow one-handed persons to enjoy this activity.[7] For patients with lower-extremity weakness, adapted microswitch controls for the sewing machine can be mounted so the patient can operate the machine using his chin or any other part of his body over which he has voluntary motor control and sensation while freeing both hands to guide the material.[7] An adaptation has been devised to enable an upper-extremity amputee to crochet.[10]

Games

Games are competitive and, as such, absorb the person's attention even if the person is an observer. For participants, they activate perceptual and intellectual abilities to the level needed to meet the challenge. Usually games are social interactions, especially if a club is organized. Board games such as checkers, chess, monopoly, and scrabble can be modified by enlarging or reducing the size of the board or the pieces. The pieces

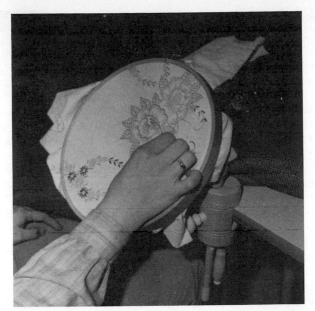

Figure 19.1 Frame that permits a person with use of one hand to do needlework.

can also be weighted, altered in shape, magnetized, or held in place with Velcro to allow persons with limited range, strength, or coordination to play.[7] Supine patients can use magnetized or Velcroed pieces that allow the playing board to be fastened in an upright or upside-down position. Prism glasses that allow viewing of something held perpendicular to the person may be needed. The glasses allow the patient whose eyes look directly ahead to see what is at or towards his waist or feet. Card games are popular and can bridge generations and bring together people of various backgrounds who share equal enthusiasm. Playing cards can be large, small, marked in braille, magnetized, shuffled by machines, or held in card holders.[7] Card holders hold the hand of cards so each card is visible to the card player; they can be purchased commercially or made by cutting slots in a piece of wood, by using an upended scrub brush, or by using the edges of a book held closed by an elastic band.

Electronic versions of chess, checkers, scrabble, poker and fantasy logistical games have been developed, some of which enable disabled persons to play these games without the need to actually handle the playing pieces. These types of games have also been computerized, enabling patients with severe upper-extremity disability to play. By adapting the computer-patient interface, whatever control function the patient has can be used to operate the computer. Many styles of switches and other types of interfaces, including voice activation, are commercially available[11,12] or can be developed by rehabilitation engineers.[12]

Electronic and computerized games offer a fine opportunity for interaction and friendly competition between the disabled person and his nondisabled friends as well as providing "challenging" solitary pastimes.

Hobbies

A hobby pursued with enthusiasm can put the person in contact with other people, disabled and nondisabled, who share the same interest through magazines, clubs, and organizations that spring up related to a certain hobby. Hobbies can range from the usual solitary interests such as reading, collecting, or calligraphy to those that involve other people such as ham radio, camping, or travel, to the more daring interests for those with adventurous spirits. Personal computers are expanding the leisure time (and vocational) choices for the severely disabled. Creative writing can be done more easily using word processing on a computer than on a typewriter. For those whose hobby interest is financial planning, programs exist to assist or record transactions. Computers with modems also offer opportunities for electronic mail "pen pals."

Talking books and magazines are available for the visually and physically disabled from participating libraries throughout the United States. The playback equipment is loaned free to the reader.[13]

Project Magic, developed by David Copperfield, magician, in conjunction with Julie DeJean, O.T.R., has for the past 5 years been motivating patients to feel good about themselves.[14] For those inspired to continue to develop magic as a hobby, it provides the opportunity for sharing with others.[1,15]

Camping for handicapped adults and children is becoming more possible with the greater emphasis and awareness of the need to reduce architectural barriers in all types of environments.[16,17] Travel is also becoming easier for the wheelchair bound[18,19] and offers the challenge the adventuresome are seeking.[20-22] Planning the trip and reliving it afterwards with friends via photographs are part of the pleasure of travel. Photography is possible for persons with limited hand use with care in selection of equipment and by adaptive methods of holding the camera and releasing the shutter.[7,23,24]

For those with determination, nothing seems impossible. One man, who is a high-level paraplegic from birth, pilots his own plane while lying on a special gurney and using hand controls.[25] Another paraplegic pilots a helicopter and does aerial photography.[26] Equally implausible, however less daring, was the development of an authors group among young severely disabled persons with articulation problems so severe they were not easily understood. It resulted in their learning to produce creative writing pieces that were published and sold and in their becoming better listeners and speakers through the discussions.[27]

Gardens can be adapted for enjoyment by the blind by marking the exhibits in braille, by raising the flower beds to near hand level, and by clearly demarcating the walkways by raised edging. Fragrant flowers and herbs would be a great pleasure. Raised garden beds or flower pots or planters enable a wheelchair patient to garden comfortably.[7] Involvement in garden clubs and competitions can add another dimension to the pleasure of gardening.

Sports

Both team and individual sports are engaged in by disabled persons of all types. Some become champions, some do it for fitness, and others do it for the challenge. The sports have rules and equipment suitable to the players.

Those with physical disabilities have the need for exercise to maintain good cardiovascular health just as the nondisabled do. Basketball, swimming, and long-distance wheelchair races fulfill the requirements needed for good cardiovascular training because they are dynamic exercises, use many muscle groups, require intensity of over 50% maximum capacity, and are performed over a relatively long performance time.[5,28] The Arthritis Foundation has produced an exercise videotape, featuring Jane Powell, for arthritics.[29] Martial arts classes for quadriplegics, using Uechi-Ryu Okinawan Karate, which lends itself to the sitting position, have been successfully instituted in several Veterans Administration Medical Centers.[30] These programs offer exercise as well as contribute to improved self-esteem.

Basketball,[31] softball,[32] track and field,[3] swimming,[3] table tennis, fencing,[7] weight lifting, archery,[33] dartchery, and marathoning[34] are all sports for which there are organized competitions. College- and industry-sponsored wheelchair teams engage in competition with each other.[35] Also there are games with "normal" teams who use wheelchairs for the event. Both teams use special sports chairs that are designed for maximum maneuverability.

The ParaOlympics are held every 4 years following the Olympic games.[36] As in any competition, categories of player abilities ensure that the competition is among persons of equal ability and is, therefore, fair, i.e., a paraplegic does not compete against a quadriplegic. There are national competitions for the various Para-Olympic sports to select the best representatives from the U.S.A. to compete with the best wheelchair athletes from other countries.

Kayaking, roller skating, and skate boarding are all possible by some daring amputees or spinal cord-injured persons.[32] Horseback riding has been found physically and psychologically beneficial as part of the rehabilitation program of patients diagnosed with cerebral palsy, poliomyelitis, arthritis, stroke, trauma, or blindness.[37,38] Contraindications to this sport that were cited include epilepsy with uncontrolled seizures, severe mental retardation, susceptibility to decubitus ulcers, or progressive neuromuscular disease that affects the upper extremities needed to control the horse.[38]

Adaptations have been devised to enable persons with certain handicaps to fish (pole holders for an upper-extremity amputee[7] or a stroke patient[39]); to hunt (gun mount for a quadriplegic)[40]; to do boating (open-ended sailboat with swivel seat and window shade type sail for lower-extremity disabled persons)[41]; to ride motorcycles (hand controls and side car for wheelchair for paraplegic)[42]; to ski (adapted ski poles for lower-extremity amputees, tandem skiing for the blind, and others)[43,44]; to bowl (device to propel the ball for person with upper-extremity weakness)[45]; and to play baseball or do archery (special terminal devices used in place of a hook or hand for an upper-extremity amputee).[7]

STUDY QUESTIONS:
Leisure Time Activities for the Physically Disabled

1. Why are play or leisure time pursuits important in a person's life?
2. What is the role of the occupational therapist regarding leisure pursuits by adult patients?
3. Motivation to participate depends on many factors. What might these be and how can the occupational therapist influence them?

References

1. Flanagan, J.C. Measurement of quality of life: current state of the art. *Arch. Phys. Med. Rehabil.*, 63(2): 56–59, 1982.
2. Gunn, S.L. Play as an occupation: implications for the handicapped. *Am. J. Occup. Ther.*, 29(4): 222–225, 1975.
3. Wheelchair sports. One avenue to a happy, healthy life. *Accent on Living*, 25(2): 36–41, 1980.
4. Rogers, J.C., and Figone, J.J. The avocational pursuits of rehabilitants with traumatic quadriplegia. *Am. J. Occup. Ther.*, 32(9): 571–576,1978.
5. Jochheim, K.A., and Strohkendle, H. The value of particular sports of the wheelchair-disabled in maintaining health of the paraplegic. *Paraplegia*, 11: 173–178, 1973.
6. Brinkmann, J.R., and Hoskins, T.A. Physical conditioning and altered self-concept in rehabilitated hemiplegic patients. *Phys. Ther.*, 59 (7): 859–865, 1979.
7. Lowman, E., and Klinger, J. *Aids to Independent Living: Self Help for the Handicapped*, chapters 56–60. New York: McGraw-Hill (Blakiston Division), 1969.
8. Zatlin, C. R., et al. Guitar capo for a bilateral upper-extremity amputee. *Am. J. Occup. Ther. 35* (11): 736, 1981.
9. Mailhot, A. Musical instruments for upper-limb amputees. *Interclinic Information Bulletin, 13* (10): 9–12,14–15, 1974.
10. Matsushima, D. S. Crochet aid for the amputee. *Am. J. Occup. Ther., 40* (7): 495–496, 1986.
11. ComputAbility Corporation, 101 Route 46, Pine Brook, NJ 07058.
12. Preston, J. Project leader. *Directory of Research and Development Projects on Controls to Operate Assistive Devices.* Rehabilitation Engineering Center, Children's Hospital at Stanford, 520 Willow Rd., Palo Alto, CA 94304, 1981.
13. *Facts.* National Library Service for the Blind and Physically Handicapped. The Library of Congress, Washington, DC 20542, 1985.
14. After five years "Project Magic" still going strong. *Occupational Therapy News* [official newspaper of The American Occupational Therapy Association, Rockville, MD], 41(5): 3, 1987.
15. Can magic work miracles? *Accent on Living*, 30 (2): 52–55, 1985.
16. Scouting, camping opening up for disabled youths and adults. *Accent on Living* 21(2): 88–92, 1976.
17. Shotwell, R. Addicted to camping. *Accent on Living*, 30(4): 74–75, 1986.
18. Annand, D. Sail away on the Love Boat. *Accent on Living* 25(4): 50–54, 1980.
19. Pietkiewicz, P. Seeing America. *Accent on Living*, 25(1): 78–86, 1980.
20. Jaffe, D. Traveling Europe: next stop USA. *Accent on Living*, 31(4): 66–69, 1987.
21. Ferris, B. It's thumbs out. *Accent on Living*, 26(1): 30–37, 1981.
22. Exploring caves highlight of trip. *Accent on Living*, 30(3): 58–59, 1985.
23. Have fun with photography. *Accent on Living*, 21(3): 68–73, 1976.
24. Taking pictures. *Accent on Living*, 31(3): 50–52, 1986.
25. Miller, H. L. How this paraplegic flies an airplane. *Accent on Living*, 25(2): 74–75, 1980.
26. Powers, J. M. How this paraplegic flies a helicopter. *Accent on Living*, 25(2): 76–78, 1980.
27. Fearing, V.G. An authors group for extended care patients. *Am. J. Occup. Ther.*, 32(8): 526–527, 1978.
28. Corcoran, P. J., et al. Sports medicine and the physiology of wheelchair marathon racing. *Orthop. Clin. North Am.*, 11(4): 697–716, 1980.
29. Ilgen, L. Update: fitness—move over Ms. Fonda. *Weight Watchers Magazine*, February 1987, p. 10.
30. Pandavela, J., et al. Martial arts for the quadriplegic. *Am. J. Phys. Med.*, 65(1): 17–29, 1986.
31. Pykare, J. 30th wheelchair basketball games. *Accent on Living*, 23(1): 82–83, 1978.
32. Accent on pictures. *Accent on Living*, 25(4): 58–59, 1981.
33. Kenoyer, M. and Kenoyer, N. Bullseye! *Accent on Living*, 25(1): 22–25, 1980.
34. Marathon for fast and fit. *Accent on Living*, 25(2): 42–46, 1980.
35. Arnett, C. All work and no play: until after the games. *Accent on Living*, 30(3): 72–75, 1985.
36. Lipton, B. The role of wheelchair sports in rehabilitation. *Int. Rehabil. Rev.*, 21(2): 1970.
37. Disabled on horseback? *Accent on Living*, 23(1): 88–93, 1978.
38. Woods, D. Horseriding catching on as therapy for the disabled. *Can. Med. Assoc. J.*, 121(5): 631–634, 650, 1979.
39. Crewe, R.A. Fishing for the hemiplegic. *Br. J. Occup. Ther.*, 38(9): 195, 1975.
40. Szeto, A. Y. J. Hunting rifle for quadriplegic patients. *Arch. Phys. Med. Rehabil.*, 60(9): 425–427, 1979.
41. Lundberg, Lasse. Personal communication, Goteburg, Sweden.
42. World champion paraplegic motorcyclist talks about 8,000 mile ride to speed cure of spinal cord injury. *Accent on Living*, 21(3): 88–92, 1976.
43. Skiing on one leg! *Accent on Living*, 21(3): 56–63, 1976.
44. Thrills and spills on the downhill run. *Accent on Living*, 25(3): 38–39, 1980.
45. Bowl with your feet. *Accent on Living*, 22(1): 94–95, 1977.

Supplementary Reading

American Occupational Therapy Association. *Adaptive Equipment Rehabilitation Technology Information Packet.* Rockville, MD: American Occupational Therapy Association, 1986.

Arnetz, B. B. Gerontic occupational therapy: psychological and social predictors of participation and therapeutic benefits. *Am. J. Occup. Ther.*, 39(7): 460–465, 1985.

Garcia, S., and Greenfield, J. Dynamic protractible mouthstick. *Am. J. Occup. Ther. 35*(8): 529–530, 1981.

Gordon, S., et al. Adaptive device for the quadriplegic golfer. *Arch. Phys. Med. Rehabil.*, 66(7): 475–476, 1985.

Mouthstick handles small, light items. *Accent on Living*, 24(3): 86–87, 1979.

Overs, R. P. Avocational evaluation and work adjustment: a deterrent to dependency. *J. Rehabil.*, 42(6): 21–24, 40, 48, 1976.

Shein, G. F., and Mandel, A. R. Large area flap switch to control battery-operated toys. *Am. J. Occup. Ther.*, 36 (2): 107–110, 1982.

Truong, X. T., Erickson, R., and Galbreath, R. Baseball adaptation for below-elbow prosthesis. *Arch. Phys. Med. Rehabil.*, 67(6): 418, 1986.

Selected Resources

American Wheelchair Bowling Association, N54W15858 Larkspur Lane, Menomonee Falls, WI 53051.

Blind Outdoor Leisure Development (BOLD), 533 East Main St., Aspen, CO 81611.

Boating for the Handicapped, Guidelines for the Physically Disabled, by Eugene Hedley, Ph.D. Available from: Products Manager, Human Resources Center, I.U. Willets Rd., Albertson, NY 11507.

Breckenridge Outdoor Education Center, P.O. Box 697, Breckenridge, CO 80424.

Disabled Artists' Network, P.O. Box 20781, New York, NY 10025.

Handicapped Boater's Association Magazine, P.O. Box 1134, Ansonia Station, NY 10023.

Mobility International, P.O. Box 3551, Eugene, OR 97403.

National Association of Sports for Cerebral Palsy, 66 East 34th St., New York, NY 10016.

National Foundation of Wheelchair Tennis, 4000 MacArthur Blvd., Newport Beach, CA 92660.

National Handicapped Sports and Recreation Association, Capitol Hill Station, P.O. Box 18664, Denver, CO 80218.

National Inconvenienced Sportsmen's Association (NISA), 3738 Walnut Ave., Carmichael, CA 95608.

The National Wheelchair Athletic Association, 40-24 62nd St., Woodside, NY 11377.

New England Handicapped Sportmen's Association, 26 McFarlin Rd., Chelmsford, MA 01824.

North American Riding for the Handicapped Association (NARHA) Thistlecroft, Park St., Mendon, MA 01756.

Personal Computers & Special Needs. Sybex Books, 2344 Sixth St., Berkeley, CA 94710.

Project Magic, c/o Julie DeJean, O.T.R., Box 100, Inglewood, CA 90306.

Riding for Rehabilitation, a Guide for Handicapped Riders and Their Instructors, by Joseph Bauer. Available from: Can Ride, 209 Deloraine Ave., Toronto, Canada M5M 2B2.

Senior Olympics, 5670 Wilshire Blvd., Los Angeles, CA 90036.

Society for the Advancement of Travel for the Handicapped (SATH), 26 Court St., Suite 1110, Brooklyn, NY 11242.

Spinal Cord Injury Life. Official publication of the National Spinal Cord Injury Association, 149 California St., Newton, MA 02158.

Therapeutic Horsemanship, Inc., Mrs. Sandy Rafferty, M.A., O.T.R., Director, Route 1, Valley Road, Pacific, MO 63069.

The United States Association for Blind Athletes, 55 W. California Ave., Beach Haven Park, NJ 08008.

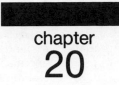

chapter

20

Environmental Evaluation and Community Reintegration

Catherine A. Trombly and Hilda Powers Versluys

Occupational therapists believe that the individual has the basic right to achieve maximum potential and to control his own life through educated choices, in interaction with the environment.[1] The ultimate objective of rehabilitation is to enable the patient to live successfully and independently, to be reintegrated into the family and community, and to find contributory and self-satisfying roles.[2] Occupational therapists join with other rehabilitation professionals and with disabled consumers to facilitate a continuum of services that support independent living.[1] In the in-hospital phase of rehabilitation, only basic activity of daily living (BADL) skills and compensatory techniques can be adequately learned. Therefore, rehabilitation must be viewed as a long-term learning process that continues postdischarge.[2,3] Part of rehabilitation must be a transitional process in which problem solving and coping skills are learned and self-esteem is heightened so that the disabled person who expects to be active in the community can act confidently and take charge. A transitional reintegration program should include learning to correct or bypass barriers to independent living. The barriers are environmental (architectural, societal attitudes), personal (taking charge, feeling confident and in control), social (putting the nondisabled at ease, asking for information or help from strangers, being assertive), and economic (funding for housing and equipment and for maintaining a family).[4-6]

The Independent Living Movement

Independent living is defined as noninstitutional living in which the individual has primary responsibility for his own choices, decision making, and performance of self-care and home-community activities within the limits of his physical, emotional, social, mental, and economic capabilities.[1]

Based on the Comprehensive Rehabilitation Services Amendment of the Rehabilitation Act of 1973, Title VII Public Law 95-602, services to increase the quality of life for disabled citizens were established.

These included access to medical care and educational and vocational opportunities. The role of the consumer as a self-advocate and coplanner of his own rehabilitation was stressed. This marked the beginning of the Independent Living Movement (ILM).[7] The ILM, modeling itself on the civil rights movement from which it drew inspiration, was first concerned with eradicating direct discrimination.[8] It addressed a major truth slow to be accepted: the disabled are not unable.[9] The ILM was strengthened by a growing number of articulate severely disabled individuals who networked and raised consciousness among the disabled themselves.[9]

The beginning goals of the ILM were to facilitate independent living through Independent Living Centers established to provide referral and direct services relating to housing, attendant care, transportation, and social-vocational counseling. These centers are important in light of the fact that modern family life is changing. Families are smaller and more mobile; both spouses work; people live longer and may live a distance from their grown children; the divorce rate is high. The family is ill-equipped to deal with members with permanent handicaps.[10] Therefore, many handicapped persons have to rely on their own resources or be institutionalized. The Independent Living Centers are meant to enhance their resources. Centers for Independent Living are unique community-based, nonprofit, nonresidential programs that are consumer oriented and are substantially controlled by consumers who are disabled.[11] They provide a diversity of resource and referral services that may include assistance in locating accessible housing or in hiring personal-care attendants; advice on sports and recreational resources and on purchase of equipment such as vans and lifts; and provision of vocational counseling. ILM programs now serve 20,000 individuals in 290 sites across the country.[4,11,12]

In a self-report, quadriplegic patients stated a concern with the transfer of skills acquired within hospital treatment programs to community settings. They requested more practice experiences and training programs involving actual community experiences before discharge.[13] Such patient reports and other observations made it clear within the rehabilitation sector that in-hospital rehabilitation alone was inadequate to prepare for independent community living. Reintegration programs were established to help the patient bridge the gap from rehabilitation center to community living.

Reintegration Programs

Successful community reintegration requires not only traditional hospital-based rehabilitation but also advanced living skill programs. In the initial hospital phase of treatment, the role of the occupational therapist includes training in basic ADL skills, use of adaptive equipment, and psychosocial intervention. The therapist is concerned with values clarification, development of obtainable life goals, and instillation of positive attitudes toward advanced, transitional programs, independent living, and use of community resources.[4,5]

Advanced living skills refer to those experiences and activities that combine basic performance segments into more complex daily routines and roles and also require feasible use of time and preplanning.[14] Performance skills are motoric task skills (transfers, use of equipment, cooking, shopping, personal care), cognitive skills (organization, problem solving), and social-communication skills. Advanced living skill programming fits within an education-action-training model that includes direct, intense skill practice and encourages the transfer of learning between the hospital and the community.[2] Topic areas of advanced programming include crisis management and stress reduction; time management; first aid, emergency medical procedures, and emergency egress procedures; sexuality; hiring and management of personal-care attendants and home health aides;[15] resources for and practice of recreational and leisure interests; financial management; dealing with architectural barriers; consumer rights laws; learning interactional skills that put the nondisabled at ease; and the development of ability to handle stares and personal questions.[4,16-19]

The patient is encouraged to develop personal learning objectives, contribute to the design of the learning experience, research personal life-style requirements, and take responsibility for planning and implementing community out-trips.[2,3]

Programs that prepare for discharge allow the person to practice overcoming architectural and transportation barriers and to develop understanding of the attitudes of the general public with the opportunity to discuss the successes, failures, and frustrations with peers and rehabilitation personnel. Realistic activities encourage skill practice in various environments, encourage the patient to develop solutions to problems and barriers, and diffuse fear of community reintegration through rehearsals and anticipatory guidance. Examples of such bridging activities are: shopping with family, friends, or alone; attending community programs and activities; job interviewing; attending educational classes; doing errands; and visiting independent living centers.[2] Patients learn, for example, to plan ahead, to allow enough time, to inquire by phone about accessibility of a building, and to arrange for special parking and for help at the entrance if necessary. In the practice sessions, the patient is put into situations that are within his capabilities but present problems so that he can learn to anticipate and solve problems. He assumes as much responsibility as he can at the time in arranging and conducting the outing. The therapist takes up the slack in responsibility if necessary and is there to provide assistance in unexpected situations.

Since the needs of a patient population are diverse, the occupational therapist must be inventive and realistic in problem solving around issues of housing, transportation, home and equipment adaptations, and family. Presentations can be provided by experts on the law, finances, vocational exploration, adapted housing, first aid, and emergency procedures. Those experienced disabled who model confidence, success, and resourcefulness should be invited to present to patient groups. The experienced disabled can provide invaluable information about architectural barriers, transportation, clothing selection, owning a car, adapting the home interior, adapted equipment, and recreational possibilities. For example, one person's suggestions for marketing from a wheelchair included: choose an accessible store by visiting several beforehand to determine the one where shopping can be done with least effort; shop on a slow day; and ask for help when necessary, but do not allow the helper to take over the shopping.[20]

The use of videotapes are valuable in living skill training. Scenes on the training tapes can be imitated, provide models for community practice, or pose problems for discussion and problem-solving sessions.

One approach to comprehensive transitional programming is the use of *role-focused group therapy* that treats role disorders during the hospital phase of rehabilitation and links the patient to former family, work, and community roles and relationships. Objectives of such a group include role maintenance during hospitalization; evaluation of the need for change in role; analysis of components of each major role and of the patient's interests and past experiences relative to role substitutions; the redefinition and redesign of roles; and the opportunity to practice and internalize the new role concepts. The group format includes member problem solving and a variety of sequenced educational and intervention modules.[21]

Family group programming is also important and should include the opportunity to share difficult feelings and fears, increase knowledge of the effects of the disability, and allow for a discussion of future plans after discharge.[22] A group format that is designed for patients and families improves communication and provides an opportunity to express feelings attendant to discharge.[23]

EXAMPLES OF REINTEGRATION PROGRAMS

Research studies and clinical investigations graphically present the case for community reintegration programs including follow-up programs after discharge. Patients involved in follow-up services that emphasized skill training, identification of interests, social and recreational activities, and family counseling showed a significant improvement in performance of ADL and mobility as compared to a control group.[24,25]

The need for reintegration programs is further supported by a survey that was conducted among disabled and nondisabled college students.[26] It was found that there was a significant difference in feelings of confidence between the two groups in these areas: problem-solving skills related to managing money, conserving physical energy, and finding a place to live; school-vocational skills of finding a job, interviewing and applying for a job, planning a school program, and talking with teachers or employers; home skills; and community mobility skills. There was no difference in feelings of confidence regarding abilities to manage activities of daily living, which would indicate that traditional rehabilitation is effective; however it is "clear that provision of traditional rehabilitation services alone does not guarantee life satisfaction."[26]

Examples are as follows. A transitional family activity group was formed to strengthen family relationships and encourage the continuation of the patient's roles within the family. Emphasis was on action programming that provided opportunities for family members to observe the patient's abilities: for example, eating, organizing activities, and researching and presenting information at group meetings. Activities for such groups can include dinners, trips, music, plays, sports, and social events. Through observation of family interaction patterns, the therapist can identify potential problem areas and plan interventions.[21]

A sensitivity training group was designed to assist patients in coping with feelings about community reentry, relating to the nonhandicapped community, being visible in the community, and dealing with stigma. Emphasis was on the assignment of experimental community tasks, follow-up reports to the group on the community experience, and identification of feelings and reactions. The group provided feedback, support, and suggestions on solving problems encountered in community interactions, travel, access, and in regaining poise in public and social situations.[21]

A training model was devised to teach spinal cord-injured patients to anticipate architectural barriers within the home environment. The method was an audiovisual presentation of wheelchair mobility requirements, standards of accessibility, and common problems encountered by wheelchair-bound persons in homes. There was a statistically significant difference between the experimental and control subjects in their ability to notice and circumvent environmental problems in an actual test home.[27]

A learning skills program model with inherent demands for adult role behavior and an educational structure emphasizing personal responsibility for behavior, learning, and the use of time was successful in remotivating disabled adults to acquire independent living skills. Such programs are seen as critical in the maintenance of rehabilitation gains and in continued social and physical development.[28]

A transitional training apartment within a community contributed to earlier and more successful discharge and an increased rate of independent living success. Goals were to assist the client in decreasing separation anxiety, regaining confidence, and initiating positive relationships among family members. The patients contracted to assume responsibility for all maintenance tasks (meals, cleaning), self-medication, personal care, and community contacts (such as shopping, equipment repair) and were evaluated on their ability to carry out task responsibilities. An occupational therapist organized the experience and acted as liaison between the hospital and apartment program.[29]

Simulated practical experiences to prepare for out-trip training experiences are important. A remedial gym class was designed with the objective of increasing the patients' sense of independence and confidence in their abilities. The minimum criterion for membership was the ability to stand independently. Some of the exercises were practice on all types of stairs; getting on and off a simulated bus platform in a crowd and within time limits; games to prepare for walking on uneven surfaces and with noise, hubbub of traffic, and people introduced; obstacle courses; and practice in getting up from the floor.[30]

A program of community outings was rated as very useful by rheumatoid arthritic patients in increasing their self-confidence.[31] The program was designed to evaluate a patient's functional abilities to do skills that are required out of hospital and to assess each patient's problem-solving skills in relation to his own disability regarding architectural barriers, joint protection techniques, the avoidance of decubiti, etc. Minimum criteria for participation included mobility and ADL independence to the level expected. A COTA (certified occupational therapy assistant) planned the outing with the patient, based on the patient's needs. If the patient was expecting to be active post discharge, the outings were to markets, banks, restaurants, and sometimes to the job. If not, less ambitious outings were planned. A checklist was used to evaluate the experience.

Reports such as these suggest ideas for development of community reintegration programs. They should be continually monitored to ensure that current concerns of policymakers and funding bodies are being addressed, such as whether these programs meet national standards and enable the disabled individual to continue to remain successfully in the community and to reach vocational goals and/or to contribute to family and community. A methodology for measuring long-term effects of independent living programs has been described.[32] Methods of evaluation of quality assurance by occupational therapists providing community services have been published.[28] Standards to gauge successful delivery of such services to the disabled in the community also have been identified.[28]

Barriers to Independent Living

ATTITUDINAL BARRIERS

At the time of discharge, the patient faces formidable hurdles including the response of society to his disability. The patient may experience staring, rejection, and intimate personal questioning concerning the disability, or intrusive assistance that he has not requested and does not need.

The most insidious barriers that the disabled, like any minority, need to overcome are attitudinal barriers—stubborn misconceptions and prejudices that block the channels for greater integration and more equal opportunity.[9] Anything that serves to exclude a person or foster dependency on others is an obstacle holding someone back.[9]

Prejudice toward the disabled is manifested in diverse ways: for example, critical judgments based on the limitations, assumptions of disability in all areas of functioning instead of specific areas,[33,34] or patronizing and overly sympathetic attitudes.[35,36] The disabled individual within the community may experience a confusing kind of limited friendliness.[37] Origins of prejudicial and fearful attitudes toward the disabled may stem from a variety of sources and are complex, largely unconscious, and firmly entrenched. Healthy acceptance of the disabled is related to qualities in the nondisabled such as positive self-image and personal confidence and secure concepts of body image and self-worth that enable development of sound, stable interpersonal relationships.[38,39]

There is a tendency on the part of the nondisabled viewer to deny the extent of the injury and its functional loss. Thus, prejudice is found to be modified by cosmetic appearance, the severity of visibility of the disability, and the degree of competence and social ability shown by the disabled. Modern adaptive devices, such as electric wheelchairs, somewhat mask the extent of helplessness of the disabled, allowing the viewer to feel more comfortable and enter into a relationship of social interaction.

The less confident and inexperienced patient will find it a devastating experience to face the community and to handle those constant vibrations of rejection. The successfully rehabilitated and more experienced patient may shrink from the experience but will have developed the social skills and the confidence to handle the community, maintain his sense of worth, and manipulate social situations.[38,39] Becoming comfortable with one's handicap and developing a positive attitude toward living with one's disability can ward off nega-

tive reactions and/or allow overlooking callous remarks as being a manifestation of the able-bodied person's disabled personality rather than relating to the physically disabled person's worth at all.[33] Better social skills on the part of the disabled in relating to the able-bodied may help break down these attitudinal barriers.[40]

ARCHITECTURAL BARRIERS

Persons who are paralyzed and must use wheelchairs or ambulatory aids, who are blind and need orienting aids, or who are old, have low endurance, or are unable to move quickly or negotiate rough terrain or stairs are prevented from use of public buildings, parks, and other facilities unless architectural barriers are eliminated. The international symbol of access (Fig. 20.1) indicates that a facility meets standards of accessibility for the handicapped, including wheelchair users. The American National Standards Institute[41] has adopted and published specifications (ANSI A117.1-1986) for making buildings and facilities accessible to, and usable by, the physically disabled. This is a voluntary standard that has formed the basis of many governmental regulations and standards. The standard is based on adult dimensions and anthropometrics and therefore would need to be modified for making buildings accessible to disabled children.

The Public Buildings–Handicapped Persons Act of 1968, also known as the Architectural Barriers Act, provided that all federally owned, financed, or leased buildings and transportation facilities constructed since 1968 be fully accessible to the handicapped.[42,43] The Uniform Federal Access Standards (UFAS) published in 1984 are in effect for design, construction, and alteration of federal buildings in accordance with the

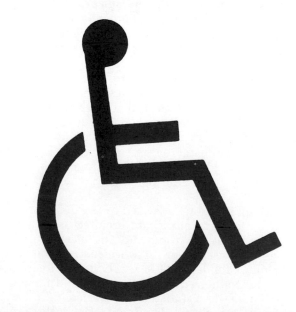

Figure 20.1 International symbol of handicapped accessibility.

Architectural Barriers Act of 1968.[44] The Rehabilitation Act of 1973 created the Architectural and Transportation Barriers Compliance Board (ATBCB) and charged it with enforcing the legislation.[43] In 1976, Congress passed an amendment to the Architectural Barriers Act of 1968 providing that any building or facility built or altered with federal funds must be accessible (P.L. 94-541, Title 2).[43] The Comprehensive Rehabilitation Services Amendments (P.L. 95-602), passed in 1978, expanded the responsibilities and clout of the ATBCB.[7] In 1982, the ATBCB published its Minimum Guidelines and Requirements for Accessible Design (MGRAD), which closely follow the ANSI 1980 revised standards.[43] The MGRAD set baseline requirements the UFAS must meet,[44] thereby making enforcement of the law more manageable.

The common barriers encountered in public buildings and private homes and their solutions are listed here. Most barriers are against the use of wheelchairs, with stairs and curbs the most common ones. Elevators eliminate the stair barrier inside buildings. However, many public buildings that are wheelchair accessible are not designed for emergency exiting in case of fire because elevators do not operate during fires. It is important that the disabled person who will be independent in the community be trained in protective procedures during a fire emergency.[45]

Outside entrances can be ramped or a lift can be installed if a ramp is not possible.[46] To enable a wheelchair-bound person to negotiate a ramp independently, there should be a ratio of 12 inches of ramp length for each 1 inch of rise.[41] For example, if a door entrance is 24 inches from the ground, the ramp must extend 24 feet. The ramp may need to zigzag if the required length would extend it into the street or extend it longer than 30 feet. A ramp that has a rise greater than 6 inches must have two railings.[41] All ramps should have a nonskid surface, fireproof construction, and landings 5 feet square at the beginning, end, and at each turn in a zigzagging ramp.[41] A canopy or automatic snow-melting equipment should be provided for outdoor ramps in snowy locations.

Stairs for the ambulatory disabled should have bilateral railings and uniform riser height of 7 inches maximum and tread depth of 11 inches.[41]

Curbs are eliminated at crosswalks by curb cuts using the 12:1 ratio, but not greater than 10:1, for proper rise. A cut that is set back into the sidewalk and ends at the street is safer for wheelchair users than a ramp that starts at the curb edge and continues into the street.[41] Street crossing lights should be set slow enough to allow safe crossing. They should be equipped with sound alarms for the blind.

With more wheelchairs being used on public ways, there is a need to establish their legal status. It is recommended that wheelchairs that travel at pedestrian speeds be classified as modified pedestrian status, not as motor vehicles.[47] The wheelchair user should consider himself a pedestrian and use the roadways as a pedestrian would, i.e., travel on the same side of the road as oncoming traffic.[47] To promote the safety of wheelchair users on the streets, reflectors that outline the wheelchair from back, front, and sides and lights should be required if the wheelchair will be used for night travel.[47]

Heavy doors are barriers to the disabled as they are to many able-bodied persons. Revolving doors are impossible for wheelchair users. Doors that open out are difficult for them to manage. Power-assisted or low-energy power-operated doors[41] are good alternatives. The timed electric-eye automatic sliding doors are excellent. Thresholds should be as flush as possible. Room identification, elevator buttons, and building or shopping mall layouts should be in standard tactile characters or symbols for the blind.[41] Doors that open to dangerous areas, such as the boiler room, should be identified for the blind by special signals such as knurled doorknobs.[41]

All doors should be 32 inches wide to accommodate wheelchairs.[41] A clear space of 60 inches in diameter or a T-shaped space of 36 inches minimum is required for a wheelchair to make a 180° turn. Adequate turning radius is also necessary for access to a public toilet stall.

In public bathrooms the stall doors must allow the person to go into the stall, close the door behind, and then open the door and go out of the stall; that usually means an outwardly opening door. The stall must be wide enough (36 inches) and long enough (56 inches in the case of wall-mounted toilet) to accommodate the chair.[41] Safety grab bars complying to standards need to be available. The toilet can be wall- or floor-mounted so that the seat is 17–19 inches from the floor. The lavatory faucets should be the lever or push-on type with mixer spout. The soap dispenser should be operable by pushing it.

Water fountains should be operable with one hand and should not require tight grasping, pinching, or twisting of the wrist and should require no more than 5 pounds of force.[41]

Telephone booths should be mounted low enough for a seated person to reach the highest operable part. The cord length should be 29 inches minimum. Push buttons should be provided if service for such equipment is available. One phone should have an amplifier device for the hard of hearing.[41]

Parking spaces for the handicapped must be wide enough for the car or van, as well as an additional 4 to 8 feet for the transfer, with or without a lift.[41]

Public recreation areas and schools should have showers with padded seats for use by spinal cord-injured patrons and others with similar disability.

Wheelchair areas in auditoriums and assembly areas should be an integral part of any fixed seating plan and should be distributed throughout the seating area.[41] They should adjoin an accessible route that can be used to egress in case of fire.[41]

Although the standards do not address barriers in commercial businesses, supermarkets are becoming better designed and equipped for the handicapped. In the less aware markets, the checkout areas can be barriers, groceries can be displayed out of reach, assistance is scarce, and the narrow fence openings to prevent theft of shopping wagons also prevents access to wheelchairs. In the more aware markets, these barriers have been removed and special carts are provided and reserved for wheelchair shoppers.[20]

Since most public transportation systems were built before 1968, the law does not apply. Therefore, making transportation accessible to the handicapped has lagged behind the advances that have been made in building accessibility in the United States. However, the National Mass Transportation Assistance Act of 1974 amended the Urban Mass Transportation Administration Act of 1964 to state in part that it is "national policy that elderly and handicapped persons have the same right as others to utilize mass transportation facilities and services."[48] Busses and rapid transit cars have seats designated for preference for the handicapped and elderly, although enforcement rarely seems to be attempted. Some inconveniences experienced by the handicapped are due to the indifference of the able-bodied who are unhelpful, especially during rush hour[49]—every commuter's lament. Several systems have made an attempt to comply and make public transportation accessible to wheelchairs and allow realistic commuting by wheelchair-bound persons.[49,50] Newer busses purchased in many areas are equipped with hydraulic lifts to allow wheelchair access (Fig. 20.2).

Guides to public facilities accessible by the disabled are now available for most cities from the chamber of commerce of the city. It is also common now for newspaper notices of special events or restaurant reviews to mention handicapped access. *AccessLine*, operated by a rehabilitation center of a major city, makes leisure information—both accessibility information for such things as theaters, museums, restaurants, Nautilus programs, campgrounds, etc., and buyer's guide information for such things as suitable games and toys for specific disabilities—available by telephone.[8]

A survey form, originally developed for use in preparing city guides for the handicapped, is published here (Table 20.1) because it also can be helpful during the reintegration educational process. Other forms are available to suit specific purposes such as to select accommodations for meetings that disabled persons will attend.[51]

Home Evaluation

The living quarters to which the patient will be discharged also may have architectural or safety barriers. A home evaluation is necessary for every patient returning home with a residual disability and expectations of independent functioning on some level. It is done at about the time of discharge when the patient has reached his peak in rehabilitation skills. Sometimes the evaluation can be done by interview with the patient and family, preferably after a home visit. If the problems are complex, the evaluation is done by visit. For a patient who has had to learn adapted methods of self-care and mobility, the visit is usually done by the occupational and physical therapist together. The patient and responsible family members are present in the home during the visit. The patient has all ambulation aids that he customarily uses. Whether by visit or interview, preparation for the evaluation requires the therapist to list the disabilities and probable areas of difficulty for this particular patient.

As a result of a postevaluation audit, it was also recommended that the patient and therapist together identify the expected problems to guide the home evaluation and to better address the concerns of patient and family.[52] In general, specific targets of observation include architectural barriers; hazards such as inadequate lighting in key areas; entryways; stairs; carpets; safety with kitchen appliances; safety in the bathroom; placement of electrical outlets; and accessibility of storage areas, telephones, and emergency exit.[52] An example of a problem list for a poststroke patient who uses a cane and has not regained use of the upper extremity might include ambulation on various surfaces in the home, stairs, ability to carry things safely, ability to work in the kitchen and do other home care chores, and ability to get in and out of the bathtub. The therapists would need to be alert to check these tasks specifically. By using a form such as the one developed by Rita Lefkovitz, M.O.T., and published here (Table 20.2), the evaluation proceeds by reenacting the patient's daily routine and noting what cannot be done and why. The problems are solved or noted as they arise during the course of the visit.

The most common changes that need to be made in the home are installation of a ramp or railings to enter and exit the home, removal of scatter rugs and extraneous furniture, removal of thresholds, addition of tub or toilet safety grab bars, rearrangement of furniture,

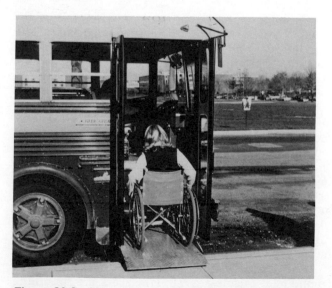

Figure 20.2 Bus with hydraulic lift, University of Illinois.

Table 20.1
BUILDING SURVEY TO DEVELOP GUIDES FOR THE HANDICAPPED

National Society for Crippled Children and Adults, 2023 W. Ogden Ave., Chicago, IL 60612

Name and Type of Building _____ Phone Number _____

Street Address _____ City _____ State _____

Person Interviewed _____ Title _____

1. Offstreet Parking

   a. Is an offstreet parking area available adjacent to building? . . . . Yes   No
   b. If adjacent offstreet parking is not available, identify and give location of nearest and most convenient
      parking area.
      _____
   c. Are parking area and building separated by a street? . . . . Yes   No
   d. Is the surface of the parking area smooth and hard (no sand, gravel, etc.)? . . . . Yes   No

2. Passenger Loading Zone

   a. Is there a passenger loading zone? . . . . Yes   No
   b. If yes, where is it located in relation to selected entrance?_____
      _____

3. Approach to Selected Entrance

   a. Which entrance was selected as most accessible?_____
   b. Is the approach to the entrance door ground level?. . . . . Yes   No
   c. Is there a ramp in the approach to or at the entrance door? . . . . Yes   No
   d. If there are any steps in the approach to or at the entrance, give total number of steps. . . . . _____
   e. If there are steps, is there a sturdy handrail on at least one side or in the center?. . . . . Yes   No

4. Entrance Door

   a. What is the width of the entrance doorway (with door open)?. . . . . _____
   b. Is the door automatic? . . . . Yes   No
   c. Are there steps between entrance and main areas or corridor? . . . . Yes   No
   d. If yes, what is the total number of steps? . . . . _____
   e. If there are steps, is there a sturdy handrail in the center or on at least one side?. . . . . Yes   No

5. Elevator

   a. Is there a passenger elevator? . . . . Yes   No
   b. Does it serve all essential areas? . . . . Yes   No

6. Essential Areas (areas to which access is essential if building is to be used)

   Area 1_____ Area 2_____

   Area 3_____

7. Access from Entry to Essential Areas

	(1)	(2)	(3)
a. Is the usable width of corridors and aisles at least 32 inches?	Yes No	Yes No	Yes No
b. Is the narrowest clear doorway with door open 28 inches wide or more?	Yes No	Yes No	Yes No
c. If not, what is the width?	_____	_____	_____

8. Interior of Essential Areas

	(1)	(2)	(3)
a. Are there any steps between essential areas not served by elevators?	Yes No	Yes No	Yes No
b. Does each flight of steps have a sturdy handrail on at least one side or in the center?.	Yes No	Yes No	Yes No

Table 20.1—*continued*

9. Public Toilet Rooms

	Men		Women	
a. Where are toilet rooms located? .. Men_____				
Women_____	**Men**		**Women**	
b. Would one need to go up or down steps to get to toilet room?	Yes	No	Yes	No
c. If so, how many?				
d. If there are steps, does each flight of steps have a sturdy handrail on at least one side or in the center?	Yes	No	Yes	No
e. What is the width of toilet room entrance doorway (with door open)?				
f. Is there a free space in the room to permit a wheelchair to turn?	Yes	No	Yes	No
g. What is width of widest toilet stall door?				
h. Does this stall have handrails or grab bars?	Yes	No	Yes	No

10. Public Telephone

   a. Where is the most accessible phone located?_____
   b. What type (booth, wall, desk)?_____
   c. If phone is in a booth, what is width of booth door (with door open)? ....
   d. Is the handset 48 inches or less from the floor? ....   Yes   No
   e. Does the phone have amplifying controls for the hard of hearing? ....   Yes   No

11. Interior (auditorium, church, restaurant, etc.)

   a. What is the distance from floor to edge of restaurant table? ....
   b. If there are booths, can a wheelchair be placed at the open end of the booth? ....   Yes   No
   c. In theaters, public halls, churches, etc., can persons remain in wheelchairs? ....   Yes   No
   d. If yes, where?_____
   e. Can arrangements be made to reserve wheelchair space? ....   Yes   No

12. Assistance and Aids Available

   a. Is there an attendant who will take cars? ....   Yes   No
   b. Is there help available for those needing assistance in entering (doorman, porter)? ....   Yes   No
   c. If not, is help available for those needing assistance if arranged for in advance? ....   Yes   No
   d. Who to call in advance for assistance_____
   _____
   e. Telephone number_____
   f. Are wheelchairs available? (at airports, hotels, museums, etc.)? ....   Yes   No

13. Motel or Hotel Guest Rooms

   a. What is width of the entrance door to guest room (with door open)? ....   _____
   b. What is width of entrance door to bathroom (with door open)? ....   _____
   c. Are there handrails or grab bars near the toilet? ....   _____
   d. Are there handrails or grab bars for the bath and shower? ....   _____

raising the bed height, moving the telephone near to the bed, putting a center pull on dresser drawers, rearrangement of kitchen storage, and lowering the clothes in the closet by use of a suction spring rod or a dowel hung by rope from the bar above.[53] These changes need not give the home a hospital atmosphere.[54]

The ability to respond in an emergency is an important independent living skill that does not receive enough emphasis in rehabilitation training probably because it is viewed as being too infrequent a need to justify the time spent on training.[55] Two safety skills a person absolutely needs are the ability to perceive an emergency situation and the ability to summon assistance.[55] Physical ability for self-protection is important but not as crucial as the first two. In assessing

the home, emergency exits need to be identified and the communication system needs to be accessible, available, and usable by the disabled person. The patient needs to be assessed concerning his ability to perceive an emergency and to communicate it to another. The responder system of the community needs to be assessed (fire, police, call-in service to a hospital or health agency, neighbor, relatives, etc.) and the specific person or agency to be called for help should be identified.[55]

Suggested specifications for an ideal wheelchair kitchen are listed here[56] since this is one room that needs major modifications if the homemaker is wheelchair bound. Sometimes, funding for remodeling is available from the Rehabilitation Services Administra-

Table 20.2
HOME EVALUATION

Type of Home

_____ Apartment: What floor does patient live on? _____

Is elevator available? _____

_____ Single family home: Number of floors _____ Which are used by the patient?

Entrances to Building or Home

1. *Location*—Front, Back, or Side (Circle One)
   a. Which entrance is used most frequently or easily? _____
   b. Can patient get to entrance? _____

2. *Stairs*—Does patient manage outside stairs? _____

   a. Width of stairway _____
   b. Number of steps _____ Height of steps _____
   c. Railing present as you go up. R _____ L _____ Both _____
   d. Is ramp available for wheelchair patient? _____ length _____ height of rise _____

3. *Door*

   a. Can patient unlock, open, close, lock door? (Circle for yes)
   b. Is doorsill present, give height _____ and material _____
   c. Width of doorway _____
   d. Can patient enter _____ leave _____ via door?

4. *Hallway*

   a. Width of hallway _____
   b. Are any objects obstructing the way? _____

Approach to Apartment or Living Area (Omit if not applicable)

1. *Hallway*

   a. Width _____
   b. Obstructions? _____

2. *Steps*

   a. Does patient manage? _____
   b. Width of stairway _____
   c. Number of steps _____ Height of steps _____
   d. Railing present as you go up. R _____ L _____ Both _____
   e. Is ramp available? _____ Length _____ Height of rise _____

3. *Door*

   a. Can patient unlock, open, close, lock door? (Circle one)
   b. Doorsill? Give height _____ Material _____
   c. Width of doorway _____
   d. Can patient enter _____ leave _____ via door? _____

4. *Elevator*

   a. Is elevator present _____ Does it land flush with floor? _____
   b. Width of door opening _____
   c. Height of control buttons _____
   d. Can patient manage elevator alone? _____

Table 20.2—_continued_

Inside Home

Note width of hallway and of door entrances.
Note presence of doorsills and height.
Note if must climb stairs to reach room.

1. Can patient move from one part of house to another?
   a. Hallways
   b. Bedroom
   c. Kitchen
   d. Bathroom
   e. Living room
   f. Others

2. Can patient move safely? _____
   a. Note loose rugs
   b. Electrical cords
   c. Faulty floors
   d. Highly waxed floors
   e. Sharp-edged furniture
   f. Animals

3. Note areas of potential danger for patient.

Bedroom

1. _Light Switch_—Accessible? _____ Can patient open and close windows? _____

2. _Bed_

   a. Height _____ Width _____
   b. Both sides of bed accessible? _____ Headboard present? _____ Footboard? _____
   c. Is bed on wheels? _____ Is it stable? _____
   d. Can patient transfer wheelchair/bed _____ and bed/wheelchair? _____

3. Is _night table_ within patient's reach from bed? _____ Is telephone on it? _____

4. _Clothing_—Are patient's clothes located in bedroom? _____
   Can patient get clothes from dresser? _____
   Closet? _____ Elsewhere? _____

Bathroom

1. Does patient use wheelchair _____ walker _____ in bathroom?

2. Does wheelchair _____ walker _____ fit into bathroom?

3. Light switch accessible? _____ Can patient open and close window? _____

4. What materials are bathroom walls made of? _____

   a. If tile, how many inches does it extend from the floor beside the toilet?
   b. How many inches from the top of the rim of the bathtub? _____

5. Does patient use toilet? _____

   a. Can patient transfer independently to and from toilet? _____
   b. Does wheelchair wheel directly to toilet for transfers? _____
   c. What is height of toilet seat from floor? _____
   d. Are there bars or _sturdy_ supports near toilet? _____
   e. Is there room for grab bars to be installed? _____

6. Can patient use sink? _____ What is height of sink? _____

   a. Able to reach and turn faucets? _____
   b. Is there knee space beneath sink? _____
   c. Is patient able to reach necessary articles? _____

Table 20.2—_continued_

7. _Bathing_

   a. Does patient take tub bath? _____ Shower? _____ Sponge bath? _____
   b. If uses tub, can patient transfer safely without assistance? _____
   c. Bars or sturdy supports present beside tub? _____
   d. Is equipment necessary? (tub seat, handspray attachment, tub rail, no-skid strips, grab rails, other _____)
   e. Can patient manage faucets and drain plug? _____
   f. Height of tub from floor to rim _____
   g. Is tub built-in _____ or on legs _____?
   h. Width of tub from the inside _____
   i. If uses separate shower stall, can patient transfer independently and manage faucets? _____
   j. If patient takes sponge bath, describe method.

Living Room Area

1. Light switch accessible? _____ Can patient open and close window? _____

2. Can furniture be rearranged to allow passage of wheelchair? _____

3. Can patient transfer from wheelchair to and from sturdy chair? _____ Height of chair seat _____

4. Can ambulatory patient sit and rise from chair? _____ Sofa? _____

5. Can patient manage TV, radio or other devices? _____

Dining Room

1. Light switch accessible? _____

2. Is patient able to use table? _____ Height of table _____

Kitchen

1. What is the table height? _____ Can wheelchair fit under? _____

2. Can patient open refrigerator door and take food? _____

3. Can patient open freezer door and take food? _____

3. _Sink_

   a. Can patient be seated at sink? _____
   b. Can patient reach faucets? _____ turn them on and off? _____
   c. Can patient reach bottom of basin? _____

4. _Shelves and cabinets_

   a. Can patient open and close? _____
   b. Can patient reach dishes, pots, silver, and food? _____
Comments:

5. _Transport_

   a. Can patient carry utensils from one part of kitchen to another? _____

6. _Stove_

   a. Can patient reach and manipulate controls? _____
   b. Light pilot on oven? _____
   c. Manage oven door? _____
   d. Place food in oven and remove? _____
   e. Manage broiler door? _____
   f. Put food in and remove? _____

Table 20.2—*continued*

7. *Other Appliances*

    a. Can patient reach and turn on appliances? _____

    b. Can patient use outlets? _____

8. *Counter space*—Is there enough for storage and work area? _____

9. *Diagram:*

    (Include stove, refrigerator, sink, table, counters, others if applicable)

Laundry

1. If patient has no facilities, how will laundry be managed?

2. Location of facilities in home or apartment, and description of facilities present:

3. Can patient reach laundry area? _____

4. Can patient use washing machine and dryer? _____

    a. Load and empty? _____

    b. Manage doors and controls? _____

5. Can patient use sink? _____

    a. What is height of sink? _____

    b. Able to reach and turn on faucets? _____

    c. Knee space beneath sink? _____

    d. Able to reach necessary articles? _____

6. Is laundry cart available? _____

7. Can patient hang clothing on line? _____

8. Ironing board

    a. Location:

    b. Is it kept open? _____

    c. If not kept open, can patient set up and take down ironing board? _____

    d. Can patient reach outlet? _____

Cleaning

1. Can patient remove mop, broom, vacuum, pail from storage? _____

2. Use equipment? (Mop, broom, vacuum, etc.) _____

Emergency

1. Location of telephones in house:

2. Could patient use fire escape or back door in a hurry if alone? _____

3. Does patient have neighbors', police, fire, and M.D. phone numbers? _____

tion. If not, the changes must be prioritized and implemented when the budget permits. A U-shaped or corridor-type layout is better than a large square kitchen, which requires much moving around from appliance to appliance. A 60-inch minimal clearance between the counters and appliances that are arranged in a U-shape is required.[41] Counters that are at least 30 inches wide should be lowered to 30 inches in height with space underneath to accommodate the wheelchair. The top cabinets should be lowered so the bottom shelf is no higher than 48 inches above the floor.[41] An eye-level oven with a drop front and self-cleaning feature is better than a traditional stove. Westinghouse produces a built-in oven that has a swing-open door. A countertop cook stove should be installed in one of the counters with lowered/insulated roll space beneath. Alternatively to the conventional cook stove configuration, four burners can be installed in a row if reaching to the back of a stove would be a problem. In either case, controls should not require reaching across the burners.[41] A shallow sink (6½ inches maximum depth[41]) is ideal for the person who must sit to use it. If there is a basement, the garbage disposal can be installed below floor level so that it will not interfere with rolling under the sink. A side-by-side refrigerator-freezer is the best choice for a wheelchair homemaker.

The therapist must explain why each recommendation is made. Sometimes families are reluctant about making changes in the home. When the therapists sense this, they must remember that they are guests in the home and should refrain from actually rearranging. The therapists should teach the person to be as independent as possible within the limitations or make clear how the patient would be limited with the present arrangements. If the patient needs assistance, the family member is taught how to assist him safely using the proper body mechanics.

At the end of the evaluation, a report is written to the patient and his family. It is worded for understanding and acceptance of the ideas presented. The report contains a list and description of every important suggestion made. Source, cost, and description of equipment that is needed are specified. The cost of this equipment must be within the family's budget, or sources of financing must be sought; usually, the social service department of a rehabilitation facility assumes this responsibility. If modifications are necessary, they are listed with specifications. If the family agrees to these, help may be appreciated in locating a tradesman to do the work. Therapists can develop knowledge of such resources by talking to former patients who made modifications in their homes.

A summary report of the recommendations, including the therapists' judgment of the wisdom of discharging the person home, is sent to the referring physician and included in the medical record.

If the patient is returning to work, a similar environmental evaluation may be necessary at the place of employment. In addition to the points already mentioned, special attention should be paid to how the arrangement of the working space affects the disabled worker's energy consumption and posture. Comfortable forward reach distance for a person seated in a standard wheelchair is approximately 25 inches; reach height is 48 inches from the floor; and horizontal work surface reach is 30 inches.[41] Working within limits of easy reach conserves energy. Consideration also should be given to the likelihood of developing cumulative trauma disorders through repetitive movements or prolonged postures required by the job that stress the patient's muscles, ligaments, or peripheral nerves, an issue which is discussed in chapter 21.

STUDY QUESTIONS
Environmental Evaluation and Community Reintegration

1. What are the barriers to independent living for the disabled?
2. Define independent living.
3. What did Public Law 95–602 provide for?
4. What services do Independent Living Centers offer consumers?
5. Why are transitional community reintegration programs needed?
6. What type of programming is included in reintegration programs? What are the methods used by occupational therapists in this type of treatment?
7. What does the international symbol of access indicate?
8. What is the value of the American National Standards specifications?
9. Describe ramp design and construction for a house that has a 15-foot front yard and a front door that is 20 inches from the ground.
10. What is the required door width for a standard wheelchair?
11. What is the space requirement for a wheelchair to make a 180° turn?
12. What are the procedures involved in a home evaluation?
13. Describe the layout and characteristics of the major appliances of an ideal kitchen for a wheelchair-bound homemaker.

References

1. American Occupational Therapy Association. Official position paper: occupational therapy's role in independent or alternative living situations. *Am. J. Occup. Ther., 35*(12): 812–814, 1981.
2. Versluys, H. P. Community reintegration: the value of education-action-training models. *Rehabil. Lit., 45*(5–6): 138–145, 1984.
3. Wright, B. A. Value-laden beliefs and principles for rehabilitation. In *Rehabilitation: 25 Years of Concepts, Principles, Perspectives.* Edited by S. J. Regnier and M. Petkovsek. Chicago: National Easter Seal Society, 1985.
4. Frieden, L., and Cole, J. A. Independence: the ultimate goal of rehabilitation for spinal cord-injured persons. *Am. J. Occup. Ther., 39*(11): 734–739, 1985.
5. Neistadt, M. E., and Marques, K. An independent living skills training program. *Am. J. Occup. Ther. 38*(10): 671–676, 1984.
6. Brady, J. P. Social skills training for psychiatric patients. I. Concepts, methods, and clinical results. *Am. J. Psychiatry, 141*(3): 333–340, 1984.
7. Ross, E. C. New rehabilitation law. *Accent on Living, 23*(3): 23, 1978.
8. Spaudling Rehabilitation Hospital. *NEWS.* Boston: January 1987, pp. 1–3.
9. Kennedy, T. Our right to independence. *Parade Magazine,* November 23, 1986, pp. 4–7.
10. Zisserman, L. The modern family and rehabilitation of the handicapped. *Am. J. Occup. Ther., 35*(1): 13–20, 1981.
11. Johnson, J. Centers for independent living: a new concept in promoting independence. *American Occupational Therapy Association Physical Disabilities Special Interest Section Newsletter, 9*(3): 4–5, 1986.
12. Frieden, L. Independent living models. *Rehabil. Lit., 41*(8): 169–173, 1980.
13. Rogers, J. C., and Figone, J. J. Psychological parameters in treating the person with quadriplegia. *Am. J. Occup. Ther., 33*(7): 432–439, 1978.
14. Keilhofner, G., and Burke, J. P. Components and determinants of human occupation. In *A Model of Human Occupation: Theory and Applications.* Edited by G. Keilhofner. Baltimore: Williams & Wilkins, 1985.
15. Rush, W. L. PCA's. *Accent on Living, 32*(1): 76–80, 1987.
16. Mauras-Corsino, E., Daniewicz, C. V., and Swan, L. C. The use of community networks for chronic psychiatric patients. *Am. J. Occup. Ther., 39*(6): 374–378, 1985.

17. Ogren, K. A living skills program in an acute psychiatric setting. *American Occupational Therapy Association Mental Health Special Interest Section Newsletter*, *6*(4): 1,4, 1983.
18. Decker, S. D., and Schulz, R. Correlates of life satisfaction and depression in middle-aged and elderly spinal cord-injured persons. *Am. J. Occup. Ther.*, *39*(11): 740–745, 1985.
19. Kutner, B. Milieu therapy. *J. Rehabil.*, *34*(2): 14–17, 1968.
20. Davies, J. This little wheelchair went to market. *Accent on Living*, *29*(4): 86–88, 1985.
21. Versluys, H. P. The remediation of role disorders through focused group work. *Am. J. Occup. Ther.*, *34*(9): 609–614, 1980.
22. Rohrer, K., et al. Rehabilitation in spinal cord injury: the use of patient-family groups. *Arch. Phys. Med. Rehabil.*, *61*: 5, 1980.
23. D'Afflitte, J. G., and Weitz, B. G. W. Rehabilitating the stroke patient through patient-family groups. In *Coping with Physical Illness*. Edited by R. Moos. New York: Plenum Medical Book Co., 1977.
24. Belcher, S. A., Clowers, M. R., and Cabanayan, A. C. Independent living rehabilitation needs of post discharge stroke persons: a pilot study. *Arch. Phys. Med. Rehabil.*, *59*(9): 404–409, 1978.
25. Anderson, T. P., Baldridge, M., and Ettinger, M. G. Quality of care for completed stroke without rehabilitation: evaluation by assessing patient outcomes. *Arch. Phys. Med. Rehabil.*, *60*(3): 103–107, 1979.
26. Burnett, S. E., and Yerxa, E. J. Community-based and college-based needs assessment of physically disabled persons. *Am. J. Occup. Ther.*, *34*(3): 201–207, 1980.
27. Wittmeyer, M. B., and Stolov, W. C. Educating wheelchair patients on home architectural barriers. *Am. J. Occup. Ther.*, *32*(9): 557–564, 1978.
28. McColl, M. A., and Quinn, B. A quality assurance method for community occupational therapy. *Am. J. Occup. Ther.*, *39*(9): 570–577, 1985.
29. El-Ghatit, A. Z., Melvin, J. L., and Poole, M. A. Training apartment in the community for spinal cord injured patients: a model. *Arch. Phys. Med. Rehabil.*, *61*(2): 90–92, 1980.
30. Whycherley, J. Group therapy in the treatment of the hemiplegic patient. *Nursing Mirror*, 73–76, 1974.
31. Kales-Rogoff, L. Community skills experience for rheumatic disease patients. *Am. J. Occup. Ther.*, *33*(6): 394–395, 1979.
32. DeJong, G., and Hughes, J. Independent living: methodology for measuring long term outcomes. *Arch. Phys. Med. Rehabil.*, *63*(2): 68–73, 1982.
33. Anderson, H. Don't let the stares get you down. *Accent on Living*, *28*(1): 59–64, 1983.
34. Johnson, J. H. Practice patience with the severely nondisabled. *Accent on Living*, *32*(1): 46–48, 1987.
35. Zola, I. K. Social and cultural disincentives to independent living. *Arch. Phys. Med. Rehabil.*, *63*(8): 394–397, 1982.
36. Tucker, S. J. The psychology of spinal cord injury: patient-staff interaction. *Rehabil. Lit.*, *41*(5–6): 114–160, 1981.
37. Steenma, J. Expressions. *Rehabil. Lit.*, *45*: 383, 1984.
38. Wright, B. A. *Physical Disability—A Psychological Approach*, 2nd edition. New York: Harper & Row, 1983.
39. Safilios-Rothschild, C. *The Sociology and Social Psychology of Disability and Rehabilitation*. New York: Random House, 1970.
40. Frederick, L. L. Can you give more than you should? *Accent on Living*, *31*(3): 90–92, 1986.
41. *American National Standard for Buildings and Facilities: Providing Accessibility and Usability for Physically Handicapped People*. New York: American National Standards Institute, 1986.
42. Silver, M. Federal compliance board under fire. *Accent on Living*, *22*(1): 24–31, 1977.
43. Martin, L. M. Wheelchair accessibility of public buildings in Utica, New York. *Am. J. Occup. Ther.*, *41*(4): 217–221, 1987.
44. Accessibility: two standards. *Accent on Living*, *31*(4): 104–105, 1987.
45. Schroeder, C., and Benedict, P. Brief or new: egress during fire—wheelchair exiting in an emergency. *Am. J. Occup. Ther.*, *38*(8): 541–542, 1984.
46. Upstairs downstairs. *Accent on Living*, *32*(1): 40–44, 1987.
47. Breed, A. L., and Ibler, I. The motorized wheelchair: new freedom, new responsibility and new problems. *Dev. Med. Child Neurol.*, *24*: 366–371, 1982.
48. Transportation for the disabled. *Accent on Living*, *20*(1): 36, 1975.
49. Tanaka, T. BART: how accessible? *Accent on Living*, *25*(1): 58–61, 1980.
50. Transportation: Denver busing its disabled. *Accent on Living*, *28*(1): 86–89, 1983.
51. What makes a meeting site accessible? *Accent on Living*, *21*(3): 28–34, 1976.
52. Mason, M. The home visit: a step from hospital to home. *Occupational Therapy in Health Care*, *2*(1): 39–49, 1985.
53. Lowman, E., and Klinger, J. *Aids to Independent Living: Self Help for the Handicapped*. New York: McGraw-Hill (Blakiston Division), 1969.
54. Brodigan, J. Use imagination: it's your home. *Accent on Living*, *30*(2): 44–47, 1985.
55. Gaines, B. J. Emergency response: a neglected treatment area. *Occupational Therapy Forum*, *2*(22): 1, 3–4, 1987.
56. Webb, C. Tips on making your kitchen accessible. *Accent on Living*, *23*(3): 104–109, 1978.

Supplementary Reading

Accessibility and Architectural Modifications Information Packet. Rockville, MD: American Occupational Therapy Association, 1987.

Barris, R. Environmental interactions: an extension of the model of occupation. *Am. J. Occup. Ther.*, *36*(10): 637–644, 1982.

Baum, C. M. Nationally speaking: Independent living—a critical role for occupational therapy. *Am. J. Occup. Ther.*, *34*(12): 773–774, 1980.

Block, J. Income tax deductions for home improvements. *Accent on Living*, *21*(3): 36–37, 1976.

Bracciano, A. Medicare reimbursement of occupational therapy in home health care. *American Occupational Therapy Association Gerontology Special Interest Section Newsletter*, *8*(4): 3,6, 1985.

Cary, J. R. *How to Create Interiors for the Disabled: A Guidebook for Family and Friends*. New York: Pantheon Books (Division of Random House), 1978.

Colvin, M. E., and Korn, T. L. Eliminating barriers to the disabled. *Am. J. Occup. Ther.*, *38*(11): 748–753, 1984.

Dardick, G. Removing barriers: a do-it-yourself plan that's working. *Accent on Living*, *29*(3): 96–99, 1984.

DeJong, G. *Independent Living and Disability Policy in the Netherlands: Three Models of Residential Care and Independent Living*. World Rehabilitation Fund, 400 East 34th Street, New York, NY 10016, 1984.

Lewis, L. How to win the parking space battle: a practical guide for the handicapped driver. *Accent on Living*, *25*(3): 92–94, 1980.

Living Independently: A Consumer's Guide About Personal Care Attendants. Concepts of Independence, Inc., 853 Broadway, Suite 1920, New York, NY 10003.

Shortridge, S. D. Facilitating attitude change toward the handicapped. *Am. J. Occup. Ther.*, *36*(7): 456–460, 1982.

Symington, D. C., and MacLean, J. Environmental control systems in chronic care hospitals and nursing homes. *Arch. Phys. Med. Rehabil.*, *67*(5): 322–325, 1986.

Wittmeyer, M. B., and Peszczynski, M. Housing for the disabled. In *Orthotics Etcetera*, 3rd edition. Edited by J. B. Redford. Baltimore: Williams & Wilkins, 1986.

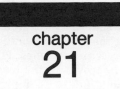

chapter
21

Employment for the Physically Disabled

Catherine A. Trombly

Historical Perspective of Occupational Therapy and Work

The concept of work is fundamental to our profession. The definition of work has varied over the extent of our history but has primarily been broadly defined to view crafts as work done for such goals as intrinsic productivity and personal fulfillment rather than for financial renumeration. "Real vocational education" was considered beyond the scope of occupational therapy, although crafts were used during World War I as a means of prevocational evaluation of injured soldiers. In the 1950s work was redefined as employment for renumeration and crafts were seen as unrelated to the vocational demands of the contemporary world.[1] The 1954 amendments to the Vocational Rehabilitation Act established prevocational evaluation as part of rehabilitation and became an impetus to therapists to offer this service.[2] Gainful employment became the focus of therapy. Work evaluation programs were established using work samples that reflected specific jobs. Therapists who specialized in work evaluation matched evaluated skills of the patient with job skills. Industrial therapy placed patients temporarily in jobs in the institution to assess job readiness and to provide some skills training.

Occupational therapists offer services to disabled persons who need to establish or reestablish salable skills and abilities; to the injured worker to restore function and to recover capacities needed to return to his job; to the nondisabled worker to prevent injury or illness at the workplace; and in the not-so-distant future, as a result of a move away from an industrial/agricultural society to an information/service society, therapists will be working with those who are displaced or retired early from work to help them reestablish their sense of productivity and worth. These people will be treated by those therapists who have adopted a generalist view and interpret work in terms of the intrinsic sense of competence or mastery that a person achieves as a result of engaging in activity.[1] Activity is recognized as a major life role, and work is seen as encompassing all forms of productive activity regardless of reimbursement.[1,3]

Employment/Unemployment

For some people, work (that is, employment) is one of the most important social roles a person fulfills in a lifetime. Work provides economic security, intellectual or physical challenge, and friendships; helps promote life satisfaction[4]; and helps define the person and his estimate of his worth. Others value work simply as a means to earn money in order to participate in other aspects of life that they find more meaningful. Patients who value work for whatever reason are eager to participate in vocational rehabilitation. Some patients who do value work are not ready at the time of discharge from the rehabilitation center to consider return to work or to work through the process of determining abilities for work because they are still in a period of mourning for their loss. These persons need to know where to go for these services when they are ready.

There are some disabled persons for whom work after disability is not possible, despite its positive value to them. Those with frequent concurrent illnesses that would result in absenteeism are not good candidates unless their illnesses can be controlled. For example, a spinal cord-injured patient prone to urinary tract infections needs to have that condition corrected before seeking employment. Persons with brain damage that severely interferes with learning or appropriate social behavior would also not be candidates. When it is determined that these persons are indeed unemployable, they need to be taught satisfying avocational pursuits, if possible, to enhance the quality of their lives.

Older workers may have difficulty returning to work. Going back to a former job or learning a new one through on-the-job training is preferred for the older worker because few older workers are interested in investing the time in retraining. Neither do the insurance companies and state departments of rehabilitation want to invest the money for training programs. It is important to identify the person's transferable skills if he must change jobs. In addition to analyzing the job demands in relation to the patient's work capacities and developing assistive devices or methods to improve function, the occupational therapist also should address the psychological needs of the older person, i.e., his decision to work or not, based on realistic appraisal of his abilities; whether depression is present; and the need for support during the job search.[4]

There are also those who find no value whatever in work and actually see it as an interruption of their "true life." People in this latter category easily accept the limitations of the disability relative to work and prefer to receive compensation from insurance companies or federal social security.

Unemployment is common among the disabled. According to a survey of 1,000 disabled workers done by Louis Harris & Associates, commissioned by the International Center for the Disabled in cooperation with the National Council on the Handicapped, employment is one of the most important concerns of the disabled at this time. Yet only 25% of disabled persons have full-time jobs, with another 10% having part-time jobs. Of those not working, 60% receive benefits as their primary source of income, and the majority of these persons are the primary wage earners in their households.[5]

There are probably many reasons for underemployment of the disabled. One reason may be that disabled persons are unwilling to jeopardize their social security Supplemental Security Income benefits, which include Medicare, although the 1980 Social Security Amendments were meant to enable disabled persons to have a trial at gainful employment without loss of benefits.[6] Another problem may be the lack of knowledge on the part of able-bodied employers about the capabilities of disabled workers. The unwillingness of some insurance companies to insure small private industries who hire physically disabled workers is another problem. Section 504 of the Rehabilitation Act of 1973 prohibits discrimination against hiring the handicapped for jobs they can be judged capable and safe to perform, i.e., for which they are qualified. Section 503 of that Act provides for affirmative action in hiring the handicapped. However, both of these laws apply only to companies or contractors who do more than $2,500 worth of business for the U.S. government or receive federal grants.[7]

The level of motivation of the individual is probably the greatest determining factor concerning return to work after injury. Motivation refers to a person's determination or persistence in pursuing a goal. When no motivation exists or can be generated, the rehabilitation specialists must realize that vocational planning-evaluation-training will be unsuccessful. For those patients motivated by earning power and/or personal satisfaction, more opportunities than ever exist for employment. Although the physically disabled are often limited to sedentary jobs, electronic technology is making more of these types of jobs available to them. In the next decade, the demand is expected to increase for workers in technical, professional, and clerical jobs [8] that use the new technologies. However, a major problem in unemployment is the low level of education and training many have in comparison to what is needed for the types of jobs most suited for disabled persons. This problem is not limited to the disabled; however, the job market is very competitive for the disabled.[8] Based on predictions of the types of jobs that will be most available in the future, it seems that the nonqualified disabled will miss opportunities for employment.

Because awareness of the job opportunities that some disabled persons have found for themselves sparks ideas for others, a loose compilation is published here. Homebound workers operate service agencies that rent out specialized labor.[9] Disabled experienced actors are sought for TV and films.[10,11] The National Theater of the Handicapped in New York has established a training program for qualified persons to prepare for careers as professional actors.[12] Dramatic experience can also be gained from community or college theater, just as it is by the able-bodied. Severely disabled people are meeting the demand for micrographic technicians to microfilm documents and other material produced by the information explosion.[13] The American Association for the Advancement of Science has established an Office of Opportunities in Science to study the needs and contributions of disabled scientists and science students.[14] Other jobs done by severely disabled persons include parking code enforcement personnel of the police department ("Quad Squad"),[15] vocational counselor,[16,17] comedian,[18,19] disk jockey,[20] dentist,[21,22] anaesthesiologist,[23] physiatrist,[24] medical student,[25] computer programmer,[26,27] accountant,[28,29] owner-manager of boutique and decorator service,[30] owner-inventor of medical products company,[31] orthotist, farmer, [32,33] fashion designer, [34] executive directors of nonprofit agencies, and occupational therapists.

The job should fit a person's realistic self-image and values regarding work. Discussions during early phases of vocational rehabilitation concerning work-related issues, e.g., job versus career, pay versus personal satisfaction, office work versus physical work, small company or large, etc., help the person not only to clarify his values but also to develop realistic attitudes and self perceptions.

Roles of Occupational Therapists in Vocational Rehabilitation

The occupational therapist-work evaluator assists injured workers to develop work readiness and the physical capacities necessary for working productively. Specifically, the roles and responsibilities of the occupational therapist to the individual involved in the vocational rehabilitation process include the following.[2]

1. *Screening* to obtain a history of occupational performance related to work, self-maintenance, leisure, and social roles.

2. *Evaluation* to identify individual capacities and deficits in motor, sensory, cognitive, psychological, and social components of performance.

3. *Treatment*—the use of selected activities, assistive devices, and educational techniques—to restore the patient to the highest level of functioning (increase range of motion, etc.) and to improve working habits, psychosocial work skills, and adapted work skills.

4. *Prevocational Interview Assessment and Counseling* to identify the client's vocational interests and goals. How the individual values work in general and type of work in particular needs to be determined. A person who once held a managerial position may not be able to emotionally accept employment at a job that he views as less prestigious. A manual laborer who has a limited view of his abilities to do other types of work may be too emotionally insecure to accept a more intellectually, but less physically, demanding job. Each type of reaction needs careful therapy to facilitate acceptance of this new aspect of the self concept.

5. *Prevocational Evaluation* to assess and predict work behavior and vocational potential through application of practical, reality-based assessment techniques. Prevocational assessment should begin at the outset of the rehabilitation program and should logically develop into vocational planning, programming, and follow-up.[35] The plan must be flexible and alterable as the rehabilitation program progresses and the patient's physical functioning, resources, and understanding of impairment change.[35] This is a specialized field needing postgraduate training.

6. *Work Adjustment Services* for those without work habits and skills needed to function adequately in formal vocational training or active employment. This is an experiential educational experience for the patient.

7. *Work Activity Services* to provide purposeful and functional vocational or supportive programming for nonemployable persons.

8. *Vocational Evaluation, Training, Placement.*

9. *Postplacement Services* including job analysis, work simplification training, and assistive devices to enable effective job performance.

A total of 10.3% of the (1982) American Occupational Therapy Association members reported being involved in helping patients prepare for employment. Most occupational therapy programs were reported to include the following components: personality adjustment training, work capacity evaluation, physical tolerance or work tolerance screening, job simulation, work hardening, and ergonomic job analysis.[36] Programs to prevent industrial injury or reinjury have more recently been added to the services offered by occupational therapists.

PERSONAL ADJUSTMENT TRAINING

Personal adjustment training refers to that part of the process in which the therapist works on helping the patient to develop behaviors and skills required for future vocational tasks and job placement, including job search skills and job retention skills.

The preparation for work starts from the beginning of the rehabilitation process with training to improve function. Independence in self-care and mobility are generally prerequisites to being able to work outside of the home. Therapy to improve strength, range of motion, coordination, perception, etc., that is done to improve the person's independence in self-care and mobility also improves the person's work-related skills. Ability to manipulate objects in the environment and/or problem solve are other prerequisite skills addressed in occupational therapy.

Personal skills that are prerequisite to employment need to be evaluated for those who were never employed, have a poor work history, or have suffered brain damage. Personal skills refer to the ability to behave appropriately, a sense of time and responsibility, the ability to read, write, and handle money, acceptable personal hygiene, the ability to accept and use supervision, the ability to make friends and get along with others, and other developmental tasks.[37]

Treating the developmental deficits is a goal of the occupational therapist, who usually becomes aware of these in the course of treating the patient for other reasons. Self-care training, therapeutic activity and sports, group discussions, or group projects all generate pieces of information concerning the person's readiness for employment. Special situations may need to be devised, however, to gather information or to allow the patient to practice basic skills such as promptness, thoroughness, neatness, safety, accuracy, use of supervision without dependency or resentfulness, acceptance of responsibility, and tolerance for working a full day. The nature of occupational therapy provides an ideal laboratory experience for such learning to take place.

Psychotherapy to address the emotional issues of returning to work with a physical disability may be considered a part of prevocational training also.

To facilitate the client's emotional adjustment, group therapy, as described in chapter 2, is used. Goals are to assist the patient to accept himself as a worthy person, though changed; to value his working ability, although skills that may have been a source of pride to him are now impossible; to develop realistic expectations of himself and the working community; to redevelop his former level of motivation for work; and to explore new career possibilities. The group discussions could be organized around information presented by former patients with similar diagnoses, by group interviews of experts in the fields of interest to find out what the job requirements actually are, or by discussion of published information. The group discussions should help the person realize that work for the disabled is no longer stereotyped, for example, watchmaking for paraplegics and broom-making for the blind, but that there are a large variety of jobs that are being done successfully by even the most severely disabled, limited only by drive and imagination.

The patient who has never worked before may need assistance in learning job acquisition skills. All persons seeking a job for the first time after disability need to learn that in addition to the usual behavior of any job applicant (good grooming, knowledge about the particular business, a definite job goal, evidence of dependability, and a well-composed resumé or reference list), he needs to take the initiative to put the interviewer at ease regarding the disability and how it relates to the job sought.[38,39] This would prevent a naive interviewer from refusing the job on the basis of preconceived ideas. The person needs to act confidently and let the interviewer know what skills he expects to bring to the company.[38,39] Role playing in occupational therapy can provide the opportunity to learn good job interview skills.

In summary, the occupational therapist contributes to prevocational training by (1) facilitating the client's emotional adjustment to the change in self-concept or need to change careers; (2) remediating the cognitive-perceptual-motor deficits that limit job opportunity; and (3) treating developmental deficits that would interfere with the person's ability to work or to seek employment in a competitive market. The training that the occupational therapist does with the patient to prepare him to live as independently as possible also contributes to the likelihood of his employability.

WORK CAPACITY EVALUATION

Residual physical disability requires the person to either change his type of employment or to resume previous employment using adapted tools or methods. In either case, the person's ability to work safely and efficiently must be determined. Work capacity evaluation is defined as a comprehensive process that systematically uses work, real or simulated, to assess and measure an individual's physical abilities to work.[36,40] Practical, reality-based assessments are used to evaluate work abilities related to specific job tasks.[2] Testing by use of concrete functional tasks is especially important to obtain more accurate knowledge of a brain-damaged patient's abilities than use of standardized tests, which require him to cope with complex, abstract concepts.[41]

Commercially available prevocational tests that test a person's ability to do competitive manual work have been devised to help in counseling, training decisions, and placement of patients. The types of tasks and opportunities for behavioral observation under work conditions that these tests afford are similar to other occupational therapy evaluations. Three of fourteen tests that have been thoroughly reviewed and compared by Botterbusch[42] will be mentioned here. The reader is referred to the original source for greater detailing of these and for information on the other tests. Botterbusch states that most work sample systems are technically inadequate in that validity, reliability, and norms are poorly established, if at all.[42] The COATS (Comprehensive Occupational Assessment and Training System) and Micro-TOWER Systems seem to be the only ones with reliability, validity, and a data base

completed. The TOWER System, developed by the Institute for Crippled and Disabled (ICD) in New York, is the oldest complete work evaluation system.[42]

The COATS system consists of four sections, each with three program levels: the Job Matching System, which matches the person's preferences, experiences, and abilities to employment and/or training opportunities based on the *Dictionary of Occupational Titles* (DOT); the Employability Attitudes System, which allows the client to evaluate his attitudes and compare them to the attitudes seen as important by employers for hiring, promoting, and firing of employees; the Work Sample System, which contains 26 work samples that are representative of tasks common to types of trades; and the Living Skills System, which tests those skills needed to be functionally literate in contemporary society. The instruction is given by way of audio-visual cartridges.

The Micro-TOWER System was devised by ICD to be used for general rehabilitation patients of average intelligence. The system contains 13 work samples that measure 8 specific aptitudes, plus general learning ability. The samples are organized into five major groups: motor, spatial, clerical perception, numerical, and verbal. The results are related to specific jobs in the 4th edition of the DOT. The cost depends on how many people are being tested at a time; each person needs a set of equipment, as does the evaluator.[42]

The TOWER System was originally developed by ICD for use with physically disabled persons, but it is now also used with other types of clients, such as the emotionally disabled. The system contains 93 work samples organized into 14 job training areas: clerical, drafting, drawing, electronics assembly, jewelry manufacturing, leather goods, machine shop, lettering, mail clerk, optical mechanics, pantograph engraving, sewing machine operation, welding, and workshop assembly. Within each major area, the work samples are graded in complexity. The recommendations that can be derived from the results are limited to jobs that relate to the work samples and do not relate to DOT classifications. The system was normed on disabled persons, and no industrial norms are available. It is a useful system for thorough evaluation in limited areas. Each facility must build its own work samples; ICD estimates the initial cost to be approximately $5000.

Another prevocational test system used by occupational therapists is the Valpar Component Work Sample Series, which consists of 16 subtests to measure those worker characteristics that have been found to be basic indicators of success within numerous job families.[43] It is keyed to the worker traits listed in DOT. Norms derived from various groups are provided including Employed Worker Norms, Skill Center Norms, Special Disability Group Norms, and norms derived from Method's Time Measurement. The 16 subtests are as follows:

1. *Small Tools (mechanical)* measures the person's ability to understand and work with small tools.

This task is related to jobs in small appliance repair, bicycle, and auto repair, jewelry making, and assembly tasks in a wide variety of manufacturing settings.

2. *Size Discrimination* measures a person's ability to perform work tasks requiring visual size discrimination such as grading and sorting jobs, performing work with close supervision using guages, calipers, and other tools, and working within prescribed standards and tolerances.

3. *Numerical Sorting* measures a person's ability to perform work tasks using numbers or numerical series; the tests are sorting, filing, and categorizing. This test relates to occupations dealing with data and things such as examining, grading and sorting, keeping records and receipts, recording or transmitting verbal or coded information, and posting verbal or numerical data on stock lists.

4. *Upper-Extremity Range of Motion* measures work tolerance related to the upper torso. It is meant to isolate the client's pain and fatigue as related to the physical requirements that a worker must meet in the completion of particular work tasks. It is closely related to the following job task factors: reaching, handling, fingering, feeling, and seeing.

5. *Clerical Comprehension and Aptitude* measures both the person's ability to do and ability to learn these types of tasks. The areas measured include telephone answering, alphabetical filing, bookkeeping, and typing. This sample best relates to those occupations dealing with data, people, and things.

6. *Independent Problem Solving* measures a person's ability to do tasks requiring visual comparison and proper selection of a series of abstract designs. This sample best relates to jobs such as verifying computations, checking items for accuracy and consistency, and record keeping.

7. *Multilevel Sorting* measures a person's ability to make decisions while performing tasks requiring physical manipulation and visual discrimination of colors, numbers, letters, and a combination of these. Jobs that this sample best relate to include laboratory tester, insurance sales agent, hair stylist, sales route driver, etc.

8. *Simulated Assembly* measures a person's ability to do a task requiring repetitive physical manipulation and bilateral use of the upper extremities. Jobs related to this sample include operating and monitoring automatic assembly machines.

9. *Whole Body Range of Motion* measures the agility of a person's gross body movements as they relate to the functional ability to perform job tasks. It is a fatiguing sample that estimates the person's work tolerance. It measures the evaluee's ability to stoop, kneel, crouch, reach, handle material, and finger material, which are basic abilities required by many occupations.

10. *Tri-Level Measurement* measures the person's ability to perform very simple to very precise inspection and measurement tasks. Jobs related to this sample include machinist, metal fabrications inspector, press operator, plumber and glazier, etc.

11. *Eye-Hand-Foot Coordination* measures in addition to these factors the person's ability to concentrate, his reaction time, and his planning and learning capacity as these relate to the task. Work activities related to this sample include starting, stopping, and observing the functions of machines; perceiving relationships between moving objects, fixtures, and surfaces; and planning the order of successive operations. Jobs related to this sample include shoe repairer, heavy-equipment operator, milling-machine operator, offset-press operator, etc.

12. *Soldering and Inspection–Electronic* measures the person's ability to acquire and apply basic skills necessary to perform soldering tasks that vary in difficulty. Observation of the client also allows judgments concerning his ability to follow directions, eye-hand coordination, dexterity, ability to measure accurately, visual acuity, frustration tolerance, attentiveness, and judgment. Jobs related to this sample include jewelry solderer, electronic assembler and tester, etc.

13. *Money Handling* measures a person's skills in dealing with monetary concepts from basic money recognition to consumer economics. Jobs related to this sample include cashier, teller, post office clerk, sales clerk, loan counselor, budget consultant, etc.

14. *Integrated Peer Performance* has been designed to allow evaluation of worker interaction during assembly tasks.

15. *Electrical Circuitry and Print Reading* measures a person's ability to understand and apply principles of electrical circuits and to use pictorial materials such as blueprints, schematics, and drawings. Jobs related to this sample include electrical appliance repairer, electrician, electronics mechanic, etc.

16. *Drafting* measures ability from minimal expertise to sophisticated, high-level performance.

There are no prevocational tests for evaluating professional or executive-type business skills. Special testing situations would need to be devised to determine if the person were able to do all essential physical components of the job safely. Evidence of good judgment and normal intellectual and perceptual abilities would be gathered from psychological and occupational therapy testing and observation of the patient. If these minimal requirements were met, then the patient's ability to do the more subtle aspects of the job would need to be evaluated in actual work situations by persons knowledgeable about the performance standards.

For those just entering a profession, college education is required. Testing to meet the usual university and departmental entrance requirements would have to be done. If the profession required the person to handle instruments or other people, the applicant would have to show evidence that he could do this with or without adaptation.

Work Capacity Evaluation, as conceived by Matheson,[44,45] considers aptitudes, interests, and vocational skills as secondary factors. Primary evaluation factors are those that comprise general "work-ability," i.e., employment feasibility and work tolerance. Feasibility is concerned with those basic factors that affect worker acceptability to an employer in the labor market: worker productivity, safety, and interpersonal behavior. It functions as a "gatekeeper" to triage clients into those who are able and unable to benefit from the vocational rehabilitation process. Those who are unable to benefit may be able to in the future after utilizing prevocational services designed to optimize their potential. The Work Capacity Evaluation certifies that the person possesses those basic attributes necessary for employment somewhere in the labor market and can buoy spirits during subsequent repeated unsuccessful attempts to secure employment. Initial work tolerances are evaluated after feasibility has been determined. These include the general factors that affect the worker's physical competence to perform basic work tasks, i.e., strength, energy reserve, flexibility, and the effect on task performance of pain and other limiting factors. Training programs are held for learning the administration of the Work Capacity Evaluation.[44]

Results of patient's performance on the functional work capacity evaluation are compared to the demands of the job, which are found in the *Dictionary of Occupational Titles: The Classification of Jobs According to Worker Trait Factors*. If there is a deficit affecting performance of the job, then an action plan is formed. This plan can involve placement of the worker in a modified work situation, participation in a work-hardening program to develop the needed capacities demanded by the job, referral to another specialty treatment center for treatment (pain clinic, etc.), or comprehensive vocational evaluation if the patient cannot return to his previous job. The therapists need to be currently aware of the legal rules and the expectations of the Worker's Compensation System to efficiently plan and direct the return to work program.[46] Functional capacity evaluation, using the Smith Physical Capacities Evaluation, which has 154 performance items measuring the 20 physical demands identified by the Department of Labor for jobs in the national competitive labor market, was studied as a predictor of reemployment of the physically disabled worker. It was found to be 86.5% accurate in prediction of employment status.[47,48] This result must be accepted with caution because the respondents represented only 41% of the invited sample,[47] but it does model one type of research needing to be done concerning work capacity evaluations.

In a study of 66 chronic back pain patients, the results indicated that quantitative functional capacity evaluation can give objective evidence of patients' physical abilities and degree of effort and can significantly guide treatment programs.[49] Chronic back pain may involve medical, legal, psychological, and socioeconomic problems, making it a difficult and complex phenomenon to evaluate.[49]

PHYSICAL TOLERANCE OR WORK TOLERANCE SCREENING

Work tolerance is defined as the ability to sustain a work effort for a prolonged period of time, the ability to maintain a steady flow of production at an acceptable pace and an acceptable level of quality, and the ability to handle a certain amount of pressure.[44,50]

Work tolerance screening is a work simulation process that incorporates principles of biomechanics, ergonomics, kinesiology, and industrial psychology.[44] Work tolerance screening evaluation serves as a stepping stone to vocational exploration that is consistent with a worker's physical abilities. In addition the data provide useful information when the occupational therapist is consulting with employers about how to modify a job so that a worker can remain within his physical work tolerances and still be productive. For example, if the therapist has objective data regarding physical capacities required in a job, she can then offer recommendations for modifying the job situation or for assisting the worker in using proper body mechanics, movement patterns, and pacing techniques to prevent reinjury.[51]

The Baltimore Therapeutic (BTE) Work Simulator is a computerized measuring device that allows measurement of repetitive upper-limb motions against measurable resistance over a specified amount of time. It quantitatively documents the work output of the user.[52] It can be used to estimate work tolerance and cardiac and pulmonary stress and for work hardening with feedback. The interchangeable handles simulate the physical demands of most jobs, such as grip, pinching, lifting, carrying, reaching, etc.

Many patients who have suffered a myocardial infarction or have undergone coronary artery bypass surgery do not return to work due to unwarranted medical restrictions or apprehension on the part of the patient, family, or employer. Satisfactory performance on a test of activities that simulate work can help the physician, patient, family, and employer gain confidence in the patient's tolerance for work. One program conducted by an occupational therapist and exercise physiologist included job analysis, graded dynamic exercise testing, and simulated work testing. The metabolic equivalent (MET—see chapter 30) level of the person's job is estimated from published MET tables. At the end of the convalescent phase of recovery an exercise test is done to estimate the patient's peak MET level based on cardiovascular response to dynamic leg effort. Simulated work testing in occupational therapy provides important information about upper-extremity lifting and carrying, which can produce greater cardiovascular changes than leg effort alone. The most physically demanding component of the person's job is evaluated while the patient is monitored for heart rate and rhythm and blood pressure responses. Before the test, the patient is reminded about proper body mechanics and cautioned against doing a Valsalva maneuver (holding the breath during effort, which causes a significant rise in blood pressure). Average energy expenditure required by a job should not exceed 40% of the patient's peak MET capacity, as determined by exercise testing. On the job, the patient uses pulse rate monitoring to be sure that special circumstances and conditions at the moment do not cause the job demands to exceed his heart rate prescription.[53]

Following evaluation, certain types of jobs can be eliminated from consideration by virtue of their physical demands and the patient's expected maximum ability in that area. Others can be eliminated by virtue of their intellectual demands in light of the patient's capacities. Selection will continue to be narrowed, based on interest, aptitude, realistic appraisal of the training required, and the person's willingness to invest time and effort.

WORK HARDENING AND JOB SIMULATION

Work hardening is a work-oriented treatment program, the outcome of which is measured in terms of improvement in the client's productivity.[45] The ultimate goal is to help the person achieve a level of productivity that is acceptable in the competitive labor market. The present form of work hardening originated at Rancho Los Amigos Hospital in Downey, California, in the late 1970s. A large majority of the current programs in the United States were established by occupational therapists. The programs serve injured workers as their primary population.

Improvement in productivity is achieved through increased work tolerances, improved work rate, mastery of pain, improved work habits, increased confidence, and proficiency with work adaptations or assistive devices. It involves the client in highly structured, simulated work tasks in an environment where expectations for basic worker behaviors (timeliness, attendance, and dress) are in keeping with workplace standards. Work-hardening programs use work capacity evaluation devices as the primary treatment tools. This is a new class of evaluation equipment that allows presentation of tasks that simulate job tasks and that can be graded in difficulty or length of time involved. Most of the devices in use are "homemade," although many are becoming commercially available. Some therapists use traditional craft activities in treatment of industrial injuries to simulate job requirements and to develop work tolerance. In a program for 292 patients in a hand rehabilitation center, 80% of the patients returned to work within 6 weeks after entering the work tolerance program.[54]

The patients who benefit from this type of programming are those who are seriously deconditioned after an impairment caused by an injury or disease. In addition, people who have major discrepancies between their symptoms and objective findings and those whose impairment is limited to the dominant upper extremity substantially benefit from work hardening.[45]

Occupational therapy in one rehabilitation center offers low back pain patients a supportive environment where the patients can practice and improve the execution of work-related activities they need to perform their jobs while they are learning to live with or control their symptoms. Monitors and workstations have been especially designed and developed to evaluate and develop work tolerances. Treatment includes patient education through discussion, demonstration, active participation, and visual aids. Topics include anatomy of the spine, body mechanics, energy conservation, relaxation techniques, and weight reduction, if appropriate. Relaxation techniques include progressive relaxation techniques, meditation, increased body awareness, and control of breathing and muscle tension. The patient begins with activities that simulate his work environment. Treatment time is gradually increased to equal his premorbid work schedule. Modalities used include a balance monitor that provides feedback on weight bearing and symmetry of posture. A multiworkstation simulates construction jobs. The truck simulator uses a truck cab along with a computerized video road screen to simulate and measure the driving process. A computerized pneumatic lift has been designed to simulate the lifting process. An upper-extremity work simulator, similar to the BTE, is used to simulate various upper-extremity work tasks. Patients maintain an activity log to develop a sense of responsibility for their own rehabilitation and pain control. No outcome statistics for this program were provided.[55]

For further information applicable to treatment preparatory to return to work, see chapter 25, "Hand Therapy," for information on treatment of cumulative trauma disorders of the hand and wrist and chapter 26, "Orthopedic Conditions," for information on back schools.

VOCATIONAL TRAINING

Vocational training refers to the actual training program that the worker will undergo to learn the trade or profession that he has decided on. The training prepares the person for competitive job seeking. Whereas the disabled will not be blatantly discriminated against, they will not be preferentially hired either. They must be qualified. Training for some is done in a few special rehabilitation centers in the United States, such as the Woodrow Wilson Rehabilitation Center in Virginia, or in sheltered workshops throughout the country, such as Goodwill Industries or the Society for the Blind Workshops. Many patients do not need to be trained in these special settings and can be mainstreamed into community vocational-technical high schools and colleges,[56] especially since these are being made more accessible. The training is done by persons expert in the trade or profession. The cost of training may be funded by the Rehabilitation Services Administration, as finances permit.

The vocational counselor finds the training program to suit the patient's needs and may help place the patient in a job, once trained.

The only role the occupational therapist would have at this stage of vocational rehabilitation is to evaluate the patient's need or design for the necessary adaptations that the person will need to do the job for which he is training.

ERGONOMIC JOB ANALYSIS

Ergonomic job analyses are done to classify jobs according to the qualifications and physical demands that they require to determine whether or not an individual is capable of safely doing the job. Job analyses are done to determine whether a disabled person can return to his old job or could apply for a certain new job. They are also done to prevent biomechanical cumulative trauma disorders of employed workers. Ergonomics refers to the characteristics of people that need to be considered in arranging things that they use so that the people and things will interact most effectively and safely.[57]

To do a job analysis the therapist must know what the components of the job are. The *Dictionary of Occupational Titles: The Classification of Jobs According to Worker Trait Factors*[58] can serve as a useful reference to identify the components of the job. It provides a comprehensive description of job duties for over 20,000 occupations. A comprehensive explanation of common physical demands is given in *A Guide to Job Analysis*.[59] Standard demands include walking, jumping, running, balancing, climbing, crawling, standing, reclining, turning, twisting, stooping, crouching, kneeling, sitting, reaching, lifting, carrying, throwing, pushing, pulling, handling, fingering, feeling, talking, hearing, seeing, color vision, field of vision, depth perception, and visual accommodation. The physical demands are rated into five categories: sedentary, light, medium, heavy, and very heavy. These ratings are determined by the amount of weight lifted or carried, frequency of the lift, and the amount of standing or walking required.[44] Additional criteria used in assessing physical demands of particular jobs include duration of static or dynamic posture, repetitive motion over time, and the nature of the posture itself; force required to adjust a knob, engage a press, etc; distance of reach, carry, and push-pull; shape, size, and contour of objects and tools; weight of parts and tools; heights and direction of placement; number of repetitions and/or production quotas (work speed); and variations in routine.[60]

During the job analysis a clinical assessment of the patient's abilities and physical status are compared to the physical demands of the job. For efficiency's sake, the analysis should be limited to critical work demands as defined by the patient's diagnosis and limiting symptoms.[60] To assess a job, it is important to actually try it to appreciate the demands since experienced workers give an effortless-appearing performance in very demanding jobs.[60]

Suggested equipment for conducting job site analyses includes a portable videocamera that operates well in low light to record worker performance and to allow detailed study of the job tasks; a 50-foot retractable steel tape measure to measure lift and reach distances; a wheeled measuring device to measure carry distances; a push-pull gauge capable of measuring 250 pounds to measure forces that need to be exerted; and a 2-foot welded chain with a locking link at one end and a minimum pull strength of 250 pounds to use with the push-pull scale.[60] Also recommended are a 3-foot steel cable with formed loops at each end; a scale for weighing; one pair each of wide- and narrow-jaw vise-grip pliers; heavy-duty work gloves and hand towel; a clipboard, pencil, and graph paper; a stopwatch; and a case to transport these items.[60]

A procedure for work site evaluations that focuses on biomechanical hazards posing a risk to the neuromusculoskeletal system of workers has been devised by the National Institute of Occupational Safety and Health (NIOSH).[61,62] Principles and practices of ergonomics (human factors engineering) are used to determine whether or not certain work activity causes an observed incidence of cumulative trauma disorders. The procedure has three facets: (1) A structured oral interview is used to identify the worker's perceptions of hazards and sources of physical discomfort. (2) Medical screening techniques—including measures of sensation, strength, and range of motion—are used to obtain a clearer picture of the nature and severity of the health complaints. The screening is especially helpful when the worker's complaints suggest preclinical stages of disease and when there are still few documented cases of musculoskeletal injuries related to a certain job within a company. (3) A job analysis is done to determine the relationship between work patterns and musculoskeletal impairment. The ergonomic analyses are confined to three major areas: work methods, workstation design and worker posture, and handle and tool design.

Work method analysis is concerned with determining what the worker must do to perform the task successfully. Such a determination requires recording of arm and hand positions, computing the number of repetitive movements in a given work cycle, and measuring or estimating the forces required by the job. In the case of hand and wrist injuries, suspected problematic postures are noted and documented. These are full extension of the fingers and wrist, full flexion of the wrist with grasp, forceful pinch, and ulnar and radial deviation. The amount of time that the extremity is maintained in a certain stressful posture is important to note because the stress on the structure accumulates. Also considered are the speed, intensity, and pace at which the worker must perform to meet production or quality standards.

Analysis of the workstation examines the relationship of the worker and workstation features as they relate to postures required, especially stressful ones. Proper workstation design has been studied to relieve musculoskeletal problems of video display terminal operators.[63] The factors that were considered in the recommendations present good suggestion for therapists' evaluation of other types of work sites. These include chair height, back support, head angle, viewing distance, document holder placement, display angle, arm support, leg room, foot rests, display height, keyboard location, and working height.[63]

Analysis of handle and tool design is important as it is the most common cause of hand and wrist disability. The most common problem is that the handle of the tool is too short for the worker's hand, causing inflammation of the tendons and obstruction of the flow of blood in the palm and necessitating the use of smaller muscles.[61,62,64] Constant pressure may also obstruct blood flow to the hand or fingers and increase the strain on the tendon or tendon sheaths.[61]

Tichauer has redesigned many tool handles used by assembly workers to improve kinesiology and prevent stress that results in cumulative trauma disorders.[64] As a general rule, tools or tasks should be designed so that the wrist is maintained in the neutral position.[61,64] A combination of flexed wrist with significant grip force requirements and repetitive movements are biomechanical stresses commonly associated with cumulative trauma disorders of the hands and wrists.[61] Creative tool adaptations are required to protect the worker.[61]

Instructing patients in good body mechanics and ergonomic principles is helpful in managing their symptoms. They can be taught that decreasing the horizontal distance to lift, enlarging a tool handle so the distal phalanges of the fingers and thumb overlap, or lowering work surfaces so elbows are not abducted more than 30° from the torso are preventative measures.[60] For hand tasks it has been suggested that dynamic work forces should not exceed 50% of the maximum dynamic strength for short durations or more than 30% of the maximum dynamic strength for long periods. Static forces should not be greater than 15% of the maximum static strength. If job demands exceed these limits, the chance for trauma or deterioration is increased. Static forces of the hand are considered to be a significant physical demand if a high level of effort is sustained for 10 sec or more, if moderate effort is required for 60 sec or more, or if slight effort is exerted for 4 min or more.[60]

PREVENTION PROGRAMS

Prevention programs focus on the prevention of work-related injuries and the early return to work of injured employees. The majority of workers seen are those at risk for back injury or cumulative trauma disorders of the hand and wrist.

Regional musculoskeletal diseases are exceedingly common in industry. It has been assumed, from anecdotal reports, that such entities are use-associated, although there is too little formal proof at this time that pattern of usage alone causes or precipitates any regional musculoskeletal disease.[65] Other as-yet-unidentified variables seem to interact with the high usage on the job to cause cumulative trauma disorders.[66] Low back pain accounts for millions of days lost from work and millions of dollars of lost productivity as well as compensation claims. Most patients with back disease are involved in materials handling and lifting.[65] Tenosynovitis, seen increasingly in industry, seems precipitated by the initiation of intense repetitive stereotyped usage. One type of tenosynovitis, DeQuervain's disease, is associated with performance of repetitive manual tasks involving a firm grip together with a deviated wrist.[65,67] Carpal tunnel syndrome is associated with tight pinching in combination with wrist flexion or maintained wrist flexion.

A recent survey of members of the American Society of Hand Therapists revealed an expanding role for the therapist in the treatment of industrial hand injuries. Therapists are beginning to identify relationships between specific injuries and work that produced them. This enables development of primary prevention screening programs to prevent the injury-producing event from occurring and secondary prevention programs to detect disease, deficit, deviation, dysfunction, and disability early followed by appropriate intervention to prevent progression to a more serious or chronic condition.[52]

Services offered are tailored to the needs of the particular company. One service offered is a comprehensive job analysis in which the occupational therapist analyzes tasks from an ergonomic perspective. For companies whose workers are required to handle materials, the analysis concentrates primarily on lifting tasks using the NIOSH Lifting Risk Guide[68] to determine if the lifting task places the worker at risk for injury. For companies whose workers are primarily engaged in assembly tasks, the analysis focuses on the stressful positions of the hand and wrist, the forces required, the number of repetitions required, and the tool design. The therapist recommends job or tool modification and/or the minimal worker capacities required of those assigned to a particular job. This type of recommendation guides decisions regarding return of a worker to that job.[68]

Another service offered in a prevention program is job modification and work site adjustment.[69] For example, redesign of tool handles has been found to eliminate the need for working with the wrist out of neutral during grip or pinch,[64] which in turn can decrease the prevalence of tenosynovitis at the wrist.

Another service offered is an education and training program that is job specific rather than a generalized presentation of principles. Such a program involves demonstration and practice of biomechanically correct techniques that have been presented to the workers previously by lecture/discussion. The program can also include feedback to the workers at the work site and positive reinforcement regarding the use of body mechanics and safe work postures. This coaching is best done a few weeks after the classroom presentation to give the worker time to practice the new methods. This lag time enhances the learning process.

Behavior modification techniques should continue after the onsite coaching by providing training sessions to managers and supervisors so that they will continue to reinforce safe work habits.[68] This type of education should be more effective than the usual brief presentation. One study tested the effectiveness of a brief presentation format on changing the practices of food service workers. Results indicated that the group that received instruction in proper body mechanics performed significantly better on a novel lifting task, but that there was no carryover of the information to the actual job site. The instruction was via a 1-hour body mechanics course that emphasized the high-risk work style factors and the importance of maintaining a straight back during lifting and lowering of objects. Lecture, use of a visual aid (model of the back), actual practice of the principle during a lift, videotaping of the lift, and critiquing it in the group were the teaching methods.[69]

Wellness Programs

Wellness programs focus on health promotion through education for noninjured workers. Wellness is perceived as a dynamic way of life in which good health habits are incorporated into one's life-style to improve both health and the quality of life.[70] It is an emerging concept that reflects the individual's responsibility for health and well-being.[70] Health promotion programs are being offered now by companies or organizations to enhance wellness of their members through education, behavior change, and cultural support.[70]

Keeping people well and promoting a healthy lifestyle will be the focus of the future. Employee assistance programs are being instituted by many companies. A role for occupational therapists in these programs is advocated.[71] Major contributions could be providing employee services in the areas of analysis and enhancement of daily living skills for maintenance of productivity; leisure and home/family management; assessment of and recommendations on adapting work and home environments to improve health and well-being; task analysis and instruction in work simplification to reduce stress and strain on body parts; and conservation of energy and time to improve job performance. Other areas of service for occupational therapists could include identification of architectural barriers; instruction in the use of adaptive devices; modification of the work unit for the worker injured or disabled on the job; promotion of a milieu supportive of occupational role performance through interpersonal skill development; and support group processes and activities such as health and fitness promotion, stress reduction, and retirement and leisure planning.[71]

STUDY QUESTIONS:
Work

1. What are the roles of occupational therapists in vocational rehabilitation?
2. What is prevocational evaluation?
3. What is personal adjustment training and for whom is it appropriate?
4. What is work capacity evaluation?
5. Describe one test system that can be used to evaluate work capacity.
6. Define work tolerance.
7. What is included in work tolerance evaluation?
8. What is work hardening?
9. What is vocational training and what is occupational therapy's role in this?
10. Why are ergonomic job analyses done?
11. How is a job analysis done?
12. What types of services are offered by occupational therapists in prevention programs in industry?

References

1. Harvey-Krefting, L. The concept of work in occupational therapy: a historical review. *Am. J. Occup. Ther., 39*(5): 301–307, 1985.
2. American Occupational Therapy Association. Official position paper: the role of occupational therapy in the vocational rehabilitation process. *Am. J. Occup. Ther., 34*(13): 881–883, 1980.
3. Keilhofner, G. Occupation. In *Willard and Spackman's Occupational Therapy,* 6th edition. Edited by H. Hopkins and H. Smith. Philadelphia: Lippincott, 1983.
4. Kemp, B., and Kleinplatz, F. Vocational rehabilitation of the older worker. *Am. J. Occup. Ther., 39*(5): 322–326, 1985.
5. National survey examines quality of life for disabled individuals in 1980s. *Occupational Therapy News,* October 1986, p. 24.
6. Greenberg, R.M. Amendment supports SSI recipient's efforts to be self-supporting. *Accent on Living, 26*(1): 50–52, 1981.
7. Turned down because of your handicap? *Accent on Living, 23*(1): 34–39, 1978.
8. Job market for disabled: good and bad news! *Accent on Living, 21*(2): 63, 1976.
9. Lamb, S. Is good service hard to find? *Accent on Living, 25*(1): 20–21, 1980.
10. Vallero, S. Talent agency promotes experienced disabled actors. *Accent on Living, 25*(1):57, 1980.
11. Two-time Oscar winner makes a comeback. *Accent on Living, 25*(3): 64, 1980.
12. Showbiz—not for actors only. *Accent on Living, 32*(1): 56–59, 62, 1987.
13. Disabled learn microfilming techniques in special class. *Accent on Living, 23*(4):84–85, 1979.
14. Disabled scientists getting it together. *Accent on Living, 23*(4):92–93, 1979.
15. Heilpern, N. Quad squad. *Accent on Living, 24*(3): 26–28, 1979.
16. Kasper, R. An overnight success—in only 23 years. *Accent on Living 25*(3): 20–21, 1980.
17. Quad named Massachusetts Rehab Commissioner. *Accent on Living, 22*(1):43, 1977.
18. Haffner, T.E. More than show 'n tell. *Accent on Living, 25*(3): 76–78, 1980.
19. Higgins, M. Comedy routines: stand-up and sit-down style. *Accent on Living, 25*(4):84–85, 1981.
20. Lynn, R. Disc jockey by braille. *Accent on Living, 25*(3):87–90, 1980.
21. Olive, R. Disabled dentist back in practice. *Accent on Living, 25*(3): 100, 1980.
22. Bosco, A. They practice the healing arts from wheelchairs: wheelchair dentist. *Accent on Living, 22*(2): 58–59, 1977.
23. Alsofrom, J. They practice the healing arts from wheelchairs: wheelchair doctor. *Accent on Living, 22*(2): 59–61, 1977.
24. Medicine is his bag. *Accent on Living, 28*(1): 104–107, 1983.
25. Rosenkoetter, R. Quad accepted by medical school. *Accent on Living, 24*(2): 24–26, 1979.
26. Good salaries available to disabled who qualify. *Accent on Living, 23*(1): 44–47, 1978.

27. Linthicum, S. Technical training for the severely disabled: a model. *Rehabil. Lit.*, 38(11–12):373–375, 1977.
28. Hanna, J. Business booming thanks to computer. *Accent on Living*, 25(4): 93–95, 1981.
29. Accountant gets job done with custom computer office. *Accent on Living*, 29(4): 24–25, 1985.
30. Guthertz, A. T. Quad runs bed and bath boutique. *Accent on Living*, 23(3): 24–27, 1978.
31. Butcher, L. Paralyzed from the waist down, Wayne Nelson runs a $100,000 a year business. *Accent on Living*, 22(1): 63–65, 1977.
32. Brinkman, G. Double amputee makes successful farmer. *Accent on Living*, 25(2): 66–70, 1980.
33. *Breaking New Ground: A Newsletter for Farmers with Physical Disabilities*. Department of Agricultural Engineering, Purdue University, West Lafayette, IN 47907.
34. Dardick, G. Accessibility activist to fashion designer. *Accent on Living*, 30(3): 44–46, 1985.
35. Kanellos, M. C. Enhancing vocational outcomes of spinal cord-injured persons: the occupational therapist's role. *Am. J. Occup. Ther.*, 39(11): 726–733, 1985.
36. AOTA Practice Division. I'm glad you asked. *Occupational Therapy Newspaper*, April 1985, p.6.
37. Ryan, P. A. Widening their horizons: a model career development program for severely physically disabled youth. *Rehabil. Lit.*, 40(3): 72–74, 1979.
38. Your job interview. *Accent on Living*, 23(1): 40–43, 1978.
39. Hopkins-Best, M. How to answer the unasked questions. *Accent on Living*, 32(1): 32–35, 1987.
40. Holmes, D. The role of the occupational therapist-work evaluator. *Am. J. Occup. Ther.*, 39(5):308–313, 1985.
41. Weiss, L. Vocational evaluation: an individualized program. *Arch. Phys. Med. Rehabil.*, 61(10): 453–454,1980.
42. Botterbusch, K.F. *A Comparison of Commercial Vocational Evaluation Systems*. Menomonie, WI: Materials Development Center, Stout Vocational Rehabilitation Institute, University of Wisconsin-Stout, 1980.
43. *Catalogue*. Valpar Corporation, 3801 East 34th Street, Tucson, AZ 85713.
44. Matheson, L. N. *Work Capacity Evaluation: A Training Manual for Occupational Therapists*. Trabuco Canyon, CA: Rehabilitation Institute of Southern California, 1982.
45. Matheson, L. N., et al. Work hardening: occupational therapy in industrial rehabilitation. *Am. J. Occup. Ther.*, 39(5): 314–321, 1985.
46. Bear-Lehman, J., and McCormick, E. I'm glad you asked. *Occupational Therapy News*, March 1986, p.8.
47. Smith, S. L., Cunningham, S., and Weinberg, R. Predicting reemployment of the physically disabled worker. *Occup. Ther. J. Res.*, 3(3): 178–179, 1983.
48. Smith, S. L., Cunningham, S., and Weinberg, R. The predictive validity of the functional capacities evaluation. *Am. J. Occup. Ther.*, 40(8): 564–567, 1986.
49. Mayer, T. G., et al. Objective assessment of spine function following industrial injury. *Industrial Injury*, 10(6): 481–493, 1985.
50. *Vocational Evaluation and Work Adjustment Standards with Interpretative Guidelines and VEWAA Glossary*. Menomonie, WI: Materials Development Center, Stout Vocational Rehabilitation Institute, Dictionary of Wisconsin-Stout, 1977.
51. deRenne-Stephan, C. Industry and injuries: arena for occupational therapists. *Occupational Therapy in Health Care*, 2(1): 127–134, 1985.
52. Bear-Lehman, J., and McCormick, E. The expanding role of occupational therapy in the treatment of industrial hand injuries. *Occupational Therapy in Health Care*, 2(4): 79–88, 1985-1986.
53. Wilke, N. A., and Sheldahl, L. Use of simulated work testing in cardiac rehabilitation: a case report. *Am. J. Occup. Ther.*, 39(5): 327–330, 1985.
54. Baxter-Petralia, P., and Beaulieu, D. Therapeutic activity in treatment of industrial injuries. *American Occupational Therapy Association Physical Disabilities Special Interest Section Newsletter*, 9(4): 3, 6, 1986.
55. Bettencourt, C. M., et al. Using work simulation to treat adults with back injuries. *Am. J. Occup. Ther.*, 40(1): 12–18, 1986.
56. Improved opportunities for disabled college students goal of new national group. *Accent on Living*, 24(2): 29, 1979.
57. Mish, F. C., editor-in-chief. *Webster's Ninth New Collegiate Dictionary*. Springfield, MA: Merriam-Webster, 1984.
58. Field, T. and Field, J., editors. *The Dictionary of Occupational Titles: The Classification of Jobs According to Worker Trait Factors*, 4th edition supplement. U.S. Department of Labor. Athens, GA: VDARE Service Bureau, 1986.
59. U.S. Department of Labor. *A Guide to Job Analysis*. Menomonie, WI: University of Wisconsin Materials Development Center, 1982.
60. Heck, C. Job-site analysis for work capacity programming. *American Occupational Therapy Association Physical Disabilities Special Interest Section Newsletter*, 10(2): 2–3, 1987.
61. Habes, D. J., and Putz-Anderson, V. The NIOSH program for evaluating biomechanical hazards in the workplace. *J. Safety Res.*, 16(2): 49–60, 1985.
62. Putz-Anderson, V. *Cumulative Trauma Disorder Manual: For the Upper Extremity*. Cincinnati, OH: National Institute of Occupational Safety and Health, 1987. (draft copy)
63. Arndt, R. Working posture and musculoskeletal problems of video display terminal operators: review and reappraisal. *J. Ind. Hyg. Assoc.*, 44(6): 437–446, 1983.
64. Tichauer, E. R. Some aspects of stress on forearm and hand in industry. *J. Occup. Med.*, 8(2): 63–71, 1966.
65. Hadler, N. M. Industrial rheumatology: clinical investigations into the influence of the pattern of usage on the pattern of regional musculoskeletal disease. *Arthritis Rheum.*, 20(4): 1019–1025, 1977.
66. Trombly, C. A. Boston University-AT & T Technologies, Inc. Hand Project, in process.
67. Chandani, A. Tenosynovitis of hand and wrist: a literature review. *Br. J. Occup. Ther.*, 49(9): 288–292, 1986.
68. Holman, C., and Becker, V. Occupational therapists design work injury programs. *O.T. Week*, April 9, 1987, pp. 8–9.
69. Carlton, R. S. The effects of body mechanics instruction on work performance. *Am. J. Occup. Ther.*, 41(1): 16–20, 1987.
70. Johnson, J. A. Wellness and occupational therapy. *Am. J. Occup. Ther.*, 40(11): 753–758, 1986.
71. Maynard, M. Health promotion through employee assistance programs: a role for occupational therapists, *Am. J. Occup. Ther.*, 40(11): 771–776, 1986.

Supplementary Reading

American Occupational Therapy Association Prevocational/Vocational Information Packet. Rockville, MD: American Occupational Therapy Association, 1986.
Bear-Lehman, J. Factors affecting return to work after hand injury. *Am. J. Occup. Ther.*, 37(3): 189–194, 1983.
Bell, E., and Ford, L. (AOTA Commission on Practice). Work hardening guidelines. *Am. J. Occup. Ther.*, 40(12): 841–843, 1986.
Dictionary of Occupational Titles. U.S. Government Printing Office, Washington, DC 20402.
Fleishman, E. A. Toward a taxonomy of human performance. *Am. Psychol.*, 28(12): 1127–1149, 1975.
Flower, A., et al. An occupational therapy program for chronic back pain. *Am. J. Occup. Ther.*, 35(4): 243–248, 1981.
Frederick, B. B., et al. *Body Mechanics Instruction Manual: A Guide for Occupational Therapists*. Redmond, WA: Express Publications, 1979.
McWilliams, P. A. *Personal Computers and the Disabled*. Garden City, NJ: Quantum Press/Doubleday, 1984.

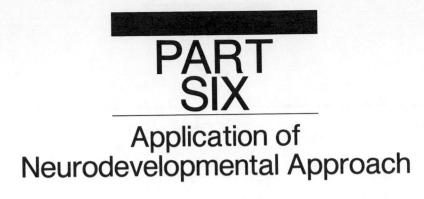

PART SIX
Application of Neurodevelopmental Approach

The *Neurodevelopmental Approach* is appropriately applied to the restoration of motor control in those patients with central nervous system disorders who have lost normal motor control and functional ability. The *Rehabilitative Approach* is used in conjunction with the Neurodevelopmental Approach so that the person may improve the quality of his life through compensation for unremediable deficits.

Some commonly seen diagnoses are presented here as examples of application of these approaches. Stroke, as representative of circumscribed brain injury; traumatic brain injury, as representative of diffuse brain injury; and selected degenerative diseases representative of cerebellar, basal ganglia, brain stem, and progressive spinal cord lesions are included in this section. Ideas presented in these chapters are applicable to other diagnoses involving the central nervous system.

Treatment for patients with neurological deficits is highly complex and multifaceted. Expertise develops through analysis and reflection on daily practice in conjunction with continuing study and supervisory guidance. Treatment procedures are based on hypotheses derived from basic research in the neurosciences. Neuroscientists are continually discovering more about how the human nervous system operates under normal or diseased conditions. Occupational and physical therapists need to modify treatment procedures as knowledge grows and new hypotheses are proposed. Therapists specializing in treatment of patients with central nervous system dysfunction need to stay up to date with neurophysiological, neuropsychological, and human-movement science information. It is also recommended that they attend continuing education programs and/or graduate school.

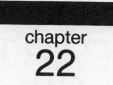

chapter
22

Stroke

Catherine A. Trombly

Stroke, or cerebrovascular accident (CVA), is caused by infarct of brain tissue secondary to oxygen deprivation. As a result of the CVA, the patient may be paralyzed (hemiplegic) or weak (hemiparetic) on the side of the body opposite to the site of the CVA. Neurological deficits of all types may occur in addition to the motor signs. The exact site and extent of the lesion in the brain determines which neurological deficits will be manifested poststroke.[1]

Although this chapter will focus on therapy for stroke patients, many of the same neurological manifestations occur due to trauma, gun shot, or disease (tumor) and can be treated similarly.

Stroke is the single most common diagnosis among patients seen by the occupational therapist in clinics for the treatment of physically disabled adults or in home care practice. Although awareness of preventative health measures on the part of the general public has increased and the percentage of persons suffering stroke has decreased, it is estimated that 400,000 persons suffer CVAs each year in the United States.[1,2] Over 200,000 of these survive and join the over 2 million other stroke survivors.[2] The incidence of stroke increases with age.[1]

Thrombosis, or total occlusion of a blood vessel due to atherosclerosis, is the most common cause of CVA, accounting for an estimated 53% to 58% of cases.[1] Embolism, a moving clot that blocks a vessel, accounts for 19% to 31% of all strokes.[1] There is a greater tendency for those who have suffered an embolic stroke, and to a lesser degree a thrombotic stroke, to have a recurrence within 5 years.[3] Hemorrhage—secondary to hypertension,[4] arteriovenous (A-V) malformation, or aneurysm—accounts for 16% to 21% of the cases.[1] Hypertension is the cause usually seen in the elderly, whereas the other two causes are seen in the young. Hemorrhage more likely results in death during the first month after onset.[1,3]

Symptoms of Stroke

Strokes cause anoxic damage to nervous tissue that is manifested by various symptoms depending on where the blood supply was lost.[4] Functions subserved by the affected brain tissue are either temporarily disrupted or permanently lost depending on the etiology and extent of nervous tissue damage. The symptoms produced by damage to the major arteries are presented below.[3-5] If the occlusion or hemorrhage affects only a small branch of one of these major arteries, then the symptoms would reflect only loss of the function controlled by the area affected. If collateral circulation is established or resorption of edema occurs, recovery reflects this.

INTERNAL CAROTID ARTERIES

Each internal carotid artery branches to form the anterior and middle cerebral arteries of one hemisphere of the brain. Occlusion of the carotid artery would result in symptoms of both middle and anterior artery damage. The middle cerebral artery is the most vulnerable to stroke.

Middle Cerebral Artery

Contralateral hemiplegia and sensory loss (especially affecting the face, tongue, and upper extremity) and contralateral homonymous hemianopsia result from a disruption of the flow of blood in this artery. Other symptoms depend on which hemisphere is infarcted: if the nondominant hemisphere is involved, visuospatial disturbances and cortical sensory disturbances with loss of spatial and discriminative sensibility resulting in mislocation or extinction of stimuli will be seen; if the dominant hemisphere is involved, expressive and/or receptive aphasia will be seen.

Anterior Cerebral Artery

After occlusion or hemorrhage of this artery, the contralateral lower extremity is more involved than the upper extremity. There is sensory loss of the cortical type, especially of the lower extremity. Aphasia and apraxia may result if the artery on the left side of the brain is involved. Confusion, homolateral amaurosis (blindness), and occasionally a grasp reflex of the upper extremity may occur.

BASILAR ARTERY

The basilar artery divides to form the two posterior cerebral arteries. This system serves the brain stem, cerebellum, medial and inferior aspects of the temporal lobe, the occipital lobe, and the thalamus. Since not all tracts have crossed in areas served by the artery, ipsilateral and contralateral signs can be mixed. Damage can result in any of the following: hemiplegia, quadriplegia, ipsilateral ataxia, thalamic syndrome (burning pain), contralateral disturbances of touch, pain, and temperature awareness, contralateral cerebellar asynergia, and tremor.

Posterior Cerebral Artery

If the posterior cerebral artery of only one hemisphere is involved, the symptoms may include contralateral homonymous hemianopsia with macular sparing, visual agnosia, visual memory disturbance, homolateral cerebellar ataxia, dysphonia, dysphagia, Horner's syndrome, facial paralysis, and contralateral loss of pain and temperature awareness. If the pyramidal tract is involved, a contralateral hemiplegia will occur.

The exact site of the stroke in most patients who have suffered a stroke is determined by one of the several computerized diagnostic systems now available such as CT (computerized tomography) scan, PET (positron emission tomography), or nuclear magnetic resonance imaging.[6] Yet no systematic classification of strokes exists.[7,8] The reliance on stereotyped models of stroke leads to generalized and often inappropriate therapy.[7] Studies are needed to correlate differences in effectiveness of treatment methods to site of lesion. Such information would allow greater precision in treatment planning and prediction of treatment outcomes. However, even in patients with the same neurological deficit, the impact of the disability is different, depending on the patient's life situation.[2] Stroke rehabilitation should consider the patient's entire lifestyle, not merely focus on the specific neurological deficits.[2]

Prognosis and Recovery of Function

In 494 persons who survived 6 months poststroke, 47% were totally independent; 9% were dependent (scored 45 or less on Barthel Index); and 44% were partially independent (scored 50 to 95 on the Barthel).[9] It is estimated that of those patients who survive 2 to 5 years poststroke, 40% to 60% become functionally independent, 10% to 25% remain dependent, and the rest become partially independent.[3]

Spontaneous recovery of function may occur in a stroke patient because edema subsides or nonfunctional but viable neurons reactivate.[3,10] Recovery may also occur due to physiological reorganization of the neural connections[11] and/or development of new behavioral strategies.[6] Individual differences in neural connections and learned behaviors play a major role in functional recovery.[11,12]

Continued urinary and fecal incontinence forecasts poor rehabilitation potential.[13] On the other hand, rehabilitation potential is high for those who can reestablish informational inputs to the sensory association areas of the brain that direct or redirect motor programs.[6] It is believed that with proper training to reestablish the patient's ability to process information that the learning process associated with neuromuscular reeducation can be a continuation of normal adaptive motor programming.[6] Because anatomical connections reorganize during recovery, motor patterns need to be relearned but they rarely return to the prestroke level, especially those patterns involving distal muscles,[12,14] which are more likely to be directly innervated by corticospinal motorneurons.[10,15] See chapter 5 for further discussion.

Prognosis for recovery of function is greater in young patients,[13,16] possibly because their cognitive functioning was better than that of older patients before the stroke,[16] because the young brain is more plastic, and/or because the young are generally in better physical condition. Traumatic brain injury that causes damage equivalent to that caused by a CVA portends greater hope for recovery over a longer period of time than that expected for a post-CVA patient, possibly because the blood vessels are not diseased so collateral circulation can be established more effectively. Heart disease, obesity, peripheral vascular disease (PVD), and hypertension are all common in patients who have cerebrovascular disease and mitigate against optimal functional recovery.

It is generally believed that recovery of function occurs, on average, within 3[3,17] to 6 months,[18] although this belief could be due to the insensitivity of measuring instruments used to evaluate recovery.[17] Recovery of arm function continues for 1 year after an initial rapid change during the first 3 months.[17]

Gowland[19] has made an attempt to develop clinically useful formulae to predict probable outcomes for individual stroke patients based on initial evaluation data. To predict the degree of arm function recovery, the values for the recovery stage of the arm and for the leg at admission[19,20] and weeks poststroke at initiation of treatment are used in the equation. Predicted arm recovery = [0.41 + 0.86 (Brunnstrom's stage of recovery of the arm) + 0.27 (Brunnstrom's stage of recovery of the leg) − 0.01 (weeks)]. For example, a patient whose arm is in stage 3 and whose leg is in stage 5 and who is 4 weeks poststroke [0.41 + 0.86(3) + 0.27(5) − 0.01(4)] would be predicted to achieve arm recovery to stage 4.3 ± 0.76 (confidence level determined by the study).[19] This formula accounted for 81% of the variance related to recovery seen in a sample of 332 subjects.[19] One hundred percent accuracy in prediction of function or rate of return in a given stroke patient may not be possible due to individual variability of anatomy and extent of brain damage as well as differences in types of CVA, learning ability, premorbid personality and intelligence, and motivation. However, general estimates of final level of function may be made based on such formulae or on observations of many patients over time. Those patients with good sensation, minimal spasticity, some selective motor control, and no fixed contractures seem to make the greatest improvements in functional abilities.[21] On the other hand, if the patient lacks a concept of his affected side and cannot localize stimuli to the affected side, the outlook for independence is poor.[21]

Left hemiplegics improve with rehabilitation, but show a lesser degree of improvement in self-care independence, social adjustment, and recovery of motor function 6 months poststroke than do right hemiplegics, presumably because of unilateral spatial neglect.[22] However, this difference is not confirmed by all,[15,23,24] indicating that other unidentified variables may be interacting with the affected side to cause different results in separate studies.

The natural course of return of motor function is from proximal to distal and from mass, patterned, undifferentiated movement to fine, isolated movement.[12,25] If return of function deviates from the proximal to distal pattern, a peripheral nerve injury (brachial plexus injury) should be suspected; this commonly occurs secondary to traction (pulling) on the weak shoulder[2] by those trying to help the patient move in bed or transfer.

Usually, the recovery of upper- and lower-limb motor control follows the sequence as outlined by Brunnstrom (chapter 6, part C) based on the work of Twitchell.[12] This sequence of recovery has also been confirmed in a longitudinal study of 20 hemiplegic patients followed from the first week of stroke to 1 year poststroke.[26] Therapy is aimed at facilitating this process, but the recovery of motor control can unpredictably stop at any point.[12] Patients often do not regain full function of the upper extremity. The least likely motor function to recover is finger extension[27] because it is the most cortically controlled upper-extremity function[15,282] and fine motor coordination requires intact sensation. If the patient is able to move voluntarily but sensation is lost, then the limb will be used only when the patient pays attention to it.[21] It is a good prognostic sign for functional recovery if the patient uses his affected limbs spontaneously, even if he moves only in patterned movements.

In summary, many factors affect outcome including stage of recovery at the time of starting therapy[7,29]; site, type, and extent of lesion; environmental and social influences; the premorbid state including age, fitness, and cardiovascular history; cognitive and emotional states; secondary complications[7]; and effectiveness of therapy program.

Evaluation

The occupational therapist's goal is to increase the stroke patient's independence in occupational performance tasks. The necessity for occupational therapy, administered early after the stroke, has been demonstrated in a controlled study.[30]

As seen by the lists of symptoms associated with damage to any of the arteries serving the brain, the stroke can cause many deficits that interfere with function. No two stroke patients will display the same symptoms to the same degree. Even if the same brain sites were infarcted, the deficits could vary due to individual anatomical, genetic, and environmental differences.[11] Careful evaluation must be done to reveal the deficits and their probable interrelatedness. However, if the therapist were to administer all tests needed in order to discover all possible deficits before starting treatment, the patient would be discharged before treatment began! Therefore, rather than use an inductive reasoning process, the therapist must use a deductive one by starting with the self-care evaluation. Every stroke patient is evaluated for level of independent functioning in self-care tasks. Observation of performance during this evaluation suggests to the therapist probable deficits that limit independent functioning. Those probabilities are then tested directly by administration of selected tests. Evaluation also indicates residual abilities, which will be the key to restoration of function.[31]

Evaluation may include measurement of sensation, muscle tone, automatic postural adjustments, voluntary motor control, perception, and cognition. If motor control is intact, the therapist will evaluate muscle strength and dexterity. Additionally, information concerning other factors that affect the ability of the person to progress or learn must be gathered. These factors include the presence of speech and language disorders or visual deficits. The presence, or potential for developing, secondary motor deficits that will limit function also must be evaluated. Emotional status of the patient and level of adaptation to the stroke by the patient and his family will affect outcome and need to be evaluated, as does the patient's degree of motivation to recover. Motivation plays a major role in functional recovery.[11]

An evaluation form that allows recording of the results of all evaluations helps in treatment planning. Such forms are usually developed by each occupational therapy department to reflect its philosophy regarding treatment of the stroke patient; some of these have been published.[21]

LEVEL OF INDEPENDENT FUNCTIONING

The patient's ability to perform the self-care, recreational, and vocational tasks that he hopes to continue postrehabilitation are evaluated by observation[9,31] using the methods described in Part Five. It is important to observe patient performance because there is a discrepancy between what the patient can do and what he does do[9] and also between what he believes he can do and what he can do. As mentioned above, the self-care evaluation is administered early in the patient's rehabilitation (chapter 16). Evaluation of other areas of occupational performance is done as warranted by the patient's improvement. All aspects of daily life in which the patient intends to engage after discharge should be evaluated prior to the patient's discharge to ensure that he can do them successfully and safely.

A home evaluation will be necessary (chapter 20). Prevocational evaluation and possibly a job site evaluation (chapter 21) will be required for the patient who plans to resume work.

SENSORY DEFICITS

Sensory losses with concomitant syndromes of parietal lobe dysfunction have been found to be of major significance in affecting the degree of recovery of independence in self-care and ambulation[32] and ability to relearn normal movement.[33] The main significance of impaired sensation is not necessarily the actual loss but the fact that it is closely associated with the presence of less easily recognized parietal lobe syndromes of unilateral neglect, spatial and body disorientation, and bilateral ideomotor apraxia, all of which are serious impediments to rehabilitation success.[32] In one study, 64% of left hemiplegic patients with discriminatory sensory losses and 72% of those with hemianesthesia or hypesthesia had concomitant parietal lobe syndromes.[32]

Primary sensory awareness and discriminatory sensory perception are tested using procedures described in chapter 3. When evaluating a hemiplegic patient's sensation, the uninvolved limbs are evaluated first to gauge expected levels of response for the involved extremities of the particular patient,[32] although the so-called normal extremities may also be involved to a lesser degree following a CVA.[34] Kinesthesia and proprioception are especially important to test in all patients who will be treated for primary motor deficits because of their importance in control of nonprogrammed (unlearned, dexterous) movement. Regaining motor control is a process of learning to combine limb synergies into normal movement patterns.[35]

In testing sensation of a person who has expressive aphasia, it is necessary to establish a means of communication with the patient. This may be a nod of the head or other facial expression[36] or the use of two distinct sounds within the capability of the patient to mean "yes" or "no." When it is necessary to name an object, as in testing for stereognosis, the patient with expressive aphasia may be presented with a small array of objects from which he selects the stimulus object. The degree of discrimination can be tested by making the objects in the array more or less similar. Testing a patient with receptive aphasia is questionably valid, and the therapist must be sure not to overestimate the person's ability to understand.[37] One method used to check the level of understanding is to say one thing and gesture another; the patient's response will give a clue to his understanding.[37]

PERCEPTUAL AND COGNITIVE DEFICITS

Patients may have perceptual and/or cognitive losses that render them less able to get around in their world and/or to manipulate the components of their environment for normal functioning. Discriminatory sensory losses are often perceptual losses. Methods to evaluate cognitive/perceptual function are detailed in chapter 7. To ensure valid testing, choice of neuropsychological tests should control for the problems of the patient that could impinge on results. For example, stroke patients evidence physical and communication deficits; therefore, tests chosen to measure cognitive/perceptual abilities must not rely on these modes for response.[38] One neuropsychological test is not a pure measure of a single function. The basis for diagnosing a specific functional deficit is that the performance on a test or group of tests is consistently depressed in relation to performance on others.[38]

Some norms for persons aged 40 to 89 have been published for tests that measure parietal lobe function,[39] including the Parietal Lobe subtests of the Boston Diagnostic Aphasia Examination (drawing construction, finger gnosis, right-left orientation, arithmetic ability, and topographical orientation); the Hooper Visual Organization Test; and the Poppelreuter Superimposed Figures Test.[39]

It is difficult to separate cognitive and perceptual deficits because cognitive processes are used in the process of perceiving.[40] Clinically these can be differentiated; e.g., if the patient is unable to attend to, remember, or solve problems involving visual information but can do so using auditory information, then he has a visual perceptual deficit, not a cognitive deficit, because he is able to operate cognitively once he perceives the information.[40] Cognitive functions to be tested include orientation, conceptualization, comprehension abilities (concentration, attention span, and memory), cognitive integration abilities including generalization (application of specific concepts to a variety of related situations), and problem solving (ability to define the problem, organize a plan, make decisions or judgments, implement the plan in logical sequence, and evaluate the outcome).[41] Conditions that facilitate performance or under which performance deteriorates are as important to know as the test score.[40] Special note should be made of the strategies the patient uses and their effectiveness.[40] Ideally test items are arranged in an hierarchy, starting with those that have minimal processing requirements. Such an hierarchical battery of O.T.-relevant test items has not yet been developed. In fact, such a test battery for use by neuropsychologists is still in the developmental stages.[38] Using a test that arranges abilities in an hierarchy assists treatment planning because treatment would begin at the breakdown point in performance.[40]

EVALUATION OF PRIMARY MOTOR DEFICITS

The motor deficits caused by cortical lesions include changes in muscle tone (positive symptom) and loss of skilled movement (negative symptom). See chapter 5 for a discussion of motor deficits caused by cortical lesions. The motor loss is not one of weakness but the inability to control each limb joint in isolation or to direct the limb in other than stereotyped, reflex-based movement. The negative symptoms seem to be the overriding deficit in stroke patients. It is as if the person cannot remember, generate, or execute the proper motor program to meet the environmental demand (levels II to IV of the model in chapter 5).

Electromyographic (EMG) analysis of 16 patients with upper motor neuron lesions (12 CVAs) and 8 normal subjects led Sahrmann and Norton[42] to the conclusion that "impairment of movement is not due to antagonist stretch reflexes [spasticity], but rather to limited and prolonged recruitment of agonist contraction and delayed cessation of agonist contraction at the termination of movement,"[42] in other words, lack of ability to control activation and deactivation of motor units. Some patients also exhibit poor trunk stability and/or loss of automatic postural adjustments, although these symptoms are less frequently seen[43] because of subcortical control of automatic reactions and bilateral innervation of the trunk and postural muscles.

Methods for evaluating muscle tone have been described in chapter 4 and chapter 6, part B. Notice should be made of changes in tone due to the various attitudinal (brain stem level) reflexes,[44] as well as other variables mentioned in chapter 4.

The evaluation of automatic and voluntary motor control may be done using methods described in chapter 4 and/or by using Brunnstrom's or Bobath's procedures and scoring methods detailed in chapter 6, parts B and C. It will be helpful for treatment planning if during the evaluation of motor control the therapist notices such things as the following: is there a difference in the patient's ability to do automatic versus voluntary movement, indicating preservation of subcortical motor control functions but loss of cortical ones? A patient in whom automatic movement is preserved will easily adjust to disturbances of balance (equilibrium reactions) and his body will follow as his head moves (righting reactions). Do proximal segments (neck, trunk, shoulder, hip) stabilize as needed to provide firm support for movement of the distal parts? If not, treatment must begin here. Is the patient able to do a habitual movement sequence but not a new sequence of movements? This may indicate preservation of old motor programs but difficulty with learning new motor patterns in which case treatment methods need to emphasize motor learning techniques. Or this difference could reflect sensory loss or disturbances because programmed movement relies less on external sensory guidance than on an autonomous internal system of control, whereas new skills are guided externally by sensory feedback. Sensory deficits would need to be ruled out to allow the therapist to decide on a course of action in therapy.

The evaluations in chapters 4 and 6 are commonly used observational, nonscored tools. However, quantified evaluations are preferred and are required for documentation of treatment effectiveness. It is important for therapists to use quantifiable tests because not only can individual progress in motor recovery be better documented, but, over time, the scores of many patients can be correlated with scores of a quantified activities of daily living (ADL) test, and the relationship between upper-extremity function and ADL independence can be established for stroke patients. Also, the natural history of recovery can be documented, which could guide treatment by indicating the average score required in a lower category before moving to the next higher level.

Fugl-Meyer and colleagues[26] have standardized and quantified Brunnstrom's method for evaluating motor control in stroke patients. The evaluation of the upper extremity is divided into 33 details; each detail examined is graded 0 (unable), 1, or 2 (performed faultlessly or within normal limits, as defined for each specific task), resulting in a maximum total score of 66 points.[26,45] (See Table 1.) In the full Brunnstrom–Fugl-Meyer (B–F–M) evaluation, motor function of the lower extremity, balance, sensation of light touch, joint position and motion sense, and pain are included. The Fugl–Meyer assessment has internal validity in that actual recovery of stroke patients parallel the test items[26,45,46] and has high intrarater reliability ($r = 0.99$) as well as interrater reliability that ranged from $r = 0.96$ to 0.99 for the upper-extremity function test.[47]

When motor recovery, as expressed in the B–F–M test, is compared to functional recovery, as measured by the Action Research Arm (ARA) test developed by Lyle,[48] there is a positive and strong correlation ($r_s = 0.91$ at 2 weeks and $r_s = 0.94$ at 8 weeks). Both are valid and reliable tests that provide ordinal level scores and appear to measure arm-hand function equally well.[45]

The ARA test is hierarchical in the sense that if the patient passes the top item in each category, he will be able to do the other items within that category and these need not be tested. This feature means that test administration can require very little time (8 min versus 11 min for the B–F–M test in one study[45]). However, the ARA test requires equipment such as a trolley (wheeled cart), wooden cubes, a cricket ball, sharpening stone, washer and bolt, water glasses, marbles, and ballbearings.[45] It is subdivided into four tests: grasp, grip, pinch, and gross movement. It consists of 19 items overall, graded on a 4-point scale: 0 = unable; 3 = normal; 1 = partial performance; and 2 = full performance but slow or done with difficulty, for a total of 57 points. The intrarater and retest reliability of the ARA test are +0.99 and +0.98, respectively.[48]

Often the control of the affected extremity is compared to that of the "normal" extremity as baseline; however, the so-called normal extremity has been found deficient as compared to those of neurologically unimpaired subjects.[49,50]

MUSCLE STRENGTH, ENDURANCE, AND ASSISTIVE HAND FUNCTION

These are evaluated using procedures described in chapters 4 and 8. Muscle strength is tested only in those few patients who regain total isolated control of muscles.

SPEECH AND LANGUAGE DISTURBANCES

Aphasia is a disturbance of language, of the symbolic use of the spoken or written word. Expressive aphasia, also called Broca's aphasia, is the inability to express verbally what one desires to say due to a lesion in the anterior speech cortex.[51] A patient with expressive aphasia may be able to sing or speak in other automatic ways, such as praying[52] or swearing. A person who

Table 22.1
BRUNNSTROM-FUGL-MEYER TEST: ASSESSMENT OF
MOTOR FUNCTION OF THE UPPER EXTREMITY IN
HEMIPLEGIA[45]

Test 1. Reflex activity (can reflexes be elicited or not?):
   1. Flexors
   2. Extensors

Test 2. Dynamic flexor and extensor synergies:
   3. Scapular retraction
   4. Scapular elevation
   5. Shoulder abduction
   6. Shoulder external rotation
   7. Elbow flexion
   8. Forearm supination
   9. Shoulder adduction and internal rotation
   10. Elbow extension
   11. Forearm pronation

Test 3. Motions that mix the flexor and extensor synergies:
   12. Hand to lumbar spine
   13. Shoulder flexion from 0° to 90°
   14. Pronation and supination of the forearm with the elbow actively flexed to about 90°

Test 4. Volitional movements with little or no synergy dependence:
   15. Shoulder abduction from 0° to 90°
   16. Shoulder forward flexion from 90° to 180°
   17. Pronation and supination of the forearm with the elbow straight and the shoulder flexed

Test 5. Normal reflex activity:
   18. Scored as being hyperactive or not

Test 6. Three different functions of the wrist:
   19. Wrist stability (shoulder 0°; elbow 90°)
   20. Wrist flexion/extension (shoulder 0°; elbow 90°)
   21. Wrist stability (shoulder 30°; elbow 0°)
   22. Wrist flexion/extension (shoulder 30°; elbow 0°)
   23. Circumduction of the wrist

Test 7. Seven details of function of the hand:
   24. Mass flexion of the fingers
   25. Mass extension of the fingers
   26. Grasp with extended metacarpophalangeal joints of digits 2–5 and flexion of the proximal and distal interphalangeal joints (hook grasp)
   27. Grasp with pure thumb adduction (lateral prehension of a playing card or paper)
   28. Grasp with opposition of the thumb pulp against the pulp of the index finger (palmar pinch of a pencil)
   29. Grasp of a cylinder-shaped object
   30. A spherical grasp (tennis ball)

Test 8. Coordination and speed: Finger to nose test is applied five times in succession, as rapidly as possible. The following details are assessed:
   31. Tremor
   32. Dysmetria
   33. Speed

learned English as a second language may be aphasic for English but able to speak his native language. Usually, however, the patient is aphasic in both languages. Agraphia is the inability to express in writing what one wishes to say. A person with Broca's aphasia may have agraphia also. Receptive aphasia, also called Wernicke's aphasia, is the inability to understand spoken language due to a lesion in the posterior speech cortex. Alexia is the inability to understand written language and therefore the inability to read. A combination of receptive (sensory) and expressive (motor) aphasia is called global aphasia.[53]

Dysarthria is a slurring of speech due to paralysis or incoordination of the speech musculature. The patient is able to understand and express symbolic language.

The speech pathologist evaluates these functions. The occupational therapist needs the results of the evaluation to evaluate, instruct, or communicate effectively with the patient.

VISUAL DEFICITS

The most common visual disturbances are hemianopsia and impaired depth perception. Hemianopsia is a visual field defect in which the patient is unable to see part of his visual field while looking straight ahead. Right homonymous hemianopsia means that the patient has lost the perception of vision in the nasal half of the left eye and the temporal half of the right eye and is unable to see to the right of midline.[5]

When hemianopsia is combined with sensory loss of the affected side, the patient may neglect the side altogether. However, he may also do this in the absence of these two symptoms due to a malfunction in the central processing system of the right parietal lobe.[54]

Hemianopsia may be tested in several ways. Two commonly used tests are:

1. Draw a horizontal line on a blackboard. With the patient positioned in exact center of the line and with his head held so that he looks straight ahead, give him the chalk and ask him to bisect the line.

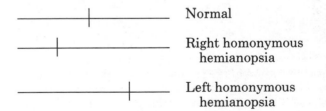

Normal

Right homonymous hemianopsia

Left homonymous hemianopsia

2. Stand in front of the patient, who is looking straight ahead so that he will not compensate for the loss by turning his head. Hold two new pencils at the 180° limits of peripheral vision. Keep your arms and hands down below his level of vision so that he does not get extra cues by watching your arms. Simultaneously move the pencils in an arc toward the patient's midline. He is to indicate when he sees each of them. If he fails to notice the pencil on the affected side, it is necessary to rule out the possibility that the patient is extinguishing one stimulus. A patient with brain damage may have sensory and perceptual deficits that limit him to perception of only one stimulus of a similar nature at a time. To rule that out, the patient is tested again by presenting the stimulus only to the defective side.

Depth perception can be tested by holding two pencils in front of the patient's face at eye level and at different distances. One pencil is slowly moved toward the other until the patient indicates when they are parallel with each other. Another way to test depth perception is to place one block farther away from another on a table, which is raised to approximately eye level to eliminate the cues obtained from looking down on the blocks, and to ask the patient to identify which is closer.

SECONDARY MOTOR DEFICITS

Secondary motor deficits that may occur as a result of the paralysis and spasticity include contractures and subluxation of the shoulder and shoulder-hand syndrome (reflex sympathetic dystrophy), which may lead to a frozen shoulder.

Measurement of passive range of motion, as described in chapter 9, is done when moderate to severe spasticity or beginning contractures are present in order to document status before therapy. When these conditions are not present, an estimate of passive range of motion without actually measuring is enough. Subluxation is noted by observation of whether a space exists between the acromion process and head of the humerus, indicated by an indentation just below the acromion. The amount of subluxation is estimated in "finger breadths," i.e., the size of the space is reported by how many fingers can be placed between the acromion and the humerus. This condition will be verified by x-ray. Reflex sympathetic dystrophy or shoulder-hand syndrome is an autonomic reaction that is manifested by pain in the shoulder and hand as well as nonpitting edema of the hand.

EMOTIONAL ADJUSTMENT

Evaluation of the patient's and his family's adjustment to the stroke, to rehabilitation, and to the prospect of living with the aftermath of the stroke can be done through conversation and observation (chapter 2).

Interpretation of the results of the evaluations leads to the development of a problem list and to the statement of goals. The occupational therapy goals for poststroke patients may include: (1) to improve independence in daily life tasks, (2) to prevent deformities, (3) to re-educate sensation or compensate for sensory disturbances, (4) to restore motor control, (5) to improve cognitive and perceptual skills or to compensate for lost abilities, (6) to compensate for visual defects, (7) to prevent development of secondary motor deficits, and (8) to facilitate emotional adjustment and to motivate participation in the rehabilitation program.

Treatment

Treatment is facilitated in an atmosphere of low stress. One source of stress to aphasic patients is their inability to communicate their wants and thoughts. Providing nonstressful opportunities for communication is an adjunct to the patient's progress. One method of reducing the stress of communication is to phrase questions so that the patient has to answer by "yes" or "no" rather than by descriptive phrases and allowing time for the patient to process the information and respond. Talking loudly to the aphasic patient is not useful and increases his stress. Of course, displaying annoyance or frustration at being unable to communicate with the patient is nontherapeutic.

The type of therapy program will be influenced by the patient's age, type of stroke, and expected prognosis for life and recovery. The Rehabilitative Approach may be best for some patients, the elderly in particular, whereas the greater time, expense, and effort required by the Neurodevelopmental Approach directed at the recovery of perceptual and/or sensorimotor functions may be warranted for others, especially the young stroke patient.

Therapy begins as soon as the patient's medical condition has stabilized.[2] Early therapy is delivered at bedside because the stroke patient is unpredictably apt to deteriorate neurologically early on, to be disoriented or easily become disoriented, to have unstable blood pressure, to be lethargic, and/or to be incontinent.[55] The goals of early treatment are preventative. The effects of prolonged bedrest and immobility are counteracted. Contractures are prevented through positioning (see Bobath Neurodevelopmental Approach: chapter 6, part B) and range of motion. Endurance and strength (in limbs under the patient's control) are maintained through activity. To prevent sensory deprivation, the room should be arranged so that the patient with hemianopsia or lateral inattention is facing the action with his unaffected side. As the patient is able, skills for self-care are begun, starting with feeding, grooming, and bed mobility. Coming to a sitting position on the side of the bed and bed-to-wheelchair transfers are taught as soon as the patient is able. Throughout, the patient and family are offered psychological support and are educated about stroke.[2]

The acute-care stage only lasts an average 10 days poststroke due to the influence of the new federal prospective payment system.[55] The patient begins a rehabilitation program when he demonstrates neurological stability; urinary and fecal continence or conformity to a bowel and bladder control program; and potential to progress.[55]

OCCUPATIONAL PERFORMANCE TASKS

The occupational therapist's goal is to improve independence in occupational performance tasks and hence to improve the patient's quality of life. It is controversial as to whether the patient should be taught compensatory one-handed techniques for self-care independence before regaining motor control of the involved upper extremity and relearning to do the tasks bilaterally. It is the opinion of some[56,57] that should the compensatory choice be made too early, the effectiveness of restorative treatment will be lessened since the patient will fail to learn symmetrical movements and will instead learn unilateral habits. They believe that preferential use of the sound side of the body for weight bearing and functional tasks increases the spasticity, making development of normalized motor control less possible.[56] Others restate the view by saying that in order to develop versatility in the patient's performance, the underlying sensorimotor processes that result in dependence must be attacked and that "splinter skill training" of self-care skills will only result in stereotyped performance. Yet another view is that ADL training results in success at a faster rate and is therefore more economical and more satisfying to the patient, who again feels competent.[31] Because of the psychological importance of being independent of others for basic self-care and because of the reduced hospitalization time available to stroke patients under the government's new prospective payment plan, in my opinion, the patient should be taught compensatory methods of ADL from the beginning. These use the principle of stabilizing objects being worked on to substitute for loss of one side of the body and are found in chapter 17. The patient must practice to learn these new techniques of self-care because, due to his altered condition, he cannot rely on his old habitual methods. Of course the patient must have requisite hand skills in the noninvolved upper extremity.[50] Therapy aimed at improving hand skill may be required prior to progressing with ADL training.[50] Early poststroke, even before the patient is ready to actively participate, training begins by the nurses talking the patient through the process as they assist him with his daily care. For example, when the nurse puts on or removes his hospital gown, she says aloud "affected limb in first and out last."

Several studies discerned an hierarchy of achievement of self-care skills.[9,58] In the study of 494 stroke survivors, 47% of whom became independent by 6 months poststroke, dressing unaided was regained late in recovery and bathing independently was the most difficult task.[9] Both of these skills require the patient to reach to and move all parts of his body and require learning special techniques.

Rehabilitation is a learning process and if the patient is capable of receiving and processing sensory input, then motor skills can be relearned. Left hemiplegics (right CVA) have a primary problem with information received through the visual modality, whereas right hemiplegics have a problem processing information received through the auditory modality.[59] But, since each half of the brain attends to different aspects of the same experience, the patient with unilateral brain damage will be able to relearn functional tasks if the therapist teaches him using the system that remains intact. (See Table 7.2.)

Pantomime and demonstrated instructions confuse the patient with right cerebral damage but he can understand verbal or written instructions.[31,37,60] Additionally, the patient with right hemisphere damage tends to omit or minimize problems and to perform a task too quickly without paying attention to detail.

Left hemiplegic patients (right CVA or RCVA) need to be slowed down and their attention focused in order to improve the quality of their performance.[31,61]

The performance of visuospatial tasks by the patient with left cerebral hemisphere damage is generally free from error, and he understands pantomime, but he may not be able to understand verbal or written instructions.[31,37,60,62] Left CVA (LCVA) patients are cognizant that a problem exists and perform tasks very slowly in an effort to perform correctly. Right hemiplegic patients (LCVA) should be encouraged to persist in performing a task, although they require more than the normal amount of time and need frequent specific feedback that they are proceeding correctly.[37]

In a study of 1665 patients in one city, 88% of the patients receiving rehabilitation were discharged home and only 11% were discharged to long-term-care facilities.[63] A study of 105 discharged poststroke subjects indicated that those living with another adult performed less of their own activities of daily living but socialized more than those who lived alone,[63] who were more independent in ADL tasks. Home activity, outside activity, and social interaction were severely limited (less than 50% of normal) in both groups,[63] whereas cognition and ADL, though limited, were less so, perhaps reflecting the emphasis on these aspects of function during rehabilitation.

As the patient improves and discharge planning progresses, occupational performance tasks other than ADL tasks may need to be taught. Homemaking skills that the patient would be likely to do are taught to those patients with sufficient cognitive and perceptual abilities to enable success and safety in these tasks (chapter 18). Patients who choose to retire from work as a result of the stroke, or who have hobbies they wish to continue, should be taught adapted methods of avocational tasks (chapter 19). For those who expect to resume working, prevocational evaluation and work hardening, if warranted, need to be done (chapter 21). Those factors found generally predictive of likelihood to return to work included independence in self-care, younger age, greater education, stable marital status, and high cognitive capacities.[64] In particular, the variables that differentiated those that did return to work from those that did not were the verbal-cognitive and communicative deficits of the right hemiplegics and the nonverbal abstract reasoning deficits and disregard or disuse of the affected upper extremity of the left hemiplegics.[64]

The ability to drive rates high on a person's list of everyday skills.[65] Those who want to drive should be evaluated by the occupational therapist specializing in driver evaluation. Evaluation is necessary not so much because of the paralysis but rather the cognitive/perceptual losses and slowed motor reactions may be too disabling to permit it. These can be measured by an off-road driver's evaluation involving measurement of foot reaction time and ability to track using a computerized simulated driving experience (chapter 17), followed by an on-road driving test, if warranted.[65] Interestingly, the results of one program in New Zealand indicated no significant difference in pass/fail rates of right or left stroke patients in a sample of 91 patients. Twenty-six (14 RCVA and 12 LCVA) passed with full satisfaction; 23 others (10 RCVA and 13 LCVA) received a borderline rating that was less than satisfactory, but not sufficient to warrant restriction.[65]

When the opportunity arises as part of ongoing occupational therapy treatment, the occupational therapist should reinforce speech therapy. This is important because of the value of language to the individual. In this, the occupational therapist is guided by the speech therapist. Reinforcement of speech therapy involves requiring written or verbal responses of the patient at the level of which he is capable.

THERAPY FOR SENSORY DEFICITS

In a study of 271 hemiplegic patients, 82 showed sensory defects and these patients remained in a more dependent category of achievement in rehabilitation.[32] Kinesthesia and proprioception are important in relearning normal movement patterns.[35] Tactile sensation enables coordinated, dexterous movement and is important in spontaneous use of the limb. Stereognosis improves functional ability.

Treatment for sensory dysfunction of stroke patients has not been systematically developed, although therapists attempt remediation as well as compensation for these deficits. Remedial treatment involves the presentation of the stimulus, response by the patient, exact feedback, and practice.[67] Compensatory treatment involves substituting intact senses for those lost or dysfunctional.

Recalibration of proprioception is attempted by getting the patient to attend to the limb through tactile stimulation and then focusing the patient's awareness on the location of the limb while, with vision occluded, he tries to move to a target. A stick-on dot can be used to designate the target. He then opens his eyes to get feedback on how exact his movement was. Practice starts with the patient moving the arm to designated targets on his own body and then, as he becomes consistently successful, the targets are located away from the body. Electrogoniometric biofeedback may also be useful in recalibrating kinesthesia. The patient moves a certain range of motion, with vision occluded; then if he is successful, the feedback signal will operate.

One technique to restore tactile awareness is vigorous rubbing of the limb with terry toweling while the patient watches,[32] followed by repetitive movement of the limb. Such treatment should be done with care to avoid increasing spasticity.[66] Weight bearing on the affected hand on different surface textures such as foam, carpeting, sand, or toweling and handling objects of various textures have been suggested to facilitate touch sensation.[66] Another method of retraining sensory (tactile) awareness used was to require the patient to point to corresponding places on a manikin placed in front of him after he had been touched on his back.[67]

One method used to improve stereognosis is to have the patient feel the object first with the eyes closed, make a guess of what the object is while concentrating on its features, and then open the eyes for immediate feedback and reinforcement.[68]

Treatment for sensory deficits is discussed further in chapter 3. Restoration of sensory awareness is a relearning process requiring much practice under many different conditions. If the patient cannot or does not want to invest the time and effort required for retraining, he is taught to compensate for lost sensation through the use of the remaining senses. Visual compensation is the most natural and often used, although auditory monitoring may be used in certain instances. The patient is taught to watch his limbs as they move or to remind himself in some way of their location. If he is capable, he is taught to use a mental checklist that includes locating the anesthetic limb before moving. Noisy bracelets on the wrist or ankle provide an auditory reminder. Success in compensatory methods is limited if the patient is hemianoptic, has unilateral neglect, or is confused.

COGNITIVE AND PERCEPTUAL FUNCTION

The O.T.R. is the rehabilitation professional who is assigned to provide remediation and compensation for cognitive and perceptual deficits to permit greater independence in occupational performance tasks. Neither type of deficit can be treated in isolation.[40] Cognitive abilities such as attention and problem solving are of higher order than praxis and visuospatial perceptual abilities, which in turn are higher order than sensory reception and awareness abilities.[38] Each level of the hierarchy processes information with increasingly more abstraction and interrelatedness.[38,40]

Perceptual deficits of body image or body scheme, space perception, unilateral neglect, and constructional apraxia, in spite of average or above-average intelligence, correlate to failure to progress in ADL training.[54,69,70] Although these relationships have been noted, the minimal cognitive-perceptual requirements for occupational performance tasks unfortunately have not been identified. This seems to result in too little or too much therapy. Whether the cognitive-perceptual skills transfer directly to ADL has not been tested, although the skills can be taught directly in relation to ADL tasks if necessary.[67] For example, scanning in a systematic way can help the patient to perform ADL better; e.g., systematically scanning the face in the mirror according to a plan repeated each time ensures that the patient will shave both sides of the face.[67] Without the learned system the patient is apt to neglect the need to shave one side.[67]

Whether to treat the adult patient's perceptual deficits neurophysiologically, educationally, or by means of compensation remains a question. These options are discussed in chapter 7. One group found that improved perceptual abilities due to pencil and paper training tasks was related to improved driving performance.[71] This study is not definitive, however, because it was done on a small (n = 8), heterogenous sample of stroke patients, the order of improvement for both types of tasks appears small, and no comment was made regarding the practical significance of the changes.

Compensatory education is the alternative to remediation, although brain-damaged patients have difficulty substituting use of other senses when perception through one sense (e.g., visual) is affected.[67] It was found that successful treatment of one perceptual defect led to uncovering others; perceptual defects seem to be layered.[67]

One method of compensation is to structure the environment to increase the patient's chance to succeed. An example of this is for the patient with figure-ground deficit to use sheets of contrasting color on the bed so that the top sheet can be distinguished from the bottom when making the bed. Another method of compensation is to teach the patient "attack skills" using his cognitive abilities. Some of these are the use of cues to chain an activity, i.e., one step of an activity cues the next; organizing things according to color, shape, size, function, etc., using logical, sequential thinking; the use of categorizing skills in which the patient cognitively describes the object to himself in order to categorize it, e.g., "this object has three angles and three straight sides, therefore it is a triangle"; and the use of verbal memory by which the patient learns a verbal sequence and cues himself to perform sequential tasks by repeating the sequence aloud.

The overriding defect accounting for a particular patient's incapacity may be a change in intellect; paralysis alone may contribute little to his incapacity.[61] Brain damage causes deficient learning in which there is difficulty in receiving and processing incoming information, assimilating or retaining information, associating new information with previous information, or retrieving information from memory to effect behavior. Each patient will have a particular learning requirement depending on the site of lesion. Because information processing is slowed in brain-injured patients,[72] instruction should be brief, concrete, and standardized. Delivering one instruction at a time may be necessary for some patients.

Brain-damaged persons have difficulty structuring and organizing information.[40] Since they do not automatically use efficient strategies to process information, they need to be taught strategies to attend to relevant features of a task, to group similar items together, to formulate a plan, or to break a task down into its steps.[40] Strategies are organized sets of rules that operate to select and guide information processing.[40] For example, when you shop for a new blouse, you do not need to try on each blouse on the rack; you have an organizational strategy that lets you select the few that meet your rules of color or style that are "you."

Therapy involves use of learning principles to ameliorate deficiencies by using activities that systematically and gradually increase demand on the information processing system.[40,73] Gradations are from simple to complex, from automatic to effortful, and from the ability to respond to the external environment to the ability to manipulate the external environment.[40] Characteristics of activity that can be manipulated to change the processing demands include: rate of presentation and required response (slower is easier); amount of items in the presentation (few are easier); duration of task requiring attention, concentration, etc. (shorter time is easier); sensory modality through which the stimulus is presented (easier is that not affected by stroke, i.e., visual for right hemiplegics and auditory for left hemiplegics); and complexity or degree of difficulty in terms of familiarity and abstractness (easier are familiar, concrete habitual daily tasks).[40] An activity that requires cues 50% or more of the time is too advanced for the patient's level.[40]

Task conditions influence the success of brain-damaged persons in performing a task. In a normal person, for example, peripheral stimuli facilitate performance, whereas in brain-damaged persons excess stimuli may impede it.[62,74] If the patient seems to be having difficulty completing a task, the task conditions could be modified by reducing the stimuli in the environment to the point that the patient is able to perform successfully. Gradually over time as the task becomes learned, the stimuli should be reinstated if possible. The patient needs to be able to perform in natural situations rather than be dependent on adapted ones.[62,74]

Methods of retraining and/or compensating for lost cognitive abilities are described in chapter 7.

REDEVELOPMENT OF MOTOR CONTROL

Therapy to regain motor control involves treatment of the positive as well as the negative symptoms. It is not entirely clear whether one must be treated before the other, that is, whether tone must be normalized before eliciting voluntary motor responses; or whether they must be treated simultaneously, that is, whether spasticity must be inhibited at the same time that voluntary motor responses are elicited; or whether treatment should be aimed directly at the negative symptoms to redevelop motor control, which coincidentally might lead to normalization of the positive symptoms.

Enhanced performance is not necessarily directly related to reduction of spasticity. This was demonstrated in a study of 20 hemiplegics patients in whom improved function was observed following exercise and biofeedback therapy, but no significant concomitant change in spasticity, as measured by EMG, was observed.[75] Whereas in the past spasticity was considered the major motor problem, it may not be so.

In another study that compared motor output and pattern of 10 hemiparetic and 10 normal subjects electromyographically, the hemiparetic subjects' inability to generate motor unit recruitment was confirmed. But also confirmed was the patients' inability to move through full unresisted range despite the ability to generate the same amount of motor unit activity generated by the normal subjects during unresisted finger extension.[76] Whether this inability was due to excess neural or biomechanical aspects of tone or to lost patterns of movement could not be discerned from that experiment.[76]

A review of literature suggests that factors such as decreased convergent impulses on motor cells in the spinal cord and prolonged agonist action may be as important or perhaps more important than antagonistic spasticity in limiting voluntary movement.[77]

If tone is excessive, movement may be prevented if the muscles antagonistic to the spastic ones are also weak. Excessive tone is inhibited using the previously described procedures (chapters 5 and 6). As mentioned in chapter 12, EMG biofeedback also can be used to teach the patient to control spasticity. If tone is low, movement may not occur because too few motor units are sufficiently excited in response to supraspinal commands since they lack this background of excitation. Therapists use various sensory stimulation techniques described in chapters 5 and 6 to facilitate tone. Another technique used exclusively with stroke patients is the dynamic sling (Fig. 13.64) to facilitate tone in the elbow extensors, key muscles needed to reach forward.

Redevelopment of motor patterns is a matter of relearning motor control on a continuum from reflex, mass movements to voluntary, isolated movements to voluntary automatically controlled movements rather than strengthening of muscles, per se. Learning is a conscious and organized process.[6] The therapist gives information to the patient and helps him process it (attend to it, manipulate it); provides feedback; structures practice so that it is functionally related and interesting; and sets finely spaced, attainable goals to give a sense of accomplishment.[6] Retraining requires active patient involvement in which he attends to retraining information (the signal) while disregarding extraneous information (the noise) not related to motor control.[6] The goal is to increase the signal-to-noise ratio.[6]

The feedback provided can be knowledge of performance (KP) or knowledge of results (KR). KP is knowledge about the movement pattern produced rather than the outcome.[78] KR is information about the outcome. KP is important for patients during the relearning process because, although they can see the outcome (correct or incorrect) they are often unaware of the process needed to accomplish the outcome correctly. Instead of giving feedback such as "reach was 2 inches too short" (KR), feedback such as "straighten your elbow" (KP) helps the patient learn to control the many variables that need to be constrained for the appropriate outcome to occur.[78] Those with impaired sensation need extrinsic feedback (verbal cueing from the therapist or biofeedback). Those with intact position sense but impaired motor control need extrinsic feedback to direct attention to the inherent feedback[78]— how it felt to move. Extrinsic feedback provides information, acts as a reinforcer, and motivates the patient.[78] Closed-loop control mechanisms make conscious use of feedback, whereas open-loop control processes use the feedback unconsciously. (See chapter 5 for a discussion of these control systems.) Therefore, once the patient has learned a response (that is, once it has become programmed or controlled in an open-loop mode), then continuing to provide extrinsic KP feedback is inappropriate and interferes with performance and continued learning.

Another factor that may interfere with learning is the influence of brain stem level reflexes.[79] It may be that following hemiplegia the individual needs to use these reflexes to add stability to movement against gravity as a reaction to the stress placed on the person by the loss of higher-level automatic gravity-adjusting mechanisms, the righting and equilibrium reactions.[79] Use of brain stem level reflexes should be viewed as a normal response to nervous system distress rather than a symptom of pathology.[79] In that context, the appearance of primitive reflexes is a signal that the person is experiencing uncontrollable stress caused by gravity (fear of falling, effort to move), by the complexity of the movement asked for, or by the body position required by the activity in combination with intricate skilled movements at the peak or slightly beyond the peak of a person's capability. Modifying the requirements for the patient will decrease the primitive response. Treatment then should be aimed at improving the person's postural adaptation so that he does not have to rely on primitive reflexes to make an adaptive response to the environment.[79]

Redevelopment of motor control should not be done in the abstract. That is, newly relearned patterns of movement should be made part of ADL training and practiced in that context.[56,80] Acquisition of motor skills requires much repetition,[80,81] high motivation, and perseverance.[82] Enriched environments should be used to provide sensory stimulation from which motivation arises and to stimulate the patient to attempt to interact with the environment.[82]

Procedures described in chapters 5 and 6 are used to restore motor control.

A study of a small number of stroke patients showed a trend that indicated attention, feedback, and practice in combination with activities to elicit high percentages of motor unit recruitment are beneficial to improve finger extension.[29] Persons capable of some voluntary control at the start of the treatment seemed to benefit more from this therapy.[29] Extremely high variability of scores was seen among subjects, indicating the presence of unidentified controller variables that need to be identified.[29]

Kimura[83] studied the ability of post-CVA patients to learn a sequence of three tasks on a manual test box using the ipsilateral ("nonaffected") hand. Sixteen RCVA and 29 LCVA (14 aphasic and 15 nonaphasic) patients were studied. Six LCVA patients failed to learn the sequence. Of the patients who did learn, the nonaphasic LCVAs and the RCVAs did not differ significantly on number of trials needed to achieve the criterion nor on the time needed to perform the task. The aphasic LCVAs required significantly more trials to learn the task than did the nonaphasic LCVAs or the RCVAs. Kimura concluded that LCVA patients are impaired in acquisition and subsequent performance of a motor skill that involves sequencing several changes in hand and limb posture using the ipsilateral hand in which strength and tapping ability are within normal limits. The types of errors that significantly distinguished LCVA from RCVA patients were of the decision-making type involving motor planning: making wrong or unrelated movements or perseverating. Jason[84] enlarged on Kimura's study in order to sort out the deficiencies and concluded that the LCVA patients were impaired in remembering the sequence of the acts, not in the performance of the sequence, which they could do with visual prompting.

Other treatments have been tried to improve motor control. One is functional electrical stimulation (FES). FES is defined as electrical stimulation of muscle, both smooth and striated, deprived of nervous control with a view to providing muscular contraction to produce a functionally useful movement.[85] (See chapter 13.) FES has been found useful in increasing strength of muscles antagonistic to spastic ones and in increasing range of motion. Three ½-hour periods of passive cyclical (7 sec on; 10 sec off) electrical stimulation 7 days a week for 4 weeks to the wrist and finger extensor muscles of 16 hemiplegic patients resulted in gains of passive range and strength of contraction of wrist and finger extensors, but no definite trend of reduction in spasticity or changes in sensation were seen.[86]

Biofeedback therapy is another treatment choice (chapter 12). Patients are often eager to use the equipment and therefore are motivated to relearn movement control using it.[82] EMG biofeedback presents an opportunity for a patient to know the result of his efforts to perform a certain contraction. By obtaining correct sensory information, the patient can gain new sensorimotor strategies.[6,82] Biofeedback is most appropriately used during the early, cognitive stage of motor learning.[78] By combining this external source of KP[78] with an internal source of feedback, such as proprioceptive sensation and visual observation of movement, if movement occurs, the patient may redevelop motor patterns.[87] This treatment has been found as effective as the Bobath treatment for patients classified as early-severely impaired (severe upper-extremity dysfunction of <4 months' duration) and those classified as late-mildly impaired (4 or more months poststroke).[88] Some patients did not improve, and further study of controller variables is under way.[88] Using EMG biofeedback, the patient can be taught to voluntarily initiate and stop activity of the agonist and antagonist during movement.[77] Control over initiation and cessation times of both agonist and antagonist will prevent the abnormal prolongation of contraction of both muscles, which is seen as bursts of EMG in studies of motor control in stroke patients.[77]

STRENGTH, ENDURANCE, AND HAND FUNCTION

When the patient has gained voluntary control of isolated movement, strengthening of weak muscles may be done using the methods of the Biomechanical Approach listed in chapter 9.

At first the patient's endurance may be too low for function. If no cardiac contraindications exist against increased activity, endurance may be improved by using principles outlined in chapters 9 and 30.

The unaffected upper extremity may require therapy to increase strength and coordination since it must now become the preferred, dexterous one. The need to retrain skill in the right hand of left hemiplegics is not often stressed, since the right hand is most often the dominant one and considered "normal." However, Bell et al.[50] report severe disability in hand skill of left hemiplegics using their "normal" right hand.

Methods to increase coordination and dexterity of the unaffected upper extremity follow the principle of selecting activities the patient is just able to do coordinately (quickly and accurately) and then grading the activities to require increased amounts of speed and/or accuracy.

If a change of hand preference is involved, considerable time will be spent in writing training if the patient is not agraphic. The paper is stabilized so the lower corner is about at the midline of the patient. Writing practice begins with exercises of continuous circles and progresses to connected up and down strokes.[31] These exercises first are done using large strokes and a large pencil or crayon if necessary; then the stroke and writing tools are graded smaller and smaller. Later, the alphabet and words are practiced. The patient should at least be able to sign his name before this therapy is discontinued.

COMPENSATION FOR VISUAL DEFECTS

Therapy is aimed at retraining the patient to scan his environment. Visual deficits that are not complicated by sensory/perceptual deficits are often overcome with training. Compensation for hemianopsia may be taught by reminding the patient to turn his head to view the scene on his affected side or by having the patient do activities that require him to turn his head in order to complete them. Exercises that require motor crossing of the midline often force and also reinforce visual crossing of the midline.[62] Examples of such activities include weaving on a floor loom, ironing, reading aloud, making a puzzle with some prominent pieces placed on the hemianoptic side, or playing a board game that forces scanning for pieces or place for the next move. If the patient has certain perceptual deficits, however, he will not do the activities properly and will be unaware of errors so that self-correction of his performance will not happen.

Practice in compensating for disturbances of depth perception occurs intrinsically in activities of daily living, homemaking, and other therapy. Imperceived, an object that is in the way will be knocked over and is immediate negative reinforcement. Exercises to practice depth perception may be done if necessary. An example is to place a container at the patient's arm reach at about waist level and to have him put objects into the container. Gradually raise the level of the container to eye level as the patient improves. Pouring from container to container, needle threading, and games with tall pieces, such as chess, are all interesting drills.

SECONDARY MOTOR DEFICITS

Shoulder pain is probably the most frequent complication of hemiplegia.[89] Development of a painful shoulder can interfere with the entire rehabilitation program, especially self-care activities.[90] Seventy-two percent of a group of 219 hemiplegic patients followed for 1 year poststroke had shoulder pain at least once. Shoulder subluxation and spasticity were the most frequently cited causes of the pain. Reflex sympathetic dystrophy (RSD) was present in 23% of all cases.[89]

The physical therapist may be primarily responsible for the treatment of painful shoulder. The occupational therapist must incorporate the principles of treatment into functional activities and exercise and provide orthotic devices to position the shoulder to prevent or correct misalignment.[89] Efforts to reduce pain due to shoulder spasticity should begin early by proper positioning in antispasticity positions.[89]

Subluxation of the Shoulder

Subluxation of the glenohumeral joint occurs secondarily to spasticity or flaccidity of the scapulohumeral and/or scapular muscles. Supraspinatus weakness has also been found correlated with radiographic evidence of subluxation, indicating that loading of the glenohumeral joint should be avoided as long as the affected limb is flaccid.[91] One way therapists guard against loading the affected shoulder, even by the weight of the arm itself, is to use slings. In normal shoulders the glenoid fossa is oriented upward, forward, and lateral so that the head of the humerus remains locked in contact with it.[92] The hemiplegic orientation of the glenoid fossa is downward, backward, and medial due to the scapular retraction and downward rotation that are part of the common spastic pattern. This position nullifies the "locking mechanism"[93] and allows gravity to pull the head of the humerus out of the fossa. A treatment goal should be improvement of scapular mobility with emphasis on restoring the normal orientation of the glenoid fossa.

Slings, arm boards, and lapboard wheelchair trays are all used by occupational therapists to provide a positive upward force to the hemiplegic shoulder.[89] Choice depends on the needs of each patient and the characteristics of each support.[94] Some examples are described in chapter 13.

Prevention of Contractures

Contractures are detrimental to function and hygiene and are therefore to be avoided. Contractures develop when limbs remain in one position. Because of the spasticity, the hemiplegic patient who develops contractures usually develops them in a typical hemiplegic pattern: shoulder adduction and internal rotation, elbow flexion, forearm pronation, and wrist and finger flexion.

Deforming contractures are prevented by moving the limb through range of motion at least once daily and positioning it opposite to the typical position of deformity. Precautions, as described in chapter 9, are followed when moving the hemiplegic shoulder through range of motion. The goal should be maintenance of pain-free functional range of motion in each joint, not necessarily "full range of motion."[95] Functional shoulder range of motion is defined as shoulder flexion to 100°, abduction to 90°, lateral rotation to 30°, and medial rotation to 70°.[95] Passive movement to which the patient is not attending has no place in the early care of the stroke patient, according to Carr and Shepherd.[57] The patient needs to relearn movement by feeling and thinking about movement.[57] See chapter 6, part B, and chapter 9 for specifics of technique for moving the hemiplegic shoulder through range of motion. Care must be taken that the motions are done correctly. Upward rotation of the scapula minimizes soft tissue injury, as does humeral rotation.[95] The humerus should be internally rotated during flexion and externally rotated during abduction of the arm above the horizontal to avoid rotator cuff ischemia, or tissue injury. Rotator cuff tear is associated with forceful abduction above 90° without externally rotating the humerus because the tissue becomes jammed between the humerus and the coracoacromial arch.[95,96] This tissue injury is a frequent cause of shoulder pain in hemiplegics[95,97] and often results in frozen shoulder (adhesive capsulitis[98]) because the patient refuses to move it,[96,99] although frozen shoulder can occur separate from rotator cuff tear or spasticity.[100] Evidence of rotor cuff injury was found in x-rays of all 32 hemiplegic patients evaluated[96] in one study. Range of motion should be done only by properly trained persons, including the patient himself.[95] Overhead pulleys, used in some clinics to provide for self-ranging of the shoulder, should not be used because neither correct scapular nor humeral rotation occurs and the force may be excessive. Pain is a sign of too strenuous and improper movement of the joint that has lost its rotational component.[99]

Self-administration of passive range of motion is often taught to patients in group classes. The patient holds the unaffected arm at the wrist, or by clasping the fingers of both hands, or by cradling the affected forearm with the unaffected one, or by holding onto a 1-inch dowel or a towel with both hands to help the affected arm to move in all directions. The motions frequently taught include scapular elevation by shrugging the shoulders; scapular mobility by clasping hands together and extending the arms in front and then describing a large circle; shoulder flexion by clasping the hands and raising the arms overhead; shoulder abduction and adduction in conjunction with trunk rotation, as per Brunnstrom (chapter 6, part C); elbow flexion and extension; forearm supination and pronation; wrist flexion and extension; finger flexion and extension; and thumb flexion, extension, opposition, abduction, and adduction.[101]

Positioning is used to maintain the limb in "antispastic" position or functional positions. (See chapter 6, part B.) Splinting is used to position hands; however, splinting of the spastic hand is controversial. Splinting was seen to increase the EMG output over that seen with no splint.[102] Splinting, therefore, may contribute to the problem of contracture development by increasing spasticity. This needs further study. Splint designs for the hemiplegic hand are found in chapter 13.

Serial casting of spastic limbs is a treatment choice of some therapists for stroke patients with fixed or semifixed contractures (chapter 9). By changing the casts, the limb is pulled more and more away from the spastic posture with each change, and greater range and function are obtained.[103]

Reflex Sympathetic Dystrophy (Shoulder-Hand Syndrome)

This neurovascular disorder is a disabling complication that is characterized by severe shoulder pain, along with stiffness, swelling, and pain in the hand,[2] trophic changes, and vasomotor instability.[95]

Occupational therapy objectives for shoulder-hand syndrome are to prevent it or to recognize it early and initiate treatment.[90] Prevention is by early frequent mobilization to counteract the effects of immobilization, which include edema and adhesions in the shoulder and finger joints that result in loss of the pumping mechanism to relieve the edema. Immobilization of the upper extremity can result from spasticity or decreased active movement.[90] Movements should elevate the hand above cardiac level and should activate the shoulder and hand muscles to reactivate them as pumps. If the patient is unable to move actively, bilateral activities should be used in which the nonaffected limb provides power for the affected.[90] Bathing, bilateral sanding, or polishing are examples. The occupational therapist also teaches the patient proper positioning of the limb during ADL to prevent dependent edema.[90] Prompt treatment is required to prevent permanent disability.[95] Severe shoulder-hand syndrome can be relieved by an aggressive exercise program that includes active muscle contraction, joint movement, and light weight-bearing activities. Exercise is performed within pain-free range in short bouts frequently throughout the day.[95] Hand edema must be treated aggressively and promptly to prevent irreversible hand stiffness[95] (see chapter 9). Psychological management is necessary also since the emotional state of patients associated with this syndrome may be tense, hyperresponsive to pain, overemotional, or emotionally dependent.[95]

Another possible cause of shoulder pain in hemiplegia is trauma to the brachial plexus, which is confirmed by diagnostic EMG.[90] Because of the flaccidity of the hemiplegic arm, brachial plexus injuries may not be readily identified. The occupational therapist may be the professional who first suspects it by noticing unusual patterns of return of function and/or muscle atrophy.[104] Proposed treatment is to maintain correct positioning day and night to prevent further stretch to the plexus, to maintain passive range of motion, to prevent further traction injury, and to prevent atrophy by activating still-innervated motor units using facilitation techniques.[104] The preferred position is 45° shoulder abduction, 45° external rotation, 90° elbow flexion, and 0° forearm supination. Slings should be used during ambulation, and a wedge-shaped pillow can be used to maintain the position during sleep. Mobile arm supports can also be used while the patient is sitting in his wheelchair.[104]

CARDIAC PRECAUTIONS RELATED TO EXERCISE

Ten to 12% of stroke patients have simultaneous myocardial infarction.[2] About 40% have hypertension and 60% have been found to have electrocardiographic abnormalities.[2] Therapy should be modified for patients with secondary cardiac symptoms to include warm-up and cool-down exercise. Resistive exercise should be avoided.[105] See chapter 30 for a discussion of the energy requirements of ADL and other activities. During treatment the therapist should monitor the heart rate in relation to target heart rate[2] and must attend to signs of cardiac distress such as dizziness, diaphoresis, dyspnea, excessive fatigue, or chest pain. Therapy should be discontinued if any of these are noted or if there is any indication of intolerance to exercise. In those patients with cardiac precautions, heart rate and rhythm are noted by palpation of the pulse, and blood pressure should be monitored during rest and during or within 15 sec of cessation of activity to note the patient's response to exercise. Intolerance to exercise is signified by decreased systolic blood pressure with increasing activity; diastolic blood pressure greater than 110 mm Hg; combination of decreased systolic and increased diastolic pressure with activity; decreased heart rate with activity; more than five missed beats (premature ventricular contractions [PVCs]) per minute during or immediately after activity; or more than 10 PVCs per minute at rest.[105]

EMOTIONAL ADJUSTMENT

Early poststroke, the patient may be emotionally labile.[37,106] He may cry, laugh, or express anger unprovoked by events in the external environment or to a greater degree than warranted. He needs to be told that lability is a symptom of the stroke, reassured that he is not mentally ill, and assured that his control will improve in time.[57] In the meantime, calling his name, clapping, or asking a question will interrupt and stop the emotional behavior due to organic lesion, as opposed to emotional behavior that reflects true feeling, which won't be stopped so easily.[37]

The hemiplegic patient, as with any patient who has suffered a change in his physical abilities, will need to be assisted to make a healthy emotional adjustment. His family will also need this help. In addition to supportive therapy, family group education and therapy sessions have been used in some rehabilitation centers[107]. Topics of discussion include how to communicate with an aphasic patient, how to modify the environment or task to augment functional performance, sexual counseling that focuses on coping processes within the partnership, which have been found to be the real cause for major changes in the sex life of married couples poststroke,[108] and other topics of concern. Information about conserving energy and using less stressful positions during sex and avoiding food and drink before sex should be given to the patient and his sexual partner.[2] These sessions are a rehabilitation team effort; the occupational therapist contributes to the discussion about the topics of which he/she is most informed.

Prior to discharge, the patient needs to be reintegrated into his community at the level at which he will function in it (see chapter 20). The family can share this responsibility with the rehabilitation team under their guidance as part of the family group education sessions. One concern will be patient safety. Both right and left hemiplegic hospitalized patients have been found to have more falling accidents than other patients.[109] The falling seems related to the patient's ambiguity concerning the range of what he can and cannot do without help.[109] Family members, as well as patients, need to be told clearly what the patient needs help with in order to be safe.

Effectiveness of Therapy

No definitive studies have been done to establish the effects of specific therapeutic procedures in improving the function of poststroke patients. This may be because studies to describe the natural history of the recovery of many patients need to be done first to categorize patients more precisely in order to evaluate them more specifically and treat them more effectively.[7,8] Stereotyped therapies applied to a heterogeneous population such as "stroke" patients cannot help but have dubious results.[7]

Some studies that have been reported concerning effects of rehabilitation in general include the following. Logigan et al. compared traditional (biomechanical + rehabilitative) and facilitation (neurodevelopmental) approaches to therapeutic exercise in occupational and physical therapy programs for stroke patients and found them equally beneficial in terms of functional independence and muscle strength.[110]

Dickstein et al. also compared traditional therapy involving exercise and functional activities (Biomechanical and Rehabilitative Approaches) with proprioceptive neuromuscular facilitation and Bobath treatment (Neurodevelopmental Approach) in 131 patients over a 6-week period. Improvement was noted in ADL (average 24 points on the Barthel Index) and ambula-tion nondifferentially across groups. Little to no improvement was seen in wrist or ankle dorsiflexion strength or range of motion across all treatment groups after 6 weeks. Muscle tone increased as a result of all three treatments, including the Bobath treatment, a major goal of which is reflex inhibition of spasticity.[111]

Stern et al. compared neuromuscular reeducation techniques with a program of therapy that did not include these techniques.[112] Hemiplegic patients in the population were randomly assigned to one of these two programs. Both groups improved in lower-extremity strength, overall mobility, and functional abilities.[112]

Inaba et al.[113] reported a study in which three groups of patients of a homogeneous population were randomly assigned to one of three treatment groups. Group I received functional physical therapy and selective stretching; group II received active exercise in addition to the treatment group I received; group III received progressive resistive exercise in addition to the treatment also given group I. After 1 month of treatment, progressive resistive exercise in mass extension pattern of the lower extremities (group III) was shown to significantly contribute to early increase of lower-extremity function in hemiplegics; however, after 2 months no difference was seen in the functional level of the three groups.[113]

A quantitative review of studies on the effectiveness of rehabilitation therapy for patients who have suffered a CVA indicates that the average patient who received rehabilitation services performed at a higher level than 58% to 63% of patients in comparison or control conditions.[114] Although treatment effects were small, they were practically significantly in that small improvements in independent functioning can make the difference between discharge home and institutionalization.[114] The greatest treatment effects were associated with therapy that began early poststroke and included occupational therapy.[114]

STUDY QUESTIONS:

Stroke

1. What is a stroke? What is the most common cause?
2. Which cerebral artery is most commonly affected? What are the resultant symptoms and signs resulting from a total occlusion of this artery?
3. What neurophysiological and behavioral changes enable a stroke patient to recover function poststroke?
4. What factors or variables contribute to the likelihood of full recovery of function poststroke?
5. What is the natural course of return of motor function poststroke?
6. Which evaluation is administered to every poststroke patient? How is it administered and what is the therapist looking for during the evaluation?
7. How can perceptual and cognitive losses be differentiated clinically? Would a left CVA (LCVA) or right CVA (RCVA) patient be more likely to have visuospatial perceptual deficits?

8. What are some questions the therapist needs to keep in mind while evaluating primary motor deficits in order to plan effective treatment?

9. Distinguish Broca's aphasia from Wernicke's aphasia. Would a LCVA or RCVA patient be more likely to have aphasia?

10. What precautions should be taken to prevent the poststroke patient from developing secondary motor deficits?

11. What are the occupational therapy goals for poststroke patients?

12. What are the arguments pro and con for starting activities of daily living training early poststroke?

13. What methods are appropriate to use to teach the LCVA patient? The RCVA patient? Why?

14. Along what continua are activities graded to improve cognitive functioning in poststroke patients?

15. Learning is a conscious and organized process. How does the therapist facilitate learning in the poststroke patient?

References

1. Levine, R. L. Diagnostic, medical, and surgical aspects of stroke management. In *Stroke Rehabilitation: The Recovery of Motor Control.* Edited by P. W. Duncan and M. B. Badke. Chicago: Year Book Medical Publishers, 1987.
2. Schuchmann, J. A. Stroke rehabilitation: minimizing the functional deficits. *Postgrad. Med., 74*(5): 101–111, 1983.
3. Mossman, P. L. *A Problem Oriented Approach to Stroke Rehabilitation.* Springfield, IL: Charles C Thomas, 1976.
4. Branch, E. F. The neuropathology of stroke. In *Stroke Rehabilitation: The Recovery of Motor Control.* Edited by P. W. Duncan and M. B. Badke. Chicago: Year Book Medical Publishers, 1987.
5. Bannister, R. *Brain's Clinical Neurology,* 4th edition. New York: Oxford University Press, 1973.
6. Bach-y-Rita, P., and Balliet, R. Recovery from stroke. In *Stroke Rehabilitation: The Recovery of Motor Control.* Edited by P. W. Duncan and M. B. Badke. Chicago: Year Book Medical Publishers, 1987.
7. Basmajian, J. V., and Gowland, C. Commentary. The many hidden faces of stroke: a call for action. *Arch. Phys. Med. Rehabil., 68*(5): 319, 1987.
8. Gordon, E. E. Editorial: toward a rational approach to motor disorder. *Arch. Phys. Med. Rehabil., 68*(5): 265–266, 1987.
9. Wade, D. T., and Hewer, R. L. Functional abilities after a stroke: measurement, natural history and prognosis. *J. Neurol. Neurosurg. Psychiatry, 50*: 177–182, 1987.
10. Braun, J. J. Time and recovery from brain damage. In *Recovery from Brain Damage: Research and Theory.* Edited by S. Finger. New York: Plenum, 1978.
11. Moore, J. C. Recovery potentials following CNS lesions: a brief historical perspective in relation to modern research data on neuroplasticity. *Am. J. Occup. Ther., 40*(7): 459–463, 1986.
12. Twitchell, T. E. The restoration of motor function following hemiplegia in man. *Brain, 74*: 443–480, 1951.
13. Bourestom, N. C. Predictors of long-term recovery in cerebrovascular disease. *Arch. Phys. Med. Rehabil., 48*(8): 415–419, 1967.
14. Brodal, A. Self-observations and neuro-anatomical considerations after a stroke. *Brain, 96*: 675–694, 1973.
15. Lawrence, D., and Kuypers, H. Pyramidal and non-pyramidal pathways in monkeys: anatomical and functional correlation. *Science, 148*(May 14): 973–975, 1965.
16. Wade, D. T., and Hewer, R. L. Stroke: associations with age, sex, and side of weakness. *Arch. Phys. Med. Rehabil., 67*(8): 540–545, 1986.
17. Skilbeck, C. E., et al. Recovery after stroke. *J. Neurol. Neurosurg. Psychiatry, 46*: 5–8, 1983.
18. Moskowitz, E., Lightbody, F., and Freitag, N. Long term followup of the poststroke patient. *Arch. Phys. Med. Rehabil., 53*(4): 167–172, 1972.
19. Gowland, C. Predicting sensorimotor recovery following stroke rehabilitation. *Physiotherapy Canada, 36*(6): 313–320, 1984.
20. Gowland, C. Recovery of motor function following stroke: profile and predictors. *Physiotherapy Canada, 34*: 77–84, 1982.
21. Caldwell, C. B., Wilson, D. J., and Braun, R. M. Evaluation and treatment of the upper extremity in the hemiplegic stroke patient. *Clin. Orthop., 63*: 69–93, 1969.
22. Denes, G., et al. Unilateral spatial neglect and recovery from hemiplegia. *Brain, 105*: 543–552, 1982.
23. Wade, D. T., Hewer, R. L., and Wood, V. A. Stroke: influence of patient's sex and side of weakness on outcome. *Arch. Phys. Med. Rehabil., 65*(9): 513–516, 1984.
24. Mills, V. M., and DiGenio, M. Functional differences in patients with left or right cerebrovascular accidents. *Phys. Ther., 63*(4): 481–488, 1983.
25. Brunnstrom, S. *Movement Therapy in Hemiplegia.* New York: Harper & Row, 1970.
26. Fugl-Meyer, A. R., et al. The post-stroke hemiplegic patient. I. A method for evaluation of physical performance. *Scand. J. Rehab. Med., 7*: 13–31, 1975.
27. Shah, S. K. Volition following hemiplegia. *Arch. Phys. Med. Rehabil., 61*(11): 523–528, 1980.
28. Brinkman, J., and Kuypers, H. Splitbrain monkeys: cerebral control of ipsilateral and contralateral arm, hand and finger movements. *Science, 176*(May 5): 536–538, 1972.
29. Trombly, C. A., et al. The effectiveness of therapy in improving finger extension in stroke patients. *Am. J. Occup. Ther., 40*(9): 612–617, 1986.
30. Smith, M. E., et al. Therapy impact on functional outcome in a controlled trial of stroke rehabilitation. *Arch. Phys. Med. Rehabil., 63*(1): 21–24, 1982.
31. Sine, R. D., et al. *Basic Rehabilitation Techniques: A Self-Instructional Guide,* 2nd edition. Rockville, MD: Aspen Systems Corporation, 1981.
32. Anderson, E. K. Sensory impairments in hemiplegia. *Arch. Phys. Med. Rehabil., 52*(7): 293–297, 1971.
33. Michels, E. Motor behavior in hemiplegia. *Phys. Ther., 45*: 759–767, 1965.
34. Gersten, J., Jung, A., and Brooks, C. Perceptual deficits in patients with left and right hemiparesis. *Am. J. Phys. Med., 51*: 79–85, 1972.
35. Leo, K. C., and Soderberg, G. L. Relationship between perception of joint position sense and limb synergies in patients with hemiplegia. *Phys. Ther., 61*(10): 1433–1437, 1981.
36. Ornstein, R. *The Psychology of Consciousness.* San Francisco: W. H. Freeman, 1972.
37. Fowler, R. S., and Fordyce, W. E. Stroke: why do they behave that way? (50-035-A) Dallas: American Heart Association, 1974.
38. Reinvang, I., and Sundet, K. The validity of functional assessment with neuropsychological tests in aphasic stroke patients. *Scand. J. Psychol., 26*: 208–218, 1985.
39. Farver, P. F., and Farver, T. B. Performance of normal older adults on tests designed to measure parietal lobe functions. *Am. J. Occup. Ther., 36*(7): 444–449, 1982.
40. Abreu, B. C., and Toglia, J. P. Cognitive rehabilitation: a model for occupational therapy. *Am. J. Occup. Ther., 41*(7): 439–448, 1987.
41. AOTA Commission on Uniform Reporting System Task Force. *Uniform Terminology for Reporting Occupational Therapy Services.* Rockville, MD: American Occupational Therapy Association, 1979.
42. Sahrmann, S. A., and Norton, B. J. The relationship of voluntary movement to spasticity in the upper motor neuron syndrome. *Ann. Neurol., 2*: 460–465, 1977.
43. Shah, S. K., Harasymiw, S. J., and Stahl, P. L. Stroke rehabilitation: outcome based on Brunnstrom recovery stages. *Occup. Ther. J. Res., 6*(6): 365–376, 1986.
44. Brennan, J. B. Clinical method of assessing tonus and voluntary movement in hemiplegia. *Br. Med. J., 1*(March 21): 767–768, 1959.
45. DeWeerdt, W. J. G., and Harrison, M. A. Measuring recovery of arm-hand function in stroke patients: a comparison of the Brunnstrom-Fugl-Meyer test and the Action Research Arm Test. *Physiotherapy Canada, 37*(2): 65–70, 1985.
46. Fugl-Meyer, A. R. Post-stroke hemiplegia assessment of physical properties. *Scand. J. Rehab. Med., Suppl 7*: 85–93, 1980.
47. Duncan, P. W., Propst, M., and Nelson, S. G. Reliability of the Fugl-Meyer assessment of sensorimotor recovery following cerebrovascular accident. *Phys. Ther., 63*(10): 1606–1610, 1983.
48. Lyle, R. C. A performance test for assessment of upper limb function in physical rehabilitation treatment and research. *Int. J. Rehab. Res., 4*(4): 483–492, 1981.
49. Jebsen, R. H., et al. Function of "normal" hand in stroke patients. *Arch. Phys. Med. Rehabil., 52*(4): 170–174, 1971.
50. Bell, E., Jurek, K., and Wilson, T. Hand skill: a gauge for treatment. *Am. J. Occup. Ther., 30*(2): 80–86, 1976.
51. Penfield, W. Speech perception and the uncommitted cortex. In *Brain and Conscious Experience.* Edited by J. C. Eccles. New York: Springer-Verlag, 1966.
52. Goodglass, H., and Kaplan, E. *The Assessment of Aphasia and Related Disorders.* Philadelphia: Lea & Febiger, 1972.
53. Levenson, C. Rehabilitation of the stroke hemiplegia patient. In *Handbook of Physical Medicine and Rehabilitation,* 2nd edition. Edited by F. H. Krusen, F. J. Kottke, and P. M. Ellwood. Philadelphia: W. B. Saunders, 1971.

54. Anderson, E., and Choy, E. Parietal lobe syndromes in hemiplegia: a program for treatment. *Am. J. Occup. Ther., 24*(1): 13–18, 1970.
55. Gallagher, S. Treating the acute stroke patient. *Physical Therapy Forum, 5*(9): 1, 3, 1986.
56. Bobath, B. Treatment of adult hemiplegia. *Physiotherapy, 63*(10): 310–313, 1977.
57. Carr, J., and Shepherd, R. *Early Care of the Stroke Patient: A Positive Approach.* London: William Heinemann Medical Books, 1976.
58. Katz, S., et al. Studies of illness in the aged. The index of ADL: a standardized measure of biological and psychosocial function. *J.A.M.A., 185*(12): 914–919, 1963.
59. Diller, L., and Weinberg, J. Differential aspects of attention in brain-damaged persons. *Percept. Mot. Skills., 35:* 71–81, 1972.
60. Fordyce, W. E., and Jones, R. H. The efficacy of oral and pantomime instructions for hemiplegic patients. *Arch. Phys. Med. Rehabil., 47*(10): 676–680, 1966.
61. Non-paralytic motor dysfunction after strokes. *Br. Med. J., 1*(6121): 1165–1166, 1978.
62. Diller, L. Perceptual and intellectual problems in hemiplegia: Implications for rehabilitation. *Med. Clin. North Am., 53*(3): 575–583, 1969.
63. Schmidt, S. M., et al. Status of stroke patients: a community assessment. *Arch. Phys. Med. Rehabil., 67*(2): 99–102, 1986.
64. Weisbroth, S., Esibill, N., and Zuger, R. R. Factors in the vocational success of hemiplegic patients. *Arch. Phys. Med. Rehabil., 52*(10): 441–446, 486, 1971.
65. Jones, R., Giddens, H., and Croft, D. Assessment and training of brain-damaged drivers. *Am. J. Occup. Ther., 37*(11): 754–760, 1983.
66. Eggers, O. *Occupational Therapy in the Treatment of Adult Hemiplegia.* London: William Heinemann Medical Books, 1983.
67. Weinberg, J., et al. Training sensory awareness and spatial organization in people with right brain damage. *Arch. Phys. Med. Rehabil., 60*(11): 491–496, 1979.
68. Vinograd, A., Taylor, E., and Grossman, S. Sensory retraining of the hemiplegic hand. *Am. J. Occup. Ther., 16*(5): 246–250, 1962.
69. Lorenze, E. J., and Cancro, R. Dysfunction in visual perception with hemiplegia: its relation to activities of daily living. *Arch. Phys. Med. Rehabil., 43:* 514–517, 1962.
70. Warren, M. Relationship of constructional apraxia and body scheme disorders to dressing performance in adult CVA. *Am. J. Occup. Ther., 35*(7): 431–437, 1981.
71. Sivak, M., et al. Improved driving performance following perceptual training in persons with brain damage. *Arch. Phys. Med. Rehabil., 65*(4): 163–167, 1984.
72. Benton, A. Reaction time in brain disease: some reflections. *Cortex, 22:* 129–140, 1986.
73. Carter, L. T., Howard, B. E., and O'Neil, W. A. Effectiveness of cognitive skill remediation in acute stroke patients. *Am. J. Occup. Ther., 37*(5): 320–326, 1983.
74. Nemec, R. E. Effects of controlled background interference on test performance by right and left hemiplegics. *J. Consult. Clin. Psychol., 46*(2): 294–297, 1978.
75. Takebe, K., et al. Biofeedback treatment of foot drop after stroke compared with standard rehabilitation techniques (part 2): effects on nerve conduction velocity and spasticity. *Arch. Phys. Med. Rehabil., 57*(1): 9–11, 1976.
76. Trombly, C. A., and Quintana, L. A. Differences in response to exercise by post-CVA and normal subjects. *Occup. Ther. J. Res., 5*(1): 39–58, 1985.
77. Nwaobi, O. M. Voluntary movement impairment in upper motor neuron lesions: is spasticity the main cause? *Occup. Ther. J. Res., 3*(3): 131–140, 1983.
78. Winstein, C. J. Motor learning considerations in stroke rehabilitation. In *Stroke Rehabilitation: The Recovery of Motor Control.* Edited by P. W. Duncan and M. B. Badke. Chicago: Year Book Medical Publishers, 1987.
79. Warren, M. L. A comparative study on the presence of the asymmetrical tonic neck reflex in adult hemiplegia. *Am. J. Occup. Ther., 38*(6): 386–392, 1984.
80. Carr, J. H., and Shepherd, R. B. *A Motor Relearning Programme for Stroke.* Rockville, MD: Aspen Systems Corporation, 1987.
81. Swenson, J. R. Therapeutic exercise in hemiplegia. In *Therapeutic Exercise,* 3rd edition. Edited by J. V. Basmajian. Baltimore: Williams & Wilkins, 1978.
82. DeSouza, L. H. The effects of sensation and motivation on regaining movement control following stroke. *Physiotherapy, 69*(7): 238–240, 1983.
83. Kimura, D. Acquisition of a motor skill after left-hemispheric damage. *Brain, 100:* 527–542, 1977.
84. Jason, G. W. Hemispheric asymmetries in motor function. I. Left-hemisphere specialization for memory but not performance. *Neuropsychologia, 21*(1): 35–45, 1983.
85. Gracanin, F. Functional electrical stimulation in control of motor output and movements. *Contemp. Clin. Neurophysiol. (EEG Suppl No. 34):* 355–368, 1978.
86. Baker, L. L., Yeh, C., Wilson, D., and Waters, R. L. Electrical stimulation of wrist and fingers for hemiplegic patients. *Phys. Ther., 59*(12): 1495–1499, 1979.
87. Nafpliotis, H. Electromyographic feedback to improve ankle dorsiflexion, wrist extension, and hand grasp. *Phys. Ther., 56*(7): 821–825, 1976.
88. Basmajian, J. V., et al. Stroke treatment: comparison of integrated behavioral-physical therapy vs traditional physical therapy programs. *Arch. Phys. Med. Rehabil., 68*(5): 267–272, 1987.
89. Van Ouwenaller, C., Laplace, P. M., and Chantraine, A. Painful shoulder in hemiplegia. *Arch. Phys. Med. Rehabil., 67*(1): 23–36, 1986.
90. Andersen, L. T. Shoulder pain in hemiplegia. *Am. J. Occup. Ther., 39*(1): 11–19, 1985.
91. Chaco, J., and Wolf, E. Subluxation of the glenohumeral joint in hemiplegia. *Am. J. Phys. Med., 50*(3): 139–143, 1971.
92. Basmajian, J. V., Regenos, E. M., and Baker, M. P. Rehabilitating stroke patients with biofeedback. *Geriatrics, 32:* 85–88, 1977.
93. Basmajian, J. V., and DeLuca, C. J. *Muscles Alives: Their Functions Revealed by Electromyography,* 5th edition. Baltimore: Williams & Wilkins, 1985.
94. Smith, R. O., and Okamoto, G. A. Checklist for the prescription of slings for the hemiplegic patient. *Am. J. Occup. Ther., 35*(2): 91–95, 1981.
95. Griffin, J. W. Hemiplegic shoulder pain. *Phys. Ther., 66*(12): 1884–1893, 1986.
96. Najenson, T., Yacubovich, E., and Pikielni, S. S. Rotator cuff injury in shoulder joints of hemiplegic patients. *Scand. J. Rehab. Med., 3:* 131–137, 1971.
97. Cailliet, R. *The Shoulder in Hemiplegia.* Philadelphia: F. A. Davis, 1980.
98. Wadsworth, C. T. Frozen shoulder. *Phys. Ther., 66*(12): 1878–1883, 1986.
99. Jensen, E. M. The hemiplegic shoulder. *Scand. J. Rehab. Med., Suppl 7:* 113–119, 1980.
100. Rizk, T. E., et al. Arthrographic studies in painful hemiplegic shoulders. *Arch. Phys. Med. Rehabil., 65*(5): 254–256, 1984.
101. Cripe, L., Lanier, D., and Palazon, A. *Occupational Range of Motion Guide.* Chicago, IL: Rehabilitation Institute of Chicago, undated.
102. Mathiowetz, V., Bolding, D. J., and Trombly, C. A. Immediate effects of positioning devices on the normal and spastic hand measured by electromyography. *Am. J. Occup. Ther., 37*(4): 247–254, 1983.
103. King, T. I. Plaster splinting as a means of reducing elbow flexor spasticity: a case study. *Am. J. Occup. Ther., 36*(10): 671–673, 1982.
104. Meredith, J., Taft, G., and Kaplan, P. Diagnosis and treatment of the hemiplegic patient with brachial plexus injury. *Am. J. Occup. Ther., 35*(10): 656–660, 1981.
105. Baumgarten, J. Hands on: stroke. Importance of physiological screening to occupational therapy assessment. *American Occupational Therapy Association Physical Disabilities Specialty Section Newsletter, 3*(3): 1–2, 1980.
106. Fordyce, W. Psychological assessment and management. In *Handbook of Physical Medicine and Rehabilitation,* 2nd edition. Edited by F. H. Krusen, F. J. Kottke, and P. M. Ellwood. Philadelphia: W. B. Saunders, 1971.
107. Bouchard, V. C. Hemiplegic exercise and discussion group. *Am. J. Occup. Ther., 26*(7): 330–331, 1972.
108. Fugl-Meyer, A. R., and Joasko, L. Post-stroke hemiplegia and sexual intercourse. *Scand. J. Rehab. Med., Suppl 7:* 158–166, 1980.
109. Diller, L., and Weinberg, J. Evidence for accident-prone behavior in hemiplegic patients. *Arch. Phys. Med. Rehabil., 51*(6): 358–363, 1970.
110. Logigan, M. K., Samuels, M. A., and Falconer, J. Clinical exercise trial for stroke patients. *Arch. Phys. Med. Rehabil., 64*(8): 364–367, 1983.
111. Dickstein, R., et al. Stroke rehabilitation: three exercise therapy approaches. *Phys. Ther., 66*(8): 1233–1238, 1986.
112. Stern, P. H., et al. Effects of facilitation exercise techniques in stroke rehabilitation. *Arch. Phys. Med. Rehabil., 51*(9): 526–531, 1970.
113. Inaba, M., et al. Effectiveness of functional training, active exercise, and resistive exercise for patients with hemiplegia. *Phys. Ther., 53*(1): 28–35, 1973.
114. Ottenbacher, K. J. The efficacy of rehabilitation for stroke patients. In *Outcomes of Stroke Rehabilitation: Research Resources and Implications for Occupational Therapy.* Edited by P. C. Ostrow, D. Lieberman, and S. C. Merrill. Rockville, MD: The American Occupational Therapy Association, 1985.

Supplementary Reading

American Occupational Therapy Association Practice Division. *CVA (Stroke)*. Rockville, MD: American Occupational Therapy Association, 1983.

Barbour, R. Jar holder lends a hand. *Accent on Living, 30*(2): 62–63, 1985.

Carr, J. H., et al. Investigation of a new motor assessment scale for stroke patients. *Phys. Ther., 65*(2): 175–180, 1985.

Davies, B., and Knapp, M. A treatment for the hemiplegic arm. *Br. J. Occup. Ther., 49*(7): 225–226, 1986.

DeSouza, L. H., Hewer, R. L., and Miller, S. Assessment of recovery of arm control in hemiplegic stroke patients. 1. Arm function tests. *Int. Rehab. Med., 2:* 3–9, 1980.

Dudgeon, B. J., DeLisa, J. A., and Miller, R. M. Optokinetic nystagmus and upper extremity dressing independence after stroke. *Arch. Phys. Med. Rehabil., 66*(3): 164–167, 1985.

Haaland, K. Y., and Delaney, H. D. Motor deficits after left or right hemisphere damage due to stroke or tumor. *Neuropsychologia, 19:* 17–27, 1981.

Harlowe, D., and Van Deusen, J. Construct validation of the St. Mary's CVA evaluation: perceptual measures. *Am. J. Occup. Ther., 38*(3): 184–186, 1984.

Harlowe, D., and Van Deusen, J. Evaluating cutaneous sensation following CVA: relationships among touch, pain, and temperature tests. *Occup. Ther. J. Res., 5*(1): 70–72, 1985.

Johnstone, M. *Restoration of Motor Function in the Stroke Patient.* New York: Churchill Livingstone, 1983.

Jongbloed, L. E., Collins, J. B., and Jones, W. A sensorimotor integration test battery for CVA clients: preliminary evidence of reliability and validity. *Occup. Ther. J. Res., 6*(3): 131–150, 1986.

Logigan, M. *Adult Rehabilitation: A Team Approach.* Boston: Little, Brown & Co., 1982.

Lord, J. P., and Hall, K. Neuromuscular reeducation versus traditional programs for stroke rehabilitation. *Arch. Phys. Med. Rehabil., 67*(2): 88–91, 1986.

Malkmus, D. Integrating cognitive strategies into the physical therapy setting. *Phys. Ther., 63*(12): 1952–1959, 1983.

Matyas, T. A., Galea, M. P., and Spicer, S. D. Facilitation of the maximum voluntary contraction in hemiplegia by concomitant cutaneous stimulation. *Am. J. Phys. Med., 65*(3): 125–134, 1986.

National Stroke Association. *The Road Ahead: A Stroke Recovery Guide.* Denver, CO: The National Stroke Association, 1986.

National Stroke Association. *Open Channels* (newsletter). Denver, CO: The National Stroke Association.

Ostendorf, C. G., and Wolf, S. L. Effect of forced use of the upper extremity of a hemiplegic patient on changes in function. *Phys. Ther., 61*(7): 1022–1028, 1981.

Ryerson, S. D. Hemiplegia resulting from vascular insult or disease. In *Neurological Rehabilitation.* Edited by D. A. Umphred. St. Louis: C. V. Mosby, 1985.

Selley, W. G. Swallowing difficulties in stroke patients: a new treatment. *Age Aging, 14:* 361–365, 1985.

Sharpless, J. W. *Mossman's A Problem-Oriented Approach to Stroke Rehabilitation.* Springfield, IL: Charles C Thomas, 1982.

Siev, E., Freishtat, B., and Zoltan, B. *Perceptual and Cognitive Dysfunction in the Adult Stroke Patient: A Manual for Evaluation and Treatment.* Thorofare, NJ: Slack Incorporated, 1986.

Trombly, C. A., and Quintana, L. A. The effects of exercise on finger extension of CVA patients. *Am. J. Occup. Ther., 37*(3): 195–202, 1983.

Twist, D. J. Effects of a wrapping technique on passive range of motion in a spastic upper extremity. *Phys. Ther., 65*(3): 299–304, 1985.

Van Deusen Fox, J. Construct validation of occupational therapy measures used in CVA evaluation: a beginning. *Am. J. Occup. Ther., 38*(2): 101–106, 1984.

Van Deusen, J., and Harlowe, D. Continued construct validation of the St. Mary's CVA evaluation: Brunnstrom arm and hand stage ratings. *Am. J. Occup. Ther., 40*(8): 561–563, 1986.

Van Deusen, J., and Harlowe, D. Continued construct validation of the St. Mary's CVA evaluation: bilateral awareness scale. *Am. J. Occup. Ther., 41*(4): 242–245, 1987.

vanRavensberg, C. D., et al. Visual perception in hemiplegic patients. *Arch. Phys. Med. Rehabil., 65*(6): 304–309, 1984.

Wade, D. T., et al. The hemiplegic arm after stroke: measurement and recovery. *J. Neurol. Neurosurg. Psychiatry, 46:* 521–524, 1983.

Wilson, D. J., Baker, L. L., and Craddock, J. A. Functional test for the hemiparetic upper extremity. *Am. J. Occup. Ther., 38*(3): 159–164, 1984.

Woodson, A. M. Proposal for splinting the adult hemiplegic hand to promote function. *Occupational Therapy in Health Care, 4*(3/4): 85–96, 1987.

chapter
23

Degenerative Diseases

Catherine A. Trombly and Anna Deane Scott

Degenerative diseases involve pathology that leads to progressive disability. This chapter will describe the evaluation and treatment of degenerative diseases commonly seen in rehabilitation programs. Multiple sclerosis is representative of diseases in which cerebellar signs of ataxia and intention tremor are often prominent. Parkinson's disease is representative of basal ganglia disorders with rigidity, akinesia, and resting tremor. Amyotrophic lateral sclerosis is a degenerative disease of the upper motor neurons as well as the lower motor neurons of the spinal cord and brain stem. Post polio syndrome involves the lower motor neurons of the spinal cord and brain stem. Weakness is the outstanding problem that patients with these diseases have.

The goal of treatment is to delay the degenerative effects of the disease and to maintain a level of function. Treatment is directed toward management of existing symptoms, prevention of deformity, and compensation for lost abilities to maintain independence in occupational performance tasks. Periodic reevaluations are done to determine whether there has been any decline in function, or whether function is being maintained.

Multiple Sclerosis

Multiple sclerosis (M.S.), or disseminated sclerosis, involves patches of demyelination in the white matter of the brain and/or spinal cord followed by the overgrowth of glial cells that form sclerotic plaques creating focal lesions of the central nervous system. It usually begins between the ages of 20 and 40 years. Although the cause remains unknown, some related factors have been identified and much of the current literature reflects continuing research efforts to identify the cause.[1] Multiple sclerosis is more prevalent in Canada, northern Europe, and northern United States. There is a familial tendency to develop the disease, but the explanation for this appears to be common exposure to an environmental factor rather than heredity.[2] Some precipitating factors include influenza and upper respiratory tract infections, pregnancy, sur-

gery, tooth extraction, and electric shock.[1] Current theories regarding etiology suggest that M.S. could be a rare sequel of a childhood viral infection, because patients with M.S. have a high antibody titer to measles and herpes viruses.[1] It is suspected that a childhood virus with a long latency is activated by a secondary factor later in life and that M.S. is an autoimmune reaction that attacks the myelin.[2,3] However, there is still not enough evidence to confirm either a viral cause or that M.S. is an autoimmune reaction.[1,2]

The disease may have an acute onset beginning with one or more focal lesions or the onset may be subacute usually involving slowly progressing lower-extremity weakness, spasticity, ataxia, and sensory loss.[1] Lesions continue to develop after onset. The course may be acute, with rapid decline of function, or it may be slowly progressive. Remissions and exacerbations are characteristic of M.S., but the intervals between episodes are highly variable and unpredictable.[1] Deterioration of movement control continues even when a relapse cannot be clinically identified.[4,5]

Symptoms reflect the location of the plaques or areas of demyelination. Therefore, each patient has a unique constellation of symptoms that may include one or more of the following. Incoordination (dysmetria, dyssynergia, ataxia, and intention tremor) due to loss of cerebellar control is a common sign. Muscle weakness and spasticity, especially of the lower extremities, indicate plaques within the spinal cord. Cerebellar hypotonia can also be manifested as weakness. Sensory involvement may include anesthesia, paresthesia, and/or loss of a particular modality, especially proprioception and stereognosis due to plaques in the sensory tracts. Diplopia and nystagmus reflect brain stem involvement. Other visual impairments may include decreased acuity or blurring. Dysarthria ("slurring speech") and dysphagia may be seen. Frontal lobe signs of mild dementia with loss of judgment, intellect,[6] and/or recent memory[6-8] can be seen in some patients, as can emotional lability or euphoria, a false sense of well-being.[9] Patients who are mentally aware may be anxious, depressed, or irritable.[10] There may be bladder incontinence, but bowel incontinence is seldom a problem.[2,7]

EVALUATION

Possible symptoms must be carefully evaluated because of the uniqueness of each patient's constellation and because the patient, due to euphoria, may fail to recognize changes in physical status.[1] Muscle tone, coordination, sensation, cognitive function, emotional status, range of motion, muscle strength if voluntary movement is preserved, endurance, and performance of occupational performance tasks, including work and leisure time activities, should be evaluated using the procedures described throughout this book. If visual symptoms are not evaluated by other professionals, the occupational therapist needs to do so because visual defects will affect decisions concerning adaptations as well as teaching methods. Throughout the evaluation the therapist should attend to strengths and assets that can be used in training the patient to compensate for losses and can serve as a basis for alleviating feelings of depression and hopelessness.

Fatigue must be avoided[1] because relapses are related to exhaustion[11] and other stresses. To reduce the stress on the patient, only those functions suspected to be diminished—from observation of how the patient moves and interacts with the environment—should be formally tested. The evaluation should be planned so that rest periods are given and position changes kept to a minimum to prevent fatigue, which is both detrimental to the patient and affects the validity and reliability of evaluation results.[12]

Interpretation of evaluation data results in a problem list from which goals are developed. Treatment goals must be realistic and directed toward relief of the debilitating effects of existing problems, prevention of additional problems, and maintenance of current abilities and level of functioning. Goals may include: (1) to improve coordination, (2) to increase or maintain strength and endurance, (3) to prevent contractures and decubiti, (4) to facilitate emotional adjustment to the disability and its uncertain course, (5) to improve cognitive strategies and safety, and (6) to improve or maintain performance of daily life tasks.

TREATMENT

Precautions must be observed concerning fatigue, heat, or other physical or psychological stress. During acute exacerbations the treatment of choice is essentially no treatment with complete bed rest and avoidance of all exertion.[13] At other times, scheduling of treatment by all members of the rehabilitation team is done in such a way as to avoid generalized fatigue. More patients become fatigued in the afternoon, but each person's peak time for activity is different and should be taken into consideration.[14] Localized muscle fatigue must also be avoided since it can lead to decreased muscle strength. High body temperatures can result in an exacerbation of the disease; therefore, treatment should be done in cool, nonhumid places.[14,15]

It is important to note that vigorous exercise can raise body temperature just as weather and infection do.

Motor Control/Coordination

Those patients who show cerebellar symptoms of incoordination are able to do planned movement but are unable to control the smoothness and accuracy of the movement. These patients have intact motor programs, in contrast to patients with cortical lesions, but there is a timing problem.[16,17] The cause for this is as yet unknown. Hypotheses are the following: (1) The feedback is too slow to guide the output or there is a problem integrating the feedback with the output command.[17] (2) The output command reaches antagonistic muscles at abnormal times so that the muscles contract out of normal sequence during smooth movements.[17,18] (3) There is a delay in the selection of the program, as demonstrated by increased reaction time, especially premotor time, in cerebellar patients.[17] (Premotor time is that time from the signal to move to the initial activation of muscle. It is considered processing time during which the meaning of the stimulus and the selection of the response are determined.) (4) Incoordinated patients may have too many motor memories related to one movement.[19] In the process of learning a movement, reafference (feedback of movement) did not fully match the efference (motor command) to confirm the correctness of the command. Therefore, the next time such a task was attempted, a new movement program was generated so no movement program was actually practiced enough to build up one strong engram that became the main program for that task. According to this hypothesis, what the patient has, then, are many programs for the same task and his output fluctuates among them.

How these hypotheses can direct treatment is still obscure. None has sufficient support to adopt it as the basis for treatment. However, they do suggest innovative approaches to treatment of cerebellar problems usually considered unamenable to improvement. Few controlled studies, and no definitive studies, have been done on treatments to restore motor control in patients with cerebellar deficits or to tap alternate behavior strategies to promote functional recovery.[4] It has been generally believed that motor control could not be relearned or recovered by these patients. Treatment, therefore, concentrated on teaching the patient to compensate for his motor problems while offering restorative treatment to stem the tide of debility due to inactivity. Based on the above hypotheses, therapists might be inclined to investigate whether providing visual or auditory feedback would improve movement (see chapter 12), or whether repeated movement within a guided track would result in development of a given motor program and enhanced coordination by ensuring similarity of motion and therefore feedback.

Treatments that have been devised serendipitously or from reflection on other hypothesized bases for the manifested motor problems include the following. *Cooling of the extensor surface* of the forearm markedly reduced intention tremor in 8 of 13 patients of various cerebellar diagnoses.[20] A 0° C water bottle was applied on the extensor surface for a period that varied between 7 and 30 min. After 30 min of cooling, one patient was tremor free for 30 additional min. Neither cooling of the flexor surface nor warming of either surface reduced tremor, but warming of the extensor surface actually increased the tremor in almost half of the patients tested.[20] No follow-up research appears to have been done to validate these findings or to determine what variables were associated with improvement in the 8 patients but not the other 5.

Based on an hypothesis that circulatory insufficiency in the white matter of the brain and spinal cord causes ischemia, which influences the formation of plaques, *a rest and exercise program (R.E.P.)* was devised with the aim of increasing circulation to these areas.[11] Positive results were reported for 69 patients placed on the program, which consisted of alternating rest and exercise. The R.E.P. started with 24 hours of total rest and then two to three rest periods of 10 to 20 min each day, with stressful exercises carried out before, or sometimes after, the rest period. The exercises were of the aerobic type and included push-ups, calisthenics on the mat, running, cycling, sports, gardening, or weight lifting, depending on the patient's degree of disability. Signs of increased circulation (dyspnea, increased heart rate, flushing of the skin on the face, head, and neck) were sought as a result of the exercise. The hypothesis of the R.E.P. program is interesting and although successes have been reported by the group that originated the program, no further reports have been seen. Because fatigue is a serious precaution, very careful monitoring of patients needs to be done if a program such as this is tried.

Weighted cuffs and utensils are regularly used to compensate for intention tremor during daily activities. *Adding weight to the limb* is also being studied as a treatment to improve motor control. Two studies have found a reduction of intention tremor in 36% and 64% of patients of various cerebellar diagnoses.[21,22] The weights used were 60-gm pieces of lead that fitted into a wrist band so that the weight was distributed around the wrist as opposed to the flexors or extensors exclusively. An optimal weight, ranging from 600 to 840 gm, was found for each patient independent of severity of tremor. Interestingly, increasing the weight above optimum value produced no further improvement and in fact increased tremor in some patients, reduced limb function when there was weakness, and increased fatigue even when there was no weakness.[21,22] The mechanism for improvement is unknown. The hypotheses include increased awareness and attention to the weighted limb; increased momentum of the limb resulting in increased tension in the antagonists to improve agonist/antagonist timing; or increased inertia of the system that damps the oscillations.[22]

Another treatment program was based on the assumption that motor control can be regained through learning and that only voluntary movement and effort can result in *learning, or relearning of movement strategies.*[4] The movement and its relevance for everyday activities are taught together, similar to the Carr and Shepherd Approach (chapter 6, part E). Active assistive movement is used if the patient is grossly disabled. The patient is guided by voice rather than by therapist's hands so that movement control is seen by the patient as a product of his own efforts rather than the manipulation skill of the therapist. This approach gives patients a sense of control, important in overcoming depression.[4] No reflex-based procedures, such as proprioceptive neuromuscular facilitation (PNF) and sensory stimulation described by Rood, are used in this program.[4] Also, when the patient shows no progress in therapy, it is considered a period of consolidation of learning and is used to reinforce previous learning; it is not considered an indication for discontinuing therapy,[4] which is a positive, refreshing attitude in the treatment of these patients.

In summary, there are no proven treatments to improve motor control in patients with cerebellar dysfunction. Several interesting ideas and hypotheses have been presented and may be worth trying. In any degenerative disease of unknown etiology, delay of the degenerative effects of the disease remains the primary treatment objective while efforts continue to discover treatment methods to effect an essential change in symptoms. If motor control cannot be improved, then compensatory methods described in Part Five of this book will need to be taught to the patient and/or family.

Strength and Endurance

Decreased muscle strength resulting from anterior horn cell destruction or motor tract involvement, which is associated with spasticity, cannot be significantly improved, but weakness and reduced endurance secondary to inactivity or disuse can be improved.[15] Activities to increase strength follow the principles of applying graded resistance to stress the muscle within the limits of fatigue (chapter 9), whereas those to increase endurance follow the principle of increasing the duration (chapter 9) or increasing the metabolic equivalent level requirement of activities (chapter 30).

Prevention of Contractures

Contractures limit range of motion, which hinders functional abilities. Two symptoms seen in M.S. patients, spasticity and weakness, unless treated prophylactically, can result in deforming contractures. Daily movement of each joint through the full range[13,15] with gentle stretching of tight muscles,[12] together with splinting to maintain range or to provide a slight sustained stretch[13] are used to prevent contractures (chapters 9 and 13).

Prevention of Decubiti

Prevention of decubiti is another important goal of treatment for all disciplines working with the patient. The occupational therapist should ensure that during activity or when using splints or equipment that trauma, heat, cold, and pressure are avoided on skin areas where there is sensory loss. The patient should be reminded to change position at least every 2 hours[15] whether in bed or in a wheelchair. A wheelchair cushion (chapter 3) and push-ups to relieve pressure (chapter 28) are important.

Emotional Adjustment

Psychological support is important in all rehabilitation programs,[15] and it has been noted that patients with M.S. respond favorably to the interest and encouragement given by all therapists.[11] The best protection against depression is an internal locus of control tempered by a realistic assessment of disease-related limits.[10] The occupational therapist can help the patient to identify life goals and values and encourage him to realistically take control to direct his rehabilitation and life toward these goals. Training in activities of daily living (ADL) using acceptable modifications that enable independence will help the patient to limit his sense of inability and disablement. Group activity therapy that includes skill development activities and tasks related to work, home maintenance, and leisure interests and that focuses around problem solving and sharing of experiences and reactions offers the patient physical and psychological benefits.[23,24] See chapter 2 for group therapy ideas and procedures.

Patient education concerning management of daily life by balancing exercise with relaxation and making the patient aware of the relationship of exercise to function[4] diminishes the patient's depressive responses to the disease. Because M.S. patients with spinal cord involvement are liable to experience sexual problems similar to those described for the spinal cord-injured patient (chapter 28), sexual counseling should be available for those who desire it. Informing the patient's spouse of the effects of the disease and compensatory methods for sexual satisfaction is suggested.[13]

Cognitive/Perceptual Functions

Although euphoria and poor safety judgment have been observed by therapists for a long time, no attempt has been made to treat these symptoms since they are considered unalterable manifestations of the disease process. Further study of these patients suggests that memory and other neuropsychological functions are also impaired. Short-term memory, recall of both verbal and visual information, and learning in both modalities have been found impaired in patients in early and middle phases of M.S.[8] They were found to require more trials to learn than normal subjects did, but even after learning occurred they were less able to recall bits of information than normal subjects.[8] After evaluating the patient to determine his specific deficits, remediation using methods suggested in chapter 7 could be attempted. If improvement does not occur, then compensatory methods of approaching or coping with daily life tasks (chapter 7) will need to be taught to the patient and/or family members.

Performance of Occupational Performance Tasks

Compensation to enable independence will address whichever symptoms the patient has that interfere with performance. Adapted methods and equipment available to assist the patient in compensating for deficits that limit independence in self-care, homemaking, work, and leisure pursuits are found in Part Five and in chapter 7. Ideas suggested in chapter 28 pertaining to compensation for weakness and in chapter 30 pertaining to low endurance are applicable to patients with M.S. also.

Depending on the severity of the disease, the patient may need adaptations and training for tasks requiring fine coordination such as eating, writing, using fasteners, etc., or, if the disability is more extensive, training for whole body tasks such as mobility and transfers. The need for mechanical aids increases as the disease progresses. The severely disabled patient can activate the television, radio, lights, and other electronic devices using an environmental control unit[15]; the control unit may need an adapted switch to enable the patient to utilize it.

Compensation for problems of incoordination involves stabilization. Stability can be gained by widening the base of postural support, by reducing the number of linkages to be controlled, or by the use of weights. Stabilizing the proximal part of the extremity reduces the number of joints needing control, which limits need for control to the distal part of the limb. The upper arms can be stabilized by holding them against the sides of the body or by holding the elbows or forearms against the table. The distal part can be stabilized directly for fine activities such as writing by holding one wrist with the other hand. Use of weighted tools or a weighted wrist cuff also directly stabilizes the distal part of the limb.

Patients who have a tendency to rush to complete tasks during periods of "energy high"[14] should be taught to pace activities and to balance activity with rest. Energy conservation methods are appropriately used with these patients.

A patch over one eye can be used to eliminate the problem of double vision; this is beneficial even at the sacrifice of depth perception.[13,15]

If decreased judgment resulting from euphoria or denial interferes with the patient's safety for independent living, especially in relation to the use of the stove, bathtub, knives, or automobile, and if retraining does not improve the situation, then the patient must be discharged to a supervised living situation and prohibited from undertaking tasks that threaten his or others' safety.

The National Multiple Sclerosis Society has helpful literature available to patients and their families. Local chapters offer many services including education, referral to community resources, and assistance with obtaining direct care.

Parkinson's Disease

Parkinson's disease (P.D.) is characterized by slowing and diminution of voluntary and emotional movements, rigidity, and resting tremor,[1,7,25,26] although the prominence of each of these symptoms differs from patient to patient. It is caused by ideopathic degeneration of neurons in the substantia nigra. Normally neurons from the substantia nigra pass to the striatum, which has the highest dopamine content in the brain. When these neurons are destroyed, dopamine content of the substantia nigra is reduced. There is an upset in the balance between dopaminergic activity (inhibitory) and cholinergic activity (excitatory) on the cells of the basal ganglia. This condition can be somewhat corrected by administering dopamine, in the form of L-dopa, to the parkinsonian patient.[1]

Infections or toxic agents also may cause this disorder.

Onset may be abrupt but generally is insidious.[27] It usually occurs after age 60, with no preference for sex, race, or climate.[7,26] The disease progresses slowly[26] to complete immobility and death. The rate of deterioration varies from 2 years up to 20 years.[1,28] Patients with tremor as the major symptom have a better prognosis than patients with rigidity and slowness of movement.

The appearance of patients with P.D. reflects the triad of clinical signs: resting or nonintention tremor, akinesia or bradykinesia, and rigidity. The first symptom to appear is tremor, which begins in the hand or foot and may spread throughout all limbs.[27] Tremor at rest is increased by stress, decreased by fatigue, and eliminated during sleep.[29] Rigidity develops, especially in the flexor muscles of the trunk and limbs,[12] to produce the typical stooped posture: head bowed; body bent forward; elbows, knees, and hips flexed; thumbs flexed across the palms;[27] and metacarpophalangeal joints flexed with interphalangeal joints extended. Akinesia is the basis of the characteristic festinating gait of small, fast, shuffling steps[2,30] that propels the body (which inclines more and more forward as the disease progresses) forward until the patient hits a wall or falls in order to stop. Arm swing is lost or diminished.[30] Akinesia results in reduced frequency or rate of certain movements and contributes to the clinical picture seen, for example: lack of facial expression, reduced eye movements, and drooling.[7] Automatic balance and equilibrium adjustments are not made in patients with akinesia.[26] Speech is characteristically monotone with low volume[31] and shows lack of emotional expression, tremulousness, and blocking,[31] all of which parallel motor problems seen in the rest of the body. Effects of autonomic dysfunction are excessive sweating, greasy skin, bladder dysfunction, and flushing of the skin.[25,28]

The basal ganglia, in general, are responsible for execution of maturationally acquired anticipatory postural reflexes and the automatic running of learned motor plans.[32,33] Patients retain simple motor programs, but automatic execution of whole motor sequences is disturbed.[32,33] Patients exhibit delay in initiation of movement, slowness in execution, inability to smoothly move from sequence to sequence within a total motor action,[34] and inability to do two tasks at once since each requires full attention[32] (see chapter 5). Akinesia is the term given to impaired ability to initiate voluntary and spontaneous motor responses.[35] It is characterized by hesitance to begin a movement, inability to gradually halt a movement, or

the interruption of performance of an ongoing movement ("freezing")[26] when attention is distracted. Bradykinesia refers to slowness or decreased velocity of movement. There are multiple mechanisms potentially responsible for bradykinesia[35] that are under study.

Although patients with P.D. have difficulty initiating movement, particularly in the absence of an external trigger,[36] from the findings of one study it appears that they are able to select correct motor responses indicating that they do not have a disorder of the perceptual or decision-making systems.[35] They do seem to lack a sufficient arousal level that normally keeps the motor system ready to react on command or at will. They are less quick to correct their false moves than normal persons, which suggests an impairment of proprioceptive monitoring.[35] Some patients do seem able to use prior information to guide ongoing movement, once initiated, and do not have to rely totally on visual feedback[36] to compensate for proprioceptive inattention. P.D. patients also require more time to complete movements, which may indicate faulty transmission from the decision-making system to the upper motor neuron motor apparatus[35] or a need to repetitively activate small motor programs. They have been found unable to do large-scale ballistic movements. However, the centrally programmed triphasic activity pattern of the agonist-antagonist-agonist,[37] characteristic of ballistic movement, is preserved. They can successfully do small ballistic movements but fall short of the target in large movements, necessitating many cycles of this pattern.[37] There appears to be a reduction in the number of motor units activated for each cycle.[37]

It is hypothesized that patients with P.D. abnormally process mechanoreceptor sensory input utilized in the generation and execution of movement.[38] Results of a study in which P.D. patients and controls were compared on their ability to track various waveforms displayed on an oscilloscope indicated that (1) the patients had a decreased repertoire of movements; (2) ballistic (preprogramed) movements were slow; (3) the movements were broken into two or more smaller movements once a given amplitude was exceeded; (4) visual feedback was required, suggesting that sensory input from mechanoreceptors was not sufficient to maintain the movement's course; and (5) the patients' performance did not improve with repetition.[38]

Neuropsychological deficits, although not previously suspected, are being investigated in patients with P.D. In one study that looked at apraxia in P.D., there was a significant inability to do unfamiliar, nonrepresentational gestures as compared to representational gestures. Both types were found to be done significantly worse by P.D. patients than by normal subjects, suggesting a perceptual spatial deficit-based apraxia.[39] Another possible perceptual deficit was found in P.D. patients' ability to trace and do construction tasks. However, the difficulty was thought to be a deficit in sequential and predictive movement, rather than spatial perception, *per se*.[40] Studies need to be done to test perceptual spatial abilities separate from motor abilities in order to determine whether P.D. patients actually have perceptual deficits. Tests known to reveal frontal lobe damage were administered to 30 mildly disabled P.D. patients and no abnormalities of general intelligence or memory were found.[41] There were significant differences in the ability to shift conceptual sets and in the number of perseverative errors compared to the test results for normal subjects, however.[41]

EVALUATION

The selection of the evaluation procedures to be completed is based on knowledge of typical symptoms. Commonly used evaluations include range of motion, muscle tone, righting reactions and other automatic postural movements, speed and accuracy of voluntary movement, and functional performance in daily living tasks. Sensory testing done under conditions of full attention to stimuli and distracted attention may help the therapist determine procedures to use to increase movement or to guide patient education regarding compensation.

Ongoing evaluation of the effect of medication on function is done, since therapists who work with these patients daily are in a good position to observe behavior indicative of side effects that might otherwise be missed.[42] One medication, L-dopa, administered to restore the balance between dopamine and acetylcholine, is effective in the treatment of parkinsonism and is therefore commonly used. It is particularly effective in decreasing bradykinesia and rigidity,[1,25,28] but ameliorates all symptoms to some degree.[42-44] The side effects include gastrointestinal symptoms such as nausea, vomiting, and anorexia; cardiovascular changes such as dizziness, orthostatic hypotension, and irregular heart rhythm; or central nervous system changes such as involuntary dyskinetic movements, confusion, agitation, depression, hallucinations, or drowsiness.[28,42,45]

A problem list is developed from those evaluation data that indicate function is in jeopardy and treatment goals are developed. Occupational therapy goals, in general, for patients with P.D. include (1) to increase mobility and prevent deformities, (2) to improve initiation of movement and to increase the amplitude and velocity of ongoing movement, (3) to improve psychosocial status, and (4) to improve or maintain independent performance of daily life tasks.

TREATMENT

Treatment suggestions listed here need study to determine their effectiveness. Until such documentation is available, treatment remains on a trial-and-error basis.

Increase Mobility/Prevent Deformities

Rigidity and akinesia produce a stiff, inanimate patient. Mobility of the neck and trunk are important because head movements lead body movements in the quick adjustments needed in response to disturbances of equilibrium. Acceleration, deceleration, and rotation are vestibular stimuli recommended by Rood to mobilize the neck and trunk.[46] PNF techniques such as chopping, lifting, and unilateral diagonal patterns also may be beneficial in improving trunk mobility (chapter 6, part D). Biofeedback to relax the rigidity might help mobilize the trunk or proximal joints of the limbs (chapter 12).

To relate neck and trunk rotation (which also tends to neutralize excess truncal tone) to function and to promote mobility responses of the proximal joints of the upper extremities, activities that incorporate reaching from side to side could be used. Rapid, rhythmical movements rather than resistive ones are most appropriate for developing mobility responses (see chapter 5). Music can be used to establish and maintain the rhythm.

The Rood Approach (chapter 6, part A) addresses problems of the parkinsonian patient with the goals of increasing protective, mobility responses of the face and increasing proximal mobility and distal stability.[46] Sharp smells, such as that of vinegar, can be used to activate a protective, withdrawal response of facial muscles. Grasp of an object provides distal stability that reduces tremor. Many activities, such as leather punching and hammering, involve resisted grasp. Since resistance produces stability, it should be avoided in treatment of the trunk and proximal parts of the limbs.

Treatment to prevent deformities beyond increasing the patient's general level of active mobility is the same as listed above and in chapters 9 and 13.

Initiation of Movement and Enhancement of Ongoing Movement

Tactile, visual, or auditory cues to evoke movement and/or "pumping up" may be needed to enable the patient with P.D. to initiate movement. The PNF technique of "pumping up" is one in which the body part to be used in an activity is moved several times passively and rhythmically through the pattern of movement sought.[47] Then the patient is asked to assist in the movement.[47] After several more repetitions, the therapist withdraws and allows the patient to move independently.

Several treatment programs designed to improve initiation and movement quality have been published and are cited here. One program of therapeutic exercise was administered to 50 patients in conjunction with L-dopa treatment.[28] The goals were to increase mobility and to improve the speed and coordination of movement. Active exercises followed PNF patterns, and the PNF techniques of rhythmic initiation and slow reversal were also used (chapter 6, part D). Neck and trunk rotation exercises were done to increase mobility and improve balance. Hanging from an overhead bar to put prolonged stretch on upper-extremity flexors and exercises involving prone extension with particular emphasis on the shoulder abduction component were done to help correct the typical fixed posture. Breathing exercises, gait training, and group therapy to increase socialization and improve motivation toward independence were also included in the program. Heavy resistance, which decreases mobility,[28] was used to reduce the tremor by having the patient grasp an object while exercising. Improvement in initiation of movement, controlling movement direction, and mobility were seen as a result of this program.[28]

Based on the idea that integration of sensory information is an essential aspect of development of preprogrammed (ballistic) movements and that P.D. patients have a defect in their capacity to use kinesthetic feedback to predict the subsequent course of movement[38] and seem to ignore proprioceptive input,[26] treatments involving sensory stimuli other than proprioceptive stimuli have met with some success. In one study on the influence of sensory stimuli on the initiation of motion, 10 P.D. patients were compared to 5 normal subjects. The elapsed time between application of a stimulus and initiation and completion of movement were measured. Two motions were tested (90° of elbow flexion and 90° of elbow extension of the dominant arm) under four stimulus conditions. Stimuli included a light, a click, a shout, and a touch on the shoulder. All subjects completed the eight tests to establish a baseline. The patients were then placed on a 3-week exercise program in which the same stimuli were used to initiate movement. Posttest scores showed a significant improvement in the mean time for patients on seven of the eight tests. When compared to normal subjects on the pretest, the patients had scored significantly worse than the normal subjects, but they did not significantly differ on the posttest. This study supports the use of sensory stimuli to increase speed of initiation of movement.[48,49] Improvement also was noted in all patients in areas of performance other than arm movements, including speech and ambulation.[48,49]

Whether the patient can ever develop voluntary initiation or must remain dependent on another for premovement stimuli has not been documented.

Improve Psychosocial Status

The parkinsonian patient is faced with several psychosocial problems: physical isolation imposed by the disability, social isolation imposed by the inactive face and voice, and depression. Feedback from a mirror can be used beneficially to help the patient become aware of his facial expression and to make an effort to appear more animated, which is important to facilitate social interaction and to increase feelings of belonging. Counseling for the family is important so that they understand the patient's problems because the lack of facial expression and the slowness of movement can be misinterpreted as lack of interest or stubborness.

Not to be overlooked is the beneficial effect of interest and attention that active participation in a well-planned and well-supervised group program provides. Suggestions for group therapy to help the patient deal

th the progressive, disabling nature of the disease can be found in chapter 2. Day treatment programs can keep the patient active and interacting with others to alleviate depression as well as improve function.

One group program was constituted with the goal of maintaining the functional status of patients.[34] The program was tested using a two-group, experimental design in which 16 patients were randomly assigned to treatment or control conditions. They were evaluated on ADL, dexterity, physical and motor signs of the disease, and sense of well-being four times: before the program and immediately, 6 months, and 1 year after the program concluded. The entire experiment was repeated four times with four different groups of patients. The rehabilitation group treatment consisted of 10 2-hour sessions (2 per week). Each session followed this format: welcome and socialization, mobility activities, rest and socialization, dexterity activities, functional activities, educational activities, and departure and socialization.[34] To address the problems of initiation and slowness of movement, they used imitation and mirror feedback, visual and auditory cues as triggers, music with regular rhythm, a metronome, and verbal suggestions and reinforcement from their therapist. Mobility exercises included balance, walking with good posture, range of motion, and facial mobilization. Rhythm, music, singing, and dancing were used to facilitate performance. Dexterity tasks used games, writing exercises, and crafts. The functional activity period used discussion, demonstration, and practice of all indoor and outdoor ADL identified as difficult by the group. Educational activities included programs to facilitate better understanding of the disease. A home program was included; the patients were given books with lists of exercises and activities to do at home, summaries of the lectures attended, and literature on Parkinson's disease.

Fifty-nine patients completed the study through the 1-year follow-up reevaluation, 30 of whom participated in the treatment program. The experimental and control groups were comparable on all measures prior to the program. As a result of the program, the treated group maintained their ADL performance while the control group had deteriorated. Dexterity did not change in either group. The treated group had a heightened sense of well-being in that they felt the symptoms of their disease had regressed; the control group did not. As far as the physical and motor signs were concerned, the treated group's bradykinesia decreased, whereas it did not change in the control group. Ten patients of the treated group were reclassified to a stage of lesser disability following the program, but this did not happen for any control subject. The treated group had knowledge of the disease, increased self-assurance, better physical appearance, and less egocentricity following the program.[34] The conclusion was that group treatment is recommended for patients with chronic degenerative disease to prevent their tendency toward depression and social isolation. Group treatment is also a cost-effective method of servicing patients.[34]

Performance of Daily Life Tasks

In the early stage of P.D., activities requiring trunk mobility and postural reflexes, such as transfers or working in the kitchen, are affected. Later, manipulation and dexterity problems appear and affect ability to dress, wash, feed, etc. [34] Patients report that tremor at rest has negligible effects on occupational performance tasks, but postural instability is a major element in disability at home and work.[34]

Akinesia also presents a major difficulty for achievement of independence in occupational performance tasks. Sensory stimuli to evoke movement or use of such techniques as "pumping up" can facilitate performance; however, whether the patient ever becomes independent of the person who provides the stimuli is doubtful.

Extensive experience led some therapists to conclude that learning to compensate for akinesia does not occur[26] in P.D. patients. They devised a compensatory treatment program that uses sensory input to evoke or maintain motor output during functional activities. They report from clinical observation that the treatments appear promising for reasons as yet not understood. The treatments are verbal and tactile cueing, rhythm, imitation (visual cueing), and visualization or imagination.[26] Verbal cues such as a one-stage command given abruptly and commandingly ("reach!") alone or in combination with a light, directing touch to the shoulder may initiate the movement. Rhythm may be useful to initiate and maintain movement. Counting, cadence, and music with a beat are all examples of ways to impose rhythm on movement. Use of a portable radio or tape recorder with earphones may be useful to the patient during ongoing reciprocal activities such as walking. If experiencing difficulty in doing an activity, such as lifting a fork to his mouth, the P.D. patient can use imitation. He observes and copies the movement of another person; e.g., observing someone else at the dinner table using a fork may be sufficient to get the patient started. Visualization (focusing on) or imagining an object so that movement is directed at reaching for or clearing the object may enable the patient to move. By attending to stepping over a beam from a flashlight or the design in a carpet, he may be able to walk forward. With practice, imagination of the object alone may be enough to replace the actual object.[26]

Amyotrophic Lateral Sclerosis

Amyotrophic lateral sclerosis (ALS), or motor neuron disease, is a progressive degenerative disease that involves upper and lower motor neurons and may include brain stem involvement.[50] Nerve cells are lost in the anterior horn, brain stem, and motor cortex, and there is degeneration of the corticospinal tracts.[2] There is a progressive inability to move, speak, swallow, or breathe.[51] Mentation, sensation, and sphincter control are preserved.[51]

The average age of onset is 57 years, and it affects men 1 1/2 times more often than women.[51] The course of the disease is rapidly progressive and in the majority of cases death occurs before the third year due to respiratory problems and complications such as choking, aspiration, or pneumonia.[51]

The etiology is unknown,[51] but possibilities include that it is a viral, autoimmune disease or is the result of lead or mercury poisoning.[7]

Early symptoms include muscle weakness with atrophy, cramping, and fasciculations.[7,51] Initial involvement may be in the hands, in the lower extremities, or in the shoulders. In the hands, the thenar and hypothenar eminences, as well as the interossei, atrophy.[7] Finger extensors become weakened before the flexors. In the lower extremities, foot drop progresses to weakness of the gastrocnemius and quadriceps muscles. If initial weakness is in the shoulders, involvement gradually spreads distally.[7] Early weakness of neck musculature may accompany shoulder weakness.[50] In some patients, the upper extremities may become almost useless while the patient is still ambulatory.[2] No matter where it begins, weakness spreads quickly to other muscle groups, and corticospinal tract signs develop: spasticity and hyperactive tendon reflexes[7] with presence of clonus.[52] The triad of upper-extremity weakness, lower-extremity spasticity and hyperreflexia throughout, and the absense of sensory loss lead to certainty regarding this diagnosis.[2] In some patients, bulbar signs occur initially, and rapid progression occurs.[7] Bulbar signs result from weakness of cranial nerve-innervated musculature[50] with symptoms of difficulty speaking, coughing, swallowing, and breathing[7,50] Pseudobulbar palsy from brain stem upper motor neuron involvement may occur and results in symptoms of a positive sucking reflex, hyperactive gag reflex,[50] and emotional lability with mood swings and outbursts of crying.[50,52]

EVALUATION

Occupational therapy evaluation of ALS includes measurement of range of motion, muscle strength, and muscle tone as well as estimation of functional performance of daily life skills and emotional status. Feeding is carefully assessed to include ability to chew and swallow as well as other problems associated with dysphagia (chapter 22).

TREATMENT

Treatment planning depends on recognition of existing symptoms and anticipation of the effects of rapid degeneration. Treatment is individualized because the initial symptoms and the degenerative process are highly variable, but potential needs should be anticipated, especially when purchasing expensive equipment.[53] Goals include maintaining full range of motion and preventing contractures, maintaining muscle strength, avoiding fatigue, promoting independence in all important areas of functional performance, and emotional support.

Goals change as the disease progresses. One center has identified four clinical stages of ALS.[51]

Stage I. "The patient is able to perform normal life activities, although mild discomfort or limitations of performance and endurance may be apparent"[51] (p. 305). The goals for this stage include maintenance of joint mobility, maintenance and increase of strength of the unaffected musculature, and compensation for weakness and reduced endurance during daily life tasks.[51] Strenuous exercise to maintain strength is not recommended; rather mild, aerobic exercises for general conditioning should be used.[51] As a guideline, muscles that grade above fair plus can be strengthened using gradually increasing resistance, but the patient must be monitored carefully for signs of fatigue and increasing weakness.

Simple adaptive devices and orthoses may be needed.[51] From the outset, patients and their families should be involved in the choice of adapted method and/or equipment.[54] Some suggestions for adaptations for weakness are found in chapter 17. To prepare the patient and family to constructively meet future losses of abilities and movement, a problem-solving approach to adaptation should be encouraged.[54] The most commonly prescribed hand splints at this stage are the short opponens splint to substitute for atrophied thenar muscles and the wrist cock-up splint to substitute for weak wrist extensors.[54] See chapter 13 for a description of these.

Stage II. "The patient demonstrates muscle imbalance, increased muscle fatigue caused by excessive energy expenditure, decreased mobility and function)"[51] (p. 305). Exercise continues to maintain strength and endurance within the limits of the disease process, but is done in several short bouts rather than in one prolonged period.[51] Patients are taught pacing to balance activity with rest and other energy conservation techniques if they do not already know how to do this. Passive range of motion or stretch to prevent or decrease contractures resulting from the muscle imbalances may be necessary.[51]

Weakness progresses despite therapy and orthotic devices. It will be necessary first to assist function and then to provide function (chapter 13). Molded or soft neck collars may be needed to support the head due to weak neck extensors.[51,54] Depending on the extent of the lost upper-extremity function, proximal and/or distal orthoses may be required. Suspension slings relieve painful stretch on weak shoulder muscles[53] while providing shoulder function. Mobile arm supports are preferred for compensation for proximal weakness in the upper extremities because they require less energy and muscle power to operate if balanced properly (chapter 13) and provide more function than suspension slings do. They also promote respiration by allowing the patient to move his arms in wide arcs horizontally, which expands and contracts the chest. Externally powered flexor hinge hand slints provide wrist support, opposition, and functional palmar pinch.

Adaptations for independence in areas of function important to the patient should incorporate work simplification and energy conservation measures.[51] One example is use of extended handles to increase the leverage and reduce the force necessary to operate knobs, dials, faucets, etc. An adjustable-height chair will make getting up from a sitting position easier for a person with weak knee and hip extensors. For similar reasons, a raised toilet seat may be needed.[54] Other aids appropriate to problems of muscle weakness and low endurance can be found in Part Five and chapters 28 and 30.

Stage III. "This stage is characterized by progressive weakness of axial muscles and deterioration of mobility and endurance. The patient requires a wheelchair to go long distances and later in this stage, becomes wheelchair-bound"[51] (p. 306). A standard wheelchair for long-distance locomotion is required at first and then a reclining wheelchair with head support. Eventually, a powered wheelchair is needed.[53,54]

Breathing, relaxation, and range of motion exercises are continued by occupational or physical therapists.[51]

Compensatory methods may become necessary when speech is severely involved. An electrolarynx may be helpful for voice amplification[53,55] or aids that substitute for speech may be needed such as a magic slate for writing,[53] a communication board with useful phrases,[53,55] or even a signal system using eye blinks[55] or electronic communication aids.

Patients with swallowing deficits may be unable to swallow saliva, and suctioning may be needed.[53] Methods to compensate for swallowing deficits found useful include a long-stemmed spoon that permits food to be placed far back in the pharynx to increase likelihood of swallowing[51,53] and blended, finely chopped foods or formula diets.[52,53]

Psychological support is an important part of treatment for patients with this disease and their families, especially at this stage. Death in the forseeable future is inevitable, and all professionals will need to help the patient to deal with this as well as deal with it for themselves (See chapter 2).

Stage IV. The patient is totally ADL dependent. A chest respirator may be used. If swallowing is diminished, a tracheostomy may be done to enable suctioning to prevent aspiration and/or to facilitate respiration by some form of respiratory assistance. The use of artificial respiratory assistance becomes the decision of the patient.[51] Gastrostomy[51,53] or cervical esophagostomy[52] may become necessary for feeding when swallowing is lost.

Post Polio Syndrome

Polio is preventable by immunization; fewer than 15 cases a year are reported in the United States now compared to 28,000 in 1955, the year prior to use of the vaccine.[56] The patients with post polio syndrome were among those affected in the major outbreaks of polio in the United States, in the 1940s and 1950s.[56] Survivors were left with weakness that ranged from involvement of all muscles innervated by spinal or bulbar lower motor neurons, including respiratory muscles, to weakness of one limb or part of one limb.[56] Life-saving methods were good enough at the time to keep even those with bulbar paralysis alive.[56]

Polio does not cause sensory losses, upper motor neuron signs, or cognitive/perceptual changes. Until recently, the disease was considered stable.[57] After the febrile stage, some recovery of strength was made, and compensatory methods and devices were employed by these people to enable performance of occupational performance tasks to the extent of their capability. No further deterioration of function was expected. Within the past years, approximately 20% to 25% of post polio survivors have been experiencing losses in function 20 to 30 years after infection.[57] At first it was thought the increased weakness was due to the normal aging process affecting muscles, ligaments, and joints.[56,57] However, a constellation of symptoms has been identified that includes fatigue, weakness in muscles previously affected and not affected, muscle pain, joint pain, breathing difficulties, and cold intolerance.[57] Progressive post polio muscular atrophy (PPMA) is the term given to progressive weakness of affected muscles.[56] The cause is unknown.[57] It is known that anterior horn cell populations decline up to 20% between the ages of 60 and 90 years,[56,58] but this magnitude of loss does not cause clinical weakness in normal persons. However, in polio patients, following the death of anterior horn cells during the febrile stage, many muscle fibers served by those anterior horn cells were reinnervated due to sprouting of the terminal axons of neighboring healthy motor neurons.[59,60] These motor neurons supplied larger numbers of muscle fibers than they were originally designed for.[60] Due to overwork, these anterior horn cells may experience the aging process earlier.[59,60] Because these cells control a greater than normal percentage of muscle function,[59] these age-related losses are enough to produce weakness that interferes with function.[56,59] Exercise-induced damage to the motor units is an additional explanation.[61] The post polio syndrome is not caused by reinfection or activation of a latent virus.[56]

The discovery of this syndrome started with an article published in 1979 in the *Rehabilitation Gazette*.[56] Since then, conferences have been called to study it and to inform patients and physicians. An effort is also being made to enlighten insurance companies to provide payment for additional assistive devices and treatment and the Social Security Administration to allow for disability claims.[62]

Treatment recommendations are according to best estimates without having much data on outcome.[57] One precaution is known and all treatment is guided by it. That is *overuse weakness*, which is a loss of maximum muscle force persisting for days, weeks, or longer following strenuous activities or exercise.[56] Cause is unknown,[56] although it seems related to use beyond the normal limits of a given muscle. In the absence of sufficient motor units, as is the case with post polio patients, overwork contributes to muscle damage.[61] Overuse weakness can occur in neurologically normal individuals as well who exceed their limits in very intense exercise.[56] Early symptoms of overuse, before lasting weakness occurs, are transient postexercise fatigue, transient postexercise weakness, or pain in specific muscles after exercise.[56] Throughout this text, the student therapist has been cautioned against fatiguing weak muscles. It was through the experience of the therapists who treated patients during the polio epidemics that we became aware of this precaution.

Treatment goals for post polio survivors are (1) to improve functional independence and to facilitate life-style changes, (2) to maintain strength and improve endurance, and (3) to alleviate emotional distress.

Life-style changes are necessary to avoid overuse of muscles and to accommodate the weakness and fatigue.[56,57,63] The occupational therapist may be requested to see these patients to evaluate them for revision of adapted techniques for their daily life tasks and/or to teach work simplification and energy conservation methods.[56] The only approach validly used with this group of patients is collaborative problem solving with the patient, who has lived successfully and productively up to this time in spite of the disability[56] by gradually adding to the adaptations he was originally taught during his first course of rehabilitation. The difference now is that many adaptations must be made at once, and the patients need support as well as ideas. Also, newer devices are available than those they may be aware of. Adapted methods are preferred to devices.[56] Patients need to learn their limits of strength and endurance and avoid going to those limits.[56] It is imperative that they learn to conserve energy and the importance of rest.[56] Methods for increasing independence will compensate for the patient's weakness and low endurance (see Part Five and chapters 28 and 30). Adaptations need to be based on joint and muscle protection principles (chapter 27), because due to muscle imbalances, joints have been stressed and there is a possibility that some of the pain experienced by these patients is due to osteoarthritis.[56,63] Splinting may be needed to protect joints or to place them in alignment to prevent stretch and to improve the mechanical advantage of weak muscles.[61]

Home and job site evaluations may be required [56] as may prevocational exploration if a job change is indicated.[64]

Exercise programs may address problems of weakness as well as endurance, although this is not entirely agreed upon.[61,63,63] Conditioning aerobic exercises to maintain or improve cardiovascular endurance is important for polio survivors.[56,64] Swimming, in which the buoyancy of the water removes stress from the joints and tendons, is an especially good conditioning exercise.[56,64] A vigorous strengthening exercise program is contraindicated because weak muscles respond poorly to such a program [61] and because the basic problem of these patients is overuse, not disuse.[63] A mild exercise program for strengthening in which resistance is very gradually increased can lead to modest but significant improvement in strength.[56,61] The increases are guided by the patient's level of fatigue or pain, which are indications of overuse. When either of these occurs, the activity or exercise is modified or discontinued and rest time is increased.[56] The exercise program should focus on functionally important muscles,[56] exclusive of markedly denervated muscles for which exercise is futile since they are already overworked as a result of ordinary daily activity.[61]

Depression results from the feelings of loss generated by the deteriorating condition and resultant decreased independence, as well as the developmental need to adjust to midlife changes.[56,64] Group support is beneficial (chapter 2), as is adapted recreation (chapter 19).[64] Putting patients in touch with peer support groups if they are not already active in one is important. Gazette International Networking Institute is the association for polio survivors.[65] Two publications that would be particularly helpful to these patients are *Rehabilitation Gazette*[65] and *Accent on Living*.[66]

Conclusion

For any other degenerative diseases, the process involved in treatment planning follows the same sequence. First, the disease process is studied to determine the possible cause and symptoms. Then, evaluations selected on the basis of potential symptomatology are done, and a treatment program is planned that will help to correct problems noted. Reevaluations are done periodically to measure the effectiveness of treatment and to record changes. Finally, it is important to keep up with advances in research on causes and beneficial treatment programs and to report any treatment found to be effective.

STUDY QUESTIONS:

Degenerative Diseases

1. What are the goals of the therapy, in general, for patients with degenerative diseases?
2. What is the characteristic motor deficit(s) that patients with multiple sclerosis display?
3. What are the goals of treatment for patients with multiple sclerosis?
4. What treatments have been suggested to improve motor control in patients with cerebellar intention tremor?
5. What symptoms of multiple sclerosis will interfere with the patient's psychosocial adaptation to life situations?
6. What are the goals of treatment for patients with Parkinson's disease?
7. What are the characteristic motor deficits that patients with Parkinson's disease display?
8. What are the hypothesized neurophysiological bases of bradykinesia?
9. What treatments are used in an attempt to overcome akinesia and bradykinesia to increase independent functioning?
10. What are the symptoms of amyotrophic lateral sclerosis (ALS) that will be treated or affect treatment by the occupational therapist?
11. What are the occupational therapy treatment goals for stage II of ALS?
12. What adaptations and/or orthoses will patients with ALS need to use for feeding in early stage III of the disease?
13. What is the hypothesized basis for muscular weakness seen in post polio syndrome?
14. Define overuse weakness. What are the early symptoms of overuse weakness?
15. What treatment would an occupational therapist likely offer to a post polio patient?

REFERENCES

1. Bannister, R. *Brain's Clinical Neurology*, 4th ed London: Oxford University Press, 1973.
2. Adams, R. D., and Victor, M. *Principles of Neurology*. New York: McGraw-Hill, 1977.
3. Dean, G. The multiple sclerosis problem. *Sci. Am.*, 223(1): 40-46, 1970.
4. DeSouza, L. H. A different approach to physiotherapy for multiple sclerosis patients. *Physiotherapy*, 70(11): 429-432, 1984.
5. Patzold, U., and Pocklington, P. R. Course of multiple sclerosis. First results of a prospective study carried out on 102 M.S. patients from 1976-1980, *Acta Neurol. Scand.* 65: 248-266, 1982.
6. Fink, S. L., and Houser, H. B. An investigation of physical and intellectual changes in multiple sclerosis. *Arch. Phys. Med. Rehabil.*, 47(2): 56-61, 1966.
7. Gilray, J., and Meyer, J. S. *Medical Neurology*, 3rd edition. New York: Macmillan, 1979.
8. Grant, I., et al. Deficient learning and memory in early and middle phases of multiple sclerosis. *J. Neurol. Neurosurg. Psychiatry*, 47: 250-255, 1984.
9. Weinstein, E. A. Behavioral aspects of multiple sclerosis. *Mod. Treatment*, 7(5): 961-968, 1970.
10. Halligan, F. R., and Reznikoff, M. Personality factors and change with multiple sclerosis. *J. Consult. Clin. Psychol.*, 53(4): 547-548, 1985.
11. Russell, W. R., and Palfrey, G. Disseminated sclerosis: rest-exercise therapy—a program report. *Physiotherapy*, 55: 306-310, 1969.
12. Abrams, H.M. A comprehensive physical therapy program for the treatment of multiple sclerosis patients. *Phys. Ther.*, 48(4): 337-341, 1968.
13. Schneitzer, L. Rehabilitation of patients with multiple sclerosis. *Arch. Phys. Med. Rehabil.*, 59: 430-437, 1978.
14. Beisel, K. Multiple sclerosis—factors that affect activity performance: a patient survey. *The American Occupational Therapy Association Physical Disabilities Special Interest Section Newsletter*, 6(1): 1-2, 1983.
15. Block, J. M., and Kester, N. C. Role of rehabilitation in the management of multiple sclerosis. *Mod. Treatment*, 7(5): 930-940, 1970.
16. Murphy, J. T., et al. Physiological basis of cerebellar dysmetria. *Can. J. Neurol. Sci.*, 2(3): 279-281, 1975.
17. Beppu, H., Suda, M., and Tanaka, R. Analysis of cerebellar motor disorders by visually guided elbow tracking movement. *Brain*, 107: 787-809, 1984.
18. Hallet, M., Shahani, B. T., and Young, R. R. EMG analysis of patients with cerebellar deficits. *J. Neurol. Neurosurg. Psychiatry*, 38:1163-1169, 1975.
19. Hein, A., and Held, R. A neural model for labile sensorimotor coordination. In *Biological Prototypes and Synthetic Systems*, Vol.I Proceedings of the Bionics Symposium, Ithaca, NY, August–September 1961. Edited by E. E. Bernard and M. R. Kare. New York: Plenum Press, 1962.
20. Chase, R. A., Cullen, J. K., and Sullivan, S. A. Modification of intention tremor in man. *Nature*, 206: 485-487, 1965.
21. Hewer, R. L., Cooper, R., and Morgan, M. H. An investigation into the value of treating intention tremor by weighting the affected limb. *Brain*, 95: 579-590, 1972.
22. Morgan, M. H., Hewer, R. L., and Cooper, R. Application of an objective method of assessing intention tremor—a further study on the use of weights to reduce intention tremor. *J. Neurol. Neurosurg. Psychiatry*, 38: 259-264, 1975.
23. Power, P. W., and Rogers, S. Group counselling for multiple sclerosis patients: a preferred model of treatment for unique adaptive problems. In *Group Counselling and Physical Disability*. Edited by R. C. Lasky and A. E. Dell Orto. Duxbury, MA: Duxbury Press, 1979.
24. Lewis, F. An outpatient M.S. group. *The American Occupational Therapy Association Physical Disabilities Special Interest Section Newsletter*, 6(1): 3, 1983.
25. Herbison, G. J. H-reflex in patients with parkinsonism: effect of levodopa. *Arch. Phys. Med. Rehabil.*, 54: 291-295, 301, 1973.
26. Quintyn, M., and Cross, E. Factors affecting the ability to initiate movement in Parkinson's disease. *Physical & Occupational Therapy in Geriatrics*, 4(4): 51-60, 1986.
27. Thomas, C. L., editor. *Taber's Cyclopedic Medical Dictionary*, 12th edition. Philadelphia: F. A. Davis, 1973.

28. Wroe, M., and Greer, M. Parkinson's disease and physical management. *Phys. Ther.*, 53(8): 849-854, 1973.
29. Ackmann, J. J., Sances, A., Jr., Larson, S. J., and Baker, J. B. Quantitative evaluation of long-term Parkinson tremor. *IEEE Trans. Biomed. Eng.*, 24(1): 49-56, 1977.
30. Webster, D. D. Critical analysis of the disability in Parkinson's disease. *Mod. Treatment*, 5(2): 257-282, 1968.
31. Hoehn, M. M., and Yahr, M. D. Parkinsonism: onset, progression, and mortality. *Neurology*, 17(5): 427-442, 1967.
32. Marsden, C. D. The mysterious motor function of the basal ganglia. *Neurology, 32*: 514-539, 1982.
33. Marsden, C. D. Movement disorders and the basal ganglia. *Trends Neurosci., 9*: 512-515, 1986.
34. Gauthier, L., Dalziel, S., and Gauthier, S. The benefits of group occupational therapy for patients with Parkinson's disease. *Am. J. Occup. Ther.*, 41(6): 360-365, 1987.
35. Angel, R. W., Alston, W., and Higgens, J. R. Control of movement in Parkinson's disease. *Brain, 93*: 1-14, 1970.
36. Bloxham, C. A., Mindel, T. A., and Frith, C. D. Initiation and execution of predictable and unpredictable movements in Parkinson's disease. *Brain, 107*: 371-384, 1984.
37. Hallett, M. and Khoshbin, S. A physiological mechanism of bradykinesia. *Brain, 103*: 301-314, 1980.
38. Tatton, W. G., et al, Defective utilization of sensory input as the basis for bradykinesia, rigidity and decreased movement repertoire in Parkinson's disease: a hypothesis. *Can. J. Neurol. Sci., II*: 136-143, 1984.
39. Sharpe, M. H., Cermak, S. A., and Sax, D. S. Motor planning in Parkinson patients. *Neuropsychologia, 21*(5): 455-462, 1983.
40. Stern, Y., Mayeux, R., and Rosen, J. Contribution of perceptual motor dysfunction to construction and tracing disturbances in Parkinson's disease. *J. Neurol. Neurosurg. Psychiatry, 47*: 983-989, 1984.
41. Lees, A. J., and Smith, E. Cognitive deficits in the early stages of Parkinson's disease. *Brain, 106*: 257-270, 1983.
42. Blonsky, E. R. The changing picture of parkinsonism. Part 1. Neurological modifications resulting from administration of L-dopa. *Rehabil. Lit., 32(2)* : 34-37, 1971.
43. Gersten, J. W., et al. External work of walking and functional capacity in parkinsonian patients treated with L-dopa. *Arch. Phys. Med. Rehabil., 53*(12): 547-553, 1972.
44. Peterson, C. R., et al. Quantitative analysis of the effects of L-dopa on gait in 26 patients with parkinsonism. *Phys. Med.,51*(4): 171-181, 1972.
45. Meunter, M. D., and Tyce, G. M. L-dopa therapy of Parkinson's disease: plasma L-dopa concentration, therapeutic response, and side effects. *Mayo Clin. Proc.*, 46(4): 231-239, 1971.
46. Stockmeyer, S. A. An interpretation of the approach of Rood to the treatment of neuromuscular dysfunction. *Am. J. Phys. Med.*, 46(1): 953-954, 1967.
47. Knott, M. Report of a case of parkinsonism treated with proprioceptive facilitation technics. *Phys. Ther. Rev.*, 37(4): 229, 1957.
48. Minnigh, E. C. Changing picture of Parkinsonism. Part II. The Northwestern University concept of rehabilitation through group physical therapy. *Rehabil. Lit., 32*(2): 38-39, 50, 1971.
49. Stefaniwsky, L., and Bilowit, D. Parkinsonism: facilitation of motion by sensory stimulation. *Arch. Phys. Med. Rehabil., 54*: 75-77, 1973.
50. Carpenter, R. J., McDonald, T. J., and Howard, F. M. The otolaryngologic presentation of amyotrophic lateral sclerosis. *Otolaryngology, 86*(3; Part I): 479-484, 1978.
51. Janiszewski, D. W., Caroscio, J. T., and Wisham, L. H. Amyotrophic lateral sclerosis: a comprehensive rehabilitation approach. *Arch. Phys. Med. Rehabil.* 64(7): 304-307, 1983.
52. Norris, F. H., Sang, K., Denys, E. H., Archibald, K. C., and Lebo, C. Letter: amyotrophic lateral sclerosis. *Mayo Clin. Proc.*, 53(8): 544-545, 1978.
53. Sinaki, M., and Mulder, D. W. Rehabilitation techniques for patients with amyotrophic lateral sclerosis. *Mayo Clin. Proc.*, 53(3): 173-178, 1978.
54. Takai, V. ADL and adaptive equipment for ALS patients. *The American Occupational Therapy Association Physical Disabilities Special Interest Section Newsletter, 6*(2): 1-2, 1983.
55. Adams, M. R. Communication aids for patients with amyotrophic lateral sclerosis. *J. Speech Hearing Dis.*, 31(3): 274-275, 1966.
56. Laurie, G., et al. *Handbook on the Late Effects of Poliomyelitis for Physicians and Survivors.* St. Louis: Gazette International Networking Institute, 1984.
57. Halstead, L. S., and Wiechers, D. O. Introduction. In *Late Effects of Poliomyelitis.* Edited by L. S. Halstead and D. O. Wiechers. Miami, FL: Symposia Foundation, 1985.
58. Tomlinson, B. E., and Irving, D. The number of limb motor neurons in the human lumbosacral cord throughout life. *J. Neurol. Sci. 34*: 213-219, 1977.
59. Dalakas, M. C., et al. Neuromuscular symptoms in patients with old poliomyelitis: clinical, virological and immunological studies. In *Late Effects of Poliomyelitis.* Edited by L. S. Halstead and D. O. Wiechers. Miami, FL: Symposia Foundation, 1985.
60. Weichers, D. O. Pathophysiology and late changes of the motor unit after poliomyelitis. In *Late Effects of Poliomyelitis.* Edited by L. S. Halstead and D. O. Wiechers. Miami, FL: Symposia Foundation, 1985.
61. Herbison, G. J., Jaweed, M. M., and Ditunno, J. F. Clinical management of partially innervated muscle. In *Late Effects of Poliomyelitis.* Edited by L. S. Halstead and D. O. Wiechers. Miami, FL: Symposia Foundation, 1985.
62. McDonnell, J. M. New medical problems associated with polio. *American Physical Therapy Association Progress Report*, July/August 1985, pp. 1, 10.
63. Perry, J. Orthopedic management of post-polio sequelae. In *Late Effects of Poliomyelitis.* Edited by L. S. Halstead and D. O. Wiechers. Miami, FL: Symposia Foundation, 1985.
64. Owen, R. R. Polio residuals clinic and exercise protocol: research implications. In *Late Effects of Poliomyelitis.* Edited by L. S. Halstead and D. O. Wiechers. Miami, FL: Symposia Foundation, 1985.
65. Gazette International Networking Institute. 4502 Maryland Avenue, St. Louis, MO 63108.
66. *Accent on Living.* Cheever Publishing, Inc., Gillum Road and High Drive, P.O. Box 700, Bloomington, IL 61701.

Supplementary Reading

Berardelli, A., Sabra, A. F., and Hallett, M. Physiological mechanisms of rigidity in Parkinson's disease. *J. Neurol. Neurosurg. Psychiatry, 46*: 45-53, 1983.

Bohannon, R. W. Documentation of tremor in patients with central nervous system lesions: a clinical report. *Phys. Ther. 66* (2): 229-230, 1986.

Braile, L. E. Support for the drooping head. *Am. J. Occup. Ther. 35* (10): 661-662, 1981.

Cooke, J. D., Brown, J. D., and Brooks, V. B. Increased dependence on visual information for movement control in patients with Parkinson's disease. *Can. J. Neurol. Sci. 5*(4): 413-315, 1978.

DeLisa, J. A., Stolov, W. C., and Troupin, A. S. Action myoclonus following acute cerebral anoxia. *Arch. Phys. Med. Rehabil. 60*(1): 32-36, 1979.

Palmer, S. G., et al. Exercise therapy for Parkinson's disease. *Arch. Phys. Med. Rehabil., 67*(10): 741-745, 1986.

Romsaas, E. P., and Rosa, S. A. Occupational therapy intervention for cancer patients with metastatic disease. *Am. J. Occup. Ther. 39*(2):79-83, 1985.

Takai, V. L. Case report: the development of a feeding harness for an ALS patient. *Am. J. Occup. Ther. 40*(5): 359-361, 1986.

Yasuda, Y. L., Bowman, K., and Hsu, J. D. Mobile arm supports: criteria for successful use in muscle disease patients. *Arch. Phys. Med. Rehabil. 67*(4): 253-256,1986.

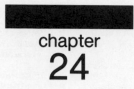

chapter
24

Traumatic Brain Injuries

Patricia Weber Dow

The incidence of traumatic brain injury[a] has steadily increased over the years. The National Institute of Neurological and Communicative Disorders and Stroke reports more than 400,000 new head-injured, people admitted to hospitals each year.[1] Males are twice as likely as females to incur traumatic brain injuries, with the highest risk age group from 15-29 years.[2] Motor vehicle accidents and falls are the most common causes of head injuries.[2] Approximately half of these new head injuries each year are classified as moderate or severe, involving loss of consciousness and hospitalization. Improved emergency medical treatment has increased the survival rate of persons with severe traumatic brain injuries from 10% 25 years ago to approximately 50% today.[1,3] With this increased survival comes the challenge to therapists and the medical team to rehabilitate these severely injured patients to the fullest possible degree.

Mechanisms of Injury

PRIMARY EFFECTS

A traumatic brain injury is usually caused by a dynamic loading or impact to the head from direct blows or from sudden movements produced by impacts to other body parts. This loading can result in any combination of compression, expansion, acceleration, deceleration, or rotation of the brain inside the skull.[2,4] Actual stretching or tearing of neural structures, brain white matter, or vascular structures may occur.[2,5,6] Vascular tearing can produce a hematoma within the brain (intracerebral) or between the brain and the skull, which can cause increased pressure on the brain and further injury. A rotational component is believed essential for diffuse brain injury, whereas linear movement of the head leads to focal lesions at the site of impact (coup) or on the opposite side of the brain (countercoup).[2,4,7] Focal lesions involve one area of the brain; diffuse lesions involve several areas.

The brain may also suffer contusions or lacerations as it is moved by the impact across or into the bony prominences of the skull, i.e., the sphenoid wings, the petrous bones, or the orbital bones. Such contusions commonly involve the poles of the temporal and frontal lobes, the undersurfaces of the temporal lobes, and the orbital cortex.[3,5,6] The occipital and parietal lobes, covered by smooth skull surfaces, are less likely to incur damage. The folds of the dural membranes (especially the falx cerebri and the tentorium) can also cause damage to the brain stem, the medial aspect of the occipital lobe, or the superior surface of the cerebellum.[4,5]

The skull may fracture from the force of the impact in the area of or at a distance from the impact.[5] The type of fracture depends on the force of the blow and ranges from a linear fracture to a stellate fracture and, lastly, to a depressed skull fracture, which is frequently seen and is the result of the most forceful blow.[4,5] A basilar skull fracture, occurring 21% of the time,[2] frequently involves the petrous portion of the temporal bone and thus can result in cranial nerve damage. Cranial nerves I, II, III, VI, VII, and VIII are most frequently damaged in traumatic brain injuries, because of their position and course within the skull.[5,6] The patient with a brain injury from a motor vehicle accident or a fall may have other systemic trauma, such as fractures of the extremities, shoulder girdle, pelvis, or face; cervical fractures with possible spinal cord injury; abdominal trauma; or pneumothorax or other chest cavity trauma.

---

[a]A shift in the terminology for this area has recently begun. Increasingly, the more precise term "traumatic brain injury" (TBI) is being used by researchers and practitioners to describe the condition previously labeled "head injury" or "closed head injury" (CHI). To reflect this transition in terminology and to familiarize the reader with the variety of terms seen in currently available literature, this chapter will use the following terms interchangeably: severe head injury, brain injury, head injury, closed head injury, and traumatic brain injury.

SECONDARY EFFECTS

Secondary effects of the traumatic brain injury can occur immediately or develop within hours or days.[5,6] Trauma can abolish or disrupt autoregulation of cerebral blood flow, the blood-brain barrier, and vasomotor functions resulting in disordered cerebral energy metabolism, intracranial hypotension, cerebral vasospasm, and increases in intracranial pressure (ICP) and in cerebral edema.[6,8] Other secondary effects of brain trauma include intracranial hemorrhage, ischemic brain damage, uncal herniation resulting in brain stem compression, general systemic reactions to the neural impairment, electrolyte abnormalities, altered respiratory regulation, intracranial infection, or abnormal autonomic nervous system responses.[2,3,8] Usually by the time the patient is stabilized and therapy ordered, the secondary effects of brain trauma are already present and will be a factor in the patient's ability to respond to therapy.

Initial Medical Evaluation and Treatment

Once the severely brain-injured patient is brought to an emergency room, several measures are taken immediately. An adequate airway, if not present, must be established through intubation or tracheostomy (trach). Assisted ventilation may be required. The extent of extracranial injuries, such as fractures, abdominal trauma, or pneumothorax, is assessed. A neurologist or neurosurgeon will evaluate the patient to determine the level of consciousness, severity and extent of the injury, and the presence of intracranial hematomas. Computer tomography (CT) scanning, cerebral angiography, and/or skull x-rays may be utilized to determine presence of hematomas and indications for immediate craniotomy to evacuate a hematoma.[6]

LEVEL OF CONSCIOUSNESS

A brain-injured person may exhibit any of a number of states of altered consciousness, depending on the severity of the injury. Consciousness, unconsciousness, and coma are best viewed on a continuum from complete consciousness to death or complete absence of consciousness. It is important to realize that coma is not a stable state. A person in a coma can fluctuate spontaneously or from stimulation along the continuum towards, and indeed into, varying levels of consciousness.[2] Complete consciousness, the first level, is defined as an awareness, a cognition of self and the surrounding environment; consciousness implies perception, interpretation of this perception, and an appropriate response.[9] Such consciousness is a function of an intact cortex. A lesser type of consciousness, arousal, is a state of wakefulness and attention to the environment on primarily a survival and basic function level. Arousal is governed by the ascending reticular activating system (RAS) and may occur despite complete destruction of cerebral hemispheres.[2] The next level on the continuum, clouding of consciousness, is a state of reduced wakefulness, reduced clarity of thought with possible confusion, decreased attention span, and memory lapses. The following stage, stupor, involves unresponsiveness from which the person is aroused only by vigorous stimulation. In the comatose stage, the person cannot be aroused by sensory stimulation, has eyes closed, and demonstrates an absence of observable interaction with the environment.[2,10] Coma results from interruption of communication from the RAS to the cerebral hemispheres.[2] It is possible for a person to function in a "vegetative state" but without consciousness, i.e., the deeper brain stem structures regulating breathing, reflexes, and heart rate are intact, but the cortex is completely impaired.[4]

SEVERITY OF INJURY

Neurological evaluation to assess the extent and severity of the brain damage usually includes evaluation of motor response to stimulation, brain stem reflexes such as pupillary reactions and oculovestibular reflexes, and the presence of various pathological reflexes, such as Babinski's sign (extension of the large toe and fanning of the other toes following stroking stimulation of the plantar surface of that foot from heel to toe), snouting (exaggerated contraction of lips following sharp tap of mid-upper lip), rooting, and ankle clonus (rapid flexion/extension of the foot following quick dorsiflexion of the foot).[2,6,11] These pathological reflexes are primitive responses that are normally inhibited by the cerebral cortex. Presence of such responses indicates release of lower centers from higher-level influence.

Motor Responses to Stimulation

Patients in the very deepest level of coma will show no observable change in behavior, no movement, no muscle tone changes, and no eye opening in response to painful, auditory, tactile, or proprioceptive stimulation. Such stimulation consists of pressure on the fingernail bed or sternum, voices of the family or loud noises, touch on the body or face, or being moved. The motor response will be flaccid. No reflexive movement will be produced either, with the possible exception of purely spinal cord level reflex arcs.[2,12] No pupillary reactions will be present.[12] The damage producing this lack of response is thought to be below the vestibular nuclei in the brain stem, i.e., the pontomedullary area.[12]

In the next higher level of coma, the patient responds to internal or external stimulation, such as loud noises, painful stimulation, or quick position changes, with a generalized motor reflex known as decerebrate rigidity or extensor posturing.[13] The patient's hips and shoulders extend, adduct, and internally rotate; knees and elbows extend; the forearm hyperpronates; the wrist and fingers flex; the feet plantarflex and invert; the trunk extends; and the head retracts, sometimes exhibiting opisthotonos.[10,14,15] This motor picture is thought to be caused by damage in the upper midbrain and the lower pons,[11,12] sparing the vestibular nuclei; in effect, removing the lower pontine structures from more rostral neural influences.[9,10,14] Pupillary reactivity and oculovestibular reflexes may or may not be present.[12] Spinal level reflexes and lower brain stem reflexes, such as the asymmetrical tonic neck reflex (ATNR), the tonic labyrinthine reflex (TLR), and the positive supporting reaction, may be seen in their entirety, or might simply be influencing the patient's muscle tone.[14] The vestibular reflexes are usually operable and assist in the production of increased tone in antigravity (extensor) muscles. The grasp reflex and sucking reflex may also be elicited at this stage of coma (see chapter 4).

The third higher level of coma entails a response to stimulation known as decorticate rigidity or flexor posturing. This stereotyped pattern of movement consists of adduction, internal rotation, and slight flexion of the shoulder; elbow flexion; forearm pronation; and wrist and finger flexion.[9,10,15] The patient's lower extremities extend, adduct, and internally rotate as they do in decerebrate rigidity. If flexion of the hip and knee is elicited by painful stimulation, this is a spinal reflex, known as triple flexion, which indicates damage to the descending motor tracts.[16] The decorticate response is thought to indicate damage in the internal capsule or cerebral hemispheres, causing an interruption in the corticospinal pathways.[2,10] Midbrain reactions, i.e., neck and body righting reactions, may be elicited at this stage of coma for use in treatment.[14]

The fourth possible motor response to stimulation is withdrawal, which includes shoulder abduction and is a more rapid movement than decorticate posturing. For example, the patient withdraws the entire limb when his hand is stimulated. The patient may also show spontaneous, nonpurposeful movement of his limbs. Withdrawal is thought to indicate some function present in the cerebral hemispheres.[2]

The fifth level motor response to stimulation is localization. At this stage, the patient may be said to be "lighter," that is, he is still comatose, but not as deeply. His responses to stimulation are quicker and becoming more appropriate. The patient may reach over and brush the painful stimulation away, move just the part being stimulated, blink in response to strong light or visual threat, turn toward or away from auditory stimulation, and/or visually track a moving object.[13] Cortical equilibrium reactions or protective extension reactions may be elicited at this stage. According to Finkelstein and Ropper,[16] limb abduction, or movement away from the body midline (present at this level), is the only movement that is always purposeful and indicates an intact connection from the cortex to that limb.

The sixth and highest level motor response of the patient to stimulation is an appropriate response, i.e., not withdrawing from all touch and stimuli, but only from that which is noxious or irritating, and following simple requests or initiating purposeful activity.

The patient could demonstrate any combination of these responses, depending on which areas of the brain were damaged.[6] For example, he may exhibit decerebrate rigidity with his right limbs and localizing response with his left side. He could exhibit bilateral decerebrate posturing. He may initially evidence decorticate posturing on one side and then sink to decerebrate rigidity or flaccidity on that side, which indicates a deterioration in his condition. He may exhibit hemiplegia on one side and normal muscle tone on the other. The terms decerebrate and decorticate can be easily confused. Some physicians prefer the respective description of abnormal extension or abnormal flexion in response to pain,[6] or a description of the limb movement without the label. In the stages of recovery described below, the first three levels of these motor responses to stimulation are seen in stage I, the fourth and fifth levels (withdrawal and localization) are seen in stage II, and the sixth level motor response would be seen in stages III and IV.

Various scales have been proposed to facilitate consistent description of coma among the medical team and between research centers, to assess the depth of coma and the inferred severity of the head injury, to monitor and delineate change in the patient's condition, and to eventually predict the patient's outcome as early as possible.[6,17-20] The most widely used scale is the Glasgow Coma Scale (GCS) (Table 24.1), which assesses the following parameters: eye opening in response to a variety of stimuli, best motor response to pressure on the nail bed and to supraorbital pressure, and best verbal response. Two other scales, the Maryland Coma Scale and the Comprehensive Level of Consciousness Scale, include such additional areas as eye movements and eye position at rest, brain stem reflexes, posturing and more detailed motor responsiveness, orientation, and intensity of stimulation necessary to elicit motor and verbal responses.[19,20] These authors feel their scales provide a more sensitive assessment of the subtle changes in a patient's level of consciousness than does the GCS.[19,20] Dr. Jennett him-

TABLE 24.1
Glasgow Coma Scale[a]

Eye opening	Spontaneous	E	4
	To speech		3
	To pain		2
	Nil		1
Best motor response	Obeys	M	6
	Localizes		5
	Withdraws		4
	Abnormal flexion		3
	Extensor response		2
	Nil		1
Verbal response	Oriented	V	5
	Confused conversation		4
	Inappropriate words		3
	Incomprehensible sounds		2
	Nil		1
Coma score (E + M + V) = 3 to 15			

[a] Reprinted with permission from Jennett, B. and Teasdale, G. *Management of Head Injuries*. Philadelphia: F. A. Davis, 1981.

self records information on motor response of all four limbs, pupil reaction and size, eye movements, and respiration patterns in addition to assessing the GCS score.[6] Specific scales to assess coma in children differ primarily in the criteria of assessment of verbalization, ocular response, and motor response, or in the addition of brain stem assessment.[17,18]

Another scale for assessing a patient's level of consciousness or cognitive functioning, developed by Rancho Los Amigos Hospital (Rancho), describes levels of a comatose patient's reaction to stimuli or the environment,[21] abridged as follows:

Level I—no response: unresponsive to stimuli.

Level II—generalized response: nonspecific, inconsistent, and nonpurposeful reaction to stimuli.

Level III—localized response: response directly related to type of stimuli, yet still inconsistent and delayed.

Level IV—confused-agitated: response heightened, severely confused and could be bizarre.

Level V—confused-inappropriate: some response to simple commands, but confusion with more complex commands. High level of distractibility.

Level VI—confused-appropriate: response more goal directed, but cues necessary.

Level VII—automatic-appropriate: response robotlike, judgment and problem-solving lacking.

Level VIII—purposeful-appropriate: response adequate, subtle deficits persist.

INTENSIVE CARE UNIT (ICU) TREATMENT

Following emergency assessment and stabilization, the comatose brain-injured patient is usually taken to ICU. The patient will typically then have additional diagnostic procedures, continued monitoring, and treatment of systemic and cerebral function, nutrition, and fluid and electrolyte balance in an attempt to minimize the secondary results of the head injury.[2,6] Diagnostic procedures may include an electroencephalogram or evoked potentials, such as visual, auditory, or somatosensory, to analyze cerebral dysfunction; measurement of cerebral blood flow; or biochemical analyses.[2,6,22] The cardiorespiratory system may be monitored and assisted via frequent vital sign checks, arterial lines, heart monitors, or a ventilator. The ICP can be monitored with a subarachnoid bolt or an intraventricular catheter. Other measures will include a urinary catheter, a nasogastric (n/g) tube for nutrition and medication, and various intravenous lines (IVs) for medications and management.

The therapist working in ICU should become familiar with equipment mentioned above and with medications used in treatment to control systemic injuries, ICP, spasticity, or seizures, since therapy and patient movement may be limited by the equipment or IVs, or the patient's response may be decreased by the drugs. The therapist can consult the physician and nurse to see if a change can safely be made in equipment or drugs to facilitate therapeutic intervention with the patient.

Early intervention is crucial to address tone, positioning, stimulation, and the family's concerns. Therapists can familiarize ICU nurses with the necessity of such services, and thus improve the promptness of referrals.

Prognosis and Outcome

In recent years, as the number of patients surviving severe traumatic brain injuries has increased, research has focused on factors that would predict the outcome of such injuries. The reasoning has been that if outcome can be predicted early in coma, expensive medical treatment or rehabilitation could be directed to patients who had the best chance for survival with fewer residual deficits, the effectiveness of medical treatment in decreasing secondary damage could be evaluated, the family could be better prepared to make informed, realistic decisions on immediate and long-term care, and society might be spared the expense of supporting severely impaired survivors.[2,6,12,23,24] There are many studies attempting to assess the predictive power of age, clinical observations (such as the GCS, pupillary reactions, and eye movements), data from a CT scan, presence of a surgical lesion, length of posttraumatic amnesia (i.e., the length of time after the accident before the return of continuous memory), presence of brain stem dysfunction, evoked potentials, increased ICP, or a combination of these factors.[2,4,6,19,22–26]

No predictive factors have been located that can classify patients within the first week or so following head injury into two categories, death or survival, with 100% accuracy. There are falsely pessimistic and falsely optimistic predictions; accuracy ranges from 68% to 98%.[4,6,12,22,25–27] The GCS predicts outcome most accurately in those patients with GCS scores of under 5 or over 7. The outcome of patients with scores between 5 and 7 cannot begin to be accurately predicted.[2]

Outcome scales have been developed to allow physicians to correlate "final" recovery levels to early treatment and prognostic indicators.[6,20,28] The Glasgow Outcome Scale (GOS) is widely used. Its categories are death, vegetative state, severe disability (conscious but dependent), moderate disability (independent but disabled), and good recovery (able to participate in normal social life and could return to work), with 90% accurate assessment of prognosis possible at 6 months postinjury.[2,6] The GOS does assess some aspects of mental function as well as physical function in assigning outcome categories.[29] Some researchers feel more detailed neuropsychological or social factors need to be considered in determining outcome in the above categories.[2,23,28,30] When these factors are added, more residual disability is identified than by the GOS and improvements in levels of disability are identified more accurately.[30] Addition of these factors also allows assessment of continued subtle recovery to be made beyond 6 or 12 months post injury.[1,23,24,30,31]

The therapist is not required to predict, but will consider the predictive factors listed above when deciding on treatment goals or length of rehabilitation efforts. Cognition, personality, and motivation, all of which may substantially affect quality of survival,[23,29] are also considered in determining treatment goals. In addition, it behooves the entire medical team to be aware of the possibility of error in prediction. Outcome predictions are based on groups of patients, not on individuals who may have family and character strengths that cannot be measured, which allow them to recover more completely than anticipated. The therapist's communication with the physician, whose time spent observing the patient's responses is usually limited, is vital to assure more comprehensive assessment of patient prognosis. For further discussion of these issues and prognostic factors, the reader is referred to the references.[2,6]

Occupational Therapy Evaluation

The evaluation may need to be done in several brief sessions because of the patient's reduced endurance, other scheduled procedures, or the therapist's decision to gather a representative sample of the patient's responses. The patient can fluctuate between levels of response during the day. He may be at a higher level in the morning and regress with fatigue, or he may evidence brief responses of higher level scattered throughout predominantly lower-level neurological responses. The therapist's observations may differ from those of the physicians, nurses, or other allied health team members as each discipline is assessing different aspects of the patient's responsiveness and function. In the process of recovery, not all patients will experience all the stages of recovery described below, as some may show initial responses of a higher neurological level. Still other patients may stop at one level and plateau there indefinitely. Verbal skills usually return before nonverbal or performance skills; the patient may be able to understand more than he can demonstrate.[6] The occupational therapy evaluation components will change depending upon the patient's stage of coma.

Precautions

The brain-injured patient may be referred for therapy before he is completely medically stable. Due to systemic injuries, secondary effects of the brain injury itself, disturbance of basic body regulatory systems, and the life-support equipment utilized to treat the patient, precautions may be numerous and must be heeded by the therapist. Typical precautions are described below; other precautions may also be necessary and should be ascertained from the nurse, physician, or patient's chart before initiation of the evaluation.

If the patient is within a month of his injury, the therapist must be alert to drastic systemic changes in response to stimulation.[32,33] A major concern with acute brain trauma is control of ICP. Increased ICP sustained above a certain level can be fatal.[6] The patient with an ICP monitor can be readily checked during stimulation sessions; a patient not on a monitor must be closely observed for pupil changes, decreased neurological responses, abnormal brain stem reflexes, flaccidity, behavioral changes, vomiting, or changes in pulse rate, blood pressure, or respiration rate.[11,32,33] Fluids may be restricted or the patient's head may be positioned in neutral at 30° elevation in an attempt to regulate his ICP.[17] Turning the patient's head to one side may obstruct the internal jugular vein and result in a sudden increase of ICP.[33,34] The neck should not be flexed when the patient is positioned on his side. Changes in the patient's blood pressure and respiration also must be monitored and kept within ranges designated by the physician.

Early posttraumatic epilepsy occurs in 5% of patients with brain injuries, and late epilepsy in 20% of those with prolonged unconsciousness, depressed skull fracture, or intracranial hematoma.[6,35] To reduce the chance of a seizure occurring during treatment, tactile and vestibular stimulation and icing are begun slowly and distally to assess the patient's physiological response. His heart rate, blood pressure, and facial color are monitored, as well as any autonomic changes such as sudden perspiration or increased restlessness. As the therapist becomes more familiar with the patient's responses, intensity of stimulation is gradually increased. A padded tongue blade is kept at the patient's bedside. If a seizure does occur, the therapist should position the patient safely, insert the padded tongue blade or a small rolled towel between his teeth if possible, and summon medical assistance. The patient's limbs should not be restrained during a seizure.

If the patient has had a craniotomy for evacuation of a hematoma, the bone flap may be left off, and the brain may be covered only by scalp to allow the brain to expand. Direct pressure to this site must be avoided.

The patient may have a tear in the dura with subsequent cerebrospinal fluid leak. In this case, the patient initially is treated by observation, head elevation, antibiotics, and precautions against nose blowing.[6,35]

If the patient has other systemic trauma, such as fractures or chest cavity trauma, appropriate precautions must be taken when stimulating or moving him. Care must also be taken to avoid disturbing i.v. sites, a trach, an n/g tube, endotracheal or respirator tubes, or traction for extremity fractures.

BACKGROUND INFORMATION

The first step in evaluation of a newly referred brain-injured patient is to read his medical chart, carefully noting the areas of brain damage, other medical problems, surgical procedures, any precautions that will restrict the evaluation or future therapy, significant past medical history, and current medications. The daily physician's progress notes and the nursing notes are reviewed for the patient's current status and the procedures around which therapeutic evaluation and intervention must be scheduled.

After perusal of the chart, the therapist should talk with the patient's nurse of that day, especially if the patient is in ICU. The nurse will be an invaluable source of information about precautions, patient status and level of responsiveness, the schedule for tests and procedures, and the patient's family's concerns. The nurse will also be crucial in therapeutic follow-through.

Following the prior two steps, the therapist begins observing any spontaneous patient movement. The patient's eyes may be open or closed. Most traumatic brain injury patients open their eyes spontaneously or to stimulation within the second to fourth week post injury.[2,4,24] Nonpurposeful, roving eye movements or other abnormal movements may be present.[2,6] Primitive automatic responses of facial grimacing, teeth clenching and grinding, and/or rhythmic chewing may occur spontaneously or in response to stimulation.[4,10] Spontaneous decerebrate or decorticate posturing or patterned movements are noted. The therapist then proceeds with specific data gathering as detailed below. During the evaluation and treatment, the therapist describes the procedures to the patient (i.e., what is being done, what movements his body will be taken through, etc.).

PASSIVE AND ACTIVE RANGE OF MOTION

Joint motion of the upper extremities (UEs), face, jaw, and neck are assessed with the patient in supine. If the patient's tone is severely abnormal, accurate range of motion (ROM) measurements may require two therapists and/or some tone-inhibiting techniques (chapter 6). During passive range of motion (PROM), the therapist also begins to assess the patient's muscle tone, presence of spasticity, reactions to touch and movement, and nature of any joint limitations discovered.[6] Contractures are noted as discussed in chapter 8. The therapist may discover fractures or dislocations that have not been identified previously. Heterotopic ossification (HO), the formation of bone in soft tissue and periarticular locations, is a relatively common occurrence in those severely brain-injured patients with limb spasticity who are in prolonged coma. Early clinical signs of HO are warmth, swelling, pain, and decreased joint motion.[36] Common joints for HO, in order of frequency of involvement, are the shoulder, elbow, hip, and knee.[36]

SENSORY AWARENESS

The therapist assesses the patient's basic sensations by presenting the sensory stimulus and observing any motor response, decrease or change in ongoing posturing or in facial movements, a startle reaction, eye opening, or changes in heart rate, blood pressure, or respirations. The therapist checks the response from both UEs, the right and left sides of the face, and the upper trunk, and may change the patient's position to see if the response can be altered or magnified. One interesting study describes the different posturing patterns elicited from the same comatose patient depending on the stimulus location and limb position. Initial arm flexion with a painful stimulus produced significantly higher abnormal flexion, whereas initial arm

extension produced significantly higher abnormal extension.[37] Motor responses may be charted as appropriate, delayed, localized, generalized, abnormal posturing, or absent; increased in frequency; or changed in nature secondary to stimulation.

The therapist evaluates the patient's response to pain using pinprick and pinches on the arm. Tactile input consists of a variety of textures, touch, and rubbing. Auditory stimuli are loud bells, tapes of familiar voices, hand claps, calling the patient's name, or talking to him. Visual skills such as eye opening, blink to threat, tracking, and focus are assessed using familiar photos, movements, or commands. Visual field neglect and higher-level perceptual skills are difficult to assess before the patient is moving spontaneously or responding specifically to stimulation.[2]

Olfactory evaluation is done with pleasant and unpleasant odors. Ammonia and vinegar irritate the trigeminal nerve and are avoided.[38] Musk, lemon, almond, fruity, or floral scents can be used.[38]

Proprioception and kinesthetic evaluation is grossly done by observing the patient's responses to movement of his head, UEs, and trunk. More discrete testing of these sensations, stereognosis, two-point discrimination, and tactile localization (chapter 3) will need to be deferred until the patient is more cognitively alert, approximately level V or above of the Rancho scale[21], or stage III in this chapter. Cranial nerve function must be evaluated continually throughout treatment, as it may influence prognosis and treatment. For example, one traumatic brain injury patient, who suffered bilateral cranial nerve VII damage, was judged unresponsive and cognitively impaired by his physician long after he was cooperating with commands in therapy, because of his lack of facial expression and difficulty forming words.

NEUROMUSCULAR SKILLS

Assessment of the patient's neuromuscular function includes evaluation of strength, coordination, muscle tone, presence and strength of spasticity, and reflex integration. Traditional muscle strength and coordination tests (chapters 4 and 8) are usually inappropriate for the head-injured patient with spasticity or abnormal muscle tone, or with decreased alertness and ability to cooperate. Instead, observation of spontaneous movements or movements elicited during position changes is necessary to determine muscle strength in early stages of recovery. Isolated motor control and its quality cannot be assessed until stage II or III, or level IV or V of the Rancho scale.[21] At this stage, the therapist can begin to observe whether the patient moves in response to command, spontaneously, or only in reaction to a stimulus; whether the movement is in a synergy or is selective; whether the movement is purposeful or not; whether cerebellar dysfunction is present (chapter 4); and whether there is a disturbance in praxis (chapters 5 and 7). Isolated motor control can be evaluated within a neurodevelopmental framework (chapter 6), or, in later stages of recovery, with specific tests (chapter 8) and with tests of coordination such as the Minnesota Rate of Manipulation Test (chapter 4) or the Bennett Hand Tool Test.

Muscle tone is assessed both passively and during position changes through normal transition postures (chapter 6) and charted as described in chapter 4. From handling the patient, the therapist determines whether his head movements are coordinated with his trunk and whether touch and movement increase abnormal tone, posturing, or reflexes. Muscle tone is usually increased in a patient with some level of motor response to stimulation. Decreased muscle tone may indicate a lower motor neuron lesion.[2]

Types of abnormal posturing have been described above. Abnormal reflexes commonly found upon evaluation are the ATNR, the symmetrical tonic neck reflex (STNR), the TLR, the positive supporting reaction, and the extensor thrust [21] (see chapter 4). Equilibrium, righting, and protective extension reactions are generally decreased or absent in early stages, as are coordination and control of the head and trunk in static and dynamic positions.[2] The TLR, STNR, and ATNR will influence ROM, strength of spasticity, and the potential for isolated movement.[2] The patient who exhibits increased flexor tone in supine and increased extensor tone in prone (in contrast to the typical TLR) may be reacting more to exteroceptive stimuli and tonic stretch. The position and posture of the patient must be controlled to obtain an accurate assessment of reflexes and motor control. Assessment of reflexes and equilibrium reactions is done in supine or sitting as described in chapters 4 and 6.

ORAL MOTOR EVALUATION

A prefeeding evaluation is done if the patient shows some response to stimulation.[21] This evaluation includes assessment of tone and motor function of individual facial muscles and tongue movements; jaw mobility; facial, tongue, and mouth sensation; sucking and swallowing; and presence of normal and abnormal oral reflexes. During evaluation and treatment, the patient should be positioned in sitting with neck slightly flexed and with hips and knees in flexion. Pressure to the back of the head is avoided; pillows are placed at shoulder height if head control can be obtained in this way. If the patient cannot be optimally positioned in sitting, this should be noted in the evaluation, and consideration should be given by the therapist to the influence of abnormal limb reflexes or poor head and trunk control on observed oral motor function.

Reflexes

The presence of a primitive bite reflex is ascertained by tactile stimulation with a padded tongue blade on the patient's gums, teeth, or tongue.[38] Fingers are not used. The bite reflex, although diminished in severity, can continue in patients even after they are independent feeders. If the patient exhibits a tonic bite reflex, further testing of the tongue and oral cavity will be difficult, if not impossible. Presence of the rooting reflex and snouting are determined. The presence and

strength of cough and gag reflexes, frequently observed during respiratory treatment, are assessed. Continued presence of an endotracheal tube or n/g tube will usually decrease the gag reflex.

Motor and Sensory

Cranial nerves V, VII, IX, X, XI, or XII may have been injured, with resulting paresis or paralysis of facial muscles, lips, tongue movements, and/or soft palate movements and possible sensory impairment.[14,39] Selective muscle movement of facial musculature, lips, and tongue is assessed if the patient is able to follow commands.[40] If not, maintained touch, light touch, and pressure are applied to facial musculature to observe any motor responses to this stimulation, spontaneous facial expressions are noted, and manual palpation of tone is done, if safe. The cheeks and lips are evaluated for their mobility, response to tactile stimulation on outside and inside, and ability to close. The cheeks need to hold against the teeth to decrease pooling of food and to create negative pressure for swallowing and bolus progression; the lips need to close to swallow normally.[39] Jaw opening and closing is assessed, especially noting the ability of tongue to move without association with the jaw. Soft palate elevation, elicited by light touch on the inferior edge of the soft palate near the uvula, is assessed if the bite reflex is not present.[39]

If the tonic bite reflex is not present, the sensitivity of the tongue to tactile (tested with a cotton swab), temperature (tested with an eyedropper with hot and cold water), and taste (sugar, salt, lemon, and quinine) input is assessed.[11] Anterior and posterior tongue movements, tongue tone and symmetry, lateralization ability, and tongue tip elevation are evaluated. The tongue should not be a single movement unit, but should be able to take on several different postures, i.e., the posterior part of the tongue should elevate, the tongue should extend out of the mouth without humping posteriorly, the anterior portion of the tongue should be able to assume a relaxed position in the bottom of the mouth at times, and tongue thrust should not be present. The tongue also normally functions to mix saliva with food. The patient who has little or no saliva (secondary to injury or medications) will have difficulty preparing the food to swallow.[39]

Swallowing

Spontaneous swallowing in control of saliva or a swallow elicited by stretch of the digastric and geniohyoid muscles is assessed visually for coordination, completeness, and symmetrical, adequate elevation of the laryngeal area, and the therapist listens for quietness and sound quality of the swallow. The swallow is also assessed manually as the therapist places a hand on the patient's throat and under the chin, with no pressure, but only a light touch to feel the initiation of tongue movement and laryngeal movement.[39]

Feeding

If the patient is not aspirating (i.e., taking fluids into his lungs) and if the physician consents, the patient's ability to swallow is assessed. Small quantities (1/3 teaspoon) of a liquid thickened with gelatin[40] or a food with a consistency between liquid and paste[39] are used. In general, the patient with a cuffed trach should have the cuff inflated by his nurse prior to the feeding evaluation; for a trach without a cuff, a nurse should stand by to suction the patient if necessary. A cough or gargling noise in a patient without a trach would indicate aspiration and further evaluation would be deferred until the physician was consulted. Many patients are silent aspirators and do not make the usual sounds of coughing, gagging, or gargling when aspirating.[39] It is therefore advisable to have x-rays done during actual swallowing to determine possible aspiration. During this evaluation with food, the therapist observes the total oral manipulation of the food by the lips and the tongue, and during the swallow itself.

SENSORY INTEGRATION

Sensory integration cannot be formally evaluated in the patient who is only responding to stimuli in a generalized or localized fashion. However, the therapist can utilize observation of the patient moving spontaneously to infer possible deficits in this area.[2] The ability to cross the midline, neglect of an extremity, decreased tracking and focus into all visual quadrants, or uncoordinated movement of the body through space would alert the therapist to possible visual-spatial and body integration deficits. Once the patient has begun to respond specifically to external stimuli, his performance during "automatic" physical daily living tasks may indicate possible body schema dysfunction or dyspraxia; his figure-ground and position-in-space awareness and his visual-motor integration may be observed during reaching for objects on a table or reaching for the bed rail; and his neglect of space or body parts can be observed during spontaneous movement. The patient can also be given gross table top activities such as sorting or matching, pegboards, simple imitation of block designs, or shape, color, or form puzzles to evaluate perceptual deficits more exactly.

Specific tests of sensory integration generally can only be done when the brain-injured patient is responding at stage IV (level VII of the Rancho scale), i.e., when he is no longer confused. He then has the attention span and short-term memory to understand and follow testing instructions. Tests of perceptual skills include the Beery-Buktenica Test of Visual Motor Integration, the Motor Free Visual Perception Test, the Baylor Adult Visual-Perceptual Assessment, the Perceptual Motor Evaluation for Head Injured and Other Neurologically Impaired Adults, and others.[2,41] (See chapter 7.)

COGNITIVE COMPONENTS

As with sensory integrative deficits, specific cognitive deficits cannot be evaluated in a patient who is exhibiting a generalized, localized, or agitated response to stimulation and the environment. The therapist can observe the presence or absence of certain cognitive skills in patients who are confused, i.e., stage III. Initia-

tive, length of attention span, concentration, rate of and ability to do information processing, problem solving, sequencing, and appropriateness of response to environmental stimuli can be initially assessed at this time by observing the patient's approach to functional tasks and to simple therapeutic tasks.

The patient is usually able to cooperate with standardized tests of cognition after he has recovered some memory function and is no longer confused. His responses may continue to be inappropriate, however, when task complexity exceeds his cognitive ability. Neuropsychological testing is usually done at this time to fully assess higher-level cognitive deficits.[2] The occupational therapist is concerned about aspects of cognitive functioning primarily as they impede the patient's skills in independent living and daily living tasks. Particular aspects of concern include the patient's judgment, ability for new learning, problem solving, abstract thinking, selective attention, and memory.

INDEPENDENT LIVING/DAILY LIVING SKILLS

Physical Daily Living Skills

Assessment of these skills can only begin when the patient is responding more locally to the external environment. When the patient is confused and agitated, he may respond to simple functional tasks such as moving from the bed to the wheelchair or brushing his teeth, but be unable to complete enough of the task to offer a true assessment of his physical daily living skills. Once the patient is not agitated, evaluation may be initiated (see chapter 16). As much as possible, evaluation of these skills is done in the morning to avoid adding to a patient's temporal disorientation. This evaluation is usually the first opportunity for the therapist to begin investigating the patient's perceptual and/or cognitive function.[21] Patient performance in physical daily living skills may be decreased by physical limitations of motor control or tone, low endurance, dyspraxia, poor head control, oral motor dysfunction, sensory integrative dysfunction, behavioral and cognitive disturbances, or lethargy.[2,21]

Work and Community Involvement Skills

The skills of the patient in these areas cannot be evaluated until the patient is responding fairly appropriately to his environment (i.e., stage IV, or level VII of the Rancho scale). Evaluation checklists for home and community skills are then useful[42] (see chapters 16 and 20). In addition, the therapist will need to carefully assess the amount of supervision and structuring necessary secondary to the patient's decreased judgment and problem solving ability. The patient's wheelchair mobility, body control, and/or balance during functional tasks in the kitchen or in the community need to be assessed carefully. The patient's ability to bend over and get something from a lower cupboard, climb on an escalator, cross the street safely, organize his time adequately, manage his finances, and interact with others in a functional manner must be evaluated to determine the patient's ability to function independently in the community.[2] The Rehabilitation Institute of Chicago has developed a community skills evaluation, as has Santa Clara Valley Medical Center.[15,43]

Driving. The patient's residual physical, cognitive, perceptual, and visual dysfunction must be thoroughly assessed in determining his ability to drive safely. The patient's psychosocial status, including self-control, impulse control, and frustration tolerance, must be carefully considered. A complete history of the patient's medical status, current medications, and previous driving record is also taken. Simulated driving situations on a computer are helpful, if available. Adaptations can be made on a car to compensate for some physical problems (chapter 17), and the patient can be trained to compensate for visual field neglect. However, no compensation can be made for slowed reaction to emergency situations, lack of judgment or problem-solving ability, spatial or directional confusion on the road, deficit in depth perception, or decreased endurance.[2,44] Following evaluation, if the patient appears suitable for driving, an on-the-road test, covering all driving situations, is performed in a dual-control car or the patient's own car, with the assistance of an adaptive driving instructor.[44] The therapist performing a driving evaluation should be familiar with the Department of Motor Vehicle regulations applicable in that state or area.

Employment Preparation. A prevocational evaluation is performed as described in chapter 21. If modification of standardized tests is required, the standardized scoring cannot be used, but the results can be described.

SUMMARY

The evaluation results for a deeply comatose patient would consist of the nature, location, frequency, and duration of patient response to various types of stimulation; PROM measurements; evaluation of muscle tone and abnormal posturing; and evaluation of oral motor function and abnormal reflexes. As the patient begins to emerge from a deep coma, the therapist would reevaluate those areas and begin to evaluate aspects of daily living skills and elementary sensory integration and cognitive skills. As the patient becomes less confused, more formal evaluation of sensory integration, cognition, and independent living skills can be done.

Occupational Therapy Treatment

In determining goals of treatment from the evaluation results, the therapist must consider the interplay of the physical and cognitive deficits identified. Physical deficits will limit independent functioning in the community less than will cognitive deficits, which may reduce the patient's ability for new learning, for problem solving in new unstructured situations, or for learning to compensate for sensory or neuromuscular deficits.[2,6,23] The therapist must also consider the severity of the patient's brain injury and coma, as well as preinjury per-

sonality, drive, intelligence, and the positive or negative aspects of the patient's family dynamics, which will all influence recovery.[2,21,23] Goal formulation should be a team effort, with good team communication a necessity. Once goals are initially determined, the therapist and team will need to revise the goals as the patient continues to recover, and as constant reassessment reveals further strengths and more specific deficits. Goals can be derived according to a particular theory of treatment, such as rehabilitative or neurodevelopmental (chapter 1). Examples of long-term goals and short-term goals will be given below for each stage of recovery.

STAGE I: ABSENT OR GENERALIZED RESPONSE TO STIMULATION

The goal of occupational therapy with the deeply comatose patient, who exhibits flaccidity or posturing, is to provide the patient with organized stimulation that attempts to elicit an increasingly higher level, and more frequent, motor response from the patient. This patient exhibits little spontaneous response to the environment, so the therapist attempts to simplify, structure, and heighten the stimuli to increase the chance of a response being elicited.[21] Each stimulus is thus provided with a desired motor response in mind. The response is verbally requested and/or implied through the therapist's handling. For example, certain oral-motor stimulation implies the desired motor response of lip closure, and certain positional changes imply the desired motor response of head righting. As the patient responds more consistently, the therapist attempts to channel those responses into more appropriate patient interaction with his body and environment. The therapist also begins treating oral motor dysfunction, establishes a positioning program, and provides splints or casts as deemed necessary. Joint occupational therapy/physical therapy sessions are often scheduled to provide optimal treatment, inhibition of abnormal tone, and handling through transitional postures. Frequency of treatment sessions must be carefully coordinated.

Specific Sensory Stimulation

Tactile, vestibular, olfactory, kinesthetic, proprioceptive, auditory, and visual stimuli are utilized. Gustatory stimulation may be used if the patient's oral motor status permits. Both pleasant and unpleasant and familiar and unfamiliar stimuli are used; stimuli with emotional significance to the patient may be more likely to elicit a response. Organized stimulation periods are done frequently throughout the day for 15 to 30 min each, or until a deterioration in the quality of the patient's responses occurs. These sessions must be spaced to allow for rest and nursing care. Stimulation consists of one or two modalities presented in a consistent and meaningful manner; i.e., the patient is told what the therapist is doing and what is expected of him.[21,45] Stimulation can be presented according to developmental sequence (as listed above).[38] It is helpful in ICU to draw the curtain around the bed to reduce competing visual and auditory stimuli. Simple, clear verbal feedback is given on every response elicited: "Good, you are pushing your arm forward," or "Your lips are closing, close them more." The patient's response to stimulation may be quite delayed, as CNS processing is slowed by the damage sustained, if not prevented altogether. The therapist should wait for a response to the stimulation and, if necessary, repeat the stimulus.

Desired responses in this stage will be that of the patient localizing the stimulus (i.e., turning toward a noise, a change in facial expressions, or increased sucking to olfactory stimuli), making a more normal motor response (pushing painful stimuli away), or evidencing a change in muscle tone. Responses are noted to determine any pattern of more consistent, timely responses. If a particular type of stimulation (especially vestibular or olfactory) causes an increase of posturing or large fluctuations in the patient's status (see Precautions section), the precipitating stimulation is reduced in intensity or stopped. The goal is to improve the patient's level of response, not upset his fragile homeostasis.

Tactile stimulation includes rubbing the patient's skin with items of various texture or temperature, applying vibration, and using a firm or moving touch on the patient's limbs with verbal cues to orient the patient to his body.[38,45] The daily bath and other physical daily living tasks are excellent sources of varied cutaneous input, especially if verbal orientation to body parts being washed or moved is included. Moving touch at the T10 dermatome may be used with a decerebrate patient to facilitate a flexor pattern in the legs. This touch is applied from midline to lateral, with up to five repetitions as necessary.[38]

Gentle vestibular stimuli are provided by body position changes (from supine to sitting, sitting to sidelying), head and neck movements, rolling, tilting the bed to sitting, side-to-side or anterior-posterior movement of the patient in bed or on a mat, slow spinning, or rocking. Inversion of the head (leaning over while seated, or lying over a large therapy ball) helps reduce hypertonicity. However, this, and other forms of vestibular stimulation, may be contraindicated in a patient with a trach, elevated ICP, or seizures. Patient reaction must be closely monitored during and after all vestibular stimulation, and used with extreme caution only by a therapist who is very familiar with the neurophysiology of vestibular stimulation.[38] Precautions and desired ranges of heart rate, ICP, and blood pressure must be adhered to during stimulation.

Olfactory stimulation can be attempted with noxious or pleasant odors such as sulfur, spices, almond, vanilla, banana, lemon, perfumes, coffee, or other smells familiar to the patient. This stimulation may be more effective when done prior to the patient's being fed. The therapist must have an effective concentration of the odor. Saturated cotton balls or a sniff bottle are held close to, but not touching, the patient's nose for 2–5 sec.[38] This cranial nerve is sometimes injured in head trauma, and thus olfactory stimulation might not be effective.[6] In addition, the presence of a trach or an n/g tube or both, will eliminate or reduce the air passing through the nostrils, and thus reduce the effectiveness of olfactory stimuli.

Auditory stimulation consists of tapes of favorite music or familiar voices, bells, loud alerting noises such as clapping hands, direct conversation to the patient, verbal commands, explanations, and feedback. A normal but firm voice is used; a comatose patient does not need to be soothed. During therapy sessions, radios, TVs, or other noises should be eliminated as much as possible so that voice commands for motor responses or the selected auditory stimuli are the most prevalent auditory input to the patient. TVs and radios should not be left on all day, or the patient may adapt to the input.

Visual stimulation to elicit attention, focus, and visual tracking is provided by brightly colored objects, mobiles over the bed, mirrors, lighting changes during the day and night, using a flashlight in a darkened room, the family members, or by pictures of family, friends, and the patient. Pictures are labeled by the family to assist in orienting the patient to them. Environmental changes from the bed to therapy room, or from indoors to outdoors, are important sources of visual stimulation. It is important to get the patient upright and well positioned in a wheelchair in order to encourage typical visual orientation, provide more normal kinesthetic input to the patient, and facilitate more normal muscle tone.[14,21]

Specific Therapeutic Procedures to Improve Neuromuscular Skills

Specific therapeutic facilitation techniques to stimulate the patient's kinesthetic, vestibular, and proprioceptive senses include neurodevelopmental treatment (NDT), proprioceptive neuromuscular facilitation (PNF), and Brunnstrom's movement therapy. (See chapter 6.) Such techniques (or modifications thereof) can be combined with quick stretch, tapping over the muscle belly, joint approximation, and the request for an appropriate motor response, thus providing additional tactile and auditory stimulation to the patient.[38,46] Quick ice also can be used to facilitate an individual muscle response when applied to the muscle belly[46] (see chapter 5 and chapter 6, part A) or can be used for directionality of motion. ("I am going to put ice on your hand. Pull away from the ice"). Quick ice is perceived as a distinct noxious stimulus when applied to the face, soles of the feet, or palms.[46] Normal precautions with use of ice are observed as described in chapters 5 and 6.

The head, neck, and trunk receive special emphasis in early treatment, in accordance with the cervicocephalocaudal, proximal-to-distal nature of development, and also because of the crucial contribution of these areas to development of visual-spatial awareness and body integration.[45] The comatose patient is told in advance of any body position changes performed or elicited to decrease the possibility of posturing and other stereotypic reactions. If the stimulation causes an increase of posturing, it is stopped temporarily and resumed after the patient has rested.

NDT positions, weight shifting, weight bearing, and transitional movements between positions can be used to selectively increase or decrease muscle tone in a developmental progression of movement, or can be used to elicit beginning righting reactions.[2,15,45,47] (See chapters 5 and 6.) Supine, side-lying, prone, and sitting positions are the most feasible to use with a patient at this level. The prone position may need to be modified for a patient with a trach. Prone and sitting in particular are best done on a firm surface, such as a mat, and may not be possible if the patient cannot be treated in the therapy department. The therapist can, however, incorporate the techniques of weight shifting and weight bearing into treatment in ICU to change muscle tone and work to normalize the patient's proprioceptive input.[15,47]

If using PNF or Brunnstrom patterns, the therapist would first treat the arm responding to stimulation with a higher level motor reaction. The patient may only be able to respond in one part of a muscle's range, so the shortened or slightly lengthened positions must each be tried. Verbal instructions to the patient must be consistent, simple, and as noncortical as possible. The patient is instructed to "reach," or "look up," or is simply facilitated into the position and the desired motor response is shaped. Modifications of these techniques may be necessary when working with a patient in ICU with restrictions on his movement.

Since isolated, well-controlled movements in the arms or trunk will not be visible in this stage of coma, the therapist must feel the muscle tone changes that signify the beginnings of a voluntary effort. As the therapist handles the comatose patient and becomes more familiar with his pattern of muscle tone, changes occurring in that tone will be more obvious. Movement or pressure in a range where there was no movement before might represent the beginnings of voluntary movement. A sustained push felt near the end of the range is not likely to be the result of quick stretch, which elicits a phasic response (chapter 5).

Specific maneuvers to inhibit tone may be necessary with the comatose patient who is posturing. One such inhibition method is axial rotation of the trunk. While the patient is positioned in side-lying, the therapist attempts to rotate the thorax on the pelvis, thus breaking up the typical trunk tightness and immobility. This rotation, and inhibition of trunk tone, will be necessary later for rolling with appropriate patterns of head and neck, for moving from prone to sitting, for UE function, and eventually for equilibrium reactions. Extensor tone can be somewhat lessened by maintenance of hip and knee flexion, avoidance of resistance to the back of the head, and avoidance of the supine position itself. Other methods would include lateral elongation of the trunk in supine with shoulders kept steady, followed by wiggling of the pelvis to obtain anterior pelvic tilt on the elongated side, followed by repetition of this technique on the other side; maintained touch or pressure in the perioral or abdominal areas; neutral warmth or wrapping; weight bearing; or the principles of reflex inhibiting patterns.[15,38,45] (See chapter 6.) The speed of the therapist's movements and the patient's response to frequent hand position changes should be considered in altering procedures to decrease the patient's tone. Immediately following successful inhibition of tone, the therapist would attempt to facilitate more normal movement in a functional pattern. For example, if trunk extensor tone was reduced while the patient was side-lying, the therapist might choose to facilitate upper trunk initiation of rolling to prone, reaching with upper arm, or coming up from side-lying to partial sitting.

Prefeeding Stimulation

In this stage, the prefeeding treatment would consist of decreasing abnormal sensitivity, tone, and reflexes, and facilitating more normal oral movements with the patient positioned in sitting in a wheelchair or in bed. Hypersensitivity is reduced by applying maintained pressure to the inside of the cheeks, lips, external surface of the gums, and the posterior portion of the tongue (if severe bite reflex is absent). The therapist utilizes glycerine swabs, padded tongue blades, a soft toothbrush, or gloved fingers to apply pressure. Hypertonia of cheeks and lips is reduced by handling, taking each of the facial muscles through their normal range, "shaking" out the cheek with one finger on the inside and one on the outside of the cheek and ending by crossing the midline,[14] and other types of inhibitory techniques.

If a bite reflex is present, firm rubbing on the external surface of the gums and/or firm stroking from the side of the nose to the mouth is done to inhibit this reflex.[14] Bite reflex inhibition may not be obtained if the patient is posturing severely. The therapist may need to continue inhibition during further stages of recovery until the bite reflex is reduced. If decrease of the bite reflex is achieved, a rubber seizure stick is used to give midline maintained pressure of 3–5 sec to the posterior two-thirds of the tongue to reduce tongue hypersensitivity and increase posterior tongue movement.[38] After reduction of hypersensitivity in the oral area and tongue, tongue thrust or abnormal retraction is reduced if present.

The therapist must be familiar with the normal oral motor sequence of swallowing and the correct head/neck/trunk posture for swallowing in order to work towards normalizing a patient's oral motor tone and movements. Appropriate lip closure and jaw stability are facilitated through quick stretch, pressure, tapping, and manual vibration on appropriate muscles.[14,38] Facilitation of appropriate tongue movements and swallowing is usually not possible with a deeply comatose patient, especially if posturing is severe. Caution is essential with the use of vibration and ice around the face.[38] Further information may be found in references 15, 38, and 39.

Gustatory stimulation may be initiated if there is access to the patient's tongue, palate, and mucosa of the lips and cheeks, and if there is minimal risk of aspiration. Again, with severe posturing, this stimulation may need to be deferred until stage II. The patient would need to be positioned in a wheelchair or propped up in bed, as oral control is more difficult and risk of aspiration is greater if the patient is supine.[38] Stimuli would include a very small amount of salty, sweet, bitter, sour, or favorite tastes of the patient's. The stimuli are presented in a water solution, and are placed via a cotton swab or eyedropper on the part of the tongue or oral area most sensitive to that flavor.[15] A rinse with sterile water or with a lemon glycerine swab is recommended between different flavors.[38] If the patient has a risk of aspiration, the rinse would be reduced or eliminated, and the amounts of stimuli would be reduced. Oral feeding is generally not done with patients in this stage.

Positioning

Early implementation of positioning designed to prevent or reduce contractures, foot drop, or abnormal patterns of muscle tone is essential.[2,6,14] Some typical abnormalities in position seen in patients with severe traumatic brain injuries are abnormally forward head, protracted and forward tipped scapulae with or without elevation, posterior pelvic tilt with unilateral retraction and/or elevation, severe trunk tightness with lack of trunk dissociation from neck and head, hip flexor and adductor tightness, foot plantar flexion, and inversion with lack of dissociation of hindfoot from forefoot.

Patient positioning must be reevaluated frequently. Assistive positioning supports are used intermittently and removed as the patient's neuromuscular status improves. The staff at Elizabethtown Hospital have developed a reusable, adaptable seating system for patients, which reduces the expense and time of fabrication and provides immediately available seating for patients.[48] For further positioning suggestions, the reader is referred to references 15 and 38.

The nursing staff and the patient's family must be made aware of the desired bed and wheelchair positioning and of the splint-wearing schedule. For abnormal tone to be reduced and contractures to be reduced or prevented, the positioning must continue throughout the day and night.

In Bed. Side-lying or semiprone, with good body alignment, is preferable to supine if the patient is exhibiting abnormal posturing.[14,38] The supine position triggers the TLR extensor response. The head, resting on a small pillow, should be in neutral, midline, and aligned with the trunk; the bottom UE in scapular protraction and humeral external rotation; the top UE with scapular protraction, slight shoulder flexion, and resting on a pillow to avoid horizontal adduction; the bottom elbow flexed, the top elbow extended; wrists in extension; and cones in hands to decrease spasticity and maintain thumb web space. Slight hip and knee flexion of the upper leg may need to be maintained with pillows or sandbags, with a pillow between the knees to decrease hip internal rotation and adduction. The lower leg also may need pillow support to be aligned with the thigh. The lower hip and knee are flexed only slightly. Elongation of the lower side of the trunk between the shoulder and pelvis is desirable. Side-lying trunk position may need to be maintained by a pillow or sandbag behind the back and shoulder. Footboards are avoided as they elicit extensor thrust. Splints or special shoes[38] are used that are cut to avoid pressure to the ball of the foot but still maintain ankle flexion to 90° and reduce foot drop. The foot drop splint pictured in chapter 13 would need to be modified for the comatose patient. The splint would have to be cut down below the ball of the foot to avoid stimulating an extensor thrust.

If the patient must be positioned in supine, a small pillow under the head is used, with small rolled pillows under that pillow to keep head in midline (if the patient cannot do so); small pillows are placed under the scapulae to protract them; shoulders are positioned in slight abduction and external rotation; elbows are extended; and cones or finger spreaders are used for positioning the fingers.[15] If the pelvis is retracted on one side, a small folded towel is placed behind it and that leg positioned in neutral rotation. Some knee flexion should be encouraged by a small towel roll placed under the distal thigh just above the knee joint.

In Wheelchair. Early and correct upright positioning in a wheelchair is helpful in inhibiting abnormal tone, providing normal proprioceptive input, and reducing the likelihood and/or extent of contractures and complications from prolonged bed rest.

The pelvis must be positioned correctly before addressing other areas. The pelvis should be in a neutral position or slight anterior pelvic tilt and symmetrical without one side retracted or elevated. Weight bearing equally through both buttocks is essential to attainment of more normal tone. Solid seat and back inserts are necessary, as the typical wheelchair seat and back sag and actually facilitate posterior pelvic tilt, unequal weight bearing through both hips, and hip internal rotation and adduction. A small, flat lumbar roll is placed wherever necessary, above the pelvis and below the scapula, to facilitate anterior pelvic tilt in that patient. If the pelvis is retracted on one side, wedged back pieces may be helpful for positioning. If unequal weight bearing is occurring with habitual elongation of one side of the trunk, an insert under the habitual weight-bearing buttock may be helpful. The back of the chair may be reclined 10–15° to position the trunk and head more appropriately. Hip flexion should be 90° and can be achieved by a wedge cushion with the high end at the distal thigh. The seat belt should come from the corners of the seat at a 45° angle and fasten over the lower pelvis/hip area to help maintain the anterior pelvic tilt and equal weight bearing through the buttocks.

To assist leg and pelvis position through slight abduction and external rotation, wide soft straps can be utilized that come from the side of the chair, under the patient's upper thigh, and around the top of that thigh to the hip joint (Rona Alexander, unpublished information). These straps should not come from the chair corners, but from the side somewhere along the patient's thigh, and are made separately for each thigh. The patient may need firm pads on the outer aspect of the thighs to reduce excessive abduction, or a knee abductor to decrease excessive adduction. If the seat belt cannot keep the patient from scooting forward in the chair, a removable padded bar may need to be placed close to the pelvis and femurs.

The trunk, positioned next, should be symmetrical, and in midline with shoulders over pelvis in sagittal, frontal, and horizontal planes. Lateral trunk supports can be used to decrease lateral trunk flexion. Experimentation with the positioning is essential, as patients differ in their trunk control. The therapist must not provide too much trunk support, but only enough to facilitate the patient's normal movement and control. With a solid seat and back, the patient may not require additional trunk supports.

A harness, shoulder straps, or a chest strap may be necessary if the patient exhibits forward trunk flexion. These should not fasten directly on top of the shoulders, but should extend a little higher up before going through the seat back to fasten. An additional seat belt can also be used, placed horizontally across the anterior superior iliac crests to provide backward pressure.[15]

Knees and ankles are flexed to 90°, heels slightly behind the knees in sitting, feet in neutral pronation/supination and inversion/eversion. The footplate should be large enough to support the whole foot. Ankle straps can encourage increased plantar flexion in some patients; a foot wedge, heel loops, an insert behind the foot, special shoes, toe guards, or a combination may be helpful in decreasing abnormal tone and in achieving weight bearing in the heel.

The ideal UE position is neutral scapular elevation or depression with scapulae in slight protraction, slight shoulder external rotation, slight flexion and abduction, elbows in comfortable flexion, forearm in pronation, wrists in neutral flexion/extension and ulnar/radial deviation, fingers relaxed, and thumb radially abducted. Excessive scapular retraction may require contouring of the seat back or reclining the seat unit by about 10°. Position of shoulder straps, chest straps, or lateral trunk supports may be helpful in obtaining adequate shoulder position.

A lapboard, positioned at the proper height to allow good UE weight bearing, is helpful. The lapboard should not be positioned against the patient's trunk, but far enough away so the patient can flex forward slightly at the hips. There should be a cutout so that the lapboard fits around the patient, and the lapboard needs to be large enough to accommodate the whole arm. A V-shaped piece of dense foam can be positioned behind the patient's elbow to decrease elbow flexion and retraction of the arm off the back of the lapboard. A contoured surface for the hands may be added to the lapboard. Hand fixation usually causes the patient to pull back against the fixation.

The head ideally should be in midline, with cervical elongation, chin tucked slightly, and horizontal eye gaze. There should be no chin jutting or neck hyperextension. Head positioning is very difficult. The position of the patient's shoulders and upper trunk will have an influence upon head position. A Philadelphia collar is usually not successful, as the patient sinks or pushes down into it, and it hinders normalization of oral motor tone and movement. Chin straps also have not been successful. A customized head support or U-shaped support may be required.[38] Pressure directly to the occipital area of the head elicits increased extensor tone of the head and trunk. Therefore, the pressure to right the head is applied up from the occipital process (to each side of midline) and around the forehead in a back and downwards pressure. Such a head support would need to be fastened to a head rest, which is recessed so that the patient's head could not push or rest against it. Lateral head supports may be necessary to adequately position the patient's head.

Passive Range of Motion

PROM can be difficult with this patient. Sudden stretch and inappropriate stimulation and handling should be avoided. Scapular mobility should be addressed before UE PROM is done to facilitate normal scapular/humeral movement during the rest of PROM. PROM and positioning are helpful in minimizing the effects of heterotopic ossification.[21]

Splinting and Casting

The goals of splinting or casting are to decrease abnormal tone and increase the patient's functional movement. Splints and casts are therefore changed as necessary to meet these goals. The patient's quality of movement is constantly reassessed to determine continued necessity of the splints. Splints can assist in positioning flaccid patients, but should be very carefully monitored when used with severely spastic or posturing patients, as abnormal tone can be aggravated and pressure areas created quickly.

Splints to provide maintained pressure and stretch between the thenar and hypothenar eminences or to stretch the fingers in abduction (chapter 13) may be helpful. The splint should simulate the position of the hand and wrist in weight bearing. With severe tone in elbow, hand, knee, ankle, or foot, serial casting may be indicated.[21] Serial cylinder casting provides neutral warmth, more even skin pressure, and allows for less movement than do splints. Casts are usually left on up to 7 days.[2,21] Drop-out casts (casts leaving a portion of the limb free to relax out of a tightly contracted position), bivalved casts (casts for maintaining a position that are split in two, with moleskin protecting the edges, so they can be removed during therapy or nursing procedures), and weight-bearing inhibitory casts (casts fabricated to approximate the ideal weight-bearing posture of the foot or hand) can also be utilized.[14,21]

Therapy Related to Family Needs

The family of these patients usually indicates its need to be involved in the patient's care, to feel they can do something to promote his recovery. Family members can be shown simple PROM exercises to do with the patient. The importance of periods of organized sensory stimulation followed by rest is explained to the family. Auditory and tactile stimulation can be provided by the family, as their voices and touch will be more familiar to the patient at first and may elicit more response than unfamiliar voices.[31] Positioning is described and demonstrated to the family, with their participation urged.

The team members also must cope with the family's need for hope and optimism, the reality of the patient's situation, and his probable outcome and residual deficits.[2] Consistency of team members' interactions with the family is essential. Family members may express severe anxiety, a sense of isolation, fear about their ability to cope with any future deficits, helplessness, or prolonged denial. Timing of intervention by the team is crucial. The family will not be able to hear and understand the team members' realistic assessment until they are ready.[2] Conversations and instructions will have to be repeated frequently, as the family is under considerable stress and flux.[49]

Goals for Patients in Stage I of Recovery

Evaluation of the patient at this stage would likely indicate severely decreased movement and responsiveness in specific sensory systems, presence of abnormal tone and reflexes, and presence of abnormal oral motor function.

Possible long-term goals would be to normalize the patient's abnormal tone, increase the amount of voluntary movement, and increase the level of responsiveness to sensory stimulation.

Examples of short-term goals with this patient would be to increase his level of awareness to tactile sensory stimuli as measured by increased head turning or withdrawal responses, decrease his extensor tone through positioning and appropriate sensory stimuli, increase his flexor response to stimuli and facilitation, maintain ROM by implementation of optimal positioning and appropriate sensory stimulation during treatment and nursing tasks, and improve his ability to keep his head in midline.

STAGE II: LOCALIZED RESPONSE TO STIMULATION

The occupational therapy goal is to refine and direct the patient's response to stimulation once the patient begins to respond to stimulation with a more localized and adaptive behavioral response. Such localization is seen when the patient pulls at his n/g tube or catheter, focuses on something briefly, or turns his head away when his cheek is stimulated. The therapist attempts to obtain greater consistency in localizing responses and avoiding stereotypic movements, more variety in the patient's response, and a decreased interval between stimulation and response.[21] The therapist also attempts to increase the patient's ability to follow simple commands, to attend to an activity, and to use common objects such as a spoon, comb, or washcloth.

At this stage of coma, the therapist may be able to more precisely identify motor or sensory deficits by observing the patient's spontaneous repositioning in bed; his periods of restlessness; his neuromuscular response to stimuli of light touch, temperature, pain, sounds, and proprioception; his facial movements in response to family, friends, or stimuli; or his spontaneous response to, or manipulation of, utensils. Specific evaluation and tests are still inappropriate, as the patient is unable to consistently attend to a task or follow commands and has decreased periods of alertness.

Sensory Stimulation

Sensory stimulation as described above would be continued with the goal of refining the patient's motor responses. For example, visual stimulation would attempt to increase the length of the patient's attentiveness and improve tracking skills. More active vestibular stimulation may be possible at this level. Prone or semiprone inversion over a large therapy ball with visual stimulation may increase head and neck control; however, optimal position of the shoulder girdle must be maintained to avoid hyperextension of the neck with elevation of the shoulders. Reduction of the extent of positioning supports (splints, casts, wheelchair modifications, and bed positioning) would be done as possible.

Procedures to Improve Neuromuscular Skills

Treatment of neuromuscular skills continues with NDT, PNF (with resistance applied proximally if necessary to get less associated reactions), Brunnstrom techniques, and facilitation to specific muscles and areas. If the patient has an n/g tube, caution must be taken that the patient's head remain above stomach level to avoid regurgitation and aspiration.[2] At this level, mat activities for the developmental stages of head and neck control, rolling, and sitting may be more feasible. The patient can be more readily facilitated into positions or transitional movements such as prone, from prone to prone on elbows (for weight bearing through forearms and hands, inhibition of hypertonus, and feedback into the shoulder girdle),[15] prone on elbows with weight shifting side-to-side and coordinated trunk shortening, from prone on elbows to sidelying and back, rolling from prone to supine and back, and sitting with weight shifting in sagittal and frontal planes to facilitate appropriate trunk and UE reactions. The sitting position can be used with UE weight bearing onto a table in front, or onto the mat at the patient's side. If the patient has increased hip adduction, he may be positioned in sitting over a bolster with weight bearing onto hands in front or on the bolster.[15] The patient's feet must have weight bearing throughout the soles, with hip flexion at 90° or more.[14] The above positions are developmentally important to attain head and neck, shoulder girdle, and upper trunk control, to free the arms for function, and to develop righting reactions and protective responses. Two therapists may be needed to handle the patient and facilitate appropriate body alignment through the positions. If the patient's motor skills are more intact, simple "automatic" games such as throwing or hitting a large ball may be tried. Due to the patient's limited alertness, his praxis cannot be fully assessed at this level.

Redevelopment of Physical Daily Living Skills

Rudimentary skills of feeding, face washing, and light grooming are now begun. These basic tasks are overlearned and may draw automatic responses from the patient. Such tasks are normally relegated to subcortical direction,[21,45] which may not have been impaired.[7] The attention of the patient is focused on the end result, rather than the process, to tap this subcortical direction.[45] The therapist may simply hand a wet washcloth to him, or put it in his hand and bring it to his face. The therapist assists as necessary, so that the patient can initiate as much as possible and receive the sensory feedback from the task. These tasks are done at appropriate times of the day to orient the patient. Rest periods are essential, as he fatigues rapidly. He is treated in a quiet environment, with minimal and consistent instructions. The variables in the task are reduced and the tasks are simplified drastically. For example, one dish and one spoon are used in feeding, and the rest of the tray is put out of sight; the patient is not required to bathe himself entirely, but merely to wash his face. Once the patient is more consistent and successful at a part of the task, the task can be gradually expanded and made more complex.

Feeding. Oral motor treatment continues as detailed above in order to desensitize the oral area, decrease abnormal reflexes, normalize the gag reflex, increase endurance of oral motor area, and elicit normal movements necessary in eating and swallowing.

Tongue movements (lateralization, protraction, retraction, cupping, tip elevation, and posterior elevation) and the swallowing mechanism usually can be treated at this level, if the bite reflex has been reduced. Pressure, resistance, or quick stretch to the tongue movements, and quick ice or vibration by the therapist's hand to the laryngopharyngeal musculature to facilitate swallowing are done, along with continued facilitation of normal lip, jaw, and cheek movements.[38] Improved head and neck control will improve the patient's oral motor function.

Oral feeding is begun only when the patient has been assessed to have an adequate swallow, good oral con-

trol, and strong gag and cough reflexes. The patient is positioned upright with head tilted forward slightly. Environmental distractions are reduced. Mouth care, suctioning of oral area and around the trach, and inflation of a cuffed trach are done by the nurse prior to therapy. Some therapists feel it is better to deflate a cuffed trach during treatment to decrease irritation with laryngeal elevation during swallowing.[39] However, the patient's physician must be consulted, as he may feel the patient's risk of aspiration is too high and the cuff should be inflated. The therapist monitors the patient closely for any sign of aspiration. The nurse should be present at first to suction if necessary. To decrease the risk of aspiration, the patient may be encouraged to cough, to hold his breath during swallowing, and/or to clear his throat after each swallow; however, patients at this level may not be cognitively alert enough to follow these instructions. The patient should also be given time in between each swallow to allow the food to clear the passageways. If the patient is aspirating some of each bite, the therapist would discuss this with the physician. Oral feeding may be discontinued; however, reflex facilitation, bolus control exercises, swallowing practice without food, and tongue, lip, and cheek exercises may be continued if the patient is able to cooperate.[39]

In choosing the food to use, several factors are considered: flavor, texture, temperature, and density or consistency. The food should not be too bland; sweet, sour or salty flavors elicit mastication and a swallow; sweet liquids and toothpaste elicit salivation. Ice cream and milk products tend to increase secretions, which makes swallowing more difficult. Oily liquids, such as beef broth, thin mucus secretions. Lemon flavoring tends to stimulate sucking. Texture is important to stimulate the oral sensation; for example, applesauce is preferable to a thoroughly pureed baby food. Temperature should be slightly warmer or cooler than body temperature. If the food is tepid, it will not create a different sensation to signal its presence in the mouth; if the food is too cold, it will numb the oral area and its musculature. Density is crucial. The tongue, palate, and laryngeal muscles may require food of a particular weight to provide slight "resistance" and "stretch" to facilitate function.[14] These decisions are made on the basis of evaluation of the patient's oral motor function, sensitivity, and prior food preferences.

A thin paste-like consistency is good for patients who have reduced tongue control or delayed triggering of the swallow reflex.[39] Liquids are generally difficult for the brain-injured patient to swallow at first, as the tongue must cup around liquids and seal them against the hard palate prior to swallowing. Jello and ice chips tend to melt to a liquid too quickly in the mouth, and thus are not easily managed at first. Liquids can be thickened with clear gelatin. Typically, the therapist would begin with a thin "paste" consistency food such as applesauce, pureed fruit, oatmeal, pudding, mashed potatoes, or chowder. These foods can be mixed with baby cereal to increase their consistency. Food coloring can be added to assist determination of aspiration when the patient is suctioned or coughing during or after the session. As the patient begins to handle these foods, thick liquids are introduced. If the patient has a strong sucking reflex, the therapist may choose to begin with thickened liquids and then progress to foods with paste consistency.

The amount of food or liquid used for each swallow is approximately 1/3 teaspoon.[39] Before each bite, the therapist focuses patient attention and facilitates stabilization of the head and mouth opening. Using a tongue blade or a small spoon, the therapist places the food with slight pressure on the side of the mouth with more function and sensitivity. Placement of food on the side of the mouth will encourage tongue lateralization. Appropriate oral movements of tongue, cheeks, lips, and jaw are facilitated after each placement.[38,39]

Before progressing to foods requiring chewing, the patient's tongue and jaw movements are reassessed. He must be able to keep food in between his teeth for chewing, gather it back into a bolus, move it to the back of his mouth, and elevate his tongue for swallowing. To work on chewing, the therapist would begin with canned or diced peaches or fruit, which are sweet to stimulate mastication and which slip down readily.[14] The next type of food might be egg salad and then ground chicken. Scrambled eggs are often too dry and too difficult to maintain in a bolus. Ground beef is harder to chew than ground chicken. The ground food must be moist, or it will tend to disperse throughout the mouth. Brain trauma patients may show impulsivity and lack of thorough chewing, and thus advancing them to foods that require chewing may be inappropriate. If the patient is able to bring the spoon up to his mouth with minimum or moderate physical assistance, a more automatic oral response may be elicited and the feeding training facilitated.

Following a feeding session, the patient should remain upright for 10–15 min to allow the food to be totally swallowed. Oral care and suctioning should be done. Functional self-feeding will probably not occur at this stage, but during stage III, when the cognitive status of the patient and his ability to follow instructions have improved.

Sensory Integration and Cognition

Cognitive and sensory integrative functioning cannot be formally evaluated at this point in the recovery process; such functioning must be inferred from the patient's performance of simple physical daily living skills and his motor responses to the environment. Observation will indicate if the patient notices visitors or objects on both sides of him or if he exhibits signs of homonymous hemianopia; if he seems to use objects appropriately when handed to him or needs to be shown; if he watches the therapist demonstrating usage of objects; if he visually tracks people and movement; if he is

able to sustain attention to a specific task; if he can reach across midline and position himself at midline; and if his spatial and depth perception appears impaired when reaching for objects.

The patient may still have his eyes closed most of the time. If his eyes are open and tracking, he is usually highly distractible and demonstrates a very short attention span and no memory. At this stage, the patient will not show carryover of new learning from treatment session to session. Memory entails attending to the relevant stimuli of an experience, encoding them, storing them appropriately, and then retrieving them. Any or all of these processes can be disrupted by a diffuse, severe traumatic brain injury.[2] The temporal lobes and hippocampus appear to be primarily involved in the encoding of memory, and these areas are frequently damaged.[6,7] The patient with a brain injury will usually not remember day-to-day activities until he is able to produce fairly consistent appropriate responses to external stimulation. Until then, he exists in a fugue-like, confused state.

Treatment of these areas may include simple perceptual activities such as color, form, or shape matching and sorting; simple gross motor catching and throwing games; basic sensory integration activities (within precautions noted above); and simple self-care tasks.

Treatment of the Agitated Patient

Once the patient begins localizing stimuli, he may become quite agitated and restless as he becomes acutely aware of internal discomfort, pain, internal cognitive confusion and disruption, and external restraints. The patient will usually tear at tubes and restraints, show decreased ability to cooperate with treatment, and may become aggressive.[21,50] Not all brain trauma patients pass through this phase; those who do may experience this phase for a few days or up to 4 weeks.[21,50,51] A restless or agitated patient has been found to be more likely to show greater physical improvement than an immobile or sluggishly moving patient.[50] Medication to calm the patient should be avoided whenever possible, since the large doses that are necessary slow the patient's cognitive recovery.[51] However, in some cases, behavior becomes violent and aggressive enough for drug treatment to be considered.[51] It is important to remember that the patient is not accountable for the agitation, hostility, or aggressiveness. He is responding to internal cognitive confusion, not specifically to the person who happens to be in the situation with him.

The goals of occupational therapy during this phase are to decrease the patient's agitation as much as possible by reducing stimuli that agitate the patient and increasing situations or stimuli that calm the patient, to continue to focus his attention on the external environment through engaging his participation in self-care and other "automatic" tasks, and to attempt to have the patient follow simple commands. Patient cooperation, motivation, and follow-through are minimal. He cannot focus cognitively on his environment and interpret it.[21] Therefore, he cannot learn at this stage. Removal of noxious stimulation, whenever possible, assists in decreasing agitation. Limb restraints are removed during therapy sessions and at other times of constant supervision. The patient is not left alone if contact decreases his agitation. Loud noises and external confusion may heighten agitation. An unchanged daily routine can provide structure and predictability and reduce patient confusion.

Inhibitory techniques of repetitive or sustained touch, warmth, rocking, slow rolling, slow vestibular stimulation, and use of the therapist's voice and presence to soothe the patient are helpful.[21,38,45] A change of environment to a quieter place with less stimulation; a drink of juice or a snack (if the patient has normal oral motor activity); tapes of family voices; explanation to the patient that this is a stage of recovery that will pass; and continual orientation of the patient to where he is, why, and what the therapist is doing with him can also assist in decreasing his agitation. Acknowledgment of the discomfort and gentle redirection of the patient's attention to tasks is useful.

Treatment is done in an individual or structured group setting, using simple and familiar gross motor or daily living tasks, such as face washing, walking, stationary cycling, catching a large ball, throwing beanbags, moving from supine to sitting, and putting on simple clothes such as a T-shirt or pull-on pants. The therapist changes the activity frequently as the patient grows restless or agitated. The patient may also have decreased tolerance to one person working with him; therapist assignment to the patient at this stage may need to change during a treatment session.[21] Tasks requiring concentration or fine motor precision, such as pegboards and form boards, are avoided during periods of agitation or restlessness.[15,21] The patient will most likely need maximum assistance with self-care tasks because of his short attention span, although his agitation may increase his independence in bed mobility. He also may begin transfers now, depending on his level of muscular involvement.

The patient's orientation may be assessed if he is verbally responsive. However, such assessment should not be pursued if it further agitates the patient. Patients can be aware of their situation early in the recovery process. This awareness may be simply a knowledge that something is wrong even if it cannot be defined, that they should remember something but that they don't. These patients have undergone a total loss of control of their body and actions. Each action is isolated because the patient cannot remember what came before, yet he struggles to make cognitive sense out of each moment. At this point, the patient needs the therapist to provide consistency and predictability, feedback on reality, calmness, quietness, confidence, acceptance, and consideration of his communications, however nonsensical, inappropriate, or nonverbal. The therapist can gather information on the patient's cognitive status by observing the patient functioning in tasks or by watching his social interactions.

Goals for Patients in Stage II of Recovery

The patient at stage II is more responsive to internal and external stimuli, but he still does not initiate activities or remember events and is dependent in most physical daily living skills. He may be moving and repositioning in bed secondary to restlessness, but he continues to require assistance for transfers and other forms of motor activity.

Examples of long-term goals for this stage would be to increase and to channel the patient's responsiveness and alertness, increase his ability to move independently, and increase his self-care skills.

Short-term goals might be to continue to provide appropriate positioning through splints and casts to maintain PROM; increase the consistency, variety, and quality of response to stimulation; continue normalizing muscle tone through neurorehabilitation techniques; develop more normal movements in head, neck, and trunk during transitional movements; decrease agitation through calming, inhibitory activities or simple repetitive tasks; improve oral motor function through reduction of abnormal oral reflexes; and continue evaluation of cognition and sensory integration.

STAGE III: CONFUSED AND INAPPROPRIATE (OR APPROPRIATE) RESPONSE TO STIMULATION/ENVIRONMENT

As the patient's agitation decreases, he will respond more to the external environment. His responses will be confused and inappropriate at first.[19] He is unable to process information at a normal rate or produce an appropriate response to all environmental situations. Later, his response to a given situation may be appropriate but still not completely correct due to poor short-term memory, difficulty in learning new tasks (such as one-handed methods of dressing), persistent confusion, decreased attention span, visual-spatial dysfunction, dyspraxia, and/or inconsistent orientation.[2,15,21]

Occupational therapy goals in this stage are to increase attention to more specific tasks and salient stimuli; increase the process of sequential organization; increase immediate and short-term memory (i.e., memory of events for up to one hour); and increase analysis, association, and categorization.[52,53] Treatment continues to emphasize improvement of the patient's neuromuscular skills, improvement of his perceptual skills, and his increased ability to do simple physical daily living and homemaking tasks. The therapist continues to structure the patient's environment for him because of the patient's difficulty in structuring the environment himself. Complexity and duration of the tasks are reduced to the patient's level of ability, distractions are reduced, his immediate environment and schedule are kept as unchanged as possible, and visual memory aids, such as a written daily schedule on the arm of the wheelchair, are provided.[2,15,21,52]

Redevelopment of Physical Daily Living Skills

Self-care training continues as described above in stage II. The task is simplified until the patient is consistently successful in performing it, and then the complexity is gradually increased while the externally provided structure is gradually decreased. Environmental distractions are reduced. Adaptive equipment is provided if necessary. The therapist gathers the items to be used and sequences the task by providing the patient with the appropriate item at the proper time and by giving simplified directions at each step. For example, in dressing, the therapist would first hand the patient his undershorts and then give simple verbal instructions and physical cueing as necessary to have the patient put the shorts over his legs and pull them up. The therapist would not present the patient's T-shirt until the shorts were finished. The clothes chosen initially would be solid colors with minimal fastenings to decrease perceptual confusion. The therapist may also choose to limit the task by having the patient do only one or two steps of the entire task (e.g., put on T-shirt only) if the patient has very low endurance, low frustration tolerance, or limited hip or trunk flexion. The therapist should structure the task and method so that the patient is not reinforcing abnormal movement patterns during his self-care. The position of the patient (i.e., dressing in bed, sitting in the wheelchair, or sitting on the edge of the bed) and the method of dressing would have been selected according to the patient's neuromuscular function.

Gradually as the patient becomes more successful in dressing, the therapist decreases verbal and physical cueing, gives the patient more than one piece of clothing at once, or increases the speed of the activity.[21] Hygiene training, feeding, and transfer training are structured in the same fashion. The therapist would begin with whichever self-care task was most meaningful to the patient and would not add more tasks until reasonable success had been achieved.[15]

The patient usually continues to require moderate assistance, even if he has only minimal physical deficit, because of cognitive impairment. The therapist is prepared to verbalize the task steps repeatedly or to rephrase instructions if the patient appears confused. The anticipated outcome is that the patient will begin to absorb the structure provided to him by the therapist and internalize it.[21] Generalization of the structure to other tasks is not expected, however, as the patient continues to have comprehensive cognitive deficits and decreased memory at this stage.

Procedures to Improve Neuromuscular Skills

At this stage, therapy to restore motor function can include muscle facilitation and/or strengthening exercises for UE and hand musculature to address isolated dysfunction or overall weakness; activities to develop UE stability, mobility, and function; and/or appropriate NDT, PNF, and Brunnstrom techniques. Head control, midline orientation, trunk mobility and rotation, scapular mobility and function, weight bearing, weight shifting, and dissociation of head, neck, and trunk movements are all worked on in therapy until the patient's movement is more normal.[2,15,47] (See chapter

6.) Following this, activities combining trunk movements and rotation with UE reaching and functional patterns, weight shifting and weight bearing with coordinated UE movements, and righting and equilibrium reactions are worked on.

Once the patient is exhibiting a confused but appropriate response to stimulation, more detailed sensory and motor evaluations can be done using simplified instructions with traditional tests (chapters 3, 4, and 8).

Sensory Integration

Treatment at this level of recovery may consist of matching; sorting; discrimination of differences and similarities in color, size, or shape; very simple three- or four-piece puzzles; tracing; simple figure-ground and visual-motor coordination worksheets; and simple design copying. Sequencing tasks, coding tasks, visual scanning tasks, and more complicated design copying or figure-ground tasks may be done with the patient who is confused but responding appropriately. Formal perceptual testing is usually not possible at this level, but can be done in the following stage.

Cognition and Behavior

Formal assessment of the patient's neuropsychological and behavioral deficits by the team psychologist or neuropsychologist is useful in planning occupational therapy treatment to correspond to and not overtax the patient's current memory status and cognitive abilities. Clinical observations by team members can also assist in informally determining the patient's cognitive status and behavioral problems.

Behavioral sequelae may hamper therapy at this stage. As the patient becomes more alert, his awareness of his situation may increase his irritability, his uncooperativeness, or his mood fluctuations. The patient may be impulsive, easily frustrated, perseverative, and dependent on his family.[2] He is confused and disoriented at times, and doesn't remember why he is in the hospital. Specific techniques that have been utilized at this level to reduce confusion and increase more acceptable behavior are behavioral modification programs[2] and reality-orientation peer groups.[2,21] The patient may also begin to display secondary behavioral disturbances in response to the stress of coping with his suddenly altered life-style, such as denial, depression, dependence, or isolation.[2,21,52] Preinjury characteristics of the brain-injured patient, family support and dynamics, and preinjury educational level of the patient are important contributors to postinjury behavioral sequelae and to the extent of cognitive recovery.[2,21,54,55]

Tests of the duration of posttraumatic amnesia can begin when the patient is responding verbally in a comprehensible fashion; neuropsychological tests, however, usually require the patient to be appropriate in his responses (i.e., toward the latter part of this stage or the beginning of stage IV).[56] Assessment using standardized tests can be given when the patient is confused. Results are not definitive, but can provide a preliminary baseline and possible deficit areas upon which to base the therapy approaches.[21]

Most tests of posttraumatic amnesia are given daily and include questions on basic biographical data, orientation in time and space, last memory before and first memory since the accident, and naming of familiar objects with recall requested the following day.[57] Eson et al.[56] designed a neuropsychological recovery assessment based on developmental stages of perception and cognition, which begins with 0-4 year old cognitive abilities; then tests ability to follow instructions, organize perceptual arrays, process information, selectively attend, and analyze; and finally covers the activities necessary for functioning in the community, such as following road signs and reading a want ad section. Dr. Ben-Yishay and Dr. Diller[2] at the Institute of Rehabilitation Medicine in New York City assess baseline levels of attention, speed of reaction, visual-motor integration, perceptual motor functioning, daily living skills, the patient's understanding of his disability, immediate and short-term memory, academic skills, abstract reasoning, various interpersonal social skills, and the patient's appraisal of his own personality. Results of these tests indicate the patient's ability and willingness to profit from cognitive and interpersonal remediation. These tests are given before intervention is begun and after it has ended. Cognitive deficits have also been measured with such tests as the Wechsler Adult Intelligence Scale or the Wechsler Intelligence Scale for Children, the Halstead-Reitan Neuropsychological Test Battery, the Revised Benton Visual Retention Test, and the Wechsler Memory Scale.[2,54,58] Some of these tests may only be administered by personnel qualified to do so, usually neuropsychologists.

The patient at this stage usually displays severe immediate (up to 1 min), short-term (up to 1 hour), and long-term (over 1 hour) memory impairment. He is, therefore, unlikely to demonstrate carryover of new learning from day to day or from one setting to another, but he may begin to show carryover of overly familiar tasks of self-care.[21] He appears alert but is highly distractible; he does not initiate functional tasks; he has difficulty solving problems related to basic daily living skills, such as making a phone call; he displays poor judgment. The patient's language response may include jargon, word finding difficulty, confabulation, or lack of relevance to the conversation.

Ultimately, the goal of cognitive remediation is to prepare the patient for greater independence in living, through maximum improvement in the cognitive skills underlying independent psychosocial, community, and vocational functioning, and successful planning of activities leading toward a goal.[2] Thus, all cognitive remediation, including that done through computer programs, is related to functional skills and practical application.[59,60] In treating cognitive impairment, specific tasks such as simple organizational tasks, map usage, beginning paper and pencil tasks such as word

recognition or letter cancellation, abstract verbal skills, visual memory tasks, selective attention tasks, and memory drills of letters or numbers may be utilized.[21,61] The patient may be asked to verbalize all the steps involved in a specific task such as making a sandwich, brushing his teeth, or getting ready to go home on a weekend pass.

Cognitive remediation can be done in individual or in group sessions. The groups must be well structured and guided by the leader as necessary, with good group cohesiveness.[21,52] The organization and format of one such group in occupational therapy is described by Lundgren and Persechino.[53] Group games suitable for this level would be gross motor games combined with orientation games (i.e., the patient has to answer an orientation question in turn), outdoor games such as darts or relays, simple board games, or auditory memory games.

Computers. Recently, computers have been increasingly utilized as a tool with brain-injured patients to attain the goals of cognitive remediation. Computers will not be applicable to every patient. The therapist must carefully assess the patient's abilities and needs and determine the most appropriate tool for optimal cognitive remediation.

The choice of computer programs is governed by the following factors: the skills that the patient needs to improve, the level and consistency of difficulty in the program, the ease of the instructions, the program capacity for keeping data on the patient's performance, the type and amount of feedback provided to the patient, the motivational effect of the program, a consistent response format, the amount of supervision needed from the therapist (which may be as high as 75% of the computer use time),[60] and the control of the variables (speed of task, length of display time, size of stimulus items, nature of prompts).

For treatment at this stage, computer programs would primarily be selected that would work on retraining the patient's ability to focus his attention, increase visual scanning, increase his reaction time and improve his visual-motor coordination, improve simple problem-solving skills, and increase frustration tolerance.[59] Specific programs found useful for patient's at this stage include Space Invaders, Caverns of Mars, and Pole Position (games for the Atari that work on eye-hand coordination and reaction time)[62] and the PC Coloring Book for IBM[63] and the Captain's Log Computerized Cognitive Training System, which both address attention span, visual scanning, and other visual motor skills, sequencing, and color discrimination.

Goals for Patients in Stage III of Recovery

A patient at this stage may require almost maximum assistance for independent living skills, exhibit significant neuromuscular deficits, need maximum cueing to orient himself, display severe memory impairment and possibly confused verbal and mental processes, and show little carryover of new learning. Perceptual deficits may be more apparent and identifiable and preliminary cognitive function can be assessed by observation.

Long-term goals might be to increase the patient's independent functioning in physical daily living and homemaking skills, evaluate equipment needs, increase the patient's ability to cognitively structure his environment, and to store information properly and retrieve it appropriately.

Short-term goals might be to improve the patient's voluntary selective movement through continued facilitation of transitional movements and functional positions; increase fine motor control through manipulative activities and exercises for specific muscles; improve motor control of the UEs to enable the patient to feed himself with minimal supervision; increase independence in hygiene and dressing through daily training; evaluate sensory integrative skills more precisely; improve attention and memory through specific cognitive activities and functional tasks; determine the nature of equipment the patient may need upon discharge for more independence in daily living skills; and do a home visit to assess architectural barriers and equipment needs.

STAGE IV: CONSISTENTLY APPROPRIATE RESPONSE TO STIMULATION/ENVIRONMENT

When the patient demonstrates fairly consistent appropriate responses to the external environment, the occupational therapy goals are to gradually decrease the external structuring of the patient's environment, increase his purposeful goal-directed behavior, increase his initiation of independent living and daily skills, and increase his responsibility for doing those tasks and for the consequences of his actions.[15,21] The patient is gradually made responsible for coming to therapy sessions on time, gathering the necessary materials and initiating his own exercise program, planning more advanced homemaking and meal preparation activities, dressing and grooming himself appropriately, making his own bed, and keeping a detailed daily log of events. His participation in the decision-making process of his therapy program is increased. He needs to become aware of his physical and cognitive limitations and realistically plan for his future vocational and leisure activities. In addition, therapy concentrates on improving the quality of his neuromuscular skills, cognitive skills, social interactions, and his ability to problem solve in different and new situations.

Procedures to Improve Neuromuscular Control

Motor problems seen at this stage can include problems of quality of movement as well as continued problems of ataxia, fluctuating tone, or residual spasticity. The patient may exhibit dyspraxia, decreased fine motor control, delayed protective extension or equilibrium reactions, and/or other movement problems. The

therapist would continue addressing these problems as necessary with specific facilitation or strengthening techniques, fine motor coordination and dexterity activities, motor sequencing activities, balance activities, and/or timed repetitions to improve the speed of a motor response.[15] Group games or situations can be useful in refining motor responses while providing peer feedback for maladaptive behavior.[15,52,64,65]

Sensory Integration, Cognition, Behavior

More formal cognitive and perceptual testing and retraining can be done now, as the patient can follow simple directions. Sensory integrative skills are tested and treated as indicated in chapter 7. Visual memory, visual-motor integration, visual discrimination, and spatial relations are assessed and treated, along with other perceptual areas.

Cognitively, the patient's ability to integrate, categorize, sequence, and analyze multiple inputs is assessed.[2] Immediate, short-term and long-term, and verbal memory are also evaluated by a neuropsychologist or psychologist.[23] In this stage of recovery, the patient may demonstrate specific deficits in short-term and long-term memory, reasoning, conceptualization, comprehension, abstract thinking, information processing speed, organization of information, simplification of problems, judgment, or problem solving.[2,15,61,66] He may display decreased attention during attempts to store information, decreased use of mental imagery, decreased new learning, inability to locate the salient or relevant details, decreased ability to structure or associate incoming information appropriately, and decreased cognitive flexibility.[2,65] These deficits will affect the patient's ability to make coherent decisions, to plan realistically, to structure his behavior or his leisure time, and to make safe decisions in the community.[2,21]

Cognitive remediation at this stage emphasizes increasing the patient's ability to concentrate on specific tasks, to organize and utilize information, to remember increasing amounts of information, and to be mentally flexible. The therapist must delineate the patient's cognitive impairment and choose the most appropriate way to remediate the impairment and monitor improvement, as well as assess the patient's ability to benefit from such training.[67] The patient's motivation and his ability to understand the relevance to his personal life are crucial.[2] Cognitive remediation must include systematic use of activities to develop skills, repeated practice by the patient, careful selection and teaching of compensatory cognitive methods and cueing strategies to improve the patient's cognitive skills, and constant, systematic feedback to the patient on his performance. The cognitive remediation program described by Ben-Yishay and Diller[2] is carefully structured and hierarchically arranged in areas of attentional demands (from arousal to cortical content), choice of materials (from simple eye-hand integration to verbal reasoning functions), locus of processing (external buttons and lights to internal processing in the brain), and difficulty level of tasks (easy to hard).

Tasks used by therapists in cognitive remediation at this level may include more complex reading and mathematical tasks or tasks involving increasing analysis of information such as summarizing paragraphs, interpreting proverbs, or ascertaining the meaning of stories or poems. Other examples of tasks are sequential cards depicting an activity such as a picnic, washing a car, or getting ready for school; number or letter sequences; word scrambles; visual memory activities; map reading; simple riddles; jigsaw puzzles; and auditory memory tasks with verbal or written responses requested. Also useful are board games, card games, games or tasks emphasizing problem solving in emergency, social, or community-encountered situations (such as going to a concert, assessing the transportation route, and choosing which friends to call and invite), or planning a trip to two different types of restaurants and discussing the procedures for each in terms of clothing, tipping, and ordering.[21,53,68,69]

Computer programs carefully matched to the patient's specific deficit areas can be helpful.[59] Such programs dealing specifically with retraining perceptual and memory skills are increasingly available[62] (see also Supplementary References). Some advantages of computer use in cognitive retraining are that repetition and drill become challenging due to the program's format, feedback is immediate and consistent, the patient's "failures" are witnessed only by the computer, data can be tabulated to quantify the patient's improvement, and many programs are available to challenge the patient. Some disadvantages are that computers do not provide social interaction or verbal problem solving, they can only lead to very limited generalization about real life situations, and the therapist still needs to monitor the patient's work and progress on the various programs.

Behaviorally, the patient may be experiencing continued withdrawal, anger, depression, or denial of his injury.[2] The therapist can help by letting the patient express his feelings, acknowledging the validity of his feelings, showing empathy, supporting the patient within reason, encouraging him to continue to strive for recovery, remaining accessible to the patient, and avoiding judgmental responses to the patient's expressions of anger or depression. Other behavioral changes may include lack of drive or initiation, decreased social restraint, passivity, or decreased frustration tolerance.[1,2,6,23]

Behavior modification programs may be necessary to address behaviors that are hindering rehabilitation efforts.[2] Group or individual counseling by the social worker or psychologist may be useful in providing a forum for patients to express their feelings and learn interpersonal social skills. Family counseling may also be necessary, since the family may be experiencing these same feelings and need to resolve them to cope with the reality of the patient's abilities.[2,21,49] Often this takes months or years, and occurs only after the patient has been discharged from the hospital.[21,49] A study demonstrated deterioration of relatives' psychiatric and social functioning in the year after the patient's brain injury, in direct correlation to the level of the patient's voiced subjective complaints. These relatives had twice as many psychiatric disturbances as in the normal population.[49]

Community Skills

When physical daily living skills and homemaking tasks (such as cleaning, meal preparation, laundry, solving daily household problems) are being done consistently, the patient must be reintroduced to the community and necessary survival skills. The patient needs to learn how to manage money, write checks, go shopping, use the bank and post office, move in crowds, handle architectural barriers, and go to restaurants; he needs to be able to utilize public transportation, the telephone, the newspaper, and the phone book; he should know the use and care of his equipment or splints; he needs to use crosswalks and obey traffic lights.[43] Goals of community integration of the patient are to provide increased reality testing and better preparation for an unstructured environment.[21] To incorporate memory strategies into the planning of a community outing, a form stating answers as to where, why, when, what time, what items are necessary to bring, and the method of transportation to be used is filled in by the patient.[69]

The patient also needs to be reintroduced to avocational interests and time management. Patients may have residual neuromuscular dysfunction that interferes with resumption of previous leisure activities. His lack of initiative and his cognitive inflexibility may hinder independence in play/leisure skills. The patient can participate in anticipating problems he will face in these areas and in organizing solutions. Driver training, prevocational skills, and/or vocational skills are taught, if appropriate.[21,44] A variety of job placements, such as an adaptive learning program, volunteer work, a sheltered workshop, or the patient's former job with modifications, should be considered.

Social skills must also be considered and treated by the whole team, since the postrehabilitation progress of the patient with a traumatic brain injury depends greatly on his family and other social contacts.[2,55]

Discharge Planning

After hospitalization, the patient could be discharged to a number of different settings. The functional outcome of the patient, the family's ability to care for the patient, and the wishes of the patient and family are all considered in the team's recommendations. Early in the rehabilitation process, the patient's need for equipment, such as a wheelchair or adaptive equipment, must be assessed. A home evaluation, to determine and discuss necessary modifications and to ascertain what skills need to be taught to the patient to move safely about the home environment, must be made if the patient will return to the family's home (chapter 20). Therapeutic passes give the family a "preview" of what care will be necessary and also a chance to have the team's help solving any unanticipated problems that arise with the patient in the home.

As the patient becomes ready to go home, he may still be evidencing decreased responsiveness when fatigued, difficulty operating safely in unfamiliar situations, little flexibility in cognitive processing, concrete and literal interpretation of situations, a shortened attention span, and difficulty in learning new information or tasks.[68,70] The patient may need continued cognitive rehabilitation after discharge, since recovery in this area has been shown to continue for 2 or more years postinjury.[23,31,66] Personality or behavioral changes also may still be present at discharge, for example, disinhibition, low frustration or stress tolerance, reduced insight or judgment, labile affect, irritability, and impulsivity. In the extreme, the patient may experience paranoia, phobias, confusion, or delusional ideation.[13,23] Mental, emotional, and behavioral deficits or changes are more difficult to adjust to than are physical deficits and interfere with successful reintegration into the family, social activity, and community.[23,29,55] The brain-injured patient also must cope with loss of independence and control over his life, embarrassment over residual physical or speech impairment, or decreased self-esteem.

Goals for Patients in Stage IV of Recovery

At this level, the patient continues to exhibit cognitive and behavioral deficits, decreased independence in independent living skills, and inability to function in the community and in unstructured situations.

Long-term goals might be to increase the patient's ability to respond appropriately to and interact with the environment in social, personal, educational, and vocational areas and to enable him to seek employment in a sheltered workshop or another modified job situation.

Examples of short-term goals might be to increase the patient's assumption of responsibility for his own personal needs and decrease external structuring; improve his cognitive skills and perceptual skills and teach compensation skills as necessary through specific spatial and scanning tasks, memory tasks, and organizational tasks; increase his ability to initiate and finish a task; improve his dexterity and his refined balance reactions; improve his praxis through obstacle courses or scooter board activities; increase his social interaction and its quality through use of groups for social, physical, and community tasks; and plan discharge and coordinate with family and community agencies.

Community Programs

Until recently, following the months of acute rehabilitation, the head-injured patient was discharged home with his family, or to a nursing home if he required more care and physical supervision. Sometimes, he would continue outpatient therapy for a while, but scant attention was paid to the persistent cognitive and behavioral deficits that prevented the patient from achieving a higher level of function in the society.[71]

Fortunately, that has begun to change. Several alternatives are now being developed for the patient with a traumatic brain injury. Long-term rehabilitation programs are available in nursing homes or residential schools. Transitional living programs in a nonmedical setting are designed to increase development of those skills needed for the patient to live independently in progressively more complex living environments, i.e., moving from a small group family house to a supervised group apartment to an independent apartment and independent functioning in the community with help still available from the staff.[2,72] Day care/day treatment centers are available that emphasize increased independence and preparation for further education or vocational rehabilitation.[2,73] Centers for Independent Living are community-based programs providing or coordinating services to the patient, such as psychosocial evaluation and training, counseling, cognitive retraining, job and education reorientation, or respite care.[74]

Self-help groups have been organized to help the patient cope with his psychosocial problems following discharge.[2,70] The National Head Injury Foundation, formed in 1980, now has become a valuable resource with many state associations and local chapters to assist patients and their families, to disseminate information nationwide on head injuries, and to increase awareness of the needs and advocate improvement in the ongoing treatment of this population.[75]

Studies of the Effectiveness of Therapy

There is very little agreement or evidence concerning when to initiate rehabilitation for comatose brain-injured patients, or what rehabilitation measures would be included at various stages of recovery.[2,6,14,76] Most of the available literature on traumatic brain injury has concentrated on proposed medical treatments and assessment of their efficacy[4,12] and on factors predictive of outcome of severe head injury.[22,24-27,50] Recently, more articles and books describe the mental and behavioral sequelae of the injury and discuss the implications of these sequelae.[2,6,58] Articles on cognitive rehabilitation and studies on memory are also becoming more readily available.[2,23,53,59,61,62,67,77] Unfortunately though, articles documenting the effectiveness of specific rehabilitative procedures with the brain-injured patient are scarce. The studies found that focus on the rehabilitation of such a patient primarily contain statistics on the outcome of the patients correlated to duration of coma or other factors and measured by return to work, social interaction, or degrees of independence in independent living skills.[13,29,78] These articles contain only the authors' opinions on the usefulness and necessity of rehabilitative measures, and little experimental documentation of different procedures.

Stover and Zeiger[78] found no evidence that rehabilitation initiated in the period of coma decreased the duration of that coma, but still concluded that it was important to begin then to prevent contractures and pulmonary, gastrointestinal, and urinary complications. Rusk et al.[79] found that 46% of the patients studied returned to some form of gainful employment after rehabilitation. These authors decided that severe disability can usually be helped by an intensive rehabilitation program, but they did not describe such a program nor offer statistics on a control group. Forer and Miller[80] studied progress made by patients with various diagnoses after discharge from a rehabilitation hospital. It was discovered that patients with traumatic brain injuries did not make significant gains in independent living skills after leaving the hospital, but did make significant gains in cognition, speech, and language comprehension. The authors did not document the source of these gains.

A study done by an occupational therapist[42] documented the sequence of recovery of functional skills (dressing, transfers, gross and fine hand function, wheelchair mobility, basic daily living skills, kitchen skills, and community skills). Recovery sequences of two groups of head-injured patients (one group in coma for 14 days or less, the other in coma over 14 days) were compared over a period of 2 years postinjury with significant differences in the groups' performance on 6 of 8 skills at 1 year. The recovery pattern was found to be gross hand function preceding basic daily living skills, followed by social and community skills, and lastly fine finger dexterity. No description of the rehabilitation program was offered.

There are a few authors who have described the rehabilitation programs used with patients and presented statistics on the outcome of those patients. Most of these studies had no control groups or other aspects of an experimental design. Najenson et al.[31] studied the outcome of 169 patients with severe brain injury who underwent a program utilizing postural reflexes, self-care tasks, locomotor tasks, and communicative training. The statistics presented showed that 84% of the patients were independent in daily living skills upon discharge. The authors found recovery continuing up to 3 years after injury and stressed the need for continued follow-up of these patients after discharge from a rehabilitation hospital. Rosenbaum et. al.[81] described an intensive therapeutic community setting for vocational and cognitive retraining, and offered preliminary conclusions on the importance of such a program. Gerstenbrand[76] described a rehabilitation program beginning in the acute stage after trauma that included use of reflexes to influence muscle tone and more active mobilization and socialization techniques later. He briefly stated his results with 170 patients in terms of being back at work and concluded that rehabilitation at full intensity was essential.

Brink et al.[13] studied 344 children with severe closed head injury, comatose over 24 hours, who had begun rehabilitation within 3 to 6 weeks postinjury. These authors found that 73% became independent in ambulation and self-care, 10% were partially dependent, and 17% were totally dependent. The nature of the rehabilitation techniques was not specifically described in this article. The study was carried out at Rancho Los Amigos Hospital in Downey, California, and, presumably, utilized the Rancho rehabilitation program described in literature of the same period. Jellinek et al.[82] investigated the patient's adjustment to the behavioral and cognitive sequelae of the injury in relation to his independence in daily living skills postdischarge. These researchers discovered that patients who were more independent in self-care and mobility experienced less distress and better adjustment than more dependent patients. Cole et al.[73] described a postdischarge day treatment program and reported 47% of the group attained an improved level of functioning. However, the level to which these patients improved is not specified in terms of community functioning. Mercer and Boch[64] offered clinical observations but no quantitative measures of improved quality of movement following their sensorimotor integration class with head-injured patients.

Postlesion experience in a mildly stressful, active environment has been found to be more facilitatory to behavioral and motor recovery than a more neutral, passive environment.[6,45,83,84] Other authors have emphasized the increased effectiveness of such experience when begun as soon postinjury as possible.[85,86] Cope and Hall[87] studied two groups of patients with severe brain injuries who were admitted for rehabilitation early (under 35 days postinjury) and later (more than 35 days postinjury), comparing the time required for rehabilitation and the outcome. They concluded that those admitted later required twice as much rehabilitation as those admitted early despite the similarity of initial injury severity. Outcome at 2 years postinjury was not significantly different between groups.

There are experimental studies utilizing control groups that document some of the subtle cognitive deficits caused by a brain injury.[23,54,58,66] However, again, few studies have investigated the efficacy of cognitive retraining with such patients.[2,67] A few case studies of specific cognitive retraining strategies for patients with head injury are available in the literature.[61,69] A few studies of larger groups are also available, but document only changes in patient status, not the efficacy of the therapeutic procedures utilized. Scherzer[65] studied three groups of patients with severe brain injuries who were given physical, cognitive, perceptual, social, and prevocational training and counseling at least one year after coma. He determined that the greatest improvement was shown in areas of attention, memory, and complex reasoning, with significant improvements noted also in home life. Prigatano et al.[54] observed some improvement in a group treated with a neuropsychological program compared to a control group in the areas of performance and memory scores on the

Wechsler Adult Intelligence Scale and documented reduced emotional distress in the treated group.

Even fewer studies have been done exploring the effects of sensory stimulation or therapeutic techniques on comatose patients. McGraw and Tindall[32] found changes in heart rate, respiratory rate, and ICP in 50% of their comatose patient population in response to tactile, auditory, and painful stimulation. No gross movements were noted with these changes, but increased electrical activity was recorded in some patients' cervical muscles. Boortz-Marx[34] and Parsons et al.[33] found changes in ICP in response to oral and hygienic nursing procedures with brain-injured patients. Weber[88] studied three comatose patients and found significant differences in the patients' cortical activity measured after therapy periods compared to that measured after periods of unstructured stimulation and/or activity. The therapy in this study consisted of selected PNF patterns, quick icing, joint approximation, and verbal requests for a motor response.

Documentation of specific treatment techniques has begun, but the studies contain little experimental manipulation of the variables. Baker et al.[89] presented a case study of a head-injured patient who, in addition to other rehabilitation measures, received neuromuscular electrical stimulation to increase ROM and to facilitate voluntary movement. The patient's status improved from wheelchair dependent to independent ambulator for short distances with a quad (4 pronged) cane. Booth et. al.[90] offered descriptive results only of the effects of serial casting on ROM and muscle tone in brain-injured patients.

As is evident, very few controlled studies on patients with traumatic brain injury are available that investigate the time of initiation of rehabilitation, the extent and intensity of rehabilitation necessary, the specific procedures utilized, or if these techniques affected the outcome of the injury.[2,6,23] Several factors contribute to such a lack of research: difficulty in finding and matching large numbers of patients for control and experimental groups by lesion and symptoms, the long-term period of possible recovery from brain injury, the possibility that some recovery occurs because of motivation and a "mind-body" interaction that is difficult to measure and assess, and the difficulty in quantifying and defining the nature of recovery, outcome, and quality of life.[2,6,86,91] Extraneous variables such as patient-family or patient-therapist interaction are also difficult to quantify. In addition, researchers face the philosophical dilemma of withholding therapy from a control group of patients. However, these difficulties need to be surmounted, and research needs to be conducted on the efficacy of the therapeutic procedures used with head-injured patients, their effect on the long-term outcome of the injury, the patient's subsequent quality of life, and the optimum time during the recovery period for therapeutic procedures.

Acknowledgment. I wish to acknowledge the contribution of Katherine Mason, M.E.D., O.T.R., from Louisiana State University, whose suggestions proved invaluable in this revision.

STUDY QUESTIONS:

Traumatic Brain Injuries

1. Describe the primary and secondary damage caused by a brain injury, and the residual physical, mental, and emotional/behavioral deficits that can result.
2. Discuss briefly six possible motor responses to stimulation that may be seen in a comatose patient during various stages of recovery.
3. Describe abnormal reflexes typically seen in brain-injured patients and their effect on the patient's motor responses and oral motor functioning.
4. List goals of occupational therapy treatment for stages I to IV of recovery from a traumatic brain injury.
5. List the types of sensory stimulation used to treat the stage I patient and give brief examples of each.
6. Discuss the difference in treatment for neuromuscular deficits in the four stages described in this chapter.
7. Describe appropriate wheelchair positioning, considering the pelvis, trunk, upper extremities, lower extremities, and head.
8. Discuss the progression of treatment of oral motor dysfunction and feeding.
9. When would sensory integration and cognitive treatment begin and what would it consist of, briefly?
10. Discuss the specific independent living and basic daily living skills that might be performed at each of the four stages of recovery.

References

1. National Institute of Neurological and Communicative Disorders and Stroke. *Head Injury: Hope Through Research.* Bethesda, MD: National Institutes of Health, 1984.
2. Rosenthal, M., Griffith, E. R., Bond, M. R., and Miller, J. D., editors. *Rehabilitation of the Head Injured Adult.* Philadelphia: F. A. Davis, 1983.
3. Lillehei, K. O., and Hoff, J. T. Advances in the management of closed head injury. *Ann. Emerg. Med., 14:* 789–795, 1985.
4. Bakay, L., and Glasauer, F. E. *Head Injuries.* Boston: Little, Brown, 1980.
5. Yano, J. Head injuries. *J. Neurosurg. Nurs., 16:* 173–180, 1984.
6. Jennett, B., and Teasdale, G. *Management of Head Injuries.* Philadelphia: F. A. Davis, 1981.
7. Ommaya, A. K., and Gennarelli, T. A. A physiopathologic basis for noninvasive diagnosis and prognosis of head injury severity. In *Head Injuries, Proceedings of the Second Chicago Symposium on Neural Trauma.* Edited by R. L. McLaurin. New York: Grune & Stratton, 1976.
8. Miller, J. D. Head injury and brain ischaemia—implications for therapy. *Br. J. Anaesth., 57:* 120-130, 1985.
9. Miller, B. L. and McIntyre, H. B. Evaluation of the comatose patient. *Primary Care, 11:* 693-706, 1984.
10. Plum, F. and Posner, J. *The Diagnosis of Stupor and Coma,* 2nd edition. Philadelphia: F. A. Davis, 1972.
11. Chusid, J. G. *Correlative Neuroanatomy and Functional Neurology,* 15th edition. Los Altos, CA: Lange Medical Publications, 1973.
12. Davis, R. A., and Cunningham, P. S. Prognostic factors in severe head injury. *Surg. Gynecol. Obstet., 159:* 597-604, 1984.
13. Brink, J. D., Imbus, C., and Woo-Sam, J. Physical recovery after severe closed head trauma in children and adolescents. *J. Pediatr., 97:* 721-727, 1980.
14. Carr, J. H., and Shepherd, R. B. *Physiotherapy in Disorders of the Brain.* London: William Heinemann Medical Books, 1980.
15. Charness, A. L. *Stroke/Head Injury: A Guide to Functional Outcomes in Physical Therapy Management.* Rehabilitation Institute of Chicago Series. Rockville, MD: Aspen Systems, 1986.
16. Finkelstein, S., and Ropper, A. The diagnosis of coma: its pitfalls and limitations. *Heart Lung., 8:* 1059-1064, 1979.

17. Turner, M. S. Pediatric head injury. *Indiana Med., 78:* 194-197, 1985.
18. Morray, J. P., Tyler, D. C., Jones, T. K., Stuntz, J. T., and Lemire, R. J. Coma scale for use in brain-injured children. *Crit. Care Med., 12:* 1018-1020, 1984.
19. Salcman, M., Schepp, R. S., and Ducker, T. B. Calculated recovery rates in severe head trauma. *Neurosurgery, 8:* 301-308, 1981.
20. Stanczak, D. E., White, J. G., Gouview, W. D., Moehle, K. A., Daniel, M., Novack, T., and Long, C. J. Assessment of level of consciousness following severe neurological insult. *J. Neurosurg., 60:* 955-960, 1984.
21. Malkmus, D., Booth, B. J., and Kodimer, C. *Rehabilitation of the Head Injured Adult: Comprehensive Cognitive Management.* Los Angeles: Professional Staff Association of Rancho Los Amigos Hospital, 1980.
22. Newlon, P. G., and Greenberg, R. P. Evoked potentials in severe head injury. *J. Trauma, 24:* 61-66, 1984.
23. Benton, A. Behavioral consequences of closed head injury. In *Central Nervous System Trauma Research Status Report.* Edited by G. L. Odom. Bethesda, MD: National Institutes of Health, 1979.
24. Bricolo, A., Turazzi, S., and Feriotti, G. Prolonged posttraumatic unconsciousness: therapeutic assets and liabilities. *J. Neurosurg., 52:* 625-634, 1980.
25. Braakman, R., Gelpke, G. J., Habbema, J. D. F., Maas, A. I. R., and Minderhoud, J. M. Systematic selection of prognostic features in patients with severe head injury. *Neurosurgery, 6:* 362-370, 1980.
26. Karnaze, D. S., Weiner, J. M., and Marshall, L F. Auditory evoked potentials in coma after closed head injury: a clinical-neurophysiologic coma scale for predicting outcome. *Neurology, 35:* 1122-1126, 1985.
27. Lipper, M. H., Kishore, P. R. S., Enas, G. G., da Silva, A. A. D., Choi, S. C., and Becker, D. P. Computed tomography in the prediction of outcome in head injury. *Am. J. Roentgenol., 144:* 483-486, 1985.
28. Warren, J. B. and Peck, E. A. Factors which influence neuropsychological recovery from severe head injury. *J. Neurosurg. Nurs., 16:* 248-252, 1984.
29. Jennett, B., Snoek, J., Bond, M. R., and Brooks, N. Disability after severe head injury: observations on the use of the Glasgow Outcome Scale. *J. Neurol. Neurosurg. Psychiatry, 44:* 285-293, 1981.
30. Hall, K., Cope, D. N., and Rappaport, M. Glasgow outcome scale and disability rating scale: comparative usefulness in following recovery in traumatic head injury. *Arch. Phys. Med. Rehabil., 66:* 35-37, 1985.
31. Najenson, T., Mendelson, L., Schechter, I., David, C., Mintz, N., and Grosswasser, Z. Rehabilitation after severe head injury. *Scand. J. Rehabil. Med., 6:* 5-14, 1974.
32. McGraw, C. P., and Tindall, G. T. Cardio-respiratory alterations in head injury: patients' response to stimulation. *Surg. Neurol., 2:* 263-266, 1974.
33. Parsons, L. C., Peard, A. L. S., and Page, M. C. The effects of hygiene interventions on the cerebrovascular status of severe closed head injured persons. *Res. Nurs. Health, 8:* 173-181, 1985.
34. Boortz-Marx, R. Factors affecting intracranial pressure: a descriptive study. *J. Neurosurg. Nurs., 17:* 89-94, 1985.
35. Schaffer, L., Kranzler, L. I., and Siqueira, E. B. Aspects of evaluation and treatment of head injury. *Neurol. Clin., 3:* 259-273, 1985.
36. Spielman, G., Gennarelli, T. A., and Rogers, C. R. Disodium etidronate: its role in preventing heterotopic ossification in severe head injury. *Arch. Phys. Med. Rehabil., 64:* 539-542, 1983.
37. Barolat-Romana, G., and Larson, S. J. Influence of stimulus location and limb position on motor responses in the comatose patient. *J. Neurosurg., 61:* 725-728, 1984.
38. Farber, S. D. *Neurorehabilitation: A Multisensory Approach.* Philadelphia: W. B. Saunders, 1982.
39. Logemann, J. *Evaluation and Treatment of Swallowing Disorders.* San Diego: College-Hill Press, 1983.
40. Winstein, C. J. Neurogenic dysphagia: frequency, progression, and outcome in adults following head injury. *Phys. Ther., 63:* 1992-1997, 1983.
41. Occupational Therapy Department. *Perceptual Motor Evaluation for Head Injured and Other Neurologically Impaired Adults.* San Jose, CA: Santa Clara Valley Medical Center, 1985.
42. Panikoff, L. B. Recovery trends of functional skills in the head-injured adult. *Am. J. Occup. Ther., 37:* 735-743, 1983.
43. Practice Division. *Head Injury Information Packet.* Rockville, MD: American Occupational Therapy Association, 1985.
44. Jones, R., Giddens, H., and Croft, D. Assessment and training of brain-damaged drivers. *Am. J. Occup. Ther., 37:* 754-760, 1983.
45. Moore, J. C. Neuroanatomical considerations relating to recovery of function following brain lesions. In *Recovery of Function: Theoretical Considerations for Brain Injury Rehabilitation.* Edited by P. Bach-y-Rita. Baltimore: University Park Press, 1980.
46. Stockmeyer, S. An interpretation of the approach of Rood to the treatment of neuromuscular dysfunction. *Am. J. Phys. Med., 46:* 900-956, 1967.
47. Scherzer, A. L., and Tscharnuter, I. *Early Diagnosis and Therapy in Cerebral Palsy.* New York: Marcel Dekker, 1982.
48. Keener, S. M., and Sweigart, J. E. Early use of adaptable seating for patients with head trauma. *Phys. Ther., 64:* 206-207, 1984.
49. Livingston, M. G., Brooks, D. N., and Bond, M. R. Patient outcome in the year following severe head injury and relatives' psychiatric and social function. *J. Neurol. Neurosurg. Psychiatry, 48:* 876-881, 1985.
50. Reyes, R. L., Heller, D., and Bhattacharyya, A. K. Traumatic head injury: restlessness and agitation as prognosticators of physical and psychologic improvement in patients. *Arch. Phys. Med. Rehabil., 62:* 20-23, 1981.
51. Rao, N., Jellinek, H. M., and Woolston, D. C. Agitation in closed head injury: haloperidol effects on rehabilitation outcome. *Arch. Phys. Med. Rehabil., 66:* 30-34, 1985.
52. Hill, J., and Carper, M. Greenery: group therapeutic approaches with the head injured. *Cognitive Rehabil., 3:* 18-29, 1985.
53. Lundgren, C. C., and Persechino, E. L. Cognitive group: a treatment program for head-injured adults. *Am. J. Occup. Ther., 40:* 397-401, 1986.
54. Prigatano, G. P., Fordyce, D. J., Zeiner, H. K., Roueche, J. R., Pepping, M., and Wood, B. C. Neuropsychological rehabilitation after closed head injury in young adults. *J. Neurol. Neurosurg. Psychiatry, 47:* 505-513, 1984.
55. Oddy, M., and Humphrey, M. Social recovery during the year following severe head injury. *J. Neurol. Neurosurg. Psychiatry, 43:* 798-802, 1980.
56. Eson, M. E., Yen, J. K., and Bourke, R. S. Assessment of recovery from serious head injury. *J. Neurol. Neurosurg. Psychiatry, 41:* 1036-1042, 1978.
57. Levin, H. S., O'Donnell, V. M., and Grossman, R. G. The Galveston orientation and amnesia test: a practical scale to assess cognition after head injury. *J. Nerv. Ment. Dis., 167:* 675-684, 1979.
58. Chadwick, O., Rutter, M., Brown, G., Shaffer, D., and Traub, M. A prospective study of children with head injuries. II. Cognitive sequelae. *Psychol. Med., 11:* 49-61, 1981.
59. Bracy, O., Lynch, W., Sbordone, R., and Berrol, S. Cognitive retraining through computers: fact or fad? *Cognitive Rehabil., 3:* 10-23, 1985.
60. Trexler, L. *Cognitive Rehabilitation: Questions and Answers.* Framingham, MA: National Head Injury Foundation, 1984.
61. Gianutsos, R. What is cognitive rehabilitation? *J. Rehabil., 46:* 36-40, 1980.
62. Lynch, W. J. Computer-assisted cognitive retraining. *J. Head Trauma Rehabil., 1:* 77-78, 1986.
63. Skinner, A. D., and Trachtman, L. H. Brief or new: use of a computer program (PC coloring book) in cognitive rehabilitation. *Am. J. Occup. Ther., 39:* 470-472, 1985.
64. Mercer, L., and Boch, M. Residual sensorimotor deficits in the adult head-injured patient. *Phys. Ther., 63:* 1988-1991, 1983.
65. Scherzer, B. P. Rehabilitation following severe head trauma: results of a three-year program. *Arch. Phys. Med. Rehabil., 67:* 366-374, 1986.
66. Dikmen, S., Reitan, R. M., and Temkin, N. R. Neuropsychological recovery in head injury. *Arch. Neurol., 40:* 333-338, 1983.
67. Diller, L., and Gordon, W. A. Interventions for cognitive deficits in brain-injured adults. *J. Consult. Clin. Psychol., 49:* 822-834, 1981.
68. Anderson, J., and Parenté, F. Training family members to work with the head injured patient. *Cognitive Rehabil., 3:* 12-15, 1985.
69. Milton, S. B. Compensatory memory strategy training: a practical approach for managing persisting memory problems. *Cognitive Rehabil., 3:* 8-15, 1985.
70. Scanlon-Schilpp, A. M., and Levesque, J. Helping the patient cope with the sequelae of trauma through the self-help group approach. *J. Trauma, 21:* 135-139, 1981.
71. Gloag, D. Services for people with head injury. *Br. Med. J., 291:* 557-558, 1985.
72. Centrella, J. *South Valley Ranch: A Community Re-Entry Program for Head Injured Adults.* Gilroy, CA: Learning Services Corporation, 1985.
73. Cole, J. R., Cope, D. N., and Cervelli, L. Rehabilitation of the severely brain-injured patient: a community-based, low-cost model program. *Arch. Phys. Med. Rehabil., 66:* 38-40, 1985.
74. Epperson-Sebour, M. M., and Rifkin, E. W. Center for living: trauma aftercare and outcome. *Md. Med. J., 34:* 1187-1192, 1985.
75. *National Head Injury Foundation Annual Report.* Framingham, MA: National Head Injury Foundation, 1984.
76. Gerstenbrand, F. The course of restitution of brain injury in the early and late stages and the rehabilitative measures. *Scand. J. Rehabil. Med., 4:* 85-89, 1972.
77. Bracy, O., editor. *Cognitive Rehabilitation.* Indianapolis: B. and B. Publishing, 1985.
78. Stover, S. L., and Zeiger, H. E. Head injury in children and teenagers: functional recovery correlated with the duration of coma. *Arch. Phys. Med. Rehabil., 57:* 201-205, 1976.
79. Rusk, H. A., Block, J. M., and Lowman, E. W. Rehabilitation following traumatic brain damage. *Med. Clin. North Am., 53:* 677-684, 1969.

80. Forer, S. K., and Miller, L. S. Rehabilitation outcome: comparative analysis of different patient types. *Arch. Phys. Med. Rehabil., 61*: 359-365, 1980.
81. Rosenbaum, M., Lipsitz, N., Abraham, J., and Najenson, T. A description of an intensive treatment project for the rehabilitation of severely brain-injured soldiers. *Scand. J. Rehabil. Med., 10*: 1-6, 1978.
82. Jellinek, H. M., Torkelson, R. M., and Harvey, R. F. Functional abilities and distress levels in brain injured patients at long-term follow-up. *Arch. Phys. Med. Rehabil., 63*: 160-162, 1982.
83. Herdman, S. J. Effect of experience on recovery following CNS lesions. *Phys. Ther., 63*: 51-55, 1983.
84. Walsh, R. N., and Cummins, R. A. Neural responses to therapeutic sensory environments. In *Environments as Therapy for Brain Dysfunction.* Edited by R. N. Walsh and W. T. Greenough. New York: Plenum Press, 1976.
85. Teuber, H. L. Recovery of function after brain injury in man. In *CIBA Symposium 34, Outcome of Severe Damage to the Central Nervous System.* Amsterdam: Elsevier, 1975.
86. Bach-y-Rita, P. *Brain Plasticity as a Basis of the Development of Rehabilitation Procedures for Hemiplegia.* Martinez, CA: VA Medical Center, 1981.
87. Cope D. N., and Hall, K. Head injury rehabilitation: benefit of early intervention. *Arch. Phys. Med. Rehabil., 63*: 433-437, 1982.
88. Weber, P. L. Sensorimotor therapy: its effect on electroencephalograms of acute comatose patients. *Arch. Phys. Med. Rehabil., 65*: 457-462, 1984.
89. Baker, L. L., Parker, K., and Sanderson, D. Neuromuscular electrical stimulation for the head-injured patient. *Phys. Ther., 63*: 1967-1974, 1983.
90. Booth, B. J., Doyle, M., and Montgomery, J. Serial casting for the management of spasticity in the head-injured adult. *Phys. Ther., 63*: 1960-1966, 1983.
91. Bach-y-Rita, P. Brain plasticity as a basis for therapeutic procedures. In *Recovery of Function: Theoretical Considerations for Brain Injury Rehabilitation.* Edited by P. Bach-y-Rita. Baltimore: University Park Press, 1980.

Supplementary Reading

Imes, C. Cognitive rehabilitation of brain-damaged patients: an annotated bibliography. *Cognitive Rehabil., 3*: 8-16, 1985.

Kraus, J. F., and Fife, D. Incidence, external causes, and outcomes of work-related brain injuries in males. *J. Occup. Med. 27*(10): 757-760, 1985.

Lynch, W. J., and Mauss, N. K. Brain injury rehabilitation: standard problem lists. *Arch. Phys. Med. Rehabil., 62*(5): 223-227, 1981.

Manzi, D. B., and Weaver, P. A. *Head Injury: The Acute Care Phase.* Thorofare, NJ: Slack Incorporated, 1987.

Resources

Yehuda Ben-Yishay, Ph.D., N.Y.U. Medical Center, I.R.M. Head Trauma Program, 400 East 34th Street, R. R. 119, New York, NY 10016.

Cognitive Educational Software Series, Rehabilitation Programs, 353 East State Street, Long Beach, NY 11561.

Jeffrey S. Kreutzer, Ph.D., Director of Rehabilitation, Psychology and Neuropsychology, Medical College of Virginia, Richmond, VA 23229.

Lambert Software Company, 664 Via Curvada, Chula Vista, CA 92010.

William Lynch, M.D., VA Medical Center, Brain Injury Rehabilitation Unit, 3801 Miranda Avenue, Palo Alto, CA 94304.

Neuroscience Publishers, 6555 Carrollton Avenue, Indianapolis, IN 46220. For *Cognitive Rehabilitation* journal.

Robert Sbordone, Ph.D., 8840 Warner Avenue, Fountain Valley, CA 92708. For computer use with brain-injured patients.

Michael Shipp, M. Ed., Louisiana Tech University Center for Rehabilitation and Biomedical Engineering, Ruston, LA 71272. For handicapped driving program.

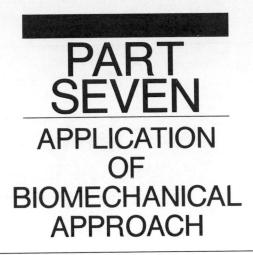

PART SEVEN

APPLICATION OF BIOMECHANICAL APPROACH

The *Biomechanical Approach* is appropriately applied to those patients who have lost range of motion, strength, or endurance due to illness or trauma that affects muscles, joints, skin, or other connective tissue, peripheral nerves, heart, lungs, or spinal cord. In all cases the brain is intact and motor control is normal as long as the sensory receptors and muscles are in communication with the brain. In cases where the brain is no longer receiving input from the periphery or the muscles receiving direction from the brain, as in spinal cord injury, for example, no motor control is expected and care is directed at prevention of secondary problems that result from loss of movement and anesthesia.

If there is residual disability when the patient's recovery has plateaued, then the *Rehabilitative Approach* should be applied to enable the person to compensate for lost function.

Some commonly seen diagnoses are presented here as examples of application of these approaches. In addition, the particular problems and an introduction to specialized treatment developed for each diagnosis are presented. Treatment for patients with any of these diagnoses is complex. Expertise is developed through reflective, analytical experience in conjunction with supervisory guidance, continuing education, study of published developments, and eventually graduate study.

chapter
25

Hand Therapy

Cynthia A. Philips

The recent advances in hand surgery, including microvascular surgery, joint implants, and staged tendon repair, require a specialized approach to patient care. The occupational therapist and physician must work closely together in a well-organized therapeutic program.

The therapist must have an intimate knowledge of normal hand anatomy and must adhere to the basic principles of wound healing to determine the choice and timing of basic therapeutic modalities. Careful thought must be given to the biomechanical principles of splinting to ensure that the intended purpose of the splint is fulfilled.

Exercises must be done gently and always within the patient's tolerance. Forced passive motion or painful therapy sets up a vicious cycle of further injury leading to increased edema and further scarring and fibrosis. Psychologically the patient becomes fearful and will not exercise. All of this leads to a stiff, useless hand.

Hand therapy should be directed by an experienced therapist who has specialized hand therapy training. A therapist interested in hand therapy should become proficient in general rehabilitation skills and then should seek out specialized hand therapy training. This chapter is meant only as a guideline to the treatment of some of the more common hand diagnoses. Treatment procedures will vary depending upon the particular patient's circumstances.

Evaluation

Before treatment can begin, a baseline evaluation is necessary to determine a plan of treatment, monitor the patient's progress, and judge the effectiveness of treatment procedures. An evaluation can be divided into subjective and objective information.

SUBJECTIVE INFORMATION

Subjective information is obtained through speaking with and listening to the patient and by observing and palpating the hand. This type of information is important from a treatment and diagnostic standpoint, but cannot be used to make valid statements for research or to accurately assess therapeutic management. Subjective information may include the following:

1. History of illness or injury and other pertinent medical information.
2. The posture of the hand. Normally the wrist is in slight dorsiflexion; the digits lie with increasing flexion toward the ulnar side of the hand; and the index and middle fingers are slightly supinated. The fingers normally lie in the direction of the scaphoid bone; tendon injuries or certain fractures will disrupt this posture.
3. The condition of the skin. Has there been skin loss? Has there been previous injury that has caused scarring? Is the skin thin and fragile?
4. The color of the skin.
5. Edema. Is the edema soft and pitting, or is it hard and brawny?
6. The sensibility of the hand. The patient would be asked to describe the way the hand feels. This would include any pain, numbness, tingling, etc.
7. Any deformity.
8. Palpation of the hand will reveal:
   a. Any masses or nodules present.
   b. Temperature of the skin.
   c. Texture of the skin (i.e., dry, wet, soft, rough, scarred).
9. The patient's hand dominance.
10. The patient's family, work, and avocational history.[1]

OBJECTIVE INFORMATION

Objective measurements lay the foundation for baseline data to determine effectiveness of treatment, to provide a basis for research, and to facilitate more accurate communication among professionals. Objective measurement includes range of motion, grip and pinch strength, edema measurements, sensory evaluation, muscle testing, and various functional tests to help assess activities of daily living, dexterity, strength, coordination and endurance.[2,3] The clinical assessment committees of the American Society of Hand Therapists and the American Society for Surgery of the Hand have provided recommendations for evaluation of range of motion, strength, sensation, volume, dexterity, and coordination.[4,5]

Range of Motion

Range of motion evaluation with a goniometer is very important in monitoring a patient's progress. Both active and passive range of motion should be noted. If there is a discrepancy between active and passive motion, the problem may be with tendon continuity or tendon glide, which could be impeded by adhesions or other tendon pathology, rather than the joint or its periarticular structures. Goniometer range of motion is recorded following the standards supplied by the American Academy of Orthopedic Surgeons[6] as cited in chapter 8.

The American Society for Surgery of the Hand also recommends the recording of total active motion (TAM) and total passive motion (TPM).[4] Total active range of motion is the sum of the angles of the metacarpophalangeal, proximal interphalangeal, and distal interphalangeal joints when the hand is in maximum active flexion, minus any deviation from full extension. Total passive range of motion is the sum of the angles formed by the metacarpophalangeal, proximal interphalangeal, and distal interphalangeal joints when the hand is in full passive flexion, minus any passive extension deficit.

A particular patient's situation (for example, in the case of severe rheumatoid arthritis) may preclude the usually accepted method of measurement and will require an alternative technique. It is important that one document the changes, and continue to be consistent with that technique throughout each reassessment.

Grip Strength

Grip strength is generally recorded with a Jamar dynamometer as described in chapter 8. Pinch strength is recorded with a standard pinchmeter as described in chapter 8. Lateral, 3 jaw chuck (palmar), and pulp pinch (thumb pad to index finger pad) are recorded.

Manual Muscle Testing

Manual muscle testing, described in chapter 8, should be done as a necessary part of a total assessment battery.[7]

Sensory Evaluation

Sensory evaluation is described in chapter 3 and will be discussed further in this chapter.

Measurements of Edema

Edema can be evaluated by recording circumferential measurements or volumeter measurements as described in chapter 8. Since reducing edema is a key element in the treatment of the injured hand, it is important to monitor this parameter along with those previously described.

Functional Evaluations

Functional evaluations include both nonstandardized and standardized tests that help assess the person's functional capacity. Standardized tests are those tests that have documented validity and reliability when the operationally defined procedures are adhered to during administration. Standardized tests represent more sophisticated tools and give the therapist the best objective measurement of the patient's abilities. It should be remembered, however, that the standardized test loses its reliability if it is also used as a practice tool.

The nonstandardized tests used in the evaluation of the injured hand include various activities of daily living evaluations and some currently available hand evaluations. Standardized tests include tests for dexterity, coordination, strength, and endurance. Standardized evaluations for dexterity and coordination include such tests as the Jebsen Hand Function Test,[8] the Minnesota Rate of Manipulation Test, the Purdue Pegboard, and the O'Connor Peg Test. The O'Connor Peg Test can be obtained with or without tweezers. Other tests, such as the Bennett Hand Tool Test and the Crawford Small Parts Dexterity Test, add the component of working with tools. These tests require a higher level of hand function, including sufficient strength to manipulate and control the tools. See chapter 4 for a description of some of these tests.

The Valpar Work Samples provide a standardized means of determining the patient's ability to do a variety of tasks or perform various motions necessary to adequately perform his or her job. The Valpar component work samples are a series of 17 workstation modules that require a wide range of manipulative and cognitive skills, depending on the work sample being used (see chapter 21).

In most busy clinics, it is not possible to perform a number of objective tests. Therefore, one must choose a battery of tests that is the most appropriate and the most helpful in obtaining the type of data required for planning treatment for a particular patient. Reevaluation should be done on an ongoing basis throughout the patient's treatment program. The frequency of reevaluation would depend on the patient's individual circumstances.

Treatment

JOINT INJURIES

Injuries to the joints and their supporting soft tissue structures are among the most common hand injuries. Unfortunately, the full implication of these injuries is not always appreciated. This can often lead to needless disability.

When one is attempting to mobilize joint injuries, there are some aspects of the rehabilitation program that are common to all the injuries to be discussed. All exercises must be done gently and within the patient's tolerance. Exercises should not, under any circumstances, increase pain or swelling. In some cases, when swelling of the joint persists, an ice pack or an ice massage may be a useful tool in controlling edema and pain, even after the acute period. Proximal interphalangeal joint injuries tend to remain swollen for long periods of time.[9] Therefore, edema control needs to be a part of the general hand therapy program for these and other joint injuries. These injuries often cause a great deal of swelling and pain within the whole hand as well. Therefore, exercises to maintain mobility of the rest of the hand and shoulder should be done. If the rest of the hand is not exercised, stiffness and fibrosis may be the result.

One should also pay particular attention to the intrinsic muscles of the hand. Because of the intimate relationship between the injured structures and the intrinsic muscles, exercises to these muscles should be started as soon as it is safe to do so. These exercises can be done in such a way as to prevent undue stress to the injured structures. When exercising the proximal interphalangeal joint, it may be useful to splint the distal joint temporarily, as well as to block the metacarpophalangeal joint (prevent it from flexing). This helps to concentrate the flexion and extension power at the proximal interphalangeal joint. Following proximal interphalangeal joint exercises, the distal joint splint is removed and the distal joint is exercised. With proximal interphalangeal joint injuries, it is important that the distal joint also be exercised. The oblique retinacular ligament may become tight, causing decreased distal joint motion. It should be remembered that although at first glance these injuries may look benign, they are serious injuries. Recovery from these injuries is often prolonged and requires the cooperation and active participation of the patient. The therapist and the physician must educate the patient to maximize his cooperation. Above all, patience and encouragement are necessary throughout the treatment period.

Discussion of joint injuries will be divided into ligamentous injuries, volar plate injuries, and dislocations.

Ligamentous Injuries

Incomplete proximal interphalangeal joint injuries probably occur most frequently. An incomplete tear of the ligament implies that the injured joint has enough capsular support remaining to prevent displacement of the joint when adequately stressed.[10]

Of course, the occupational therapist's goal is to maintain joint mobility. However, before one can begin motion, a period of rest in the most advantageous position for proper ligamentous healing is required. The joint is immobilized for 10–14 days in approximately 15° to 20° of flexion using a dorsal aluminum splint[11-13] (Fig 25.1). The dorsal splint allows the palmar surface to be free and does not block the metacarpophalangeal joint or the distal interphalangeal joint. The dorsal splint also provides better support, and is less likely to be worked loose than a volar splint.[14] In some cases, it may be wise to put the whole hand at rest for a few days until the initial pain and swelling have subsided.[13] Then only the involved joint is immobilized. The exact length of time for immobili-

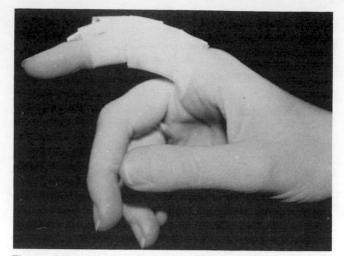

Figure 25.1   Dorsal aluminum splint to support injured proximal interphalangeal joint in the proper position.

zation depends on the amount of pain and swelling and the joint's response to the period of rest.[9,10,13] If the joint shows instability to stress, immobilization for 3 weeks is required, since this may indicate more extensive damage.[10] Following this period of immobilization, the injured finger may be taped to an adjacent digit to provide support for another 1-2 weeks.

Metacarpophalangeal joint ligamentous injuries of the digits occur with much less frequency than the proximal interphalangeal joint ligament injuries.[9,10,15] It is often the radial collateral ligament that is injured.[9-13,15] The mechanism of injury is usually hyperextension of the metacarpophalangeal joint.[10] These injuries often cause large amounts of edema and ecchymosis over both the dorsum of the hand and volar into the palm. The treatment initially is immobilization of the hand. The hand is immobilized from the proximal interphalangeal joint to the mid forearm. The metacarpophalangeal joints are placed in about 45° to 50° of flexion.[9-13,15] Immobilization is continued for approximately 2-3 weeks before exercises are started. The exact period depends on the degree of pain and swelling.

Collateral ligament injuries to the metacarpophalangeal joint of the thumb most often occur to the ulnar side and are handled differently than those of the digits.[9-11] It may be necessary to surgically repair the ligamentous injuries of the thumb metacarpophalangeal joint since soft tissue can become interposed between the bone and the ends of the ligaments.[9-13] Without surgical intervention, healing of the ligament would be prevented. The thumb is immobilized for 5-6 weeks following repair.[9] The goal is to provide a good stable joint for pinch. Active and active-assisted exercises are started following the immobilization period and are gradually increased as tolerated by the patient. Ligamentous injuries may not be considered stable for as long as 10 to 12 weeks. However, the patient may experience some discomfort and weakness for as long as 6 to 12 months following the injury. Therefore, the level of activity allowed is determined on an individual basis.[9-11] Any exercise program should be designed with this in mind and should progress accordingly.

Volar Plate Injuries

Volar plate injuries are caused by hyperextension forces against the extended finger.[9-13] A poorly treated volar plate injury can result in a symptomatic swan neck deformity (hyperextension of the proximal interphalangeal joint and flexion of the distal interphalangeal joint). Initially, the finger is splinted with the proximal interphalangeal joint in about 20° of flexion for 2 weeks. When motion is started, a dorsal block splint is used for an additional 1–2 weeks to further protect the volar plate (Fig. 25.2). In old volar plate injuries that have developed symptomatic swan neck deformities, surgery may be done. These cases would require immobilization for 3 weeks. Extension block splinting is again used for 1–2 more weeks.[9,12,13]

Dislocations

Dislocations of the proximal interphalangeal joints often occur during contact sports. The joint can become dislocated in a dorsal direction, a lateral direction, or a volar direction.[9-13] One should remember that when a dislocation occurs, there is always associated soft tissue damage. The structures injured depend on the mechanism of the injury. When a dorsal dislocation occurs, the major damage is to the volar plate.[9,11] There may be an avulsion of a small bone fragment along with the volar plate. In these cases, the joint is splinted in 20° to 30° of flexion for about 3 weeks.[11] An active exercise program is then started. A dorsal block splint may be used for an additional week or two. It is important that proper splinting be done, since the sequela of a

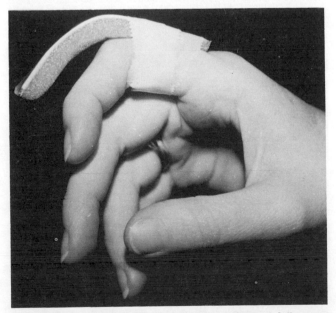

Figure 25.2 Dorsal block splinting to prevent full extension while permitting flexion.

poorly treated dorsal dislocation may be a swan neck deformity.

Another possible complication may be a proximal interphalangeal joint flexion contracture. This may occur if the joint is left in flexion for too long a period of time. Proximal interphalangeal joint flexion deformities are difficult problems. It takes a long time to correct them through either a series of cylinder splints, dynamic splints, or a combination of both. Some may ultimately require corrective surgery. For those patients that have surgery, we have found that continued monitoring may be necessary for at least 6 months postoperatively to prevent recurrence of the deformity. It is also necessary to maintain a program of extension splinting during this time. The patient is progressed from extension splinting except for exercise to intermittent splinting for specified periods of time. A night splint is recommended for an additional few weeks, since it is a person's natural tendency to sleep with the fingers in a flexed position.

Lateral dislocations are caused by torsion, angular, or shearing forces placed on the finger that rupture one of the collateral ligaments and a portion of the insertion of the volar plate.[10] The finger is splinted with the proximal interphalangeal joint in approximately 20° of flexion for about 2 weeks. Following this period of immobilization, the finger is protected for another 1–2 weeks with taping to the adjacent finger next to the side of the ruptured ligament.[10] It may be necessary to use a dorsal blocking splint to protect the volar plate.[9] Joints that are stable to active motion, but show instability to lateral stress, need to be immobilized for 3 weeks.[10]

A volar dislocation involves either incomplete or complete protrusion of the head of the proximal phalanx through the dorsal apparatus (extensor mechanism).[9-11] This injury is splinted in extension for 4–6 weeks to allow the dorsal apparatus to heal.[11] A splint used at night and/or in between exercises may be continued for another 1–2 weeks after the therapy program of active exercises has been started. It is again important that proper splinting be done, since the resulting complication of this injury may be a boutonniere deformity (flexion of the proximal interphalangeal joint and hyperextension of the distal interphalangeal joint) or a proximal interphalangeal joint flexion contracture. Therefore, when exercising the injured joint, extension is emphasized along with gentle flexion exercises. The therapist should carefully observe whether the patient can extend the finger well with each repetition of the exercise. If the patient has difficulty with extension, further splinting is necessary.

When a fracture dislocation occurs, the treatment varies depending on the size of the fragment.[9,10] Surgery is required to repair the joint and soft tissue damage if the fragment is large, causing the joint to be unstable. Postoperatively, the joint is held in plaster with the proximal interphalangeal joint in about 30–35° of flexion for approximately 3 weeks before beginning a therapy program. When exercises are begun, a dorsal blocking splint is used for another week. On about the 5th week postoperatively, gentle controlled extension exercises are allowed. If after 8 weeks the patient has not gained full extension, a dynamic splint may be used to aid in achieving full extension[9-15] (Fig. 25.3). If a closed reduction can be done and joint stability and alignment are satisfactory, the joint is immobilized for 10 days to 2 weeks. A dorsal block splint is then used for another week before full extension is allowed.[9-11] Closed reduction is the process of manipulating the parts of a fractured bone to align them without surgical intervention.

Dislocations of the metacarpophalangeal joints are rare. When they do occur, it is usually to the index or 5th fingers. The dislocation is often dorsal and more frequently requires open reduction (surgical intervention), since soft tissue may become caught in between the joint spaces.[9,10,12] Following repair, the joint is immobilized for 3 weeks. Active flexion is started but extension is not allowed for 4 weeks.[10] Dislocation of the thumb metacarpal results in a major disruption of the soft tissue structures.[9-13] These dislocations are generally reduced closed and are held for 3–4 weeks before initiating a therapy program. A dislocation of the carpometacarpal joint of the thumb usually occurs with such force that the metacarpal shaft is fractured, producing the Bennett's fracture dislocation.[9-13] The fracture may be reduced closed and a Kirschner wire may be placed percutaneously to maintain the reduction. The joint is immobilized for 4 weeks. Gentle exercises are begun at this time and are progressed gradually over the next few weeks.

The mallet deformity deserves mention at this time. It is a common injury to the distal interphalangeal joint, resulting from elongation, laceration, or rupture of the terminal tendon of the dorsal apparatus.[16,17] There may be an interarticular fracture of the distal phalanx in which the tendon avulses a fragment of bone.[17] The distal joint drops into flexion. Generally, the treatment is splinting of the distal joint in extension for 8 weeks.[14,16,17] The patient is instructed in how to change the splint and how to care for the skin to prevent skin breakdown. When the splint is changed, the patient is instructed to be very careful to maintain the joint in extension[14,16,17] (Fig. 25.4). If the joint drops into flexion, the splinting must be started all over again. During the immobilization period, exercises to the proximal interphalangeal joint are done. The result of an untreated mallet deformity may be a swan neck deformity brought about by muscle and tendon imbalance. Therefore, following the immobilization period, careful monitoring is required to be sure that extension is maintained. If an extension lag (failure to fully extend) is noted, further splinting is indicated.

JOINT IMPLANT ARTHROPLASTY

When a joint has been irreparably damaged through either trauma or arthritis, it is possible to reconstruct the joint using the various implants now available. The ones most commonly used are the Swanson flexible hinge implants. These implants are made of silicone rubber and act as joint spacers, while the new capsuloligamentous system forms during the healing process.[18-21] Swanson refers to this as the process of encapsulation.[20,21] The following is a guideline to the postoperative management of these patients. It should be kept in mind that each patient is unique, and treatment may vary.

Metacarpophalangeal Joint Interpositional Arthroplasty

Metacarpophalangeal joint arthroplasty is most often done in patients with rheumatoid arthritis. Preopera-

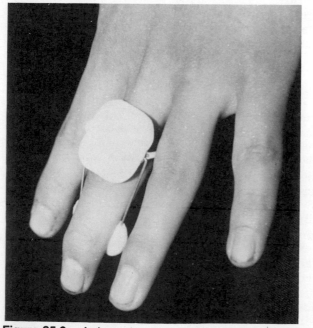

Figure 25.3 A dynamic splint used to aid in achieving or maintaining finger extension.

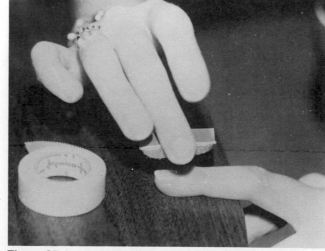

Figure 25.4 Patient changing the aluminum splint, used to maintain extension of the distal interphalangeal joint when a mallet deformity occurs.

tively, certain types of deformities are seen. Millender and Nalebuff[19] have described a classification system for these deformities. Postoperatively, the hand is initially held in a bulky dressing with a plaster splint that supports the metacarpophalangeal joints in extension and some radial deviation to maintain desired joint alignment. If, preoperatively, the patient has limited flexion and minimal or no ulnar deviation, the fingers may be held in some flexion postoperatively.[22] On days 1 and 2 following the surgery, the exercises consist of gentle finger pumping (gentle range of motion) to help reduce edema and provide gentle active metacarpophalangeal joint motion. On days 3–5, exercises consist of active and active-assisted range of motion to the metacarpophalangeal joints. Metacarpophalangeal joint flexion is stressed by teaching the patient to bring the metacarpophalangeal joints into a shelf-like position and then curl the interphalangeal joints into the palm. When the patient has good proximal interphalangeal joint motion, he may attempt to substitute this motion for metacarpophalangeal joint flexion. If such substitution is allowed to continue, the patient's final range of motion could be severely compromised. In cases where this is a problem, the proximal interphalangeal joints can be immobilized during exercise sessions to concentrate flexion and extension at the metacarpophalangeal joint.[20,21] The proximal interphalangeal joints may be immobilized either with Alumafoam splints or pieces of splinting material (Fig. 25.5). Usually on about the fifth to seventh postoperative day, depending on the amount of pain and swelling, a dynamic splint is fabricated.[18-22] It is usually an ulnar gutter splint to provide good wrist support as well as good carpometacarpal support to the mobile fourth and fifth digits. The outrigger is placed in a radial direction to give the metacarpophalangeal joints a gentle, continuous radial pull.[22] The elastics must have appropriate tension to provide adequate extension and radial deviation, but should not be so tight as to restrict flexion. Hyperextension of the metacarpophalangeal

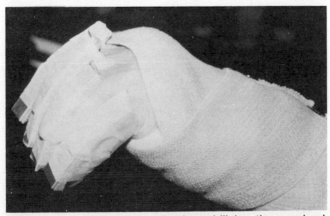

Figure 25.5 Aluminum splint immobilizing the proximal interphalangeal joints to aid in achieving better metacarpophalangeal joint motion following metacarpophalangeal joint arthroplasty.

joints must be avoided. To be sure that the patient gets full flexion, he may be instructed to remove the cuffs for short periods of time at each exercise session.[22]

If the patient is not achieving what we would consider good range of motion (60° to 65° of flexion), a volar outrigger may be attached to the splint to provide a flexion pull at the metacarpophalangeal joints.[22] The flexion outrigger is then worn alternating it with the extension outrigger. The dynamic splint is worn all day for approximately 6–8 weeks. The elastics are adjusted, and the splint is modified whenever necessary to maintain proper functioning. At night, the patient wears a plaster resting splint to maintain the position of the hand. This splint is also adjusted as necessary during the postoperative period. The night splint is often worn for another 2 weeks after the dynamic splint has been discontinued. The exact length of time that the patient is involved in the splinting program depends on the condition of the soft tissue at the time of surgery. Patients with rheumatoid arthritis often have poor soft tissue. As a result, exercise programs must be modified and the splinting program increased. One should keep in mind that it is the soft tissue that provides the joint stability.

The exercises are done approximately 4 times a day for brief periods, approximately 5 min, at each session. Several brief sessions of exercise spread out over the entire day are less likely to cause tissue reaction than one long session.

After two to three weeks, the patient is allowed to begin using the hand for light activities, such as eating, with the dynamic splint on the hand. At six to eight weeks, mild resistance may be added to the exercise program for strengthening. Functional use of the hand is also increased at that time. It should be kept in mind that the patient with rheumatoid disease is weakened to begin with. Therefore, one cannot expect the implant to provide normal strength, although strength in many cases is improved. The patient is generally allowed to use the hand for all daily activities at 3 months. This is a gradual active process and is progressed according to the patient's tolerance. Joint protection principles are taught to the patient during the course of the treatment to allow the person to use the newly reconstructed joints safely.

There are some considerations when treating patients with metacarpophalangeal joint arthroplasties. In some patients, the fifth finger is more difficult to mobilize than others. One must be sure that the elastic on the splint for the fifth finger is not too tight. In some cases, it may not be necessary to use an elastic on the fifth finger. Of course, this has to be decided on an individual basis.

Another consideration is the proper alignment of the digits. In the normal hand, there is some supination of the digits. Following metacarpophalangeal joint arthroplasty, the index finger, especially, may tend to assume a more pronated position.[20,21] For this situation, a serpentine-type finger splint made of splinting material may be wrapped around the finger to maintain the digit in some supination (Fig. 25.6). This splint is at-

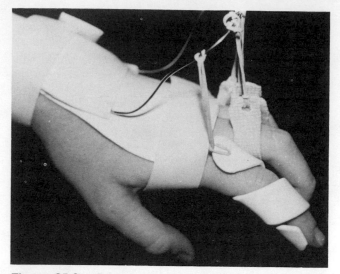

Figure 25.6 Postoperative metacarpophalangeal joint arthroplasty splint with serpentine-type splint attached to help supinate the index finger.

tached to the outrigger with the elastic and is used in place of the usual finger cuff. Another way to maintain supination is with two finger cuffs exerting tension in opposite directions to provide a force couple.

Proximal Interphalangeal Joint Arthroplasty

Much of the postoperative hand therapy management of the patient who has undergone proximal interphalangeal joint arthroplasty depends on the soft tissue surgery that is done at the time of the arthroplasty.[23] Therefore, the time when motion is begun has to be determined on an individual basis. Proximal interphalangeal joint arthroplasty may be done for the following reasons:

1. To reconstruct a stiff, painful proximal interphalangeal joint damaged by trauma, rheumatoid disease, or degenerative joint disease.
2. To reconstruct a boutonniere deformity.
3. To reconstruct a swan neck deformity (rarely done).

Stiff Proximal Interphalangeal Joint. When the proximal interphalangeal joint arthroplasty is done for pain and stiffness, gentle interphalangeal joint motion may be started as soon as 2–3 days postoperatively, depending on the amount of pain and swelling. The patient is held in a plaster splint that supports the proximal interphalangeal joint in extension in between exercise sessions. In cases where postoperative stiffness appears to be a problem, the proximal interphalangeal joint may be taped down into flexion for at least part of the time in between exercise sessions.[23]

Boutonniere Repair. When an arthroplasty is done to repair a boutonniere deformity, the extensor mechanism is repaired as part of the procedure. Therefore, the extensor mechanism must be protected in extension, usually with an Alumafoam splint. Gentle

active motion is started about 10–14 days, postoperatively.[20,21,23] Between exercise sessions, the finger is placed back in the extension splint. The splint is worn for 4–6 weeks or until the position of the finger has stabilized. It may be necessary in some cases to delay exercises as long as 4 weeks.

Swan Neck Repair. Although rarely done, this procedure is undertaken in combination with tendon reconstruction. The finger is held in approximately 20–30° of flexion to prevent a recurrent hyperextension deformity.[20,21] In this situation, a slight proximal interphalangeal joint flexion contracture may be desirable. Range of motion allowing flexion and protected extension may be started about 3–5 days postoperatively. The finger is then splinted in between exercise sessions until the position of the joint has stabilized.

General Exercise Considerations. Initially, active and active-assisted exercises are done and then increased to gentle passive motion as tolerated by the patient. Care must be taken to always support the metacarpophalangeal joint in extension. This allows all the flexion and extension forces to be placed at the proximal interphalangeal joint. Blocking of the metacarpophalangeal joint into extension may be done by the patient with the other hand or with a piece of splinting material padded with moleskin. Splinting material works well since it is rigid but also thin enough not to block any proximal interphalangeal joint motion. The hand can be positioned over a book or the edge of a table. When this method is used, one must be sure that the proximal interphalangeal joint motion is not being prevented. Usually at 6–8 weeks postoperatively, resistance may be added to the program to improve strength. Functional use of the hand should gradually be increased during this time. At 3 months postoperatively, the patient is usually allowed to use the hand for all activities of daily living.

Silastic Wrist Implant Arthroplasty

The postoperative therapy for wrist arthroplasty begins the first day following surgery, when the drain is removed, the dressing is changed, and both volar and dorsal plaster wrist splints are made. At this time, finger range of motion is begun to maintain digital motion. The pumping action of the fingers aids in reducing postoperative edema. The volar and dorsal wrist splints are kept in place for 4–6 weeks.[24] During this time, no wrist motion is allowed. If any laxity of the wrist is noted, the wrist will be held longer. Often, a distal ulnar excision is done in conjunction with the wrist arthroplasty. An ulnar head implant may or may not be used in these cases. When a distal ulnar excision is done, the forearm is held in supination for 2–3 weeks with either a sugartong splint or another form of plaster splinting to ensure good capsular healing.

Generally, wrist exercises are begun at 4 weeks. The goal of the surgery is a stable, pain-free wrist. Motion, therefore, is purposely limited to 25–30° of dorsiflexion, and 25–30° of palmar flexion. Exercises are done carefully with that goal in mind. For the first week following initiation of the exercise program, the exercises are gentle, protected, active-assisted motion. Exercises are then progressed to active and gentle passive range of motion. Gradually, after approximately 6–8 weeks postoperatively, resistance can be added to the exercise program for strengthening. Generally at this point, splinting is discontinued and the patient can begin using his hand unprotected for light activities of daily living. Activities of daily living are gradually increased as strength returns. In special cases, when any laxity of the wrist is noted, a dynamic wrist splint is fabricated to provide controlled, protected motion (Fig. 25.7). This splint is worn during the day, and a resting wrist splint is worn at night. At approximately 12 weeks, the patient may resume normal activities. However, to prevent too much stress to the wrist, it is recommended that the patient wear a wrist cock-up splint indefinitely whenever he performs heavier tasks.

Thumb Carpometacarpal Joint Implant Arthroplasty

Arthroplasty of the carpometacarpal joint of the thumb is often done in patients with osteoarthritis. When evaluating these patients for surgery, it is important that the other joints of the thumb be evaluated as well. For example, an adduction deformity of the metacarpophalangeal joint of the thumb may be an associated problem in patients with carpometacarpal joint arthritis.[20] If the adduction deformity is severe, the adductor pollicis may have to be released to ensure proper balance and seating of the implant. A hyperextension deformity of the metacarpophalangeal joint of the thumb also may contribute to the adduction deformity.[20] If the metacarpophalangeal joint of the thumb is hyperextended, it may be necessary to surgically correct this problem to prevent dislocation or subluxation of the implant. Postoperatively, the thumb is held in a plaster splint in palmar abduction for 4–6 weeks to ensure good capsular healing.[20] During this time, range of motion of the fingers is encouraged. When the splint is removed, the patient begins opposi-

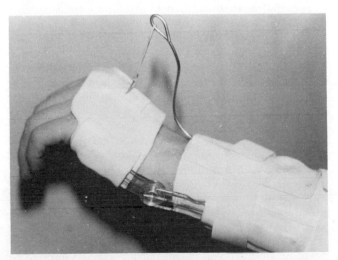

Figure 25.7 Postoperative wrist arthroplasty splint.

tion, abduction, and circumduction exercises. Hyperextension of the thumb should be avoided. Dexterity activities are then added to the program and are increased as strength begins to return. Unrestricted use of the thumb is generally allowed in about 12 weeks. Strength takes considerably longer to return. In fact, it may take up to one year before the patient feels that he has adequate strength.

PERIPHERAL NERVE INJURY

Sensibility of the hand is a very complex subject. Obviously, without functioning nerves, one would have an essentially useless appendage. Sensibility of the hand encompasses the very essence of human experience. We require sensibility of the hand for self-expression, prehension, identification, and evaluation of objects, to protect us from harmful stimuli, and to enable us to manipulate our environment. Therefore, every effort must be made to help people with peripheral nerve injuries regain as much useful function as possible.

The type of injury greatly influences treatment, as well as later regeneration and the degree of recovery of sensibility and motor control. Age is also a factor in the final results. Children recover a much higher level of sensibility than do adults, given the same injury.

The radial, ulnar, and median nerves supply sensibility and motor function to the hand. Injury to any one of them can cause significant hand dysfunction. The median nerve supplies sensation to the thumb, index finger, middle finger, and one-half of the ring finger. Loss of this nerve is significant, since the radial side of the hand is used primarily for precision grip and pinch. Loss of sensibility here leaves the hand unable to perform precise activities. Although most of the thenar muscles are also controlled by the median nerve, the motor loss is less significant in a median nerve injury than is the loss of sensation. However, the reverse is true with ulnar and radial nerve injuries. The ulnar nerve provides sensation to the fifth finger and ulnar one-half of the ring finger. The radial nerve supplies sensation to the radial three-quarters of the dorsum of the hand and the dorsum of the thumb. It also supplies the dorsum of the index and middle fingers and the radial one-half of the ring finger distally to each of the proximal interphalangeal joints. It should be kept in mind that nerve innervations vary.

Evaluation

The initial evaluation should be done in a quiet, relaxed atmosphere. It should not cause pain and therefore should not be done on hypersensitive or painful hands.

The patient's active and passive ranges of motion are recorded, and a muscle test is administered. Grip strength and pinch strength should be recorded for both hands as a comparison.

It is often helpful to first make a drawing of the hand on a piece of paper, noting the location of lacerations and any calluses or other injuries such as burns that would indicate lack of protective sensation. It may be advantageous to actually map out the areas of dysfunction on the patient's hand. The patient then is asked to describe how the hand feels,[25,26] including identification of where on the hand the sensibility changes. In this way the therapist obtains information about the degree of sensibility and also may gain insight into the patient's ability to adapt to the altered sensibility. The patient's description also may indicate his motivation for sensory reeducation.

Except for electrodiagnostic studies, there are no standardized tests currently available for evaluating sensibility. Therefore, the information obtained is subjective. However, certain information must be obtained to evaluate sensory function. It must be measured and recorded so that it can be reproduced for later comparison.

Nerve regeneration is generally thought to take place at the rate of approximately one inch per month.[27,28] Therefore, reevaluation following nerve injury should be done approximately every 4 to 6 weeks.[28]

Sensory testing should include touch (Semmes-Weinstein monofilaments), two-point discrimination, functional sensibility (dexterity and stereognosis as measured by the Moberg Pick Up Test), proprioception, and finger and point identification.

Semmes-Weinstein Monofilaments. The Semmes-Weinstein pressure aesthesiometer tests light touch and deep pressure perception (see chapter 3 and Fig. 3.2). Testing proceeds distal to proximal but is varied periodically to avoid patient anticipation.[25,26] Testing with the monofilaments begins with filaments in the normal threshold range (2.36 to 2.83) and progresses to filaments of increasing pressure until touch is identified by the patient. The numbers equal Log_{10} F_{mg}.[29] Filaments 1.65 through 4.08 are applied three times to the same spot. This is because one touch may not reach the required threshold of these lighter monofilaments. All filaments are applied within 1.0 to 1.5 sec and are held for 1.0 to 1.5 sec. They are then lifted, and the procedure is repeated twice more in the same manner. Filaments 4.17 through 6.65 are applied only once per trial. It is important to carefully control the speed of application, since a quickly applied stimulus will be more easily perceived than an equal amount of pressure placed more slowly.[25,26] During the application of the monofilaments, the patient should have his eyes closed and the hand well supported. The patient is then asked to open his eyes and to point to the spot on the skin touched with the monofilaments to determine point localization.[26,30,31] This should be recorded on the evaluation sheet. It is important to first do an assessment of the uninvolved hand to determine what the normal range is for that patient.

Two-Point Discrimination. The purpose of the two-point discrimination test is to determine if the patient can distinguish between being touched by one point or two points and at what distance this can be appreciated. Moberg has written that 6 mm of two-point discrimination is required for winding a watch, 6.8 mm is required for sewing, and 12 mm is required for manipulating precision tools.[32]

Again, the patient's other hand is tested to determine a baseline and to help the patient become familiar with the testing procedure. Testing with vision occluded proceeds in a random fashion across the hand and distal to proximal, alternating one and two points (see chapter 3). One should pause 5 sec between point application. Testing is stopped at 15 mm if responses are still incorrect at that level.

The results obtained with two-point discrimination and the Semmes-Weinstein aesthesiometer do not necessarily correlate. It is, for example, possible to have two-point discrimination recorded within normal range but still show diminished protective sensation when tested with the Semmes-Weinstein monofilaments.[25]

Moberg Pick Up Test. This test is used to help determine the patient's functional level of sensibility. The test is most appropriate in cases of median nerve injury or combined median and ulnar nerve injuries. The test consists of a group of small objects that are placed on a table. The patient is then asked to pick these objects up as quickly as possible and drop them into a small container.[30,32] The activity is timed using a stop watch. Both hands are tested. Following this procedure, the patient is blindfolded and asked to repeat the test. While blindfolded, the patient is asked to identify the objects[30,32] (see chapter 3). The time of both procedures is recorded. With vision occluded, the time is generally increased if there is a decrease in sensibility.[32] The number of objects remains constant, but the objects themselves are varied to help prevent patient learning from altering the results. It must be remembered that this is not a standardized test, and it is presented only as a useful tool for evaluating sensibility in the median nerve or in cases of combined median and ulnar nerve lesions.

Dellon has modified Moberg's pick up test by standardizing the objects used.[29] He also has added the requirement of object identification. The objects he chose are of similar material to avoid giving the patient cues by temperature or texture. The objects are graded to require increasing ability to discriminate (see chapter 3).

Moving Two-Point Discrimination. This test was devised by Dellon,[29,33] who believes that since fingertip sensibility is highly dependent on motion, the stimulus for discrimination testing should be moving. Normal moving two-point discrimination is considered to be 2 mm. Testing is stopped at this point (see chapter 3).

Proprioception. The patient's finger is supported by the examiner and then passively moved from ½ to 1 cm in different directions. The patient is then asked to identify in what direction the finger has been moved (see chapter 3). Omer states that an interphalangeal joint requires 5° to 10° of passive motion before recognition of the position is possible.[30]

Finger and Point Identification. Using the point of a pencil, the finger is touched just enough to indent the skin but not enough to cause blanching. The patient is then asked to both identify the finger touched and the point on the finger where it was touched.

Sensory Reeducation

Dellon et al. have shown that the quality of functional sensibility can be improved through a program of sensory reeducation.[29,34-38] Not only does this reeducation process appear to improve the level of sensibility, but it also seems to aid in helping the patient recalibrate altered sensibility, thus improving the patient's functional capacity.[28,29,34-39]

Sensory reeducation is begun as soon as possible following the injury. One begins training when light touch has returned to the palm and proximal phalanx.[28,29,34-37] At this stage, stimulation of the area is done by the patient himself with either a finger of the other hand or an eraser on a pencil.[28,29,34-37] Large objects of various shapes that can be grasped or placed in the palm are next introduced.[28,29,34-37] The patient also is instructed to immerse his hand in substances such as sand or rice. These activities are also done with the normal hand to help the patient in the educational process.[28,29,34-37] As the return of sensibility progresses distally, smaller objects are introduced. These are manipulated with both the normal and injured hands and include such things as nuts and bolts, coins, keys, and other everyday objects.[28,29,34-37] Various textures are added to the program as the patient progresses. Activities of daily living such as buttoning clothing and tying shoes also are encouraged.[28,29,34-37] If the injured hand is the dominant hand, writing skills and manipulation of eating utensils are practiced. As the level of sensibility improves, common objects can be buried in rice or sand. The patient must then try to find these objects and identify them.[28,38] When possible, tools the patient uses at work are introduced into the treatment program. If the patient's injury is severe and return of protective sensation is not expected, the therapist must instruct the patient in how to care for the hand to prevent further injury, such as burns.

Motor Reeducation

After nerve repair, the wrist and fingers are positioned so as to prevent tension on the repaired area.[27,40] The exact position would depend on the available length of the nerve and is determined by the surgeon at the time of operation. The nerve repair is immobilized from 3–5 weeks before motion is allowed.[27,40,41] During this period of immobilization, it may be possible to gradually bring the wrist and hand into a more neutral position, while they are protected in the splint. The nerve is adversely affected by tension. Rapid stretch will cause the nerve to exceed its elastic limits and may lead to interneural fibrosis.[42] Therefore, it is recommended that the joint not be extended more than 10° per week.[40,42]

Following immobilization, gentle active exercise should be started along with gentle passive motion to the paralyzed joints to maintain full joint mobility. Exercises for the rest of the extremity also are important to maintain strength of the uninvolved muscles and improve circulation and nutrition in the extremity.[28] Light massage is beneficial for circulation and is relaxing and pleasurable for the patient. Massage also maintains the skin in good condition. Any stretching exercises are generally delayed until 8 weeks following the repair.[28] Splinting is often necessary to prevent deformity that may be caused by muscle imbalance brought about by the nerve injury. The type of splint used depends on the nerve injured and the muscles affected by the loss of nerve function (see chapter 13). Great caution must be taken to be sure that the correct splint is used. A poorly designed or ill-conceived splint can lead to irreversible deformity. Static or dynamic splints may be used to maintain position as the joints are gradually brought into their normal positions.

Atrophy of denervated muscles will often take place regardless of good therapy or intermittent electrical stimulation. Currently the only way to prevent atrophy is to reinnervate the muscles.[43] Functional electrical stimulation, however, may be helpful to maintain muscle tone while reinnervation takes place.

TENDON TRANSFERS

When irreversible nerve and/or tendon damage occurs, it is possible to restore muscle balance and improve function through tendon transfers. Tendon transfers redistribute the remaining muscle power so that it can be used in the most effective functional combinations. The type of transfers used would, of course, depend on the muscles available for transfer. Certain conditions, however, must exist before tendons can be transferred successfully.[28,44-49] First, joints in the area of the transfer must have adequate passive mobility. In the preoperative stage, it is the responsibility of the therapist to maintain joint mobility through exercise and splinting. Second, soft tissue also must be well healed and in good condition. The therapist may help here by using massage and active exercise to uninvolved muscles and joints. This helps to improve circulation and nutrition to the extremity and maintain strength of the normal musculature. In some cases, restoration of the soft tissues through various plastic procedures may be necessary before tendon transfers can be done. Third, the proposed transferred muscle must have adequate strength to perform the desired function. Although it is generally agreed that it is easier to train a transferred tendon when synergistic muscles are used, that factor is no longer thought to be a major consideration.[44-46,49] The direction of the pull of the transfer is believed to be far more important for the success of the training.[44-49]

Following the transfer, the hand is immobilized for 3–4 weeks. Extensor tendons are generally held at least 4–6 weeks because of the force that is placed on them by the much stronger flexors.[44] A protective splint is then used for an additional 2–3 weeks between exercise sessions. The exact period of immobilization depends on the stress to be placed on the transferred tendon. Exercises begin with controlled active motion, and any forced manipulation must be avoided. Massage and other edema control treatments, such as the use of elevation and Coban® wrap (an elastic type material that gives gentle compression) or Tubigrip® (an elastic stockinette), are done. Active motion of the rest of the extremity also is encouraged. The therapy program should then progress to gradually increasing resistance for strengthening. When progressing the program, the therapist should watch for any signs of inflammation that would require that the intensity of the exercise be decreased. Proprioceptive neuromuscular facilitation patterns are quite helpful in training certain transferred tendons.[28] Functional activities are introduced into the program at about 4–6 weeks following cast removal[50,51] (Fig. 25.8). These encourage functional use of the hand and improve strength. In patients who are having difficulty with the retraining process, biofeedback may be a very useful adjunct to the treatment programs (See chapter 12). The exact timing for the introduction of various modalities is determined by the surgeon. Generally, the relearning progresses quickly and with very little difficulty.

TENDON REPAIR

Tendon lacerations are among the more common types of hand injuries. Rehabilitation of patients with these injuries offers a special challenge to the therapist. New advances in research on tendon healing and new microsurgical techniques are exciting and make the area of tendon rehabilitation very dynamic for both the surgeon and the therapist.

Flexor Tendon Repairs

Categorizing flexor tendon injuries can best be done by dividing the hand into five zones.[52-61] Zone 1 is the area distal to where the superficialis divides. Zone 2 is the area that begins at the proximal part of the flexor tendon sheath, proximal to the metacarpophalangeal joint, and extends to the middle portion of the middle phalanx. This is an especially difficult area in which to restore smooth tendon gliding. Both flexor tendons pass through a tight fibro-osseous canal. This leaves very little room for any scarring. Even a small amount of adhesion formation can disrupt the gliding mechanism and cause decreased range of motion. Zone 3 is the area from the origin of the lumbricals to, but not including, the carpal tunnel. Zone 4 includes the carpal tunnel. Repairs in this area may necessitate placing the wrist in neutral or slight dorsiflexion because of the repair of the transverse carpal ligament. This wrist placement would require the metacarpophalangeal joints to be blocked at about 45° to 60° to ensure that no tension is placed on the repair.[55] In zones 2 and 3 metacarpophalangeal joints are placed in about 35° to 40° of flexion with the distal interphalangeal joints at 0°. Zone 5 extends from the distal forearm to the wrist, proximal to the transverse carpal ligament.

Another consideration is the position of the hand at the time of injury. If the finger was flexed, the actual laceration of the tendon will be distal to the skin laceration. If the finger was in extension at the time of injury, then the skin laceration would correspond to the tendon laceration.[53,54]

One also should know how to test individual tendon function. To test for superficialis function, support all the fingers in extension except the one being tested (Fig. 25.9). If the superficialis is intact, the proximal interphalangeal joint should be able to flex. This may not be true, however, for the fifth finger. Baker et al. concluded that the fifth finger superficialis is functionally deficient in a large portion of the population.[58] To test for profundus function, put the finger in extension and ask the patient to flex the distal joint (Fig. 25.10). If the profundus is intact, he will be able to do so.[53,56]

Postoperative Management. The use of dynamic traction for early controlled mobilization adds another dimension to the management of tendon repairs in zones 2 and 3. Duran and Houser have shown that 3–5 mm of extension of the repaired tendon done in a controlled, passive exercise program is generally

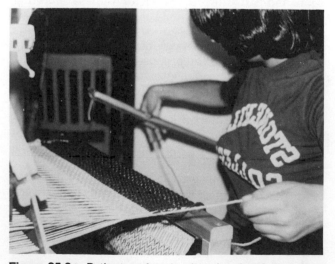

Figure 25.8 Patient performing functional activities to aid in tendon transfer training.

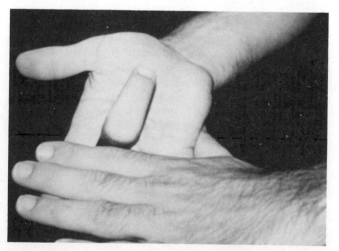

Figure 25.9 Testing for superficialis function.

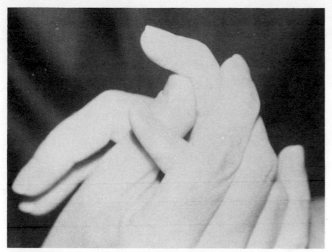

Figure 25.10   Testing for profundus function.

enough to prevent the formation of firm adhesions in zone 2 repairs.[57,59] Postoperatively, the wrist is held in about 20–45° of flexion, and the metacarpophalangeal joints are held in 35–40° of flexion using a dorsal block splint[54,55,57] (Fig. 25.11). The interphalangeal joints are positioned in 0° of extension to prevent proximal interphalangeal joint flexion contractures. An elastic is attached to the fingernail of the involved finger by means of a suture placed in the nail by the surgeon at the time of the repair. The elastic is attached proximally to the wrist with a safety pin that is fastened to the Ace bandage. When the finger is flexed, there should not be any tension on the elastic.

The exercise program begins on days 2–5. At this time, the patient is instructed to actively extend the finger within the limits of the splint. He then passively brings the digit into flexion with his other hand. Active finger flexion or passive extension is not permitted.[53,55–57,59–61] With the Duran method, only passive motion within the splint is allowed.[57,59] Kleinert et al. instruct patients to actively extend the finger within the splint and then to allow the elastic to bring the finger into flexion[60,61] It has been shown, using electro-

myography, that during active extension, the flexors reciprocally relax.[60] At 3½ to 4 weeks, the dorsal splint is removed, and the traction is attached to a wrist cuff or Ace wrap. At this time, active exercises are started, but the patient is not allowed to use the hand for any strong grasping or any passive extension.

At about 6 weeks, dynamic traction is generally discontinued. Very mild resistance may be added at 6–8 weeks to enhance tendon pull-through if there is moderate to severe adherence of the tendon. If a flexion contracture of the proximal interphalangeal joint appears to be developing, assistive extension and dynamic and static splinting may be started at 8–10 weeks.[54–56] Generally, the patient is allowed to resume normal activities at about 12 weeks following repair. It should be noted that because early motion inhibits the formation of firm scar tissue, one complication of early motion is tendon rupture. Therefore, if the patient has good motion early on, the progression of the program should be slowed.[55,56] The fact that the tendon is gliding well indicates that the scarring has been light. Therefore, the tendon juncture is vulnerable to rupture at this point.

In cases of flexor tendon grafts, the hand is immobilized for 3 weeks.[56] At this point, gentle controlled active exercises are begun to provide tendon pull-through. Protection in the splint in between exercises is continued for another 1–2 weeks. At 4 weeks, the wrist may be brought into neutral and individual blocking exercises can be initiated. Dorsiflexion of the wrist is done gradually so as not to place stress on the graft. If there is a flexion contracture of the proximal interphalangeal joint, an extension assist splint may be used intermittently at about 8 weeks. The extension assist splint also may provide mild resistance against flexion. Light massage is used at this time to help soften and maintain the skin in good condition. It is important to note that when training the patient, the more proximal joints must be blocked or held in extension, to place the flexor power at the joint being exercised. For example, when exercising the proximal interphalangeal joint, the metacarpophalangeal joint should be blocked. When exercising the distal interphalangeal joint, the metacarpophalangeal joint and the proximal interphalangeal joint should be blocked. This can be achieved by using a Bunnell block or by having the patient hold the joint with the other hand. Blocking exercises are usually started at 4–5 weeks.[55,56] For part of the exercise program, the proximal interphalangeal joint should be exercised with the metacarpophalangeal joint supported in flexion to provide tendon glide in this range.

Staged Tendon Reconstruction.   In cases of a severely damaged tendon system, tendon reconstruction may be done in two stages. This technique of staged tendon surgery has improved the results of flexor tendon grafting. Dr. James Hunter developed a method of implanting a flexible silicone rod around which a pseudosheath grows.[62–64] Later, the rod is removed and a tendon graft is placed within the sheath, providing a

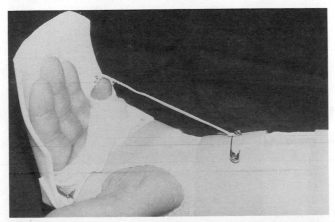

Figure 25.11   Elastic traction used for early flexor tendon mobilization.

reconstructed tendon system. A necessary part of the pseudosheath formation is an organized program of passive gliding of the prosthesis. The implant is generally left in place for approximately 3 months before grafting is undertaken. This technique also may be used in some cases for damaged extensor tendons.

Stage One. Evelyn Mackin, L.P.T., and Dr. Hunter have given us careful guidelines to follow in the care of these patients.[62-68] When this surgery is undertaken, the flexor tendons are excised, leaving a stump of the profundus about 1 cm long, attached to the distal phalanx. A silicone prosthesis is implanted in the finger and sutured to the distal end of the profundus. All potential material for pulley reconstruction is preserved at the time of surgery. Following the surgery, the wrist is placed in about 30–35° of flexion with the metacarpophalangeal joints in about 60–70° of flexion and the interphalangeal joints in 0° of extension. The hand is maintained in this position in a dorsal block splint for 3 weeks. During the first week, gentle controlled, passive flexion of the finger is started. Finger trapping also may be done. Finger trapping is the taping of the finger to the adjacent finger or using the adjacent finger to help achieve passive motion.[65-67] The therapist must be careful to note any signs of synovitis in the finger. Exercises that are done too vigorously will result in swelling and pain. If these occur, the finger must be rested and infection or failure of the implant must be ruled out.[62-68] Therefore, the surgeon and the therapist must maintain close communication. At 3 weeks, the protective dorsal splint is removed. If no sign of synovitis is present at 6 weeks, the patient is allowed to return to his normal activities. Generally, 3 months is allowed between stages 1 and 2.

Stage Two. The stage 2 procedure is the introduction of the tendon graft. Following surgery, the patient is protected in a dorsal splint with the hand in the same position as for stage 1. At about 5–7 days, with the hand still carefully protected in the dorsal splint, gentle passive flexion of the finger is done. Ten repetitions are done four times per day. The therapist must monitor for the development of flexion contractures of the proximal interphalangeal joint. At about 4–6 weeks, the pull-out wire is removed, and the active exercise program is increased.[65-67] It may be possible at this time to discontinue wearing the dorsal splint.[65-67] In some patients, however, it is necessary to protect the hand a bit longer in the dorsal splint in between exercises. This is decided on an individual basis, depending on the patient's circumstances. At about 8–10 weeks, the patient may be allowed to begin a program of graded activities to improve strength. This would include use of therapeutic putty and finger-blocking exercises. At 10 weeks, further resistance can be added. Heavy resistance is not allowed until 3 months.[65-67]

Before a staged flexor tendon reconstruction, it is important that the therapist see the patient to improve the general condition of the hand by improving passive mobility of the injured finger and active and passive mobility of the uninvolved digits. Every effort must be made to improve the condition of the soft tissue as much as possible before surgery.

Extensor Tendon Repairs

Laceration of the extensor tendon is a significant injury and can have a serious effect on hand function. Not only could the patient lose full extension, but because of scarring and a decrease in tendon excursion, he also could lose flexion. The extensor tendons, in contrast to the flexor tendons, do not glide in a synovial sheath except at the wrist.[69,70] At the wrist, the synovial sheath extends about 1 inch above and one inch below the extensor retinaculum. The blood supply to the extensors comes from soft tissue and paratenon rather than from vincula, which is the source of the blood supply for flexor tendons.[69,70]

Lacerations of the extensor tendons at the level of the distal joint result in a mallet deformity. Management of this injury has been previously discussed.

Extensor tendon injuries that occur at the level of the proximal interphalangeal joint can result in a boutonniere deformity, since the central slip of the extensor digitorum is often lacerated at that level.[69,70] The treatment for this injury is immobilization of the proximal interphalangeal joints in full extension for 5–6 weeks.[69,70] Active motion of the metacarpophalangeal joints and the distal interphalangeal joints is allowed during this time. When active proximal interphalangeal joint motion is started, extension of the proximal interphalangeal joints must be monitored carefully, to be sure that no extensor lag develops. Further splinting would be necessary if a lag does occur.

Extensor tendon injuries to the rest of the hand are immobilized for approximately 4 weeks.[69,73] The hand is immobilized in a volar splint that extends from the proximal interphalangeal joints to two-thirds up the forearm. The wrist is held in about 20° of dorsiflexion with the metacarpophalangeal joints in extension.[69,70] The proximal interphalangeal joints are free to move. Following this period of immobilization, active and active-assisted exercises are started. At 5 weeks, gentle active flexion is allowed, but it must be done carefully. Since the flexors are much stronger than the extensors, vigorous flexion could disrupt the repair. If only the wrist extensors are lacerated, the digits may be left free, and just the wrist immobilized. Immobilization is continued for 4 weeks.[69,70]

An exercise found helpful in regaining extension after extensor tendon repair is to tape the proximal interphalangeal joints into flexion (Fig. 25.12, 25.13). The patient then flexes and extends the metacarpophalangeal joints with the hand in the described position. This helps to isolate the long extensors and place the extensor power at the level of the metacarpophalangeal joints. One must remember that the excursion of the extensor tendons can be decreased due to the adherence of the extensor tendons to the surrounding tissues. Therefore, when safe to do so, gentle exercises to

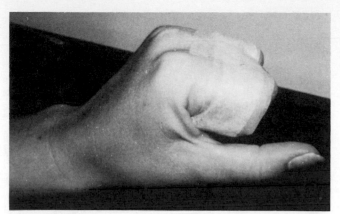

Figure 25.12 Taping exercise in flexion.

stretch the extensors should be done. In some cases, a dynamic splint to aid in stretching may be necessary. In cases in which an extensor tendon lag persists, a dynamic splint is fabricated to support the fingers in extension. In some cases, biofeedback may be useful in treating these injuries.

In carefully selected cases of complex extensor injuries in zones 5, 6, and 7 (from the metacarpophalangeal joints to the wrist), early passive motion has been used successfully. It has been found that resting the joints of the fingers in full extension helps to prevent extensor tendon lag. Active flexion allows enough metacarpophalangeal joint motion to prevent collateral ligament shortening and enough tendon glide to lengthen adhesions as they are forming, reducing the possible need for tenolysis at a later time.[73]

Generally the patient with extensor tendon injuries can expect a good result with careful monitoring.

Extensor Tendon Ruptures in Patients With Rheumatoid Arthritis.   Extensor tendon rupture is a serious complication of rheumatoid arthritis. It requires a prolonged rehabilitation program, up to 3–4 months or longer to reach the end result. There are thought to be several causes of spontaneous tendon rupture in patients with rheumatoid arthritis.[74-78] First

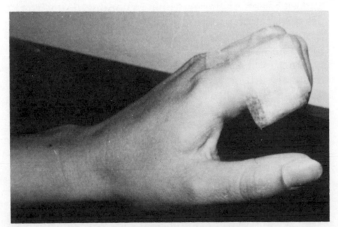

Figure 25.13 Taping exercise in extension.

is attrition rupture, when a tendon ruptures on a piece of bone, usually the distal ulna; second is tenosynovitis that infiltrates the tendon; third is pressure from a hypertrophied synovial membrane beneath the tight dorsal retinaculum; and fourth is multiple steroid injections.

Single tendon ruptures cause a minimal extension lag because of the junctura tendonae that connect the tendons over the metacarpophalangeal joints.[76,77] Patients will often have very little disability and may not even see a physician. However, when two tendons rupture, the disability becomes more obvious. Any acute extensor tendon rupture is treated with urgency, since a single tendon rupture is followed by a second or a third.[76,77] In patients with rheumatoid arthritis, either tendon transfer (usually the extensor indicis proprius) or adjacent tendon suture is often used to restore tendon function.[74,77] For more complicated ruptures, wrist extensors or the flexor digitorum superficialis tendon may be used. Generally, the poor condition of the soft tissue and the time elapsed between the actual rupture and the surgical repair prevent end-to-end suture. The final results of the repair are, of course, influenced by the number of tendons ruptured and the status of the surrounding joints and soft tissue.[76,77] Following the transfer, the hand is immobilized for 3½ weeks, with the wrist in slight extension and the metacarpophalangeal joints in extension. The proximal interphalangeal joints are free to move. At 3½ weeks, the patient is started on gentle, assisted, active and passive extension and controlled active flexion. Exercises are increased gradually over the next few weeks, including the previously described taping exercise. In some cases, it may be necessary to fabricate a dynamic splint to support the tendons in extension during the day. At night, the patient would wear the resting splint.

Tenolysis

In some patients in whom therapy has failed to restore tendon gliding, it may be necessary to perform a tenolysis following a tendon graft or repair. As has been previously mentioned, sometimes scar tissue binds down the tendon and prevents it from gliding freely. The tenolysis frees the tendon from the scar tissue.[56,79,80] Generally, the surgeon waits 3–6 months before performing tenolysis to see if the patient is able to obtain tendon pull-through without further surgery.[56,79]

Hand therapy after a tenolysis begins on the day after the surgery.[56,79,80] Range of motion is done briefly three times per day. Care must be taken to teach the patient to exercise gently so as not to increase swelling. The patient is carefully monitored over the next several weeks. During tenolysis, there is an interruption of the blood supply to the tendon. This makes the tendon more vulnerable to rupture. Therefore, no resistive activities are generally allowed before 6–8 weeks.[56,79] The exact time frame is determined by the surgeon and depends on the condition of the tendon at the time of surgery.

PAIN PROBLEMS

Problems of pain are among the most challenging, and without a doubt, often the most frustrating for all concerned. This is primarily because we, as professionals, still do not understand fully the mechanisms of pain and how to adequately control it.

Reflex Sympathetic Dystrophy

Reflex sympathetic dystrophy appears to be the result of an abnormal response of the autonomic nervous system to trauma. This response triggers a cycle of pain, immobility, swelling, and vasospasm that eventually leads to a stiff, nonfunctioning hand if not treated.[81-87] This condition has been called different names: minor causalgia, minor traumatic dystrophy, shoulder-hand syndrome, major traumatic dystrophy, and major causalgia. These, however, all can be classified under the heading of reflex sympathetic dystrophy.[81-87] This affliction was described in 1864 by Silas Weir Mitchell.[81-87] He reported this condition during the Civil War in soldiers who sustained gunshot wounds involving injuries to nerves. He termed the resultant pain as causalgia. We know now that this syndrome does not necessarily result from nerve injury. It can result from carpal tunnel compression, release of Dupuytren's contracture, a crush injury, or fractures. It can be a devastating complication of a Colles' fracture.[81-87] It may also be a sequela of a very minor injury. The predominant symptoms of reflex sympathetic dystrophy are pain and swelling that are out of all proportion to the injury. The patient often describes this pain as burning and stinging.[81-87] He also may describe it as a constricting or pressure-type pain. This pain often may be exaggerated by motion. As the dystrophy progresses, the hand becomes stiff from lack of motion. There is usually a change in skin color, which often progresses from redness to a waxlike appearance. Often, one sees either excessive sweating or dryness of the skin. The hand may at first feel warm, but in later stages will feel cool. There will also be progressive atrophy of the skin and muscles. Changes in hair growth and nail growth also may be noted. X-rays of the hand in the late stages may show demineralization of bone and narrowing of joint spaces.[81-87] The pain may become so intense that even a breeze across the arm will be unbearable, and it may progress to previously uninvolved areas.

These patients often manifest psychological problems and are angry and fearful.[81-87] Sometimes pushed from doctor to doctor, they may be suspicious and therefore not always able to cooperate in their treatment. They expect the medical team to "make it better." These patients need to be shown that someone cares about them. They need a lot of emotional support. All treatment must be well-coordinated with no inconsistencies among the professionals involved. Because these patients tend to be very suggestible, constant, positive reinforcement is beneficial. Various treatment procedures are used in an effort to relieve these unfortunate patients of their pain. Sympathetic blocks are frequently used by the physician to try to break the sympathetic arc. In some cases, it may be necessary to permanently interrupt the sympathetic arc by performing surgical sympathectomy.[81-88]

The main goals in treating these patients are first to help decrease the pain and second to help increase their range of motion. However, before these goals can be accomplished, a trusting relationship between the therapist and the patient must be established.

The program of hand therapy should begin with modalities that will decrease pain. Hot packs or paraffin may be helpful in providing relief and may be used prior to exercises or activities. Some patients may also respond well to ice, either through massage or ice pack. Contrast baths that alternate hot and cold bathing of the extremity also may help to break the pain cycle. In some cases, a trial of transcutaneous nerve stimulation (TENS) is given.

The electrode placement of the TENS unit depends on the area of the pain, the cause of the pain, and the nature of the pain. The electrodes may be placed over the trigger points, the location of the greatest pain, distant or contralateral locations, specific dermatomes or spinal segmental levels, points along the peripheral nerves, or linear pathways.[89-93] In some cases, alternative placement of electrodes may be necessary to produce pain relief. If pain relief is obtained with TENS, the patient may rent or purchase a unit to be used at home.

Naturally, once the pain is decreased, a program to improve motion and the general condition of the extremity is much easier to implement. Active exercises and activities are done by the patient insofar as he can tolerate them. Therapy that increases pain is counterproductive and only adds to the patient's anxiety. Splinting to help correct deformities and improve mobility is used as soon as it can be tolerated by the patient. Edema control through elevation, massage, and compression gloves when necessary, in conjunction with active exercise, is also an important part of the treatment. Massage is always done by the patient. In combination with massage, the patient is put on a program of systematic desensitization (see chapter 3).

In cases of painful neuroma, the use of percussion and vibration of the neuroma in conjunction with the desensitization program may be successful in relieving pain in selected patients. In most cases, however, the neuroma will need to be surgically removed.

Functional activities are also important in the treatment of pain patients and are introduced as soon as possible. Since these patients often withdraw from social contact, group activities are helpful in getting them back into the mainstream of life(see chapter 2). These people often have been out of work for long periods of time. Therefore, vocational counseling and vocational training may be necessary before the patient is able to reenter the work force (see chapter 21).

CUMULATIVE TRAUMA DISORDERS

Another group of patients seen regularly by the hand therapist are those diagnosed with cumulative trauma disorders.[94-98] This encompasses a variety of disorders including various types of tendinitis, tenosynovitis, tennis elbow, thoracic outlet syndrome, carpal tunnel syndrome, and other pain syndromes and muscle "cramps." Repetitive activities done over prolonged periods of time may produce biomechanical stress. These syndromes often may be seen in assembly-line or clerical workers, athletes, and musicians who, over time, are engaged in repetitive activities and are expected to perform at a high level. Treating these people involves good communication among the patient, the therapist, the physician, and, when applicable, the patient's supervisor at the workplace.

Initial treatment involves a thorough evaluation of the patient to obtain baseline data. It is important to get a good work and avocational history from the patient, including motions required and body positions necessary to complete the work or activity. It may also be necessary to verify the patient's job requirements with the patient's supervisor and also through the *Dictionary of Occupational Titles*. In the case of athletes and musicians, it is necessary to discuss with them their practice procedures, the types of equipment they use, and the length of time that they spend practicing or training in their specific area of endeavor.

A medical workup by the patient's physician also may be helpful in ruling out any underlying disease process. The therapist should record range of motion, grip, and pinch strength. Circumferential measurements of the upper extremity as well as volumeter measurements should be taken to assess edema. A sensory evaluation also may be needed for some patients (see chapter 3). The therapist must elicit from the patient information concerning the nature of the pain, the exact site of the pain, when it occurs, what causes it to increase, and what helps to relieve it. It is also important to carefully observe the patient's posture. Poor posture can lead to many problems that may be helped by instruction in postural exercises.

The treatment of these patients can be divided into three phases. The first phase, the acute phase, is geared toward decreasing pain and inflammation. The modalities used include splinting to rest the inflamed area and gentle range of motion of the whole extremity to prevent joint stiffness. Ice and other cold modalities also are used during this period to help reduce inflammation. Ultrasound, phonophoresis, and other electrical modalities used by the physical therapist may be helpful in reducing inflammation, as well as having an analgesic effect. Massage may be used for edema control and reduction of pain. Phase two is the subacute phase. At this stage the patient is more comfortable. Usually there is full range of motion. The pain is generally gone, but there may be discomfort at the end range or if the patient attempts to stress the extremity. The use of splints during this phase is gradually decreased, and light activities that do not cause pain are added to the patient's program. Massage is continued during this phase to aid in pain reduction and in maintaining tissue mobility.

When the patient is able to perform his activities of daily living without any significant discomfort, he is progressed to the final phase, which is that of conditioning or work hardening. Here, the patient continues to work on flexibility and gradually increasing strength and endurance. One of the modalities that can be used at this stage is the BTE work simulator (Fig. 25.14). This piece of equipment, developed by the Baltimore Therapeutic Equipment Co., has various attachments that simulate a variety of work or life tasks and is computerized to allow collection of accurate records of work performed. The BTE work simulator may be used with other modalities to increase strength and endurance. During this time, it is important, when necessary and when possible, to suggest work site modifications that would help prevent reinjury. These ergonomic modifications might include a different type of handle on a tool or a change in the height of a work table. Ergonomic considerations should be worked out with the patient and his employer. Also, any return-to-work instructions should be well coordinated and communicated to both the patient and his supervisor to prevent misunderstandings. This is particularly true when the patient has been released to do light duty. This could mean different things to different employers and must be specifically outlined to prevent reinjury to the patient. Once the patient has returned to work, it is important to monitor him periodically to make sure that his problem has not recurred.

Psychological Implications

It must be kept in mind that people who sustain hand injuries or develop hand problems have to make a number of psychological adjustments to their disability. Their daily lives are interrupted, and their functioning is altered. In many cases, the disability is temporary, and the person eventually will return to his regular routine. However, with more serious problems, the person's life may be permanently changed. He may be unable to perform his usual work or to pursue his various avocational interests. A person may lose self-esteem and become depressed when unable to do regular work. Often, a person who appears to lack motivation is re-

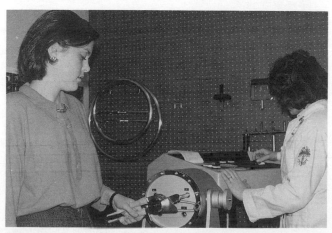

Figure 25.14 Patient being treated on the BTE work simulator.

ally depressed or may be fearful of returning to a machine on which the injury occurred. The therapist can help the patient set realistic goals and can act as a resource for needed information or referrals to outside agencies. Some patients may require professional psychiatric help to deal with the issues their disability raises. However, the supportive hand therapy environment and the encouragement (not false hope) provided by the therapist can help make the adjustment period much smoother and less traumatic.

STUDY QUESTIONS:
Hand Therapy

1. Explain the difference between standardized and nonstandardized tests. List three standardized tests used to document hand function.
2. What are the goals of early treatment of joint injuries?
3. What structures are most commonly injured in a dorsal dislocation of the proximal interphalangeal joint? In a volar dislocation of the PIP joint?
4. What deformities could develop if proper treatment is not provided for volar or dorsal proximal interphalangeal joint dislocations?
5. The process of encapsulation describes a process that occurs following what type of surgery? Describe this process and its implications for rehabilitation.
6. What is the goal of dynamic splinting following metacarpophalangeal arthroplasty?
7. Describe the goals of metacarpophalangeal and proximal interphalangeal arthroplasty. How do they differ from the goals of wrist arthroplasty?
8. What do the Semmes-Weinstein monofilaments test?
9. Describe the process for sensory reeducation.
10. Following a nerve injury, what are the treatment goals?
11. Why are tendon transfers done?
12. What is the position of hand and wrist splinting immediately following flexor tendon repair? What is the reason for placing the hand and wrist into this position?
13. What is the theory behind early controlled mobilization of flexor tendons in zones 2 and 3?
14. What are the two stages of a two-stage flexor tendon reconstruction?
15. What are the causes of extensor tendon rupture in rheumatoid arthritis?

REFERENCES

1. Aulicino, P. L., and Dupuy, T. E. Clinical examination of the hand. In *Rehabilitation of the Hand*. Edited by J. M. Hunter, L.H. Schneider, E. J. Mackin, and A. D. Callahan. St Louis: C. V. Mosby, 1984.
2. Fess, E. E. Documentation: essential elements of an upper extremity assessment battery. In *Rehabilitation of the Hand*. Edited by J.M. Hunter, L. H. Schneider, E. J. Mackin, and A. D. Callahan. St Louis: C.V. Mosby, 1984.
3. Rothstein, J. E., editor. *Clinics in Physical Therapy Vol. 7. Measurement in Physical Therapy*. New York: Churchill Livingstone, 1985.
4. American Society for Surgery of the Hand. *The Hand: Examination and Diagnosis*. Aurora, CO: The American Society for Surgery of the Hand, 1978.
5. Fess, E., and Moran, C. *Clinical Assessment Recommendations*. Indianapolis: American Society for Hand Therapists, 1981.
6. American Academy of Orthopedic Surgeons. *Joint Motion: Method of Measuring and Recording*. Chicago: American Academy of Orthopedic Surgeons, 1965.
7. Kendall, H., Kendall, F., and Wadsworth, G. *Muscle Testing and Function*. Baltimore: Williams & Wilkins, 1971.
8. Jebsen, R., et al. An objective and standardized test of hand function. *Arch. Phys. Med. Rehabil.* 50: 311–319, 1969.
9. Millender, L. H. Joint injuries. In *The Practice of Hand Surgery*. Edited by S. W. Lamb and K. Kuczynski. Boston: Blackwell Scientific Publications, 1981.
10. Eaton, R. G. *Joint Injuries of the Hand*. Springfield, IL: Charles C Thomas, 1971.
11. Burton, R. I. Acute joint injuries. In *Acute Joint Injuries: A Multispecialty Approach*. Edited by F. G. Wolfort. Boston: Little, Brown & Co., 1980.
12. Nalebuff, E. A., and Millender, L. H. Skeletal and ligamentous injuries of the hand. In *Trauma Management*. Edited by E. Cave and E. Boyd. Chicago: Year Book Medical Publishers, 1974.
13. Belsky, M. R., Ruby, L. K., and Millender, L. H. Injuries of the finger and thumb joints. *Contemporary Orthopedics* 7. (4): 39–48, 1983.
14. Burton, R. I., et al. The jammed finger or thumb. *Contemporary Orthopedics*, 3(4): 56–81, 1979.
15. Dray, G., Millender, L. H., and Nalebuff, E. A. Rupture of the radial collateral ligament of a metacarpophalangeal joint to one of the ulnar three fingers. *J. Hand Surg.* 4(4): 346–350, 1979.
16. Rosenthal, E. A. The extensor tendons. In *Rehabilitation of the Hand*. Edited by J. M. Hunter, L. H. Schneider, E. J. Mackin, and J. A. Bell. St. Louis: C. V. Mosby, 1978.
17. Beasley, R. W. *Hand Injuries*. Philadelphia: W. B. Saunders, 1981.
18. Madden, J. W., DeVore, G., and Arem, A. J. A rational post operative management program in metacarpophalangeal joint implant arthroplasty. *J. Hand Surg.* 2(5): 358–366, 1977.
19. Millender, L. H., and Nalebuff, E. A. Metacarpophalangeal joint arthroplasty utilizing the silicone rubber prosthesis. *Orthop. Clin. North Am.* 4(2): 349–371, 1973.
20. Swanson, A. B. *Flexible Implant Resection Arthroplasty in the Hand and Extremities*. St Louis: C. V. Mosby, 1973.
21. Swanson, A. B., Swanson, G., and Leonard, J. Postoperative rehabilitation in flexible implant arthroplasty of the digits. In *Rehabilitation of the Hand*. Edited by J. M. Hunter, L. H. Schneider, E. J. Mackin, and A. D. Callahan. St Louis: C. V. Mosby, 1984.
22. Philips, C. A., McCann, V. H., and Quigley, T. R. Preoperative and postoperative management: the role of the allied health professional. *Orthop. Clin. North Am.* 6(3): 881–906, 1975.
23. Nalebuff, E. A., and Millender, L. H. Personal communication.
24. Goodman, M. J., et al. Arthroplasty of the rheumatoid wrist with silicone rubber: an early evaluation. *J. Hand Surg.* 5(2): 114–121, 1980.
25. Bell, J. A. Sensibility evaluation. In *Rehabilitation of the Hand*. Edited by J. M. Hunter, L. H. Schneider, E. J. Mackin, and J. A. Bell. St. Louis: C. V. Mosby, 1978.
26. Callahan, A. D. Sensibility testing: clinical methods. In *Rehabilitation of the Hand*. Edited by J. M. Hunter, L. H. Schneider, E. J. Mackin, and A. D. Callahan. St Louis: C. V. Mosby, 1984.
27. Parry, E. G. Nerve injuries. In *Acute Hand Injuries, a Multispecialty Approach*. Edited by F. G. Wolfort. Boston: Little, Brown & Co., 1980.
28. Wynn Parry, C. B. *Rehabilitation of the Hand, 3rd edition*. London: Buttersworth & Company, 1973.
29. Dellon, A. L. *Evaluation of Sensibility and Re-Education of Sensation in the Hand*. Baltimore: Williams and Wilkins, 1981.
30. Omer, G. E. Sensibility testing. In *Management of Peripheral Nerve Problems*. Edited by G. E. Omer and M. Spinner. Philadelphia: W.B. Saunders, 1980.
31. Werner, J. L., and Omer, G. E. Evaluating cutaneous pressure sensation of the hand. *Am. J. Occup. Ther.*, 24(5): 347–356, 1970.
32. Moberg, E. Objective methods for determining the functional value of sensibility in the hand. *J. Bone Joint Surg.*, 40B(3): 454–459, 1958.
33. Dellon, A. L. The moving two-point discrimination test: clinical evaluation of the quickly adapting fiber/receptor system. *J. Hand Surg.*, 3: 474–481, 1978.
34. Curtis, R. M. and Dellon, A. L. Sensory re-education after peripheral nerve injury. In *Management of Peripheral Nerve Problems*. Edited by G. E. Omer and M. Spinner. Philadelphia: W. B. Saunders, 1980.
35. Dellon, A. L., Curtis, R. M., and Edgerton, M. T. Re-education of sensation in the hand after nerve injury and repair. *Plast. Reconstr. Surg.*, 53: 297–305, 1974.
36. Maynard, C. J. Sensory re-education following peripheral nerve injury. In *Rehabilitation of the Hand*. Edited by J. M. Hunter, L. H. Schneider, E. J. Mackin, and J. A. Bell. St. Louis: C. V. Mosby, 1978.
37. Dellon, A. L., Curtis, R. M., and Edgerton, M. T. Evaluating recovery of sensation in the hand following nerve injury. *Johns Hopkins Med. J.*, 130: 235–243, 1972.
38. Callahan, A. D. Methods of compensation and re-education for sensory dysfunction. In *Rehabilitation of the Hand*. Edited by J. M. Hunter, L. H. Schneider, E. J. Mackin, and A. D. Callahan. St. Louis: C. V. Mosby, 1984.

39. Almquist, E. E. The effect of training on sensory function. In *Traumatic Nerve Lesions of the Upper Extremity*. Edited by J. Mickon, and E. Moberg. New York: Churchill Livingstone, 1975.

40. Braun, R. M. Epineural nerve repair. In *Management of Peripheral Problems*. Edited by G. E. Omer and M. Spinner. Philadelphia: W. B. Saunders, 1980.

41. Smith, J. W. Peripheral nerve surgery—retrospective and contemporary techniques. *Clin. Plas. Surg., 13*(1): 249–254, 1986.

42. Schultz, R. J. Management of nerve gaps. In *Management of Peripheral Nerve Problems*. Edited by G. E. Omer and M. Spinner. Philadelphia: W. B. Saunders, 1980.

43. Ducker, T. B. Pathophysiology of peripheral nerve trauma. In *Management of Peripheral Nerve Problems*. Edited by G. E. Omer and M. Spinner. Philadelphia: W. B. Saunders, 1980.

44. Omer, G. E. Tendon transfers for reconstruction of the forearm and hand following peripheral nerve injuries. In *Management of Peripheral Nerve Problems*. Edited by G. E. Omer and M. Spinner. Philadelphia: W.B. Saunders, 1980.

45. Schneider, L. H. Tendon transfers in the upper extremity. In *Rehabilitation of the Hand*. Edited by J. M. Hunter, L. H. Schneider, E. J. Mackin, and J. A. Bell. St. Louis: C. V. Mosby, 1978.

46. Verdon, C. The general principles of tendon transfer in the hand and forearm. In *Tendon Surgery of the Hand, G.E.M. Monograph 4*. Edited by C. Verdon. New York: Churchill Livingstone, 1979.

47. Beasley, R. W. Basic considerations for tendon transfer operations in the upper extremity. In *American Academy of Orthopedic Surgeons Symposium on Tendon Surgery in the Hand*. St. Louis: C. V. Mosby, 1975.

48. Omer, G. E. Techniques and timing of tendon transfers. *Orthop. Clin. North Am., 5*(2): 243–252, 1974.

49. Schneider, L. H. Tendon transfers in the upper extremity. In *Rehabilitation of the Hand*. Edited by J. M. Hunter, L. H.Schneider, E. J. Mackin, and A. D. Callahan. St Louis: C. V. Mosby, 1984.

50. Kalumban, S. L. Preoperative and postoperative management of tendon transfers. In *Rehabilitation of the Hand*. Edited by J. M. Hunter, L. H. Schneider, E. J. Mackin, and A. D. Callahan. St Louis: C. V. Mosby, 1984.

51. Toth, S. Therapist's management of tendon transfers. *Hand Clinics, 2*(1): 239–246, 1986.

52. MoKay, D. Flexor tendon injuries. In *Acute Joint Injuries: A Multispecialty Approach*. Edited by F. G. Wolfort. Boston: Little, Brown & Co., 1980

53. Jaeger, S. H., and Mackin, E. J. Primary care of flexor tendon injuries. In *Rehabilitation of the Hand*. Edited by J. M. Hunter, L.H. Schneider, E. J. Mackin, and A. D. Callahan. St Louis: C. V. Mosby, 1984.

54. Nissenbaum, M. D. Early care of flexor tendon injuries: application of principles of tendon healing and early motion. In *Rehabilitation of the Hand*. Edited by J. M. Hunter, L. H. Schneider, E. J. Mackin, and J.A. Bell. St. Louis: C. V. Mosby, 1978.

55. Schneider, L. H., and McEntee, P. Flexor tendon injuries: treatment of acute problems. *Hand Clinics, 2*.(1): 119–131, 1986.

56. Schneider, L. H. *Flexor Tendon Injuries*. Boston: Little, Brown & Co., 1985.

57. Duran, R. J., et al. Management of flexor tendon lacerations in zone 2 using controlled passive motion postoperatively. In *Rehabilitation of the Hand*. Edited by J. M. Hunter, L. H. Schneider, E. J. Mackin, and A.D. Callahan. St. Louis: C. V. Mosby, 1984.

58. Baker, D. S., et al. The little finger superficialis: a clinical investigation of its anatomic and functional shortcomings. *J. Hand Surg. 6*(4): 374–378, 1981.

59. Duran, R. J., and Houser, R. G. Controlled passive motion following flexor tendon repair in zones 2 and 3. In *American Academy of Orthopedic Surgeons Symposium on Tendon Surgery in the Hand*. St Louis: C. V. Mosby, 1975.

60. Kleinert, H. E., Kutz, J. E., and Cohen, M. J. Primary repair of zone 2 flexor tendon lacerations. In *American Academy of Orthopedic Surgeons Symposium on Tendon Surgery in the Hand*. St Louis: C. V. Mosby, 1975.

61. Kleinert, H. E., and Weiland, H. E. Primary repair of flexor tendon lacerations in zone II. In *Tendon Surgery of the Hand, G. E. M. Monograph 4*. Edited by C. Verdon. New York: Churchill Livingstone,1979.

62. Hunter, J. M. Two stage flexor tendon reconstruction: A technique using a tendon prosthesis prior to tendon grafting. In *Tendon Surgery of the Hand, G. E. M. Monograph 4*. Edited by C. Verdon. New York: Churchill Livingstone, 1979.

63. Hunter, J. M., and Salisbury, R. E. Flexor tendon reconstruction in severely damaged hands. *J. Bone Joint Surg. 53A*(5): 829–857, 1971.

64. Hunter, J. M., and Schneider, L. H. Staged flexor tendon reconstruction: current status. In *American Academy of Orthopedic Surgeons Symposium on Tendon Surgery in the Hand*. St Louis: C. V. Mosby, 1975.

65. Mackin, E. J. Physical therapy and staged tendon graft: preoperative and postoperative management. In *American Academy of Orthopedic Surgeons Symposium on Tendon Surgery in the Hand*. St Louis: C. V. Mosby, 1975.

66. Mackin, E. J., and Mairano, L. Postoperative therapy following staged flexor tendon reconstruction. In *Rehabilitation of the Hand*. Edited by J. M. Hunter, L. H. Schneider, E. J. Mackin, and J. A. Bell. St. Louis: C. V. Mosby, 1978.

67. Mackin, E. J. Therapist management of staged flexor tendon reconstruction. In *Rehabilitation of the Hand*. Edited by J. M. Hunter, L. H. Schneider, E. J. Mackin, and A. D. Callahan. St. Louis: C. V. Mosby, 1984.

68. Hunter, J. M. Staged flexor tendon reconstruction. In *Rehabilitation of the Hand*. Edited by J. M. Hunter, L. H. Schneider, E. J. Mackin, and A. D. Callahan. St. Louis: C. V. Mosby, 1984.

69. Jabaley, M. E., and Heckler, E. D. Extensor tendon injuries. In *Acute Hand Injuries: A Multispecialty Approach*. Edited by F. G. Wolfort. Boston: Little, Brown & Co., 1980.

70. Rosenthal, E. A. The extensor tendons. In *Rehabilitation of the Hand*. Edited by J. M. Hunter, L. H. Schneider, E. J. Mackin, and A. D. Callahan. St. Louis: C. V. Mosby, 1984.

71. Lee, V. H. Rehabilitation of extensor tendon injuries. In *Rehabilitation of the Hand*. Edited by J. M. Hunter, L. H. Schneider, E. J. Mackin, and A. D. Callahan. St. Louis: C. V. Mosby, 1984.

72. Tubiana, R. Injuries to the extensor apparatus on the dorsum of the fingers. In *Tendon Surgery of the Hand. G.E.M. Monograph 4*. Edited by C. Verdon. New York: Churchill Livingstone, 1979.

73. Evans, R. B. Therapeutic management of extensor tendon injuries. *Hand Clinics, 2* (1): 157–169, 1986.

74. Egloff, D., and Verdon, C. Spontaneous tendon ruptures at the wrist in rheumatoid arthritis. In *Tendon Surgery of the Hand. G.E.M. Monograph*. Edited by C. Verdon. New York: Churchill Livingstone, 1979.

75. Gshwend, N. Tendon involvement in rheumatoid arthritis. In *Tendon Surgery of the Hand, G.E.M. Monograph 4*. Edited by C. Verdon. New York: Churchill Livingstone, 1979.

76. Nalebuff, E. A. The recognition and treatment of tendon ruptures in the rheumatoid hand. In *American Academy of Orthopedic Surgeons Symposium on Tendon Surgery in the Hand*. St Louis: C. V. Mosby, 1975.

77. Nalebuff, E. A. Surgical treatment of tendon rupture in the rheumatoid hand. *Surg. Clin. North Am., 49*(4): 811–822, 1969.

78. Cantero, J., and Chamay, A. Extensor tendon lesions on the dorsum of the hand and wrist. In *Tendon Surgery of the Hand, G.E.M. Monograph*. Edited by C. Verdon. New York: Churchill Livingstone, 1979.

79. Schneider, L. H., and Hunter, J, M, Flexor tenolysis. In *American Academy of Orthopedic Surgeons Symposium on Tendon Surgery in the Hand*. St Louis: C. V. Mosby, 1975.

80. Verdon, C. Tenolysis. In *Tendon Surgery of the Hand, G. E. M. Monograph 4*. Edited by C. Verdon. New York: Churchill Livingstone, 1979.

81. Omer, G. E. Management of pain syndromes in the upper extremity. In *Rehabilitation of the Hand*. Edited by J. M. Hunter, L. H. Schneider, E. J. Mackin, and J. A. Bell. St. Louis: C. V. Mosby, 1978.

82. Clark, G. L. Causalgia: a discussion of chronic pain syndromes in the upper limb. In *Rehabilitation of the Hand*. Edited by J. M. Hunter, L. H. Schneider, E. J. Mackin, and J. A. Bell. St. Louis: C. V. Mosby, 1978.

83. Erickson, J. C. Evaluation and management of autonomic dystrophies of the upper extremity. In *Rehabilitation of the Hand*. Edited by J. M. Hunter, L. H. Schneider, E. J. Mackin, and J. A. Bell. St. Louis: C. V. Mosby, 1978.

84. Lankford, L. L. Reflex sympathetic dystrophy. In *Management of Peripheral Nerve Problems*. Edited by G. E. Omer and M. Skinner. Philadelphia: W. B. Saunders, 1980.

85. Morgan, J. E. Sympathetic dystrophy. In *Acute Hand Injuries: A Multispecialty Approach*. Edited by F. G. Wolfort. Boston: Little, Brown & Co., 1980.

86. Lankford, L. L. Reflex sympathetic dystrophy. In *Rehabilitation of the Hand*. Edited by J. M. Hunter, L. H. Schneider, E. J. Mackin, and A. D. Callahan. St. Louis: C. V. Mosby, 1984.

87. Lankford, L. L. Reflex sympathetic dystrophy. In *Operative Hand Surgery*. Edited by D. P. Green, New York: Churchill Livingstone, 1982.

88. Kleinert, H. E., Norberg, H., and McDonough, J. J. Surgical sympathectomy of the upper and lower extremity. In *Management of Peripheral Nerve Problems*. Edited by G. E. Omer and M. Spinner. Philadelphia: W. B. Saunders, 1980.

89. Lampe, G. N. Introduction to the use of transcutaneous electrical nerve stimulation devices. *Phys. Ther. 58*(12): 1450–1454, 1978.

90. Mannheimer, J. S. Electrode placements for transcutaneous electrical nerve stimulation. *Phys. Ther. 58*(12): 1455–1462, 1978.

91. Mannheimer, J. S., and Lampe, G. N. *Clinical Transcutaneous Electrical Nerve Stimulation*. Philadelphia: F. A. Davis, 1984.

92. Wolf, S. L., Gersh, M. R., and Kutner, M. Relationship of selected clinical variables to current delivered during transcutaneous electrical nerve stimulation. *Phys. Ther.* 58(12): 1478–1485, 1978.
93. Wolf, S. L. Perspective on central nervous system responsiveness to transcutaneous electrical nerve stimulation. *Phys. Ther.* 58(12):1443–1447, 1978.
94. Hersherson, A. Cumulative injury: a national problem. *J. Occup. Med.* 21(10): 674–676, 1975.
95. Granjean, E. *Fitting the Task to Man: An Ergonomic Approach.* London: Taylor and Francis, Ltd., 1981.
96. Habes, D. J., and Putz-Anderson, V. The NIOSH program for evaluating biomechanical hazards in the work place. *J. Safety Research* 16(2):49–60, 1985.
97. Dobyns, J. H., Sim, F. H., and Linscheid, R. L. Sports stress syndromes of the hand and wrist. *Am. J. Sports Med.* 6(5): 236–254, 1978.
98. Tubiana, R. Crampes: professionnelles du membre superieur. *Annales De Chirurgie De La Main* 2(2): 134–142, 1983.

Supplementary Readings

Bell, J. A. Light touch-deep pressure testing using Semmes-Weinstein monofilaments. In *Rehabilitation of the Hand.* Edited by J. M. Hunter, L. H. Schneider, E. J. Mackin, and A. D. Callahan. St. Louis: C. V. Mosby, 1984.

Boscheinen-Morrin, J., Davey, V., and Connolly, W. B. *The Hand: Fundamentals of Therapy* Boston: Butterworths, 1985.

Cromwell, F. S., and Bear-Lehman, J., editors. *Hand Rehabilitation in Occupational Therapy.* New York: The Haworth Press, 1987.

Fess, E. E. The effects of Jamar dynamometer handle position and test protocol on normal grip strength. Proceedings of the American Society of Hand Therapists. *J. Hand Surg. 7:* 308, 1982.

Pryce, J. The wrist position between neutral and ulnar deviation that facilitates maximum power grip strength. *J. Biomech. 13:* 505, 1980.

Waylett, J., and Seibly, D. A study to determine the average deviation accuracy of a commercially available volumeter. *J. Hand Surg. 6:* 300, 1981.

Orthopedic Conditions

Lillian Hoyle Parent

This chapter describes orthopedic conditions most often seen by occupational therapists for evaluation and treatment to maintain the patient's independence. These include fractures and their sequelae, elective surgery of the hip, and low back pain.

Orthopedics refers to the branch of medicine that preserves and restores function of the skeletal system, its articulations, and supporting structures.[1] The four main problems treated by orthopedists are loss of independent mobility, deformity, neurological problems that result from disease or injury to the musculoskeletal system, and pain that may result from fractures and neuromuscular injury.[2]

Fractures

As long as orthopedists have been treating fractures, there has been a controversy between the "movers" and the "resters." The physicians prescribing rest as a fracture treatment keep patients immobilized for long periods of time in traction or plaster.[3] Currently, the goal in fracture treatment is to mobilize the injured structures as quickly as is compatible with the healing process and to return the patient to independence in work and leisure activities.[4]

A fracture is an interruption of the continuity of bone or an epiphyseal plate, usually caused by trauma. A direct blow to the extremity often causes a transverse fracture, whereas a twisting force causes a spiral fracture. A crushing injury often results in a comminuted fracture, one with multiple bone fragments. Symptoms of a fracture are pain and loss of function. The presence of a fracture is confirmed by x-rays.[5] An open fracture is characterized by skin and soft tissue wounds, whereas a closed fracture does not interrupt the skin. A pathological fracture is one that occurs spontaneously because of an abnormal condition such as osteoporosis or metastatic disease that causes bone to weaken.[6]

The goal of fracture treatment is to prevent malunion by reducing the fracture. That is, the bone fragments are brought together in as close an anatomical position as possible to create the environment needed for the fracture to heal. Closed reduction is done by manipulation, and the result is confirmed by x-ray. The injured part is then immobilized in a plaster cast or a fracture brace. Surgery is used to reduce open fractures and those closed fractures where the bone fragments cannot be approximated accurately by closed reduction. In open reduction, the bone fragments are brought into a closer anatomical position by insertion of an internal fixation device such as an orthopedic nail, pin, screw, rod, or compression plate. Surgical repair also can involve prosthetic devices that are implanted to restore joint motion.[5] Fracture healing, when the part is immobilized by a cast or fracture brace, is accomplished through formation of immature woven bone or external callus that splints or immobilizes the injured bone. The woven bone consolidates and remodels so that the fracture is repaired with lamellar bone.[5,6] When more complete immobilization of the bone is achieved with internal fixation, external callus does not form and direct healing occurs. This requires more time than healing by external callus formation.[6] Research has shown that small repetitive movements of the fracture site can increase callus formation and that this occurs with immobilization in plaster casts or fracture braces.[7]

Fracture healing has a general timetable that is confirmed by repeated x-rays during the course of treatment. Consolidation or complete repair of the fracture has occurred when the callus is ossified, the fracture site is no longer tender and painful, and there is no movement when the fractured bone is manipulated.[5] There is no known way to shorten the time of fracture healing.[6] The general estimate of healing time for uncomplicated fractures is as follows[5]:

Upper-extremity spiral fracture,	6 to 8 weeks.
Upper-extremity transverse fracture,	12 weeks.
Lower-extremity spiral fracture,	12–16 weeks.
Lower-extremity transverse fracture,	24–30 weeks.

The goal of fracture rehabilitation is to return the patient to the previous level of function. Rehabilitation begins as soon as the fracture is immobilized. The supporting soft tissue structures such as muscle, nerve, and skin should be active from the start of fracture immobilization, which is when the plaster dries or within a day or two after surgery for open reduction. The amount and kind of activity depends on the place and kind of fracture, the method of fracture reduction selected by the orthopedist, and in some instances the age of the patient.[4]

Current approaches to treatment indicate that early but specific use of immobilized extremities fosters bone healing. Early movement of tissues around the fracture and movement of the joints above and below the fracture diminishes, or in some instances eliminates, the need for treatment after immobilization. Early movement prevents the unwanted side effects of immobilization: stiff joints, disuse atrophy, and weakness.[4]

Because many upper-extremity fractures are seen in an emergency room where reduction and immobilization are done immediately, at any hour, patients may not be referred to occupational therapy and may not be taught a home treatment program designed for their needs. If occupational therapists are to receive referrals for these patients it is necessary to set up treatment protocols and referral mechanisms with the orthopedic surgeons and emergency room physicians. Patients whose fractures are treated in outpatient clinics otherwise may not know that muscular exercise is beneficial while the fracture heals. Written instructions for therapeutic activities can be issued, and routine outpatient visits to change the program can be scheduled as necessary.

Evaluation is done for active range of motion of any joint available for testing. Also, if fingers are not included in the immobilization, pinch evaluation can be done. The treatment program is planned to prevent disuse and stiffness. It is better to try to prevent the conditions that result from inactivity during immobilization rather than to wait until the cast is removed and then to have to treat those unwanted residual effects of immobilization. A program based on personal daily living skills (chapter 17) and work modalities will cause the patient to use the muscles repeatedly. The occupational therapy goal is to teach the patient that movement and use of the involved extremity is more desirable than inactivity. However, older patients, because of pain and familiarity with older treatment regimens, may be fearful of early mobilization of fractured extremities. The occupational therapist needs to emphasize the benefits of movement and to teach the patients how to move the extremity.[5,8]

UPPER-EXTREMITY FRACTURES

As soon as pain of a fracture diminishes, the patient with an upper extremity immobilized by plaster or a fracture brace or placed in a sling should be taught to do daily active movement of all uninvolved joints. This is especially important for the elderly, who must mobilize the shoulder and fingers because they lose range of motion quickly. The goal is to decrease atrophy and maintain muscle function and range of motion in any joint not immobilized.[9]

Shoulder Fractures

Fractures of the shoulder area are immobilized briefly. However, because immobilization quickly results in stiffness, active motion of the shoulder is begun as soon as the acute pain diminishes. All motion should be active motion. Passive motion is contraindicated, particularly in the elderly.[10] Isometric exercises are a stimulant for fracture healing and callus formation. These should be done during and after immobilization.[9]

Codman's exercises provide gentle active motion that is used to reestablish function following upper-extremity fractures and dislocations. Codman's pendulum exercises are done by having the patient bend over at the waist, either standing or sitting, so that the trunk is parallel to the floor. The arm is allowed to assume a position away from the body, as much as pain and stiffness permit, either with or without a sling. In this position the shoulder is in a gravity-minimized position, and the patient can move the arm forward in flexion or back in extension more easily than trying to do the movements in the upright position. Shoulder flexion is strengthened by voluntary movement forward until 90° is achieved. If a humeral fracture is involved, voluntary abduction can begin then, and later all shoulder motions.[10,11]

The Codman exercises can be incorporated into an activity if the patient is seated and leans forward. An activity to encourage these motions might be a game board that has been placed on a low stool on the floor. Perhaps parts of a puzzle could be positioned posteriorly for movement into place anteriorly, or a tile project could be assembled by picking up tiles posteriorly and moving them to a project anteriorly.

Codman's exercises should not be used with an edematous upper extremity. An overhead suspension sling would permit gravity-minimized shoulder movement while the edematous upper extremity is elevated.

Elbow Fractures

Supracondylar fractures of the humerus may be treated in plaster following open reduction. The elbow is placed in 90° to 100° of flexion with a plaster slab or splint, and the arm is supported in a collar and cuff sling.[12] This sling is a circle of material that is placed around the neck. The forearm is placed in the circle and supported only at the wrist. The length of the sling should place the radial side of the wrist just below the nipple line.[5] After the first week, the plaster slab is removed daily for gentle, nonresistive active motion and then reapplied between activity sessions. Active motion for fractures around the elbow emphasizes flexion rather than extension. Active exercise can be done in a gravity-minimized position.[11]

Treatment following dislocation of the elbow or fracture of the humerus, radius, or ulna in the immediate vicinity of the elbow emphasizes active movement. Passive motion should not be done because of the possibility of myositis ossificans occurring, which would cause further limitation.[5,11] An injury in this area may result in some permanent limitation in elbow extension. However, many patients with injuries in this area achieve close to full range of motion after 6 months to a year without specific treatment.[5,10] A complication of supracondylar fractures may be Volkmann's ischemia or peripheral nerve injury.[5] (See chapter 25.)

Complex fractures of the elbow are often treated with open reduction and with well-secured fixation. Active motion can begin within 5 days. Fractures of the elbow are usually splinted in flexion rather than extension because in flexion the hand can be raised to the face and head for personal daily living skills.[10] In the elderly, elbow fractures are often treated in a collar and cuff sling, described above, and mobilized early. Otherwise the joints become stiff and painful. A useful arc of motion for daily activities can be regained, although full range of motion is not always achieved.[8]

Forearm Fractures

There are many varieties of fractures involving the radius and the ulna and their articulations. If the fractures can be reduced and held in place with a plaster cast, that is done. However, many of these fractures require internal fixation, which is removed after bony union has been achieved. For some forearm fractures, the plaster is removed after 12 days and a functional arm brace of thermoplastic material is applied.[10,13]

A Colles fracture, a common fracture of the distal radius, is immobilized in a long or short arm plaster cast or in a short arm splint or functional brace. Whatever the choice, the design is such that full finger motion is permitted. The cast usually places the hand in pronation because the hand is more functional in that position.[5,14] A variety of dysfunctions result from Colles fractures. They include loss of range of motion of the shoulder, elbow, and digits. These are preventable sequelae if the cast is not so tight as to cause edema, which could result in ischemia of the intrinsic muscles of the hand, and if the cast allows the metacarpophalangeal joints to have full range of movement. Additionally, the patient must be taught to move the shoulder and elbow and to elevate the hand to prevent or reduce edema.[5]

Wrist Fractures

Various fractures to the carpal bones are immobilized for healing. Most of these injuries require some form of rehabilitation. Measures to reduce edema and prevent functional disuse of the hand include teaching the patient to use the muscles around the bones that have been immobilized. Also, all uninjured joints should be moved. As soon as immobilization ends, the patient must be taught how to perform active range of motion for all wrist motions: flexion, extension, radial and ulnar deviation, and circumduction. During the final stages of healing, the patient may need a static splint to hold the wrist in neutral or slight dorsiflexion until healing is completed. Then functional activities and resistive exercises will be necessary to restore functional strength to the forearm and hand muscles.[14]

Precautions. Although fracture braces are often used in the treatment of both upper- and lower-extremity fractures, during the first 2 weeks after injury the patient's extremity will be immobilized in a plaster cast. Patients wearing casts must be observed for signs of edema forming within the extremity inside the cast, particularly if it is a recent injury. Soft tissue damage associated with a fracture results in extracellular edema. Unless this condition is treated quickly, the extracellular fluid will gel and bind down all the tissue with adhesions, a condition that retards restoration of movement and function.[5,15] The best treatment for this condition is muscular contraction to pump away the edema fluid.[16] Elevation is another method to reduce edema. The upper extremity can be elevated using an overhead sling, an arm sling, or some other method to support or to suspend the extremity with the hand held above the level of the heart, while avoiding acute flexion of any joint that would impede the flow of fluid back toward the heart.[17]

If a patient in a cast complains of burning pain under the cast, or there are signs of ischemia, the physician should be notified because the pain may be a signal that pressure is developing and the cast needs refitting to prevent problems. A well-made, properly fitted cast or fracture brace should provide comfort, never pain.[5]

Excessive edema can damage arterial circulation or result in compression of nerve and muscle. Nerve will regenerate, but muscle can survive ischemia for only 6 to 8 hours and cannot regenerate. Arterial occlusion, if complete in the upper extremity, results in Volkmann's ischemia, which can be caused by edema or acute elbow flexion that compresses an artery against bone. If occlusion is complete, gangrene can result. Signs of ischemia are pale bluish color of skin, absence of forearm radial pulse, or decreased hand sensation accompanied by severe pain. Any of these signs indicate that arterial circulation may be compromised. The patient's physician must be notified immediately. If not treated quickly, muscles become fibrosed and contracted, leaving deformity, stiffness, and perhaps sensory loss to the hand. This typically results in a claw hand deformity: proximal interphalangeal and distal interphalangeal flexion with metacarpophalangeal extension. Tenodesis action can provide some grip to a hand with this deformity, but such a hand is needlessly weak and severely impaired from a preventable condition.[5,9,10]

Ischemia of the hand can follow forearm injuries and result in adhesions of the intrinsic muscles, leaving a deformity of metacarpophalangeal flexion and interphalangeal extension with the thumb held in adduction. Lower extremities can be subject to ischemia following fractures of the lower leg or ankle with similar residual effects in the foreleg and foot.[5]

Other possible complications of a fracture include venous thrombosis and pulmonary embolism. Tetanus can occur following an open fracture.[10] Muscles, tendons, and nerves may be damaged by an open fracture of the humerus; this is particularly true in the supracondylar area because the radial, median, and ulnar nerves are in close proximity to the humerus before they enter the forearm.[5] Nerve and tendon injuries that accompany a fracture and fractures of the hand should be treated according to methods described in chapter 25.

HIP FRACTURES

Approximately 200,000 hip fractures occur annually in the United States, most in elderly women. These patients should be mobilized early because if they remain in the recumbent position for long periods calcium is lost, which diminishes bone strength, and disuse atrophy of muscle increases. The cost of caring for these patients exceeds $750 million annually. The need for long-term care for these patients increases costs because many of them were independent prior to the hip fracture.[18]

Elderly women are a population at risk for falls often without apparent cause. Sensorimotor abilities seem to deteriorate, and the elderly are slow to react in an emergency such as tripping or missing the last step in descending stairs. The elderly who fall tend to show changes in gait made in order to gain stability but at the expense of efficiency. Speed and length of step decrease, and the length of the steps varies markedly. It is suggested that there may be some loss of central control over automatic stepping.[19]

Hasselkus reports that in some elderly patients the more primitive protective response patterns tend to reappear, which may interfere with refined equilibrium responses of the normal adult.[20] Patients who are to be ambulatory, or non-weight-bearing or partially weight bearing, after hip surgery should have these reactions evaluated and be trained in modified techniques. Although physical therapists are responsible for postsurgical training in lower-extremity movement techniques, the occupational therapist's role is to teach the patient how to perform activities of daily living within the imposed mobility limitations to achieve the best surgical result and long-term improvement of patient function. Methods for personal daily living skills are described in chapter 17.

The patient with lower-extremity fractures learns gait training, transfer, and other gross mobility activities in physical therapy. Once the patient has learned the basic techniques, often cognitively and consciously, occupational therapy programs can provide the opportunity to apply mobility skills so that mobility becomes automatic while the patient concentrates on personal daily living skills, homemaking activities, or activities preparatory to return to work.[4,21]

Early reacquisition of personal daily living skills after a hip fracture makes a statistically significant difference in the patient's outcome following discharge from the hospital. Prognostic indicators for elderly patients to return home after a hip fracture, in addition to age and general medical condition, include whether they lived with someone and had a preinjury pattern of social contacts outside of their home. Also, those patients who were ambulated early in the hospital and could manage dressing, personal hygiene, and toileting during the first 2 postoperative weeks were statistically more likely to return home. Physical therapists' ratings on weight bearing and strength of the uninvolved lower extremity, endurance, balance, mental clarity, and evidence of motivation also were indicators of individual rehabilitation potential.[22]

Orthopedic surgical procedures for the hip are divided into emergency surgery for hip fractures and elective surgery for relief of pain and restoration of range of motion and function. The orthopedist's selection of a treatment method for a fracture will depend on the history of the patient's activities immediately prior to the injury, the type of fracture, and the anticipated level of activity after recovery.[23] These and other fractures of the lower extremity may be treated with closed reduction by immobilization in plaster or open reduction with internal fixation or intramedullary nailing.[10] The goal is to return the patient to function as quickly as possible.[4] Occupational therapists will receive referrals for these patients for training and provision of assistive devices to enable lower-extremity dressing and bathing.

Partial joint replacement is the treatment for some fractures of the neck and head of the femur. An Austin-Moore prosthesis is used, particularly in the older patient, to ensure quick postsurgical mobilization. After excision of the head of the femur, the metal prosthesis is inserted into the femur and it articulates with the normal acetabulum. Thus, there is no bone to heal. This procedure has tended to be replaced in some institutions by the total hip arthroplasty. The postoperative procedures when an Austin-Moore prosthesis is used are similar to those described below for elective surgery.[24]

LOWER-EXTREMITY ELECTIVE SURGERY

A hip fracture is considered an emergency and is an acute problem requiring immediate and definitive care. Other conditions of the hip joint may have an insidious progressive onset. Surgical correction for relief of pain is an elective procedure. Some hip joint problems, for which surgery is an elective procedure, are congenital hip disease, rheumatoid arthritis, and osteoarthritis or degenerative joint disease. Osteoarthritis is a common form of arthritis of unknown etiology, which results in the inability of the joint cartilages to repair themselves as quickly as they degenerate. Osteophytes form on the joint surface, leaving an uneven surface, which results in painful joint movement. The onset is gradual and may involve one or a few joints. The hip joint is a common site of osteoarthritis, where the condition leads to a painful limp that can cause great restriction of a person's activities over time. Abnormal body mechanics in which weight is displaced from painful joints to other joints can produce overload or stress on otherwise satisfactory joints.[25]

Conservative treatment of degenerative joint disease of the hip includes reduction of activities, use of a cane, walker, crutches, or a wheelchair to protect weight-bearing joints, weight control, and use of analgesics.[24] Energy conservation techniques are taught to reduce the kind and amount of homemaking and personal daily living skills in order to conserve energy for vocational and leisure activities. Disabling pain is usually the reason for the patient's final decision to seek surgical correction.[25,26]

There are a number of surgical procedures for reduction of hip disability and pain. They include osteotomy, arthrodesis or hip fusion, THARIES (total hip articular replacement with internal eccentric shells), and total hip arthroplasty (THA). In selecting the procedure, the orthopedic surgeon will consider the degree of the deformity and the amount of bone stock available, as well as the patient's age, occupation, life-style, and potential for cooperation in postoperative rehabilitation. Also, the patient's weight and activity level must be considered in conjunction with what is known of the selected procedure's ability to provide a predictably good result with a decreasing chance of failure.[26] Involved in the choice of any orthopedic procedure is consideration of the patient's personal daily living activities, including occupation and leisure activities. In younger patients, work activities are considered carefully. For the older patient, who may not be employed, it is important to survey the living arrangements and social support system to which the patient will return following a given procedure.[8] Also, the surgeon may select the least radical procedure in order to make possible another procedure later, if this should become necessary.

Osteotomy

Intertrochanteric osteotomy is a procedure to change the alignment of the femur to relieve weight bearing on the hip joint. This may be the surgery of choice if it is done in the early stages of the osteoarthritic process. When this procedure is done, compression plates are used to stabilize the bone, and the patient can begin early postoperative mobilization with passive movement. The knee especially should be mobilized. However, no active, resisted exercise is permitted for the lower extremity for the first postoperative weeks. Only partial weight bearing can be done for 6 months because this increases pressure on the hip joint. A successful outcome of a hip osteotomy depends on this long non-weight-bearing period.[28]

Arthrodesis

An arthrodesis of the hip fuses the hip joint at about 30° of flexion and in neutral abduction and rotation. It results in a stable, pain-free joint. This procedure is considered for patients under age 60 who are in good physical condition and have one painful osteoarthritic hip. Preoperative assessment for an arthrodesis will consider the physical requirements of the patient's occupation and life-style and the kind of disability caused by the pain. The patient must have full range of motion of the knee on the side to be operated and full hip and knee range of motion on the opposite side for this surgery to be done.[5,29]

The patient with a hip arthrodesis, fixed by a metal plate, is mobilized about a week after surgery and is allowed gradual weight bearing up to full weight bearing in 2 months. Some patients may use a cane for ambulation for a long time after surgery. The patient with an arthrodesis of the hip sits with a curved lumbar spine. In the early postoperative stages, these patients require assistive devices for lower-extremity dressing and bathing. The patients may ultimately be able to put on a sock and shoe when seated, by bending the knee and reaching behind to pull them onto the foot using touch without visual guidance. Although it may seem that this procedure leaves the patient with residual disability, it does give him a strong, stable, pain-free hip that is adequate for the endurance needed for standing at work. Follow-up studies indicate that many of these patients participate in active sports such as walking, hiking, sailing, and horseback riding.[29]

Hip Arthroplasty

A procedure used with younger patients with painful stiff hips is the Smith-Petersen cup arthroplasty. A metal cup is placed over the head of the femur and the acetabulum is shaped to fit the cup. Postoperative training must be done carefully, and no weight bearing is allowed on the operated leg for more than 6 months because it requires that long for fibrous cartilage to regenerate on both sides of the metal cup. All movements of the hip are done without pressure to enhance the development of the cartilage for better function. Because of the long non-weight-bearing period, the patient and his life-style must be evaluated carefully before a decision is made to do this surgery. Once this procedure is done, the occupational therapist can teach the patient personal daily living skills that do not involve weight bearing on the operated side.[30]

THARIES

Total hip articular replacement by internal eccentric shells is a procedure that saves more of the femur by placing a shell over the prepared head of the femur that articulates with an acetabular component. It is considered a useful procedure for younger active patients to buy time while waiting for development of improvements in the technology of hip surgery. Because bone is retained, further revision can be done later. The hip must be protected, and the bone interface must not be stressed early in the postoperative period.[31]

Postoperative care includes immediate muscle setting (isometric contractions) of the quadriceps, gluteus maximus, and hamstring muscles. On the second or third day, active flexion, rotation, and extension of the hip begins. On the fourth day the patient is progressed to a walker for touchdown weight bearing, which means that he is allowed momentarily and lightly to touch the floor with the foot of the operated leg. Only partial weight bearing is allowed for 2 months. Hip flexion contracture occurs more easily with the THARIES procedure and must be prevented. Also, these patients should not do any heavy lifting. The rehabilitation procedures and precautions are similar to those for THA.[32]

Total Hip Arthroplasty

THA, or total hip replacement, is a procedure developed by Sir John Charnley in England. The technique became available in the United States in 1971 when the Food and Drug Administration approved the use of methyl methacrylate, a self-curing acrylic resin, to cement the plastic acetabular cup to the pelvis and the metal prosthetic femoral head into a hollowed-out femur.[33] The Charnley prosthesis is usually reserved for older adults even though there is a 20-year experience with the procedure. The head and neck of the femur are removed to place the Charnley prosthesis, which leaves the surgeon fewer options if a second operation should become necessary. Before the procedure is selected for younger patients, all medical and social aspects are considered, and the patient is made aware that there are specific restrictions on activity once this surgery is performed.[25] However, the procedure can be used at any age if the hip disease is severe enough.[26]

Success of the THA depends on a special operating room environment to decrease the incidence of infections, the greatest cause of failure of this procedure, exacting surgical technique, and very careful postoperative mobilization of the patient. To date, the success rate is about 90% for patients receiving the Charnley procedure for relief of pain and to increase functional ability.[25,26]

If a patient has other disabilities, such as arthritis involving numerous joints, a careful plan for sequential surgeries and patient preparation must be made. Arthritic patients with multiple joint involvement may require four to six procedures to become ambulatory and independent.[34] It is important that surgeons, occupational therapists, and physical therapists carefully evaluate and plan together the sequence of surgeries and rehabilitation procedures for severely involved patients. The patient with THA needs strength in the upper extremities for postoperative crutch walking, an important part of THA rehabilitation. Therefore, patients being considered for multiple joint replacement, such as hips and knees, must be evaluated for upper-extremity function because patients with multiple involvements of the upper extremities have more problems in rehabilitation. Also, without hip and knee flexion adequate to climb stairs or rise from a chair, the patients are less able to compensate for diminished abilities.[35]

Postoperative Treatment for Total Hip Arthroplasty A specific treatment program follows THA, and the first 2 months of activity are critical for protection and function of the new joint. During the Charnley procedure for THA, the greater trochanter is removed with muscle attachments intact and is reflected back for a surgical approach to the hip joint. After the prosthetic placement, the trochanter is wired back into place.[26] The postsurgical program is designed to allow for healing of the trochanter and soft tissues and for development of a capsule around the joint for future stability. Postoperatively when supine, the patient's hips are held abducted with a splint or foam wedge.[36] Some centers use a balanced sling suspension postoperatively.[32] Hip flexion beyond 70° to 80° is avoided for the first 2 months postsurgery until soft tissue healing is secure. Passive motion is never used with THA. The postsurgical program also is a time for muscle reeducation to gain strength and stability needed for walking.[36]

The artificial hip joint design permits only 90° of hip flexion, which may equal 120° when combined with abduction. This is adequate for most functional activities. Patients who are candidates for this surgery usually have had a limited range of hip flexion prior to surgery. About two-thirds of that motion is regained through walking during the first 3 weeks postsurgery.[36]

An occupational therapy evaluation is done prior to surgery to estimate the capabilities and other disabilities the patient may have. The patient should be evaluated for personal daily living skills, home environment, home responsibilities, and the social network available for posthospital events. What are the requirements for the patient to do homemaking, drive a car, etc.? A patient with a painful hip comes to surgery after an insidious onset of pain and reduction of activities. The therapist finds out what the patient has not been able to do. Postoperatively it will be necessary to teach the patient safe methods of performance of those activities to promote independence while protecting the operated hip. It may be possible to rehearse some of the activities for remediation prior to surgery. At the least, the occupational therapist can describe what the occupational therapy program for the patient will be after surgery.

Following surgery, the physical therapist mobilizes the patient quickly to promote walking. The patient learns to transfer from supine to standing without flexing the operated hip, by keeping the knees apart with the hips abducted, and sliding out of a raised bed to take weight on the unoperated leg. The patient is then encouraged to bear full weight on the operated leg from the beginning of ambulation training, which may start by using a walker. There is a quick progression to crutches, which are used for about 6 weeks, and then a cane is recommended until the Trendelenburg gait disappears. Older patients may use a walker or cane for extended periods for safety or reassurance.[36]

The patient is urged not to try to gain hip flexion motion too quickly after surgery. During the early postoperative period the patient should avoid sitting on low chairs or stools because this flexes the hip acutely and has resulted in dislocation of the prosthesis. He should not lean over to pull on socks and shoes.[36] Patients who sit upright in the hospital bed too soon after surgery risk dislocating the prosthesis. If dislocation occurs, the hip is realigned, and the patient is placed in a hip spica cast for 3 weeks, thus delaying rehabilitation.[26]

When the patient gains about 55° of hip flexion, usually about the second week after surgery, the patient may sit in a chair with a seat that has been elevated by use of a cushion or raised legs. Armrests are useful to help the patient get out of the chair. The raised chair is to avoid passive hip flexion caused by sitting in an upright position. The patient should sit with the hip extended, and the knee should be kept in extension,[36] thus breaking up the hip-knee flexion pattern. Sitting on a firm wedge cushion promotes hip extension and comfort for the patient. A wedge cushion can be cut of firm foam, 20 inches (50 cm) across for the chair width, 10 inches (25 cm) for the chair depth, and 6 inches (15 cm) deep. The cushion should taper from the 6-inch thickness on the long side to nothing on the opposite side to make the wedge. The thick edge is placed at the back of the chair.[37] It also can be used as a back rest that keeps the patient from sitting back in the chair at 90° if the 6-inch side is placed flat on the chair seat. If this cushion is covered and a handle is attached, the patient can carry it easily to any place that he will be sitting to remind him to keep the hip extended. This is particularly important during the first 2 months after surgery.

When the patient can sit, modified techniques can be taught for lower-extremity dressing and hygiene, such as showering or bathing using a tub seat. For any activity, the patient must be reminded that the hip is not to be passively flexed or the leg adducted.[36] He should not lean over to pull on socks, shoes, or trousers. To get into a bathtub to take a standing shower, the patient should stand with his feet parallel to the tub and with his weight on the unoperated leg while stabilizing his body by holding onto a grab bar or counter. With the operated leg in hip extension, he flexes the knee on the same side and abducts it over the edge of the tub, then he extends the knee and places the foot on a secure nonskid mat. When balance is secure and weight is transferred to the operated leg, he lifts the unoperated leg over the edge of the tub and places the foot in the tub. To get out, the patient needs to turn around carefully to face the opposite direction and repeat the procedure to avoid unnecessary adduction of the operated hip.

Since the operated hip should not be adducted, it should not be crossed over the other leg in either sitting or standing position. Passive hip flexion such as occurs when sitting in a straight chair also is to be avoided. The patient should not lean forward to get closer to a table or desk because this is equivalent to hip flexion. The patient must be taught to place the chair closer to the table to allow leaning back or to use the wedge cushion, which helps to maintain the proper reclining position. Adapted equipment used by THA patients includes a raised toilet seat with a cut out for the surgical side, a sock donner, a long-handled shoe horn, a reacher, and a long-handled bath brush for feet and legs. Ideally their use should be taught prior to discharge from the hospital.[38]

The patient with THA needs to be upright and to walk more than sit because sitting tends to flex the hip, whereas walking actively improves hip motion and strength. Simple walking is the most important activity at home because it improves hip motion and strength. The patient can stand at the kitchen or bathroom counter or home workbench. Practicing side stepping in abduction for getting around when working at counter heights is a good activity for the hip. However, adduction of the operated side should never be carried across midline.[36]

Usually patients do not receive outpatient therapy following THA. After receiving the appropriate training in ambulation and personal daily living skills in the hospital, the patient is discharged with a written list of what he can do or should not do. During the hospital stay, the patient should have been taught the ambulatory skills he will need in physical therapy and how to use reachers and other adapted equipment for lower-extremity dressing and bathing in occupational therapy. The preoperative evaluation of the patient's home environment and responsibilities should have indicated which skills the patient will need most.

The therapist may want to advise that the patient arrange for someone to reorganize household storage so that things to be used for the next 6 months are placed in the midrange of neither too high overhead nor too close to the floor so that the patient can get to them. This is especially true for items stored in the kitchen, bathroom, and closets.

Although a reacher is a better solution, patients can be taught to reach something on the floor in an emergency. The patient should use a stable piece of furniture to hold onto for balance, and then extend the operated leg posteriorly into hyperextension while flexing the other hip and knee to get closer to the floor with the hand.

If a patient must sit in a regular-height chair, he should be taught to stand up without overflexing the operated hip, which can lead to dislocation of the hip prosthesis. In a regular chair with armrests, the patient should scoot to the front edge of the chair, keeping the hip extended, and then use the armrests to push straight up without bending forward at the hip. In a chair without armrests, the patient can move to the side of the chair so that the operated thigh is over the edge with the foot placed back to the midline of the chair. This places the foot closer to the center of gravity and enables standing up without excessive hip flexion to gain momentum. The same technique can be used for rising from a regular-height toilet seat.[11] In public facilities, a patient should use the wheelchair accommodation because it often has a raised toilet seat.

When sleeping in supine position, the patient should keep a pillow between the legs to prevent hip adduction. The patient should not sleep on the operated side, but can sleep on the unoperated side if a pillow is placed between the knees to prevent adduction.[36] To facilitate getting in or out of bed at home the first few months (to avoid acute hip flexion) the height of the bed can be raised by placing blocks or other extenders under each leg of the bed or by putting another mattress on the bed.

Patients are advised not to use a car with bucket seats for the first few months. To enter an automobile with a bench-type seat, the patient stands with his back to the front seat, sits down, and then scoots toward the middle of the car seat. Then the patient swings his legs around to face the front of the car without too much hip flexion.[36] Resumption of driving will depend on the surgeon's approval and the side of the operation. For example, a patient who has a car with an automatic transmission and a THA on the left side will be able to resume driving sooner than a patient with a THA on the right side.

Social dancing can be done if the precautions about hip flexion and adduction are observed and the dance is moderate, such as a slow waltz. However, very vigorous dance activity should not be done.[39]

Physical problems related to presurgical sexual expression are pain, stiffness, and limited hip motion rather than loss of libido, and these can cause marital stress. THA is a more enabling procedure for sexual activity than other hip procedures. The hip arthrodesis, for example, greatly limits function for women in coition.[40] Following THA, sexual activity, which may begin 2–3 months postsurgically, is no problem for the patient in the supine position. Pillows can be used to position the operated leg to prevent excessive hip internal rotation and adduction. Kneeling should be avoided for any activity for 3 to 4 months after surgery.[25,36,41] Patients surveyed thought that written information about hip procedures and sexual activity would be helpful if supplied to a patient and his sexual partner.[42]

Between the second and third month postsurgically, all routine daily activities can be resumed with the restrictions about too much hip flexion and no adduction or internal rotation still applicable. Strenuous sports such as tennis, skiing, or jogging should not be encouraged. The Charnley prosthesis is designed for walking, not running or other athletic activities. One problem that has occurred is the loosening of the femoral components of the prosthesis. Patients who put too much stress, through work or recreational activities, on the prosthetic-cement-bone components tend to have a higher incidence of loosening. Even with x-ray evidence of loosening, the signs may not progress if the patient reduces his activity level and loses weight. Failures of THA reported in the literature followed walking on uneven ground daily at work, climbing ladders, and long-distance running. Probably the procedure should not be considered for the patient who is highly motivated to perform activities that will cause daily stress to the hip replacement. No failures have been reported with moderate levels of swimming, hiking, or horseback riding.[25,42-46]

Four-year follow-up studies of THA patients showed that most patients have dramatic relief of pain and improved functional performance by 6 months after surgery. At the end of 2 years, most functional activities showed improvement that was maintained through the 4-year period of the study. Some patients reported slight pain when beginning walking, but the pain decreased as they continued the activity. Patients who developed ossification around the prosthetic head had reduction of hip flexion and internal rotation, which made lower-extremity dressing a bit more difficult but not impossible.[47]

For some patients lower-extremity dressing is a problem for quite a while after surgery but one that is solved through the use of adapted equipment. Postsurgically, mobility for the THA patient can be estimated by the ability to put on stockings and tie shoes, while stability can be estimated by the ability to do cleaning and shopping.[48]

Porous Surface Implant

Another type of implant used for hip replacement is a porous-surfaced metal implant that allows for bone growth into the implant for fixation. This hip plant is indicated for active individuals over 40 years of age with strong healthy bone, generally the patients for whom the cemented implant is not indicated.[49]

The follow-up care for the patient with this type of implant is different from that for the patient who has had a Charnley THA. Patients with the porous-surfaced implant should not do active hip range of motion or full weight bearing on the operated leg for 14 weeks. At 6 weeks, touchdown weight bearing using two crutches is allowed, followed 4 weeks later by use of one crutch, and then 4 weeks later by the use of a cane for support. When this procedure is done through a posterior approach, the patient is not permitted to bend over to pick up things from the floor, should not flex his hip past 70°, and should not internally rotate the operated hip for 8 weeks.[49] Before hospital discharge these patients will need instruction in personal daily living skills with equipment similar to that used by patients who have had THA.

Pain

Orthopedists treat patients with pain that results from musculoskeletal disorders. Two common pain problems referred to occupational therapists are arm and hand pain,[50] usually following trauma (see chapters 3 and 25), and low back pain from specific and nonspecific causes.

Kirkaldy-Willis writes that "all pain is real."[51] Pain that lasts for months or years results in personality changes in the patient. Thus, pain may have both a physical and a psychological component.[52,53] The goal is to alleviate the pain early to prevent affective changes in the patient. Programs to alleviate pain are based on the gate control theory of pain. According to the theory, pain perception occurs when a summation of impulses from small sensory nerve fibers subserving nociceptors activate transmission cells of the substantia gelatinosa in the dorsal horns of the spinal cord. When a series of pain impulses overcomes the threshold in the cells, the impulses are able to reach the cortex, where pain is perceived. Impulses from large sensory nerve fibers subserving mechanoreceptors stimulate the transmission cells to inhibit the perception of pain. The mechanoreceptors increase inhibition in response to active and passive movement of the muscle and joints. The reticular formation of the brain stem exerts an inhibitory effect on pain by closing the gate, or inhibiting the pain via the reticulospinal tract.[51,54] The inhibitory effect is enhanced by concentration on work or other activity. One way the theory is implemented in therapy is by requiring movement of the joints and muscles augmented by concentration on work or other activity; studies have shown this method inhibits pain.[51]

LOW BACK PAIN

Back pain is a leading cause of industrial disability in the 19–45 year age group.[53] The most common cause of low back pain (LBP) is soft tissue strain,[55] which affects 50–80% of the people in modern industrial society.[53] Most episodes of LBP are self-limiting and people recover within 3 months. However, recurrences are frequent, and patients with back pain lasting longer than 6 months have only a 50% chance of returning to work.[55] Injury to the lumbar spine results from poor posture, from minor but repeated injuries such as twisting, and from falling on the buttocks.[56] There is no definitive test to establish the diagnosis of most low back pain.[55]

Fractures of the vertebral bodies and ruptured disks are emergency conditions. Treatment following fractures of vertebral bodies that result in extensive nerve damage is described in chapter 28 on spinal cord injury. Ruptured disks may be treated conservatively with traction and rest, or surgically.[5] The follow-up care can be accomplished in back school programs.

Back School for Treatment of Low Back Pain

The back school concept for educating patients about their back and body mechanics began in Sweden.[55] In the United States a back school team usually consists of a physician, a physical therapist, an occupational therapist, and in some instances a social worker or psychologist. The back school is based on the premise that the LBP patient should be taught to be responsible for his own health.[55,57-59] The patient is taught anatomy and function of the spine and proper body mechanics for personal daily living and leisure activities. Assertiveness training is included to help the patient reduce stress and take responsibility for maintenance of his own back health.[59] To be successful, the patient must be an active participant in the process.[60] The patient must be taught to heal himself and how to avoid injury in the future by keeping his back fit.[59] In industry the physically fit have fewer back problems.[56]

Many back schools involving occupational therapists have been described.[58-65] After medical evaluation establishes that the patient can participate in the back school program, the patient begins a series of classes. It has been found that a class of 6 to 12 patients meeting for four or five sessions is more effective than smaller groups.[59] In the first class the physical therapist may give instruction on anatomy, structure and function of the spine, spinal biomechanics, and the degenerative processes related to the spine. After the occupational therapist evaluates the patient's use of his body in personal daily living, work, and leisure activities, she instructs the patient in basic body mechanics that should be used for reaching, pushing, pulling, or lifting. The patient is asked to practice the activities; this may be done through use of a series of simulated workstations where the patient performs activities and the performance is recorded by the occupational therapist.[59,60]

At the second class, the physical therapist describes muscles and ligaments of the spine and their role in LBP. Patients perform simple maintenance exercises for the back and are given general fitness and recreation guidelines because many leisure activities require movements that can cause back pain. In the third class the occupational therapist instructs patients in proper posture for personal daily living and work activities. Structural stress in various body positions is described by the occupational therapist, and patients are taught to avoid movements and positions that are most likely to cause injury. Patients practice personal daily living skills demonstrating proper body mechanics. The class members are asked to critique each other's performance as a means to check individual learning. Some back school programs also help the patients to analyze their leisure and recreational activities so that they can learn to perform them safely to prevent further back problems.[59]

In the fourth class stress identification and stress management techniques are taught to the patients.[58,59] The patient must understand that through his thoughts and attitudes, he can control the risks to his back.[58] Many patients with chronic back pain become preoccupied with the pain to the elimination of other interests. They may develop coping mechanisms and pain behaviors that restrict their life-styles and work activities. The back school program is designed to help reduce these maladaptive behaviors through stress management and by teaching the patients how to care for their backs and to prevent exacerbation or reinjury.[52]

The results reported for back school programs have been a decrease in frequency and intensity of pain, as well as changes in patients' attitudes and improved understanding of their own needs.[59]

Body Mechanics. The objective in teaching body mechanics is to show the patient how to help himself. Patients do not become free of back pain until they are moving normally; the use of good body mechanics is the way to start. The occupational therapist teaches body mechanics related to standing, sitting, reaching, weight shifting, pushing, lifting, lying down, and getting in and out of beds and cars. The body mechanics used under these conditions are then applied to personal daily living skills and work, and leisure activities.

The principles of body mechanics involve analysis of the load placed on the spine in the various positions and determination of the safest methods of moving for patients with back pain to reduce the stress on back structures. Compression or twisting of the spine is to be avoided, as are attempts to exert force in positions where the spine is poorly supported. The lowest load on the spine is in the supine position; side-lying offers the next greater load. Standing places a moderate load on the spine, whereas sitting places the greatest load of all.[66] Therefore, standing to work is probably safer if the patient puts one foot on a step stool to rotate the pelvis anteriorly to relax the lower back.[56] During episodes of acute back pain the patient should schedule several rest periods a day supine on a firm surface.

In general, activities should be done facing forward without twisting or bending the trunk. The legs are used to turn to face work or activity. The legs are used to help move toward the floor or rise from the floor.[67] Bending over at the waist is avoided.[56]

Standing. The patient should use a relaxed posture with knees slightly bent. When he must stand for longer periods, such as in the kitchen, or bathroom or at a workbench, it is useful to alternate feet on a small step stool to anteriorly rotate the pelvis. To avoid the need to twist, the patient should face the work being done.[67]

Sitting. When sitting down, the patient should flex the knees and hips, without bending forward at the hips. He should sit slightly reclined, using a foot stool, and move the chair close to the work surface to avoid bending over the work from the waist.[68]

The patient should use his hands to lower himself into the chair if necessary. When standing up from a chair, the patient should move toward the front edge of the chair, place his hands on the chair armrests, and keeping his back straight, push up to stand.

Weight Shifting. When standing and working with a tool, such as a broom or vacuum cleaner, the patient should use the proprioceptive neuromuscular facilitation upper-extremity diagonal patterns of motion (see chapter 6) because of their functional correlation with trunk movement[53] to avoid twisting and bending.

Push Versus Pull. When pushing, the patient should face the object, one foot in front of the other, bend at the hips and knees, and walk forward. He should avoid the need to pull a heavy object, but if necessary the same method can be used when walking backward.[67]

Lifting. For lifting objects from the floor to intermediate heights, the patient's choice of position depends on the size of the object. For small, lightweight objects, the patient should face the object and bend his hips and knees into a partial squat while keeping his back straight and not bending over at the waist. When lifting a large object, the patient should face the object, get close to it to bring the mass near to his center of gravity, and assume a half-kneeling position with one knee bent and the hip in extension and the other hip and knee flexed. The object should be grasped firmly and securely. The knee on the floor should be used to help push up, and then both legs can extend to lift the weight while the object is kept close to the body. In the upright position, the patient should achieve balance before carrying the object. If possible, the object should be lifted to an intermediate height such as a chair, rested, and then lifted from there for carrying. When in doubt about the weight of the box or one's ability to lift, the patient should be taught to get another person to help with the lifting.[67]

Lying Down. When lying supine, small pillows under the head and knees are recommended. Another recommendation is to place small pillows under the head and between the knees when side-lying. When side-lying, the hips and knees should be flexed.[68]

To get into bed, the patient sits on the edge of the bed with the knees bent. He uses his arms to lower his trunk to the bed gradually and then brings his legs onto the bed while lying down. He then rolls onto his back with his knees bent. To get up from the bed, the patient reverses the procedure by lying on his side, flexing his hips and knees, and then letting his legs over the edge of the bed as his arms push his trunk to an upright position.[68]

Sitting in a Car. To get into a car, the patient should stand with his back to the car seat. He should bend his hips and knees and lower his body carefully onto the seat, holding onto the door if necessary. He should bend his head slightly to avoid bumping it on the car roof. He should use his hands and arms to press down on the seat as he lifts his legs into the car and turns his trunk to face forward. The procedure is reversed for getting out of the car. The patient should be taught to avoid driving when his back is especially painful. When he does drive, he should bring the seat close to the wheel so that his hips and knees are flexed. The use of a small pillow or rolled-up towel behind the low back offers support.[68]

Patients taught proper body mechanics can learn how to avoid further injuries and exacerbations of low back pain and can become responsible for the state of their back health. Patients with this knowledge tend to have fewer recurrences of low back problems.[55,56]

In addition to body mechanics, all of the occupational therapy back school programs emphasize the occupational therapy premise that movement and activity are important for physical conditioning and mental health.[56] They adhere to Fordyce's maxim:, "Those who have something better to do don't hurt as much."[69]

STUDY QUESTIONS

Orthopedic Conditions

1. List three physical problems treated by orthopedists.
2. List three major kinds of fractures. What is the orthopedist's goal in fracture treatment?
3. What are the symptoms of a fracture?
4. What are the unwanted side effects of immobilization of any fracture? How can they be prevented?
5. What is a major treatment goal for any patient with an upper-extremity fracture?
6. Why is passive motion not used in the treatment of fractures of the elbow?
7. What is the occupational therapist's responsibility if a patient complains of burning pain under a cast? Why?
8. Why should patients with a fractured hip be referred to occupational therapy?
9. What techniques can an occupational therapist teach a patient with hip pain for whom conservative treatment is recommended?
10. What major skills can an occupational therapist teach a patient with a hip fracture or total hip arthroplasty?
11. List precautions that must be taught to a patient with a total hip arthroplasty.
12. What is the occupational therapist's role in a back school?
13. What is the ultimate goal of a back school (the premise on which it is based)?

References

1. *Pocket Medical Dictionary*, 23rd edition. Philadelphia: W. B. Saunders, 1982.
2. Newell, R. L. M., and Turner, J. G. *Orthopaedic Disorders in General Practice*. London: Butterworths, 1985.
3. Salter, R. B. Motion versus rest: why immobilize joints? *J. Bone Joint Surg. (Br)*, 64(2): 251-254, 1982.
4. Mooney, V. Major fractures. In *Orthopedic Rehabilitation*. Edited by V. L. Nickel. New York: Churchill Livingstone, 1982.
5. Apley, A. G., Solomon, L. *Apley's System of Orthopaedics and Fractures*, 6th edition. London: Butterworth Scientific, 1982.
6. Newman, F. H. New developments in fracture management. In *Recent Advances in Surgery*. Edited by R. C. G. Russell. Edinburgh: Churchill Livingstone, 1986.
7. Sarmiento, A., Latta, L. L., and Tarr, R. R. The effects of function in fracture healing and stability. In *American Academy of Orthopaedic Surgeons, Instructional Course Lectures*, Vol. 33. St. Louis: C. V. Mosby, 1984.
8. Devas, M., editor. *Geriatric Orthopaedics*. London: Academic Press, 1977.
9. Epps, C. H., Jr., and Cotler, J. M. Complications of treatment of fractures of the humeral shaft. In *Complications in Orthopaedic Surgery*, Vol. I, 2nd edition. Edited by C. H. Epps, Jr. Philadelphia: J. B. Lippincott, 1985.
10. Heppenstall, R. B., editor. *Fracture Treatment and Healing*. Philadelphia: W. B. Saunders, 1980.
11. Glazer, R. M. Rehabilitation. In *Fracture Treatment and Healing*. Edited by R. B. Heppenstall. Philadelphia: W. B. Saunders, 1980.
12. Muckle, D. S. *An Outline of Fractures and Dislocations*. Bristol: John Wright & Sons, Ltd., 1985.
13. Ross, S. D. K., and Saramiento, A. Complications of functional fracture bracing. In *Complications of Orthopaedic Surgery*, Vol. I, 2nd edition. Edited by C. H. Epps, Jr. Philadelphia: J.B. Lippincott, 1986.
14. Frykman, G. K., and Nelson, E. F. Fractures and traumatic conditions of the wrist. In *Rehabilitation of the Hand*, 2nd edition. Edited by J. M. Hunter, et al. St Louis: C. V. Mosby, 1984.
15. Colditz, J. C. Dynamic splinting of the stiff hand. In *Rehabilitation of the Hand*, 2nd edition. Edited by J. M. Hunter, et al. St Louis: C. V. Mosby, 1984.
16. Hunter, J. M., Mackin, E. J. Edema and bandaging. In *Rehabilitation of the Hand*, 2nd edition. Edited by J. M. Hunter., et al. St. Louis: C. V. Mosby, 1984.
17. Vasudevan, S. V., and Melvin, J. L. Upper extremity edema control: rationale of the techniques. *Am. J. Occup. Ther.* 33(8): 520-523, 1979.
18. Lewinnek, G. E., et al. The significance and a comparative analysis of the epidemiology of hip fractures. *Clin. Orthop.*, 152: 35-43, 1980.
19. Guimaraes, R. M., and Isaacs, B. Characteristics of the gait in old people who fall. *Int. Rehabil. Med.*, 2(4): 177-180, 1980.
20. Hasselkus, B. R., Aging and the human nervous system. *Am. J. Occup. Ther.* 28(1): 16-21, 1974.
21. Schaefer, R. Occupational therapy for lower extremity problems. *Am. J. Occup. Ther.*, 27(3): 132-137, 1973.
22. Ceder, L., Thorngren, K.-G., and Wallden, B. Prognostic indicators and early home rehabilitation in elderly patients with hip fractures. *Clin. Orthop.*, 152: 173-184, 1980.
23. Simm, F. H., and Stauffer, R. N. Fractures of the neck of the femur. In *American Academy of Orthopaedic Surgeons Instructional Course Lectures*, Vol. 29. St. Louis: C. V. Mosby, 1980.
24. Hirschberg, G. G., Lewis, L., and Vaughan, P. *Rehabilitation: A Manual for the Care of the Disabled and Elderly*, 2nd edition. Philadelphia: J. B. Lippincott, 1976.
25. Hardinge, K. *Hip Replacement: The Facts*. Oxford: Oxford University Press, 1983.
26. Eftekhar, N. S. *Principles of Total Hip Arthroplasty*. St. Louis: C. V. Mosby, 1978.
27. Coventry, M. B. Total hip replacement. In *The Hip*. Edited by L. H. Riley, Jr. Proceedings of the Hip Society Eighth Scientific Meeting, 1980. St. Louis: C. V. Mosby, 1980.
28. Morscher, E. W. Intertrochanteric osteotomy in osteoarthritis of the hip. In *The Hip*. Edited by L. H. Riley, Jr. Proceedings of the Hip Society Eighth Scientific Meeting, 1980. St. Louis: C. V. Mosby, 1980.
29. Liechti, R. *Hip Arthrodesis and Associated Problems*. Berlin: Springer-Verlag, 1978.
30. Friedebold, G. The Smith-Peterson cup arthroplasty: an analysis of failures. In *Arthroplasty of the Hip*. Edited by G. Chapchal. Stuttgart: Georg Thieme, 1973.
31. Amstutz, H. C., et al. Total hip articular replacement by internal eccentric shells. *Clin. Orthop.*, 128: 261-184, 1977.
32. Amstutz, H. C. Surface replacement of the hip. In *The Hip*. Edited by L. H. Riley, Jr. Proceedings of the Hip Society Eighth Scientific Meeting, 1980. St. Louis: C. V. Mosby, 1980.
33. Muller, M. E. Late complications of total hip replacement. In *The Hip*. Edited by W. H. Harris. Proceedings of the Hip Society Second Scientific Meeting, 1974. St. Louis: C. V. Mosby, 1974.
34. Poss, R. Total hip replacement in the patient with rheumatoid arthritis. In *American Academy of Orthopaedic Surgeons, Instructional Course Lectures*, Vol. 28. St. Louis: C. V. Mosby, 1979.
35. Jergesen, H. E., Poss, R., and Sledge, C. B. Bilateral total hip and knee replacement in adults with rheumatoid arthritis: an evaluation of function. *Clin. Orthop.*, 137: 120-128, 1978.
36. Aufranc, O. E. Postoperative management. In *Principles of Total Hip Arthroplasty*. Edited by N. S. Eftekhar. St. Louis: C. V. Mosby, 1978.
37. McKee, J. I. Foam wedges aid sitting posture of patients with total hip replacement. *Phys. Ther.* 55(7): 767, 1975.
38. Seeger, M. S., and Fisher, L. A. Adaptive equipment used in the rehabilitation of hip arthroplasty patients. *Am. J. Occup. Ther.*, 36(8): 503-508, 1982.
39. Carpenter, E. S., et al. *Information for Our Patients: Total Hip Joint Replacement*, revised edition. Downey, CA: Professional Staff Association, Rancho Los Amigos Hospital, 1979.
40. Harris, J., and Currey, H. L. F. Sexual problems due to disease of the hip joint: its relevance to hip surgery. In *Total Hip Replacement*. Edited by M. Jayson. Philadelphia: J. B. Lippincott, 1971.
41. Yoslow, W., Simeone, J., and Huestis, D. Hip replacement rehabilitation. *Arch. Phys. Med. Rehabil.*, 57(6): 275-278, 1976.
42. Todd, R. C., Lishtowler, C. D. R., and Harris, J. Low friction arthroplasty of the hip joint and sexual activity. *Acta Orthop. Scand.*, 44(6): 690-693, 1973.
43. Ling, R. S. M. Prevention of loosening of total hip components. In *The Hip*. Edited by L. H. Riley, Jr. Proceedings of the Hip Society Eighth Scientific Meeting, 1980. St. Louis: C. V. Mosby, 1980.
44. Moreland, J. R., et al. Aseptic loosening of total hip replacement: incidence and significance. In *The Hip*. Edited by L. H. Riley, Jr. Proceedings of the Hip Society Eighth Scientific Meeting, 1980. St. Louis: C. V. Mosby, 1980.

45. Stinchfeld, F. E., guest editor. Symposium—statistics in total hip replacement. *Clin. Orthop., 95*: 9–223, 1973.
46. Weaver, J. K. Activity expectations and limitations following total joint replacement. *Clin. Orthop., 137:* 55–61, 1978.
47. Murray, M. P., et al. Joint function after total hip arthroplasty: a four-year follow-up of 72 cases with Charnley and Muller replacements. *Clin. Orthop., 157:* 119–124, 1981.
48. Visuri, T., and Honkanen, R. The influence of total hip replacement on selected activities of daily living and on the use of domestic aid. *Scand. J. Rehabil. Med., 10*(4): 221–225, 1978.
49. Engh, C. A., and Bobyn, J. D. *Biological Fixation in Total Hip Arthroplasty.* Thorofare, NJ: Slack Incorporated, 1985.
50. Schultz, K. S. The Schultz structured interview for assessing upper extremity pain. *Occupational Therapy in Health Care 1*(3): 69–82, 1984.
51. Kirkaldy-Willis, W. H. *Managing Low Back Pain.* New York: Churchill Livingstone, 1983.
52. Cameron, A. J. R., Shepel, L. F., and Bowen, R. C. Psychological treatment of back pain and associated problems. In *Managing Low Back Pain.* Edited by W. H. Kirkaldy-Willis. New York: Churchill Livingstone, 1983.
53. Raj, P. P. *Practical Management of Pain.* Chicago: Year Book Medical Publishers, 1986.
54. Omer, G. E., Jr. Nerve response to injury and repair. In *Rehabilitation of the Hand.* Edited by J. M. Hunter, et al. St. Louis: C. V. Mosby, 1984.
55. Mooney, V. Low back disability. In *Orthopaedic Rehabilitation.* Edited by V. L. Nickel. New York: Churchill Livingstone, 1982.
56. Nachemson, A. L. Toward a better understanding of low back injury. In *Proceedings of the Liberty Mutual Back Pain Symposium.* Boston: Liberty Mutual, 1981.
57. White, A. H. Low back pain. *American Academy of Orthopaedic Surgeons Instructional Course Lectures,* Vol. 34. St. Louis: C. V. Mosby, 1985.
58. Mooney, V. and Cairns, D. Management in the patient with chronic low back pain. *Orthop. Clin. North Am., 9*(2): 543–557, 1978.
59. Randolph, J. W. The role of occupational therapy in back school. *Occupational Therapy in Health Care, 1*(3): 93–102, 1984.
60. Bettencourt, C. M., et al. Using work simulation to treat adults with back injuries. *Am. J. Occup. Ther., 40*(1): 12–18, 1986.
61. Caruso, L. A. and Chan, D. E. Evaluation and management of the patient with acute back pain. *Am. J. Occup. Ther., 40*(5): 347–351, 1986.
62. Clements, L. and Dixon, M. A model role of occupational therapy in back education. *Can J. Occup. Ther., 46*(4): 161–163, 1979.
63. Flower, A., et al. An occupational therapy program for chronic back pain. *Am. J. Occup. Ther., 35*(4): 243–248, 1981.
64. Rivera, A. M. Occupational therapy in the rehabilitation of low back pain. *Occup. Ther. News, 39*(7): 10, 1985.
65. Sanborn, C. P. Chronic pain management: occupational therapy role. *American Occupational Therapy Association Physical Disabilities Special Interest Section Newsletter 4* (4): 2–3, 1981.
66. Nachemson, A. L., and Morris, J. M. In vivo measurements of intradiscal pressure. *J. Bone Joint Surg. 46 A*(5): 1077–1091, 1964.
67. Frederick, B. B., et al. *Body Mechanics Instruction Manual.* A guide for therapists. Redmond, WA: Express Publications, 1979.
68. Kirkaldy-Willis, W. H. Spine education program—intensive therapy—the pain clinic. In *Managing Low Back Pain.* Edited by W. H. Kirkaldy-Willis. New York: Churchill Livingstone, 1983.
69. Murphy, K. A., and Cornish, R. D. Prediction of chronicity in acute low back pain. *Arch. Phys. Med. Rehabil. 65*(6): 334–337, 1984.

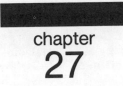

chapter

27

Arthritis

Catherine A. Trombly

Two of the many types of arthritic diseases are discussed in this chapter: rheumatoid arthritis and degenerative joint disease, also known as osteoarthritis.

Rheumatoid Arthritis

Rheumatoid arthritis (RA) is a systemic disease characterized by remissions and exacerbations that vary in severity and timing among people.[1,2] Joint inflammation is the dominant clinical manifestation of the generalized disease of connective tissue,[3] but the disease may also involve the lungs, heart, blood vessels, or eyes.[4] In countries in the temperate zones, 2.5% of the population has this disease.[3] Two to three times more women are stricken than men.[1-3] Onset is usually between the 20th to 40th year of age.[3] Etiology is unknown.[1-4] Two theories, not mutually exclusive, are being studied: the infection and the autoimmunity theories. The infection theory hypothesizes that a virus may be the cause. The autoimmune theory holds that there is a disruption of the immune process resulting in a continuous immunological response to a persistent antigen, which could be altered gamma globulin in the diseased joint.[3] In 70% of the cases a rheumatoid factor can be demonstrated by a blood test in patients who have had the disease for some time.[3] There may be a genetic predisposition to the disease.[4] Stress is not a causative factor but may precipitate the onset of symptoms and aggravate the disease once it is established.[2,3] There is no cure at this time.[2,3]

Because of the disease's chronic nature and often degenerative course, those treating patients with RA follow the philosophy applied in the care of patients with any degenerative disease: maintain the patient's physical, psychological, and functional abilities as long as possible through an ongoing, carefully planned treatment program. Integrated team management is essential[5-8] and has been found to be a statistically important factor in the improvement of patients with rheumatoid disease, although a priori differences in groups could have accounted for the detected differences.[7] The team at the successful Multipurpose Arthritic Center consisted of a rheumatologist, nurse educator, physical and occupational therapists, and social worker.[8]

Symptoms of RA are variable but include pain, stiffness and limited movement of involved joints, malaise, fatigue, wasting of the muscles around the joints, and anemia.[5] The disease begins within the joints as inflammation of the synovium.[1,5] The five characteristic manifestations of inflammation (redness, swelling, heat, pain, and loss of function) become progressively more evident.[3] Rheumatoid arthritis affects many joints (polyarthritis). The most commonly involved joints, in order of frequency, are those of the hands,[2,3] wrists, knees, elbows, feet, shoulders, and hips.[3] The distribution tends to be bilaterally symmetrical.[3] The metacarpophalangeal (MP) joints of the thumb, index, and middle fingers, the proximal interphalangeal (PIP) joints of the index, middle, and ring fingers, and the metatarsophalangeal joints of the four small toes are characteristically involved in early stages of the disease.[3]

Once the active disease process burns out, the patient is left with residual joint deformities[1,3,5] and resultant limitations of function. The primary objective of treatment is to prevent joint destruction, which is nonreversible.[2]

Occupational therapists help the patient understand his disease pathology and its effects on his life tasks.[9] Through assessment and treatment, the occupational therapist seeks to improve the patient's ability to perform daily activities, prevent loss of function, and facilitate successful adaptation.[9] The occupational therapist treats the physical and psychosocial dysfunction and helps the patient to develop the problem-solving skills needed to make adaptations throughout life.[9] Specific goals depend on the identified problems of the particular patient. These may be any or all of the following:

1. Prevent joint pain and deformity.
2. Maintain joint mobility.

3. Maintain or increase strength.
4. Maintain or increase endurance.
5. Maintain or increase functional ability.
6. Develop problem-solving skills to modify daily activities at home and at work to protect joints and conserve energy.[9]
7. Promote psychosocial adjustment to chronic disability.

EVALUATION

In response to a request for services, the occupational therapist does a screening by chart review, interview and observation of the patient, and use of screening tests to determine if referral for occupational therapy is indicated.[9] A patient who risks losing function due to pain, fatigue, loss of strength or endurance, changes in joint range of motion (ROM), or loss of coping skills, or whose function may be improved, is considered an appropriate candidate for occupational therapy.[9] Assessment includes a review of medical history and status of the patient's disease; tests to document manifestations of the disease including ROM evaluation, strength testing, and daily living skills evaluations; environmental analyses to determine the impact of the environment on the patient's ability to function; evaluation of the patient's psychosocial status; and identification of the patient's personal goals, interests, and expectations.[9] Sensory evaluation should be done if systemic involvement includes polyneuropathies or nerve compression.[1]

Joint Mobility

Changes in joint mobility result from excess joint play due to loosened ligaments and joint capsules and due to contractures of muscles and other connective tissue. Range of motion is measured as described in chapter 8.

Deformities or Their Precursors

These deformities and their precursors are evaluated by determining whether the ligaments and capsule are slack, resulting in excess joint play, whether the muscles are too tight, whether swelling or nodules are present, and whether the integrity of the tendons and joints has been preserved.

Ligamentous stability of the fingers is evaluated by placing the PIP and distal interphalangeal (DIP) joints in full passive extension (0°), stabilizing the proximal bone, and moving the distal one from side to side.[4] The amount of joint play should be little; however, normality is determined by comparison to a normal joint, since the amount of normal joint play differs among people.[4] Abnormal laxity of the radial collateral ligament at the MP joint is evaluated by placing the patient's MP joints in 90° of flexion; the therapist then pushes the digit ulnarly. The ligament is stretched if the finger can be pushed easily.

To test for shortened ulnar intrinsic muscles, the patient flexes the PIP joint while the MP joint is held in 0° of deviation. The amount of PIP flexion is measured with a goniometer. The patient then ulnarly deviates the MP joint and flexes the PIP joint again. The amount of PIP flexion is measured and compared to the previous measurement. If the ulnar intrinsic muscles are tight, there will be more PIP flexion with the MP joint in ulnar deviation than with the MP joint in 0° of deviation.[10]

Nodules are sometimes found on the extrinsic tendons of the finger muscles. Although extensor tendon nodules can be easily detected visually, flexor tendon nodules are less obvious. Nodules are more likely to form on the flexor digitorum sublimis (superficialis) than on the flexor digitorum profundus.[11] Flexor tendon nodules can be detected using the following method. If active finger flexion motion is less than normal, but passive motion is normal, then flexor tendon nodules can be suspected. To test, have the patient flex each finger; if active range of motion is limited, check passive range of motion. It will be normal, but the finger will meet a stopping point (the nodule) and have to be moved slowly to full range.[10]

Tendon rupture is uncommon,[11] but due to the disease process, may occur. If the tendon has ruptured, the full passive range of motion will be achieved without resistance. The most common tendons to rupture are those of the extensor digitorum due to rubbing of the tendons on the distal ulna. A single rupture stands out because the finger droops. Multiple ruptures become evident when the patient is asked to flex and extend the MP joints. Flexor tendon rupture can follow development of nodules on the flexor tendons and is usually preceded by the "trigger" or "locking" phenomenon of the finger with a nodule. An isolated rupture of any of the flexor tendons causes little functional loss. These can be found, however, using standard muscle testing procedures: there will be a loss of flexor motion of either the distal interphalangeal joint or the proximal interphalangeal joint of one finger while motion is preserved in the fingers unaffected by the rupture.[10]

The location of pain, hot and inflamed joints, swelling, tendon rupture, nodules, crepitus, and subluxations or dislocations are noted in such a way as to allow comparison from evaluation to evaluation. Some clinics use xerography, and others use photography to supplement written descriptions.

The severity of pain can be graded based on its occurrence during activity; it is graded mild if it occurs only with stressful activity, moderate if it occurs with active motion, and severe if it occurs even at rest.[12]

The typical deformities of the wrist and hand and the underlying mechanisms thought to produce these deformities are being described in detail not only so that they may be evaluated, but also because it is hypothesized that normal use of the hands produces forces that promote the deformities. Although one study that compared deformities of dominant and nondominant hands (based on the assumption that the dominant hand is subject to greater stress during daily activity and therefore would have significantly greater deformity) found no significant difference in the frequency or type of deformities between the two hands,[13] therapy is guided by the assumption that use increases deformity. Until studies are done that actually document the amount and type of dominant and nondominant hand usage before comparing for deformity, the direction of therapy probably ought not to change. The findings in the above study may be explained by noting that whereas the dominant hand is used more often for dexterous tasks involving pinch and grasp, the nondominant hand is used for stabilization and is therefore also equally subjected to deforming static pinch and grasp forces.

The exact cause of deformity is not yet fully understood, but it appears that hypertrophy of the synovium due to the inflammation process pushes against the joint structures from within. The ligaments become stretched, and when the swelling of the synovium subsides, the ligaments are left lax. The force moments of the tendons are changed because of the ligamentous abnormality, and their pull becomes deforming.[11]

Deformities of the Wrist. Volar subluxation of the hand in relation to the ulna is caused by erosion of the intercarpal ligaments and volar displacement of the extensor carpi ulnaris[14] which, in effect, causes this muscle to act as a flexor force.

Commonly, the wrist radially deviates due to a loss of support of the radial and ulnar ligaments[4] and forward displacement of the extensor carpi ulnaris (ECU) and predominant action of the radial muscles—flexor carpi radialis, extensor carpi radialis brevis, and extensor carpi radialis longus.[15] Loss of ligamentous support allows the carpal bones to ulnarly sublux, which results in the radial deviation.[4,16] The fingers, especially the index, then ulnarly deviate in an effort to realign the index with the radius, its normal position.[4,16] This completes the zig-zag deformity: wrist radial deviation with MP ulnar deviation. However, this sequence of events is disputed based on clinical observation that the ulnar drift of the MP joints seems to occur first, which means that factors other than wrist radial deviation influence finger deviation.[15]

Deformities of the Metacarpophalangeal Joints. Volar subluxation of the fingers appears to develop in the following way.[11] Synovitis of the MP joint stretches the extensor mechanism. The extensor hood is thinner radially, and the hypertrophied synovium tends to herniate on the radial side of the extensor tendons. The hood is pushed distally, which causes the extensor tendons to slip ulnarly off the tops of the joints to the "valleys" between. This places them below the joint axes; therefore, their force becomes a flexor force.[10,11] In addition, the large volar forces generated at the mouth of the flexor tunnels during pinch or grasp cause mechanical damage to the metacarpoglenoidal ligaments supporting them. The tunnel mouths are displaced volarly.[17] A new equilibrium of forces is established between the pull of the flexors and the supporting structure: the rim of the phalanx and the MP (collateral) ligaments. If the rim wears down, or the ligaments are stretched, the deformity of volar subluxation results.[17]

One theory is that ulnar deviation deformity develops when the tissues surrounding the joint, especially the radial collateral ligaments,[14] become permanently stretched due to the push of the synovium. Normally, the ulnar interossei exert a stronger pull than the radial ones do.[4,11,17] This, combined with the pull of the flexor tendons on the mouths of the tendon sheaths in an ulnar direction, contributes to the force that causes the dynamic ulnar deviation.[17] In time, the ulnar intrinsics become shortened, creating a constant pull toward ulnar deviation. Although it is hypothesized that a protective MP flexor response is induced in the interossei muscles as a pain avoidance mechanism, which eventually results in fibrous, fixed shortening of the intrinsics,[18] electromyographical evidence has failed to validate spasm as a possible source of this deformity and supports the findings that muscle action normally present in the hand is the cause of deformity.[17,19] Another theory is that ulnar deviation deformity results as a compensation for wrist radial deviation deformity.[20]

The Interphalangeal Joint Deformities. The deformities of the interphalangeal joints caused by rheumatoid arthritis, degenerative joint disease, and traumatic arthritis are swan neck deformity, boutonniere deformity, and fixed flexor or extensor deformities.[21]

A swan neck deformity (intrinsic plus hand) is a combination of PIP hyperextension and DIP flexion caused by tight interossei that pull abnormally on the extensor tendons and cause hyperextension of the hypermobile PIP joints.[10,14] This deformity may be flexible or fixed. To test for flexibility, support the MP joints in extension and have the patient flex the PIP joint.[10] If full flexion of the PIP joint occurs, the deformity is flexible, and the volar plate that prevents hyperextension is only slightly stretched. If PIP flexion is impossible with the MP joint extended but can be accomplished with the MP joint flexed, a fixed deformity due to tight intrinsics is present.

The intrinsic muscles are on stretch when the MP joints are extended and the interphalangeal joints are flexed. Early detection of tightness of the intrinsics is important so treatment can be instituted. Tightness can be detected by noting whether a difference exists in the amount of flexion of the PIP joints when the MP joints are flexed or extended.[4]

A fixed swan neck deformity also may be caused by sticking lateral bands. In this case, PIP flexion is impossible, regardless of the position of the MP joint.[10]

A boutonniere deformity is a combination of PIP flexion and DIP hyperextension caused by the PIP joint slipping up between the lateral bands of the extensor digitorum,[10,14] which then act to flex the PIP joint. The relationship between the flexor digitorum profundus and the extensor digitorum is changed, and the extensor acts unopposed at the DIP joint.[14] To test for shortening of the lateral bands, hold the PIP extended and passively try to flex the DIP; if this is difficult, there is shortening.[14]

Deformities of the Thumb. Interphalangeal hyperextension is caused by intrinsic-plus pull on the extensor mechanism of the hypermobile interphalangeal joint when MP extension is lost due to volar displacement of the long extensor secondary to capsular and extensor apparatus stretch caused by inflammation of the MP joint.[14]

Metacarpophalangeal hyperextension occurs in response to the pull of a tight adductor pollicis on weakened joint structures.[14]

Strength

The systemic nature of rheumatoid arthritis, along with atrophy of disuse, produces muscle weakness.[16] Use of manual muscle testing involving resistance is controversial. On the one hand, it is necessary to know the patient's strength, especially the comparative strength of muscles around a joint; on the other hand, resistance causes harm to the diseased tissue, which causes pain. Pain causes the patient to protect the part and results in an unreliable test. Some rheumatologists prohibit any resistance beyond that which is necessary for self-care due to the deforming forces of muscle contraction when joint structures are stretched and weakened.[19] Others feel that knowledge of the level of muscle strength and the effectiveness of strengthening exercises is important.[22] The muscle test should be done isometrically, not isotonically; isotonic movement against resistance tends to increase inflammation and pain in arthritic joints.[22] The metal hydraulic dynamometers and pinch meters are not used by patients with RA. Measurement of grasp and pinch strength should be done using an adapted sphygmomanometer[4] or vigorometer that is commercially available. The vigorometer compares favorably with the Jamar dynamometer, although it is not interchangeable with it due to different measurement units.[23] Norms have been published for the vigorometer.[24,25]

Endurance

Endurance is evaluated as outlined in chapters 8 and 30 or by noticing the patient's limits of endurance during daily activity. The patient must learn to evaluate this for himself, since he must learn to rest before fatigue becomes a factor in the performance of activities.

Activities of Daily Living

Activities of daily living (ADL) are evaluated as described in chapter 16. It may be useful to add two categories to the scoring criteria for "independent," one category for activity that is possible to complete independently but not entirely without pain and one category for those activities that are very difficult or painful.[26] These would clue the therapist to help the patient find alternative methods of doing these tasks since pain is to be avoided. Melvin suggests that it is good, when evaluating functional impairment, to end the evaluation with a task the patient can do in order to focus the patient on ability rather than disability. It is also suggested, in order to contain the feelings of total disablement and to help clarify the limits of dysfunction, that the patient be asked to be very specific when he reports the inability to do something.[4]

A factor analytical study of ADL/homemaking activities was done to determine if certain factors could be identified with the hope of developing a "screening approach to ADL" rather than test all items on an ADL test, which is fatiguing.[26] One possibility is to use a modified test that screens function according to each factor identified in a factor analysis. Factor analysis is a statistical method of clustering individual measurements together into factors. The measures grouped together into one factor are highly related to each other and, in essence, measure similar aspects of the factor-function. Therefore, one task from each identified factor could be tested and if the patient did not have difficulty with the tested item, other tasks within that factor would not be tested. This assumes that the tasks grouped into factors statistically are in fact not independent skills. It is a useful approach that needs further validation.[26]

Assessment of Hand Function

Hand function, and the function of the upper extremity insofar as it serves hand function, is of particular interest. Maintenance of hand function is important since the disabling nature of this disease may limit employment to a sedentary type for which good hand function is a necessity.[11] Both the prehensile and nonprehensile functions of the hand should be evaluated.[4] Prehensile functions are pinch and grasp; nonprehensile functions are those that use the hand statically held either flexed (hook grasp) or extended (e.g., tucking in clothing, smoothing sheets, sorting coins on a surface).[4] In RA, the prehensile functions are potentially deforming; therefore, if nonprehensile functions can be substituted, the joints may be protected from deformity.

A number of hand function tests exist. These tests focus on the prehensile functions. One is the Jebsen Hand Function Test,[27] described in chapter 4. Another is a method of assessing the rheumatoid hand that was proposed some years ago,[28] but further development of the battery does not seem to have occurred. The battery consists of the most useful methods of assessment chosen from 128 separate measurements.[28] The tests were (1) strength of grasp using an adapted sphygmomanometer; (2) strength of cylindrical grasp using wooden dowels ranging in diameter from ½ inch to 1⅝ inches attached to an aluminum weight pan onto which 15 pounds of disc weights were added (if the patient was unable to hold for 10 sec, the amount of weight was reduced to 10, 5, 2½, and 1¼ pounds [this seems to be a deforming task and is not recommended]); (3) pulp to pulp and lateral pinches; (4) finger flexor power and finger stability using a special device that requires the finger to push a button; (5) deformity that interferes with function as measured by the other tasks of the battery; (6) presence or absence of pain and tenderness as reported by the patient and heat and crepitus as felt by the therapist; (7) range of motion; (8) ulnar deviation measurement; (9) one-handed activities: safety pin test, button test, and scissors test; and (10) two-handed activities: knife and fork test and shoelace test.

The latter two sets of tests are timed tests of operationally defined tasks. The reader is referred to the original source for greater detail.

An electronic standardized test to measure hand movement (active and passive), strength (pinches, grip, and finger extension), and manipulative ability (holding, placing, and twisting) has been devised.[29] Values obtained for arthritic women were compared to those for normal subjects. The arthritic patients were found to be severely compromised in active motion (50% of normal), strength (ranged from 10% of normal for grip to 25% of normal for pinches), and manipulation (50% of normal).[29]

TREATMENT

Treatment addresses the problems identified by evaluation and is guided by the progress of the disease.[30] In all stages, fatigue is avoided.

Acute Stage: Synovial Inflammation and Proliferation

The goals are to prevent joint deformity and pain by resting the affected joint(s) using positioning or splinting; to maintain joint mobility; to assist the patient to cope with the unpredictable nature of the disease; and to begin energy conservation education.

Subacute Stage: Postinflammation

The goals are to maintain or increase mobility, strength,[30] and endurance; to maintain or increase functional abilities; to prevent deformity by splinting and joint protection techniques; to develop the patient's problem-solving skills relative to energy conservation and joint protection; and to assist in psychosocial adjustment to chronic pain and disability.

Chronic Stage: Burn Out of Disease; Deformity Remains

The goals are to maintain or increase mobility and strength[1]; to assist psychosocial adjustment; and to increase skill in functional tasks. Destroyed joints may be replaced surgically. See chapters 25 and 26 for a discussion of therapy following joint replacement.

An important treatment method used with RA patients throughout the course of their disease is patient education. Energy conservation principles, work simplification techniques, joint protection techniques, and exercise programs are taught to the patient, who must also learn his home program designed to continue healthy behaviors throughout his lifetime.

When instructing the patient, attention should be paid to the instructional process as well as the patient's specific needs and methods of coping with his disability.[4] A process for designing the instructional program has been described.[31] Instructional sessions should have specific goals stated in behavioral terms and should clearly present the material through discussion, audiovisuals, and demonstration. Opportunities to problem solve relative to the patient's own life tasks and to practice the principles under various conditions also should be included. After assessing what the patient has learned, the information may have to be repeated because it is not all retained at once.[5] Prior to starting, the therapist should assess the psychological readiness of the patient to learn.[4] Pain, concern with the disease, and the effects of medication may interfere with the learning process; therefore, written information is helpful for future reference.[4,5]

Encouraging but not conclusive evidence was presented in support of an instructional program that was based on use of a workbook in conjunction with group or tutorial interactive sessions.[31] The topics covered were energy conservation and joint protection techniques.[31,32] The workbook has an introduction describing the disease, and the remainder is divided into four units on positioning, rest, activity analysis for energy conservation, and joint protection. Each unit contains didactic information and illustrations of the techniques, practice assignments to apply learned techniques, and a self-evaluation section.[31,32] The instructor's guide includes suggestions for teaching the techniques and topics to emphasize in each session.[31] It is meant to be used in a 6-week program of 1½ hour group or individual sessions. Part of the success of the workbook program has to be attributed to careful delineation of behavioral objectives; for example, "patient will demonstrate inclusion of 2 daily 1-hour lying down rest periods"[31] (p.105).

Maintenance of Joint Mobility

In acute disease, passive or very gentle active-assistive motion is done for each joint daily to maintain mobility. As the disease subsides, the therapist assists less. The patient should be treated in three or four short periods per day, with different joints treated at each session.[33] Exercise is best done when pain has been diminished by drugs or heat and when morning stiffness has subsided.[34] Neutral warmth may be sufficient to reduce pain and since it avoids the rebound effect of other methods of warming, it may be preferred, although no research has been published to support that suggestion.

In the postinflammatory stage, passive range of motion to just beyond the point of pain is done to provide gentle prolonged stretch to prevent the muscles and connective tissues from shortening into fixed deformities.[33,34] Abrupt application of stretch may rupture the tissue[30] and must be avoided. Warming before the passive exercises is beneficial. If the occupational therapist is to take responsibility for passive ranging, then it should be done directly after the patient receives heat treatments in physical therapy. If the physical therapist does the ranging, that is enough. If pain persists several hours after therapy, the amount of exercise at the next session should be cut in half.[33,34] If pain persists, the joint must be rested.

Nonresistive activities that require the patient to move to full range in nondeforming motion patterns are desirable. However, repetitious use of the joints or overexercise may aggravate the disease by causing inflammation.[30,34] Therefore, signs of inflammation must be carefully monitored. Pain should not last more than 2 hours on therapy day and on the next day should be no worse than before therapy.[34] A visual analogue pain rating scale[35] is available in which the patient indicates on a continuum represented by a 10-cm line the intensity of the pain he is experiencing at the moment, with the beginning of the line signifying 0 (no pain) and the end of the line signifying 100 (most severe pain possible).[35,36]

In a trial of 30 patients with RA, an airsplint that applies constant, uniform external pressure to all portions of the hand was applied for 20 min with the wrist in neutral and the fingers in extension and then for 20 min with the fingers fisted. Inflation was 40 mm Hg. The mechanism involved in relief of hand symptoms by airsplint is not as yet known,[36] but benefit may result from forcing the fluid out of the synovium as explained by Byers.[37] Whatever the mechanism, after one such treatment mobility increased 45%, and after five treatments it increased 63%, which was a significant improvement compared to the control (contralateral) hands.[36]

Prevention of Deformity

This goal does not stem from evaluation findings but rather from the known course of the disease. Deformity is prevented by splinting and positioning, by exercise, and by joint protection techniques.

Splinting. Actively inflamed joints need local rest by splinting in functional positions.[5] The full-hand splint is usually worn at night,[38] and the hand is left free for light activity during the day. Based on the biomechanical analysis of deformity at the MP joint, it is suggested by one author that the hand be splinted with the MPs in extension with no deviation, which would protect the flexor tunnel mouths from damaging forces.[17] In this position, the joint capsule would be in the slack position (off stretch),[39] and if maintained there, it might tighten to its normal tautness. Others suggest MP flexion[11,38] and slight radial deviation.[16] One guideline for a resting hand splint is 30° to 40° wrist dorsiflexion, 70° to 80° MP flexion, and 10° to 20° PIP and DIP flexion.[38] There are no research data to support any one design over another. There are few studies on the effectiveness of splinting RA hands at all.[40]

Some advocate removing the resting splint several times a day for ranging,[5] and others say that splints can be left on up to 4 weeks without ROM exercises with no loss of mobility.[30,34] Again, these ideas are not based on research findings.

In a study of 50 RA patients splinted in full-hand resting splints, it was found at follow-up that no significant differences occurred in the range of motion between the compliant (splints worn more than 50% of the time) and the noncompliant group (splints worn less than 50% of the time).[12] The noncompliant group actually improved slightly more than the compliant group in range of motion. The patients were noncompliant when symptoms remitted or diminished and therefore freed their hands for active use.[7,12] That outcome leads one to wonder if splints need closer monitoring so that they can be discarded at the moment inflammation has subsided to allow free use of the joints to maintain the range.

During the day, if a splint is used, a design that is less confining is chosen. A wrist cock-up splint (Figs. 13.5 and 13.6) frees the hand for use while supporting the wrist.[38] It should be lightweight and constructed to put the wrist in about 5° of ulnar deviation.[16] If the MP joints need support, the splint can be extended to support them in extension with no deviation; finger interphalangeal flexion would still be possible[17] (Fig. 27.1).

In addition to using splints to rest the joint, prevent deformity, and to stabilize the joint during movement to increase function, splints also are used for correcting contractures and to assist in the postsurgical rehabilitation of the hand.[34]

Exercise. Exercise, used to maintain or increase muscle strength to help maintain joint alignment, is done with particular attention paid to minimizing stress on joints.[15]

Joint Protection. Principles of joint protection are based on the theory that forces involved in use of the hand contribute to structured joint changes and disease activity that fosters deformity.[13] The principles are[32,41]: (1) respect pain as a signal to stop the activity; (2) maintain muscle strength and joint range of motion; (3) avoid positions of deformity; (4) avoid external and internal deforming forces; (5) use the strongest/largest joints available for the job; (6) use each joint in its most stable anatomical and functional plane; (7) use correct patterns of motion; (8) avoid holding one position for any undue length of time; and (9) avoid starting an activity that cannot be stopped if it proves to be beyond capability.

The patient has to learn the application of these principles through supervised practice of specific joint protection techniques, some of which follow.

Static deforming positions, or motions in the direction of potential deformity, should be strictly avoided. Strong grasp or pinch are deforming forces in the rheumatoid hand.[10,17,19,42] For that reason, knitting, ham-

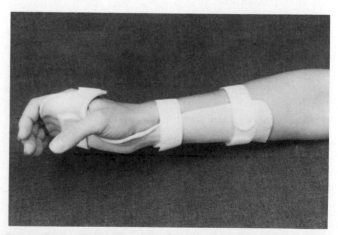

Figure 27.1 Splint to support wrist and metacarpophalangeal joints in extension.

mering, and leather lacing are examples of activities to be avoided. In fact, in all cases, motions in the direction opposite to the deformity or potential deformity are desirable. For example, looper potholder weaving from right to left using the right hand is an acceptable choice of activity because it involves minimal resistance and finger movement in a radial direction.

Avoidance of positions of deformity is a particularly important principle to be aware of when the hands are used functionally since the forces generated during grasp and pinch become increasingly deforming as resistance increases. To avoid this, the hand is used in nonprehensile functional ways if possible, or the joints are supported in a splint to counteract the deforming pull of the muscles (Fig. 13.14), or the motion is done in a way opposite to the deformity. Some examples of this principle are as follows: (a) One correct way to open jars is to stabilize the jar on a wet towel or nonskid pad, place the palm of the right hand on the jar lid, and press down and turn in a radial direction. A better solution is to use a wall-mounted jar opener (Fig. 27.2). (b) Press water from a cloth or sponge rather than wring it. (c) Hold a knife with the blade protruding from the ulnar side of the hand, which pushes the hand toward radial deviation (Fig. 27.3). The knife should be sharp to offer less resistance. (d) Hold stirring spoons so that the bowl of the spoon is on the ulnar side of the hand.

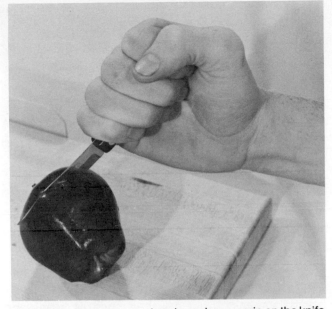

Figure 27.3 Cutting an apple using a dagger-grip on the knife to force the fingers in a radial direction during cutting.

Pressure that pushes the MP joints in an ulnar direction should be avoided. Some examples of ways to avoid it are as follows: (a) Smooth ironing, bedsheets, etc., by moving the flat hand in a radial direction. (b) Turn handles or lids in a radial direction; this may mean using the nondominant hand. (c) When using the hands to assist standing up, avoid putting pressure anywhere except on the heel of the hand and especially avoid the radial side of the index finger. (d) Use adapted tools and utensils in which the handles are angled to eliminate wrist deviation[43] or ulnar deviation of the MP joints. For example, a knife can be adapted by angling the handle 90° to the blade,[44] which prevents ulnar deviation during the cutting process by allowing a dagger grip but still keeping the length of the blade in contact with the food to be cut.

Further testing in the laboratory and clinic needs to be done to establish the effectiveness of these measures to prevent deformities.

The strongest, largest joints available should be used to do a task.[41] The proximal joints are stronger than the distal ones, and their use protects the weaker distal ones. Examples demonstrating this principle are as follows: (a) Slip a pocketbook, shopping bag, or briefcase over the forearm instead of carrying it in the hand. (b) Carry pots, casseroles, or heavy objects by putting one hand and forearm flat underneath and steadying the object with the other. (c) Use forearm platform crutches instead of standard crutches, which require the body weight to be transported by the hands during ambulation.

Use each joint in its most stable and functional plane. For example, avoid twisting the knees when standing up by standing up first and then turning. A splint can be used to hold the fingers in good alignment and to prevent ulnar deviation during hand usage (Fig. 27.4). If constructed from thermoplastic materials, the

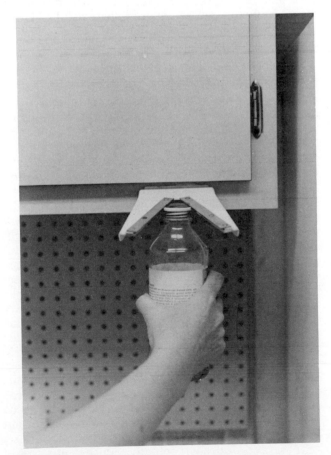

Figure 27.2 Zim jar opener.

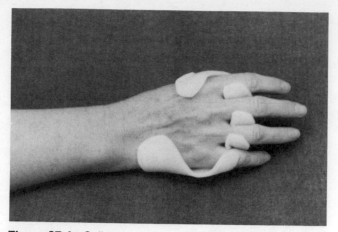

Figure 27.4 Splint to prevent ulnar deviation during hand use.

splint may hinder some activities such as writing but greatly enhance other activities such as lifting and grasping and relieve the patient from the need to constantly monitor activity from a joint protection standpoint.[40,45] Detailed, illustrated directions for construction of this type of splint have been published.[45] A soft version is also sold commercially (Fig. 13.14).

Maintenance or Increase of Strength

Exercise for strengthening is avoided during acute systemic illness[4] and during inflammation of the joints.[30] During the subacute stage, the type of exercise that causes the least pain is used.[4] That is usually isometric exercise.[4,34] One rheumatologist suggests that one maximum contraction per muscle group is enough.[30] Others recommend repetition of the isometric exercise three times per muscle group, once per day.[4,30] The goal is to maintain the static holding ability of muscle so that proper positioning can be maintained during functional activities.[30] Strengthening exercises follow a period of warm-up and are done when pain and stiffness are at a minimum.[30]

Resistive exercise for patients with RA is controversial. Some authorities advocate avoidance of resistance[42] because resistive exercise can neither improve weakened joint structures nor reposition the tendons and because the disease has changed the relationship of the tendons to the axes of movement, causing the forces during resistive isotonic exercise to be deforming. However, Swezey[30] states that there is not enough research to support whether resistive exercises are helpful or harmful in cases of myositis, but to be cautious, he defers resistive exercises until serum enzymes are normal to avoid exacerbating the myositis. Both Flatt[42] and Swezey[30] advocate graduated exercise programs and protection of supporting joint structures during exercise. The graduation of resistance is *very* gradual. In estimating the initial amount of resistance, as well as the graduated increments, it is better to err on the side of too little rather than too much.

Activities to maintain and increase strength should be gently resistive, done for short periods of time within the limits of pain and fatigue, and balanced with rest of the part. Joint protection principles should be adhered to when choosing an activity.[4] Activities that require reaching to pick up objects are good choices for the upper extremities, trunk, and neck. The joints exercised and the extent of the exercise are controlled by the location of the pieces to be picked up. An example is to place pieces for a finger weaving project (Fig. 9.9) in various locations in relation to the patient. He reaches for them and then to another plane to work each piece into the project.

It is important that the patient be kept interested in moving actively throughout the day but within limits. Care should be exercised that the repetitive exercise/activity is not exacerbating the disease. Choice of activity should be such that the activity can be done at home as part of a home program.

Maintenance or Increase of Endurance

Endurance is increased by involving the patient in interesting activities. This provides the opportunity for the patient to learn to gauge his own endurance and to rest before fatigue ensues. Fatigue not only may cause careless use of joints, but also requires a longer rest period, which means longer immobilization. The total day of the patient with RA must be examined to coordinate rest with activity. This balance of rest and activity is carried over to home planning also.

Recreational activities to maintain endurance and to overcome the depression associated with chronic disability and pain, yet which are nonstressful to joints, should be promoted. Swimming is one especially good activity for most persons.[30]

Maintenance or Increase of Skill in Functional Tasks

Principles and methods of self-care and homemaking activities for a patient with limited range of motion are described in Part Five. Essentially, the methods involve the use of long handles to extend reach, joint protection such as that provided by enlarged handles to decrease the grasp force required, and energy conservation. Some other suggestions include the following. A warm morning bath or shower helps the patient overcome stiffness. Sleeping on flannel sheets in the wintertime also may help relieve pain and stiffness in the morning. Zippers with large teeth and ring pull tabs and convex buttons on shanks used with vertical buttonholes have been found easiest to manage by women with RA in remission.[46] A chair with elevated seat height has been found to significantly decrease the stress on hips and knees when rising.[47] Patients with advanced inflammatory polyarthritis may develop such deformities and muscle weakness that a powered wheelchair becomes a necessity.[48]

It is important that the patient learn how to protect his joints during activities of daily living.[5] Any means of substituting for grasp or reducing the force required during functional activities are sought. A study needs to be done collaboratively by O.T.R.s and rehabilitation engineers to determine what handle adaptations (size, softness, and/or design) actually reduce joint stress.

Sex is a functional task and should be discussed with the patient in relation to joint protection and avoidance of pain. Sex presents difficulty to the patient with RA because of pain and joint limitations.[49] The difficulty may not only be related to the mechanics, but also may have to do with fear about the effect sex will have on the condition; guilt feelings connected to the idea that the disease is punishment for some previous wrong; role anxieties related to a change in role due to the disease; or feelings of anger and depression or a poor self-image. There is also a concern with the inability to physically obtain or use certain types of contraceptive methods. There may be worry that the disease is hereditary. Sexual counseling beyond the information concerning joint protection should be available to the patient.[49] Regarding the mechanics, it is recommended that the patient take pain medication beforehand, use cushions to support painful limbs, use positions that are found to be most comfortable,[50] and make other methods of sexual satisfaction an important aspect of intimacy.[49] It is recommended that the patient identify comfortable reclining positions for him or herself and then adapt them for sexual intercourse; the positions should minimize stress on the joints.[51] Sexual intercourse should be avoided during periods of fatigue and during flare-ups of the disease.[52]

Home evaluation and home modifications may be necessary to facilitate daily life tasks. One home assessment program sponsored by the Arthritis Foundation has been helping to remove barriers within homes in Ohio by sponsoring an O.T.R. whose job it is to evaluate the home and make recommendations for change and sources of equipment. Trained volunteers are available to help implement modifications.[53]

Gainful employment can provide the patient with psychosocial and physical benefits, as well as financial benefits.[54] The therapist works with the patient to solve problems related to joint protection and energy conservation while working. The day's routine and specific tasks are reviewed, and each is analyzed to ensure that energy is conserved and joints are protected. If modifications must be made in the work site or method of doing tasks, the patient may authorize, in writing, the O.T.R. to contact management personnel and review with them the patient's needs and requirements to facilitate the modifications to enable return to work.[54]

Living with Rheumatoid Arthritis

When the patient is systemically unwell and has generalized synovitis, he needs to increase his rest periods. However, he must not choose complete bed rest, which can result in weakness, stiffening, and loss of mobility.[5] As the disease activity decreases, he should increase his exercise.[34] In other words, the patient is taught not to push beyond his capacity, but that inactivity is equally undesirable because it starts a cycle of discouragement, depression, and further inactivity.[55]

Energy conservation must become part of the patient's new habit repertoire. Principles of energy conservation include a realization that tired muscles fail to protect damaged joints[32]; use of lightweight, energy-saving equipment; deletion of some jobs; planning ahead to balance rest with exertion; gathering all necessary equipment ahead of time; making storage convenient; and sitting to work when possible. The patient needs to be able to evaluate whether an activity is too much for him to do by noting whether it causes extreme fatigue or causes joint pain that persists for more than 1 hour, or if the activity takes longer than 20 min to complete.[32] An activity that causes too much pain or fatigue can be adjusted so rest breaks are taken during the activity to distribute energy better. Posture and methods of doing the activity can be changed to reduce energy requirements.[32]

Group therapy to deal with issues of disturbance of self-image, body image, job status, family relationships, and coping mechanisms would be useful.[52]

An essential part of the treatment program of a rheumatoid arthritic is a written and rehearsed home program of activity to maintain gains. The therapist carefully explains to the patient and family the rationale for all stages of the treatment program, including the home program. The patient's acceptance of responsibility for his own program is sought. The patient must be educated to the importance of maintaining mobility and protecting his joints throughout life. He therefore must learn the techniques prior to discharge. One outpatient therapy program to promote range of motion utilizes T'ai-Chi Ch'uen in a dance program combined with recital of relaxing verses.[56] Although the disease is characterized by unpredictable exacerbations and remissions, the patient must commit to an ongoing program that balances activity and rest. A 15-minute program of non-weight-bearing active exercise involving four repetitions of movement at each joint was used after researchers observed that joint stiffness/mobility covaried with the rest/activity pattern. The study found that evening exercise was effective in significantly decreasing morning stiffness. The reason for this is that increased synovial volume restricts movement, which is perceived by patients as stiffness, while exercise decreases the synovial volume by increasing lymph flow.[37]

Compliance in an ongoing program of health behaviors for patients with chronic disease is a problem. The more active a patient is in planning and controlling his own care, the greater the chance of successful compliance.[57]

An "Arthritis Club" run by and for persons with arthritis and their families could improve the person's chances of coping successfully with the disease on a long-term day-to-day basis. One such club is described that educates in lay terms, organizes recreational programs, and provides peer counseling and many other services.[58]

Program Examples

Programs have been published that illustrate treatment planning for the shoulders[59] and the hands[11] of RA patients.

The three stages of development of joint damage in the rheumatoid shoulder are as follows. The first stage is simple synovitis, in which there is pain and loss of movement, but the joint structures are normal. In the second stage there is more advanced involvement of the joint, and movement is painful, ROM is decreased, the joint space is narrowed, and erosions are visible on x-ray. The synovium has become proliferative. Rupture of the rotator cuff may occur. There is rarely full functional recovery from this state. The third stage involves advanced joint damage with advanced narrowing of the joint space; the humeral head may be distorted or disappear.[59]

The motions that are affected are hand to back of the head, hand to buttocks, and hand to opposite shoulder.

Treatment during the early stage consists of steroid drugs and gentle mobilizing exercise directed toward recovery of function. Isometric contractions of the shoulder muscles are done three to six times each treatment. The scapula is mobilized with the humerus held immobile as soon as the inflammation diminishes. The shoulder is positioned into abduction to avoid the typical pattern of deformity (adduction and internal rotation) that is adopted because it is comfortable. Movement is done in functional patterns to the limit of pain and without resistance. Mobility exercises and activities to encourage gentle abduction and elevation of the upper limb are used. The shoulder is supported in a sling if painful. Treatment is offered in short periods of increasing frequency to avoid fatigue. Adaptive devices, organization of the work area, support for the shoulder, elimination of tasks, and energy conservation comprise treatment in the later stages. In the final stage, the joint may be surgically replaced if deterioration severely interferes with function.

The progress of disease in the rheumatoid hand proceeds through three stages also: (1) early proliferative stage; (2) a period of regression of synovitis; and (3) stage of fixed deformity.[11] Therapy in the active proliferative stage is aimed at limiting damage caused by the synovitis. Drugs are used to reduce the bulk of the synovium, and the actively involved joints are rested in splints that hold the part in functional position, especially flexion of the MP joints. During the second stage, which is the most important stage in the management of the rheumatoid hand, the goal is to prevent progression of the deformities to a fixed status. As the swelling decreases, stretched capsule and other joint tissues result in joint laxity; in this condition, the joint is vulnerable to abnormal forces. In this stage, therapy includes exercises to encourage strength of the radial interossei, joint protection techniques by which the hands are used in the least damaging way, and extensor exercises to counteract the flexion/extension imbalance caused by stretched extensor tendons whose mechanical effectiveness has decreased. In the third stage, the stage of fixed deformity, treatment is surgical replacement of the joint(s).

Degenerative Joint Disease

Degenerative joint disease, or osteoarthritis (OA), is more common than RA, but less systemically damaging.[2] Whereas rheumatoid arthritis is a relatively recent disease, osteoarthritis is an ancient disease not confined to humans.[60] Men and women are equally likely to be afflicted with OA, but females are more likely to have moderate to severe disease.[60] There is also an increased incidence in those people who do repetitive motions in their jobs.[60]

Osteoarthritis is best characterized as "joint failure," a syndrome rather than a single disease. The pathophysiology remains largely unknown. Primary osteoarthritis, that is, OA arising as the initial disease, is the most common type.[60] This type is due to more than "wear and tear" as once thought,[1] since there are striking biochemical differences between aged cartilage and osteoarthritic cartilage.[60,61] Some of these biochemical changes are loss of proteoglycans, increased water content, decreased aggregations of proteoglycans, and abnormal link proteins.[61] The proteoglycans, which constitute 50% of the dry weight of hyaline cartilage, have great capacity for holding water and give cartilage its remarkable shock absorbancy and lubricating characteristics.[60] In early OA, the water content of cartilage increases, the proteoglycans decrease, and later the collagen is disrupted. Without protection of the proteoglycans, the surface of the collagen fibers becomes rough, resulting in friction on movement that eventually causes the cartilage to destruct. The destruction is mediated by enzymes. As cartilage destructs, compensatory changes in subchondral bone develop and marginal osteophytes (e.g., Heberden's nodes) develop. The bald surface of the subchrondral bone (without cartilaginous covering) cannot withstand stress and becomes eroded, although there is usually evidence of biochemical changes resulting from failed attempts at repair.[60] Primary OA results from an interplay among genetic factors, enzymantic changes in the cartilage, and micro/macro trauma to the joint.[60] Secondary OA develops as a result of chronic or acute trauma, mechanical derangement of the joint (dysplasia, congential abnormality), or articular lesion due to infection or other disorders that attack the articular cartilage directly.[60]

Common sites of osteoarthritis are hands, cervical spine, lumbar spine, hips, knees, ankles, and feet.[61] Treatment has three levels: nonpharmalogical or conservative, pharmalogical, and surgical. Suggestions for conservative treatment (exercise and adaptations) of the hands will be discussed here, and the reader is referred to the published source for specifics related to the other joints.[61]

Primary OA of the hands is characterized by pain and swelling affecting the DIP and PIP joints of the fingers and the first carpometacarpal (CMC) joints, especially of middle-aged, perimenopausal women.[61]

Occupational therapy treatment includes: (1) splinting to relieve pain; (2) compression to reduce swelling; (3) exercise to maintain ROM and strength; (4) joint protection techniques to prevent deformity; (5) teaching adapted techniques to maintain functional independence; (6) assistance with psychosocial adjustment to this chronic disease; and (7) splinting and remobilization after implant surgery in late stage disease.

Because osteoarthritis, in contrast to rheumatoid arthritis, may involve a single joint, splints are used to rest only the particular joint(s) that is painful. The rest position is the functional position. Splinting is also used to support a joint, especially the CMC joint of the thumb, during functional use.[4,62]

Compression can be done using a Coban® or similar bandage (see chapter 9) or using cloth stretch gloves (Isotoner®), which are most appropriately used at night. Exercise to maintain ROM is particularly directed at thumb adduction, a common deformity.[60] Active ROM exercises should be done for each motion of the hand, preferably with the hand submerged in warm water, 20 times, once or twice per day.[61] ROM exercises can be preceded by paraffin baths or warm water soaks[61] if the exercises are not done in water. Moist heat should be avoided for those with concomitant diabetes or peripheral vascular disease.[61] To maintain and increase strength, isometric, not isotonic, exercise should be done.[60] Maintaining grasp strength is particularly important because the patient has a tendency to eliminate the thumb from grasp,[60] which eliminates 50% of hand function. Practice in grasping handles of various sizes and shapes is recommended.[60] Joint protection treatment focuses on relieving the joints of stress. The therapist should obtain a careful history of hand use in order to focus this aspect of treatment. Treatment can include advising the patient to temporarily stop those motions (pinching, grasping, wringing) or those activities that aggravate the joints and/or to wear gloves while doing some tasks (dishes, gardening, etc.) to decrease microtrauma.[60] Another means of joint protection is to adapt handles of frequently used tools and utensils, as suggested above for RA, to decrease joint stress. Patient education is crucial to the success of the measures used to achieve or maintain functional independence.[61] Education should include not only the use of adapted techniques and equipment, as discussed in chapter 17, but also the need to balance moderate exercise with rest, to avoid overactivity, and to maintain daily activities within pain and fatigue tolerances. The exercise program for home use should be practiced with the patient under supervision.

Surgery is considered when significant pain and functional limitations persist despite other treatment measures.[61] In the hand, the first CMC joint of the thumb is most likely to require surgery to relieve the pain and to improve grasp. The surgical procedure may be an arthroplasty with Silastic spacer or prosthetic implant. If a strong grasp is required and ROM is secondary, an arthrodesis is done. Similar surgical options exist for the MP and PIP joints; DIP joints can only be fused.[60,61] See chapter 25 for postsurgical therapy.

STUDY QUESTIONS:

Arthritis

1. Compare and contrast the pathology of rheumatoid arthritis (RA) with that of osteoarthritis.

2. What is the philosophy of treatment of patients with chronic, degenerative diseases?
3. What are the five characteristic manifestations of inflammation?
4. What assessments are considered in the evaluation of patients with RA?
5. How is ligamentous stability of the fingers evaluated?
6. How is it determined that the intrinsic muscles of the fingers have become abnormally shortened?
7. Describe the underlying process of finger metacarpophalangeal deformities.
8. Discuss the controversy concerning use of resistance with RA patients.
9. Name some nonprehensile and prehensile functions of the hand.
10. What are the occupational therapy goals for patients with RA during the acute stage?
11. What are the goals during the subacute stage?
12. What are the positions of deformity that RA patients are educated to avoid?
13. List the joint protection principles.
14. What are the components of a home program for patients with RA?
15. What are some research studies that need to be done by occupational therapists relative to treatment of arthritic patients?
16. What are the different etiological factors between primary and secondary osteoarthritis?
17. What are the goals of occupational therapy treatment for the patient with osteoarthritis?

References

1. Rodnon, G. P., editor. *Primer on the Rheumatic Diseases*, 7th edition. Reprinted from *JAMA 224* (Suppl.5), 1973. Distributed by The Arthritis Foundation, 1212 Avenue of the Americas, New York, NY 10036.
2. National Institute of Arthritis, Metabolism, and Digestive Diseases. *How to Cope with Arthritis.* DHEW Publication No. (NIH) 78-1092. Washington, DC: U.S. Government Printing Office, 1978.
3. Salter, R. B. *Textbook of Disorders and Injuries of the Musculoskeletal System.* Baltimore: Williams & Wilkins, 1983.
4. Melvin, J. L. *Rheumatic Disease: Occupational Therapy and Rehabilitation*, 2nd edition. Philadelphia: F. A. Davis, 1982.
5. Edmonds, J. The management of rheumatoid arthritis. *Aust. Fam. Phys.,* 7(8): 925–935, 1978.
6. Barrows, D. M., Berezny, L. M., and Reynolds, M. D. Physical and occupational therapy for arthritic patients: a cooperative effort among hospital departments. *Arch. Phys. Med. Rehabil.,* 59(2): 64–67, 1978.
7. Feinberg, J. R., and Brandt, K. D. Allied health team management of rheumatoid arthritis patients. *Am. J. Occup. Ther.,* 38(9): 613–620, 1984.
8. Gross, M., et al. Team care for patients with chronic rheumatic disease. *J. Allied Health,* 15(11): 239–247, 1982.
9. AOTA Commission on Practice. Roles and functions of occupational therapy in the management of patients with rheumatic diseases. *Am. J. Occup. Ther.,* 40(12): 825–829, 1986.
10. English, C. B., and Nalebuff, E. A. Understanding the arthritic hand. *Am. J. Occup. Ther.,* 25(7): 353–358, 1971.
11. Kay, A. G. L. Management of the rheumatoid hand. *Rheumatol. Rehabil.,* 18(Suppl. 1): 76–81, 1979.
12. Feinberg, J., and Brandt, K. D. Use of resting splints by patients with rheumatoid arthritis. *Am. J. Occup. Ther.,* 35(3): 173–178, 1981.
13. Hasselkus, B. R., Kshepakaran, K. K., and Safrit, M. J. Handedness and hand joint changes in rheumatoid arthritis. *Am. J. Occup. Ther.,* 35(11): 705–710, 1981.
14. Swezey, R. L. Dynamic factors in deformity of the rheumatoid arthritic hand. *Bull. Rheum. Dis.,* 22(1 and 2): 651–654, 1971–72. The Arthritis Foundation, 1212 Avenue of the Americas, New York, NY 10036.
15. Tubiana, R., Thomine, J. M., and Mackin, E. *Examination of the Hand and Upper Limb.* Philadelphia: W. B. Saunders, 1984.
16. Pahle, J. A., and Raunio, P. The influence of wrist position on finger deviation in the rheumatoid hand. *J. Bone Joint Surg.,* 5(4): 664–676, 1969.

17. Smith, E. M., Juvinall, R. C., Bender, L. F., and Pearson, J. R. Role of the finger flexors in rheumatoid deformities of the metacarpophalangeal joints. *Arthritis Rheum., 7*(5): 467–480, 1964.
18. Swezey, R. L., and Fiegenberg, D. S. Inappropriate intrinsic muscle action in the rheumatoid hand. *Ann. Rheum. Dis., 30:* 619–625, 1971.
19. Wozny, W., and Long, C. Electromyographic kinesiology of the rheumatoid hand. *Arch. Phys. Med. Rehabil., 47*(11): 702–703, 1966.
20. Shapiro, J.S. The etiology of ulnar drift: a new factor. *J. Bone Joint Surg., 50A:* 634, 1968.
21. Swanson, A. B. Flexible implant arthroplasty for arthritic finger joints. *J. Bone Joint Surg., 54A*(3): 435–455, 1972.
22. Vignos, P. J. Editorial: physiotherapy in rheumatoid arthritis. *J. Rheumatol., 7*(3): 269–271, 1980.
23. Fike, M. L., and Rousseau, E. Measurement of adult hand strength: a comparison of two instruments. *Occup. Ther. J. Res., 2*(1): 43–49, 1982.
24. Thorngren, K. D., and Werner, D. O. Normal grip strength. *Acta Orthop. Scand., 50:* 255–259, 1979.
25. Swanson, A. B., Matev, I. B., and DeGroot, G. The strength of the hand. *Inter-Clinic Information Bulletin, 13*(10): 1–8, 1974.
26. Badley, E. M., Lee, J., and Wood, P. H. N. Patterns of disability related to joint involvement in rheumatoid arthritis. *Rheumatol. Rehabil., 18*(2): 105–109, 1979
27. Jebsen, R. H., et al. An objective and standardized test of hand function. *Arch. Phys. Med. Rehabil., 50*(6): 311–319, 1969.
28. Carthum, C. J., Clawson, D. K., and Decker, J. L. Functional assessment of the rheumatoid hand. *Am. J. Occup. Ther., 23*(2): 122–125, 1969.
29. Walker, P. S., Davidson, W., and Erkman, M. J. An apparatus to assess function of the hand. *J. Hand Surg., 3*(2): 189–193, 1978.
30. Swezey, R. L. Rehabilitation aspects in arthritis. In *Arthritis and Allied Conditions,* 9th edition. Edited by D. J. McCarty. Philadelphia: Lea & Febiger, 1979.
31. Furst, G. P., et al. A program for improving energy conservation behaviors in adults with rheumatoid arthritis. *Am. J. Occup. Ther., 41*(2): 102–111, 1987.
32. Furst, G. P., Gerber, L. H., and Smith, C. B. *Rehabilitation Through Learning: Energy Conservation and Joint Protection—A Workbook for Persons with Rheumatoid Arthritis.* Publication No. 017-045-00107-4. Washington, DC: U.S. Government Printing Office, 1987.
33. Long, C. Lecture. Highland View Hospital, Cleveland, Ohio. June 1962.
34. Glass, J. Physical medicine in rheumatology. *Aust. N.Z. J. Med., 8*(Suppl.1): 168–171, 1978.
35. Mirabelli, L. Pain management. In *Neurological Rehabilitation.* Edited by D. A. Umphred. St. Louis: C.V. Mosby, 1985.
36. McKnight, P. T., and Schomburg, F. L. Air pressure splint effects on hand symptoms of patients with rheumatoid arthritis. *Arch. Phys. Med. Rehabil., 63*(11): 560–564, 1982.
37. Byers, P. H. Effect of exercise on morning stiffness and mobility in patients with rheumatoid arthritis. *Research in Nursing & Health, 8:* 275–281, 1985.
38. Davis, J., and Janecki, C. J. Rehabilitation of the rheumatoid upper limb. *Orthop. Clin. North Am., 9*(2): 559–568, 1978.
39. Kaplan, E. B. *Functional and Surgical Anatomy of the Hand.* Philadelphia: J. B. Lippincott, 1965.
40. Hanten, D. W. The splinting controversy in rheumatoid arthritis. *The American Occupational Therapy Association Physical Disabilities Special Interest Section Newsletter, 5*(4): 1–3, 1982.
41. Cordery, J. Joint protection: a responsibility of the occupational therapist. *Am. J. Occup. Ther., 19*(5): 285–294, 1965.
42. Flatt, A. E. *The Care of the Rheumatoid Hand,* 3rd edition. St. Louis: C. V. Mosby, 1974.
43. Tichauer, E. R. Some aspects of stress on forearm and hand in industry. *J. Occup. Med., 8*(2): 63–71, 1966.
44. Moore, J. W. Adapted knife for rheumatoid arthritics. *Am. J. Occup. Ther., 32*(2): 112–113, 1978.
45. Quest, I. M., and Cordery, J. A functional ulnar deviation cuff for rheumatoid deformity. *Am. J. Occup. Ther., 25*(1): 32–37,40, 1971.

46. Dallas, M. J., and White, L. W. Clothing fasteners for women with arthritis. *Am. J. Occup. Ther., 36*(8): 515–518, 1982.
47. Burdett, R. G., et al. Biomechanical comparison of rising from two types of chairs. *Phys. Ther., 65*(8): 1177–1183, 1985.
48. Bossingham, D. H., and Russell, P. The usefulness of powered wheelchairs in advanced inflammatory polyarthritis. *Rheumatol. Rehabil., 19*(2): 131–135, 1980.
49. Greengross, W. Sex and arthritis. *Rheumatol. Rehabil., 18*(Suppl.1): 68–70, 1979.
50. Frederick, B. B. et al. *Body Mechanics Instruction Manual: A Guide for Therapists.* Redmond, WA: Express Publications, 1979.
51. Onder, J., Lachniet, D., and Becker, M. C. Sexual counselling, arthritis, and women. *Allied Health Professions Section Newsletter, 7*(3 and 4): 1–6, 1973. Distributed by the Arthritis Foundation, 1212 The Avenue of the Americas, New York, NY 10036.
52. Krawitz, M., and Wolman, T. Group therapy in rheumatoid arthritis. *Pennsylvania Med., 82*(12): 35–37, 1979.
53. Lund, N. W. Arthritis home assessment program. *The American Occupational Therapy Association Physical Disabilities Special Interest Section Newsletter, 7*(3): 3, 1984.
54. Budic, C. Arthritis and employment on-site job intervention. *The American Occupational Therapy Association Physical Disabilities Special Interest Section Newsletter, 3*(1): 1–2, 1980.
55. Schwaid, M. C. Advice to arthritics: keep moving. *Am. J. Nurs. 78:* 1708–1709, 1978.
56. Van Deusen, J., and Harlowe, D. The efficacy of the ROM dance program for adults with rheumatoid arthritis. *Am. J. Occup. Ther., 41*(2): 90–95, 1987.
57. Hasselkus, B. R. Emerging trends in geriatric care. *O.T. Week,* February 19, 1987, pp. 5–6.
58. Gatter, R. A., Richmond, J. D., and Andrews, R. P. Arthritis community outreach program. *N. Engl. J. Med., 301*(1): 52, 1979.
59. Simon, L. Rehabilitation of the rheumatoid shoulder. *Rheumatol. Rehabil., 18*(Suppl.-1): 81–85, 1979.
60. Swanson, A. B., and Swanson, G. DeG. Osteoarthritis in the hand. *Clinics in Rheumatic Diseases, 11*(2): 393–420, 1985.
61. Quinet, R. J. Osteoarthritis: increasing mobility and reducing disability. *Geriatrics, 41*(2): 36–50, 1986.
62. Barsamian, P. *More Splinting with Aquaplast.* Ramsey, NJ: WFR/Aquaplast Corp., 1983.

Supplementary Reading

Brandt, K. D. Management of osteoarthritis. In *Textbook of Rheumatology.* Edited by W. N. Kelley, E. D. Harris, S. Ruddy, and C. B. Sledge. Philadelphia: W. B. Saunders, 1985.

Brattström, M. *Joint Protection and Rehabilitation in Chronic Rheumatic Disorders.* Rockville, MD: Aspen Publications, 1987.

Burckhardt, C. S. The impact of arthritis on quality of life. *Nursing Res., 34*(1): 11–16, 1985.

Cone, D. M. Clothing needs of elderly arthritic women. *Educational Gerontology, 10:* 441–448, 1984.

Hadler, N. M. Industrial rheumatology: clinical investigation into the influence of the pattern of usage on the pattern of regional musculoskeletal disease. *Arthritis Rheum., 20*(4): 1019–1025, 1977.

Home Care Programs in Arthritis: A Manual for Patients. The Arthritis Foundation, 1212 The Avenue of the Americas, New York, NY 10036.

MacBain, K. P., Galbraith, M., and Brady, F. *Nonoperative Hand Management of Adult Onset Rheumatoid Arthritis.* The Arthritis Society, B.C. Division, 895 West 10th Avenue, Vancouver, BC V5Z1L7, 1981.

Meenan, R. F., Gertman, P. M., and Mason, J. H. Measuring health status in arthritis: The Arthritis Impact Measurement Scales. *Arthritis Rheum., 23*(2): 146–152, 1980.

Moskowitz, R. W., et al. *Osteoarthritis: Diagnosis and Management.* Philadelphia: W. B. Saunders, 1984.

University of Michigan Pilot Geriatric Arthritis Program, *Joint Protection for Osteoarthritis.*

University of Michigan Pilot Geriatric Arthritis Program, *Osteoarthritis.*

chapter
28

Spinal Cord Injury

Catherine A. Trombly

The spinal cord contains the neural connecting tracts that transmit sensory and motor impulses to and from the brain and the cell bodies of the motor neurons. Disease or injury to the spinal cord will affect the sensory motor function of the person in that lower motor neuron signs will be seen at the site of the lesion due to destruction of anterior horn cells or peripheral nerves (cauda equina), and upper motor neuron signs will be visible below the level of the lesion if the sensory and motor tracts are interrupted. Spinal cord function can be disrupted by disease, such as multiple sclerosis or amyotrophic lateral sclerosis; by tumors; by congenital deformities, such as myelomeningocele; or by trauma, such as automobile accidents, gunshot wounds, knife wounds, or diving accidents. Some causes of spinal cord dysfunction, such as multiple sclerosis, may also involve brain dysfunction. This chapter will concentrate on therapy for the traumatic spinal cord-injured (SCI) patient. Patients with only spinal cord injury do not have brain damage; therefore, cognition, perception, and voluntary control of muscles above the lesion site are intact. The ideas presented in this chapter are selectively appropriate for patients with other types of spinal cord dysfunction.

Seven to eight thousand patients survive traumatic spinal cord injury each year.[1] It is estimated that there is a population of 500,000 SCI persons in the United States[2] (30–35 per 1,000,000[3]), 53% of whom are quadriplegic.[1,3]

Unless the cord is physically cut, as in knife or gunshot wounds, the usual injury is a vertebral fracture in which the cord is squeezed by the damaged or displaced vertebrae. The injury can be complete (no function below the level of the lesion) or incomplete (sparing of sensory and/or motor function below the lesion level). Innervation of muscles is arranged in an orderly progression so that the lower the location of the lesion, the more upper-extremity (proximal to distal), trunk, and finally lower-extremity musculature is preserved. Spinal cord injury is designated by the last segmental level of the cord that is preserved. For example, C_6 quadri-

plegia (complete) designates that all motor, sensory, and autonomic functions mediated by the nervous system at the sixth cervical level of the cord and above are preserved. Injuries to the cord may be diagonal, which results in greater preservation of function on one side of the body than on the other. In this case, both levels are noted. For example, $C_{5,6}$ means that the functions of the fifth cervical segment are preserved on one side and those of the sixth on the other. There are no shorthand methods of labeling for incomplete lesions with distal sparing.

In one type of incomplete lesion, the functions of the central cord are preserved, while the functions of the peripheral cord are lost below the lesion level. This results in sparing of the lower-extremity function because of the location of the tracts serving these limbs within the cord. Sacral sparing is confirmed by evidence of perianal sensation and active toe flexion.[4]

Effective emergency and immediate care of SCI patients have increased the number of patients coming for rehabilitation and their functional potential.[10] The preservation of one additional spinal cord segment can contribute significantly to the functional capabilities of the patient (see Table 28.1). For that reason, improved handling at the accident scene and transportation techniques are now in common usage for persons suspected of having spinal injury.

Clinical Picture

Spinal cord injury is a physically and psychologically devastating disability. The injury usually precipitates an abrupt change from vigorous activity to infantile dependency that plummets the patient and his family into depression, distress, and denial.

The immediate consequence of spinal cord injury is spinal shock, which may last several days to weeks. It is characterized by areflexia of the limbs, bowel, and bladder.[5] As soon as spinal shock subsides, two types of motor responses are seen: reflex spasticity below the level of lesion and recovery of strength of muscles innervated above the level of lesion. The nervous sys-

Table 28.1

EXPECTED ACHIEVEMENT AND SUGGESTED METHODS FOR SPINAL CORD-INJURED PATIENTS

Last Fully Innervated Level and Key Muscles Added	Movements the Patient Can Do	Achievement	Technique and/or Equipment
C_1, C_2, C_3 Facial and neck muscles innervated by cranial nerves	Chew Swallow Talk Blow	Self-care None	a. Needs respirator. Phrenic nerve stimulator may be used in daytime.[4]
		Mobility 1. W/c locomotion	a. Electronically controlled electric w/c with gradual acceleration feature[11] and safety belt; can use sip and puff or microswitch controls. b. May need corset; cushion needed.
		2. Recline	a. Electronically controlled reclining electric w/c.[5]
		Communication 1. Typing	a. Electric typewriter and mouthstick or sip and puff controls. b. Paper on a roll.[48]
		2. Writing 3. Word processing	c. Mouthstick.[2] d. Microcomputer with adapted interface and help with disk loading. e. Protractible mouthstick to push buttons.[12,50]
		4. Telephoning	a. Automatic telephone dialer.[32,48] b. Speaker phone.[49] c. Operator's headset.
		Recreation 1. Games	a. Computer games. b. Electronic games.[51] c. Table games with grasp-type mouthstick.[2]
		2. Art	a. Mouthstick painting (after set up).
		3. Reading 4. Other	a. Turn pages with mouthstick.[2] a. Environmental control unit to control TV power and channel selection, stereo, electric bed, nurse call, lamp, etc.[32,49]
		Vocation	a. Minicomputer with assistance. b. Calculator. c. Mouthstick.
C_4 Diaphragm Trapezius	Respiration Scapular elevation	Self-care 1. Some feeding	a. Mobile arm supports, which may need to have a powered elbow. b. Externally powered flexor hinge hand splint for the stronger extremity.[48,49] Long opponens with double "T" bars for other, assistive extremity. c. Lapboard. A plexiglass lapboard is preferred for patients who use an electric w/c so they can see where their feet are and avoid bumping them while traveling. d. Plate guard or scoop dish so the food can be "captured." e. Long straw with a strawholder because the patient cannot pick up the glass.

Table 28.1—*Continued*

Last Fully Innervated Level and Key Muscles Added	Movements the Patient Can Do	Achievement	Technique and/or Equipment
			f. Swivel "spork" with built-up, friction handle.[48]
			g. The dish may need to be elevated off the lapboard until the patient gains skills. The dish must be stabilized by a nonskid pad or wet towel.
		Mobility Locomotion and weight shift	a. Electronically controlled w/c with reclining back; controls can be sip and puff,[5] chin switches,[32] or switches mounted on the lapboard or in a shoulder harness. A gradual acceleration accessory on the w/c to prevent sudden starts and a seat belt are good safety measures.
			b. Cushion.
			c. Trunk support if necessary.[52]
		Communication 1. Typing	a. Electric ball-type typewriter with automatic pushbutton return; can be used with a mouthstick or sip and puff controls.
			b. Self-correcting ribbon.[48]
			c. Paper in roll[48] or use a modified mouthstick to put the paper in.[48,53]
			d. Some patients use a rubber-tipped stick held in the splint to type.
			e. A good bookstand is a commercially available industrial catalogue rack.[53]
		2. Telephoning	a. Automatic telephone dialer.[32,48]
			b. Speaker phone.[48]
		3. Note taking in school or business	a. Adapted tape recorder that must have electronic switching to allow adaptation to remote pushbutton control unit.
		4. Control appliances	a. Environmental control units.[32,48,49,54] An ultrasound remote control unit that can take 16 appliances and can summon aid from nearby house has been developed.[53]
		Vocation	a. Minicomputer with assistance.
			b. Calculator.
			c. Mouthstick.
		Recreation 1. Table games	a. The same orthotic equipment used for feeding can be used to move playing pieces, which may need to be adapted as to size, shape, or texture.[55]
		2. Painting or drawing.	a. Mouthstick with brush or pencil attached. A battery-operated oral telescoping orthosis with a mouthpiece that covers the complete dentition has been developed; it has interchangeable terminal pieces.[56]

Table 28.1—*Continued*

Last Fully Innervated Level and Key Muscles Added	Movements the Patient Can Do	Achievement	Technique and/or Equipment
C₅ Biceps Brachialis[6] Brachioradialis[6] Supinator[6] Infraspinatus[6] Deltoid	Elbow flexion and supination Shoulder external rotation Shoulder abduction to 80-90° Gravity provides: shoulder adduction pronation internal rotation	All of the above tasks are done more easily.	The patient may not need some adaptations and may be able to use others. He will not need a powered elbow on the mobile arm support (MAS); some patients get strong enough to discard the MAS altogether in time. A ratchet splint can be used in lieu of external power and when functional wrist extension is lacking.[12,47,57] The controls of the electric bed can be lever type adaptations to the regular controls, which the patient operates by elbow flexion.[58]
C₆ Pectoralis major Serratus anterior Latissimus dorsi Pronator teres Radial wrist extensors	Shoulder flexion Reach forward Shoulder internal rotation and extension Shoulder adduction More respiratory reserve (accessory breathing muscles) Pronation Wrist extension (tenodesis grasp)	Self-care 1. Feeding 2. Dressing	a. May use a universal cuff, thread the utensil through his fingers ("interlacing grip"[43]), or use a wrist-driven flexor hinge hand splint; does not use MAS, but may need to initially. b. Rocker knife or very sharp paring knife for cutting. c. Does not need long straw; may use cup or mug with a large handle. d. Does not need plate guard. a. Uses flexor hinge hand splint when pinch is necessary. If wrist extension only rates P to F a SAFRA (Sequential Advancing Flexion Retention Attachment) locking mechanism can be added to a standard flexor hinge splint.[59] b. Dresses lower extremities in bed as described in chapter 17. Uses momentum and substitute movements to turn over, sit up, pull up clothing.[60] c. Uses button hook and zipper pull. d. Cannot tie shoes. e. Clothes should be of correct size or one size larger.
		3. Bathing and grooming	a. Uses bath mitt with a pocket to hold the soap. b. In a tub or shower, the patient sits on a padded shower bench. Faucets must be within reach. c. In tub or shower, uses a hand-held spray attachment to rinse and to shampoo. d. Toothbrushing, shaving, makeup can all be done using the pinch of the flexor hinge splint.
		4. Bowel and bladder care	a. Uses bowel routine, inserts suppositories with adapted device.[48] b. May be independent in transfer to toilet or commode chair. A transfer commode seat may be necessary.[61] c. Self-catherization may be an option for the patient.[5,16]

Table 28.1—*Continued*

Last Fully Innervated Level and Key Muscles Added	Movements the Patient Can Do	Achievement	Technique and/or Equipment
			d. If external drainage for urine is used, the patient learns to apply the drainage system, which usually consists of a condom, tubing, and storage bag.
			e. May need adapted means to clamp and unclamp the tubing and to empty the drainage bag.[62]
		Mobility	
		1. Locomotion	a. Pushes standard wheelchair with friction material on the rims or by using push mitt.[63] He may need projection knobs on the rims in the beginning.[11] An electric wheelchair would be required if the person had to wheel long distances.[63]
		2. Transfer	a. Uses a transfer board and partial depression or swivel transfer. Assistance may be needed.
		3. Bed mobility	a. Independent in rolling over[63] and sitting up using the method described in chapter 17.
			b. Loops attached to the overhead bed frame may be needed initially to come to sitting position.[63]
		4. Automobile	a. May be able to drive a car adapted with hand controls, and "U" shaped cuff attached to steering wheel.
			b. Will need assistance (human or mechanical) to put the wheelchair into the car.
		Communication	
		1. Writing	a. Can hold the pencil using the wrist-driven flexor hinge hand splint or a special writing splint that abducts the thumb and holds the pencil in place.[64]
		2. Typing	a. Can put paper into the typewriter.
			b. Uses an electric typewriter with push button return.
			c. May use typing splints that fit over the index fingers only[65] or use typing sticks with the flexor hinge splint or universal cuff.
		3. Note taking	a. Can use adapted tape recorder.[66]
			b. Can write short notes as above.
		4. Telephoning	a. Can use a standard phone, dialing with a pencil held in a universal cuff or threaded through the fingers.
		Recreation	a. Can turn radio, TV, etc., on and off.
			b. Can play table games with some adaptation.[67]
			c. Can participate in some w/c sports.
		Vocation	a. Homebound work is most practical.
			b. Cannot use hand tools that require strength.
			c. Electronic office machines are very well suited to these patients.

Table 28.1—*Continued*

Last Fully Innervated Level and Key Muscles Added	Movements the Patient Can Do	Achievement	Technique and/or Equipment
			d. Is able to independently relieve pressure while in the wheelchair; therefore is able to work out of the home.
			e. Homemaking: at best can be an assistive homemaker. Can only do some cooking and light cleaning with great expenditure of energy and time. Needs w/c accessible kitchen.
C_7 Triceps Extrinsic finger extensors Flexor carpi radialis	Elbow extension Active finger extension (tenodesis grasp) Wrist flexion	Self-care 1. Feeding 2. Dressing 3. Bathing and grooming 4. Bowel and bladder Mobility 1. Locomotion 2. Bed mobility 3. Transfers 4. Driving Communication Recreation Vocation	 Independent Independent with aid of buttonhook. Same as for C_6 but easier. Same as for C_6 but easier. Wheels standard chair easily. Independent. Independent using depression transfer; does push-ups to relieve ischial pressure. Uses adapted car; may need help getting the wheelchair into the car. Independent without adapted equipment. Games without adaptation; w/c sports. Same as for C_6, but easier.
C_8T_1 Intrinsics including thumb Ulnar wrist flexors and extensors Extrinsic finger and thumb flexors Extrinsic thumb extensor	Full upper-extremity control including fine coordination and strong grasp	1. Independent in feeding, dressing, bathing, bowel and bladder care, skin inspection, locomotion 2. Work 3. Housekeeping	Uses minimal adapted equipment. Homebound work or work in a building free of architectural barriers. Travel by private car, or accessible public transportation. Can do light housekeeping independently, but this is time-consuming. Needs a wheelchair-accessible house.
T_6 Top half of intercostals Long muscles of the back	Increased endurance due to larger respiratory reserve Pectoral girdle stabilized for heavy lifting Better trunk control	1. Independent in all self-care 2. Work 3. Sports 4. Housekeeping	Will use full braces (including trunk and pelvic bracing) and a standing aid for physiological standing only. Can ambulate with *great* difficulty, on level surface, but this is not practical for locomotion. Can work with tools and do fairly heavy lifting from a sedentary position. Active wheelchair sports (basketball, archery, hunting, etc.). Independent but needs help with seasonal cleaning. Needs a wheelchair-accessible house.

Table 28.1—Continued

Last Fully Innervated Level and Key Muscles Added	Movements the Patient Can Do	Achievement	Technique and/or Equipment
T_{12} Full innervations of intercostals Abdominal musculature	Better endurance Better trunk control	1. Independent in self-care, work, sports, housekeeping when architectural barriers do not prevent independence. 2. Locomotion	 Chooses wheelchair for energy conservation. Ambulates with difficulty using long-leg braces and crutches. A new lightweight KAO that can be worn with lightweight athletic shoes has been developed[68] that would reduce the energy requirement for ambulation. Can use ride-on snow plow, grass cutter, etc. if adapted with hand controls.
L_4 Low back muscles Hip flexors Quadriceps	Hip flexion Knee extension	1. Independent in all activities plus ambulation.	Uses canes to prevent deforming effects of gait (recurvatum of knee and lumbar lordosis), which could cause, in time, degenerative arthritis. Uses short-leg braces with dorsiflexion stop. Wheelchair may still be a convenience at work and at home. Bowel and bladder control is not voluntary.

tems of patients with neurological lesions undergo synaptic reorganization and rewiring, which may explain some of the recovery phenomena.[6] There is enhanced synaptic transmission within the monosynaptic stretch reflex, which contributes to spasticity, and collateral sprouting of viable neurons, which contributes to adaptive sensory and motor recovery responses.[6] Recovery continues for approximately 1 year.

In addition to the spasticity and loss of motor control below the level of lesion, there are many other sequelae, including loss of sensory awareness and discrimination below lesion level; loss of control of bowel, bladder, and sexual functions; and, in high-level lesions (16% of patients have C_1 to C_4 level lesions[2]), there is loss or dysfunction of autonomic control of body temperature and blood pressure.

Many complications can arise from these sequelae and must be carefully attended to in order to ensure that the patient does not lose potential functional ability because of their effects. Some of the complications that directly affect therapy are listed here.

In time, spasticity may develop into spasms, either clonic or tonic. Spasms are usually triggered by a certain sensory stimulus, such as infection, sudden touch, or other irritation. Mild spasms can be controlled by ensuring that the patient is free of the triggering stimuli. Clonus, spasmodic alternation of contraction of agonist and antagonist, can be stopped by holding the part steady for a few moments, which dampens the oscillations. Some patients use their spasms to accomplish certain functions, and they learn to trigger them in a controlled way. Severe spasms, however, may interfere with the achievement of independence, and medical or surgical relief may be required.

Contractures tend to develop in patterns of spasticity and in each joint that is not kept mobile by either active or passive range of motion exercises. Heterotopic ossification (paraosteoarthroplasty or POA) may occur in muscle or other connective tissue innervated below the level of lesion due to too much (or too little) exercise, although these causative factors are as yet unproven.[7,8] Common sites are elbow and hip, but it has also been reported in hands of quadriplegics.[8,9] This complication limits use of the extremity and decreases functional independence. Surgical removal provides at least temporary relief; however, there is a tendency for recurrence.

High-level lesions (C_{1-4}) damage the phrenic nerve, and paralysis of the diaphragm is the result. These patients must be artificially respirated at all times. Although chest respirators are the most common method of doing this, phrenic nerve stimulators have been developed by rehabilitation engineers and are used by some because they allow elimination of the bulky respirator during part of the day.[10] They can only be used if the anterior horn cells of the phrenic nerve are intact.[4] The stimulator paces the diaphragm with an electrical impulse to the phrenic nerve.[10] These patients and others with lesions at T_6 and above require therapy for hygiene of their lungs.[5] They are unable to cough to rid themselves of the waste in their lungs as persons with normally innervated respiratory muscles are able to do.

High-level SCI patients (above T_7)[7] suffer from severely disturbed autonomic function. An emergency associated with this is called sympathetic hyperreflexia[11] or autonomic dysreflexia[12] in which the sympathetic nervous system is bombarded with noxious impulses,[12] causing the blood pressure of the patient to rise dangerously. *It can be fatal if not treated promptly.* The patient may exhibit some or all of these symptoms: he is flushed, restless, perspiring, nauseous,[11] chilled, has increased spasticity, and headache.[13] The stimulus may be bowel or bladder distension, the latter being more common. If it should occur while the patient is in therapy, immediately check to see if the patient's catheter is unclamped and free flowing. If not, unclamp it and tap briskly once or twice over the bladder in an attempt to cause the bladder to spontaneously empty. If the catheter is unclamped, but not freely flowing, remove any kinks in the tubing and squeeze it several times in an effort to dislodge a plug. However, lose no time in calling the nurse or physician whether the crisis seems to pass or not. In the meantime, do not recline the patient because this will increase the already high cerebral blood pressure. Eventually patients learn to recognize the onset of symptoms early, what the triggering stimulus is, and how to guide the person who assists them.

High-level quadriplegic patients also cannot regulate their temperature automatically and need to be artificially kept warm in winter and cool in summer. The latter is especially important because hyperthermia may ensue. Exercise should be discontinued if air conditioning is unavailable and the patient is experiencing a rise in body temperature.

The lack of sensory awareness coupled with the reduced blood flow to tissue results in a propensity to develop decubiti from prolonged pressure.[5,11] At all times, *and for the rest of his life*, the patient must be constantly vigilant against this.

Decubiti develop in stages; therefore, recognition of early stages of decubitus formation will allow early treatment and can prevent loss of rehabilitation time. In stage I, the area stays red for 20 to 30 min and may be warm to the touch, but the skin is intact. This is the warning that whatever device is causing pressure in the area needs to be enlarged or smoothed at the reddened point or that, in the case of ischial redness, sitting pressure should have been relieved earlier and more frequently before this stage was reached. In stage II,

blisters develop and skin loss is limited to the superficial layers.[14] The wound now has become a deterrent to rehabilitation in that pressure must be kept off the area until it heals.[14] Any actual or potential infection must be treated.[14] In stage III the wound extends into the deeper layers of the skin. In stage IV, the wound extends into tendon, muscle, and bone and is draining.[14] Repair by relief of pressure in the latter two stages would take so much time that it would delay rehabilitation for months and leave the patient susceptible to contractures, loss of strength and endurance, and depression. Therefore, treatment is surgical or by electrical stimulation, an experimental wound healing treatment. Prevention is a primary goal. At first the personnel take responsibility for instructing, turning, and positioning the patient. Gradually the responsibility is shifted to the patient even if he can only direct someone else to move him. Patients at lesion levels of C_6 and below can learn to relieve pressure themselves, and achieving this becomes a major goal of therapy.

Bowel and bladder regulation can be achieved through special training and use of adaptive techniques and equipment. The rehabilitation nurse usually assumes responsibility for this aspect of the patient's rehabilitation, although others become involved as their expertise warrants. Rehabilitation engineers are working on electrical stimulation methods for micturition.[10] The occupational therapist may get involved by developing special aids to enable the patients to assume independent self-care. The bowel is regulated via diet and regular use of suppositories. Upper motor neuron lesion may result in neurogenic bladder[11] or detrusor-external urethral sphincter dyssynergia in which the urethral sphincter fails to relax as in normal voiding.[15] This results in spasmodic and incomplete voiding, potential sources of infection and embarrassment. It has been found that one way this problem can be overcome is by anal sphincter stretch during voiding, which causes a reflex relaxation of the urethral sphincter.[15] An orthotic finger appliance has been devised to assist selected C_7, C_8 quadriplegics to maintain a sustained stretch on the anal sphincter.[15] Patients with lower level lesions do not require the appliance and those with higher lesions lack the trunk balance and/or upper-extremity requirements to do the procedure. Intermittent catheterization is another method of controlling the bladder problem and is replacing the use of indwelling catheters in some patients. Intermittent catheterization can be done by patients with lesions as high as C_6 with adaptations and practice.[16]

Sexual functions are less disturbed in female than male patients. The female usually resumes menstruation within 6 months postinjury and must consider birth control if a child is not wanted.[5] There may be a reduction in reflex vaginal lubrication during intercourse,[5] which can be rectified by use of recommended lubricants. In male patients who suffer a lesion to $S_{2,3}$ or $_4$, there is a loss of erection (flaccidity).[5] In all other male patients, reflex, though not psychogenic, erection is preserved.[5] In patients with high-level lesions, erections occur frequently in response to various stimuli,[7] which is a potential source of embarrassment to the patient and needs to be dealt with as part of sexual counseling. Ejaculation occurs less often than erections; patients with levels T_{11} to L_2 preserved are more likely to have this function. Patients with incomplete lesions, especially those with sacral sparing, may have psychogenic erections with ejaculation and therefore may sire children.[12] It is otherwise rare for SCI patients to father children both because of inability to ejaculate and because of decreased and altered motility of the sperm.[5] Sexual counseling needs to be done with these patients by a knowledgeable team member. Four aspects of sexuality need to be addressed: satisfaction, including information about attitudes and methods that can be used as alternatives to genital sexual satisfaction[5]; function[5,17]; fertility; and desirability, which becomes a true concern given the values of society.[5]

The psychological complications of the injury must be addressed in therapy from the beginning. Rehabilitation can only occur in the patient whose motivation is not blocked by depression and denial.[18,19] In fact the high levels of distress and depression during early hospitalization portend a lengthy rehabilitation process and less commitment to self-care independence.[19]

The typical patient is male (82%), and the mean age is 28.7 years.[1] These facts present several problems to rehabilitation. One is that the patient is in a period of his life when physical prowess, independence, developing sexuality, and preparation for life's work are important issues. Immediately the accident renders him dependent on others for basic self-care needs, unable to move, and doubtful about his masculinity and future abilities. Another problem is that if he were a person who used physical activity to dissipate feelings of frustration and anger, that avenue may be closed to him if paralysis is extensive. Young adults often consider physical appearance of prime importance in the valuing of self or others, and patients may reject their new appearance and the use of special techniques or necessary mechanical devices, such as wheelchairs, splints, etc., on this basis.

Occupational Therapy Goals and Treatment Planning

Rehabilitation of the SCI patient is lengthy, requiring, on average, 156 days for a quadriplegic.[3,7] The rehabilitation process must be comprehensive and involve not only the restoration of and compensation for lost function but also therapy to help the patient accept and value his changed self. The patient is helped to take the responsibility for directing and carrying out his rehabilitative process. Rehabilitation of an SCI patient is complex and is effective only if a true team effort is put forth by the patient as well as the SCI unit personnel.

The primary goal of the occupational therapist in the rehabilitation of SCI patients is to teach the person to be as independent as he is able to become in all aspects of occupational performance tasks.[20] Adjunctive to increased independence is maintenance of range of motion (ROM), increase of strength and endurance, prevention of decubiti, acceptance of body image, and containment of depression and denial to within workable limits. To become independent, the person needs to learn techniques that compensate for weakness and lack of function, especially lack of hand function in quadriplegics. The person needs to learn to use gravity and leverage to handle his own body and objects.

Neurologic functions, as measured by manual muscle testing and sensation of pinprick, were found to correlate positively, at the time of discharge and at 1 year follow-up, with function defined as movement of the limbs, ability to do essential self-care, walk 50 meters on level ground, and transfers.[21] These types of observations over the years have led therapists and physicians to develop guidelines for certain expected levels of achievement in performance of daily life tasks by SCI patients. These expectations are outlined in Table 28.1. Use of such guidelines helps the therapist to know what levels of accomplishment to expect and to keep goal setting realistic. The guidelines suppose that the patient is a healthy, athletic male who is free from secondarily limiting factors, such as spasm, decubiti, contractures, an unstable fracture site, etc. They also presume that the patient has been active in therapy to develop sufficient strength and endurance equal to each task. These guidelines ought not to be considered limiting; some patients of unusual drive, strength, and resourcefulness are able to become more independent than one would expect, based on the experience of the accomplishments of other SCI patients at a similar level. However, it is psychologically crucial that the patient not be asked to try to do tasks that will cause him to experience failure.

In early treatment, if the patient is emotionally overwhelmed, goal setting may not involve active decision making on his part. However, at the earliest point that he can participate in goal setting, he should. An informative study indicates the need for closer collaboration between the occupational therapist and the SCI patient in establishing therapy goals and priorities.[22] Those considered by occupational therapists to be important for C_5, C_6 quadriplegics were different from those considered important by the patients themselves. The patients valued, in order of priority, development of work tolerance, muscle strengthening, and bowel and bladder control. They valued bathing and dressing least. The therapists prioritized goals as follows: development of adaptive devices, feeding, socialization, wheelchair mobility, driver education, and bowel and bladder control.[22]

In developing priorities for daily therapy, the therapist uses as a guide the fact that the patient needs to have prerequisite psychological attitudes and physical abilities to do daily living tasks. Therapy is aimed at establishing these prerequisites and then introducing the functional task with expectations for success. A good sequence of training is to start with light activities, such as feeding and hygiene, and progress, as strength and endurance permit, to activities that add control to the patient's life such as bed mobility, wheelchair mobility, and transfers. Then, toileting, bathing, and dressing—which require strength and agility generally equal to that required for bed and wheelchair mobility and transfers—can be instituted as prerequisite community living skills. Usually mastery of in-depth independent self-care gauges progress toward community reintegration goals, including driving and vocational preparation.

Occupational Therapy Evaluation and Treatment

Occupational therapists should interview the patient and his family about his life achievements and goals prior to the accident. Work and activity histories are particularly important for use in planning the treatment program over time. An impression of mental and emotional status can be gained over the course of several interviews,[12] and the therapist-patient relationship important to successful rehabilitation can begin to develop. Assumptions cannot be made about what the patient is feeling; it has been demonstrated that significant discrepancies exist between patients' feelings and personnel estimates of those feelings. Personnel tend to overestimate patients' sense of depression and psychological discomfort and underestimate their anxiety and sense of optimism.[23]

Evaluation includes measurements, as appropriate to the patient's lesion level, of passive range of motion, muscle strength, endurance (chapter 8), sensory awareness and discrimination (especially stereognosis [see chapter 3]), level of independence in occupational performance tasks (chapter 16), and degree of recovery of emotional equilibrium (chapter 2). The Biomechanical Approach is used to restore or maintain range of motion, strength, and endurance (see chapter 9). All muscles with any remaining supraspinal innervation are strengthened by exercise to recruit motor units and then to hypertrophy the motor fibers of the units through repetitive resistive exercise. If the lesion is complete, no hope of regaining control of the muscles innervated below the level of lesion is held. Sometimes neurodevelopmental inhibition techniques are helpful in reducing the spasticity of the muscles below the lesion, but this reduction is reflexive in nature and never develops beyond this. In patients with incomplete lesions, there may be a combination of spasticity and weak voluntary power in some muscles. The neurodevelopmental techniques may prove beneficial in these cases. Therapy for sensory loss and functional loss is compensatory (see chapter 3 and Part Five). Orthoses may be needed, especially for quadriplegics, and are suggested in Table 28.1 and described in chapter 13. Training in control and use of orthotic devices (including wheelchairs and environmental control units, as well as orthoses) are major aspects of therapy for quadriplegic patients (see chapter 13). The information in chapter 2 will assist the occupational therapist to devise an appropriate therapeutic program that inherently interweaves psychosocial programming with the program directed toward increased physical functioning.

The occupational therapy program must be part of a collaborative effort with the rest of the rehabilitation program, all of which is dictated by the recovery process.

EARLY TREATMENT PROGRAM FOR SCI PATIENTS

The period covered by the early treatment program extends from the emergency room through the period of immobilization. To maintain normal alignment of the spine, patients are immobilized in special beds or on turning frames until the vertebral fracture site is healed. Turning frames not only enable nursing staff to safely and easily turn the immobilized patient over every 2 hours, thus preventing development of decubiti over bony prominences, but also put the patient in positions that facilitate exercise and practice of functional tasks. Stryker or Foster turning frames have sectional mattresses that do not support certain areas of the patient in order to eliminate pressure on those areas that are susceptible to breakdown. The frames pivot around their longitudinal axis and turn the patient as if he were on a rotisserie.

Patients with cervical injuries may further have their necks immobilized in correct alignment by use of skeletal traction attached to the patient by cranial tongs or a head halter.[5] Halo braces also are used to provide traction and alignment.[5] Thoracolumbar injuries may be immobilized in plaster jackets or braces.[5]

The immobilization places limits on the types of therapy possible. Precautions are exercised by all personnel when handling or interacting with the patient to prevent movement of the fracture site, which could jeopardize the neurological functioning of the patient, and, in high cervical lesions, even his life. No upright, rotary, or flexion/extension movements of the spine are allowed until the orthopedist clears the patient for such movement.[5] It is important that personnel approach and address the patient within his visual field so he will not turn his head.[24]

Rehabilitation of the SCI patient should be initiated within 48 hours of admission as soon as the patient is medically stable.[24] Early intervention decreases the potential for contractures and other complications that extend the length and cost of hospitalization.[24] Goals include: (1) maintaining functional ROM; (2) promoting independent control of environment; (3) instilling hope and facilitating relief of distress and depression; (4) educating patient about prevention of decubiti and other lesions due to sensory loss; (5) increasing strength; and (6) improving functional ability and endurance.

Maintenance of ROM requires a concerted effort of therapists and nurses. The occupational therapist is particularly responsible for seeing that all joints of the upper extremities maintain adequate ROM so that future independence in daily life tasks is not precluded or limited. Attention to the upper extremity is critical from the earliest point because functional achievement depends on the upper extremities.[11] It is extremely important, however, that the finger flexors of the C_6 quadriplegic be allowed to tighten into a partially flexed position so that he will have a more effective tenodesis grasp. During ROM exercise, when the fingers are flexed, the wrist must be extended, and when the fingers are extended, the wrist must be flexed.[12,25] In this case, range is done to keep the joint capsules free,[25] not to stretch the extrinsic muscles. If the intrinsic muscles need to be stretched, that is done by flexing the interphalangeal joints with the metacarpophalangeal extended. Positioning is important between sessions of ROM exercise. Any hand splint used should protect the alignment of the fingers, thumb, and wrist for future function or dynamic splinting. For example, if the web space tightens, a flexor hinge hand splint for prehension will not fit properly for a secure palmar pinch. For C_6 patients, who will depend on their tenodesis grasp, some SCI units utilize a hand roll,[11] or a thermoplastic splint, which has a roll to support the fingers in a flexed position. The splint also preserves the width of the web space and extends over the volar wrist to protect the weak wrist extensors from being stretched (Fig. 28.1).

The patient can be set up to use an environmental control unit (ECU) if he has a source of voluntary control. One method of control available even to those with lesions of C_1 to C_4 is pneumatic control, commonly known as sip and puff.[26]

The patient, having survived the life threat, must cope with the enormity of the disability. Although a false sense of hope for full recovery should never be engendered, the patient should gain a sense of hope that recovery of function is expected to whatever degree it can realistically be expected. That sense is developed as the professionals interact and work with him in a competent and confident manner and with hope conveyed. The patient needs to relieve his anxiety[23] by trusting that although he is unable to control his life, others will do so competently and compassionately. The therapist needs to have a supportive manner while moving forward through the rehabilitation tasks at a pace consistent with the patient's emotional status and sense of involvement.

The patient is taught to compensate visually for lost sensation as a protective measure. Burns, abrasions, and pressure are all potentially dangerous to the insensitive extremities, and the patient must be alerted to avoid situations that could cause them. Some less obvious situations include dragging the body across the sheet during dressing or transfer and sitting too close to a hot radiator.

The strength of remaining musculature is increased within the limitations imposed by the patient's recumbent position and the precautions regarding immobilization and avoidance of fatigue of very weak muscles. Sling suspensions with springs can be used on the patient's bed to offer active assistive exercise for proximal muscles. These are suspended from an orthopedic frame mounted on the bed. Activities or exercise to increase forearm, wrist, and hand strength should be included if these muscles are innervated.

Those independent living activities that can be done within the limitations of position and weakness are initiated. For example, the C_7 quadriplegic patient can do self-feeding and some grooming while in the prone position on a turning frame. C_4, C_5 patients will be unable to do any functional activities in this position, however. The C_4, C_5 quadriplegic patient can begin controls training for use of his externally powered hand splint; this would be beneficial because he would then be ready to start use training when permitted to sit up. The more active the patient is, the more endurance he will develop.

INTERMEDIATE TREATMENT PROGRAM FOR SCI PATIENTS

Once the spine is stabilized by surgery or bracing and the patient is cleared to begin sitting, a new phase of rehabilitation begins.

Goals of this phase of treatment are a continuation of those of the early phase with the overall goal of increasing the patient's expertise in, and responsibility for, his rehabilitation program.[27] One center has found group therapy (i.e., classes) to expedite this process since one patient learns from another. Wheelchair skills, including community reintegration outings, activities of daily living (ADL) preparatory for the outings, skin monitoring, instructing others to assist, etc., especially lend themselves to a class approach.[27] Ad hoc grouping of patients also seems to benefit those needing to learn the same or similar ADL skills. Group treatment does not replace the patient-therapist relationship that needs to be established.[27]

SCI patients usually begin sitting at less than 90° upright and for short periods of time. A fully reclining wheelchair is used initially for quadriplegic patients to

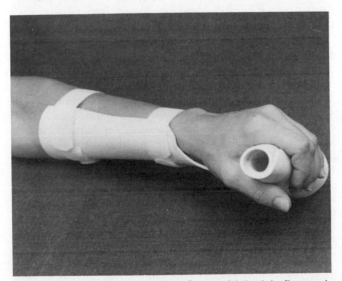

Figure 28.1 Splint to support C_6 quadriplegic's fingers in flexion, to maintain the web space, and to keep the wrist supported in neutral.

enable them to gradually develop tolerance for upright sitting. After being recumbent for several weeks, any SCI patient may experience syncope if he is moved to a sitting position too quickly. Fainting also may occur when in a sitting position because blood pools in the lower extremities due to the loss of the muscular pumping action that helps venous return. Elastic stockings and sometimes an abdominal binder or corset are worn to help alleviate this problem. If fainting or syncope occur during treatment, stand behind the locked wheelchair and tip it backward so that the patient's feet are higher than his head.[12,25] Raise the chair slowly to its upright position when the patient feels better.

Sitting tolerance is evaluated and improved until the patient can sit upright for an average day. Concurrent with development of sitting tolerance, the patient's awareness and sense of responsibility are heightened regarding ischial pressure relief. Each patient must develop the habit of using his chosen method routinely even if it means only taking the responsibility of reminding someone else to do it for him.[12,25] Prevention of decubiti requires that two factors are attended to. One is a proper cushion (see chapter 3). But since no cushion provides less than capillary pressure on soft tissue, relief of pressure by change of position must also be done.[5]

Patients with lesions of C_7 and below have the muscle innervation (triceps) to do push-ups, that is, raise the buttocks off the seat by pressing down with the extended arms. In the early stages of learning, when the patient is too unskilled and weak to lift off the surface, a push-up should be done approximately every 10 min. As a lifelong measure, push-ups should be done three to four times per hour (every 15 to 20 min) and the weight should be off the buttocks for 1 or 2 min to allow the capillaries to refill. The C_6 patient independently relieves ischial pressure by doing lateral or forward weight shifts with the aid of a web belt loop attached to the wheelchair arm to assist regaining upright position.[12,28] To do a lateral shift, which removes pressure from one buttock, he removes the arm rest, loops his forearm into the web loop, and leans to the side so that gravity assists his lateral flexion while he is prevented from falling too far by the web strap. After regaining upright position, he must then bend to the other side. Alternately, two such web loops can be attached to the uprights of the wheelchair back. With the wheelchair locked, the feet on the floor, and the arms through the loops, the patient bends fully forward for 1 min, then uses the loops to regain upright sitting.[12,25]

The C_5 patient may be able to accomplish the forward maneuver just described[12] or may need assistance in relieving pressure. Patients with lesion levels higher than C_5 will need assistance to relieve pressure. Full reclining with the legs raised to horizontal is a method used by lightweight persons. Another method is as follows: with the wheelchair locked, a person sits next to the patient, removes the armrest, and pulls the patient's trunk onto his or her lap. This posture is maintained for 1 min.[25]

The occupational therapist should reinforce the instructions of the physical therapist and rehabilitation nurse regarding push-ups and other maneuvers that the patient has been taught to use to relieve pressure. Patients who find it difficult to remember to relieve pressure can learn by using an electronic device[29] that gives off an audible signal if pressure is not relieved at preset intervals, usually beginning at 10 min apart.

The rehabilitation nurse teaches the patient methods of skin inspection and helps him to inspect his skin for reddened areas each night. Hand mirrors are used and are one way that the patient compensates visually for his sensory loss.

Not only are ischial decubiti of concern, but also any other source of decubiti, which will result from pressure greater than capillary pressure (25 to 35 mm Hg[10]). Any equipment or splint that leaves a reddened area on the skin that lasts 20 min after removal needs modification to relieve the pressure. The corrected equipment should not be used again until the reddened area disappears.

Therapy to maintain range is continued. This will be necessary as long as the patient cannot move a joint actively through full range. Patients with lower level lesions can learn to range their own limbs daily. Evaluations are done regularly to determine if passive range of motion is being preserved.

Therapy to increase the strength and the endurance of innervated musculature continues. Regular muscle tests and measures of endurance are done to document progress. The use of recreational and sports activities may engage the patient's interest and participation in therapy aimed at increasing strength and endurance, while allowing some friendly competition and socialization, which are normal life tasks of this age group. A program of progressively vigorous handling of quadriplegics with stable fracture sites was found to be psychologically beneficial in that there was less fear of falling, more body control developed, fewer feelings of fragility, and more feelings of being "touchable."[30]

For the C_{1-4} patient, therapy to increase strength and control of facial and neck muscles is used in preparation for use of mouthsticks, microswitches, or sip and puff controls.[4,11] Mouthsticks are used to turn pages, write, draw, type, and push telephone buttons and other control buttons of electronic devices such as electronic games, computers, and calculators. With adaptations, mouthsticks can be used to move playing pieces and change cassette tapes[31] or computer disks. Microswitches can be mounted so they are tongue- or chin-operated and can be used to control electric wheelchairs, environmental control units, and upper-limb orthoses. Sip and puff controls are used on electric wheelchairs, environmental control units, and electric typewriters.[32]

As the patient gains adequate strength and endurance, ADLs are taught using appropriate methods and equipment (see chapter 17). Patients with lesions at C_8 or below are expected to become independent in community living skills.[3] Patients with lesions at C_5 and above will need assistance with basic self-care.[3] Patients with lesions at C_6 and C_7 can be independent in self-care and possibly community living skills if all contributing factors (skin, bladder, general health, weight, etc.) are in an ideal state. A problem-solving, collaborative[12] approach is used to teach ADL because the person needs to be able to independently solve novel problems as they arise in his life. The more competent the patient feels in his ability to solve problems independently, the more satisfied he is with his life. This is supported by a study comparing SCI patients with normal subjects that found a positive relationship between satisfaction with performance of home-management and social/community problem-solving skills and overall life satisfaction.[33,34]

The rehabilitation nurse works with the patient to develop bowel and bladder hygiene and programs for independent care. Most male patients eventually change from indwelling catheters to intermittent catheterization or external drainage. The occupational therapist will be involved in devising ways for the patient to apply the external drainage devices, to clamp the catheter between voidings, to empty the collection bag, or to insert a catheter.

LATER TREATMENT PROGRAM FOR SCI PATIENTS

As the patient progresses through the stages of rehabilitation, discharge, and community reintegration, he assumes increased responsibility for, and control over, his own care.[5] When the patient nears his maximal strength, endurance, and self-care ability, the focus changes to development of socially productive roles and discharge planning. Vocational and recreational pursuits that he plans to engage in must be planned and prepared for. It may be necessary to explore new avenues of vocation and recreation due to the extent of the disability (see chapters 18 and 21). The occupational therapy clinic becomes a valuable laboratory for testing skills within a secure environment.

A community reintegration program is initiated that includes trips into the community to practice skills needed as a wheelchair-bound citizen (see chapter 20). In the beginning the occupational and physical therapists help work out the problems as they arise, but gradually the patient takes over the initiative.

As the patient resumes social interactions, personal grooming may become an important issue. Clothing designed for wheelchair-bound persons is available, but this need remains only partially addressed.[35] One example of adaptive clothing is the tailoring of men's suits so that the trousers do not ride up even though the person is sitting and the jacket fits neatly without bunching into the chair seat.

As part of discharge planning, living arrangements after discharge must be discussed with him and his family. Six factors have been shown to statistically predict the living status after discharge. The single most important factor in determining whether the patient will live in a less restrictive environment is being married. This fact emphasizes the importance of paying attention to lessening stress on the marital relationship as a goal of rehabilitation.[36,37] Another of the six factors found to be contributory to predicting independent living was "unmet occupational therapy needs"; that is, those who did not receive occupational therapy were more likely to be living in restrictive environments.[36,37]

An alternative living arrangement if discharge to home is not possible and a nursing home is not necessary is accessible housing sponsored by Independent Living Centers. Not all of these centers offer this service, but they do offer many services to enable independent living by the disabled, including the severely disabled. One important service some of them offer is job placement. The patient can be directed to the nearest center to negotiate his discharge plans based on his needs and the services offered. The C_{1-4} quadriplegic will require an attendant for life to take care of all dressing, bathing, grooming, transfer, toilet needs, respiratory equipment maintenance, out-of-home locomotion, and possibly feeding or set up of complicated orthotic equipment. These patients will probably be best served in a protective environment, if not living with reliable, full-time attendant care.

Shortly before the time of discharge, a home evaluation visit is done by the occupational and physical therapists. They evaluate the wheelchair accessibility of the home and help the patient and his family determine what changes need to be made to facilitate independence and to preserve the life-style of the patient as much as possible (see chapter 20). Weekend visits home during the ongoing rehabilitation process are valuable in pointing out accessibility problems prior to the home visit.

To prevent posthospitalization deterioration of physical fitness gained in rehabilitation, continued involvement in aerobic sports activities or fitness training is recommended. One study found, using monitors to record heart rate during a 48-hour period, that fitness training was needed in addition to normal ADL to maintain cardiopulmonary and muscular fitness of the rehabilitated paraplegics being studied. The ADL activities alone did not tax the heart enough for a training effect to occur.[38] Opportunities for wheelchair sports and recreation have improved for the disabled. It would be beneficial if the patient were introduced to these as part of his rehabilitation since they not only maintain physical fitness but add significantly to emotional and social rehabilitation.[39]

Before discharge, the patient should be put in touch with the local chapter of the National Spinal Cord Injury Foundation. He should also be made aware of other resources, such as *Accent on Living*, a quarterly periodical that offers realistic solutions to the problems encountered in daily life by disabled persons.

After at least 1 year postinjury when the patient has attained maximum return of strength[7,11,40,41] and maximum improvement in self-care and transfer activities,[21] and after he has been neurologically stable for 6 months,[41] one decision that he may have the opportunity to make is whether or not to have hand reconstruction surgery. Such surgery may increase the function of a C_6, C_7, or C_8 level patient and allow him to discard his orthosis.[42] Restoration is aimed at preserving the hand as a means of human contact as well as its function as a gripping tool.[43] Surgical reconstruction is still not a routine treatment, although it is beginning to be considered more of a feasible alternative to splinting.[42]

Prerequisites to reconstructive hand surgery that some surgeons look for are a realistic attitude toward the outcome; afferent input either visual or preferably two-point discrimination in the thumb, index, and long fingers of 10 to 12 mm[42,43]; strength of transferable muscles of grades 4 to 5[42,43] (G to N); and one movable joint in the thumb.[43] If the only sensory input is by visual observation of the hand, only one hand can be restored successfully.[43]

The surgical procedures performed on C_5, C_6 patients with good results are as follows[43]: Active wrist extension is achieved by use of the brachioradialis. Tenodesis thumb flexor grip (lateral pinch), which is estimated to be the preferred pincer function,[43] is achieved by allowing the flexor pollicis longus (FPL) to bowstring from the metacarpophalangeal joint to increase the moment arm and therefore decrease the power needed while tenodesing the FPL to the radius and stabilizing the interphalangeal joint. Elbow extension is provided to some patients by attaching the posterior half of the deltoid to the triceps aponeurosis and by lengthening the deltoid with free grafts from the toe extensors. Two-stage hand reconstruction surgery for grasp and pinch is a procedure used for C_6 level patients to provide grasp, lateral pinch, and tenodesis finger and thumb extension.[41] Candidates for this surgery must have normal strength in the extensors carpi radialis longus and brevis (ECRL and ECRB) and brachioradialis; G+ strength in the pronator teres; and F+ in the flexor carpi radialis (FCR). Testing the FCR provides an estimate of ECRB strength because the ECRB cannot be tested in isolation. The ECRB will become the sole wrist extensor after transfer surgery. This extensive surgery is done in two stages. Stage 1 (tenodesis extension) is done if the patient has weak tenodesis extensor action. The extensor pollicis longus, abductor pollicis longus, and extensor digitorum are tenodesed to the distal radius. At the same time an intrinsic procedure is done to prevent hyperextension of the metacarpophalangeal joints. A short protective arm cast is put on with the hand in functional position.[41] In stage 2 (active gross grasp and lateral pinch), the ECRL is sutured to the tendons of the flexor digitorum profundus for grasp, and the brachioradialis is inserted into the short thumb abductor and opponens for thumb opposition. The pronator is transferred to the flexor pollicis longus tendon for thumb flexion. A full arm cast is applied to protect the transferred tendons.[41]

Procedures used for C_7, C_8 patients are aimed at refining hand function, specifically finger flexion and opposition. To provide the finger flexion, the extensor carpi radialis longus, which is synergistic to finger flexion,[40] is transferred if the more centrally located brevis is strong.[40,42] The brachioradialis is transferred to provide thumb flexion[42] or adduction/opposition of the thumb.[40] The expected average strength of grasp is 5.5 kg and pinch is 3.0 kg.[40]

The occupational therapist provides both preoperative and postoperative treatment.[41,44] The goals of preop treatment are to educate the patient regarding the surgery, its expected outcomes, and the problems that are to be expected during the convalescent stage.[44] The major problem during that time is the inability to independently relieve ischial pressure, since the operated hand is casted or too fragile yet to withstand the stresses patients put on their hands during push-ups or other pressure-relieving maneuvers. The patient is taught alternate pressure-relief techniques, or if these are not within the patient's capabilities, he is helped to work out a plan for assistance in this crucial function during the 3 to 6 weeks of immobilization.[40-45] Post-op treatment begins when the cast is removed. A half shell is still used to protect against stretching and rupture of the healing tissue. The half shell is removed for treatment twice daily. If joint fusion has been done, e.g., carpometacarpal joint of the thumb, a splint is made to prevent movement but to allow some use of the part. Other splints may be needed, depending on the type of surgery done and healing requirements; these will be specifically ordered by the hand surgeon.

Goals of post-op therapy are to prevent edema and to increase ROM, strength, endurance, coordination, and ADL independence.[44] (see chapter 25). Therapy for range, strength, and endurance during the first month involves only active ROM exercises. Aggressive passive ROM and resistive exercise are avoided for fear the tendon(s) would be stretched or detached as a result. Evaluation of strength of pinch and grasp is made only after healing is complete. Electromyographic biofeedback is beneficial in muscle reeducation to help the patient learn to use the transferred tendon(s) in its new function (see chapter 12). First, the patient learns to contract and relax the muscle voluntarily, then to isolate each motion, and finally to combine motions.[41] Coordination is achieved through use of nonresistive hand activities. Speed is measured as an index of improved coordination. Activities of daily living are reevaluated with the purpose of discarding adaptive devices as a result of improved function following surgery.[44] Also, the need to teach new techniques that will protect the transferred tendon is also evaluated. One such new technique is the use of the hands during transfer: normally quadriplegics transfer with the fingers and wrist in full extension, but this would put too much stress on the newly arranged tendons; therefore, patients are taught to transfer with the hand fisted or with the fingers extending over the surface's edge.[44] Careful documentation of which hand functions and life tasks are enhanced and which are diminished is important for evaluation of the outcome of surgery.[46]

Follow-Up

SCI patients are followed routinely for reevaluation of medical, emotional, and functional status. The information gathered during the course of the follow-up evaluations serves as data for outcome evaluation of SCI programs. One follow-up study of 35 quadriplegic persons (20 with radial wrist extensors and 15 without), 1 to 4 years postdischarge, indicated that level of independence in self-care was generally maintained posthospitalization, especially in the areas of feeding and desk skills.[47] Regression in grooming, bathing, toileting, and lower-extremity dressing seemed to be secondary to a reordering of time and energy priorities.[47] The equipment issued at discharge and still in use was splints, universal cuffs, push cuffs (for wheelchair propulsion), and adapted catheter clamps. Other equipment, including mobile arm supports, lapboard, buttonhooks, reachers, and mouthsticks, had been abandoned.[47] In another study, 17 C_6 and 12 C_7 quadriplegics were surveyed 3 months to 4 years postdischarge to determine the level of self-care independence and change in abilities since discharge.[3] C_7 patients were more independent than C_6 patients, as expected, but both groups changed. Bed mobility, transfers, wheelchair mobility, and driving were done by more C_6 patients than at the time of discharge, whereas upper-extremity dressing was done by fewer. Bed mobility, grooming, bowel care, transfers, and driving were done by more C_7 patients, whereas dressing, especially upper-extremity dressing, was done by fewer. Reasons cited by the subjects for improved abilities included increased strength and motor ability, increased desire, an easier method found, or the existence of a home demand. The researchers speculated that those activities that decreased require considerable energy that the patient would rather use in other pursuits; therefore, he accepted assistance for these tasks.[3]

More study is needed concerning the nature and extent of rehabilitation services that should be offered to be both fiscally responsible and to afford the person with this devastating injury all the opportunity he can benefit from to regain a quality life.

STUDY QUESTIONS:

Spinal Cord Injury

1. What is the clinical picture, after shock subsides, of a person who has suffered a SCI?
2. What are the symptoms of autonomic dysreflexia and what should the occupational therapist do if the patient exhibits some of them?
3. What are the sexual abilities of a man with a complete SCI at T_{12} level?
4. What evaluations are used with SCI patients?
5. What key muscles are added and what achievements can be expected of a patient with a C_6 lesion level?
6. What factors influence expected levels of achievement of occupational performance tasks?
7. What are the occupational therapy goals for early therapy for SCI patients?
8. Describe the passive ranging process for hands and wrists of C_6 quadriplegics.
9. What is the procedure when a patient in a wheelchair faints?
10. What is a mouthstick and what is it used for?
11. Describe stage 2 of the Two-Stage Reconstruction Surgery for Grasp and Pinch.
12. What are the goals, in order, of postoperative muscle reeducation following tendon transplant surgery?
13. What key muscles are added and what achievements can be expected of T_{12} paraplegics?
14. Describe the adaptations and set up a C_4 quadriplegic college student would need to be able to write a paper for his English class.

References

1. Garber, S. L. New perspectives for the occupational therapist in the treatment of spinal cord-injured individuals. *Am. J. Occup. Ther.,* 39(11): 703–704, 1985.
2. Lathem, P. A., Gregorio, T. L., and Garber, S. L. High-level quadriplegia: an occupational therapy challenge. *Am. J. Occup. Ther.,* 39(11): 705–714, 1985.
3. Welch, R. D., et al. Functional independence in quadriplegia: critical levels. *Arch. Phys. Med. Rehabil.,* 67(4): 235–240, 1986.
4. Van Steen, H. Treatment of a patient with a complete C_1 quadriplegia. *Phys. Ther.,* 55(1): 35–38, 1975.
5. King, R. B., and Dudas, S. Rehabilitation of the patient with a spinal cord injury. *Nurs. Clin. North Am.,* 15(2): 225–243, 1980.
6. Bishop, B. Neural plasticity. Part 4. Lesion-induced reorganization of the CNS. *Phys. Ther.,* 62(10): 1442–1451, 1982.
7. Panchal, P. D. Rehabilitation of the patient with spinal cord injury. *Curr. Probl. Surg.,* 17(94): 254–262, 1980.
8. Lee, I. Y., and Rossier, A. B. Letter to the editor: Heterotopic ossification in the hand. *Arch. Phys. Med. Rehabil.,* 63(2): 96, 1982.
9. Lynch, C., Pont, A., and Weingarden, S. I. Heterotopic ossification in the hand of a patient with spinal cord injury. *Arch. Phys. Med. Rehabil.,* 62: 291–293, 1981.
10. Rozin, R. The upper limb in spinal cord injury. *Prog. Surg.,* 16: 207–220, 1978.
11. Reswick, M. B., and Simoes, N. Application of engineering principles in management of spinal cord injured patients. *Clin. Orthop.,* 112: 4–129, 1975.
12. Wilson, D. J., et al. *Spinal Cord Injury: A Treatment Guide for Occupational Therapists,* revised edition. Thorofare, NJ: Slack Incorporated, 1984.
13. Long, C. Congenital and traumatic lesions of the spinal cord. In *Handbook of Physical Medicine and Rehabilitation,* 2nd edition. Edited by F. H. Krusen, F. J. Kottke, and P. M. Ellwood. Philadelphia: W. B. Saunders, 1971.
14. Panzau, K. Recognizing a pressure sore and doing something about it is the best treatment and costs you nothing. *Accent on Living,* 31(3): 106–107, 1986.
15. Donovan, W. H., Macri, D., and Clowers, D. E. A finger device for obtaining satisfactory voiding in spinal cord-injured patients. *Am. J. Occup. Ther.,* 31(2): 107–108, 1977.
16. Dailey, J., and Michael, R. Nonsterile self-intermittent catherization for male quadriplegic patients. *Am. J. Occup. Ther.,* 31(2): 86–89, 1977.
17. Mooney, T., Cole, T., and Chilgren, R. *Sexual Options for Paraplegics and Quadriplegics.* Boston: Little, Brown, 1975.
18. Thomas, C. Rehabilitation: is it for you? *Accent on Living,* 30(4): 76–78, 1986.
19. Malec, J., and Neimeyer, R. Psychologic prediction of duration of inpatient spinal cord injury rehabilitation and performance of self-care. *Arch. Phys. Med. Rehabil.,* 64(8): 359–363, 1983.
20. Frieden, L., and Cole, J. A. Independence: the ultimate goal of rehabilitation for spinal cord-injured persons. *Am. J. Occup. Ther.,* 39(11): 734–739, 1985.
21. Bracken, M. B., et al. Relationship between neurological and functional status after acute spinal cord injury: an epidemiological study. *J. Chronic Dis.,* 33: 115–125, 1980.
22. Taylor, D. P. Treatment goals for quadriplegic patients. *Am. J. Occup. Ther.,* 28(1): 22–29, 1974.

23. Bodenhamer, E., et al. Staff and patient perceptions of the psychosocial concerns of spinal cord injured persons. *Am. J. Phys. Med.*, 62(4): 182-193, 1983.
24. Sargant, C., and Braun, M. A. Occupational therapy management of the acute spinal cord-injured patient. *Am. J. Occup. Ther.*, 40(5): 333-337, 1986.
25. McKenzie, M. W., and Buck, G. L. Combined motor and peripheral sensory insufficiency. III. Management of spinal cord injury. *Phys. Ther.*, 58(3): 294-303, 1978.
26. Stratford, C. D. NYU engineering program: clinical evaluations of electronic devices. *The American Occupational Therapy Association Physical Disabilities Special Interest Section Newsletter*, 2(3): 4, 1979.
27. Machmer, P. Group treatment in the physical rehabilitation of the patient with a spinal cord injury. *The American Occupational Therapy Association Physical Disabilities Special Interest Section Newsletter*, 2(3): 1-2, 1979.
28. Agrawal, B. K., Arnold, T., and Vicich, J. Web-belt loop for relief of pressure on buttocks. *Arch. Phys. Med. Rehabil.*, 59(7): 346-347, 1978.
29. Halstead, L. S., et al. Sit time monitor: a device for measuring wheelchair sitting time. *Am. J. Occup. Ther.*, 36(7): 463-465, 1982.
30. Gerhart, K. A. Increasing sensory and motor stimulation for the patient with quadriplegia. *Phys. Ther.*, 59(12): 1518-1520, 1979.
31. Kelly, S. N. Adaptations for independent use of cassette tape recorder/radio by high-level quadriplegic patients. *Am. J. Occup. Ther.*, 37(11): 766-768, 1983.
32. Prentke-Romich Company. *Electronic Aids for the Severely Handicapped.* Shreve, OH, 1986.
33. Yerxa, E. J., and Baum, S. Engagement in daily occupations and life satisfaction among people with spinal cord injuries. *Occup. Ther. J. Res.*, 6(5): 271-283, 1986.
34. Decker, S. D., and Schulz, R. Correlates of life satisfaction and depression in middle-aged and elderly spinal cord-injured persons. *Am. J. Occup. Ther.*, 39(11): 740-745, 1985.
35. Nessley, E., and King, R. R. Textile fabric and clothing needs of paraplegic and quadriplegic persons confined to wheelchairs. *J. Rehabil.*, 46(2): 63-67, 1980.
36. DeJong, G., Branch, L. G., and Corcoran, P. J. Independent living outcomes in spinal cord injury: multivariate analyses. *Arch. Phys. Med. Rehabil.*, 65(2): 66-73, 1984.
37. Ostrow, P. C., Lawlor, M. C., and Johnson, M. *American Occupational Therapy Association Efficacy Data Brief*, 2(1): 1-4, 1986.
38. Hjeltnes, N., and Vokac, Z. Circulatory strain in everyday life of paraplegics. *Scand. J. Rehabil. Med.*, 11: 67-73, 1979.
39. Madorsky, J. B., and Madorsky, A. Wheelchair racing: an important modality in acute rehabilitation after paraplegia. *Arch. Phys. Med. Rehabil.*, 64(4): 186-187, 1983.
40. House, J. H., Gwathmey, F. W., and Lundsgaard, D. K. Restoration of strong grasp and lateral pinch in tetraplegia due to cervical cord injury. *J. Hand Surg.*, 1(2): 152-159, 1976.
41. Ainsley, J., Voorhees, C., and Drake, E. Reconstructive hand surgery for quadriplegic persons. *Am. J. Occup. Ther.*, 39(11): 715-721, 1985.
42. Hentz, V. R., and Keoshian, L. A. Changing perspectives in surgical hand rehabilitation in quadriplegic patients. *Plast. Reconstr. Surg.*, 64(4): 509-515, 1979.
43. Moberg, E. Surgical treatment for absent single-hand grip and elbow extension in quadriplegia. *J. Bone Joint Surg.*, 57/A(2): 196-206, 1975.
44. Mathiowetz, V., and Brambilla, M. Tendon transfers for quadriplegics: implications for therapy. *American Occupational Therapy Association Physical Disabilities Specialty Section Newsletter*, 2(3): 3, 1979.
45. Zancolli, E. Surgery for the quadriplegic hand with active, strong wrist extension preserved: a study of 97 cases. *Clin. Orthop.*, 112: 101-113, 1975.
46. Bell, J., Jurek, K., and Wilson, T. Hand skill measurement: a gauge for treatment. *Am. J. Occup. Ther.*, 30(2): 80-86, 1976.
47. Rogers, J. C., and Figone, J. J. Traumatic quadriplegia: follow-up study of self-care skills. *Arch. Phys. Med. Rehabil.*, 61(7): 316-321, 1980.
48. Lowman, E., and Klinger, J. *Aids to Independent Living.* New York: McGraw Hill, Blakiston Division, 1969.
49. Parish, J. G. A study of the use of electronic environmental control systems by severely paralyzed patients. *Paraplegia*, 17: 147-156, 1979-80.
50. Garcia, S., and Greenfield, J. Dynamic protractible mouthstick. *Am. J. Occup. Ther.*, 35(8): 529-530, 1981.
51. White, G. W., Wussow, A. E., and Merritt, J. L. Videogame adaptation for patients with high-level cervical injury. *Arch. Phys. Med. Rehabil.*, 65(4): 208-209, 1984.
52. McKenzie, M., and Rogers, J. Use of trunk supports for severely paralyzed people. *Am. J. Occup. Ther.*, 27(3): 147-148, 1973.
53. Schmeisser, G., and Seamone, W. Low cost assistive device systems for a high spinal cord-injured person in the home environment—a technical note. *Bull. Prosthet. Res.*, 16(2): 212-223, 1979.
54. Sell, G. H., et al. Environmental and typewriter control systems for high-level quadriplegic patients: evaluation and prescription. *Arch. Phys. Med. Rehabil.*, 60(6): 246-251, 1979.
55. Berard, E., et al. The technical aids of tetraplegic patients. *Paraplegia*, 17: 157-160, 1979-80.
56. Cloran, A. J., et al. Oral telescoping orthosis: an aid to functional rehabilitation of quadriplegic patients. *J. Am. Dent. Assoc.*, 100(6): 876-879, 1980.
57. McKenzie, M. The ratchet hand-splint. *Am. J. Occup. Ther.*, 27(8): 477-479, 1973.
58. Smith, B. Adapted bed controls and the quadriplegic patient. *Am. J. Occup. Ther.*, 32(5): 322, 1978.
59. Bacon, G., and Olszewski, E. Sequential advancing flexion retention attachment. *Am. J. Occup. Ther.*, 32(9): 577-585, 1978.
60. Ford, J. R., and Duckworth, B. *Physical Management of the Quadriplegic Patient.* Philadelphia: F. A. Davis, 1974.
61. Bortner, E. The transfer commode seat. *Am. J. Occup. Ther.*, 33(10): 655, 1979.
62. Williams, L., and Garetz, D. Independent leg bag emptying technique for cervical five quadriplegic clients. *Am. J. Occup. Ther.*, 35(1): 40-42, 1981.
63. McGee, M., and Hertling, D. Equipment and transfer techniques used by C_6 quadriplegic patients. *Phys. Ther.*, 57(12): 1372-1375, 1977.
64. Feinberg, J. Writing device for the quadriplegic patient. *Am. J. Occup. Ther.*, 29(2): 101, 1975.
65. Craver, P. N. Typing splints for the quadriplegic patient. *Am. J. Occup. Ther.*, 29(9): 551, 1975.
66. Grahn, E. Tape recorder modifications for use by quadriplegics. *Am. J. Occup. Ther.*, 24(5): 360-361, 1970.
67. Slatter, E. R., and Gibb, M. M. A table tennis glove for tetraplegics. *Paraplegia*, 17(2): 259-261, 1979.
68. Lobely, S., et al. Orthotic design from the New England Regional Spinal Cord Injury Center. *Phys. Ther.*, 65(4): 492-493, 1985.

Supplementary Reading

Extensions for Independence: Designers and Manufacturers of Vocational Aids for the Handicapped. 635-5 N. Twin Oaks Valley Road, San Marcos, CA 92069.

Garber, S. L. Wheelchair cushions for spinal cord-injured individuals. *Am. J. Occup. Ther.*, 39(11): 722-725, 1985.

Hage, G. Two pronation splints. *Am. J. Occup. Ther.*, 39(4): 265-267, 1985.

Hotline help for spinal cord injured. *Accent on Living*, 30(3): 26-27, 1985. (1-800-526-3456)

Kanellos, M. C. Enhancing vocational outcomes of spinal cord-injured persons: the occupational therapist's role. *Am. J. Occup. Ther.*, 39(11): 726-733, 1985.

Little, J. Little talks: do super-crips have more fun? *Accent on Living*, 30(3): 80-83, 1985.

Rehabilitation Institute of Chicago. *Spinal Cord Injury: A Guide to Functional Outcomes in Occupational Therapy.* Gaithersburg, MD: Aspen Publishers, 1986.

Rogers, J. C., and Figone, J. J. Psychosocial parameters in treating the person with quadriplegia. *Am. J. Occup. Ther.*, 33(7): 432-439, 1979.

Rogers, J. C., and Figone, J. J. The avocational pursuits of rehabilitants with traumatic quadriplegia. *Am. J. Occup. Ther.*, 32(8): 571-576, 1978.

Seplowitz, C. Technology and occupational therapy in the rehabilitation of the bedridden quadriplegic. *Am. J. Occup. Ther.*, 38(11): 743-747, 1984.

Tator, C., editor. *Early Management of Acute Spinal Cord Injury.* New York: Raven Press, 1982.

Trombly, C. A. Principles of operant conditioning related to orthotic training of quadriplegic patients. *Am. J. Occup. Ther.*, 20(5): 217-220, 1966.

Wiener, M. M. Feeding device for finger foods. *Am. J. Occup. Ther.*, 39(11): 746-747, 1985.

chapter

29

Burns

Lillian Hoyle Parent

Burns are the third largest cause of accidental death in the United States.[1] An estimated 2 million Americans are seriously burned annually and about 100,000 require hospitalization.[2] Most burns occur in the home.[1] Significant advances in the care of burned patients have improved survival rates while decreasing the length of hospitalization for all types of burns.[3] These advances include improved medications to reduce or to prevent burn wound infection, improvement in many life support measures, the use of biological dressings for immediate covering in extensive burns, and vigorous rehabilitation measures to reduce the morbidity of severe burns.[4] Burn care specialists are no longer satisfied with just survival in the treatment of burns.[5] Burn care programs in the United States are similar, and most of them use occupational therapists in the rehabilitation of the burn patient.[6] The goal is to help patients reach their maximum rehabilitation status.[5]

A burned patient has an acute illness of weeks to months and requires a therapeutic regimen that may extend for 2 years after the initial trauma.[2] Immediate treatment for burns can occur in a doctor's office or in the emergency room of a hospital.[7] However, major burns require specialized hospitalization. Some hospitals have burn programs where there is a method of consistent management for burn patients. This includes special training for some staff and an available doctor who has special skills in the treatment of burns. A burn unit within a hospital refers to beds set aside for the exclusive use of burn patients, who are treated only by trained personnel. In addition, a burn center also promotes education and research.[8]

A burn wound is a tissue response to heat. The source of heat may be thermal, chemical, or electrical. The resultant problems and their resolution depend on the depth and extent of the trauma.[9] Flame burns cause the most severe burns because of their depth and extent. Scald burns from hot liquid, a common burn injury among the very young, may be superficial or deep in a limited area. Chemical burns may penetrate deeply into tissues until the substance is washed away.[10]

Electrical burns constitute a small proportion of all burns, but they have unique characteristics that cause special problems for patients. Although the extent of thermal burns can be identified and is predictable, the extent of electrical burns may not be. They usually have an entry and exit point, and the skin between those points may appear normal. However, the passage of current beneath the skin may have damaged muscles, nerves, and vascular supply between those points. Thus, the extent of damage cannot be estimated early. The distinction between necrotic and surviving tissue is slow to develop,[11] and tissue is highly susceptible to infection.[12] Edema also may compromise vascular supply, which affects muscle and nerve, resulting in peripheral nerve injury. Treatment can include fasciotomy to relieve pressure and debridement to remove necrotic tissue. The sequelae of electrical burns are progressive muscular fibrosis, contracture, and loss of function. Amputation is often necessary to save the patient's life by preventing the spread of infection or gangrene after an electrical burn.[11] Patients with electrical burns have more severe psychological problems than other burn patients[13] and often require intensive rehabilitation procedures.[11] Many of the procedures applied to the treatment of thermal burns can be applied to the treatment of electrical burns.[10]

Symptoms

The extent of a burn is estimated by percentage of total body surface area (TBSA) of the burn. The Lund-Browder[4] system adjusts percentage of burn with age of the patient. A common method of estimating TBSA of adults is the rule of nines. In adults the percentage of TBSA with second and third degree burns is calculated by this formula: head and neck equal 9%; each upper extremity is 9%, for a total of 18%; anterior trunk is 18%; posterior trunk is 18%; each lower extremity is 18%, equaling 36%; and the genitalia are 1%, for a total of 100%. The extent of a patient's burn is given in a percentage figure assessment for TBSA involved.[4]

571

Major burns are those that involve more than 25% of TBSA with deep second and third degree burns, or more than 10% third degree burns.[2] Massive burns of more than 60% TBSA have a very high mortality and only a few people survive a burn of 80% TBSA or more,[3] although there are reports of a few survivors of 100% TBSA burns.[14] Patients over age 60 with large burns are at greatest risk for death.[1]

The depth of trauma is based on the intensity of heat on the skin surface. A first degree burn involves only the superficial outer layer of the epidermis, which heals in 2 to 3 days. Sunburn is an example of this and is a painful burn.[10] A second degree burn is a partial-thickness burn, characterized by redness and blisters. It involves epidermis and some of the underlying dermis. The epithelial structure of sebaceous and sweat glands and hair follicles (because they are deep in the skin) survive and are a source of regeneration of new epidermis to reepithelialize the wound. They are painful burns that heal in 10–21 days.[2,4] Very deep second degree burns that do not heal in three weeks require grafting. Third degree burns are full-thickness burns characterized by a hard, dry surface. The entire skin thickness and deep epithelium have been traumatized. Their surfaces are inelastic and anesthetic because the sensory nerve endings are destroyed. Because there is no ability for spontaneous healing or regeneration of the epithelium, a skin graft must be placed on the area to promote healing.[4]

Comprehensive care of a burn patient requires the special skills and knowledge that come with a multidisciplinary team effort and the coordination of responsibilities of all personnel for optimum care. Since many body systems are involved in a severe burn, resulting in physical and psychosocial consequences, the burn care team includes several medical specialists, nurses, physical and occupational therapists, a nutritionist, and a social worker.[15] Treatment begins in the emergency room where resuscitation to correct fluid, electrolyte, and protein deficits is instituted to maintain fluid balance without overloading the circulatory system, which can result in excess edema formation.[16]

The patient is hospitalized to be cared for by specialists who recognize that medical complications of a burn may involve the respiratory tract from inhalation injury, cardiovascular and renal dysfunction, and/or acute gastroduodenal ulceration from stress and the hypermetabolic state characteristic of a severely burned patient. To counteract the hypermetabolism a high-calorie diet is required until skin coverage is complete and body fluids are no longer being lost.[17]

Whatever the extent of a burn, maximal therapy is administered until further evaluations can be completed. In some facilities, if the patient's condition indicates that survival is not possible, and when the patient and family accept the futility of maximal therapy, then the patient receives comfort care—a protocol that maintains the patient pain free and mentally and physically as comfortable as possible while not prolonging a difficult death.[18]

A burn injury destroys protective skin covering, leaving an open wound with the tissue becoming a medium for bacteria growth within 24 hours of the trauma. Until the burn wound is closed through healing or grafting, it is essential to prevent bacterial contamination of the wound.[19] Prevention of infection is a prime goal in burn units, where methicillin-resistant *Staphylococcus aureus* is a problem.[6] Reverse isolation or protective isolation is used by all personnel to protect burn patients from an increased risk of infection. Each institution may have its own procedures; however, the general guidelines include the following: the patient is placed in a private room, or, if on a ward, the bed is surrounded by screens or curtains; all personnel wash their hands before treating the burn patient; a gown and mask are donned before entering the patient's room and, after leaving the patient, the gown and mask are removed and placed in an appropriate receptacle and hands are washed again to prevent spread of infection between patients. Disposable equipment is used whenever possible. Other equipment, including splints, braces and occupational therapy media supplies and equipment, must be sterilized according to institutional standards before they are used with a patient.[19] Infection in a deep second degree burn can convert the wound to a third degree burn.[9]

Topical antibacterial creams and ointments are used as dressings to prevent infection, soften eschar (the coagulated burn slough), and permit movement before grafting. The primary substances are Sulfamylon and silver sulfadiazine, the latter having fewer side effects.[20] The antibacterial ointments require minimal dressings and permit the patient to move unless restricted by splints.[2] The open treatment of patients without dressings requires patients to be in a warm environment to prevent heat loss and to lower metabolic needs, a reason burn units may be kept warmer than other hospital areas.[20] Biological dressings are used as temporary cover to reduce infection and pain and to promote granulation of the wound site for autografting. Biological dressings may be allografts or homografts (skin from the same species), xenografts (skin from another species), amnion (the fetal membrane), or a recently developed synthetic skin cover, Biobrane.[21] The patient's own skin must be used for autografting because it is the only skin cover the patient's body will not reject.[22]

Deep burns result in much edema that may invade adjacent tissues, leading to ischemic necrosis and contractures. Edema begins to form within 6 hours postinjury in third degree burns and may result in capillary damage. The elasticity of the skin is lost, and the resultant eschar does not stretch, which may result in pressure great enough to cause venous occlusion or ischemia in the trunk or extremities. The pressure is relieved by escharotomy, an incision into the burned skin.[20]

Burn Care Stages

Burn care is divided into stages according to time intervals. The *emergent stage* is from 0 to 72 hours after the burn.[23] The patient is in emotional shock with emotional lability, and his adaptation in this stage may be expressed by withdrawal or protest behaviors.[24] Between 48 and 72 hours, the patient begins to recover from the physiological shock and initial emotional shock.[25]

Severely burned patients, aggravated by stress, may exhibit a variety of pain behaviors. Pain, shock, fear, and anxiety are present. A patient's response may be excitation, delirium, or hallucinations. The patient may focus on the pain. A stable, well-adjusted person may accept the treatment routine better than a frightened, immature person. When prolonged treatment is necessary, the continuing stress may lead to depression or hostility toward the personnel responsible for the patient's care.[26]

A burn patient's response to personnel may create hostility and resentment among the staff. Daily contact with emotionally distraught, disfigured, and critically ill patients may provoke strong emotions and anxiety in professionals working with them. During these times the therapist needs to accept the patient without attaching judgmental labels to behavior.[27] It is situational and represents the patient's response to the situation. Often burn team members work through their negative feelings and depression in team meetings.[25] The difficult patient behaviors are often reduced when physiological functions are stabilized.[28] Improvements in emotional stress are noted when most of the burn wounds have healed or have been covered with grafts.[24]

The *acute stage* of burn care, which is now of 4 to 7 days' duration,[23] used to last for weeks or months. Surgeons used less aggressive debridement techniques and waited for the burn wound to prepare itself for grafting. Newer medical techniques and anesthesias now permit earlier surgical treatment for burn wound closure. A topical agent, Travase is used in combination with silver sulfadiazine for enzymatic debridement to treat first and superficial second degree burns to enable autografting within 12 to 24 hours.[29]

Deep second degree burns are treated by tangential excision, the surgical removal of thin layers of burned tissue, until uniform bleeding occurs. Then split-thickness autografts are placed on the burn wound. The treatment for third degree burns is tangential debridement after which the wounds are covered with biological dressings and antimicrobial dressings. The technique promotes healthy granulation of tissue, which can be followed quickly with autografts.[29]

The *rehabilitation stage* is denoted to be from the second week through the remainder of a patient's treatment. However, rehabilitation and prevention are actually begun from the moment the patient's medical condition is stabilized. As the patient's condition permits, the patient should begin to participate in personal daily living skills such as eating and any daily hygiene permissible using adapted methods or equipment. Early involvement of the patient in his own rehabilitation is important to avoid progressive dependency and passivity and to promote self-esteem, self-reliance, and a more positive feeling for the future.[23]

Prevention of deformity is a prime consideration. Most alterations in the musculoskeletal system occur secondary to the acute injury and are not the direct result of it. It is important to anticipate potential impairment and to use measures to prevent deformity in order to ensure that these do not extend the time of hospitalization and rehabilitation. To be effective, all positioning must be enforced from the first day of treatment. The goal is to prevent deformities, which requires the patient to maintain the same positioning program and a variety of positioning devices from the time of hospital admission until discharge. After discharge, prevention of deformity requires continued positioning and splinting of the burned areas until active scar development has ended. If a patient is able to cooperate with the goals of the positioning program, that is, to avoid potentially deforming positions, devices are used only at night to maintain the desired positions.[29] Some centers do not use splints unless it is determined that the patient's condition or ability to cooperate will result in loss of range of motion or function.[23] The occupational therapist uses the protocol written for the individual burn unit or by the surgeon. Some surgeons use skeletal traction for positioning circumferential burns of the extremities, either early in treatment or at time of grafting. Other methods to position include the use of splints, braces, and other devices to maintain the burn patient in optimum position.[29] Early prophylactic use of this equipment, particularly if the skin overlying joints is burned, can decrease the development of secondary deformities.[2]

The methods for positioning and splinting to prevent deformity in each stage of burn care are similar and will be described for the acute stage. The general rule is to position the body segment opposite to the anticipated deformity. The prone and supine positions are similar, except that in prone position the forehead should be supported on a contoured piece of foam rubber to maintain an airway and to keep the neck in slight extension.[29]

The deforming position for a burn on the face, neck, or chest is neck flexion. The eyelids and mouth, as well as the neck and shoulders, can be deformed by neck flexion contractures. The antideformity position places the neck in neutral or slight extension by use of a mattress with a cutout area or use of a thermoplastic neck conformer (Fig. 29.1). The thermoplastic neck conformer reported by Willis[30] has been successful in preventing deformity.[31] In that report, the neck conformer was used in the acute phase over Sulfamylon gauze and in the postgraft phase without padding. Two neck conformers were made: one for the patient in the supine position and the other for the upright position. Since the introduction of that neck conformer, other neck conformers have been developed.[32,33] A modified version of the Willis conformer that also provides total contact to the grafted area is constructed with a removable lip conformer, thus allowing lip movement for

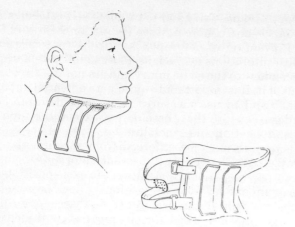

Figure 29.1 Conformer neck splint made of Orthoplast. (Reproduced with permission from Shirley Baty, illustrator, and Larson, D. L. Making the least of burn scars. *Emerg. Med., 4*: 24–35, 1972.)

speech and removal for eating and oral hygiene while maintaining pressure on the neck and chin.[34] The conformer is removed every 2 hours to cleanse and dry it before reapplication.[30]

The deforming position for a burn on the shoulder or axilla is the anatomical position with the arms at the side in adduction. To counteract this, the arm is positioned in 100° to 110° of abduction[23] and externally rotated.[35] Greater abduction may result in brachial plexus injury.[23] Placement in abduction may be maintained by use of arm troughs,[36] by placing the outstretched arms on pillows supported on a bedside table, or by use of an airplane splint (Fig. 13.16) if a contracture is developing. In the upright position, semicircular sponges are placed in the axilla and secured with an elastic wrap[29] (Fig. 29.2).

The deforming position for the elbow is elbow flexion, so the antideformity position is elbow extension with forearm in midposition. Care is taken not to hyperextend the elbow; up to 5° of flexion can be per-

mitted with the forearm in midposition.[35] Extension contractures are rare.[23] The elbow can be maintained in extension with a simple three-point extension brace[37] (Fig. 29.3) or a thermoplastic conformer placed anteriorly[23] (Fig. 29.4).

People experiencing thermal injuries tend to put their hands to their face protectively, which results in burns to the dorsum of the hand and fingers. This burn results in loss of elasticity to the dorsal surface of the hand and, without proper care and positioning, leads to deformity.

The position of deformity for the burned hand is wrist flexion, metacarpophalangeal (MP) hyperextension, and proximal interphalangeal (PIP) flexion with the thumb adducted and the palmar arch flattened. This is the "intrinsic minus" hand. The deformity can occur within a day or two if the burned hand is allowed to rest unsplinted on a bed.[29] Previous literature on burns suggested placing the hand in the "position of function" during treatment.[38] More recent descriptions of treatment for burns on the dorsum of the hand recommend the "antideformity"[35] or "safe" position.[7] This position places the wrist in 0° to 45° of extension, which allows the MP joints to fall into flexion. It is also recommended that splints position the MP joints into 70° to 90° of flexion. Most authors recommend that the PIP and distal interphalangeal (DIP) joints be placed in full extension.[8,15,23,29,35,37] (See Figure 13.7.)

A rationale for splinting the fingers in MP flexion and IP extension is proposed by James, who described the MP ligaments as being slack when the MP joint is extended. If the MP joint is positioned in extension, the slackened ligaments can become tight and unyield-

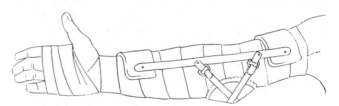

Figure 29.3 Three-point extension splint. (Reproduced with permission from Shirley Baty, illustrator, and Larson, D. L. Making the least of burn scars. *Emerg. Med., 4*: 24–35, 1972.)

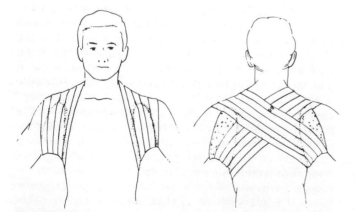

Figure 29.2 Semicircular foam pads held in place at axilla by figure of eight Ace bandage. (Reproduced with permission from Shirley Baty, illustrator, and Larson, D. L. Making the least of burn scars. *Emerg. Med., 4*: 24–35, 1972.)

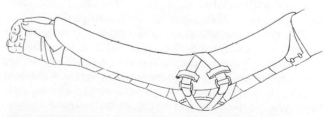

Figure 29.4 Elbow conformer splint made of Orthoplast. (Reproduced with permission from Shirley Baty, illustrator, and Larson, D. L. Making the least of burn scars. *Emerg. Med., 4*: 24–35, 1972.)

ing, further preventing MP flexion in the future. The ligaments of PIP and DIP joints are slack when placed in flexion. To correct these potential deforming forces, the MP joints are placed in flexion and the IPs in extension where all lateral ligaments are taut and less likely to shorten.[39] The thumb should be abducted and extended at the carpometacarpal (CMC) joint with the MP and interphalangeal (IP) joint extended.[8,15,23,29,35]

For burns on the volar surface of the hand, the position of choice is with the wrist in neutral (0° to 30° of extension), the MP joints in neutral (0°), and the fingers extended and abducted. The thumb is extended and abducted to prevent contracture of the flexor tendons.[23,35]

When circumferential burns involve the dorsal and volar surfaces of the hand, it will be necessary to alternate the two positions equally by using a day splint and a night splint.[23,35]

Lateral burns of the trunk may result in a hemi-thoracic scar resulting in scoliotic contracture. There is convexity of the curve toward the contralateral side. The trunk should be positioned in a straight line to prevent development of an incipient contracture toward a scoliosis-like position.[29]

The position of deformity for the hip is hip flexion and adduction. Therefore, hips are positioned in extension and 15° to 20° of symmetrical hip abduction. A severe burn over the anterior hip joint requires great vigilance to keep the hips and legs in position. A knee-positioning splint on the leg will discourage hip flexion in the supine position.[29]

A burned knee, like a burned elbow, tends to develop a flexion deformity, especially when the popliteal area is involved. The antideformity position is knee extension, which can be maintained by a three-point extension splint,[29,37] or a posterior leg splint.[23] Neither splint should hyperextend the knee to avoid injury to the popliteal nerve.[23]

The deforming position for the ankle is plantar flexion. The ankle should be maintained in neutral to allow for later weight bearing and comfortable walking. A footboard or a posterior splint can be used to support the foot.[23,29] When the patient is in prone position, if a short mattress is used, the feet can be placed over the edge to maintain the ankle joint in the neutral position.[29]

Occupational Therapy Related To Stages of Care

From the moment a burn patient enters an emergency room, the occupational therapy goals for physical restoration are established for any body segment with a burn. The goals are to prevent contracture and deformity; to maintain range of motion, muscle function, and strength; to promote physical daily living skills; and to provide emotional support. The long-range goal is to return the patient to pretrauma functional ability. From the beginning the patient should understand that he is expected to return to maximum function. The goals are accomplished by a program of position-ing and splinting to prevent contractures of joints. Active range of motion activities are used to maintain range of motion and strength.[23] Emotional adjustment is facilitated using the principles and methods described in chapter 2.

EMERGENT PHASE

The immediate care of a burn patient concentrates on relieving the shock and physiological complications of the burn to save life. Life support measures and rigid techniques that isolate the patient from infection tend to result also in social isolation, itself psychologically stressful.[24] The occupational therapist can provide some social involvement at every visit, the goals of which may be positioning for reduction of edema or fitting and adjusting splints. At that time, the therapist should always explain to the patient what is being done and why. The patient is told that the positioning and splinting are to ensure him more function when the wounds have healed or skin cover is achieved by the surgical staff. This is evidence to the patient that his recovery is anticipated. The occupational therapist can foster the patient's efforts in his own treatment from the first visit. Hope for life is a powerful ally.

Assessment

The usual occupational therapy evaluations, such as goniometric range of motion and manual muscle testing, are not feasible for a patient with acute and extensive burns. Any body segments unaffected by the injury may be evaluated and a comparison may be made with burned segments to establish an information base. Knowledge of the patient's occupation and its physical requirements, his leisure activities, and age may indicate an approximate extent of function prior to the injury. The medical history should contain information as to any preexisting conditions, such as arthritis, that might indicate less than normal strength and range of motion. If a patient's history and occupation indicate functional ability up to the time of the burn, one might assume that range of motion and strength were within normal limits. As the patient becomes able to do active motion, goniometric measures can be made. Physicians test for sensation in burn patients to discriminate between second degree and third degree burns, because it is known that second degree burns are very painful, whereas third degree burns, in which the free nerve endings are destroyed, do not cause pain. However, the patient feels pain from adjacent areas.[40] An occupational therapist probably would not want to repeat the sensory test because the findings are not useful at this stage of treatment.

ACUTE STAGE

The acute period, fourth through seventh day after the burn,[23] will begin the patient's progression through stages of burn care. The goals for preventing deformity and maintaining range of motion are consistent with each stage. In cases of extensive burns, the patient will have some full-thickness wounds in the pregraft stage, whereas other body parts are in the healing stage or in the postgraft stage. Specific procedures are used for each burned area and its stage until total skin coverage is achieved.

The burn wound is cleansed daily by nursing or physical therapy personnel. Some centers prefer to use water sprays,[2] showers[6], or an ordinary bath. In other centers the Hubbard tank continues to be used in burn care.[29] Antibacterial ointment dressings are applied daily after cleansing and this is an optimum time, while the tissues are soft and moist, for the patient to do active motion.[2] It is essential, in addition to maintaining proper positioning, for the burn patient to perform active movement from the day of admission to prevent deformity and contracture, the most disabling sequelae of burns. All nonburned areas should be exercised daily. At that time the patient may be asked to move, or is assisted to move, all joints. Splints and positioning devices are removed several times daily for the devices to be cleansed so that they do not become reservoirs for bacteria.[35] At these times active exercise should be supervised by the therapist. The patient should also be taught to move unsplinted parts every 2 hours for up to 10 repetitions of movement each time. An activity list can be kept at bedside to remind the patient and other personnel of the treatment program.

The greatest obstacle to this goal is the patient's anticipation of pain when moving a burned extremity. Although burns are painful, the pain is not constant and when at rest the patient may be comfortable. The most severe pain occurs during treatment procedures.[40] One sequence for gaining patient cooperation has been described by Evans.[41] The therapist approaches the patient and describes what needs to be done and why, meanwhile surveying the patient to identify joints without burns. Then the patient is coached to do active and active assisted motion with the unburned joints. The patient is then taught to do isometric exercises, or muscle setting, in any unburned parts. Next the patient is encouraged to do isometric contraction under burned areas. As the patient learns that some muscle contraction can be done without extreme discomfort, he should be able to begin to cooperate with maintaining muscle awareness. Then the patient is asked to perform some active, or active-assisted, motion with a burned part. Daily contraction of all muscles and movement of uninvolved joints is essential to maintain joint awareness.[41] During periods of strict positioning, before and after grafting, it is important that the burn patient be allowed to initiate some voluntary active motion of the parts that are not being immobilized, either in or out of splints. Experiments have shown that immobilization alone can result in behavioral changes involving cognition and mood, similar to those that result from being in a sensory or perceptual deprivation environment, but that exercise or simple movements decrease the behavioral changes.[42,43]

If active voluntary joint movement is too painful for the burn patient, at least isometric contractions within splints are encouraged. During the acute phase, muscle awareness, rather than strength building, is the goal of isometric contractions.[41] If a patient is allowed to be immobile for a few days, he will become fearful of moving and avoid any active or passive motion. If an unconscious patient is unable to do active motion, gentle passive motion should be done at least once a day. The diagonal patterns of proprioceptive neuromuscular facilitation are recommended for passive motion of limbs in burn patients.[44] (See chapter 6 for description of proprioceptive neuromuscular facilitation.)

Passive motion should be done slowly and gently and never beyond tissue resistance. Mild sustained motions, rather than vigorously repeated motions, are used to avoid additional damage to the wound or healing areas.[2,41]

Active motion should begin early in treatment of areas of partial-thickness burns because surgery will not be done on those areas. The motions should be done after cleansing or after analgesics, when the patient is more comfortable. Because partial-thickness burns expose nerve endings,[2] a patient with a large second degree burn may experience more pain than a patient with a deeper burn.[40] Areas with superficial second degree burns may be actively or passively exercised to maintain range of motion. Ambulation and personal daily living skills are encouraged early, depending on the extent and complications of the burn.[23]

The hand with deep second and third degree burns on the dorsum must be given special care. Burns on the dorsum of the hand may threaten the integrity of the extensor mechanism. Deep second and third degree burns can distort the joints because of thermal trauma or because of fibrosis of joint capsules and loss of continuity of the extensor tendons. Neither active nor passive motion should be allowed to place tension on the extensor mechanism. Tension is placed on the extensor mechanism when the patient actively makes a tight fist or when the therapist moves the fingers passively into total flexion. This tension can cause the extensor mechanism to split, slip, or be otherwise damaged. Acute flexion of the MP and IP joints simultaneously can result in disruption of the central slip, creating a boutonniere deformity that will require surgical repair. Splinting the wrist in neutral with only slight MP flexion and with the IP joints extended counteracts the force toward a boutonniere deformity.[35]

One method used to exercise the hand burned on the dorsum suggests that when one joint is flexed, the other joints should remain in extension. Muscle testing positions for MP, PIP, and DIP flexion may be used (see chapter 8); that is, MP flexion is done with the PIP and DIP joints in neutral or extension; the PIP joint is flexed slightly with the MP and DIP joints in neutral extension; and the DIP joint is flexed with the MP and PIP joints in neutral extension.[35] A Bunnell block can be used to assist positioning for such activity.[45,46] For thumb range of motion, the CMC joint is held in neutral while thumb MP flexion is done with the IP joint in neutral. Thumb IP flexion can be done with the CMC with the CMC and MP joints in neutral.

REHABILITATION STAGE

Grafting

With newer, more aggressive treatment to achieve wound cover, eschar is removed from burns sooner,[29] including facial burns.[47] Biological dressings or synthetic dressings are used to cover the wounds. This results in relief of pain for the patient and physiological and psychological improvement.[48] These substances are not accepted by the body and are replaced later by autografts of the patient's own skin.[49] Prior to placement of the final graft, the surgeon and the occupational therapist may confer to plan the positioning devices to be used after the grafting procedure. Splints may be made prior to surgery or in the operating room.[35] The extremity can be placed in the splint and the grafts laid over the open wound without sutures or dressings, or they may be secured with tape.[20] A splint immobilizes the part while the graft takes. The immobilization results in greater success and decreases the chance that the graft will be lost.[35]

After grafting, the wound is painless but the donor site is painful. It requires about 3 weeks to heal and should be cared for similarly to a burn.[50] To avoid the patient's disappointment at the first appearance of the graft, the patient should be told ahead of time that the skin on that area will not have the appearance it had before the burn.[20]

Postgraft Treatment

Following placement of the graft, positioning continues. The newly placed graft survives on plasma until it links up with the capillaries in the dermis. During this phase, movement can destroy the capillary linkage causing the graft to be lost; therefore any movement before 5-7 days may not be beneficial enough to warrant it.[44] The surgeon has the responsibility to decide when the grafted area can be moved. The therapist should expect that after the fourth day a determination will be made about moving the grafted part. However, it may be up to 10 days before the area should actually be moved. Active or assisted motion should continue for those joints not being immobilized for grafting procedures.[20]

As the patient's wounds heal and the grafts begin to take, it then becomes possible for the occupational therapist to obtain more formal assessment measures for range of motion, muscle strength, and pinch measurements. Reinnervation of the grafted area may begin within 2 weeks after the graft is placed, when the nerve fibers may enter vacant neurilemma sheaths of the graft. Because the return of sensation depends on the accessibility of neurilemma sheaths in the donor graft, it is not complete for some time after grafting. Touch, pain, temperature, and two-point discrimination return at varying rates.[22] Sensory testing may be informative at this time (see chapter 3).

After the grafts are healed the patient can begin a program of active motion to restore range of motion and function. All joints must be kept mobile, and the patient must be taught to avoid heat, friction, and trauma to the grafted areas.[23] In the case of hand grafts, the patient begins by moving each of the finger joints carefully. A program of hourly repetitions of these exercises is established. Games and activities are introduced to encourage development of functional strength and dexterity.[35]

Following grafting to the lower extremities, the patient is not permitted to ambulate until venous drainage has been achieved in the grafted area, or the graft may be lost. After 10 days the patient may be allowed to walk if the legs are wrapped in elastic bandages.[51]

As the patient becomes ambulatory, he may be able to attend the occupational therapy clinic where personal daily living skills can be practiced and work evaluation can begin. Specific modalities are introduced for elimination of specific deficits.[23]

Scarring and Scar Prevention

The early result of burn wound healing may be satisfactory, but in a few months smooth skin becomes contracted scar. Hypertrophic scarring and the contractures that follow closure of a deep burn wound are a frustrating sequelae of healed burns.[52] Hypertrophic scars occur in areas of deep burns that have required several weeks to heal.[53] When the deep reticular portion of the dermis is disturbed, hypertrophic scarring begins. Increased vascularity in the grafted area leaves a bright red healing wound. Collagen fibers develop to bridge the wound and begin to form a tangled mass that may take a year to mature. Continuous gentle pressure influences the arrangement of the collagen fibers so that they align in parallel rows rather then in ropelike whorls, as happens without pressure. It is thought that the pressure decreases the circulation to the area and retards scar development. As long as the scar is active it can be influenced by pressure and positioning. Immature hypertrophic scar is firm, raised, and red. Mature hypertrophic scar is pale, flat, and soft.[52] Once the scar becomes mature, only surgical correction is possible to remove the deformity. If grafts cover a joint, the hypertrophic scar tends to involve flexor surfaces. These deformities can be avoided through a program of pressure dressing and conformer splinting for a long period, sometimes more than a year, after the wounds have healed.[2,54]

In addition to flexor surfaces being subject to hypertrophic scar, full-thickness burns over the shoulder, anterior elbow, and hip have resulted in bridging of the joints with heterotopic bone. This has occurred in patients who were unable to participate in an active therapy program, or who were resistant to such participation. Heterotopic bone formation is rarely seen when patients are started in programs that emphasize early mobilization. Joints that do not yield to usual measures for increasing range of motion should be x-rayed, because if heterotopic bone is present, surgical excision is required to restore range of motion.[29] However, active motion should be encouraged in the available range until surgery can be done.[55]

After the autografts take and each body area has skin cover, the area is wrapped in elastic bandages or tubular compression bandages (Tubigrip) to prevent contracture and to control hypertrophic scar. Using the tubular compression bandage for 3 to 6 months postgraft results in decreased hypertrophy of scar tissue. Tubular compression bandage is made by Seaton Products, Montgomery, Pennsylvania, under the name Tubigrip. This product is available in continuous tubes with a selection of circumferences to fit all sizes of trunks and extremities; gloves can be made from the tubes.[56] The tubular compression bandages, used until custom-fit garments can be ordered, allow modifications and can be changed frequently. Tension of 5–10 mm Hg is not sufficient to control scarring. However, 10–20 mm Hg has been found to be sufficient pressure and is usually tolerable in the early postgraft period.[57] Although pressure garments have been used routinely for most postburn patients since mid 1970s,[52] recent studies have indicated that not all burns require the use of pressure garments. Patients with burn wounds that heal in 1 to 2 weeks are offered garments. Those whose wounds heal in 2 to 3 weeks are advised to use pressure garments. Any wound that requires more than 21 days to heal (usually a deeper burn) must be treated with pressure garments to prevent deformity and to promote remodeling of the scar.[53]

After the patient's body weight stabilizes following skin cover, custom-knit Jobskin® Pressure Covers are ordered to replace the elastic bandages or Tubigrip bandages,[56] which are used until the Jobskin® Pressure Covers are received. Isotoner gloves, with decorations removed and turned inside out to avoid seams against the skin, may be used temporarily for the grafted hand when the grafts heal enough to tolerate the force of application.[23]

The Jobskin® Pressure Covers are custom made for each patient by Jobst Institute in Toledo, Ohio.[58] The company provides instructions for measuring and ordering. Because the garments are worn continuously, two sets are ordered to permit laundering. The garments are removed only for bathing or during exercise if they interfere with exercise movements. However, for the best results they should not be removed for more than an hour at a time.[56]

Patients should be taught the necessary hygiene and cleanliness requirements for use of the garments. Patients should also be taught that nonoily skin moisturizers and sunscreens can be used to prevent skin breakdown. Skin creams should not contain oil because it causes deterioration of the elastic garments.[23,35] The splinting and positioning program continues with the use of the Jobskin® Pressure Covers, combined with thermoplastic conformers, which provide pressure in specific areas.[23]

A Jobskin® Pressure Cover mask is available to cover the head, face, and neck for burns to that area. A thermoplastic face conformer is made to provide consistent pressure to the areas of the face, particularly for scars around the nose and mouth, and is worn under

the Jobskin® garment. A transparent face mask is an alternative choice to treat facial scars.[59,60] There are also special splints for increasing the mouth opening to prevent oral microstomia secondary to burns to that area.[61]

For areas such as the shoulder, neck, and axilla, where it is difficult to fit thermoplastic materials, a flexible elastomer is available to make contour molds to wear under the elastic garments.[62] The neck conformer is applied for total contact to burns of the neck. The use of the neck conformer, following partial- or full-thickness burns,[30] has decreased the incidence and severity of neck contractures in patients with severe burns from an expected 37% to only 9%.[31]

To control hypertrophic scarring in the axilla, a Jobskin® Pressure Cover with sleeves is worn and foam crescents are secured in the axilla with elastic bandages[29] (Fig. 29.2). Contracture of the elbow by hypertrophic scar is controlled by use of an anterior thermoplastic conformer, which can be changed as elbow extension range increases[23] (Fig. 29.4). The successful use of a spring-tension device to exert prolonged low-load pressure also has been reported useful to correct elbow flexion contracture following burn rehabilitation.[63]

Jobskin® gloves are available and can be detached from the garment sleeves to permit hand washing.[64] Gloves are useful to keep the finger webs from becoming adherent and scarred. The positioning hand splint is worn at night over the Jobskin® Pressure Cover garment.[52] Elastomer molds have been used by some to improve finger and thumb web spaces[62]; others use materials graded for progressive widening of the spaces to counteract scar formation there. The materials used range from Telfa gauze to dressmaker elastic to elastic bandages stretched through the web spaces and attached to a wrist cuff volarly and dorsally.[65]

Hypertrophic scarring of the trunk can be reduced by wearing a Jobskin® Pressure Cover over the area.[23]

If hip and knee contractures are a potential problem, a three-point knee extension brace,[37] using the same principles as pictured in Fig. 29.3 for the elbow, or a posterior splint[23] can be used when the patient is supine to avoid both hip and knee flexion contractures.

Treatment for the prevention of scars in healed burns to the dorsum of the foot is by use of high tennis shoes, lined with sheepskin, laced firmly to apply pressure.[52]

Discharge Planning and Home Program

Some reports suggest that the program of splinting and positioning can be relaxed when the patient is able to maintain actively the appropriate positioning and do the range of motion programs.[23] Other studies indicate that with more recently developed surgical techniques such as early excision, the postburn treatment routines may be modified.[53] However, Linares et al. indicate that the program must be maintained as long as there is evidence that the burn scars have not matured.[52]

The occupational therapist should devise a home program for wearing splints and Jobskin® Pressure

Covers. She should educate the patient and caregiver about how to apply the Jobskin® Pressure Covers, splints, and elastomer molds correctly and how to do the prescribed exercises accurately. The education must also include the reasons for splinting, as well as an explanation of the consequences of not following the program. Written instructions for hospital and home treatment have been found to be effective for teaching patients.[66] Also, the therapist should give the patient the name and telephone number of the person at the occupational therapy department to call to have questions answered.[23]

Although prolonged use of pressure garments and splints is necessary to achieve better function and cosmesis following a burn, the wearing program as outlined appears to be an incredible burden over an extended period of 12 to 18 months for an injured patient who has already been through the rigors of all that the care of an acute or extensive burn requires. On what basis can a therapist encourage and convince a patient or a family that this treatment must be continued for a year or more? Prior to this regimen, contractures and multiple readmissions for reconstructive surgery were the common and accepted sequelae of a burn. A review of 625 patients at follow-up showed that the longer the pressure garments were worn, the fewer number of contractures and ultimate surgical releases of contractures were needed. In the population, 219 patients were treated prior to the introduction of the splint and pressure garment procedures. Of that group 92% required one or more follow-up surgeries after recovery from the burn. Of the 406 patients who were treated with splints and pressure, only 25% required one or more operations following recovery. An assessment of the length of time the garments and splints were worn showed that 70% of the patients who wore them for only 6 months required follow-up surgery, whereas only 23% of those wearing splints and garments for 6 to 12 months required surgery. Of the patients who followed the wearing program for more than 12 months only 15% required additional surgery. The savings in fewer inpatient hospitalizations and the trauma of surgery are impressive, but of greater interest is the information that the program is truly preventative and of great benefit for restoration of function following a burn.[31] Therefore, following discharge, patients should be rechecked regularly for a year or more, or until the grafts mature and there is no evidence of hypertrophic scar activity.

A large burn leaves physical and emotional scars. This is particularly true of the facially disfigured. The patients must call up coping and adapting mechanisms to get themselves through the repeated surgeries and uncomfortable procedures. Adjustment may take a long time especially for the patient with a facial burn.[24]

Although the quality of burn care, measured in survival statistics, improves yearly[3] the quality of life following a burn is only partially known. Psychosocial studies of adult burn patients indicate that about 30% of burn patients have long-term psychosocial problems, commonly anxiety and depression.[67] That percentage suggests that about 70% manage to cope and adapt following a burn, although it requires about a year for patients to resolve the depression, which seems unrelated to the extent of the burn injury.[68,69] The quality of a patient's social network system, particularly the family, has been found to relate to measures of self-esteem and life satisfaction following a burn.[67,69,70]

Occupational therapy for burn patients is primarily prevention of the deforming sequelae of the burn and maintenance of independent daily living skills and psychological and emotional coping skills. It may be difficult to realize when confronted with a severely injured burn patient that most of these patients, with current knowledge and practice, have a good prognosis for functional recovery. Occupational therapists make a substantial contribution to that functional recovery and the affirmation that the patient is a normal, acceptable person in spite of the burns.[71]

STUDY QUESTIONS

Burns

1. Define first degree, second degree, and third degree burns.
2. What is the "rule of nines"? How is it used?
3. Describe reverse, or protective, isolation techniques.
4. What is the general rule for positioning or splinting the burn patient?
5. What is the course of medical/surgical treatment of second degree burns?
6. What goals do occupational therapists pursue with patients who have second degree burns?
7. What is the course of medical/surgical treatment of third degree burns?
8. What are the goals the occupational therapist has for the patient with third degree burns?
9. Describe the safest methods of doing range of motion to the burned hand. Why are these methods preferred?
10. What is the antideformity splinting position of choice for the hand with dorsal burns? Why?
11. Why is constant pressure against healing burn scar recommended, and how is the pressure applied?
12. State two reasons you would give a patient to convince him to wear the pressure garments until they are discontinued by the physician.

References

1. Feller, I., James, M. H., and Jones, C. A. Burn epidemiology: focus on youngsters and the aged. *J. Burn Care Rehabil.*, 3(5): 285–288, 1982.
2. Helm, P. A., et al. Burn injury: rehabilitation management in 1982. *J. Burn Care Rehabil.*, 4(6): 411–422, 1983.
3. Feller, I., and Jones, C. A. Introduction—statement of the problem. In *Comprehensive Rehabilitation Of Burns*. Edited by S. V. Fisher and P. A. Helm. Baltimore: Williams & Wilkins, 1984.
4. Salisbury, R. E., Newman, N. M., and Dingeldein, G. P., Jr. *Manual Of Burn Therapeutics: An Interdisciplinary Approach.* Boston: Little, Brown & Company, 1983.
5. Dimick, A. R. Pathophysiology. In *Comprehensive Rehabilitation Of Burns*. Edited by S. V. Fisher and P. H. Helm. Baltimore: Williams & Wilkins, 1984.
6. Purdue, G. F. Reflections on modern burn care. *J. Burn Care Rehabil.*, 5(1): 58–61, 1984.

7. Hummel, R. P. Care of the burn wound. In *Clinical Burn Wound Therapy: A Management and Prevention Guide.* Edited by R. P. Hummel. Boston: John Wright, 1982.

8. Johnson, C. L., O'Shaughnessy, E. J., and Ostergren, G. *Burn Management.* New York: Raven Press, 1981.

9. Solem, L. D. Classification. In *Comprehensive Rehabilitation Of Burns.* Edited by S. V. Fisher and P. H. Helm. Baltimore: Williams & Wilkins, 1984.

10. Abston, S., and Rinear, C. Burns. In *Basic Emergency Care Of The Sick And Injured,* 3rd edition. Edited by Guy S. Parcel. St. Louis: Times Mirror/Mosby College Publishing, 1986.

11. Nichter, L. S., et al. Injuries due to commercial electric current. *J. Burn Care Rehabil.,* 5(2): 124-137, 1984.

12. Hunt, J. L. Electrical injuries. In *Comprehensive Rehabilitation Of Burns.* Edited by S. V. Fisher and P. A. Helm. Baltimore: Williams & Wilkins, 1984.

13. Mancusi-Ungaro, H. R., Jr., Tarbox, A. R., and Wainwright, D. J. Posttraumatic stress disorder in electric burn patients. *J. Burn Care Rehabil.,* 7(6): 521-524, 1986.

14. Fengxun, X., Yuanzhang, M., and Susong, P. Successful treatment for two extensive third degree burn patients. In *Recent Advances In Burns And Plastic Surgery: The Chinese Experience.* Edited by C. Tisheng, S. Jixiang, and Y. Zhijun, Lancaster, England: MIP Press Ltd., 1985.

15. DiGregorio, V. R., editor. *Rehabilitation Of The Burn Patient.* New York: Churchill Livingstone, 1984.

16. Pruitt, B. A. Fluid resuscitation. *J. Burn Care Rehabil.,* 2(5): 263-294, 1981.

17. Dingeldein, G. P., Jr. Complications of thermal injury. In *Manual Of Burn Therapeutics.* Edited by R. E. Salisbury, N. M. Newman, and G. P. Dingeldein, Jr. Boston: Little, Brown & Company, 1983.

18. Frank, H. A., and Wachtel, T. L. Life and death in a burn center. *J. Burn Care Rehabil.,* 5(4): 339-342, 1984.

19. Sheretz, R. J. Isolation practices. In *Manual Of Burn Therapeutics.* Edited by R. E. Salisbury, N. M. Newman, and G. P. Dingeldein, Jr. Boston: Little, Brown & Company, 1983.

20. Hartford, C. E. Surgical management. In *Comprehensive Rehabilitation Of Burns.* Edited by S. V. Fisher and P. A. Helm. Baltimore: Williams & Wilkins, 1984.

21. Zawacki, B. E. Temporary wound closure after burn excision. *J. Burn Care Rehabil.,* 7(2): 138-143, 1986.

22. Smahel, J. The healing of skin grafts. *Clin. Plast. Surg.,* 4(3): 409-424, 1977.

23. Reeves, S. U. Occupational therapy in burn care. In *Manual Of Burn Therapeutics.* Edited by R. E. Salisbury, N. M. Newman, and G. P. Dingeldein, Jr. Boston: Little, Brown & Company, 1983.

24. Bernstein, N. R. *Emotional Care Of The Facially Burned And Disfigured.* Boston: Little, Brown & Company, 1976.

25. Wagner, M. Pain and nursing care associated with burns. In *Pain: A Source Book For Nurses And Other Health Professionals.* Edited by A. K. Jacox. Boston: Little, Brown & Company, 1977.

26. Kolman, P. B. Managing psychopathology in burn patients. *J. Burn Care Rehabil.,* 5(3): 239-243, 1984.

27. Jones, C. A., and Feller, I. *Procedures for Nursing the Burned Patient.* Ann Arbor: National Institute of Burn Medicine, 1973.

28. Rudowski, W. *Burn Therapy And Research.* Baltimore: The Johns Hopkins University Press, 1976.

29. Evans, E. B., and Parks, D. H. Burns. In *Orthopedic Rehabilitation.* Edited by V. L. Nickel. New York: Churchill Livingstone, 1982.

30. Willis, B. The use of orthoplane isoprene splints in the treatment of the acutely burned child. *Am. J. Occup. Ther.,* 24(3): 187-191, 1970.

31. Huang, T. T., Blackwell, S. J., and Lewis, S. R. Ten years of experience in managing patients with burn contractures of axilla, elbow, wrist and knee joints. *Plast. Reconstr. Surg.,* 61(1): 70-76, 1978.

32. Sandel, E., and Khaleeli, C. R. Use of the thermoplastic total contact and the foam watusi ring neck splint. *American Occupational Therapy Association Physical Disabilities Special Interest Section Newsletter* 4(2): 3, 1981.

33. Leman, C. J. The triple-component neck splint. *J. Burn Care Rehabil.,* 7(4): 357-360, 1986.

34. Parrish, N. E. Postoperative splinting of the lower face and neck. *J. Burn Care Rehabil.,* 7(2): 148-150, 1986.

35. Salisbury, R. E., Reeves, S., and Wright, P. Rehabilitation of the burned hand. In *Rehabilitation Of The Hand,* 2nd edition. Edited by J. M. Hunter, et al. St. Louis: C. V. Mosby, 1984.

36. Heeter, K. H. Arm hammock for elevation of the thermally injured upper extremity. *J. Burn Care Rehabil.,* 7(2): 144-152, 1986.

37. Willis, B. The use of orthoplast isoprene splints in the treatment of the acutely burned child: preliminary report. *Am. J. Occup. Ther.,* 23(1): 57-61, 1969.

38. Georgiade, N. D. Management of the burn wound. In *Symposium on the Treatment of Burns,* Vol. 5. Edited by J. R. Lynch, and S. R. Lewis. St. Louis: C. V. Mosby, 1973.

39. James, J. I. P. Assessment and management of the injured hand. *The Hand,* 2(2): 97-105, 1970.

40. Perry, S., Heidrich, G., and Ramos, E. Assessment of pain by burn patients. *J. Burn Care Rehabil.,* 2(6): 322-326, 1981.

41. Evans, E. B. Orthopaedic measures in the treatment of severe burns. *J. Bone Joint Surg.,* 48A(4): 643-669, 1966.

42. Zubek, J. P. Counteracting effects of physical exercises performed during prolonged perceptual deprivation. *Science,* 142(3591): 504-506, 1963.

43. Zubek, J. P., and MacNeill, M. Effects of immobilization: behavioral and EEG changes. *Can. J. Psychiatry,* 20(3): 316-336, 1966.

44. Robson, M. C. Reconstruction and rehabilitation from admission: a surgeon's role at each phase. In *Comprehensive Approaches To The Burned Person.* Edited by N. R. Bernstein and M. C. Robson. New Hyde Park, NY: Medical Examination Publishing Company, 1983.

45. Bunnell, S. *Surgery Of The Hand.* Philadelphia: J. B. Lippincott, 1944.

46. Becker, C. G. Adaptation of Bunnell block. *Am. J. Occup. Ther.,* 29(2): 108, 1975.

47. Warden, G. D., et al. Excisional therapy of facial burns. *J. Burn Care Rehabil.,* 7(1): 24-28, 1986.

48. Shuck, J. M. Biologic dressings. In *Burns: A Team Approach* Edited by C. P. Artz, J. A. Moncrief, and B. A. Pruitt. Philadelphia: W. B. Saunders, 1979.

49. Remensnyder, J. P., and Wray, R. C. Burn and frostbite injuries. In *Acute Hand Injuries: A Multispecialty Approach.* Edited by F. G. Wolfort. Boston: Little, Brown & Company, 1980.

50. Heeter, P. K. A leg support for circumferential exposure of donor sites. *J. Burn Care Rehabil.,* 7(2): 146-147, 1986.

51. Johnson, C. L. PT/OT forum. *J. Burn Care Rehabil.,* 5(2): 113-115, 1984.

52. Linares, H. A., Larson, D. L., and Baur, P. S., Jr. Influences of mechanical forces on burn scar contracture and hypertrophy. In *Symposium On Basic Science In Plastic Surgery,* Vol. 15. Edited by T. J. Krizek and J. E. Hoopes. St. Louis: C. V. Mosby, 1976.

53. Deitch, E. A., et al. Hypertrophic burn scars: analysis of variables. *J. Trauma,* 23(10): 895-898, 1983.

54. Jensen, L. L., and Parshley, P. F. Postburn scar contractures: histology and effects of pressure treatment. *J. Burn Care Rehabil.,* 5(2): 119-122, 1984.

55. Crawford, C. M., et. al. Heterotopic ossification: are range of motion exercises contraindicated? *J. Burn Care Rehabil.,* 7(4): 323-327, 1986.

56. Bruster, J. M., and Pulliam, G. Gradient pressure. *Am. J. Occup. Ther.,* 37(7): 485-488, 1983.

57. Judge, J. C., May, S. R., and DeClement, F. A. Control of hypertrophic scarring in burn patients using tubular support bandages. *J. Burn Care Rehabil.,* 5(3): 221-224, 1984.

58. Blair, K. L. Prevention and control of hypertrophic scarring and contractures by the application of the Custom Made Jobskin® Pressure Covers. Toledo, OH: Jobst Institute, 1982.

59. Peterson, P. A conformer for the reduction of facial burn contractures: a preliminary report. *Am. J. Occup. Ther.,* 31(2): 101-104, 1977.

60. Rivers, E. A., Strate, R. G., and Solem, L. D. The transparent face mask. *Am. J. Occup. Ther.,* 33(2): 108-113, 1979.

61. Gorham, J. A. A mouth splint for burn microstomia. *Am. J. Occup. Ther.,* 31(2): 105-106, 1977.

62. Malick, M. H., and Carr, J. A. Flexible elastomer molds in burn scar control. *Am. J. Occup. Ther.,* 34(9): 603-608, 1980.

63. Richard, R. L. Use of Dynasplint™ to correct elbow flexion burn contractures: a case report. *J. Burn Care Rehabil.,* 7(2): 151-152, 1986.

64. Jobst Institute. *Burn Scar Therapy, A Treatment Method.* Toledo, OH: Jobst Institute, 1973.

65. Quan, P. E., et al. Control of scar tissue in the finger web spaces by use of graded pressure inserts. *J. Burn Care Rehabil.,* 1(2): 27-29, 54, 1980.

66. Kaplan, S. H. Patient education techniques used at burn centers. *Am. J. Occup. Ther.,* 39(10): 655-659, 1985.

67. Malt, U. Long-term psychosocial follow-up studies of burned adults: review of literature. *Burns,* 6(3): 190-197, 1980.

68. Blades, B. C., Jones, C., and Munster, A. M. Quality of life after major burns. *J. Trauma,* 19(8): 556-558, 1980.

69. Bowden, D. L., et al. Self-esteem of severely burned patients. *Arch. Phys. Med. Rehabil.,* 61(10): 449-452, 1980.

70. Davidson, T., Bowden, M. L., and Feller, I. Social support and postburn adjustment. *Arch. Phys. Med. Rehabil.,* 62(6): 274-278, 1981.

71. Mannon, J. M. *Caring for the Burned: Life and Death in a Hospital Burn Center.* Springfield, IL: Charles C Thomas, 1985.

chapter
30

Cardiopulmonary Rehabilitation

Catherine A. Trombly

Cardiac rehabilitation and treatment of chronic obstructive pulmonary disease have been combined into one chapter because, although there are special treatment regimes for each, the underlying physiology, oxygen (O_2) metabolism,[1] is the same. The occupational therapist has restorative as well as rehabilitative goals for some cardiac patients. However, for others and for chronic obstructive pulmonary disease patients, goals are rehabilitative; that is, treatment aims at enabling the person to live a satisfying life within the limits imposed by his condition. This chapter provides basic information; those who want to specialize in this area need to acquire advanced knowledge about the physiology, assessment, and management of the conditions, about electrocardiogram interpretation, and exercise physiology.[2]

Recovery from a heart attack or open heart surgery is an emotional process as well as a physical one. The occupational therapist, prepared in both physical and psychosocial rehabilitation, has much to offer the cardiac rehabilitation team. Cardiac rehabilitation seeks to return the patient recovering from an uncomplicated myocardial infarction (MI) or "heart attack" to optimal physiological, psychological, social, and emotional status.[2] Complications that preclude participation in a rehabilitation program as described here include congestive heart failure, myocarditis, pacemaker implant, or unstable angina.

The goals of cardiac rehabilitation, in general, are to increase functional capacity (ability to do activities and work without stress or symptoms) through a graded exercise program, to alleviate depression, to modify behaviors that place the patient at risk for recurrence, and to return the person to his previous work and recreational pursuits if possible.[3]

Symptoms of Heart Disease

The role of the circulatory system in exercise, including activities of daily living, is to augment delivery of metabolic substrates and oxygen needed for muscle contraction, to remove waste products, and to dissipate heat generated by contraction.[4] These functions are achieved by central and peripheral cardiovascular processes that increase, and change the distribution of, the blood supply.[4] Muscle uses energy obtained through oxidation to do work. The muscle receives oxygen from arterial blood. Skeletal muscle can work for short periods at levels that exceed O_2 supply, during which anaerobic metabolism (glycolysis)[5] produces the energy. Anaerobic work results in an O_2 debt, and the oxygen requirement is increased by this debt.

In order to function, heart muscle, like skeletal muscle, requires oxygen. Although the heart contains oxygenated blood in its chambers, the myocardium is not supplied with oxygen by this source. Oxygen is carried to the myocardium by the left and right coronary arteries. The oxygen supply must meet the oxygen demand of the myocardium. Unlike skeletal muscle, the cardiac muscle cannot work anaerobically nor can it tolerate an oxygen debt.[6,7] If the oxygen supply does not meet the oxygen demand, angina pectoris signals the discrepancy.[8] Angina pectoris is a severe, "squeezing" pain in the chest that may radiate to the neck, left shoulder, jaw, or down the left arm.[9,10] It is brought on by physical activity or emotional stress and is relieved by rest. It predictably occurs under the same demands.[6]

In coronary artery disease, the lumen of the coronary blood vessels narrows due to deposits of fat on the walls, a process called artherosclerosis.[9] Narrowed arteries reduce the flow of oxygen-carrying blood to the heart muscle.[9,10] A greater demand for oxygen than can be supplied manifests itself as angina pectoris.[6,8] Angina pectoris does not necessarily develop into an MI. If the person recognizes it as a warning and takes steps to treat the underlying condition and to modify his lifestyle to reduce the risk of developing greater cardiac disease, he may avert an MI.[11]

If a coronary artery becomes obstructed, the tissue that is supplied with oxygen by that artery dies; this is an MI. An MI is not necessarily fatal, but it always decreases the pumping efficiency of the heart.[9] Its severity depends upon the extent and location of the infarction.

Signs and symptoms of an MI include dyspnea, angina pectoris, palpitations, anxiety, diaphoresis, rapid and thready pulse, irregular heart rhythm, a low-grade fever, nausea or vomiting, and/or fatigue or weakness. In 25% of the cases, the first sign of MI is sudden death.[9]

Cardiac patients are classified according to the amount of work or kinds of activities they may safely perform. The American Heart Association's functional and therapeutic classifications of patients with disease of the heart[12] are found in Table 30.1.

Cardiac Rehabilitation Program

The cardiac rehabilitation program is ordered by the physician who, because of his ultimate responsibility for the patient's life, must approve the initiation and continuance of the program.

All personnel who participate in the program must be qualified. All must be certified in CPR (cardiopulmonary resuscitation).[13,14] Failure to have these qualifications could result in legal action against the person and institution in the event of a mishap.[13]

CPR is an emergency method of substituting for cardiorespiratory function without the use of equipment. The ABCs of CPR are to clear the Airway, Breathe for the patient, and Circulate the oxygenated blood.[9] The airway is cleared by putting the patient in a supine position, hyperextending the neck, and removing anything that may be obstructing it, including dentures. Artificial breathing is accomplished by pinching the patient's nose closed, by the resuscitator completely covering the patient's mouth with his mouth, and by then blowing into the patient's mouth with enough force so that the chest expands. Initially four breaths are given followed by cardiac compression, which is done by pressing over the sternum approximately 1½ inches above the end of the xyphoid process with the heels of both hands, one pressing over the other. Fifteen compressions, at a rate of 80/min, are done. Then two quick breaths are alternated with 15 compressions until the advanced life support team arrives or the patient revives.[15,16] Certification in CPR is available by taking courses offered by the American Heart Association or the American Red Cross. Certification must be renewed yearly.

The rehabilitation program is usually divided into phases,[2] each placing greater demand on the patient's heart function. The best results occur when the patient participates in all phases.

INPATIENT PHASE

The inpatient program begins early in the coronary care unit as soon as the patient is pain free, exhibits no arrhythmias at rest, and has a resting pulse of <100.[17] The goals of the inpatient program are to prevent deconditioning; to educate the patient about heart disease and recovery; to build patient confidence with activities[2]; to provide emotional support to the patient and his family; and to teach the patient the value of continuing the program as an outpatient, as well as developing his psychological readiness to do so.

The exercise program begins with light diversional and self-care activities for the purposes of increasing cardiac capacity and reducing anxiety, which in turn reduce cardiac stress. During the first few days following MI, when the patient is functionally classified in class IV, activities requiring a maximum of 1.5 meta-

Table 30.1
THE FUNCTIONAL AND THERAPEUTIC CLASSIFICATIONS OF PATIENTS WITH DISEASES OF THE HEART

	Functional Classification	Maximal METs
Class I	Patients with cardiac disease but without resulting limitations of physical activity. Ordinary physical activity does not cause undue fatigue, palpitation, dyspnea, or anginal pain.	6.5
Class II	Patients with cardiac disease resulting in slight limitation of physical activity. They are comfortable at rest. Ordinary physical activity results in fatigue, palpitation, dyspnea, or anginal pain.	4.5
Class III	Patients with cardiac disease resulting in marked limitation of physical activity. They are comfortable at rest. Less than ordinary physical activity causes fatigue, palpitation, dyspnea, or anginal pain.	3.0
Class IV	Patients with cardiac disease resulting in inability to carry on any physical activity without discomfort. Symptoms of cardiac insufficiency or of the anginal syndrome may be present even at rest. If any physical activity is undertaken, discomfort is increased.	1.5

	Therapeutic Classification
Class A	Patients with cardiac disease whose physical activity need not be restricted in any way.
Class B	Patients with cardiac disease whose ordinary physical activity need not be restricted, but who should be advised against severe or competitive efforts.
Class C	Patients with cardiac disease whose ordinary physical activity should be moderately restricted, and whose more strenuous efforts should be discontinued.
Class D	Patients with cardiac disease whose ordinary physical activity should be markedly restricted.
Class E	Patients with cardiac disease who should be at complete rest, confined to bed or chair.

bolic equivalents (METs) are allowed. The patient is placed in a fully supported sitting position with the proximal extremities supported so that activities or exercise are restricted to the distal parts of the extremities and utilize phasic movements[18] on a gravity-eliminated plane. An example is feeding with the elbows resting on the over-bed table which has been raised to axilla height.

The evening resting pulse rate is a guideline to rehabilitation progress. If it exceeds the morning resting rate by more than 20%, then the program may be progressing too rapidly.[17]

As a training effect becomes apparent by obtaining a lower pulse rate while the patient is doing the same activity, the frequency of the activity can be increased. The Grady Memorial Hospital program is included as a model at the end of this chapter. It should be remembered that each person should be advanced according to his particular response to exercise. As the training effect is seen for all activities within the classification, the patient is probably ready to be reclassified by the physician into class III, in which the METs are increased to 3.0. The patient may be transferred to the Progressive Care Unit[19] to continue rehabilitation. In the Progressive Care Unit, he will be monitored intermittently, usually via radiotelemetry, as his activity level is increased[19] and with decreasing frequency as his asymptomatic response to increased activity is evident.

When the patient is classified class III, use of full movement of the upper extremities while sitting, proximal stabilization without resistance, trunk balancing, and hand activities while standing are permitted.[18] For example, upper-extremity dressing and standing at the basin to shave are acceptable activities. Frequency and duration are increased as tolerated.

In class II, activities may require a maximum of 4.5 METs. Resistance can be graded, and more expansive movements utilizing the larger muscle groups are permitted. The patient is usually discharged home 14 to 20 days postonset and can be expected to have reached about 4.0 METs functional capacity.[17]

INTERMEDIATE PHASE OR OUTPATIENT PROGRAM

The intermediate or outpatient program begins as early as 3 to 4 weeks post-MI[14,17] for patients with stable angina pectoris or as late as 8 weeks.[19] The goals for the outpatient phase include continued physical conditioning through supervised exercise; behavioral counseling and life-style modification relative to risk factors; vocational counseling and evaluation; and continued psychological support.[2,14] Those patients who begin the outpatient program closer to the time of onset continue the supervised step-by-step progression gauged by pulse (not to exceed 100/min) and fatigue (disappears 10 to 20 min after activity).[17] At 8 weeks, the level of physical activity can be guided by a graded exercise test,[19] described below. Following this test, the person usually enters into a walk/jog program under medical supervision[19] in which the heart rate at-

tains 70% to 85% of maximum achieved during the stress test carried to symptomatic endpoint.[17]

COMMUNITY PROGRAM PHASE

After 4 to 6 months the patient may safely participate in a community program[19] or exercise independently if he has the self-discipline. He is discharged to this program when he achieves the functional capacity that is necessary for his occupation and life-style.[14]

The components of the rehabilitation program will be described in greater detail on the following pages.

Physical Activity/Exercise

Supervised exercise programs are beneficial to the recovery of cardiac patients for these reasons: they demonstrate to the patient that certain levels of physical activity can be done safely; depression is decreased[20]; the heart and other muscles are conditioned to enable them to handle stress and strain[9]; and weight is reduced (obesity requires the heart to work harder).

A graded exercise program is also financially beneficial both to the individual and to society. One study of 123 post-MI patients who were divided into an experimental and two control groups concluded, after examining alternate explanations, that a cardiac rehabilitation program of early mobilization and graded exercise and activities significantly reduced the length of hospitalization and improved the level of functional capacity at discharge.[21]

Exercise results in a training effect in which more blood is pumped during each beat (increased stroke volume) and the heart beats fewer times per minute (decreased heart rate) for the same amount of work, indicating improved functional capacity. A person starts an exercise program at a level of energy expenditure that puts demand on cardiac output but is safe for that person. When the training effect from activity at the initial level is experienced, the frequency, intensity, and/or duration are increased. The training effect will occur at successive levels of cardiac output up to a maximal level for a given individual.

Covert depression, which arises due to tensions and anxieties related to role and life-style changes, has been shown to decrease due to physical exercise.[22] In another controlled study of 43 normal young women, an aerobic exercise program was found to significantly decrease depression compared to relaxation training or no treatment.[20] The effect was seen in 5 weeks and exercise beyond that time did not enhance the effect.[20]

The information in this section relates not only to conditioning exercise done for a training effect, but also to all physical activity related to occupational performance tasks. The goal is to return the person to his original life-style. If he is unable to regain his original functional capacity, or if it is desirable to reduce the energy level required of daily tasks, work simplification and energy conservation techniques are taught.

Physiology. The oxygen supply to the coronary arteries is determined by cardiac output, blood flow, and the amount of oxygen in the blood. The cardiac output is the volume of blood pumped by the heart per minute.[23] It is the product of stroke volume × heart rate.[23,24] The blood flow depends on the patency of the coronary arteries; atherosclerosis or blockage of the arteries decreases or terminates the blood flow. The amount of oxygen depends on the blood's ability to carry oxygen in the hemoglobin; a decrease in hemoglobin would decrease the amount of oxygen available. An increased work load creates an increased demand for oxygen by the myocardium.

There is a maximal amount of oxygen that a person can take in and dispense to muscle during exercise; it is termed maximal oxygen uptake and abbreviated $\dot{V}O_2$ max. The $\dot{V}O_2$ max is proportional to weight, especially lean body mass.[8] It increases with physical training and decreases with bed rest and age.[8] It is a standard measure of cardiovascular fitness.[8] The $\dot{V}O_2$ max, as determined by stress testing, relates to the person's maximal MET level.[25]

One MET equals basal metabolic rate and is equal to 3.5 ml of oxygen per kilogram of body weight per minute.[9,14,26] Basal metabolic rate is the minimal amount of energy or oxygen consumption necessary to maintain metabolic processes (respiration, circulation, peristalsis, temperature, glandular function, etc.) of the body at rest.[10] The energy cost of activities or exercise can be rated using multiples of METs.[14] An exercise that is rated 4.0 METs requires 4 times the amount of oxygen per kilogram of body weight per minute than the basal rate.[14,27]

METs and calories are both used to estimate the metabolic cost of activity. Beyond the basal rate, however, METs and calories are not equivalent. The average number of calories required to sustain the basal metabolic rate of a person resting in a supine position is 1.0 calorie/kg/hour. One calorie equals approximately 200 ml of oxygen consumption.[28] METs are a convenient and reliable measure of energy cost because their calculation considers the oxygen requirements of activities without having to calculate the amount of oxygen consumed separately as one would have to do if calories were used. Although the MET level of an activity is equivalent for different persons, the oxygen requirement is not. For example, a 4.0 MET activity done by a 50-kg person requires 4.0 × 3.5 ml of O_2 × 50 kg/minute or 700 ml of O_2/minute, whereas a 70-kg person would use 980 ml of O_2/minute.

Clearly it can be seen that a person reduces the oxygen demand by reducing his weight. Beyond that, the oxygen supply must increase by increasing cardiac output.

As an immediate effect of exercise, the heart rate (HR) and stroke volume increase.[24] Heart rate increases to deliver the required amount of oxygenated blood to the active muscles. Stroke volume, or amount of blood pumped per heart beat, increases because of increased venous flow into the heart during diastole[24] (the period of muscle relaxation when the chambers fill).[10] The mechanical response of the ventricle is based on Starling's Law: the force of the contraction is a function of the degree of stretch of the muscle fibers during diastole.[24] Over time, a training effect is seen, and the HR and blood pressure (BP) are less than previously required for the same amount of work.[27]

Heart rate linearly relates to $\dot{V}O_2$ max except at the upper limits (80% to 90%) of maximal capacity.[24] For example, if a person's HR is 70% of maximal HR (HR max), that means he is using approximately 70% of $\dot{V}O_2$ max.[24] HR max is age dependent[24] and is calculated by subtracting the person's age from 220. Myocardial oxygen consumption ($M\dot{V}O_2$) can be estimated from the double product (peak systolic BP × HR).[23] Therefore, heart rate indicates how hard the heart is working or how well it is performing.[23,24] A stable heart rate during exercise indicates a steady state; that is, the right amount of O_2 is being supplied to meet the work demand.[24]

Heart rate is therefore monitored during exercise to determine the effect the exercise is having on the person's heart. In addition to rate, rhythm is also monitored in recent post-MI patients, since the tissue death often results in irritability of the remaining tissue or pacing system.

Monitoring Heart Response to Exercise. Heart rate and blood pressure change in response to exercise. In a cardiac patient heart rhythm may also change. Heart rate is monitored by taking radial or carotid pulse, by auscultation, or by counting the beats on an ECG monitor to which newly infarcted patients are often attached. Resting heart rate is taken with the patient reclined or sitting, after 5 min of rest.[29] The pulse is counted for a full minute for greatest accuracy, but can be taken for less time and the result multiplied to determine the number of beats per minute.[29] Radial pulse is felt at the wrist at approximately the level of the radial styloid. Light, firm pressure is applied using the index and middle fingers. Carotid pulse is felt lateral to the trachea; care must be exercised to prevent too great a pressure, which could occlude the artery and trigger the carotid sinus reflex, which will affect blood pressure. Or the heart rate can be counted by using a stethoscope over the heart (auscultation).

The exercise heart rate is measured very quickly after exercise. Rate drops fast; therefore, the beats are counted for 10 seconds only and multiplied to determine the rate per minute. This method is accurate to ± 6 beats per minute.[29] Another method is to time the first 10 beats and extrapolate to determine beats per minute.[28]

Blood pressure is measured during exercise testing to see if the heart is responding as it should to exercise. Systolic BP increases during dynamic exercise because there is a shunting of blood supply via vasoconstriction (which is the basis of the increased BP) from the viscera and nonexercising muscles to the exercising muscles, which need a large supply of oxygen.[5] Blood pressure is measured using a sphygmomanometer and stethoscope. The deflated sphygmomanometer cuff is applied firmly to the arm proximal to the elbow. The stethoscope is placed over the brachial artery under the edge of the cuff. The valve of the sphygmomanometer is closed and pumped up to a level above that expected for the patient. The valve is slowly opened to release the air from the cuff. Listening by stethoscope, the heart beat can soon be heard. The reading is noted; this is the systolic pressure. The air continues to be released. When the sound disappears, the reading is noted; this is the diastolic pressure. The results are recorded: systolic/diastolic, for example 120/80.

The normal heart beat, as monitored by ECG, is shown in Figure 30.1. The schematic indicates the waves or deflections from baseline of one heart beat. The P wave represents the electrical activity associated with depolarization of the atria. The P-R interval represents the time that elapses from the beginning of the atrial contraction to the beginning of the ventricular contraction. The QRS complex represents the electrical activity associated with the depolarization of the ventricles. The T wave represents ventricular recovery or repolarization.[30,31] The U wave is little understood but is thought to be the last part of ventricular recovery or the recovery wave of the Purkinje system.[31] The junction between S and T waves is called the J point.

These parts, with the possible exception of the U wave, are always present, but may appear different in orientation, depending on the lead from which the recording was made. The resting ECG is recorded from 12 leads in succession to look at the heart from many angles. There are three limb leads (I, II, III), three augmented limb leads (aVR, aVL, aVF), and six precordial leads (V_1 through V_6). The precordial leads extend from the fourth intercostal space on the right of the sternum to the left midlateral chest wall at the fifth intercostal space. Whether the deflection of the wave appears positive (upright) or negative (negative) depends on whether the electrode "sees" the advancing wave of depolarization (positive) or whether it "sees" a receding wave of depolarization.[32] For example, the recording

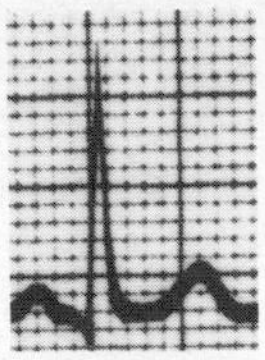

Figure 30.2 Normal electrocardiogram from V_5 lead. (Reproduced with permission from Winsor, T. The electrocardiogram in myocardial infarction. In *Clinical Symposia*. Summit, NJ: Ciba Pharmaceutical Company, Medical Education Division, 1968.)

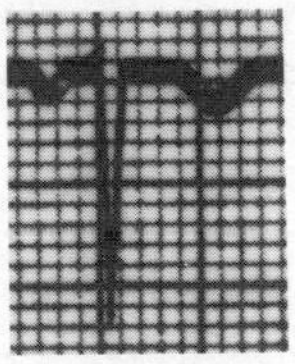

Figure 30.3 Normal electrocardiogram from aVR lead. (Reproduced with permission from Winsor, T. The electrocardiogram in myocardial infarction. In *Clinical Symposia*. Summit, NJ: Ciba Pharmaceutical Company, Medical Education Division, 1968.)

from V_5 appears like the schematic (Fig. 30.2), but the normal appearance of aVR is quite different (Fig. 30.3). During exercise testing the ECG may be monitored using the CM5 placement, a modification of the V_5 placement (Fig. 30.4). This placement is less sensitive than V_5 to detect S-T segment depression[27] but has been found to identify 89% of all S-T depression found by multiple lead systems.[24] Some choose to monitor aVF, V_1, and CM5.[24]

Heart rate can be determined from ECG by counting the time elapsed between one R-R interval and dividing that into 60 sec to determine the heart rate per minute.[31] Each five-space block (5 mm), which is marked by a heavier line on the chart paper, indicates 0.20 sec

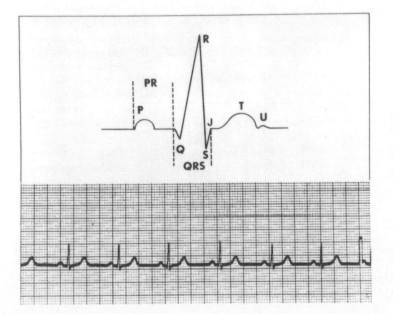

Figure 30.1 The normal electrocardiogram. (Reproduced with permission from Menard, R. H. *Introduction to Arrhythmia Recognition*. San Francisco: California Heart Association, 1968.)

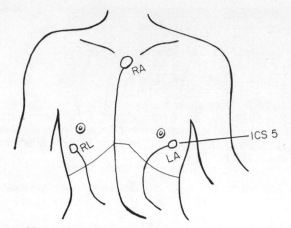

Figure 30.4 Electrode placement for exercise cardiogram. Right arm electrode (RA) is placed on the manubrium and is used as the reference. Right leg electrode (RL) is placed on the right chest and is the ground. Left arm electrode (LA) is placed on the left chest at the fifth intercostal space (ICS 5) in line with the middle of the clavicle. This setup optimizes the S-T segment display and minimizes noise. (Reproduced with permission from Erb, B. D. Physician's *Handbook for Evaluation of Cardiovascular and Physical Fitness*, 2nd edition. Nashville: Tennessee Heart Association, 1972.)

ute.[31] Each five-space block (5 mm), which is marked by a heavier line on the chart paper, indicates 0.20 sec with the paper moving at a rate of 25 mm/sec. Each 1-mm block represents 0.04 sec. Therefore, five of the large blocks or 25 of the small blocks indicates 1 sec. For example, in Figure 30.1 the time elapsed between an R-R interval is 0.8 sec, which, divided into 60 sec, equals 75 beats/minute.

Rate sticks eliminate the need for doing the mathematical calculation. The reference line of the rate stick is lined up exactly with an R peak, and three R-R intervals are counted. The heart rate is read from the value on the stick that coincides with the point of the last R peak. Another method has been described by Dubin: an R wave that falls on a dark line on the ECG paper is located; then the rate is determined by counting 300, 150, 100, 75, 60, and 50 for each successive dark line until

the next R wave that falls on a line is encountered.[33] This method has the advantage of not requiring special equipment or mathematics; however, it may require a fairly long strip of ECG. For example, the rate could not be determined for the strip in Figure 30.1 because only one R wave falls on a line.

It is important for all personnel involved in the physical activity portion of the rehabilitation program to be able to recognize abnormal rates or arrhythmias on the ECG and to know which are outside of normal limits so that the activity can be appropriately discontinued and help sought if necessary. In learning to read ECGs, one should note both the rate and rhythm. In particular, ventricular rate, ventricular regularity (same R-R interval over time), presence or absence of a P wave, association of a P wave with each QRS complex, atrial rate, and QRS width are noted.[34] If the P or P-R interval are abnormal, this indicates a disruption of the electrical flow above the bundle branches. If the QRS, S-T, or T waves are affected, this indicates that the disruption is at the bundle branches or below.

The abnormalities that are within normal limits include S-T segment depression of 1 mm or less (the J point is compared to the PQ junction to note the amount of depression)[6,24]; if the T wave, which should deflect in the same direction as the QRS, flips during exercise it is not diagnostic, but if it inverts during rest, it is abnormal[6,24]; steeply upsloping S-T segment that within 0.04 to 0.06 sec after the J point has returned to baseline[24]; and an occasional, unifocal (same shape) premature ventricular contraction (PVC).[6] A PVC is an abnormal QRS complex not preceded by a P wave, but followed by a compensatory pause (Fig. 30.5). Each focus of irritability in the ventricles produces a wave form of distinctive shape.

ECG indications of intolerance to exercise include the following.

1. Ventricular tachycardia,[11,26] defined as three or more successive PVCs[11,24,33] (Fig. 30.6). The probability of developing fibrillation increases if PVCs occur in couplets, bigeminy (every other one), or are multifocal[6,33]; therefore, exercise is terminated when any of these occur. Ventricular fibrillation (Fig. 30.7) is equivalent to

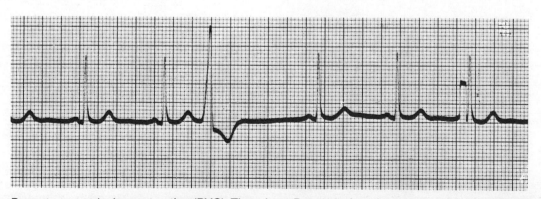

Figure 30.5 Premature ventricular contraction (PVC). There is no P wave before the abnormal PVC and there is a compensatory pause following it. (Reproduced with permission from Menard, R. H. *Introduction to Arrhythmia Recognition*. San Francisco: California Heart Association, 1968.)

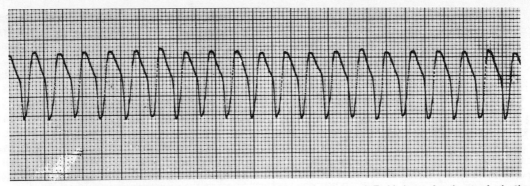

Figure 30.6 Ventricular tachycardia. (Reproduced with permission from Menard, R. H. *Introduction to Arrhythmia Recognition*. San Francisco: California Heart Association, 1968.)

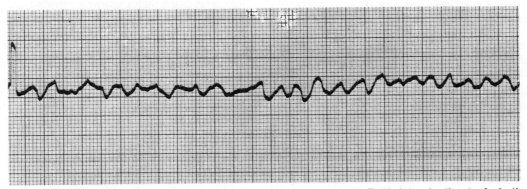

Figure 30.7 Ventricular fibrillation. (Reproduced with permission from Menard, R. H. *Introduction to Arrhythmia Recognition*. San Francisco: California Heart Association, 1968.)

cardiac standstill, and unless defibrillation and cardiopulmonary resuscitation is instituted immediately, death will ensue within minutes.[30] Cardiac arrest is indicated on the ECG by a flat line, but a disconnected or broken ECG electrode or lead may produce the same flat line in a nonemergency situation.

2. Ischemic changes (>1 mm of horizontal or downsloping S-T segment depression)[11,26,35] (Fig. 30.8A and

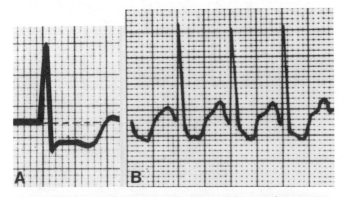

Figure 30.8 **A.** Horizontal S-T segment depression greater than 1 mm. (Reproduced with permission from Dubin, D. *Rapid Interpretation of EKG's*, 3rd edition. Tampa, FL: COVER Publishing Co., 1974.) **B.** Downsloping S-T segment depression. (Reproduced with permission from Ellestad, M. H. *Stress Testing: Principles and Practice*, 3rd edition. Philadelphia: F. A. Davis, 1986.)

B). S-T segment depression >2 mm is often accompanied by angina, a warning signal; however, in one study it was found that 72% of S-T segment depressions occurred without angina in coronary heart disease patients who were at rest or doing activity at levels below their functional capacity as determined by exercise testing.[36] This finding needs further study to determine its full implications.

3. Second or third degree heart block.[11,26,35] Impairment of conduction through the atrioventricular (AV) node is designated as a first, second, or third degree block, depending on the severity. A second degree AV block is one in which the impairment of conduction is such that some of the impulses from the atria fail to get through to activate the ventricles, resulting in skipped beats (Fig. 30.9). In a third degree AV block no impulses

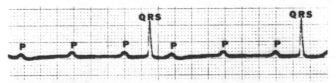

Figure 30.9 Second degree AV block. In this case, three atrial pulses are required to stimulate the ventricular response. (Reproduced with permission from Dubin, D. *Rapid Interpretation of EKG's*, 3rd edition. Tampa, FL: COVER Publishing Co., 1974.)

from the atriar each the ventricles. In order for the ventricles to contract, they must develop their own pacing system from nervous tissue within the heart, producing a very slow rate with abnormal QRS complexes (Fig. 30.10). Both the ST segment depression and the AV blocks indicate a probable impending myocardial infarction. Exercise should cease, and the physician should be notified immediately.

Neither supraventricular dysrhythmias nor bundle branch blocks (Figs. 30.11 and 30.12) are absolute contraindications to exercise, but the patient requires close supervision. In the case of a left bundle branch block (LBBB) an MI cannot be diagnosed by ECG[6,33] because the left ventricle fires late; therefore, the first portion of the QRS complex represents right ventricular activity. Q waves, indicating infarct, cannot be identified for the left ventricle.[33]

Monitoring activity during daily living activities can be done using telemetry or a Holter monitor. When using telemetry, the ECG is radioed from the battery-operated transmitter to the receiver where it is viewed and/or recorded. The person must stay within a certain range of the receiver and electrodes must be very well applied (see chapter 12 for electrode application techniques). The Holter monitor is a battery-operated receiver and tape recorder that can be worn by the person for periods up to 24 hours. The tape can later be processed to print out a 24-hour heart rate record, which is correlated with a detailed diary kept by the patient during that period.

Exercise Testing. Six to eight weeks after an uncomplicated MI, patients can be tested to determine their nonsymptomatic $\dot{V}O_2$ max, and from this, a fairly precise exercise prescription, in METs, can be given to each patient. The occupational therapist may be a member of the testing team, the composition of which varies from center to center, but which should include a physician.[14]

Graded exercise testing (GXT) is contraindicated for those persons for whom a rehabilitation program is inappropriate, as mentioned earlier, and for the acute MI patient[35] (although one study tested patients at 14.8 days, on average, without incident[37]), or patient with left bundle branch block (LBBB) abnormality.[6]

An informed consent form that explains the purpose, procedure, risks, and benefits of the GXT is given to the patient for signature.[13,14,25] The consent form does not protect the personnel from legal actions aris-

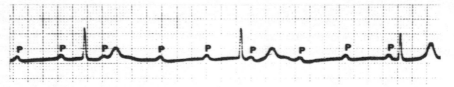

Figure 30.10 Third degree AV block. The unstimulated ventricles set their own slow independent pace. (Reproduced with permission from Dubin, D. *Rapid Interpretation of EKG's*, 3rd edition. Tampa, FL: COVER Publishing Co., 1974.)

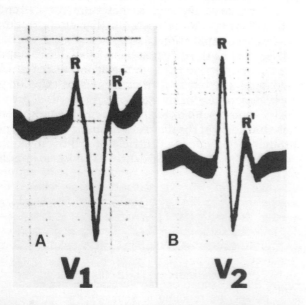

Figure 30.11 Right bundle branch block indicated in R-R' in electrocardiogram leads V₁ and V₂. (Reproduced with permission from Dubin, D. *Rapid Interpretation of EKG's*, 3rd edition. Tampa, FL: COVER Publishing Co., 1974.)

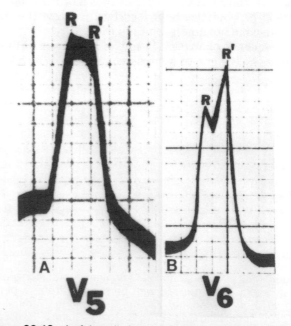

Figure 30.12 Left bundle branch block indicated by R-R' in electrocardiogram leads V₅ and V₆. (Reproduced with permission from Dubin, D. *Rapid Interpretation of EKG's*, 3rd edition. Tampa, FL: COVER Publishing Co., 1974.)

ing from negligence or malpractice, but only protects the patient's right of choice and full disclosure. The patient must also understand that he has the responsibility to report symptoms.[13]

Stress testing (exercise testing) can be done using an automated treadmill, a bicycle ergometer, or by ascending and descending a standard size and number of steps.[11,24-26] A study to test the reliability of treadmill versus bicycle ergometer concluded that they were equally reliable in a test-retest (1 year) design, but that three out of four persons preferred the treadmill.[38]

Exercise testing is preceded by a warm-up period and followed by a cool-down period of exercise.[27] The actual testing begins with a low-intensity work load estimated from the patient's body size and current activity level. He works at this level for 4 to 6 min at a controlled rate to reach a steady state of oxygen uptake,[28] although some believe 3 min is enough to reach steady state.[11] The BP and HR by ECG are recorded at the end of each minute of exercise, and the ECG is continuously monitored for arrhythmias.[28] The patient proceeds to the next work load if HR is steady and less than target HR (usually defined as 85% of HR max: $220 - age \times 0.85$) and he is free of symptoms. The symptoms that indicate endpoint of exercise testing are: dyspnea, weakness, changes in sensorium, angina, second or third degree AV blocks, S-T segment depression, decreased BP or HR for increased work load, increased ventricular arrhythmias, supraventricular tachyarrhythmias, or pallor or cyanosis.[8] The patient may signal to stop at any time. Some cardiologists believe that the endpoint of GXT should be the functional maximum or a HR of 160/min, not a target HR that may be misleading in post-MI patients.[39] Some believe that a maximal symptom-limited exercise test should be done before the patient returns to full-time work and that the average work load should be limited to one-third to one-half of the maximal capacity.[8]

At the end of the test, the patient works at a low level for a minute or two before stopping the test and then rests. ECG monitoring continues throughout the cool-down and rest periods because ECG abnormalities may occur only during these periods.[11]

If the patient is taking medication, the particular drug may alter the interpretation of the stress test. Nitroglycerin will allow the patient to exercise longer at higher levels because it decreases the $M\dot{V}O_2$.[24] Inderal (propranolol) may decrease S-T segment depression during the GXT. Many diuretics cause a loss of potassium (hypokalemia), which causes ventricular irritability and increased PVCs and other arrhythmias.

A method of testing to document the patient's cardiovascular response to activities of daily living has been devised by occupational and physical therapists at Rancho Los Amigos Hospital in California.[40,41] The procedure is also used to estimate the work requirements of functional tasks. It is used with both complicated and noncomplicated cardiac cases. Called *Monitored Task Evaluation*, it essentially stress tests the patient using activities of daily living (ADL) tasks. This evaluation starts with tasks done in supine, then sitting, and finally standing postures. Five parameters are monitored during the test: blood pressure; ECG (rhythm and ischemia) by telemetry; heart rate by auscultation; and symptoms by observation and patient report. The evaluation consists of ADL tasks graded to produce a gradual increase of cardiovascular work load. Six variables are manipulated to grade the tasks. They are (1) rate of work; (2) resistance offered by the task; (3) arm position (waist level or below, chest level, or overhead); (4) types of muscle groups used (fine versus gross); (5) involvement of trunk musculature (present during bending or when trunk stabilization is needed); and (6) isometric work producing the Valsalva effect.[41] Each task is scored as to difficulty. The scoring system assigns to each of the six variables 1 point for mild influence, 2 points for moderate influence, and 3 points for strong influence. Because of the extreme nature of the effect of certain variables on the heart, 2 additional points are added to the score if there is a strong influence of work rate, if there is a moderate influence of isometric work, and/or if there is a moderate influence of arm position.[33,34] Scores can range from 6 to 24. The higher the task is rated, the greater the cardiac response required in order to do it.

The energy expended in different positions and while performing various activities has been measured in many studies of energy metabolism. Oxygen consumption of daily living, recreational, and vocational tasks was measured, and the METs required for each task were calculated. Many charts of the metabolic cost of activities have been published. Some of these are included at the end of this chapter. Knowledge of the energy cost of activities is valuable in determining the intensity of effort required by activities. There are slight discrepancies in the amount of energy recorded for similar activities in different charts. This is a function of differing test situations or specific methods of performance of the activity. Because the method of performance is not described in these charts and because they do not take into consideration a particular person's method of doing an activity in a particular environment, the therapist can only consider the MET charts as guidelines for exercise prescription and should be conservative in selecting activities for a patient. The actual cardiac response to the task must be determined by monitoring heart rate and blood pressure.[42]

Cardiac work or stress is influenced by many factors in addition to the energy requirements of activities. *Posture* affects cardiac output. Sitting relaxed in an easy chair with the head, back, arms, and thighs supported and with the feet on the floor is the position least demanding on the heart. Sitting on the edge of the bed, sitting in a straight chair, or even relaxed standing are less demanding than lying supine or semireclined in bed.[18] *Anxiety* increases muscular tension and blood pressure and consequently places more demand on the heart.[18] The *rate* of work influences the energy requirements of an activity, and energy expenditure increases as speed of performance increases.[14,18] *Temperature* also influences cardiac stress, and a hot, humid environment increases cardiac work.[18] Other influencing factors include *drugs, fatigue, emotion, hydration,* and *time since the last meal.*[11,43] Digestion of food results in a reflex dilation of blood vessels of the alimentary canal, thereby increasing circulation there and reducing the available circulating blood to other muscles, including the heart.[44] No exercise should be done within 1 hour of finishing a meal.[17]

Contraindications for an exercise program as stated by Nanette Kass Wenger, M.D., include[35]:

New or progressive angina pectoris
Uncontrolled congestive heart failure
Impending or very recent myocardial infarction
Uncontrolled hypertension
Arrhythmias
   Second and third degree AV block
   Fixed rate pacemakers
   Ventricular tachycardia
   Uncontrolled atrial fibrillation
   Frequent premature ventricular contractions
     at rest that increase with exercise
Gross cardiac enlargement
Moderate to severe valvular disease
Outflow tract obstructive disease
Recent pulmonary embolism
Uncontrolled diabetes mellitus

For those able to participate, an individual exercise program is established taking into consideration the type of exercise, as well as the intensity, duration, and frequency of exercise, needed to produce a measurable training effect.[7,8,29] The person's exercise history, musculoskeletal integrity, motivation, and athletic ability also must be considered.[14] As with all patients, the response to therapy is carefully observed. Discontinuance or decrease of activity is indicated by one or more of the following[8,35]: (1) the appearance of chest pain or dyspnea; (2) an increase in the heart rate to over 120 beats/min; (3) a decrease in systolic blood pressure of over 20 mm Hg; (4) increased S-T segment displacement on the ECG; or (5) the occurrence of significant arrhythmias. The exercise prescription is reviewed and modified as often as is appropriate.[14]

Type of Exercise. Small muscle or arm exercise requires more energy than large muscle or lower extremity exercise.[8] Cardiac patients should avoid exercise that is primarily isometric.[8] Sustained isometric contraction produces more cardiovascular stress than dynamic contractions.[8,9] Varying levels of intensity of isometric contraction (grip) also significantly increased BP and HR of normal subjects in one study.[45] In another study of 40 normal subjects aged 19 to 30 years, there were also significant increases in BP and HR due to isometric contractions (grip, pinch, and pushing against an immovable object).[46] These responses increased with duration of contraction, which varied from 3 to 30 sec.[46] Pushing resulted in significantly greater increases than either grip or pinching. Twelve of the normal subjects in this study had to be

dropped from the study when their measured values exceeded accepted limits.[46] This occurred especially during the push activity at a 6-sec duration and would seem to confirm that this type of activity should be avoided by cardiac patients.

Static or isometric exercise (lifting weights, grasping, pushing heavy objects, etc.) produces a different cardiac response than that produced by dynamic exercise (swimming, walking, etc.). Isometric or sustained muscle contraction results in stimulation of a vagal reflex, via a neurally mediated reflex arc originating within the contracting muscle, that increases HR and BP[8] in direct proportion to the percentage of maximum voluntary contraction (MVC) of the muscle group involved.[8,47] During sustained isometric exercise at >15–20% MVC, the blood flow to the contracting muscle bed is compromised, shifting the muscle to the anerobic energy supply, which limits the duration of exercise.[8] Dynamic contractions performed at spontaneous speeds use more than seven times more oxygen per second than static contractions under the same load; at very slow speeds of dynamic activity is twice as costly, in terms of oxygen usage, as static activity.[48] Therefore, the greater cardiovascular response to physical training will be seen with dynamic exercise that uses 50% of muscle mass.[4] Dynamically exercising muscle requires an increased blood flow to supply the needed oxygen, which results in increased HR and stroke volume. Peripherally, there is a redistribution of the blood to exercising muscles, whose capillaries are vasodilated, and away from the viscera and nonworking muscles, by mild vasoconstriction.[4,5] This results in systolic BP increase and no change, or a decrease, in diastolic BP.[5]

Exercise used to increase muscle strength and endurance should be included in the program to enable the patient to do job tasks without stress. Stress decreases as strength increases.[25] Dynamic exercise is preferred to avoid the natural tendency to hold one's breath during activities that require exertion, known as the Valsalva effect[8]; this causes an increase in vagal stimulation that may add to cardiac stress above the level permitted. If a person can talk or count aloud while doing exercise, he is probably breathing correctly.

Flexibility and relaxation exercise, such as active range of motion or Yoga, should also be included in the program and can be used as warm up and cool-down exercises[25] that are part of each exercise period.[8,26]

Intensity of Exercise. The MET level of an activity is a measure of its intensity. The MET load is monitored by HR response immediately following the workout.[8,14] An indication for increasing the intensity is determination that the patient's peak exercise HR is consistently (three workouts in a row) below target HR.[8] After increasing the intensity, if the HR is more than 4 beats/min above target HR during exercise, the intensity should be decreased.

Before the patient has had a GXT, the initial MET level of activity is barely above resting and progresses as described earlier. A training effect occurs even at this low level because the patient is so debilitated. As the patient recovers, his MET level increases to the point that a regular, well-supervised dynamic exercise program can be instituted following GXT to gain a substantial training effect so that the patient's functional capacity exceeds his work and play requirements.

Exercise prescription has to be as specific as possible, since there is a dose-effect relationship just as there is with drugs.[8] As with drugs, there is a therapeutic level, a potential for overdose, contraindications, side effects, and precautions.[8]

The recommended target level of prescribed exercise in a phase II (outpatient) program is 60% to 80% of maximum,[8,29] or an average of 70%,[25] and should not exceed 90%[25] as determined by GXT. A very unfit person would see a training effect at less than 60%. An example of how to set exercise or activity prescription levels is as follows[25]:

Maximal capacity as determined by GXT = 6.0 METs.

Average conditioning intensity = 70%, therefore: $0.70 \times 6 = 4.2 = 4$ METs.

Peak intensity = 90%, therefore: $0.90 \times 6 = 5.4 = 5$ METs.

Activity or exercise that averages 4 METs but less than 5 METs would be appropriate for the person. Heart rate is used to monitor response to exercise. If HR attained at maximal capacity of GXT = 170 beats per min, then the average conditioning HR (target HR) would be $0.70 \times 170 = 119$ beats/min and peak HR should not exceed $0.90 \times 170 = 153$ beats/min.

Sex is one physical activity that both patient and spouse fear will precipitate a recurrence,[49] although the fear may not be physiologically sound. It is beneficial to the couple if the energy requirements of the sex act are explained in terms of METs, as is other physical activity. Under ordinary circumstances, the MET level is equal to about 4.7 to 5.5 METs, approximately equal to climbing two flights of stairs within 1 min[17] or vigorous walking.[50] Sexual activity is permitted when the person has reached a functional capacity of 6 METs. The couple might be advised to develop an unhurried approach to sex and to adopt positions for coitus that reduce strain on the heart patient. Normal sex in familiar surroundings[51] offers no particular risk to the average post-MI patient and may increase his self-esteem and encourage regular participation in an exercise program, which in turn improves his prognosis.[22] Like other exercise, sex should be avoided after a meal, in extremes of temperature, after ingesting alcohol, and when the patient is fatigued or under tension, and also if the conditions are illicit.[50,51]

Activities are graded not only by the intensity (METs) but also by the duration or frequency. All of these variables are interrelated and each can be graded within a given classification, but the intensity is the most critical because it is the intensity that taxes the heart. Therefore, grading should begin with frequency and duration at low METs.[28]

Duration of Exercise. This refers to the length of time or number of repetitions of exercise done. An indication of the correct duration is that the patient experiences full recovery and feels rested within an hour after the exercise period.[25] Not counting warm-up and cool-down, 20 to 30 min of exercise three times a week[25,51] is best for most on an outpatient exercise program. The duration is inversely related to the intensity.[8,25] A normal person can work almost indefinitely at 50% of $\dot{V}O_2$ capacity, whereas he would be limited to 30 to 40 min of work at 70% $\dot{V}O_2$ max.[28]

Frequency of Exercise. This refers to the number of exercise sessions within a given time period. It depends on the intensity and duration.[25] In early rehabilitation, frequency is two to three times per day for 1 to 2 min each time. In late stages of rehabilitation, the frequency is reduced to three to five times per week, but the duration is increased to 20 to 40 min. A guideline is: for patients at 3 METs, frequency is several times a day and duration is less than 5 min; for those at 3 to 5 METs, the frequency is daily and duration exceeds 5 min as tolerated; for those at ≥ 8 METs, frequency is three times a week on alternating days.[18] Exercise frequency of one to two times/week will prevent loss in $\dot{V}O_2$ max that occurs due to sedentary life-style, but three to five times/week is needed to increase $\dot{V}O_2$ max.[5]

Energy Conservation. By using the principles of work simplification and energy conservation (chapters 17, 18, 21, and 27) and electrical appliances, the person can conserve his personal energy during some tasks to use it for other activities. It has already been noted that the MET level of activity should not exceed 90% of maximal capacity[25] and that the patient should work at an average level of 50% to 70%. Average implies that some activities require less than target level and some more. The patient should be taught *pacing*, which includes rest breaks as frequent as every 10 to 15 min at first, to distribute the intensity of work over time so that average MET level is within required limits. For example, if the patient's target level is 3 METs, he might do 10 min of bed making (3.9 METS) followed by 10 min of sitting in a chair listening to the radio (1.4 METs) for an average of 2.65 METs, which is within his limits. Pacing helps to extend the function of even a severely limited patient.[40] By interspersing rest periods, the average work load can be held within very acceptable limits.

The MET values of occupational performance tasks are listed in charts such as those found at the end of this chapter.

Adapted methods of doing activities can be tested by noting if a decrease in HR actually results when the adapted method is used. Adapted methods should be devised to allow the patient to avoid stressful positions (e.g., working with the arms overhead, working in a squatting position) or motions.[52] Methods to stabilize the thing being worked on will allow the patient to avoid isometric muscle contractions.

Psychological Support

Counseling and education of the patient and his family are important aspects of cardiac rehabilitation.[14] Therapy that addresses the myths and anxieties surrounding heart function and heart disease is as important to the patient's well-being as exercise. The patient and his family have a need for information concerning the likelihood of a recurrent MI or death and the activities that the patient will and will not be able to participate in in the future. The patient also needs to learn to modify behaviors to reduce risk factors.

There are two sources of stress for the post-MI patient: (1) the threat to life during the MI and (2) the threat to life-style and livelihood that begins to develop from day 3 onward.[53] The threat to life-style produces anxiety and depression toward which the patient develops coping tactics, especially denial. Denial reduces the anxiety. The protective environment of the hospital also tends to reduce the anxiety. At the time of discharge the name and telephone number of a person to contact should be given to the patient in case he has questions.[52] This also helps to relieve anxiety. However, these do not relieve the depression, which remains "the most formidable problem in cardiac convalescence and rehabilitation."[53] Even if the depression is not noticeable, Hackett and Cassem[53] suggest that it should be assumed to be present and treated. The basis of the depression is fear of invalidism and loss of autonomy or independence; therefore, the best way to increase self-esteem and relieve depression is through activity.[53] Arts and crafts or pleasant recreational activities, chosen according to MET level permitted and the particular person's response, serve these goals. Physical activity and "physical conditioning programs are do's in a sea of don'ts and offer an affirmation of life to the patient."[53]

The educational program, whether done by occupational therapist, nurse educator, or a team, should inform the patient and his family about cardiovascular physiology in understandable terms. As a result of the educational program, the patient should be knowledgeable about safe activity selection based on MET tables that are given to him in writing and he should understand the limitations of the tables. He should be able to monitor his own response to exercise by taking his pulse. The patient should learn which symptoms are significant, how to recognize them, and what to do about them. The patient and his family need to learn about CPR and a family member should become certified.

Since 1968, deaths have dropped 27% from coronary heart disease and 48% from hypertensive disease.[54] Reasons given are a decrease in the number of people who smoke; better control of hypertension by medication, weight reduction, low sodium diet, decreased use of alcohol, and exercise; improved diets relative to low-density lipoprotein cholesterol[55] intake; stress recognition and management; and increased emphasis on exercise and fitness as part of daily life.[9,54] These are risk factors to be addressed in a patient education program.

Modification of Risk Behavior. Some coronary risk factors cannot be changed. These include family history of cardiac disease, increasing age, or being male. Risk factors that can be changed include smoking, elevated blood pressure, high levels of blood cholesterol, glucose intolerance (diabetes), a stressful life situation, and a sedentary existence.[35] There is also an association between type A behavior pattern and the incidence of ischemic heart disease.[56-58] In studies of 3,400 men and 9,097 men it was found to be a highly significant predictor of heart disease and of a second MI, even when the effects of other risk factors were statistically controlled.[57] Obesity is not a direct risk factor but it intensifies other risks: BP, cholesterol, and blood sugar levels.[9]

Each risk factor increases the probability of developing coronary heart disease two to three times; if the person has more than one risk factor, the probability multiplies.[2] If hypertension and smoking are eliminated, the risk is substantially reduced.

The occupational therapist can help the patient to alter certain risk factors: smoking, reaction to life stresses, and coronary-prone behavior pattern or type A personality[56-58] described in Rosenman and Friedman.

A behavior modification program[59] in which the goals are clearly stated in small, achievable steps and positive reinforcement is offered for successes can be used to stop or decrease smoking. The goals are expressed behaviorally to allow measurement of success. For example, instead of stating the goal as "patient will stop smoking," it is stated more specifically in terms of observable behavior and in smaller increments: "patient will not smoke before 9 AM (10 AM, 11 AM, etc.) today." Each successive short-term goal leads the person toward the long-term goal. This program needs to be accompanied by education concerning the physiology of smoking presented using audiovisual materials. A group therapy approach in which the members of the group offer support to each other is also useful.

Modern daily life consists of many stresses and strains on an individual due to frustrations. Group discussions can address alternate ways of reacting or handling situations. Putting the particular incident into perspective by asking "Is this worth dying for?"[60] may help the person develop healthier habits of reacting. Additional ways of coping with stress, some of which would provide topics for group discussion or individual reflection are: (1) establish priorities; (2) identify objective, realistic, and obtainable goals; (3) try to modify a hard-driving personality; (4) reduce frequency of stressful life change events; and (5) learn a relaxation technique and practice it daily.[60]

The type A personality is characterized by hard-driving competitiveness, time urgency, hurry and impatience, a potential for hostility,[58] or free-floating hostility.[56] Hostility has an element of destructiveness and is accompanied by feelings of anger.[58] Anger is an arousal state with expressive, subjective, visceral, and somatic components and seems to be the mediating construct linking behavior with cardiac pathogenesis.[58] The type A personality seems to be unmodifiable in persons who are at risk but who have not yet suffered an MI for several reasons, but primarily because it is a valued style and is seen as the basis for success.[56] Post-MI patients are ready to believe that the stress of trying to do too much in too little time was a risk factor and are ready for treatment.[56] The therapist needs to be a type B personality or at least a type A who is actively modifying her own behavior. The patient should trust and admire the therapist.

Before treatment begins, it is necessary to determine if both components of the type A personality are present and the degree of severity of each.[56] This is evaluated through a structured interview that allows the therapist to observe the patient's psychomotor manifestations, which are more reliable indicators than verbal responses alone.[56,57,61] The Behavior Pattern Interview used for this purpose relies on the interviewer's ability to make clinical judgments.[57] Nevertheless, the interrater reliability of this test was found to be relatively high, at least for content of patient's responses ($r = 0.85$), although where judgment enters more prominently into scoring—grading the style of the patient's responses—reliability was lower ($r = 0.50$).[57]

Those persons who are severely hostile and also exhibit time urgency, or whose general intelligence is so low that they cannot comprehend abstractions or symbolism are poor candidates for treatment.[56] Good candidates are older persons who exhibit more time urgency than hostility, who developed the behavior secondary to their milieu, who suspect their way of living needs to be changed, and who are nonegocentric.[56]

Treatment includes several facets, as described by Friedman.[56] The milieu is examined to identify and to learn to avoid stress or to reinterpret the meaning, relevance, and significance of the stressful factors. The person then learns to develop interests in things, events, and other persons outside of his own prime interests, that is, reprioritize his behavior.

Change is motivated in several ways. The fact that neither time urgency nor free-floating hostility was responsible for success and may in fact have been the basis for failures is pointed out. The valuable facets of the personality that are lost in response to type A behavior, such as leisurely participation in and enjoyment of cultural and social activities, are also pointed out. The patient's recognition of the need to redevelop value for friendship, affection, and joy is paramount to successful treatment. The person needs to learn to restructure daily events so there is enough time to do the important tasks, to eliminate the others, and to value rest time without feelings of guilt. The person needs to learn to eliminate the free-floating hostility by recognizing it, avoiding circumstances that provoke it, and substituting acts of love and affection to fill the vacuum of emotion left by not getting angry. The new behaviors need to be practiced and discussed until learned.

Group therapy has been found helpful in modifying coronary-prone behavior, although other risk factors were not significantly altered.[62]

Compliance may be a problem stemming from denial. For patients who demonstrated noncompliance with activity restrictions, a successful program was devised and reported.[63] Information was given concerning the fact that an MI actually meant death to tissue and that rest was required to allow scar formation. The patients were given the means to be in control of their disease by being taught—and allowed to establish—activity priorities within guidelines, by taking their own pulse to judge response to activity, and by requiring that they assume responsibility for reporting symptoms. Frequent positive reinforcement was offered. The program was task oriented; that is, the patient was kept busy doing tasks within his capabilities, which removed the emphasis from other activities that were restricted[63] and avoided the situation of no activity, which is depressing.

In another study of the effectiveness of group therapy using an educational approach, it was found that a significantly higher percentage of patients receiving group therapy returned to work compared to the control patients. Information given in the educational program was forgotten 1 year later, but the supportive aspects of the group program were valued by the patients.[62]

The patient may benefit, postdischarge, from contacting the local chapter of "Mended Hearts,"[64] a support group for former cardiac patients.

Prevocational and Recreational Counseling

The MET level of a patient's work and recreational activities can be determined or estimated from MET charts. If doubt exists about the patient's ability or safety to do these activities, actual response should be measured. The occupational therapist should offer a simulated work situation to test for readiness to return to previous type of work, to determine the need for and usefulness of adapted methods and/or equipment to modify the energy demands, and to help the patient improve his work skill since increased skill results in decreased stress.[65]

Many factors other than intensity stress the heart. One factor would be the need to repetitively use isometric contraction of small muscles for grasp or pinch at work. Adapted methods that transfer the demand to larger muscles or utilize devices to provide stabilization should be used. The patient also needs to be helped to develop a work/rest schedule[65] that can be adhered to at his place of employment.

Other factors that may prevent the patient from returning to the particular job he held previously or doing the recreational activity of choice are competitive situations, environmental heat or humidity or very cold temperature, stressful relationships or situations, highly time-oriented schedules, lifting or pushing heavy loads, and lack of opportunity to relax after eating. He needs to be counseled regarding the risks these factors offer and directed toward less stressful work and/or play.

Return to work is psychologically helpful to decrease depression and anxiety concerning physical status, family role, and finances. Return to certain jobs may actually require less energy expenditure than many self-care activities,[19] yet there is not a good correlation between return to work and physical capability[66] among subjects studied. After 3 months, post-MI patients are usually capable of 8 to 9 METs, which is greater than that demanded by many trade jobs (see Tables 30.3–30.7), yet only 50% to 75% return to work.[67] The self-employed individual is more likely to return to work sooner than other workers.[66] Psychotherapy and an exercise program[68] may help the patient overcome his fear of returning to work or point out secondary gains he is receiving from his condition. One secondary gain is the opportunity to be dependent on others "granted" him by the fact he has had an MI. Studies suggest that an effort must be made to identify the specific work tasks that may be potential barriers to or incentives for return to work.[69] The barriers can be simulated in occupational therapy. Satisfactory performance on an exercise test using work tasks that closely simulate the most stressful aspects of the actual work demands can help the patient, the employer, and the family gain confidence about the patient's ability to return to work.[70]

Myocardial Infarction Program at Grady Memorial Hospital, Atlanta, Georgia[35]

A 14-step program carried out under direct orders of the physician starts as the patient progresses through early recovery phases following an MI. There are four recovery phases described in this program as follows. The patient is progressed according to his particular response to activity at each step or phase.

PHASE I—CORONARY CARE UNIT

Low-energy physical activities are begun, such as those of steps 1 to 3 (see Table 30.2).

PHASE II—REMAINDER OF HOSPITALIZATION

The average hospitalization following uncomplicated MI is 21 days. Activity level is gradually increased with the goal of independent self-care, sitting, and graded rhythmic exercises progressing to walking and finally stair climbing. Patient and family education is an important part of the program. Steps 4 to 14 of the inpatient program (Table 30.2) are carried out.

PHASE III—CONVALESCENT PHASE

The patient returns home and follows a program to progressively increase physical activity to a level that will permit return to work by the 8th to 12th week after a MI. Activities include light housework, desk work, and walking, which is graded in distance and speed to approximately 1 to 2 miles a day at a rate of 3 miles per hour.

PHASE IV—RECOVERY AND MAINTENANCE

The patient returns to work at a suitable occupational or activity level. Further increase in cardiac function is encouraged by participation in community physical fitness programs. The goals of this period are to enhance function, decrease risk factors, and prevent recurrence of the disease.

PROGRAMMING FOR POSTSURGICAL CARDIAC PATIENTS

Coronary bypass and mitral or aortic valve replacement are the most common cardiac surgeries performed. The surgeon's goals for patients undergoing these surgeries include restored or improved coronary circulation, symptom-free tolerance for daily functional activities, and improved exercise tolerance. Programs for postsurgical patients are limited, although studies[71,72] are beginning to show a positive result for patients engaged in these programs. One study found that patients could begin a low-level exercise program 12 to 24 hours postbypass surgery, and it successfully prevented deleterious effects of prolonged bed rest and anxiety and depression.[72] A controlled study of two selected groups of postsurgical patients indicated that those who participated in a daily graded exercise program starting 1 day postop had increased performance on (1) a test of distance walking in 5 min; (2) an assessment of functional activities (i.e., standing calisthenics up to 3.5 METs); and (3) climbing 11 stairs at a comfortable speed.[71] A significantly shorter (1.9 days) mean length of hospitalization was found. It was expected, but not tested, that a controlled exercise program also would decrease the convalescent period postdischarge.[71]

Chronic Obstructive Pulmonary Disease

The terms chronic obstructive pulmonary disease (COPD) and chronic obstructive lung disease (COLD) encompass chronic bronchitis and emphysema.[73,74] Chronic bronchitis is a long-standing inflammation of the tracheobronchial tree accompanied by fibrotic changes in the mucous membrane,[10] producing a chronic cough usually with production of sputum. Pulmonary emphysema refers to destruction of the walls of the alveoli, which results in overdistention of these sacs and a loss of lung elasticity.[73] The lungs affected by emphysema become overstretched and progressively larger than normal so that the chest becomes "barrel" shaped.[73,75]

There is no single cause of chronic bronchitis or emphysema although a major etiological factor is cigarette smoking.[73] Prolonged dust inhalation by workers, air pollution, heredity, and aging also may be etiological factors. Specific bacterial and viral infections are not implicated.[73]

Table 30.2
GRADY MEMORIAL HOSPITAL 14-STEP PROGRAM—INPATIENT REHABILITATION AFTER MYOCARDIAL INFARCTION

	Exercise	Ward Activity	Educational & Craft Activity
Step 1	Passive ROM to all extremities (5X ea), teach pt *active* plantar and dorsiflexion of ankles to do several times per day.	Feeding self sitting with bed rolled up to 45°, trunk and arms supported by over-bed table.	Initial interview and brief orientation to program.
Step 2	Repeat exercises of Step #1.	1. Feeding self. 2. Partial AM care (washing hands & face, brushing teeth) in bed. 3. Dangle legs on side of bed (1X).	Light recreational activity, such as reading.
Step 3	Active assistive exercise in shoulder flexion and elbow flexion and extension, hip flexion, extension and rotation, knee flexion and extension, rotate feet. (4X ea).	1. Begin sitting in chair for short periods as tolerated, 2X/day. 2. Bathing whole body. 3. Use of bedside commode.	More detailed explanation of program. Continue light recreation.
Step 4	Minimal resistance, lying in bed do above ROM 5X ea. Stiffen all muscles to the count of 2 (3X).	1. Increase sitting 3X/day. 2. Change gown.	Begin explanation of what is an MI. Give pt pamphlets to read, begin craft activity: 1. Leather lacing. 2. Link belt. 3. Hand sewing, embroidery. 4. Copper tooling.
Step 5	Moderate resistance in bed at 45° above ROM exercises, hands on shoulders elbow circling (5X each arm).	1. Sitting ad lib. 2. Sitting in chair at bedside for meals. 3. Dressing, shaving, combing hair—*sitting down*. 4. Walking in room 2X/day.	Continue education about healing of heart, reasons for early restrictions in activity.
Step 6	1. Further resistive exercises sitting on side of bed, manual resistance of knee extension & flexion, (7X ea movement). 2. Walk distance to nearest bathroom and back (note if patient needs assistance).	1. Walk to bathroom, ad lib if pt can tolerate. 2. Stand at sink to shave.	Continue craft activity or supply pt with another one. Pt may attend group meetings in a wheelchair for no more than 1 hour.
Step 7	1. Standing warm-up exercises: a. Arms in extension and shoulder abduction, rotate arms together in circles (circumduction) 5X each arm. b. Stand on toes, 10X. c. May substitute abduction 5X ea leg. 2. Walk length of ward hall (50 ft) and back to room at average pace.	1. Bathe in tub. 2. Walk to telephone or sit in waiting room (1X/day).	1. May walk to group meetings on the same floor.

Table 30.2—*continued*

	Exercise	Ward Activity	Educational & Craft Activity
Step 8	1. Warm-up exercises: a. Lateral side bending, 5X ea side. b. Trunk twisting, 5X ea side. 2. Walk 1½ lengths of hall, down 1 flight of stairs, take elevator up.	1. Walk to waiting room 2X/day. 2. Stay sitting up most of the day.	Continue all previous craft and educational activities.
Step 9	1. Warm-up exercises: a. Lateral side bending, 10X ea side. b. Slight knee bends 10X with hands on hips. 2. Increase walking distance, walk down 1 flight of stairs.	Continue above activities.	Discussion of work simplification techniques and pacing of activities.
Step 10	1. Warm-up exercises: a. Lateral side bending with 1 lb weight (10X). b. Standing—leg raising leaning against wall, 5X ea. 2. Walk 2 lengths of hall and downstairs, take elevator up.	Continue all of previous ward activities.	1. Pt may walk to OT Clinic & work on craft project for ½ hr. a. Copper tooling; b. Woodworking; c. Ceramics; d. Small weaving project; e. Metal hammering; f. Mosaic tile. 2. Discussion of what exercises pt will do at home.
Step 11	1. Warm-up exercises: a. Lateral side bending with 1 lb weight leaning against wall 10X ea side; b. Standing leg raising 5X ea. c. Trunk twisting with 1 lb weight 5X ea side. 2. Repeat part 2 of Step 10.	Continue all of previous ward activities.	Increase time in OT Clinic to 1 hour.
Step 12	1. Warm-up exercises: a. Lateral side bending with 2 lb weight 10X. b. Standing—leg raising leaning against wall, 10X ea. c. Trunk twisting with 2 lb weight, 10X. 2. Walk down 2 flights of stairs.	Continue all of previous ward activities.	Continue craft activity with increased resistance.
Step 13	Repeat all exercises of Step 12.	Continue all of previous ward activities.	Complete all projects.
Step 14	1. Warm-up exercises: a. Lateral side bending with 2 lb weight 10X ea side. b. Trunk twisting with 2 lb weight 10X ea side. c. Touch toes from sitting position, 10X. 2. Walk up flight of 10 stairs and down.	Continue all of previous ward activities.	Final instructions about home activities.

The major functional abnormality of COPD is obstruction of air flow, mainly upon exhalation.[73] The typical COPD breathing pattern is rapid inspiration and prolonged expiration.[76] Maximum breathing rate during exercise is approximately 40 breaths per minute,[76] which limits exertion.

Living cells use oxygen for their metabolism and in the process produce waste products.[7] The oxygen that is transported to skeletal and heart muscle and to the brain and to other tissues is diffused from inspired air into the blood. The waste products, exchanged in the same way, are expelled out of the body in expired air.[77] The trachea splits into two bronchi, one to each lung. The bronchi branch into bronchioles, which continue branching, finally terminating in the alveoli, which are blind pouches that make up the lining of the lung.[7] Each alveolus is covered by a capillary network.[7] The diffusion of gases occurs at the alveolar-capillary interface. Chronic obstructive pulmonary disease or chronic obstructive lung disease interfere with ventilatory processes by decreasing the alveolar exchange and/or by reducing expiration.[77] If waste carbon dioxide is not expired, then oxygen intake is limited.[77]

The major disabling symptom of COPD is dyspnea on exertion. Dyspnea is the perception of shortness of breath (SOB). There is no universal definition of dyspnea, but translated from the Greek it means difficult breathing.[76] Dyspnea becomes a significant symptom when the patient reports that SOB is excessive for the level of physical activity.[76] There are several causes of dyspnea, only one of which is COPD; others are aging, obesity, anxiety, and cardiovascular disorders.[76] If the patient has several of these conditions, then SOB will be increased. Therefore, relaxation to decrease anxiety and diet to reduce weight would seem to be advantageous supplementary treatments for patients with COPD.

Although the disease process is irreversible and progressive, the patient can be taught to live more easily and productively within the limits of his pulmonary impairment.[78] As with any progressive disorder, the overall goal is to maintain function as long as possible. Rehabilitation does not alter the pathologic process[74,75,79] but increases the quality of life by giving the patient control over dyspnea and by increasing activity tolerance by producing a training effect; that is, less energy and oxygen required for a given amount of exertion.[73] The rehabilitation program focuses on breathing training and physical conditioning. A breathing pattern of slow expiration, with pursed lips, is stressed[73] and practiced during dyspnea-producing activities. Learning this gives the patient a feeling of being in control of his dyspnea.[73]

The physical therapist teaches the breathing exercises and bronchial hygiene techniques of postural drainage and assisted coughing.[80] The therapist also may apply percussion and vibration to the patient to loosen secretions.[80]

The occupational therapist reinforces the breathing techniques taught by the physical therapist, teaching the patient how to use these during functional activities. The occupational therapist also helps the patient improve his daily functional ability by teaching him how to conserve energy and simplify work.

Both physical and occupational therapists provide an exercise program. The exercise program rests on the concept that COPD patients can be conditioned and can eventually show improvement in endurance,[73] although no effect on the process of the disease is expected.[73,75,78] Studies confirm that although deterioration in ventilatory function is not slowed, there are significant improvements in exercise tolerance, which can be translated into improved activities of daily living.[74,81] Secondary benefits of the exercise program include increased feelings of self-confidence.[75]

Although dyspnea is the major focus of therapy, social or psychological reactions the patient has to this disease need to be addressed in therapy. They may include depression due to reduced abilities and the disease's progressive and fatal nature; guilt over smoking and the effect the disease has on self and family[78]; forced role change and resultant decreased self-esteem[78,79]; economic problems because of onset of the disease at a time of life (fifth or sixth decade) when high productivity is expected[78]; or reduced social interaction secondary to reduced activity level.[78,79] Because of fear of developing shortness of breath, patients tend to restrict their activities more and more.[73] The inactivity results in a vicious circle of reduced social stimulation; deterioration of strength, endurance, and sense of happiness; and increasing inactivity.[73,78] The occupational therapist helps the patient cope with these reactions and provides an opportunity to test improved exertional abilities in daily tasks of self-care, work, and play.

OCCUPATIONAL THERAPY PROGRAM

Evaluation

The evaluation should include assessment of the patient's abilities in occupational performance tasks (OPTs) (chapter 16); his strength, functional range of motion and endurance for activities rated at various MET levels (chapter 8 and Tables 30.3–30.7 in this chapter); his emotional status (chapter 2); his work and avocational history (chapters 19 and 21); and his neuropsychological status (chapter 7). The latter is necessary because increased cerebral blood flow and oxygen uptake have been shown to occur when various cortical areas become active.[82] Dyspneic patients may lack sufficient oxygen to sustain full cortical activity and may have memory, perceptual, and information-processing dysfunctions. The therapist needs to evaluate these functions as they relate to the patient's ability to understand and remember instruction and to safely and effectively interact with the environment. Evaluation of these functions should be ongoing throughout treatment because they will fluctuate with changes in oxygenation.[83]

Scoring of OPT assessments must reflect the pulmonary restrictions to successful performance. One

Table 30.3
APPROXIMATE METABOLIC COST OF ACTIVITIES[a,b]

	Occupational	Recreational
1½-2 METs[c] 4-7 ml O$_2$/min/kg 2-2½ kcal/min (70 kg person)	Desk work Auto driving[d] Typing Electric calculating machine operation	Standing Walking (strolling 1.6 km or 1 mile/hr) Flying,[d] motorcycling[d] Playing cards[d] Sewing, knitting
2-3 METs 7-11 ml O$_2$/min/kg 2½-4 kcal/min (70 kg person)	Auto repair Radio, TV repair Janitorial work Typing, manual Bartending	Level walking (3¼ km or 2 miles/hr) Level bicycling (8 km or 5 miles/hr) Riding lawn mower Billiards, bowling Skeet,[d] shuffleboard Woodworking (light) Powerboat driving[d] Golf (power cart) Canoeing (4 km or 2½ miles/hr) Horseback riding (walk) Playing piano and many musical instruments
3-4 METs 11-14 ml O$_2$/min/kg 4-5 kcal/min (70 kg person)	Brick laying, plaster-ing Wheelbarrow (220-lb or 100-kg load) Machine assembly Trailer-truck in traffic Welding (moderate load) Cleaning windows	Walking (5 km or 3 miles/hr) Cycling (10 km or 6 miles/hr) Horseshoe pitching Volleyball (6-man noncompetitive) Golf (pulling bag cart) Archery Sailing (handling small boat) Fly fishing (standing in waders) Horseback (sitting to trot) Badminton (social doubles) Pushing light power mower Energetic musician
4-5 METs 14-18 ml O$_2$/min/kg 5-6 kcal/min (70 kg person)	Painting, masonry Paperhanging Light carpentry	Walking (5½ km or 3½ miles/hr) Cycling (13 km or 8 miles/hr) Table tennis Golf (carrying clubs) Dancing (foxtrot) Badminton (singles) Tennis (doubles) Raking leaves Hoeing Many calisthenics
5-6 METs 18-21 ml O$_2$/min/kg 6-7 kcal/min (70 kg person)	Digging garden Shoveling light earth	Walking (6½ km or 4 miles/hr) Cycling (16 km or 10 miles/hr) Canoeing (6½ km or 4 miles/hr) Horseback ("posting" to trot) Stream fishing (walking in light current in waders) Ice or roller skating (15 km or 9 miles/hr)
6-7 METs 21-25 ml O$_2$/min/kg 7-8 kcal/min (70 kg person)	Shoveling 10/min (22 lb or 10 kg)	Walking (8 km or 5 miles/hr) Cycling (17½ km or 11 miles/hr) Badminton (competitive) Tennis (singles) Splitting wood Snow shoveling Hand lawn-mowing Folk (square) dancing Light downhill skiing Ski touring (4 km or 2½ miles/hr) (loose snow) Water skiing

Table 30.3—*continued*

	Occupational	Recreational
7-8 METs 25–28 ml O$_2$/min/kg 8-10 kcal/min (70 kg person)	Digging ditches Carrying 175 lb or 80 kg Sawing hardwood	Jogging (8 km or 5 miles/hr) Cycling (19 km or 12 miles/hr) Horseback (gallop) Vigorous downhill skiing Basketball Mountain climbing Ice hockey Canoeing (8 km or 5 miles/hr) Touch football Paddleball
8-9 METs 28-32 ml O$_2$/min/kg 10-11 kcal/min (70 kg person)	Shoveling 10/min (31 lb or 14 kg)	Running (9 km or 5½ miles/hr) Cycling (21 km or 13 miles/hr) Ski touring (6½ km or 4 miles/hr) (loose snow) Squash (social) Handball (social) Fencing Basketball (vigorous)
10 plus METs 32 plus ml O$_2$/min/kg 11 plus kcal/min (70 kg person)	Shoveling 10/min (35 lb or 16 kg)	Running 　6 mph =10 METs 　7 mph = 11½ METs 　8 mph = 13½ METs 　9 mph = 15 METs 　10 mph =17 METS Ski touring (8+ km or 5+ miles/hr) (loose snow) Handball (competitive) Squash (competitive)

^{a} Includes resting metabolic needs.

^{b} Reprinted with permission from Fox, S. M., et al. *Journal of the American Heart Association, 41*(4): 1972.

^{c} 1 MET is the energy expenditure at rest, equivalent to approximately 3.5 ml O$_2$/kg body weight/min.

^{d} A major increase in metabolic requirements may occur due to excitement, anxiety, or impatience, which are common responses during some activities. The patient's emotional reactivity must be assessed when prescribing or sanctioning certain activities.

Table 30.4
MINIMAL CARDIAC ACTIVITY^a

Activity	Position	METS
Leather belt assembly	Sitting at table	1.25
Leather stamping	Sitting at table	1.35
Leather tooling	Sitting at table	1.30
Listening to radio	Sitting in easy chair	1.40
Bench assembly, light	Sitting at bench	1.40
Leather lacing	Sitting at table	1.45
Chip carving	Sitting at table	1.60

^{a} Reprinted with permission from Kottke, F. J. Common cardiovascular problems in rehabilitation. In *Handbook of Physical Medicine and Rehabilitation*. Edited by F. H. Krusen, F. J. Kottke, and P. M. Ellwood. Philadelphia: W. B. Saunders, 1971.

rating method[78] suggested scoring each task 1 point for poor performance, characterized by marked breathlessness, incomplete performance, and assistance required; 2 points for fair performance, operationally defined as moderate breathlessness and needing to pause to be able to complete the task (this may make the task too time consuming for functional independence); 3 points for satisfactory performance, which is defined as complete but not entirely normal performance with mild breathlessness; and 4 points for normal

Table 30.5
LIGHT CARDIAC ACTIVITY^a

Activity	Position	METS
Eating	Sitting	1.50
Sewing	Sitting	1.60
Clerical work	Sitting	1.60
Setting type	Standing	1.60
Getting out of and into bed	Bed to chair	1.65
Leather carving	Sitting on chair	1.70
Weaving, table loom	Sitting on stool	1.70
Clerical work	Standing	1.80
Writing	Sitting	2.00
Typing	Sitting on chair	2.00
Bimanual activity test sanding, 50 strokes/min	Sitting on chair	2.00
Weaving, floor loom	Sitting on bench	2.10
Metal work, hammer	Standing	2.15
Printing, platen press	Standing	2.30
Bench assembly, moderate	Sitting	2.35
Hanging clothes on line	Standing—stooping	2.40

^{a} Reprinted with permission from Kottke, F. J.[18] Common cardiovascular problems in rehabilitation. In *Handbook of Physical Medicine and Rehabilitation*. Edited by F. H. Krusen, F. J. Kottke, and P. M. Ellwood. Philadelphia: W. B. Saunders, 1971.

Table 30.6
MODERATE CARDIAC ACTIVITY[a]

Activity	Position	METS
Playing piano		2.50
Dressing, undressing		2.50–3.50
Sawing, jeweler's saw	Sitting	1.90
Sawing, hack saw	Standing	2.55
Driving car		2.80
Bicycling, slowly		2.90
Preparing meals		3.00
Weight lifting, 10 lb lifted 15 in., 46/min	Sitting	2.80
Walking, 2.0 mph		3.20
Handsawing, wood	Standing	3.50
Warm shower		3.50

[a] Reprinted with permission from Kottke, F. J. Common cardiovascular problems in rehabilitation. In *Handbook of Physical Medicine and Rehabilitation*. Edited by F. H. Krusen, F. J. Kottke, and P. M. Ellwood. Philadelphia: W. B. Saunders, 1971.

Table 30.7
HEAVY AND SEVERE CARDIAC ACTIVITY[a]

Activity	Position	METS
Bowel movement	Toilet	3.60
Bowel movement	Bedpan	4.70
Making beds	Standing	3.90
Hot shower	Standing	4.20
Walking fast (3.5 mph)		5.00
Descending stairs		5.20
Scrubbing floor	Kneeling	5.30
Master, two-step climbing test		5.70
Weight lifting, 10-20 lb lifted 36 in., 15/min		6.50
Bicycling, fast		6.90
Running		7.40
Mowing lawn		7.70
Climbing stairs		9.00

[a] Reprinted with permission from Kottke, F. J. Common cardiovascular problems in rehabilitation. In *Handbook of Physical Medicine and Rehabilitation*. Edited by F. H. Krusen, F. J. Kottke, and P. M. Ellwood. Philadelphia: W. B. Saunders, 1971.

performance, that is, no dyspnea noted. The total score would estimate the patient's exertional level.

The ADAPT© Quality of Life Scale[84] may be useful as an inventory of interests and abilities. It lists 105 activities ordered according to estimated $\dot{V}O_2$ requirements for each. The patient is asked to check each activity as to whether he is still doing it, has quit doing it, or never did it. The activities listed include self-care, home management chores, sports, hobbies, and social activities.

Treatment

The objectives of the occupational therapy program for the COPD patient are as follows[78,85]:

1. To reinforce breathing control by teaching use of the technique during ADL, work, leisure, and all stress-producing situations. The breathing technique emphasizes slow abdominal diaphragmatic breathing[75,77] with exhalation against pursed lips, which prevents the usual collapse of the airways in these patients[77] and improves ventilatory efficiency and CO_2 elimination.[74,86] The patient needs to learn to contract the abdominal muscles during expiration and relax them during inspiration.[77] He is taught to exhale during stressful components of a motion and inhale during the return, nonstressful component of motion.[78,85]

2. To increase independence in self-care, play, and work through application of breathing training, adaptations, and coping techniques. Coping techniques are work simplification, pacing, and other energy conservation techniques.[78,79] The energy conservation and work simplification methods taught are the same as those taught to other patients with reduced endurance (see chapter 17). Additional adaptations are suggested for COPD patients: the patient is taught to avoid those movements and positions found to produce dyspnea such as bending at the waist or raising the arms over the head.[78,79,85] For example, loafer-style shoes are used in place of tie shoes that require bending over; frequently used objects are stored within easy reach; and grooming requirements are kept to a minimum by simple hair styles, sitting and propping the elbows while shaving, etc. Bathing is a particular problem needing modification since the patient may feel "suffocated" in a shower and find baths tiresome.[79] Suggestions may include the use of a bath seat, hand-held shower, and tepid water. Vigorous, fast movements such as toweling after showering are avoided.[78]

3. To provide a graded activity program to implement a training effect; to increase or maintain strength, mobility, and endurance (chapter 9); and to provide opportunities to practice coordination of breathing phases with movement. Activities should be rhythmical and repetitive.[78] Activities that start with the arms by the side and move to arms overhead help with inspiration by expanding the chest; those that start with the arms overhead and move to arms down assist expiration.[78] Examples are the lift (up) and chop (down) of proprioceptive neuromuscular facilitation (chapter 6); use of hand printing press; a loom adapted for overhead operation[78]; and calisthenics. The force required should be in the downward direction (exhalation). Activities that generate dust and those that require sustained effort overhead or stooping over should be avoided.

4. To assist the patient in recognizing the need for, and in practicing, a balanced regime of work, rest, and play as a means of improving the quality of his life. Although dyspnea may not be eradicated, it can be made less debilitating[78] by modifying life-style.

5. To facilitate a positive emotional outlook (chapter 2) by emphasizing the patient's abilities and activity options and by assisting him to see that the coping techniques he is being taught give him some control over the disease.[79] He is encouraged to take the initia-

tive and responsibility in the management of his chronic disease.[78]

6. To explore avocational interests and abilities, especially for those who must retire from work.

7. To evaluate work capacity and provide simulated work experiences, i.e., work hardening, to prepare for return to work (chapter 21). Successful return to work also may require job task analysis, adaptations of tools or procedures, and learning to pace the work so that the oxygen demand is within his limitations.

8. To reduce anxiety, which increases dyspnea,[79] through group therapy (chapter 2) and activity programs. The patient is encouraged to pace his activity by taking "resting pauses" regularly.[79] Slow, organized methods and the coordination of breathing control are stressed to reduce the patient's tendency to rush through activities in fear of developing dyspnea.[78]

9. To promote life-long adaptation to COPD, a home program of activity and exercise is established and taught to the patient.[75] The family also must be educated about the disease, the exertional restrictions, and the home program to elicit support for the patient.

STUDY QUESTIONS:

Cardiopulmonary Rehabilitation

1. Define myocardial infarction (MI). What is the relationship of angina pectoris to MI?
2. Define training effect. What is its significance?
3. What are the goals of therapy during the inpatient phase of rehabilitation?
4. Is a class III patient allowed to take a shower? Why? Relate your answer to metabolic equivalent (MET) levels.
5. Define 1 MET.
6. What is your maximum heart rate? What percentage of your $\dot{V}O_2$ max are you using at this moment?
7. What aspects of electrocardiogram (ECG) should a therapist be able to read in order to recognize problems when viewing a patient's ECG monitor during activity?
8. What are ECG indications of intolerance to exercise? What should the occupational therapist do if she notices any of these on the monitor when working with a patient?
9. You have an 11 o'clock and a 1 o'clock opening on your schedule to work with a newly assigned post-MI patient in phase I of rehabilitation. At which time should you schedule him and why?
10. How much oxygen are you consuming during ½ hour of sewing? During ½ hour of meal preparation? During ½ hour of walking (20-min mile)? Is your roommate consuming the same amount of oxygen? Why?
11. If a patient in the outpatient phase of rehabilitation has a maximum MET level of 7.5, what is the average MET level at which he should work to develop a training effect? What task(s) could he do? What tasks could he not do?
12. Select a modifiable risk factor. Describe a behavior modification program that you could use to help your patient reduce this risk. Include the short-term goals, the reinforcement(s) to be used, and the method of charting progress.
13. What is the major functional abnormality of patients with chronic obstructive pulmonary disease (COPD)? The major disabling symptom?
14. What is the expected effect of an exercise program on patients with COPD?
15. Why do cognitive and perceptual functions need to be evaluated in the COPD patient group?
16. Explain the breathing technique as it is used during activity.
17. What types of activity are used in a graded program for patients with COPD?

References

1. Whipp, B. J., and Ward, S. The normal respiratory response in exercise. In *Cardiopulmonary Exercise Testing*. Edited by A. R. Leff. Orlando, FL: Grune & Stratton, 1986.
2. Killen, K. What is cardiac rehabilitation and how does occupational therapy fit in? *Occupational Therapy News*, 40(10): 15, 1986.
3. Oldridge, N. B. Compliance of post myocardial infarction patients to exercise programs. *Med. Sci. Sports*, 11(4): 373–375, 1979.
4. Kremser, C. B., and Rajfer, S. I. The normal cardiovascular response to exercise. In *Cardiopulmonary Exercise Testing*. Edited by A. R. Leff. Orlando, FL: Grune & Stratton, 1986.
5. Littell, E. H. Support responses of the cardiovascular system to exercise. Part I. *Phys. Ther., 61*(9): 1260–1264, 1981.
6. Hartley, H. Lecture to seminar in cardiac rehabilitation, Boston University, June 1978.
7. Astrand, P. O., and Rodahl, K. *Textbook of Work Physiology: Physiological Basis of Exercise*, 3rd edition. New York: McGraw Hill, 1986.
8. Dehn, M. M., and Mullins, C. B. Physiologic effects and importance of exercise in patients with coronary artery disease. *Cardiovasc. Med.*, April 1977, pp. 365–385, 387.
9. Levy, R. L. *Medicine for the Layman: Heart Attacks*. Bethesda, MD: National Institutes of Health publication no. 80-1803, 1980.
10. Thomas, C. L., editor. *Taber's Cyclopedic Medical Dictionary*, 12th edition. Philadelphia: F. A. Davis, 1973.
11. Kattus, A. A., chairman. The Committee on Exercise. *Exercise Testing and Training of Apparently Healthy Individuals: A Handbook for Physicians*. New York: American Heart Association, 1972.
12. New York Heart Association. *Diseases of the Heart and Blood Vessels—Nomenclature and Criteria for Diagnosis*, 6th edition. Boston: Little, Brown & Company, 1964.
13. Siegel, G. H. Informed consent in exercise testing and training programs (appendix A). In *Exercise Testing and Training of Individuals with Heart Disease or at High Risk for its Development: A Handbook for Physicians*. Edited by A. A. Kattus. Dallas: American Heart Association, 1975.
14. Erb, B. D., Fletcher, G. F., and Sheffield, T. L. AHA committee report: standards for cardiovascular exercise treatment programs. *Circulation, 59*: 1084A–1090A, 1979.
15. Gordan, A. S., et al. American Heart Association committee on cardiopulmonary resuscitation and emergency cardiac care. Standards for cardiopulmonary resuscitation (CPR) and emergency cardiac care (ECC). *J.A.M.A.*, 227(Suppl.)(7): 1974.
16. Committee on Emergency Cardiac Care. *CPR in Basic Life Support*. New York: American Heart Association, 1974.
17. Mead, W. F. Exercise rehabilitation after myocardial infarction. *Am. Fam. Phys., 15*(March): 121–125, 1977.
18. Kottke, F. J. Common cardiovascular problems in rehabilitation. In *Handbook of Physical Medicine and Rehabilitation*. Edited by F. H. Krusen, F. J. Kottke, and P. M. Ellwood. Philadelphia: W. B. Saunders, 1971.
19. Cohen, B. S. A program for rehabilitation after acute myocardial infarction. *South. Med. J.*, 68(2): 145–148, 1975.
20. McCann, L., and Holmes, D. S. Influence of aerobic exercise on depression. *J. Pers. Soc. Psychol., 46*(5): 1142–1147, 1984.
21. Grant, A., and Cohen, B. S. Acute myocardial infarction: effect of a rehabilitation program on length of hospitalization and functional status at discharge. *Arch. Phys. Med. Rehabil., 54*(5): 201–206, 1973.
22. Kavanagh, T., and Shephard, R. J. Sexual activity after myocardial infarction. *Can. Med. J., 116*: 1250–1253, 1977.
23. Golding, L. A. Exercise physiology. In *Prevention and Rehabilitation in Ischemic Heart Disease*. Edited by C. Long. Baltimore: Williams & Wilkins, 1980.
24. Ellestad, M. H. *Stress Testing: Principles and Practice*, 3rd edition. Philadelphia: F. A. Davis, 1986.
25. American College of Sports Medicine. *Guidelines for Graded Exercise Testing and Exercise Prescription*. Philadelphia: Lea & Febiger, 1976.
26. Erb, B. D. *Physician's Handbook for Evaluation of Cardiovascular and Physical Fitness*, 2nd edition. Nashville: Tennessee Heart Association, 1972.

27. Fletcher, G. F., and Cantwell, J. D. *Exercise and Coronary Heart Disease: Role in Prevention, Diagnosis and Treatment*, 2nd edition. Springfield, IL: Charles C Thomas, 1979.

28. Day, W. Lecture to seminar in cardiac rehabilitation. Boston University, June 1978.

29. Lunsford, B. R. Heart rate: a clinical indicator of endurance. *Phys. Ther.*, 58(6): 705-709, 1978.

30. Menard, R. H. *Introduction to Arrhythmia Recognition*. San Francisco: California Heart Association, 1968.

31. Littmann, D. *Examination of the Heart. Part Five: The Electrocardiogram*. New York: American Heart Association, 1973.

32. Winsor, T. The electrocardiogram in myocardial infarction. In *Clinical Symposia*. Summit, NJ: Ciba Pharmaceutical Company, Medical Education Division, 1968.

33. Dubin, D. *Rapid Interpretation of EKG's*, 3rd edition. Tampa, FL: COVER Publishing Co., 1974.

34. Margolis, J. R., and Wagner, G. S. *Coronary Care: Arrhythmias in Acute Myocardial Infarction*. Dallas: American Heart Association, 1976.

35. Wenger, N. *Rehabilitation after Myocardial Infarction*. New York: American Heart Association, 1973.

36. Schang, S. J., and Pepine, C. J. Transient asymptomatic S-T segment depression during daily activity. *Am. J. Cardiol.*, 39(3): 396-402, 1977.

37. Hamm, L. F., et al. Short- and long-term prognostic value of graded exercise testing soon after myocardial infarction. *Phys. Ther.*, 66(3): 334-339, 1986.

38. Cumming, G. R. Comparison of treadmill and bicycle ergometer exercise in middle-aged males. *Am. Heart J.*, 93: 261, 1977.

39. Sutton, J. Exercise responses in post myocardial infarction patients. *Med. Sci. Sports*, 11(4): 366-367, 1979.

40. Ogden, L. D. Activity guidelines for early subacute and high-risk cardiac patients. *Am. J. Occup. Ther.*, 33(5): 291-298, 1979.

41. Ogden, L. D. Hands on: cardiac rehabilitation. Guidelines for analysis and testing of activities of daily living with cardiac patients. *American Occupational Therapy Association Physical Disabilities Specialty Section Newsletter*, 3(4): 1, 3, 1980.

42. Greer, M., et al. Physiological responses to low-intensity cardiac rehabilitation exercises. *Phys. Ther.*, 60(9): 1146-1151, 1980.

43. Corcoran, P. J. Energy expenditure during ambulation. In *Physiological Basis of Rehabilitation Medicine*. Edited by J. A. Downey and R. C. Darling. Philadelphia: W. B. Saunders, 1971.

44. Semmler, C., and Semmler, M. Counseling the coronary patient. *Am. J. Occup. Ther.*, 28(10): 609-614, 1974.

45. Ramos, M. U., et al. Cardiovascular effects of spread of excitation during prolonged isometric exercise. *Arch. Phys. Med. Rehabil.*, 54(11): 496-504, 1974.

46. Smith, D. A., and Lukens, S. A. Stress effects of isometric contraction in occupational therapy. *Occup. Ther. J. Res.*, 3(4): 222-242, 1983.

47. Ewing, D. J., Kerr, F., Irving, J. B., and Muir, A. L. Weight carrying after myocardial infarction. *Lancet*, 1(May 17): 1113-1114, 1975.

48. Monod, H. Contractility of muscle during prolonged static and repetitive dynamic activity. *Ergonomics*, 28(1): 81-89, 1985.

49. Stein, R. A. The effect of exercise training on heart rate during coitus in the post myocardial infarction patient. *Circulation*, 55(5): 738-740, 1977.

50. Tobis, J. Sex counseling for postmyocardial infarction patients. *West. J. Med.*, 131(2): 133-134, 1979.

51. Long, C. Exercise in the prevention and rehabilitation of ischemic heart disease. In *Prevention and Rehabilitation in Ischemic Heart Disease*. Edited by C. Long. Baltimore: Williams & Wilkins, 1980.

52. *Handbook for Participants*. Cardiac rehabilitation postgraduate course, University of Texas Medical Branch, 1977.

53. Hackett, T. P., and Cassem, N. H. Psychological adaptation to convalescence in myocardial infarction patients. In *Exercise Testing and Training in Coronary Heart Disease*. Edited by J. Naughton and H. K. Hellerstein. New York: Academic Press, 1973.

54. Cooper, K. H. The aerobics program for total well-being. Distinguished Lecturer Series, School of Health Studies, University of New Hampshire. November 7, 1984.

55. Medalie, J. H., Tyroler, H. A., and Heiss, G. High density lipoprotein cholesterol and ischemic heart disease. In *Prevention and Rehabilitation in Ischemic Heart Disease*. Edited by C. Long. Baltimore: Williams & Wilkins, 1980.

56. Friedman, M. The modification of type A behavior in post-infarction patients. *Am. Heart J.*, 97: 551-560, 1979.

57. Rowland, K. F., and Sokol, B. A review of research examining the coronary-prone behavior pattern. *J. Hum. Stress*, 3(September): 26-33, 1977.

58. Diamond, E. L. The role of anger and hostility in essential hypertension and coronary heart disease. *Psychol. Bull.*, 92(2): 410-433, 1982.

59. Leon, G. R. Behavior modification in reducing risk factors for ischemic heart disease. In *Prevention and Rehabilitation in Ischemic*

Heart Disease. Edited by C. Long. Baltimore: Williams & Wilkins, 1980.

60. Shearer, L. Stress and strain. *Parade*, December 19, 1976, p. 4.

61. Friedman, E. H., and Hellerstein, H. K. Influence of psychosocial factors on coronary risk adaptation to a physical fitness evaluation program. In *Exercise Testing and Training in Coronary Heart Disease*. Edited by J. Naughton and H. K. Hellerstein. New York: Academic Press, 1973.

62. Rahe, R. H., Ward, H. W., and Hayes, V. Brief group therapy in myocardial infarction rehabilitation: three- to four-year follow-up of a controlled trial. *Psychosom. Med.*, 41(3): 229-242, 1979.

63. Baile, W. F., and Engel, B. T. A behavioral strategy for promoting treatment compliance following myocardial infarction. *Psychosom. Med.*, 40(5): 413-419, 1978.

64. Mended Hearts Inc., 721 Huntington Avenue, Boston, MA 02115.

65. Brinkley, S. B. The use of exercise test results in vocational rehabilitation of cardiac clients. In *Exercise Testing and Training in Coronary Heart Disease*. Edited by J. Naughton and H. K. Hellerstein. New York: Academic Press, 1973.

66. Krasemann, E. O., and Jungmann, H. Return to work after myocardial infarction. *Cardiology*, 64(3): 190-196, 1979.

67. Muir, J. R. The rehabilitation of cardiac patients. *Proc. R. Soc. Med.*, 70(September): 655-656, 1977.

68. Hertanu, J. S., et al. Cardiac rehabilitation exercise program: outcome assessment. *Arch. Phys. Med. Rehabil.*, 67(7): 431-435, 1986.

69. Mitchell, D. K. Principles of vocational rehabilitation: a contemporary view. In *Prevention and Rehabilitation in Ischemic Heart Disease*. Edited by C. Long. Baltimore: Williams & Wilkins, 1980.

70. Wilke, N. A., and Sheldahl, L. M. Use of simulated work testing in cardiac rehabilitation: a case report. *Am. J. Occup. Ther.*, 39(5): 327-330, 1985.

71. Ungerman-deMent, P., Bemis, A., and Siebens, A. Exercise program for patients after cardiac surgery. *Arch. Phys. Med. Rehabil.*, 67(7): 463-466, 1986.

72. Dion, W. F., et al. Medical problems and physiologic responses during supervised inpatient cardiac rehabilitation: patient after coronary artery bypass grafting. *Heart Lung*, 11: 248-255, 1982.

73. Kaplan, A. S. Rehabilitation in chronic obstructive pulmonary disease. *Am. J. Occup. Ther.*, 24(3): 179-180, 1970.

74. Petty, T. L. Pulmonary rehabilitation. *Basics of RD (American Thoracic Society of the American Lung Association)*, 4(1): 1-6, 1975.

75. Sinclair, J. D. Exercise in pulmonary disease. In *Therapeutic Exercise*, 3rd edition. Edited by J. V. Basmajian. Baltimore: Williams & Wilkins, 1978.

76. Hansen, J. E. Respiratory abnormalities: exercise evaluation of the dyspneic patient. In *Cardiopulmonary Exercise Testing*. Edited by A. R. Leff. Orlando, FL: Grune & Stratton, 1986.

77. Helmholz, H. F., and Stillwell, G. K. Disorders of respiration. In *Handbook of Physical Medicine and Rehabilitation*, 2nd edition. Edited by F. H. Krusen, F. J. Kottke, and P. M. Ellwood. Philadelphia: W. B. Saunders, 1971.

78. Berzins, G. F. An occupational therapy program for the chronic obstructive pulmonary disease patient. *Am. J. Occup. Ther.*, 24(3): 181-186, 1970.

79. Barstow, R. E. Coping with emphysema. *Nurs. Clin. North Am.*, 9(1): 137-145, 1974.

80. Sessler, A. D. Chest physical therapy. In *Handbook of Physical Medicine and Rehabilitation*, 2nd edition. Edited by F. H. Krusen, F. J. Kottke, and P. M. Ellwood. Philadelphia: W. B. Saunders, 1971.

81. Alison, J. A., Samios, R., and Anderson, S. D. Evaluation of exercise training in patients with chronic airway obstruction. *Phys. Ther.*, 61(9): 1273-1277, 1981.

82. Lassen, N. A., Ingvar, D. H., and Skinhoj, E. Brain function and blood flow. *Sci. Am.*, 232: 62-71, 1978.

83. Krop, H. D., Block, A. J., and Cohen, E. Neuropsychological effects of continuous oxygen therapy in chronic obstructive pulmonary disease. *Chest*, 64: 317, 1973.

84. Daughton, D. M., et al. Maximum oxygen consumption and the ADAPT Quality-of-life scale. *Arch. Phys. Med. Rehabil.*, 63(12): 620-622, 1982.

85. Pomerantz, P., Flannery, E. L., and Findling, P. K. Occupational therapy for chronic obstructive lung disease. *Am. J. Occup. Ther.*, 29(7): 407-411, 1975.

86. Petty, T. L., and Guthrie, A. The effect of augmented breathing maneuvers on ventilation in severe chronic airway obstruction. *Respir. Care*, 16: 104, 1971.

Supplementary Reading

Alison, J. A., and Anderson, S. D. Comparison of two methods of assessing physical performance in patients with chronic airway obstruction. *Phys. Ther.*, 61(9): 1278-1281, 1981.

American College of Sports Medicine. *Guidelines for Graded Exercise Testing and Prescription*, 3rd edition. Philadelphia: Lea & Febiger, 1985.

Bachynski-Cole, M., and Cumming, G. R. The cardiovascular fitness of disabled patients attending occupational therapy. *Occup. Ther. J. Res.,* 5(4): 233–242, 1985.

Bachynski-Cole, M., and Cumming, G. R. The electrocardiographic findings of occupational therapy patients. *Occup Ther. J. Res., 4*(1): 53–58, 1984.

Chobanian, A. V., and Loviglio, L. *Boston University Medical Center's Heart Risk Book: A Practical Guide for Preventing Heart Disease.* New York: Bantam Books, 1982.

Cornett, S. J., and Watson, J. E. *Cardiac Rehabilitation: An Interdisciplinary Team Approach.* New York: John Wiley, 1984.

Frank, K. A., Heller, S. S., and Kornfeld, D. S. Psychological intervention in coronary heart disease: a review. *Gen. Hosp. Psychiatry, 1*(1): 18–23, 1979.

Friedman, M., and Rosenman, R. H. *Type A Behavior and Your Heart.* Greenwich, CT: Fawcett Publications, 1974.

Gilbert, D. Energy expenditures for the disabled homemaker: review of studies. *Am. J. Occup. Ther., 19*(6): 321–328, 1965.

Hellerstein, H., and Wenger, N. *Rehabilitation of the Coronary Heart Patient,* 2nd edition. New York: John Wiley, 1985.

Huntley, N., and Mullvain, M. A. *Basics of Cardiac Rehabilitation.* Minneapolis: Minnesota Occupational Therapy Association Cardiac Care Special Interest Group, 1978.

Mesenbourg, B., and Daniewicz, C., and Schoening, H. Occupational therapy in coronary rehabilitation. *Am. J. Occup. Ther., 24*(6): 428–431, 1970.

Peterson, L. H., editor. *Cardiovascular Rehabilitation: A Comprehensive Approach.* New York: Macmillan Publishing Co., 1983.

Quiggle, A. B., Kottke, F. J., and Magney, J. Metabolic requirements of occupational therapy procedures. *Arch. Phys. Med. Rehabil., 35*(9): 567–572, 1954.

Weidman, W. H., et al. *Recreational and Occupational Recommendations for Use by Physicians Counseling Young Patients with Heart Disease.* Dallas: American Heart Association, 1971.

Wilson, P. K., Bell, C. W., and Norton, A. C. *Rehabilitation of the Heart and Lungs.* Fullerton, CA: Beckman, 1980.

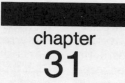

chapter
31

Amputation and Prosthetics

Anne G. Fisher

Among the adult population can be found three groups of amputees: (1) individuals born with congenital limb deficiencies; (2) individuals with acquired amputations resulting from trauma; and (3) individuals with acquired amputations who have undergone secondary amputation surgery as part of the overall management of a primary disease or disorder.

The juvenile amputee (the child with a congenital limb deficiency or an acquired amputation sustained during childhood) is beyond the scope of this chapter. Juvenile amputees represent approximately 6% of the total amputee population. Because they are fitted and trained with prostheses and/or receive activities of daily living training as children, their management is highly specialized and best carried out in one of the many regional juvenile amputee centers whose staff is trained and experienced in their care. By the time the juvenile amputee reaches adulthood, the need for services provided by the occupational therapist, beyond the occasional checkout of a new prosthesis or training in the use of a newly fitted electrically powered prosthesis, is rare.

Therefore, this chapter will be limited to a discussion of occupational therapy procedures for the individual with an acquired amputation sustained in adulthood. Principles of upper-extremity preprosthetic treatment and prosthetic fitting and training will be emphasized. The role of occupational therapy in the treatment of lower-extremity amputees and partial hand amputations will also be discussed.

Levels of Amputation[1-3]

Generally, diagnosis is descriptive and is based upon the level of amputation. An amputation that involves removal of part or all of the clavicle and scapula along with the upper limb is a *forequarter* amputation. When an amputation occurs at a joint, it is considered a disarticulation; if the clavicle and scapula are left intact but the entire humerus is removed, the level of amputation is a *shoulder disarticulation*. When the amputation is

through the humerus, the level is referred to as *above-elbow*. Amputation at the elbow is an *elbow disarticulation*, and if it is through the radius and ulna, the amputation is referred to as *below-elbow*. Above- and below-elbow amputations are further described as being very short, short, standard, or long, depending upon the relative length of the stump (residual limb). An amputation at the level of the wrist is a *wrist disarticulation* and, if through the metacarpals, the amputation is referred to as *transmetacarpal*. Transmetacarpal amputations as well as more distal amputations of the hand are generally referred to as *partial hand* amputations.

Some clinics do not adhere rigidly to the above criteria, especially when the amputation is near but not through the joint. In this instance, the diagnosis is based on the type of prosthesis that is fitted. Hence, a very high above-elbow amputee whose stump is too short to be fitted with an above-elbow prosthesis may be diagnosed as having a shoulder disarticulation. Even more commonly, the individual with an amputation just proximal to the elbow or the wrist and who is fitted with an elbow disarticulation or wrist disarticulation type prosthesis is diagnosed accordingly.

Rehabilitation of the Upper-Extremity Amputee

The goal of rehabilitation of the amputee is independence in occupational performance tasks. Ideally, prosthetic fitting and training eliminate the need to modify the environment and enable the amputee to function more normally within it. Success, in terms of high levels of prosthetic skill and awareness, return to prior occupational roles, and reintegration into society, is dependent on a comprehensive rehabilitation program that includes the fitting of a comfortable, mechanically sound prosthesis and thorough prosthetic training.

The occupational therapist is a member of a specialized rehabilitation team that also includes the patient, prosthetist, social worker, psychologist, vocational counselor, physical therapist, and physician. The occupational therapist has primary responsibility for checkout of the prosthesis, provision of prosthetic training, and provision of training in one-handed techniques. Either the occupational or physical therapist has responsibility for preprosthetic strengthening and range of motion programs. Similarly, instruction in stump care is frequently provided by other members of the team. However, the occupational therapist is an important member of the rehabilitation team; she contributes to decision making and recommends appropriate referrals to other team members at all stages in the rehabilitation process. Therefore, the occupational therapist must have knowledge of all stages of the rehabilitation process, which is illustrated in Fig. 31.1.

PREPROSTHETIC CARE AND EARLY POSTSURGICAL FITTING[1-10]

Immediate postsurgical treatment objectives are to control edema and to maintain and/or regain range of motion and strength of all remaining joints. The provision of a supportive rehabilitation environment is another important team objective.

As soon as possible following surgery, the physical or occupational therapist should initiate a program to regain and/or maintain muscle strength and range of motion. If the amputation results in loss of the preferred hand, an occupational therapy program to increase one-handed skill and coordination of the nonpreferred hand is also necessary. At best, the prosthesis can only act as an assistive extremity; the remaining limb typically assumes the role of the preferred hand. Finally, group activities that include the participation of other amputees facilitate psychological adjustments to the amputation.

Elastic stump shrinkers are preferred to more traditional elastic bandaging for the control of postsurgical edema and shaping of the stump for prosthetic fitting when immediate postsurgical rigid dressings are not applied. Elastic bandaging, even when applied correctly, can be hazardous. Uneven or excessive pressure or lack of sustained pressure restricts venous return, interferes with reduction of edema, and can cause "choke syndrome" to occur in the stump. In contrast, elastic stump shrinkers provide sustained pressure within an optimal pressure range necessary to control edema and prevent harm to the stump.

In an attempt to (1) decrease the 50% or better rejection rate of upper-extremity prostheses, (2) control edema and accelerate stump shaping, (3) prevent or reduce the painful phantom limb phenomenon, and (4) decrease the period of time the amputee is without a prosthesis to encourage the earlier development of new bilateral patterns using the prosthesis, many centers are using early postsurgical fitting of upper-extremity amputees. This technique involves the fitting of a rigid elastic plaster dressing or temporary prosthesis worn over the surgical dressing that has incorporated into it all of the appropriate prosthetic components necessary to begin prosthetic training. Prosthetic training can thereby begin within days after surgery and does not have to wait until the definitive prosthesis has been fabricated.

Studies of the benefits of immediate or early postsurgical fitting with an upper-extremity prosthesis have identified a critical 30-day "golden period." Amputees fitted within the first 30 days postsurgery have been found to have much lower prosthetic rejection rates, lower frequency or elimination of phantom limb pain, and better psychological adaptation. The results are much higher rates of return to work or to preamputation levels of activity.

Prosthetic training with an early postsurgical fitting is carried out in the same manner as with a definitive prosthesis. However, the usual preprosthetic program described above may need to be modified. The temporary prosthesis provides a source of exercise that may be sufficient to maintain and/or increase range of motion and strength. Furthermore, because the temporary prosthesis controls edema, the need for an elastic stump shrinker is eliminated.

Whether the amputee has conventional preprosthetic care or has an early postsurgical fitting, the program goals and techniques regarding range of motion, strength, coordination, and one-handed skill are based on the evaluations and treatment techniques discussed in chapters 8, 9, and 17.

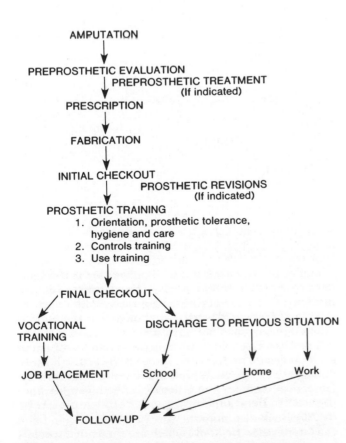

Figure 31.1 Upper-extremity rehabilitation process.

The type of prosthesis and the specific prosthetic components prescribed for the amputee primarily depend on the level of amputation. In most centers, the physician, prosthetist, and occupational therapist all contribute to the decision of what components to prescribe. The availability and extent of third-party reimbursement for prosthetic devices, the experience of the team, and the length and condition of the stump are additional factors that contribute to the decision to fit the amputee with a body-powered or an electrically powered prosthesis.

Because the description of the prescribed prosthesis traditionally lists the components in a distal to proximal order, the description of common prosthetic components begins with the terminal device and proceeds proximally. The reason for this convention may be that all prostheses have in common a terminal device, and the differences among types of prostheses progressively increase as the components become more proximal. Table 31.1 summarizes the conventional body-powered components discussed below.

Prosthetic Components[1,3,7]

Terminal Devices. There are two categories of terminal devices: the hook and the hand. Dorrance voluntary opening split hooks are the most commonly fitted hook (Fig. 31.2). Voluntary opening means that the device opens when tension (pull) is exerted on the control cable. Adult hook sizes are 5, 6, and 7. The 5, 5X, and 5XA all have canted fingers, which are designed to provide three-point prehension when grasping large, round objects. The A specifies that the hook is aluminum rather than steel, and the X specifies that the hook fingers are Neoprene lined. The 555 has lyre-shaped fingers, is aluminum, and is Neoprene lined. While the 555 is sometimes called the "housewife" hook, the 5XA is functionally superior for both men and women because of the canted fingers (Fig. 31.3). Steel hooks and those without Neoprene lining are prescribed for heavy-duty usage. As the aluminum hooks are lighter in weight, they are preferred by high-level amputees. The 6, 7, and 7LO are different from other Dorrance hooks in that the fingers are straight and the hook is L-shaped. They are all stainless steel and are designed for heavy-duty use. The 7 has two chucks, a nail holder, and a knife holder for holding objects of various shapes. The 7LO is identical, except that the opening between the hook fingers is larger to accommodate shovel or broom handles. The 6 is also like the 7, except that it has a locking mechanism that locks the fingers in the closed position.

Two more recently introduced, commercially available hooks are the CONTOURHOOK and the Grip I and Grip II. The CONTOURHOOK is aluminum with Neoprene-lined fingers. The hook fingers are designed to make it easier for the amputee to lift and hold large round objects or to slip the terminal device into confined spaces such as a pocket.

The Grip terminal devices have good prehensile surfaces that are suitable for the grasp of a large variety of objects. A disadvantage is their larger size, which precludes the ability to use them in confined spaces. The Grip I and Grip II are unique in that they are voluntary closing devices. Voluntary closing devices have several functional advantages. When the amputee exerts pull on the control cable, the terminal device closes. Therefore, the amputee receives better proprioceptive feedback regarding the amount of pinch force exerted during the grasp of objects. As the amount of force exerted determines the amount of pinch, pinch force is more precisely controlled; the amount of effort required varies according to the amount of pinch force required. Maximum pinch is determined by the amount of force the amputee can exert.

In contrast, the amputee fitted with a voluntary opening device must always exert maximal pull to open the fingers against the rubber bands or springs that close the fingers, even when grasping lightweight objects. Maximum pinch is determined by the number of rubber bands or springs.

The length of the hook from the base (wrist unit) to the tip of the hook fingers should be equal to or slightly longer than the distance from the wrist to the tip of the thumb on the sound hand (Fig. 31.4). While smaller hook sizes are available, they should not be fitted to adults, as their smaller size limits the size of the object which can be grasped.

Dorrance voluntary opening hands, like Dorrance voluntary opening hooks, are the type of hand most frequently fitted. As a voluntary opening device, tension on the control cable results in the index and middle fingers extending as the thumb abducts. The hand should be covered with a cosmetic glove of a color and style to match the characteristics of the patient's sound hand. The Dorrance hand comes in several sizes; the circumference of the hand at the metacarpophalangeal joints should be approximately ¼ inch less than the circumference of the sound hand (Fig. 31.5).

The hook is lighter in weight and more functional than the hand and is recommended for all but social occasions when the amputee may prefer to wear the hand for cosmetic purposes. The fingers of the hand are too large for precision grasp, the size of objects that can be grasped is limited, and the fingers are oriented such that excessive internal rotation and abduction of the shoulder are required to grasp objects from the table surface. Furthermore, the cosmetic glove is subject to discoloration and staining from sunlight, clothing dyes, and foods and is easily cut or torn if the hand is allowed to bang against hard surfaces.

The Otto Bock voluntary opening hand is of endoskeletal design and as such seems to be less subject to damage to the glove. While functionally similar to the Dorrance hand, many patients prefer the appearance of the Otto Bock hand.

Otto Bock also manufactures an electric hand and the Greifer electric hook, which are typically myoelec-

Table 31.1
SUMMARY OF CONVENTIONAL BODY-POWERED PROSTHETIC COMPONENTS ACCORDING TO AMPUTATION LEVEL

Component		Wrist Disarticulation	Standard Below-Elbow	Short Below-Elbow (Conventional)	Short Below-Elbow (Self-Suspended)	Elbow Disarticulation	Above-Elbow	Shoulder Disarticulation and Forequarter
Terminal device	Hook					→		
	Hand					→		
Wrist	Shape	Oval	Oval / Round →					
	Type	Constant friction	Constant friction / Manual friction / Quick disconnect →					
Forearm		Wrist disarticulation type socket	Standard below-elbow socket socket	Preflexed below-elbow socket	Muenster or NU supracondylar below-elbow socket	Forearm shell →		
Elbow		Flexible hinges	Flexible or semirigid hinges	Rigid or semi-rigid hinges →	None	Outside locking elbow	Inside locking elbow →	
Upper arm component		Triceps pad →			None	Elbow disarticulation type socket	Above-elbow type socket → Humeral section	
Shoulder		None →					Allows flexion/extension and abduction/adduction →	
Harness/Suspension		Standard below-elbow figure of eight harness →			Figure of nine harness	Standard above-elbow figure of eight harness →		Shoulder cap and chest strap
Control system		Single →				Dual →		

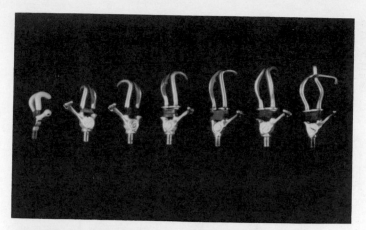

Figure 31.2 Dorrance voluntary opening split hooks in child and adult sizes. From left to right, size 12P, 10X, 99X, 88X, 5X, 555, and 7LO. The three on the right are adult sizes.

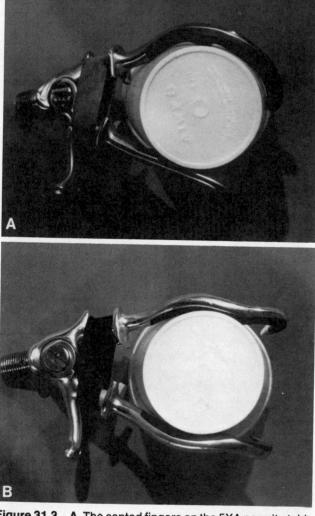

Figure 31.3 **A.** The canted fingers on the 5XA permit stable grasp of the inverted cup. **B.** The 555 only permits unstable two-point grasp.

trically controlled but can also be switch controlled. Also available is the Fidelity Electronics/VANU electric hand. The advantages and disadvantages of electrically powered devices are discussed below.

Wrist Units. The wrist unit serves as a source of attachment for the terminal device; rotation of the terminal device in the wrist unit provides for pronation or supination of the terminal device. Wrist units are round or oval; the oval wrist unit is designed for use with wrist disarticulation type prostheses. Round units are preferred when a hand is worn, as the cosmetic glove is less likely to bind when the hand is pronated or supinated. Otherwise, the shape is optional and preference varies from clinic to clinic.

Constant friction wrist units have set screws to adjust the amount of resistance to rotation of the terminal device. The amount of friction remains constant and can be adjusted by the amputee. Friction should be loose enough to allow the amputee to rotate the terminal device but tight enough to prevent terminal device rotation upon opening.

The friction on manual friction wrist units is determined by how far the terminal device is screwed into the wrist. The more the terminal device is screwed into the wrist, the more resistance is produced as a result of compression of a rubber washer. Although this type of unit is satisfactory for some patients, most amputees dislike it, since rotation of the terminal device as little as 90° can reduce the friction so far as to result in the terminal device rotating when tension is applied to the control cable for opening.

Wrist units also are available that permit quicker interchange from hook to hand when the amputee frequently changes the type of terminal device worn. These units also provide locking of the terminal device to prevent rotation when lifting heavy objects; however, some amputees find that they do not withstand heavy-duty usage. Finally, the Otto Bock Quick Disconnect permits rapid interchange of the Otto Bock electric hand and the Greifer electric hook; and the Otto Bock Hook Adapter permits interchange among a Dorrance hook, Dorrance hand, and Greifer electric hook.

Wrist units that permit flexion of the wrist are useful for higher level bilateral amputees, as they allow the amputee to reach the midline of the body in order to manage front zippers and buttons during dressing and toileting.

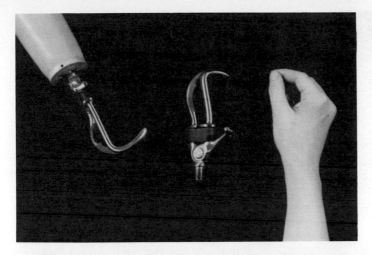

Figure 31.4 The hook correctly inserted into the wrist unit **(left)** and correct sizing of the hook when compared to the sound hand **(right)**.

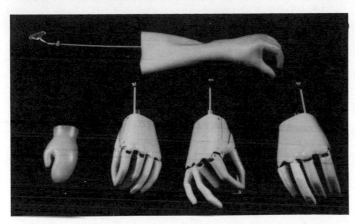

Figure 31.5 Infant passive mitt and voluntary opening hands, with and without cosmetic glove, in adult and child sizes.

Forearm. The forearm component of the wrist disarticulation or below-elbow type prosthesis is the socket. The socket is of a standard type on the long below-elbow and wrist disarticulation type prostheses. The socket on the short below-elbow is either preflexed or self-suspended (Muenster type). Myoelectric below-elbow prostheses have self-suspended sockets.

The forearm component of an elbow disarticulation, above-elbow, or shoulder disarticulation type prosthesis is the forearm shell.

Elbow. Standard wrist disarticulation, standard below-elbow, and preflexed below-elbow type prostheses have flexible, semirigid, or rigid hinges that attach the forearm socket to the triceps pad and harness. Rigid hinges (metal) provide stability when the below-elbow stump is very short. Flexible hinges (Dacron tape or leather) are used with longer stumps since they permit pronation and supination. Semirigid hinges are made of double-thickness Dacron tape or polyethylene and attach to the distal triceps pad and proximal socket. Since they are very short, they function as rigid hinges.

The standard elbow unit on the elbow disarticulation type prosthesis is the outside locking elbow. As the lock is located outside on the medial aspect of the humeral socket, the axis of rotation of the elbow is at the same level as the sound arm. The positive locking (inside) elbow is incorporated into the prosthesis distal to the humeral socket. The turntable that is part of the unit permits the amputee to preposition the prosthesis in internal or external rotation. This elbow unit is better for heavy-duty use. Although it is standard on above-elbow and shoulder disarticulation type prostheses, its use on the elbow disarticulation or very long above-elbow type prostheses results in the prosthetic elbow center being lower than the sound elbow. In addition to being undesirable cosmetically, the longer-than-normal humeral length requires that the amputee abduct excessively to use the prosthesis in bilateral table top activities.

Commercially available electric elbows include the Liberty Mutual Boston Elbow System, Fidelity Electronics/VANU Electric Elbow, NYU-Hosmer "Hush" Electric Elbow, and Utah Artificial Arm. The Boston Elbow System and the Utah Artificial Arm are designed as components of total modular systems. All of these elbows are typically used in conjunction with electric terminal devices; they are discussed in more detail below.

Upper-Arm Component. The upper-arm component of the standard below-elbow, preflexed below-elbow, and wrist disarticulation types of prostheses is the triceps pad. The triceps pad provides a source of attachment for the cable housing and the harness from which the prosthesis suspends.

The upper-arm component of the elbow disarticulation and above-elbow type prostheses is the socket. The shoulder disarticulation type prosthesis upper-arm component is the humeral section.

Shoulder. The inclusion of a shoulder joint is only necessary in shoulder disarticulation type prostheses. Although some clinics still use rigid shoulder joints or abduction hinges, a shoulder joint that permits flexion and extension, as well as abduction and adduction, is a must if the amputee is going to realize any functional benefit from the prosthesis.

Harness/Suspension and Control System

Suspension is the means by which the prosthesis is held onto the amputee. The control system refers to the method of operation of the terminal device and elbow. The control systems described in this section apply to body-powered components. Control of electrically powered components will be described below.

The wrist disarticulation, standard, and preflexed below-elbow prostheses are suspended by standard below-elbow figure of eight harnesses (Fig. 31.6). The harness also provides a source of operation of the terminal device through the single control system. Single control system means that there is only one control cable, whose only purpose is to operate the terminal device.

Like other below-elbow type prostheses, self-suspended below-elbow type prostheses have single control systems. However, because the suspension is provided by the socket, a figure of nine harness is used as the source of operation of the terminal device.

Elbow disarticulation and above-elbow type prostheses are suspended by standard above-elbow figure of eight harnesses. The harness differs from the below-elbow type, as it must provide sources of control of both the elbow lock and the terminal device-forearm lift through a dual control system (Fig. 31.7)

The suspension of the shoulder disarticulation type prosthesis is provided by the shoulder cap (socket) and a chest strap. Although a dual control system is conventional, the source of control varies. Usually, an axilla loop around the contralateral shoulder provides the source of control of the terminal device-forearm lift, whereas the cable for control of the elbow lock is incorporated into the anterior portion of the chest strap.

The basic principle for active (cable) operation of the prosthesis is that the amputee must move his body or a body part (body control motion) such that tension is applied to the control cable, and the distance between the most proximal attachment of the cable to the prosthesis and the point of attachment of the cable to the harness is lengthened. As shown in Figures 31.8 and 31.9, the body control motions for opening the terminal device are humeral flexion of the prosthetic arm and/or biscapular abduction. This applies to all but

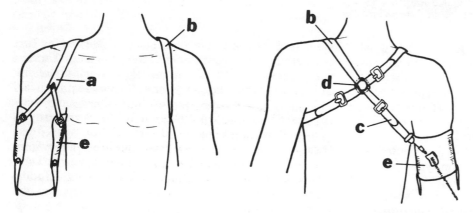

Figure 31.6 Anterior and posterior views of the standard below-elbow figure of eight harness: **(a)** anterior support strap and inverted "Y"; **(b)** axilla loop; **(c)** control attachment strap; **(d)** NU ring; and **(e)** triceps pad.

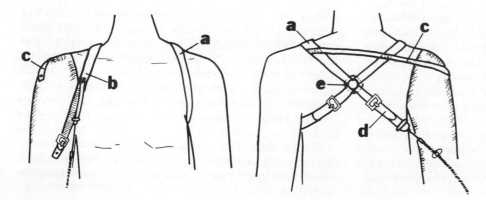

Figure 31.7 Anterior and posterior views of the standard above-elbow figure of eight harness: **(a)** axilla loop; **(b)** anterior suspensor and elbow lock control strap; **(c)** lateral suspensor; **(d)** control attachment strap; and **(e)** NU ring.

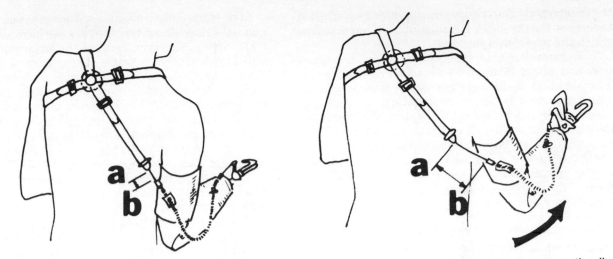

Figure 31.8 The basic body control motion of the below-elbow type prosthesis is humeral flexion, which increases the distance between the distal attachment of the cable to the harness at the cable hanger **(a)** and the proximal attachment of the cable to the prosthesis **(b)**.

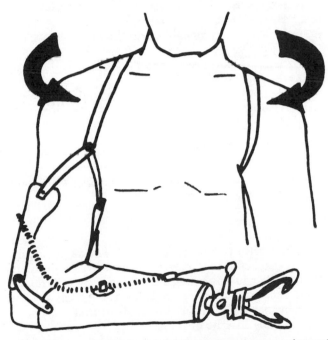

Figure 31.9 Biscapular abduction is used to supplement humeral flexion to produce terminal device opening.

shoulder disarticulation or forequarter prostheses where the motion is humeral flexion and/or unilateral scapular abduction of the uninvolved limb. In the dual control system, the same cable and body motions that open the terminal device are used for active forearm lift (elbow flexion). The elbow lock on above-elbow or elbow disarticulation type prostheses is effected by a combination of downward rotation of the scapula with simultaneous shoulder abduction and hyperextension (Fig. 31.10). The body control motion to operate the elbow lock on shoulder disarticulation type prostheses is usually chest expansion. When the elbow lock is unlocked, pull on the terminal device control cable results

in forearm lift. When the elbow lock is locked, the terminal device opens (Fig. 31.11 and 31.12).

PROSTHETIC CHECKOUT[1,11]

As soon as the amputee is fitted with a prosthesis, whether it is temporary or definitive, the occupational therapist performs a prosthetic checkout. The prosthetic checkout determines whether or not the prosthesis fits properly, appears satisfactory, and is mechanically sound. It is an evaluation of the appearance, comfort, and function of a prosthesis. Good fit and alignment are especially important with the initial fitting, as discomfort or difficulty in operation of the first prosthesis may result in the ultimate rejection of the prosthetic limb. The initial checkout is completed before the amputee begins prosthetic training; the final checkout cannot be completed until all necessary revisions to the prosthesis are made and training is initiated or completed.

The prosthetic checkout form, based upon the *Manual of Upper Extremity Prosthetics*,[11] is shown in Table 31.2 and should be referred to in the following discussion.

Sizing

The overall length and the length of the terminal device, forearm, and humeral component of the prosthesis should be the same as the length of the comparable part of the second limb. The overall length is evaluated by having the amputee stand erect with the uninvolved limb and the prosthesis extended and against the side of the body. The uninvolved limb is measured from the acromion process to the tip of the thumb. This distance should equal the distance from the acromion process or shoulder joint to the tip of the hook or thumb of the cosmetic hand. Similarly, the distance from the acromion to the lateral epicondyle and the distance from the lateral epicondyle to the tip of the thumb are compared to the distance from the acromion or shoulder

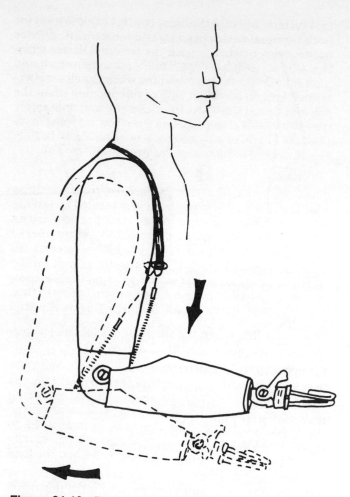

Figure 31.10 Body control motion for activation of the elbow lock on an above-elbow type prosthesis.

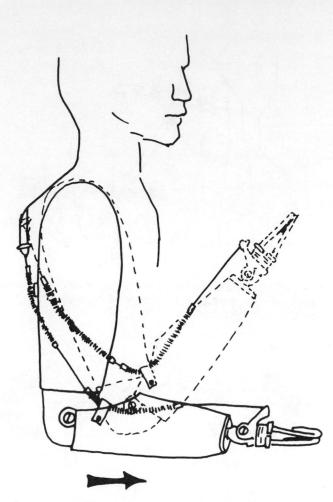

Figure 31.11 When the elbow lock is unlocked, tension on the control cable produces forearm lift.

joint to the lateral center of rotation of the elbow hinge or lock and the distance from the elbow hinge or lock center of rotation to the tip of the hook or the thumb of the cosmetic hand, respectively.

Weight

The weight of the prosthesis is evaluated using a spring scale. The weight of the prosthesis should be kept to a minimum; however, standards for weight are not available.

Terminal Device and Wrist Unit

The hook and/or hand are carefully examined for unnecessary wear, malfunction, and inappropriate sizing. If any of the listed problems are found, repair or replacement is recommended. The amputee's ability to operate the terminal device or wrist unit cannot be evaluated until the necessary training has been completed.

Control System

When checking out the prosthesis, it is important to determine whether the controls are located such that the amputee can operate them, which can only be de-

termined after training is initiated. The cable housing also is inspected to ensure that there are no problems that would cause increased friction in the control system. Increased friction reduces the efficiency and thereby increases the amount of effort that must be exerted to operate the prosthesis.

Elbow Hinges/Units and Shoulder Joint

The forearm on prostheses with dual control systems should maximally extend to 10° to 15° of initial flexion so that it is easier for the amputee to actively initiate forearm lift. The other items are self-explanatory.

Harness

Most amputees are fitted with prostheses that have an axilla loop as part of the harness. The axilla loop provides a stable point against which the amputee pulls to open the terminal device, and in the case of figure of eight harnesses, from which the prosthesis is suspended. Therefore, the harness should be properly adjusted and snug, but not so tight as to cause undue irritation under the axilla loop. When adjusting the harness, refer to the harness parts shown in Figures 31.6 and 31.7.

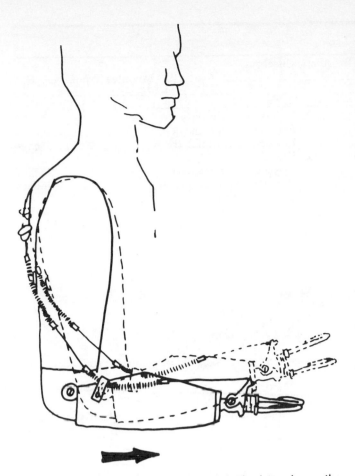

Figure 31.12 When the elbow lock is locked, tension on the control cable produces terminal device opening.

Fit

It is well to remember that a good socket fit usually results in a comfortable prosthesis, and that poor fit often results in pain or discomfort. If the prosthesis persists in causing irritation, the cause, whether medical, physical, or prosthetic in origin, must be determined. When checking for areas of irritation, pay particular attention to the socket trim line (socket edge), the acromion process on shoulder articulation type prostheses, and the opposite axilla when a figure of eight harness is used.

Range of Motion

Active and passive prosthetic range of motion are evaluated to determine whether the amputee can actively move the prosthesis through its full range of motion. To determine if the prosthesis limits the amputee's available range of motion, active motion with the prosthesis on is compared to active motion with the prosthesis off. No more than 10° of elbow flexion or 50% of forearm rotation should be lost when the prosthesis is on.

Terminal Device Opening

The single control system ensures that full terminal device opening can be accomplished regardless of the amount of elbow flexion. However, with the dual con-

trol system, because the same control cable is used for both terminal device opening and forearm lift, greater excursion is needed to open the terminal device when the elbow is flexed. The unilateral amputee should have full terminal device opening when the elbow is extended and no less than 75% of full opening when the elbow is flexed to 90°. As the unilateral amputee rarely uses the terminal device when the elbow is flexed more than 90°, little or no opening when the elbow is fully flexed should not be cause for prosthetic revision.

Forces

The force required to flex the forearm from a starting position of 90° of elbow flexion is measured by pulling on a spring scale attached to the control cable using an adapter. With the elbow lock unlocked, the number of pounds of pull that are necessary to lift the forearm are noted on the spring scale. The amount of pull on the spring scale is increased gradually so that the scale can be read at the exact moment the forearm begins to flex. The terminal device should have the fingers directed medially.

Tension stability refers to the ability of the harness/suspension to hold the prosthesis securely on the amputee when the amputee lifts heavy objects. With the prosthesis extended at the side of the body, a downward pull equal to 1/3 of the body weight, but not exceeding 50 pounds, is applied using a spring scale attached to the terminal device. The amputee is instructed to counteract the pull. The socket should not slip distally on the stump more than 1/4 to 1/2 inch when the load is applied.

The control system efficiency is a ratio of the force required to open the terminal device at the distal end of the control system (terminal device) and the force required to open the terminal device at the proximal end of the control system (cable hanger). It is a measure of the amount of friction in the control system (caused by the cable housing and the curved course of the cable). Therefore, the force needed to open the terminal device at the terminal device is generally less than the force needed to open the terminal device at the cable hanger. The force required to open the terminal device at each end of the control system is measured with a spring scale. The elbow is held in 90° of flexion (if present, the elbow lock is locked) and a small block (1/2 to 1 inch) is placed in the terminal device. The terminal device fingers are directed medially. The spring scale is first attached to the terminal device with an adapter. The spring scale is then gently pulled, keeping it in line with the normal pull of the control cable (Fig. 31.13).

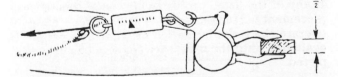

Figure 31.13 Measuring force at the terminal device. (Reproduced with permission from Santschi, W. R., editor. *Manual of Upper Extremity Prosthetics*, 2nd edition. Los Angeles: University of California at Los Angeles, 1958.)

Table 31.2
UPPER-EXTREMITY PROSTHETIC CHECKOUT FORM[a]

Upper-Extremity Prosthetic Checkout

Name_____ Age _____ Amputee Type _____ R L
Description of Prosthesis_____

Evaluation of:

_____ Old Limb
_____ New Limb—initial
_____ New Limb—final

Weight (to nearest ¼ pound):
_____ pounds

Sizing: 1. Uninvolved extremity
Acromion to epicondyle _____ inches
Epicondyle to thumb tip _____ inches
2. Prosthesis
Acromion to hinge (elbow) _____ inches
Hinge to thumb or hook tip _____ inches

Appearance

A. Terminal Device: Hook and/or cosmetic hand and glove
    1. Hook:
        _____ a. Does the hook function properly in all respects?
            _____ Are fingers sprung or worn?
            _____ Is Neoprene worn?
            _____ Does it stick or grate when passively opened or closed?
            _____ Is it noisy?
        _____ b. If Plastisol covering is used, is it undamaged and good color (not discolored or stained)?
        _____ c. Is the hook the proper size?
    2. Cosmetic hand and glove:
        _____ a. Is the hand matching (proper) size?
        _____ b. Are the springs controlling prehension too strong, preventing the amputee optimal ease in operation (opening and closing)?
        _____ c. Is the cosmetic glove satisfactory in all respects?
            _____ Proper fit?
            _____ Undamaged or stained?
            _____ Properly matched color?
            _____ Pulled completely onto hand and forearm without wrinkling?
            _____ Without gapping in palm?
            _____ Doesn't bind when hand is rotated?

B. Wrist Unit
    1. _____ Does the wrist unit operate properly in all respects?
        _____ a. Friction too loose—hook rotates when opened in pronated position?
        _____ b. Friction too tight—amputee cannot preposition terminal device (TD)?
        _____ c. Friction cannot be adjusted?
        _____ d. Wrist sticks or grates when TD prepositioned?
        _____ e. Wrist disconnect unit does not operate smoothly?
    2. _____ If wrist flexion unit is used, does it operate?
        _____ a. Will it maintain extended position when TD is pronated or
        _____ b. Does it automatically pop into flexion when TD is opened?
        _____ c. Can amputee position it in flexion and extension?
        _____ d. If wrist flexion unit has one, can amputee depress lever and position unit into different positions of flexion?

C. Control System
    1. _____ Are all active operating controls so placed as to be satisfactorily operated by the amputee?
    2. _____ Is the control cable free from sharp bends, which decrease efficiency and cause rapid cable wear?
    3. _____ Are the control cables arranged so that they do not pinch the amputee's skin?
    4. _____ If a hook is to be interchanged with a hand, is the hook-to-hand adapter the correct length and do the ball and socket connections work properly? (If complete interchangeable cable system is used, it should be evaluated as a total control system.)
    5. _____ Is the cable long enough to allow full forearm extension with full pronation of the terminal device?
    6. _____ Is the cable housing tipped with ferrules to prevent fraying?
    7. _____ Is the cable housing sprung?
    8. _____ If the cable housing is lined, is the lining properly in place and not showing any signs of wear?
  *BE 9. _____ Is the cable housing the proper length between the distal and proximal retainers? (If too long, housing will bulge out in a large loop; if too short, limits flexion or catches on hinge and damages system.)

Table 31.2—_Continued_

†AE
‡SD   10. _____ Does cable housing adequately cover cable without restricting forearm flexion?

†AE
‡SD   11. _____ Is the lift loop short enough to allow adequate terminal device operation after full forearm flexion and is it heavy enough to prevent buckling?

†AE
‡SD   12. _____ Does the lift loop pivot on screw and grip cable housing tightly enough to prevent slipping?

D. Elbow Hinges and Elbow Units

    1. _____ Does elbow function properly and smoothly without excessive force to operate?

                 _____ a. Does elbow joint bind?

                 _____ b. Is there play in joint?

                 _____ c. Is mechanism noisy?

                 _____ d. Are the screws missing at joint?

†AE/‡SD   _____ e. Is the turntable too loose, or too tight to permit the amputee to operate?

†AE/‡SD   _____ f. Does the elbow lock phase properly?

†AE
‡SD   2. _____ Is forearm set in adequate amount (10° to 15°) of initial flexion?

*BE   3. _____ If flexible or semirigid hinges are used, are they short enough to provide necessary stability, or long enough to allow forearm rotation?

E. Shoulder Joint

‡SD   1. _____ Can friction be adjusted so amputee can preposition?

‡SD   2. _____ Is friction tight enough so that the prosthesis remains in the desired position, but loose enough to permit prepositioning?

F. Harness

    1. _____ Is axilla loop and/or perineal straps and/or waist belt of such size, and so positioned, as to afford adequate support and operation?

    2. _____ Is the axilla loop, waist belt, or perineal strap comfortable to the amputee, and if necessary, is the axilla loop or perineal strap covered with felt or plastic?

    3. _____ Is control attachment strap below midscapular level, and does it remain low enough to give adequate cable travel?

    4. _____ Is harness adjusted properly for suspension and cable operation, but comfortable to amputee?

*BE
†AE   5. _____ Is the NU ring below C_7 and centered or resting toward the nonamputated side?

*BE   6. _____ Does anterior support strap pass along the deltopectoral line?

†AE   7. _____ Is elastic anterior suspensor adequate length and properly located?

*BE   8. _____ Does triceps pad fit snugly without undue gapping during forearm flexion and TD operation?

*BE   9. _____ Does triceps pad pinch patient's flesh?

   10. _____ Can any additional straps be justified (beyond conventional harness)?

G. Fit

    1. _____ Is the prosthesis the correct length?

*BE   2. _____ Do the epicondyles have sufficient space?

    3. _____ Does the socket trim line fulfill requirements of prescription and function?

    4. _____ Is socket comfortable under weight stress?

H. General Workmanship

    1. _____ Have all trimmed edges, rough spots, or uncured areas been sealed?

    2. _____ Are all rivets properly peened and all screws securely fastened?

    3. _____ Is arm color satisfactory?

    4. _____ Are all soldered joints strong and neat?

    5. _____ Are all strap ends sealed to prevent fraying?

    6. _____ Is the interior of the socket absolutely smooth?

Range of Motion (Active, A; Passive, P):

Prosthesis On		Prosthesis Off	
*BE Forearm flexion	_____ °A	*BE Forearm flexion	_____ °A
Forearm supination	_____ °A	Forearm supination	_____ °A
Forearm pronation	_____ °A	Forearm pronation	_____ °A
†AE			
‡SD Forearm flexion	_____ °A		
	_____ °P		
†AE Humeral flexion	_____ °A	†AE Humeral flexion	_____ °A
Humeral abduction	_____ °A	Humeral abduction	_____ °A
Humeral adduction	_____ °A	Humeral adduction	_____ °A

Table 31.2—*Continued*

Terminal Device Opening   (record in percentages):

———— TD Opening—complete forearm flexion
———— TD Opening—90° forearm flexion   Number of rubber bands————
———— TD Opening—full forearm extension   Prehension force   ————

Forces

†AE
‡SD Force required to flex forearm from 90°————
Tension stability (adult, 50 lb.; child, 1/3 body weight)
———— inches at———— lb
Control system efficiency
———— lb to open TD
———— lb at cable hanger

$$\frac{\text{lb to open TD}}{\text{lb at cable hanger}} \times 100 = \text{————} \text{ \% of control system efficiency}$$

Recommended Standards:
BE, above 80%
AE, above 70%
SD, above 60%

Recommendations

———————————————— Date

———————————————— Therapist

*Note: *BE   applies only to below-elbow or wrist disarticulation prostheses.
†AE   applies only to elbow disarticulation or above-elbow prostheses.
‡SD   applies only to forequarter or shoulder disarticulation prostheses.

The number of pounds of force needed to open the terminal device fingers just enough to allow the block to be moved is recorded. In a similar manner, the spring scale is then attached to the cable hanger, and the pull is applied in line with the normal pull of the control attachment strap (Fig. 31.14). The force required to just open the terminal device enough to allow the block to move is again recorded in pounds. The control system efficiency, which is stated as a percentage, is obtained by dividing the pounds required to open the terminal device at the terminal device by the pounds required to open the terminal device at the cable hanger and multiplying by 100. The standards given on the prosthetic checkout form are slightly higher than those usually given. However, rigid standards with regard to alignment of the control system and/or the use of Dacron cable with lined housings can increase the control system efficiency as much as 30%. It is well to remember ease in operation is a prerequisite for smooth and skillful use of the terminal device.

Prosthetic Training

At the initiation of prosthetic training, the amputee is oriented to the prosthesis, and a program to increase prosthetic tolerance is begun. Orientation to the prosthesis includes instruction in prosthetic hygiene and care, how to put on and remove the prosthesis, the parts of the prosthesis, and how to carry out routine maintenance such as changing cables and rubber bands, adjusting friction at joints, and adjusting the harness.

The prosthesis is cleaned with a damp washcloth using mild soap and water. The socket is wiped clean

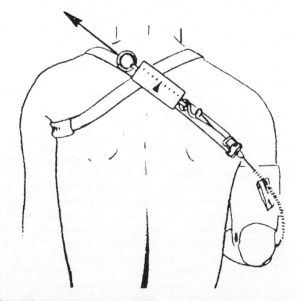

Figure 31.14   Measuring force at the cable hanger. (Reproduced with permission from Santschi, W. R., editor. *Manual of Upper-Extremity Prosthetics*, 2nd edition. Los Angeles: University of California at Los Angeles, 1958.)

daily using soap or mild detergent. Avoid abrasive cleansers as they damage the plastic lamination. Acetone (nail polish remover) or alcohol can be used to remove heavy stains on the outside of the prosthesis, but prolonged contact will soften the lamination.

The harness can be removed or left on the prosthesis and hand washed using soap, water, and a nail brush. If the harness is removed, the buckle locations are marked with indelible marker so that the harness can be correctly adjusted when reapplied.

Stump socks and a t-shirt are worn under most prostheses and harnesses to help protect the skin from irritation and to absorb perspiration. A stump sock is not worn if the amputee is fitted with a self-suspending socket; a t-shirt is not necessary. The stump sock and t-shirt are changed daily. The stump socks are washed in soap or mild detergent to prevent skin irritation.

The stump is washed twice daily with soap and water and dried thoroughly. If heavy perspiration is a problem, a small amount of unscented baby powder or cornstarch can be applied to the stump before the prosthesis is applied in the morning.

The above- and below-elbow type prosthesis is put on and removed in a manner similar to putting on a (1) front-opening or (2) slipover shirt: (1) The stump is inserted into the socket, which is held in the sound hand, and under the anteriorly fastening straps of the harness. The axilla loop is then swung behind the back as the prosthesis is raised overhead, and the sound arm is inserted through the axilla loop. (2) The prosthesis is positioned in front of the amputee, and the sound arm and stump are inserted into the axilla loop and socket, respectively. Both arms are then raised to lift the prosthesis and harness up and over the head. With either method, the harness is set with the NU ring below C_7 by using scapular retraction and depression. To remove the prosthesis, the amputee grasps the prosthesis with the sound hand and lifts the prosthesis overhead. The shoulder disarticulation prosthesis is put on using the sound hand and held in place with the chin or by leaning against the wall as the chest strap is fastened.

Prosthetic tolerance is defined as the amputee's ability to adjust to the wearing of a prosthesis. Tolerance involves the amputee's attitude toward the prosthesis, as well as the physiological acceptance of it. To develop prosthetic tolerance, the amputee begins wearing the prosthesis for 1/2 hour. The stump is checked before and after each application for areas of irritation. If there is no sign of irritation when the prosthesis is removed, the prosthesis is immediately reapplied for an additional 1/2 hour. If irritation occurs, the prosthesis is not reapplied until after the redness clears. The wearing time is increased in this manner until the amputee is able to wear the prosthesis for 2 hours without irritation. Once the prosthesis can be worn for 2 hours, wearing time can be increased to full-time wear, provided that the amputee is aware of the importance of removing the prosthesis should irritation or discomfort develop. If at any time the prosthesis persists in causing redness or irritation that lasts for more than

1/2 hour after removal, revision or relief is recommended.

Prosthetic training in the operation of the prosthesis begins with teaching the amputee to actively operate the control cables using the appropriate body control motions. This stage is known as controls training, but because it overlaps or is continuous with use training (training to develop skill in the use of prosthesis in activity), it is not a clearly defined period. In most instances, controls training is completed within one treatment session.

The body control motions are first demonstrated by passively moving the amputated limb through the correct motion. The body control motion for terminal device operation is taught first. (e.g., see Fig. 31.8 and 31.9). Once the amputee can actively open and close the terminal device, the amputee practices grasping objects of various sizes, densities, textures, and shapes.

If the prosthesis has a dual control system, the elbow lock remains locked while terminal device operation is learned. (e.g., see Fig. 31.12). Then, the elbow lock is unlocked by passively moving the prosthesis through the appropriate motion, thereby demonstrating the correct body control motion to the amputee. (e.g., see Fig. 31.10). With the elbow lock unlocked, the amputee is asked to perform the same body control motion that opens the terminal device and is shown that this motion now results in forearm lift (e.g., see Fig. 31.11). The amputee's face should initially be protected by the therapist's hand in the event that the forearm is flexed so far as to cause the terminal device to hit the face. The amputee should practice elbow lock and unlock and the forearm lift separately until they are smoothly accomplished.

The ability to combine forearm lift and elbow lock and unlock is then taught by asking the amputee to flex the forearm to varying degrees of elbow flexion and to hold the position while the elbow is locked. The elbow of above-elbow and elbow disarticulation type prostheses is more easily locked and unlocked when the forearm is flexed if only scapular depression and humeral abduction are used. This prevents the forearm from extending because of release of the tension on the terminal device control cable, which would result if the amputee also used shoulder hyperextension to operate the elbow lock (Fig. 31.10).

As the amputee develops skill in control of the terminal device, elbow lock, and forearm lift operation, manual controls, which include prepositioning the terminal device, shoulder joint, or humeral turntable using the sound hand, are taught. The amputee is then ready to begin learning to preposition the prosthesis in various positions, as appropriate for the activity. For example, to hold paper when cutting with scissors, the fingers of the hook must be parallel to the table, or horizontal. To grasp a jar, the hook fingers must be perpendicular to the table, or vertical.

By this time, the amputee has begun use training; prosthetic skill and awareness are more readily learned through the use of the prosthesis in bilateral activities of daily living appropriate for the needs and interests of the amputee. Although there are many so-called "prosthetic techniques," the best approach to use in training is based on skill in activity analysis and knowledge of prosthetic function and limitations. For example, the therapist working with an amputee for the first time might ask the patient to write his name on a piece of paper while seated at a table, without knowing how this task is accomplished using a prosthesis. The therapist should first analyze how the activity is normally accomplished. The nonpreferred extremity is positioned in approximately 45° of shoulder flexion and abduction, the elbow is flexed approximately 45°, and the forearm and hand lay flat across the paper to stabilize it while the individual writes with the writing implement in the preferred hand. This is then translated into prosthetic terms. As appropriate to the type of prosthesis, the shoulder joint is prepositioned into 45° of shoulder flexion and abduction, the elbow is flexed and locked at 45° of flexion, and the terminal device is slightly pronated such that the forearm and terminal device will lay flat across the paper and hold it securely.

The prosthesis always functions as the nonpreferred extremity did—as a stabilizer.

There are a few techniques that should be mentioned. When cutting meat, the fork is placed between the hook fingers and behind the prosthetic thumb (Fig. 31.15). The knife, as with the normal individual, is held in the sound (preferred) hand. The principles of dressing are the same as for the stroke patient: the prosthesis is dressed first and undressed last. Shoe laces can be tied in the usual manner, but if slippage of the lace in the hook fingers occurs when pulling on the lace, the hook can be opened, the lace wrapped around one of the hook fingers, and the hook closed for more secure grasp (Fig. 31.16).

With the bilateral amputee, the training procedures are the same for each limb; however, separation of controls also must be accomplished. Separation of controls involves keeping one terminal device closed to maintain grasp of an object while simultaneously opening the other terminal device. When two cable systems (one for operation of each terminal device) are attached to one harness, as they are for the bilateral

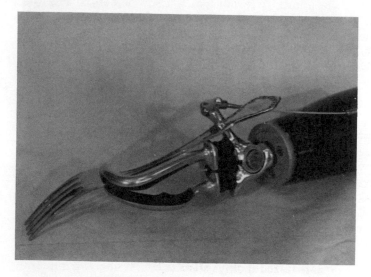

Figure 31.15 Correct positioning of the fork for cutting meat. The bilateral amputee stabilizes the knife or writing implement in a similar manner.

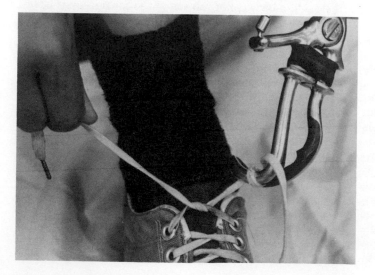

Figure 31.16 Stabilization of the shoe lace in the hook.

amputee, the patient must learn to relax one control system while operating the other. If the amputee does not do this, any attempt to open one terminal device also will open the other. The point of stability from which the amputee pulls is no longer the harness (as it should be) but rather the opposite terminal device. This ability to separate controls enables the bilateral amputee to cut with scissors with one hook while holding paper securely in the other. When the amputee is first learning to separate controls, the occupational therapist can help the amputee by cutting a rubber band in half and then placing an additional amount of rubber band on the hook used to hold or stabilize and/or loosen the control attachment strap on the same side. Both of these procedures make it more difficult for the amputee to open the nonpreferred hook; the ability to keep the hook closed improves, but the ability to use it lessens. In order to prevent this loss of skill, the amputee must eventually learn to maintain the stabilizing side extended at the shoulder to relax the tension on the control cable.

Throughout use training, the therapist tries to involve the amputee in the activity analysis process. This enables the amputee to determine how to use the prosthesis in new activities learned after discharge. It also may promote higher levels of prosthetic skill and awareness and encourage continued prosthetic use.

The rejection rate among upper-extremity amputees is high.[7] The reason for rejection can be physical or medical (weakness, incoordination, associated disability, pain, unsuitable stump for prosthetic fitting, etc.), psychological,[4] or prosthetic (poor fit, mechanical unreliability).[3,12] The prosthesis also may be rejected because the amputee develops one-handed activity patterns prior to prosthetic fitting and training that permit independence in occupational performance tasks and/or because the amputee is required to use the prosthesis when the demands of the activity exceed the functional capabilities of the prosthesis.[3,5,13] The skillful use of a prosthesis may have less of an effect on independence in daily living tasks than on enabling the amputee to function more normally utilizing two-handed activity patterns. However, the therapist and the amputee also must realize the limitations of the prosthesis. Requiring the amputee to use the prosthesis when such use is unrealistic imposes behavior on the amputee that is awkward and time consuming. Whenever it is more realistic, the principles of loss of use of one upper extremity (chapters 17 and 18) are followed.

In preparation for discharge, consideration is given to the amputee's vocational and avocational interests and prior occupational roles. A community visit with follow-up training is often indicated. Perhaps because of the limited number of commercially available components for recreational and leisure activities, participation in these activities is of special concern to upper-extremity amputees.[12] Therefore, the development of special devices or techniques that enable the amputee to participate in recreational activities is an additional occupational therapy goal. Several devices that are not commercially available have been described in the literature.

Adaptations of the bow for archery were described by Bender[1] and Zduriencik.[14] The bow also can be ordered directly from the factory with the hand grip still in block form. Pins can be added to the hand grip that insert into a female adapter designed to attach to the wrist unit. The adapter must be designed so that the bow can be aligned for direct pull on the bowstring to permit accurate aim.

A commercially available device for bowling is available through the amputee's prosthetist.[1] Redford[15] described a modification made to a Dorrance hook for holding a hockey stick, whereby metal pieces were welded to the hook fingers to make a closed loop. Sabolich[16] developed an adapter for holding a fishing rod, and Bender[1] reported an adapter for holding a golf club. More recently, occupational therapists have described adaptations for knitting,[17] crocheting,[18] and guitar playing.[19]

Most of these devices were designed to meet the special needs of the amputees who used them. Because they are not commercially available, the occupational therapist, prosthetist, and the amputee must work as a team to design and fabricate devices on an individual basis.

A commercially available alternative is the Accru-Hook. This terminal device is very similar to the Dorrance hook, but it has a small triangular hole in the lower, passive finger just distal to the rubber bands. Matching adapters are attached to virtually any hand or power tool, recreational equipment (ski poles, fishing rods, guns, cameras, etc.), or kitchen or gardening implement. The adapters insert into the triangular hole on the hook and the implement is further stabilized by the hook fingers. However, experience has demonstrated that only those amputees with high "gadget tolerance" adjust to using the Accru-Hook.

Partial Hand Amputation[20-22]

Partial hand amputations are usually the result of trauma, and management should be considered in the context of hand injuries in general. Therefore, the reader is referred to chapter 25. This chapter will be limited to a discussion of prosthetic devices for partial hand amputations.

As with all levels of amputation, cosmesis and function are both given consideration. Passive cosmetic hands or fingers are of limited cosmetic and functional benefit. Cosmetic hands are worn like a glove; the part of the hand that is missing is filled with foam, rigid, or flexible material (Fig. 31.17A and B). Although often requested initially, they are frequently rejected by the amputee. The role of the occupational therapist is generally limited to checkout of the cosmetic device and instructing the patient in prosthetic hygiene and care appropriate to the device fitted.

In contrast, because of the special skills of the occupational therapist with regard to activity analysis, fab-

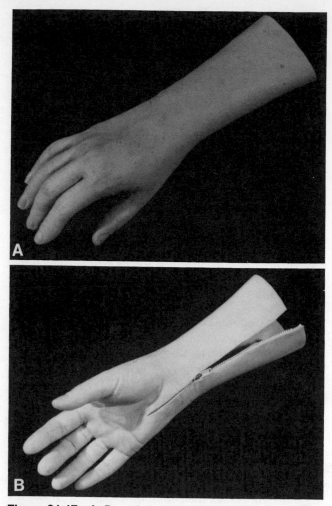

Figure 31.17 **A.** Dorsal view of a cosmetic hand. **B.** Volar view of a cosmetic hand.

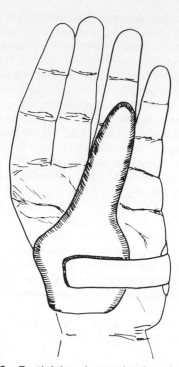

Figure 31.18 Partial hand prosthesis: plastic laminate thumb post.

rication of orthotic devices, and design of adaptive equipment, she can play a major role in designing functional partial hand prostheses. A thorough interview to determine the client's needs and a complete evaluation of residual hand function to identify functional needs can provide the basis for the design of a partial hand prosthesis.

Partial hand prostheses are usually designed to meet a specific functional need of the patient. Lack of opposition, limited strength of opposition, and inadequate stability are the most common functional problems to be overcome. Following the interview and hand evaluation, the therapist can use metal (stainless steel rods or aluminum strips) and thermoplastic splinting material to design a prototype prosthesis or opposition post. When these materials are used, the device can be easily modified until the optimal design is determined. Consideration must be given to the length, strength, and range of motion of the residual digits and to the size, shape, and weight of the objects to be picked up. Most definitive partial hand prostheses are comprised of either a plastic laminate thumb post (Fig. 31.18) or some type of stain-

less steel opposition plate covered with rubber or another nonfriction material (Fig. 31.19) and are therefore fabricated by the prosthetist or orthotist.

Phantom Limb[8,23–26]

Phantom sensation is experienced by all persons with amputations acquired in adulthood. In most cases, the phantom sensation is accompanied by feelings of cramping, shooting, burning, or crushing pain in the phantom limb. This phantom limb pain may be periodic or continuous and range from mild to severe. The phenomenon of phantom pain is poorly understood, but the cause is believed to be multifactorial with medical, physical, and psychological factors all contributing in a highly interrelated manner.

The occupational therapist may become involved in the direct treatment of phantom limb pain, and should recognize that most treatments result in only temporary relief. The only treatments found to provide significant and permanent relief are those that eliminate clearly identified sources of referred pain (e.g., prosthetic or stump problems, low back pain) and electromyographic (EMG) biofeedback and relaxation training (see chapter 12). The best "treatment" identified to date appears to be the prevention of phantom limb pain through the use of immediate or early postsurgical prosthetic fitting.

In addition to EMG biofeedback techniques, the occupational or physical therapist may use techniques that increase somatic input to the stump (e.g., vibration). (See chapter 3 for sensory desensitization programs.) Other members of the rehabilitation team may

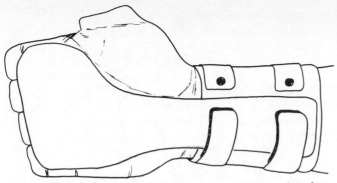

Figure 31.19 Partial hand prosthesis: opposition plate for loss of all digits (volar view).

use direct electrical stimulation or transcutaneous nerve stimulation (TENS). These latter techniques are based on the pain control theory of Melzack and Wall[24] and are believed to block ascending painful sensation.

Electrically Powered Upper-Extremity Prostheses[7,13,27-36]

Electrically powered upper-extremity prostheses or components are either switch or myoelectrically controlled. Switch control can be of two types. Switches that the amputee depresses by movement of the stump or scapula can be mounted in the socket, or pull switches that are activated by the conventional body control motions used to operate the terminal device or elbow lock can be incorporated into the harness. Simply stated, the electrical potential generated by a contracting muscle functions as a switch to activate myoelectrically powered prostheses. Whether the "switch" is a push button, pull switch, or myoelectric potential, it controls the flow of electric current from the battery to the motor.

Switch control is usually "on-off." When the switch is off, the battery is not connected to the motor, and the elbow or terminal device does not move. When the switch is on, the component moves in one direction only. Hence, one switch is needed for flexion of the elbow, and another switch is needed for elbow extension. Similarly, one switch opens the terminal device, and another closes the terminal device. Three- and five-position pull switches also are available and have the advantage of being able to control movement in two directions using a single switch. For example, with the five-position switch, no movement occurs when the switch is in position one, three, or five. The component moves in one direction (e.g., extends) when the switch is in position 2, and movement reverses (e.g., flexes) when the switch is in position 4.

Switch control of electrically powered prostheses is readily taught, provided that the switches are located in an optimal position for ease in operation. An amputee fitted with pull switches who has previously undergone training with a conventional prosthesis may not require controls training. Use training is done in the same manner as described for conventional prostheses.

Myoelectric control systems are more complex and more expensive, as the myoelectric signal must be amplified and smoothed by more sophisticated electronics. Most common is the myoelectric below-elbow prosthesis (Fig. 31.20). Either one or two electrode sites and a reference electrode are necessary to control each component. When there are two electrode sites, they are usually located over antagonistic muscle pairs; contraction of one group of muscles opens the terminal device or flexes the elbow, and contraction of the antagonist results in the reverse motion.

When there is only one electrode site, the amount or level of contraction determines which movement will occur. For example, a midrange or slow rate of contraction results in the hand closing, and a high level or fast rate of contraction results in the hand opening. When the muscle is relaxed, no movement occurs. More complex myoelectric control systems have rate (e.g., Boston Elbow System) or true proportional (e.g., Utah Artificial Arm) control of the speed of movement of the electric component.

Occupational therapy for patients with myoelectric prostheses begins with preprosthetic controls training. Depending on the system to be fitted, one or two pairs of electrodes are applied to the stump. A myotrainer, which is a specialized biofeedback unit, is used to determine the optimum electrode placement. Using trial and error, electrodes are located over superficial muscles that are capable of contracting but that do not contract during normal activity (e.g., elbow flexors and extensors in the case of the below-elbow amputee). As soon as the optimum location is determined, the patient practices using the myotrainer to develop isolated control and the ability (if necessary) to control rate or force of contraction. The electric hand and/or elbow may be connected to the myotrainer at this stage, and the amputee practices controlling the amount of opening and closing of the hand and/or flexion and extension of the elbow. Use training begins as soon as the definitive prosthesis is completed and is done in the same manner as with a conventional prosthesis.

Amputees fitted with electrically powered prostheses are also given instruction in the specialized care and maintenance of their prosthesis, which includes procedures for recharging batteries and what to do if the prosthesis requires repair.

An increasing number of electrically powered devices are being fitted, and the acceptance rate is significantly higher than with conventional prostheses. As far as is feasible, the prostheses are self-suspended and self-contained. Therefore, they require little or no harnessing and are more cosmetic, making them more acceptable to patients.

However, they are expensive and are only fitted in centers that are able to provide specialized fitting, training, and maintenance. Other contraindications for fittings with an electrically powered prosthesis include impaired cognition, lack of motivation, absence

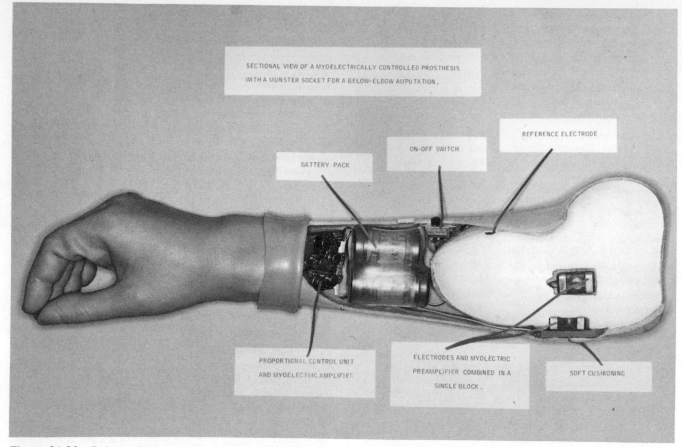

SECTIONAL VIEW OF A MYOELECTRICALLY CONTROLLED PROSTHESIS WITH A MUNSTER SOCKET FOR A BELOW-ELBOW AMPUTATION.

REFERENCE ELECTRODE

ON-OFF SWITCH

BATTERY PACK

PROPORTIONAL CONTROL UNIT AND MYOELECTRIC AMPLIFIER

ELECTRODES AND MYOELECTRIC PREAMPLIFIER COMBINED IN A SINGLE BLOCK.

SOFT CUSHIONING

Figure 31.20 Below-elbow myoelectrically controlled prosthesis with Muenster-type socket. (Reproduced with permission from Lozac, H. Y. An improved and more versatile myoelectric control. *Inter-Clinic Inform. Bull. 11*(8): 13–15, 1972.)

of a suitable EMG signal (if the prosthesis is myoelectrically controlled), or intended use in heavy-duty or dirty/greasy activities.

Although electrically powered prostheses are more cosmetic, eliminate the need for uncomfortable harnessing, and require less energy and excursion to operate, they are not without disadvantages. Reliability remains a problem; the availability of a back-up prosthesis, spare parts, and/or the ability to interchange between body-powered and electrically powered components is necessary if the amputee is going to be a regular prosthetic wearer.

Whether or not the electrically powered hand is more functional than the hook remains controversial. The greater pinch force (up to 25 pounds) and wider opening makes it functionally superior to the body-powered hand. For high-level amputees, the use of an electrically powered elbow with a body-powered hook permits the use of a single cable housing for terminal device operation. Since less exertion is needed to open the terminal device when the electric elbow is flexed, the amount of terminal device opening and/or pinch force increases. The more expensive, preferred alternative is fitting with an electrically powered terminal device (e.g., Greifer) and an electrically powered elbow.

Lower-Extremity Amputees[37–39]

Approximately 70% of acquired amputations involve the lower extremity. Most are necessary because of peripheral arterial disease or diabetes mellitus and involve individuals who are over 60 years of age. Many of these patients have the added problems of peripheral neuropathy, decreased resistance to bacterial and fungal infection, and visual impairment. Katrak and Baggott[38] found that approximately 85% of unilateral geriatric amputees were successfully fitted with prostheses and almost half of the patients who were not fitted attained wheelchair independence in activities of daily living tasks. These results were attained in a rehabilitation center that provided a comprehensive rehabilitation program, including occupational therapy.

Physical therapy assumes major responsibility for prosthetic checkout and gait training. The occupational therapist works closely with the physical therapist and provides a program that facilitates the rehabilitation process and enhances return to prior occupational roles. Specific goals of occupational therapy are to maintain and/or increase upper-extremity strength, increase standing balance and tolerance (with and without the prosthesis), achieve independence in daily living tasks (with and without the prosthesis), and to facilitate reintegration into the community. The program goals are based on an interview to determine the amputee's needs and interests and a thorough evaluation of physical and mental status.

Upper-Extremity Strengthening

Emphasis is placed on strengthening muscle groups needed for gait training and transfers. Strengthening of distal as well as proximal muscle groups is indicated, particularly if weakness is the result of a long hospitalization and/or if peripheral neuropathy is present.

Standing Balance and Tolerance

Prior to prosthetic fitting, the ability to balance on one leg and to bear weight for increasing periods of time is developed in conjunction with group, kitchen, and self-care activities. After prosthetic fitting, the amputee increases prosthetic tolerance while weight bearing in similar activities. Safety awareness also is developed.

Daily Living Tasks

Prior to prosthetic fitting, the patient is evaluated with regard to independence in dressing, toileting, bathing, kitchen, leisure, and transfer activities, and training is provided if indicated. Evaluation and treatment principles are based on those described for loss of use of one side of the body (chapters 17 and 18). Independence at this stage is particularly important, even for those amputees who are to be fitted and trained with prostheses. There are times for all prosthetic wearers when the prosthesis is not worn (i.e., at night, when repairs are needed, if stump complications develop, etc.). Therefore, the amputee needs to be safe and independent in some secondary mode of ambulation (e.g., wheelchair). Prior to and following prosthetic fitting, the development of functional mobility in conjunction with daily living tasks enables the amputee to improve self-confidence and to feel safe and comfortable during functional ambulation.

Stump hygiene, use of the elastic stump shrinker, and the ability to put on and remove the prosthesis, once fitted, are taught and reinforced by all members of the rehabilitation team. There are many types of lower-extremity prostheses, and the correct method for donning and doffing the prosthesis should be learned from the physical therapist. Dressing the prosthesis is accomplished in the same manner as with an upper-extremity prosthesis: the prosthesis is dressed first and undressed last. Many amputees find it easier to put the shoe and sock on the prosthesis before putting the prosthesis on.

Home and community visits help to identify necessary modifications to the home and/or any additional training needed in preparation for discharge. Avocational and vocational exploration and driving evaluations are also provided, if indicated.

Acknowledgement. I would like to extend my sincere appreciation to Robert Bacon, C.P., for his invaluable assistance in the preparation of this chapter.

STUDY QUESTIONS:
Amputations and Prosthetics

1. List and describe the eight levels of amputation.
2. Discuss the advantages of early postoperative prosthetic fitting.
3. Why are elastic stump shrinkers preferred to elastic bandaging?
4. What are the advantages and disadvantages of hook and hand terminal devices?
5. List the basic components of a standard (1) below-elbow prosthesis and (2) above-elbow prosthesis.
6. Discuss how an amputee uses body power to operate (1) a voluntary opening terminal device and (2) a voluntary closing terminal device.
7. Discuss the relationship between operation of the elbow and the operation of the terminal device on a body-powered above-elbow prosthesis.
8. Discuss the stages of prosthetic training. What is the relationship between use and controls training?
9. Discuss how prosthetic training for the amputee fitted with an electrically powered prosthesis differs from training for the amputee fitted with a conventional prosthesis.
10. Describe how the amputee is trained to operate (1) a myoelectric prosthesis and (2) a switch-controlled, electrically powered prosthesis.

References

1. Bender, L. F. *Prostheses and Rehabilitation after Arm Amputation.* Springfield, IL: Charles C. Thomas, 1974.
2. Steinbach, T. Upper limb amputation. *Prog. Surg., 16:* 224–248, 1978.
3. Vitali, M., Robinson, K. P., Andrews, B. G., and Harris, E. E. *Amputations and Prostheses.* London: Bailliere Tindall, 1978.
4. Bradway, J. K., Malone, J. M., Racy, J., Leal, J. M., and Poole, J. Psychological adaptation to amputation: an overview. *Orthot. Prosthet., 38*(3): 46–50, 1984.
5. Burkhalter, W. E., Mayfield, G., and Carmona, L. S. The upper-extremity amputee: early and immediate post-surgical prosthetic fitting. *J. Bone Joint Surg., 58A:* 46–51, 1976.
6. Jones, R. F. The rehabilitation of surgical patients with particular reference to traumatic upper limb disability. *Aust. NZ J. Surg., 47:* 402–407, 1977.
7. Malone, J. H., Childers, S. J., Underwood, J., and Leal, J. H. Immediate postsurgical management of upper-extremity amputation: conventional electric and myoelectric prosthesis. *Orthot. Prosthet., 35*(2): 1–9, 1981.
8. Malone, J. M., Fleming, L. L., Roberson, J., Whitesides, T. E., Leal, J. M., Poole, J. U., and Grodin, R. S. Immediate, early, and late postsurgical management of upper-limb amputation. *J. Rehabil. Res. Dev., 21:* 33–41, 1984.
9. Millstein, S., Bain, D., and Hunter, G. A. A review of employment patterns of industrial amputees: factors influencing rehabilitation. *Prosthet. Orthot. Int., 9:* 69–78, 1985.
10. Varghese, G., Hindle, P., Zilber, S., Perry, J. E., and Redford, J. B. Pressure applied by elastic prosthetic bandages: a comparative study. *Orthot. Prosthet., 35*(4): 30–36, 1981.
11. Santschi, W. R., editor. *Manual of Upper Extremity Prosthetics,* 2nd edition. Los Angeles: University of California at Los Angeles, 1958.
12. Chadderton, H. C. Prostheses, pain and sequelae of amputation, as seen by the amputee. *Prosthet. Orthot. Int., 1:* 2–14, 1978.
13. Herberts, P., Korner, L., Caine, K., and Wensby, L. Rehabilitation of unilateral below-elbow amputees with myoelectric prostheses. *Scand. J. Rehabil. Med., 12:* 123–128, 1980.
14. Zduriencik, S. Bow adapter. *Am. J. Occup. Ther., 20:* 99–100, 1966.
15. Redford, J. B. Prostheses for hockey-playing upper-limb amputees. *Inter-Clinic Inform. Bull. 14*(6): 11–15, 1975.
16. Sabolich, L. J. An adapted fishing rod for arm amputees. *Inter-Clinic Inform. Bull., 12*(2): 13–15, 1972.
17. Duncan, S. J. Knitting device for bilateral upper extremity amputee. *Am. J. Occup. Ther., 40:* 637–638, 1986.
18. Matsushima, D. S. Crochet aid for the amputee. *Am. J. Occup. Ther., 40:* 495–496, 1986.

19. Zatlin, C. R., Hemmen, E., Krouskop, T. A., and Sklan, M. Guitar capo for a bilateral upper extremity amputee. *Am. J. Occup. Ther., 35*: 736, 1981.
20. Bender, L. F. Prostheses for partial hand amputations. *Prosthet. Orthot. Int., 2*: 8–11, 1978.
21. Kramer, S. Partial hand amputation. *Orthopedics, 1*: 314, 1978.
22. Tomaszewska, A., Kapczynska, D., Konieczna, D., Dembinska, J., and Miedzyblocki, W. Solving individual problems with partial hand prostheses. *Inter-Clinic Inform. Bull., 13*(5): 7–14, 1974.
23. Berger, S. M. Conservative management of phantom-limb and amputation-stump pain. *Ann. R. Coll. Surg. Engl., 62*: 102–105, 1980.
24. Melzack, R., and Wall, P. D. *The Challenge of Pain.* New York: Basic Books, 1982.
25. Pasnau, R. O., and Pfefferbaum, B. Psychologic aspects of post-amputation pain. *Nurs. Clin. North Am., 11*: 679–685, 1976.
26. Sherman, R. A., and Tippens, J. K. Suggested guidelines for treatment of phantom limb pain. *Orthopedics, 5*: 1595–1600, 1982.
27. Agnew, P. J., and Shannon, G. F. Training program for a myo-electrically controlled prosthesis with sensory feedback system. *Am. J. Occup. Ther., 35*: 722–727, 1981.
28. Childress, D. S., Holmes, D. W., and Billock, J. N. Ideas on myoelectric prosthetic systems for upper-extremity amputees. In *The Control of Upper-Extremity Prostheses and Orthoses.* Edited by P. Herberts, R. Kadefors, R. Magnusson, and I. Petersen. Springfield, IL: Charles C Thomas, 1974.
29. Fisher, A. G. Functional results with electrically powered devices for children. In *Workshop on Children's Prosthetics.* Washington, DC: National Academy of Sciences, 1976.
30. Fisher, A. G., and Childress, D. S. The Michigan electric hook: a preliminary report on a new electrically powered hook for children. *Inter-Clinic Inform. Bull., 12*(9): 1–10, 1973.
31. Heger, H., Millstein, S., and Hunter, G. A. Electrically powered prostheses for the adult with an upper limb amputation. *J. Bone Joint Surg., 67B*: 278–281, 1985.
32. Lyttle, D., Sweitzer, R., Steinke, T., Trefler, E., and Hobson, D. Experiences with myoelectric below-elbow fittings in teenagers. *Inter-Clinic Inform Bull., 13*(6): 11–20, 1974.
33. Millstein, S., Heger, H., and Hunter, G. A review of the failures in use of the below elbow myoelectric prosthesis. *Orthot. Prosthet., 36*(2): 29–34, 1982.
34. Millstein, S. G., Heger, H., and Hunter, G. A. Prosthetic use in adult upper limb amputees: a comparison of the body powered and electrically powered prostheses. *Prosthet. Orthot. Int., 10*: 27–34, 1986.
35. Northmore-Ball, M. D., Heger, H., and Hunter, G. A. The below-elbow myoelectric prosthesis: a comparison of the Otto Bock myo-electric prosthesis with the hook and functional hand. *J. Bone Joint. Surg., 62B*: 363–367, 1980.
36. Stein, R. B., and Walley, M. Functional comparison of upper extremity amputees using myoelectric and conventional prostheses. *Arch. Phys. Med. Rehabil., 64*: 243–248, 1983.
37. Humm, W. *Rehabilitation of the Lower Limb Amputee for Nurses and Therapists,* 3rd edition. London: Bailliere Tindall, 1977.
38. Katrak, P. H., and Baggott, J. B. Rehabilitation of elderly lower-extremity amputees. *Med. J. Aust., 1*: 651–653, 1980.
39. Schafer, R. Occupational therapy for lower extremity problems. *Am. J. Occup. Ther., 27*: 132–137, 1973.

Supplementary Reading and Courses

American Academy of Orthopedic Surgeons. *Atlas of Limb Prosthetics: Surgical and Prosthetic Principles.* St. Louis: C. V. Mosby, 1981.

American Orthotic and Prosthetic Association, Washington, DC, *Orthotics and Prosthetics.*

Courses and manuals available from New York University, Prosthetics and Orthotics, NYU Post-Graduate Medical School, New York, NY: *Upper-Extremity Prosthetics* and *Lower-Extremity Prosthetics.*

Courses and manuals available from Northwestern University, The Medical School, Prosthetic-Orthotic Center, Chicago, IL: *Lower Limb Prosthetics for Physicians, Surgeons, and Therapists; Upper Limb Prosthetics and Orthotics for Physicians, Surgeons, and Therapists; Management of the Juvenile Amputee for Physicians, Surgeons, and Therapists.*

International Committee on Prosthetics and Orthotics of the International Society for the Rehabilitation of the Disabled, Copenhagen, Denmark, *Prosthetics and Orthotics International.*

Murphy, E. F., and Horn, L. W. Myoelectric control systems: a selected bibliography. *Orthot. Prosthet., 35*(1): 34–45, 1981.

Prosthetics and Orthotics, New York University Post-Graduate Medical School, New York, NY, *Inter-Clinic Information Bulletin.*

Taylor, C. L. The biomechanics of control in upper-extremity prostheses. *Orthot. Prosthet., 35*(1): 7–28, 1981.

INDEX